THE WASHINGTON MANUAL™ OF MEDICAL THERAPEUTICS

32nd Edition

THE WASHINGTON MANUAL™
OF MEDICAL THERAPEUTICS
32nd Edition

Department of Medicine
Washington University
School of Medicine
St. Louis, Missouri

Editors

Daniel H. Cooper, MD

Andrew J. Krainik, MD

Sam J. Lubner, MD

Hilary E. L. Reno, MD, PhD

Scott T. Micek, PharmD
Associate Editor for
Pharmacotherapeutics

Wolters Kluwer | Lippincott Williams & Wilkins
Health

Philadelphia • Baltimore • New York • London
Buenos Aires • Hong Kong • Sydney • Tokyo

Acquisitions Editor: Sonya Seigafuse
Managing Editor: Lauren Aquino
Project Manager: Rosanne Hallowell
Manufacturing Manager: Kathleen Brown
Marketing Manager: Kimberly Schonberger
Design Coordinator: Teresa Mallon
Cover Designer: Becky Baxendell
Production Services: TechBooks
Printer: RR Donnelley

32nd Edition
© **2007 by Department of Medicine, Washington University School of Medicine.**
© 2004, 2001 by Department of Medicine, Washington University School of Medicine.

Printed in the United States

Spiral binding:
ISBN: 978-0-7817-8125-1
ISBN: 0-7817-8125-6

Adhesive binding:
ISBN: 978-0-7817-6517-6
ISBN: 0-7817-6517-X

The Washington Manual™ is an intent-to-use mark belonging to Washington University in St. Louis to which international legal protection applies. The mark is used in this publication by LWW under license from Washington University.

Care has been taken to confirm the accuracy of the information presented and to describe generally accepted practices. However, the authors, editors, and publisher are not responsible for errors or omissions or for any consequences from application of the information in this book and make no warranty, express or implied, with respect to the currency, completeness, or accuracy of the contents of the publication. Application of this information in a particular situation remains the professional responsibility of the practitioner.

The authors, editors, and publisher have exerted every effort to ensure that drug selection and dosage set forth in this text are in accordance with the current recommendations and practice at the time of publication. However, in view of ongoing research, changes in government regulations, and the constant flow of information relating to drug therapy and drug reactions, the reader is urged to check the package insert for each drug for any change in indications and dosage and for added warnings and precautions. This is particularly important when the recommended agent is a new or infrequently employed drug.

Some drugs and medical devices presented in this publication have Food and Drug Administration (FDA) clearance for limited use in restricted research settings. It is the responsibility of the health care provider to ascertain the FDA status of each drug or device planned for use in their clinical practice.

The publishers have made every effort to trace copyright holders for borrowed material. If they have inadvertently overlooked any, they will be pleased to make the necessary arrangements at the first opportunity.

To purchase additional copies of this book, call our customer service department at (800) 639-3030 or fax orders to (301) 824-7390. International customers should call (301) 714-2324. Lippincott Williams & Wilkins customer service representatives are available from 8:30 am to 6:00 pm, EST, Monday through Friday, for telephone access. Visit Lippincott Williams & Wilkins on the Internet: http://www.lww.com.

10 9 8 7 6 5 4 3 2 1

*We dedicate this Manual to our medicine clinic director,
Dr. Jason Goldfeder, whose strength of character and dedication
to teaching inspires us all.*

CONTENTS

*W*elcome to the 32nd edition of *The Washington Manual of Medical Therapeutics*. The tradition of this publication began in 1943 as a handbook written by the Chief Residents intended for dissemination to the senior medical students and housestaff of Washington University's Department of Medicine. Wayland MacFarlane, MD, served as the first editor. In 1962, Robert Packman, MD, dramatically altered the format of the handbook, changing it from a full-page format to a pocket-sized text. His goal at that time was to provide portable, accessible knowledge for a broad range of common diseases.

Successive editions have grown in size and complexity, mirroring the practice of medicine. With the advent of portable technologies and internet resources, the *Manual* must adapt to meet the on-demand needs of physicians and students. With that in mind, we have altered the format of the *Manual* from an annotated essay to an outlined structure encompassing etiology, clinical presentation, laboratory evaluation, and differential diagnosis, while maintaining a focus on therapy. We hope that this provides information on essential pathophysiology while maintaining an emphasis on emergency therapies vital to the initial care of inpatients. Junior faculty and fellows author this text, stressing critical on-call, on-demand knowledge. Alongside the format changes, we have painstakingly updated the content of the *Manual* to keep pace with changing technologies and therapeutics.

As the best-selling medical text in the world, *The Washington Manual of Medical Therapeutics* has a tradition of excellence that we hope to uphold with this edition. We are proud to see it in the pockets of our housestaff and medical students, and on the shelves of our attendings (next to their copies of previous editions, of course).

We are grateful for the assistance of the pharmacy staff at Barnes-Jewish Hospital, particularly that of Scott Micek, whose help was essential in creating this *Manual*. We would also like to thank Lauren Aquino and the editorial staff at Lippincott Williams & Wilkins for their assistance.

We have had the honor and pleasure of serving as Chief Residents of the Shatz-Strauss, Karl-Flance, and Kipnis-Daughaday firms and the Wohl Clinic of the Department of Medicine at Washington University. To the house officers, we are moved by your fortitude and effort in what you do every day. Our Firm Chiefs, Megan Wren, William Clutter, Geoffrey Cislo, and Jason Goldfeder, have been instrumental over the course of the year, and we owe them our thanks. We would be remiss if we did not extend our thanks to our former Program Director, Daniel Goodenberger, for his help and wish him luck in all future endeavors. We owe thanks to our Program Director and Chief of Medical Education, Melvin Blanchard, and our Chairman of Medicine, Kenneth Polonsky, for guiding us through the process of publishing this text.

We would like to thank our families who have provided support and inspiration throughout the creation of the *Manual*. To Amber and Ashley; Peggy and Evan; Meghan; Shaun and Ian—our gratitude is beyond measure.

Dan Cooper, MD
Andrew Krainik, MD, MPH
Sam Lubner, MD
Hilary Reno, MD, PhD

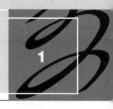

PATIENT CARE IN INTERNAL MEDICINE

Mark Thoelke and Christopher Gutjahr

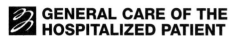

GENERAL CARE OF THE HOSPITALIZED PATIENT

- Although a general approach to common problems can be outlined, **therapy must be individualized.** All diagnostic and therapeutic procedures should be explained carefully to the patient, including the potential risks, benefits, and alternatives. This explanation minimizes anxiety and provides the patient and the physician with appropriate expectations.

PATIENT SAFETY

- The period of hospitalization represents a complex interplay of multiple caregivers that subjects the patient to potential harm by medical errors and iatrogenic complications. Every effort must be made to minimize these risks. Basic measures include:
    - Use of standardized abbreviations and dose designations
    - Excellent communication between physicians and other caregivers
    - Institution of appropriate prophylactic precautions
    - Prevention of nosocomial infections, including attention to hygiene and discontinuation of unnecessary catheters

HOSPITAL ORDERS

- **Admission orders** should be written promptly after evaluation of a patient. Each set of orders should bear the **date and time** of writing and the legible signature of the physician. Consideration should be given to including a **printed signature** and a **contact number.** All orders should be clear, concise, organized, and legible.
- To ensure that no important therapeutic measures are overlooked, the **content and organization** of admission orders should follow the outline below (**the mnemonic ADC VAAN DISML**):
    - Admitting service and location and physician responsible for the patient
    - Diagnoses pertinent to nursing care
    - Condition of the patient
    - Vital signs: type (temperature, heart rate [HR], respiratory rate, and blood pressure [BP]), frequency, and parameters for notification of the physician (e.g., systolic BP <90, HR <60, respiratory rate <10, temperature >38.3°C) specified
    - Activity limitations
    - Allergies, sensitivities, and previous drug reactions
    - Nursing instructions (e.g., Foley catheter to gravity drainage, wound care, daily weights)
    - Diet
    - IV fluids, including composition and rate
    - Sedatives, analgesics, and other PRN medications
    - Medications, including dose, frequency, and route of administration
    - Laboratory tests and radiographic studies

1

- Orders should be re-evaluated frequently and altered as patient status dictates.
  - **When changing an order,** the old order must be specifically canceled before a new one is written.
  - Orders for medications to be taken **PRN** require careful consideration to avoid adverse drug interactions. The minimum dosing interval should be specified (e.g., q4h).

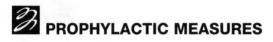

PROPHYLACTIC MEASURES

VENOUS THROMBOEMBOLISM PROPHYLAXIS

General Principles

Etiology

- **Venous thromboembolism (VTE)** is the most common preventable cause of death in hospitalized patients. Roughly 75% percent of fatal pulmonary emboli occur in non-surgical patients. **Risk factors** for VTE include advanced age, previous VTE, trauma, conditions associated with prolonged immobility (major surgery, stroke, paralysis), obesity, heart failure, malignancy, pregnancy, inflammatory bowel disease, and coagulation factor deficiency.

Prevention

- Acutely ill patients with severe respiratory disease, with congestive heart failure, or who are bedridden and have additional risk factors described above should be given **prophylactic dosing** of low-dose unfractionated heparin (UFH; 5,000 units SC q8h) or low molecular weight heparin (LMWH; enoxaparin, 40 mg SC or 4,000 units SC daily, or dalteparin, 5,000 units SC daily).
- Aspirin alone is not adequate deep vein thrombosis (DVT) prophylaxis.
- At-risk patients with contraindications to anticoagulation prophylaxis should receive mechanical prophylaxis with intermittent pneumatic compression or graded compression stockings.[1]
- **Postoperative patients** may be stratified by risk for VTE. Recommended prophylaxis is as follows:
  - Low-risk patients (minor procedure, <40 years old, and no additional risk factors): Only early mobilization is recommended.
  - Moderate-risk patients (nonmajor procedure and between 40 and 60 years old, or other risk factors, OR major procedure and <40 years old): LDUH, 5,000 units SC bid, or LMWH, <3,400 units per day.
  - Higher-risk patients (major surgery, >40 years old, and additional risk factors, OR nonmajor surgery, >60 years old, and additional risk factors): LDUH, 5,000 units SC tid, or LMWH, >3,400 units per day.
  - In highest-risk patients, medical and mechanical methods of prophylaxis should be combined.
  - Treatment of VTE is reviewed in Chapter 18, Disorders of Hemostasis.

PRESSURE ULCERS

General Measures

Epidemiology

- **Pressure ulcers** typically occur within the first 2 weeks of hospitalization and can develop within 2–6 hours. Once they develop, pressure ulcers are difficult to heal and have been associated with increased mortality.[2]

Prevention

- Prevention is the key to management of pressure ulcers. Measures include:
  - **Risk factor assessment,** include immobility, limited activity, incontinence, impaired nutritional status, impaired circulation, and altered level of consciousness
  - **Skin care,** including daily inspection with particular attention to bony prominences and minimizing exposure to moisture from incontinence, perspiration, or wound drainage.
  - Interventions aimed at **relieving or redistributing pressure,** including frequent repositioning (minimum of every 2 hours, or every 1 hour for wheelchair-bound patients), pillows or foam wedges between bony prominences, maintenance of the head of the bed at the lowest degree of elevation, and use of lifting devices when moving patients. **Pressure-reducing devices** (foam, dynamic air mattresses) and pressure-relieving devices (low-air-loss, air-fluidized beds) can also be used.

Diagnosis

Physical Examination

The National Pressure Ulcer Task Force classifies ulcers as follows:[3]

- **Stage I** (nonblanchable erythema; intact skin)
- **Stage II** (extension through epidermis, shallow crater)
- **Stage III** (full thickness without extension through fascia)
- **Stage IV** (full thickness with destruction of underlying tissue, muscle, and/or bone)

Treatment

- **Initial interventions** include use of pressure-relieving devices, occlusive dressings, pain control, normal saline for cleansing, use of topical agents that promote wound healing (DuoDERM, silver sulfadiazine [Silvadene], bacitracin zinc, Neosporin, Polysporin), avoidance of agents that delay healing (antiseptic agents, such as Dakin solution, hydrogen peroxide; wet-to-dry gauze), and removal of necrotic debris.
- **Adequate nutrition** with particular attention to protein intake (1.25–1.50 g protein/kg/d), vitamin C (500 mg PO daily) and zinc sulfate (220 mg PO daily) supplementation in the presence of deficiencies may also facilitate healing.
- For clean pressure ulcers that continue to produce exudate or are not healing after 2–4 weeks of therapy, consider a 2-week trial of **topical antibiotic** (e.g., silver sulfadiazine, double antibiotic).
- **Other adjunctive therapies** for nonhealing ulcers include electrical stimulation, radiant heat, negative pressure therapy, and surgical intervention.

OTHER PRECAUTIONS

- **Fall precautions** should be written for patients who have a history of falls or are at high risk of a fall (i.e., those with dementia, syncope, orthostatic hypotension). Falls are the most common accident in hospitalized patients, frequently leading to injury.
- **Seizure precautions** should be considered for patients with a history of seizures or those at risk of seizing. Precautions include padded bed rails and an oral airway at the bedside.
- **Restraint orders** are written for patients who are at risk of injuring themselves or interfering with their treatment due to disruptive or dangerous behaviors. Restraint orders must be reviewed and renewed every 24 hours. Physical restraints may exacerbate agitation. Bed alarms or sitters are alternatives in appropriate settings.

ADVERSE DRUG REACTIONS

Adverse drug reactions occur frequently, and the rate increases in proportion to the number of drugs taken. Adverse reactions may be allergic, idiosyncratic, or dose-related magnification of known effects.

- **Prevention.** Following the principles below may decrease the incidence of adverse drug reactions. Specific drug allergies are discussed in Chapter 10, Allergy and Immunology.
  - **Record a careful history** of previous drug reactions, including the drug involved and the specific reaction, clearly on the chart.
  - **Minimize number** of drugs used.
  - **Consider drug interactions.** New medications should be added only after careful consideration of the current medical regimen.
  - **Consider the metabolism, route of excretion, and major adverse effects** associated with each drug used. Individualize dosages according to the patient's age, weight, and kidney and liver function.
  - **Report unusual drug reactions** to the U.S. Food and Drug Administration. The MED-WATCH program provides an easy method for voluntary reporting of adverse drug reactions (www.fda.gov/medwatch/).

DISCHARGE

- **Discharge planning** begins at the time of admission. Assessment of the patient's social situation and potential discharge needs should be made.
- **Early coordination** with nursing, social work, and case coordinators/managers facilitates efficient discharge and a complete postdischarge plan.
- **Patient education** should occur regarding changes in medications and other new therapies.
- **Prescriptions** should include the name of the patient, date, name of the drug, dosage, route of administration, amount dispensed, dosage schedule instructions, and signature of the physician. The number of refills should be limited, especially for patients who appear to be self-injurious. For **narcotics**, write out all numbers in parentheses (e.g., dispense 30 [thirty], refills 2 [two]).
- **Communication** with physicians who will be resuming care of the patient after discharge is important for optimal follow-up care.

 ACUTE INPATIENT CARE

GENERAL PRINCIPLES

- New or recurrent symptoms that require evaluation and management frequently develop in hospitalized patients.
- Evaluation should generally include a directed history, including a complete description of the symptom (i.e., palliating and precipitating factors, quality of the symptom, associated symptoms, and the course of the symptom, including acuity of onset, severity, duration, and previous episodes); physical examination; review of the medical problem list; review of medications with attention to recent medication discontinuation, addition, or dosage adjustment; and consideration of recent procedures.
- Further evaluation should be directed by the initial assessment, the acuity and severity of the complaint, and the diagnostic possibilities.
- An approach to selected common complaints is presented in this section.

CHEST PAIN

- Chest pain is a common complaint in the hospitalized patient, and the severity of chest discomfort does not always correlate with the gravity of its cause. Chest pain should be evaluated to distinguish potentially life-threatening conditions such as pulmonary embolus, myocardial infarction, and aortic dissection from less serious cases.

Diagnosis

History

- History should be taken in the context of the patient's other medical conditions, particularly previous cardiac or vascular history, cardiac risk factors, and factors that would predispose to a pulmonary embolus.

Physical Examination

- Physical examination is ideally conducted during an episode of pain and includes vital signs with BP measured in both arms, a careful cardiopulmonary and abdominal examination, and inspection and palpation of the chest for possible trauma, herpes zoster rash, and reproducibility of the pain.

Testing

- Assessment of **oxygenation status, chest radiography, and ECG** is appropriate in most patients.
- If **cardiac ischemia** is a concern, initial therapy should include supplemental oxygen, chewed aspirin, and administration of nitroglycerin, 0.4 mg SL, or morphine sulfate, 1–2 mg IV, or both. Treatment of ischemic heart disease is discussed in Chapter 5, Ischemic Heart Disease.
- If a **gastrointestinal (GI) source** of chest pain is suspected a combination of Maalox and diphenhydramine (30 mL of each in a 1:1 mix) can be administered.
- **Costochondritis** typically responds to nonsteroidal anti-inflammatory drug (NSAID) therapy.
- Suspicion of **pulmonary embolism** should lead to prompt empiric anticoagulation while awaiting testing in the absence of contraindication.

DYSPNEA

- **Dyspnea** is most commonly caused by a cardiopulmonary abnormality, such as congestive heart failure, cardiac ischemia, bronchospasm, pulmonary embolus, and/or infection, and must be promptly and carefully evaluated.

Diagnosis

History

- Initial evaluation should include a review of the medical history for underlying pulmonary or cardiovascular disease, and a directed history.

Physical Examination

- A detailed cardiopulmonary examination should take place, including vital signs with comparison of current findings to those documented earlier.

Testing

- Oxygen assessment should take place promptly. Arterial blood gas measurement provides more information than pulse oximetry. Other diagnostic and therapeutic measures should be directed by the findings in the initial evaluation and the severity of the suspected diagnosis. Chest radiography is useful in most patients.

Treatment

- Therapeutic measures should be directed by the findings in the initial evaluation and the severity of the suspected diagnoses.

ACUTE HYPERTENSIVE EPISODES

General Measures

Etiology

- Acute hypertensive episodes in the hospital are most often caused by inadequately treated essential hypertension.
- Volume expansion and inadequate pain control may exacerbate hypertension and should be recognized appropriately and treated.
- Hypertension associated with withdrawal syndromes (e.g., alcohol, cocaine, etc.) and rebound hypertension associated with sudden withdrawal of antihypertensive medications (i.e., clonidine, α-adrenergic antagonists) should be considered. These entities should be treated as discussed in Chapter 4, Hypertension.
  - Evaluation and treatment decisions should consider baseline BP, presence of symptoms (e.g., chest pain or shortness of breath), and current and baseline antihypertensive medications.

FEVER

General Measures

Etiology

- Fever accompanies many illnesses and is a valuable marker of disease activity.
- Because fever can cause increased tissue catabolism, increased oxygen consumption, dehydration, exacerbation of heart failure, delirium, and convulsions, the underlying cause of fever should be ascertained as quickly as possible.

Diagnosis

Differential Diagnosis

- Infection is a primary concern; drug reaction, malignancy, VTE, vasculitis, and tissue infarction are other possibilities but are diagnoses of exclusion.
- The differential diagnosis for fever is very broad, and the pace and complexity of the workup depend on the diagnostic considerations taken in the context of the clinical stability and immune status of the host.

History

- History should include chronology of the fever and associated symptoms, medications, potential exposures, and a complete social and travel history.

Physical Examination

- Physical examination should include **oral or rectal temperature** monitoring from a consistent site. In the hospitalized patient, special attention should be paid to any rash, new murmur, abnormal fluid accumulation, intravascular lines, and indwelling devices such as gastric tubes or Foley catheters.
- In the **neutropenic patient,** the skin, oral cavity, and perineal area should be examined carefully for breaches of mucosal integrity. See Chapter 20, Medical Management of Malignant Disease, for management of neutropenic fever.

Testing

- Testing includes complete blood count (CBC) with differential, serum chemistries with liver function tests, urinalysis, and blood and urine cultures.
- Diagnostic evaluation generally includes chest radiography.
- Cultures of abnormal fluid collections, sputum, cerebrospinal fluid, and stool should be sent if clinically indicated.

Treatment

- **Antipyretic drugs** may be given to decrease associated discomfort. Not all fevers require treatment. Aspirin (325 mg) and acetaminophen are the drugs of choice (325–650 mg PO or per rectum q4h). **Aspirin should be avoided in adolescents** with possible viral infections because this combination has been associated with Reye's syndrome.
- **Tepid water baths** are effective in treating hyperpyrexia. Use of hypothermic (cooling) blankets and ice packs are uncomfortable and should generally be discouraged.
- **Empiric antibiotics** should be considered in hemodynamically unstable patients in whom infection is a primary concern and in neutropenic and asplenic patients.
- Heat stroke and malignant hyperthermia are medical emergencies that require prompt recognition and treatment (see Chapter 25, Medical Emergencies).

PAIN

General Principles

Definition

- **Pain** is subjective, and therapy must be individualized. Chronic pain may not be associated with any objective physical findings. **Pain scales** should be employed for quantitation.

Classification

- **Acute pain** usually requires only temporary therapy.
- For **chronic pain,** nonnarcotic preparations should be used when possible.
- Anticonvulsants and antidepressants are more useful than narcotics for **neuropathic pain.** If pain is refractory to conventional therapy, then nonpharmacologic modalities, such as nerve blocks, sympathectomy, and relaxation therapy, may be appropriate.

Treatment

Medications

- Acetaminophen
  - Effects
    - Acetaminophen has antipyretic and analgesic actions but does not have anti-inflammatory or antiplatelet properties.
  - Preparations and dosage
    - Acetaminophen, 325–1,000 mg q4–6h (maximum dose, 4 g/d), is available in tablet, caplet, liquid, and rectal suppository form. It should be avoided or used with caution at low doses in patients with liver disease.
  - Adverse effects
    - The principal advantage of acetaminophen is its lack of gastric toxicity.
    - **Hepatic toxicity** may be serious, however, and acute overdose with 10–15 g can cause fatal hepatic necrosis (see Chapter 17, Liver Diseases, and Chapter 25, Medical Emergencies).
- Aspirin
  - Effects
    - **Aspirin** has analgesic, antipyretic, and anti-inflammatory effects.
  - Preparations and dosages
    - Aspirin is given in a dosage of 325–1,000 mg PO q4h PRN (maximum dose, 3 g/d) for relief of pain.
    - Rectal suppositories (300–600 mg q3–4h) may be irritating to the mucosa and have variable absorption.
    - Enteric-coated tablets and nonacetylated salicylates may cause less injury to the gastric mucosa than buffered or plain aspirin.
  - Adverse effects
    - Dose-related **side effects** include tinnitus, dizziness, and hearing loss.

- Dyspepsia and GI bleeding can develop and may be severe.
- Hypersensitivity reactions, including bronchospasm, laryngeal edema, and urticaria, are uncommon, but patients with asthma and nasal polyps are more susceptible.
- **Patients with allergic or bronchospastic reactions to aspirin should not be given NSAIDs.**
- Chronic excessive use can result in interstitial nephritis and papillary necrosis.
- Aspirin should be used with caution in patients with hepatic or renal disease, bleeding disorders, and pregnancy, and those who are receiving anticoagulation therapy.
- **Antiplatelet effects** may last for up to 1 week after a single dose.

- NSAIDs
  - Effects
    - NSAIDs have analgesic, antipyretic, and anti-inflammatory properties mediated by inhibition of cyclooxygenase. All NSAIDs have similar efficacy and toxicities, with a side-effect profile similar to that of the salicylates.
  - Adverse effects
    - NSAIDs may blunt the cardioprotective effects of aspirin.
    - **NSAIDs should be used with caution in patients with impaired renal or hepatic function** (see Chapter 23, Arthritis and Rheumatologic Diseases). **Ketorolac** is an analgesic that can be given IM or IV and is often used postoperatively; however, parenteral therapy should not exceed 5 days. Nephrotoxicity is more pronounced with IM than with PO administration.

- Cyclooxygenase-2 (COX-2) inhibitors
  - Effects
    - **COX-2 inhibitors** act primarily on COX-2, which is an inducible form of cyclooxygenase and an important mediator of pain and inflammation. COX-2 inhibitors have little significant effect on the gastric mucosa. COX-2 inhibitors offer no analgesic advantage over other NSAIDs.
  - Preparations and dosages
    - The currently available selective COX-2 inhibitor is **celecoxib. Meloxicam** is also available but is less selective for COX-2.
  - Adverse effects
    - Chronic, high-dose COX-2 inhibitor use has been shown to increase death from MI.[4,5]
    - COX-2 inhibitors should not be used in patients who have allergic or bronchospastic reactions to aspirin or other NSAIDs.
    - Celecoxib is contraindicated in patients with allergic-type **reactions to sulfonamides.**

- Opioid analgesics
  - Effects
    - Opioid analgesics are pharmacologically similar to opium or morphine and are the drugs of choice when analgesia without antipyretic action is desired.
  - Preparations and dosages
    - Table 1-1 lists equianalgesic dosages.
    - Constant pain
      - **Constant pain** requires continuous (around-the-clock) analgesia with supplementary (PRN) doses for breakthrough pain at doses of roughly one third of the basal dose. Medication dosages should be maintained at the lowest level that provides adequate analgesia. If frequent PRN doses are required, the maintenance dose should be increased, or the dosing interval should be decreased.
      - **If adequate analgesia** cannot be achieved at the maximum recommended dose of one narcotic or if the side effects are intolerable, the patient should be changed to another preparation beginning at one half of the equianalgesic dose to account for incomplete cross tolerance.
      - **Oral medications** should be used when possible.

| **TABLE 1-1** | **Equianalgesic Doses of Opioid Analgesics** |

Drug	Onset (min)	Duration (hr)	IM/IV/SC (mg)	PO (mg)
Fentanyl	7–8	1–2	0.1	NA
Levorphanol	30–90	6–8	2	4
Hydromorphone	15–30	4–5	1.5–2.0	7.5
Methadone	30–60	6–8	10	20
Morphine	15–30	4–6	10	60[a]
Oxycodone	15–30	4–6	NA	30
Meperidine	10–45	2–4	75	300
Codeine	15–30	4–6	120	200

NA, not applicable.
Note: Equivalences are based on single-dose studies.
[a]An IM:PO ratio of 1:23.0 is used for repetitive dosing.

- **Parenteral and transdermal administration** are useful in the setting of dysphagia, emesis, or decreased GI absorption.
- **Continuous IV administration** provides steady blood levels and allows for rapid dose adjustment.
- Agents with short half-lives, such as morphine, should be used. Narcotic-naive patients should be started on the lowest possible doses, whereas patients with demonstrated tolerance will require higher doses.
- **Patient-controlled analgesia** is often used to control pain in a postoperative or terminally ill patient.
  - Advantages of patient-controlled analgesia include enhancement in pain relief, decrease in anxiety, and decrease in the total narcotic dose.
- **Selected drugs**
  - **Codeine** is usually given in combination with aspirin or acetaminophen. It is also an effective cough suppressant at a dosage of 10–15 mg PO q4–q6h.
  - **Oxycodone and propoxyphene** are also usually prescribed orally in combination with aspirin or acetaminophen. Available tablets include oxycodone with acetaminophen (5 mg/325 mg PO q6h), oxycodone with aspirin (5 mg/325 mg PO q6h), and propoxyphene with acetaminophen (50 mg/325 mg or 100 mg/650 mg q6h).
  - **Immediate and sustained-release morphine sulfate** preparations (immediate-release, 5–30 mg PO q2–8h; sustained-release, 15–120 mg PO q12h; or a rectal suppository) can be used. The liquid form can be useful in patients who have difficulty in swallowing pills. Larger doses of morphine may be necessary to control pain as tolerance develops.
  - **Meperidine** (50–150 mg PO, SC, or IM q2–3h) causes less biliary spasm, urinary retention, and constipation than morphine but results in more respiratory depression and is a myocardial depressant. It is **contraindicated in patients who are taking monoamine oxidase inhibitors and in individuals with renal failure** (accumulation of active metabolites causes CNS excitement and seizures). Repetitive dosing is more likely to cause seizures; therefore, chronic administration is not recommended. Coadministration of **hydroxyzine** (25–100 mg IM q4–6h) may decrease nausea and potentiate the analgesic effect of meperidine.
  - **Methadone** is very effective when administered orally and suppresses the symptoms of withdrawal from other opioids because of its extended half-life. Despite its long elimination half-life, its analgesic duration of action is much shorter.
  - **Hydromorphone** (2–4 mg PO q4–6h; 1–2 mg IM, IV, or SC q4–6h) is a potent morphine derivative. It can be given IV with caution. It is also available as a 3-mg rectal suppository.

- **Fentanyl** is available in a transdermal patch with sustained release over 72 hours. Initial onset of action is delayed. Respiratory depression may occur more frequently with fentanyl.
- **Mixed agonist–antagonist agents** (butorphanol, nalbuphine, oxymorphone, pentazocine) offer few advantages and produce more adverse effects than do the other agents.

■ Precautions
- **Opioids are contraindicated** in acute disease states in which the pattern and degree of pain are important diagnostic signs (e.g., head injuries, abdominal pain). They may also increase intracranial pressure.
- **Opioids should be used with caution** in patients with hypothyroidism, Addison disease, hypopituitarism, anemia, respiratory disease (e.g., chronic obstructive pulmonary disease [COPD], asthma, kyphoscoliosis, severe obesity), severe malnutrition, debilitation, or chronic cor pulmonale.
- Opioid dosage should be adjusted for patients with impaired hepatic function.
- Drugs that potentiate the adverse effects of opioids include phenothiazines, antidepressants, benzodiazepines, and alcohol.
- **Tolerance** develops with chronic use and coincides with the development of physical dependence.
- **Physical dependence** is characterized by a withdrawal syndrome (anxiety, irritability, diaphoresis, tachycardia, GI distress, and temperature instability) when the drug is stopped abruptly. It may occur after only 2 weeks of therapy.
- Administration of an opioid antagonist may precipitate withdrawal after only 3 days of therapy. Withdrawal can be minimized by tapering the medication slowly over several days.

■ Adverse and toxic effects
- Although individuals may tolerate some preparations better than others, at equianalgesic doses, few differences in side effects exist.
- **CNS effects** include sedation, euphoria, and pupillary constriction.
- **Respiratory depression** is dose related and is especially pronounced after IV administration.
- **Cardiovascular effects** include peripheral vasodilation and hypotension, especially after IV administration.
- **GI effects** include constipation, nausea, and vomiting. Patients who are receiving opioid medications should be provided with stool softeners and laxatives. Nausea and vomiting can be limited by keeping the patient in a recumbent position. Benzodiazepines, dopamine antagonists (e.g., prochlorperazine, metoclopramide, etc.), and ondansetron can be used as antiemetics. Opioids may precipitate toxic megacolon in patients with inflammatory bowel disease.
- **Urinary retention** may be caused by increased bladder, ureter, and urethral sphincter tone.
- **Pruritus** occurs most commonly with spinal administration.

■ Opioid overdose
- **Naloxone**, an opioid antagonist, should be readily available for administration in the case of accidental or intentional overdose. See Chapter 25, Medical Emergencies, for details of administration.
  - Side effects include hyper- or hypotension, irritability, anxiety, restlessness, tremulousness, nausea, and vomiting.
  - Naloxone can also precipitate seizure activity and cardiac arrhythmias.

Alternative Medications
■ Tramadol
  ■ Tramadol is similar to opioids but has less potential for addiction and abuse.
  ■ Preparations and dosages
  - Between 50 and 100 mg PO q4–6h can be used for acute pain. For elderly patients and those with renal or liver dysfunction, dosage reduction is recommended.

- Adverse effects
  - Because CNS effects include sedation, concomitant use of alcohol, sedatives, or narcotics should be avoided. Nausea, dizziness, constipation, and headache also may occur. Respiratory depression has not been described at prescribed dosages but may occur with overdose. **Tramadol should not be used in patients who are taking a monoamine oxidase inhibitor.**
- **Anticonvulsants** (e.g., gabapentin, valproate) **and tricyclic antidepressants** (e.g., amitriptyline) are PO agents that can be used to treat neuropathic pain.
- **Topical anesthetics** (e.g. lidocaine) may provide analgesia to a localized region (e.g., postherpetic neuralgia).

MENTAL STATUS CHANGES

General Measures

Etiology

Mental status changes have a broad differential diagnosis that includes neurologic (e.g., stroke, delirium), metabolic (e.g., hypoxemia, hypoglycemia), toxic (e.g., drug effects, alcohol withdrawal), and other etiologies.

- **Infection** (e.g., urinary tract infections, pneumonia, etc.) is a common cause of mental status changes in the elderly and patients with underlying neurologic disease.

Diagnosis

History

- **Focus** particularly on medications, underlying dementia, neurologic or psychiatric disorders, and a history of alcohol and drug use.
- Directed history should be obtained from the patient; family and nursing personnel may be able to provide additional details.

Physical Examination

- Physical examination generally includes vital signs, a search for sites of infection, a complete cardiopulmonary examination, and a detailed neurologic examination including mental status evaluation.

Testing

- Testing includes blood glucose, serum electrolytes, creatinine, CBC, urinalysis, oxygen assessment, and chest radiograph.
- Other evaluation, including culture, lumbar puncture, toxicology screen, thyroid function tests, and syphilis serologies, should be directed by initial findings and diagnostic possibilities.
- If indicated by initial findings and diagnostic possibilities, the following should be obtained:
  - Computed tomography (CT) of the head
  - Electroencephalogram (EEG)
  - Electrocardiogram (ECG)

Treatment

Management of specific disorders is discussed in Chapter 24, Neurologic Disorders.

Medications

- **Agitation and psychosis** may be features of a change in mental status. The neuroleptic haloperidol and the benzodiazepine lorazepam are commonly used in the **acute management** of these symptoms. The newer-generation neuroleptics (**risperidone, olanzapine,** quetiapine, clozapine, ziprasidone) are alternative agents that may lead to decreased incidence of extrapyramidal symptoms. All of these agents may pose risks to the elderly if given long term.

- **Haloperidol** is the initial drug of choice for acute management of agitation and psychosis. The initial dose of 1–5 mg (0.25 mg in **elderly patients**) PO, IM, or IV can be repeated every 30–60 minutes until the desired effect is achieved. Sedation is usually achieved with 10–20 mg PO or IM. **IV infusions** (1–40 mg/hr) can also be used as an alternative to bolus injections. Compared with other antipsychotics with similar efficacy, haloperidol has fewer active metabolites and fewer anticholinergic, sedative, and hypotensive effects, although it may have more extrapyramidal side effects. In low dosages, haloperidol rarely causes hypotension, cardiovascular compromise, or excessive sedation.
  - **Prolongation of the QT interval** with development of torsades de pointes may be seen with high-dose IV therapy. In patients who are receiving IV therapy, QTc and electrolytes (primarily potassium and magnesium) should be monitored. Use should be discontinued with prolongation of QTc >450 msec or 25% above baseline.
  - **Postural hypotension** may occasionally be acute and severe after IM administration. If significant hypotension occurs, administration of IV fluids with the patient in the Trendelenburg position is usually sufficient. If **vasopressors** are required, norepinephrine or phenylephrine should be used, as dopamine may exacerbate the psychotic state.
  - **Neuroleptic malignant syndrome** is an infrequent, potentially lethal complication of antipsychotic drug therapy. Clinical manifestations include rigidity, akinesia, altered sensorium, fever, tachycardia, and alteration in BP. Severe muscle rigidity can cause rhabdomyolysis and acute renal failure. **Laboratory abnormalities** include elevations in creatine kinase, liver function tests, and white blood cell count (see Chapter 24, Neurologic Disorders).
- **Lorazepam** is a benzodiazepine that is useful for agitation and psychosis in the setting of hepatic dysfunction and sedative or alcohol withdrawal, and in patients who are refractory to monotherapy with neuroleptics. The **initial dose** is 0.5–2.0 mg IV. The **key features** of lorazepam are its short duration of action and few active metabolites. The use of lorazepam, as with all benzodiazepines, is limited by excess sedation, respiratory depression, and the potential to precipitate agitation in the elderly and in patients with liver disease and low albumin.

Special Considerations

Sundown Syndrome

Definition
- **Sundown syndrome** refers to the appearance of worsening confusion in the evening and is associated with dementia, delirium, and unfamiliar environments.

Treatment
- Behavioral interventions, such as increased lighting, maintenance of a familiar environment, and reorientation, should be attempted first.
- If behavioral interventions are ineffective, short-term antipsychotic therapy may be warranted.

INSOMNIA AND ANXIETY

General Principles

Etiology
- **Insomnia and anxiety** may be attributed to a variety of underlying medical or psychiatric disorders, and symptoms may be exacerbated by hospitalization.

- Possible causes of **insomnia** to consider include mood and anxiety disorders, substance abuse disorders, common medications (i.e., beta-blockers, steroids, bronchodilators, etc.), sleep apnea, hyperthyroidism, and nocturnal myoclonus.
- **Anxiety** may be seen in anxiety disorder, depression, substance abuse disorders, hyperthyroidism, and complex partial seizures.

Treatment

Medications

- Selected medications for insomnia or anxiety, or both
  - Benzodiazepines are frequently used in management of anxiety and insomnia. Table 1-2 provides a list of selected benzodiazepines and their dosages.
    - **Pharmacology.** Most benzodiazepines undergo oxidation to active metabolites in the liver. **Lorazepam, oxazepam, and temazepam** undergo glucuronidation to inactive metabolites; therefore, these agents may be particularly useful in the elderly and in those with liver disease. **Benzodiazepine toxicity** is increased by malnutrition, advanced age, hepatic disease, and concomitant use of alcohol, other CNS depressants, isoniazid, and cimetidine. Benzodiazepines with long half-lives may accumulate substantially, even with single daily dosing. This effect is a particular concern in the elderly, in whom the half-life may be increased twofold to fourfold.
    - **Dosages**
      - **Relief of anxiety and insomnia** is achieved at the doses outlined in Table 1-2. Therapy should be started at the lowest recommended dosage with intermittent dosing schedules.
    - **Side effects** include drowsiness, dizziness, fatigue, psychomotor impairment, and anterograde amnesia.
      - The elderly are more sensitive to these agents and may experience falls, paradoxical agitation, and delirium.
      - **IV administration of diazepam and midazolam** can be associated with hypotension and respiratory or cardiac arrest.
      - **Respiratory depression** can occur even with oral administration in patients with respiratory compromise.

| TABLE 1-2 | Characteristics of Selected Benzodiazepines |

Drug	Route	Usual dosage	Half-life (hr)
Alprazolam	PO	0.75–4.0 mg/24 hr (in three doses)	11–15
Chlordiazepoxide	PO	15–100 mg/24 hr (in divided doses)	6–30
Clorazepate	PO	7.5–60.0 mg/24 hr (in one to four doses)	30–100
Diazepam	PO	6–40 mg/24 hr (in one to four doses)	20–50
	IV	2.5–20.0 mg (slow IV push)	20–50
Flurazepam	PO	15–30 mg at bedtime	50–100
Lorazepam[a]	PO	1–10 mg/24 hr (in two to three doses)	10–20
	IV or IM	0.05 mg/kg (4 mg max)	10–20
Midazolam	IV	0.01–0.05 mg/kg	1–12
	IM	0.08 mg/kg	1–12
Oxazepam[a]	PO	30–120 mg/24 hr (in three to four doses)	5–10
Prazepam	PO	20–60 mg/24 hr (in three to four divided doses)	36–70
Temazepam[a]	PO	15–30 mg at bedtime	9–12
Triazolam[a]	PO	0.125–0.250 mg at bedtime	2–3

[a]Metabolites are inactive.

- Tolerance to benzodiazepines can develop.
- Dependence may develop after only 2–4 weeks of therapy.
- A withdrawal syndrome consisting of agitation, irritability, insomnia, tremor, palpitations, headache, GI distress, and perceptual disturbance begins 1–10 days after a rapid decrease in dosage or abrupt cessation of therapy and may last for several weeks.
- Seizures and delirium may also occur with sudden discontinuation of benzodiazepines. Although the severity and incidence of withdrawal symptoms appear to be related to dose and duration of treatment, withdrawal symptoms have been reported even after brief therapy at doses in the recommended range. Short-acting and intermediate-acting drugs should be decreased by 10%–20% every 5 days, with a slower taper in the final few weeks; long-acting preparations can be tapered more quickly.
- Overdose
    - Flumazenil, a benzodiazepine antagonist, should be readily available in case of accidental or intentional overdose. See Chapter 25, Medical Emergencies, for details of administration. Common side effects include dizziness, nausea, and vomiting.
    - Flumazenil should not be used in patients with a known history of seizure disorder or if overdose with tricyclic antidepressants is suspected.
- Trazodone
    - Trazodone is an antidepressant that may be useful for the treatment of severe anxiety or insomnia.
    - Side effects
        - It is highly sedating, causes postural hypotension, and is associated with ventricular ectopy and priapism. No deaths or cardiovascular complications have been reported in patients taking trazodone alone.
        - A number of potential drug interactions can occur with trazodone.
- Nonbenzodiazepine hypnotics appear to act on the benzodiazepine receptor. These agents have been shown to be safe and effective for initiating sleep. All should be used with caution in patients with impaired respiratory function.
    - Zolpidem is an imidazopyridine hypnotic agent that is useful for the treatment of insomnia. It has no withdrawal syndrome, rebound insomnia, or tolerance. Side effects include headache, daytime somnolence, and GI upset. The starting dose is 5 mg PO every night at bedtime for the elderly and 10 mg for other patients, titrating up to 20 mg as needed. Doses should be reduced in cirrhosis.
    - Zaleplon has a half-life of approximately 1 hour and has no active metabolites. Side effects include drowsiness, dizziness, and impaired coordination. Zaleplon should be used with caution in those with compromised respiratory function. The starting dose is 5 mg PO at bedtime for the elderly or patients with hepatic dysfunction and 10–20 mg PO at bedtime for other patients.
    - Eszopiclone offers a longer half-life compared to the above agents. Side effects include headache, somnolence, and dizziness. Starting dose is 2 mg, with reduced dosing in the elderly, debilitated, and patients with liver disease.
- Antihistamines
    - Over-the-counter antihistamines can be used for insomnia and anxiety, particularly in patients with a history of drug dependence, but are only minimally effective in inducing sleep. Anticholinergic side effects limit the use of these agents.

DEPRESSION

Treatment

Protocol
- Patients with a known history of depression or in whom depression is suspected should be evaluated for the presence of suicidal or homicidal ideations.

- Patients with active ideations or a plan of action, or both, should be monitored by a 1:1 sitter and undergo immediate psychiatric evaluation.
- Psychiatric and medical conditions that may mimic or worsen depression, such as other mood disorders, substance abuse, and hypothyroidism, should be considered.
- **Psychiatric consultation** should be obtained for patients with psychotic features to determine the patient's capacity to make health care decisions.

 # PERIOPERATIVE MEDICINE

- The major focus of the preoperative evaluation of patients about to undergo surgery is to identify those at increased risk for perioperative morbidity and mortality.
- The role of the medical consultant is to risk stratify patients, determine the need for further evaluation, and prescribe possible interventions to mitigate risk.
- Though preoperative consultations often focus on cardiac risk, it is essential to remember that poor outcomes can result from significant disease in other organ systems. Evaluation of the entire patient is necessary to provide optimal perioperative care.

PREOPERATIVE CARDIAC EVALUATION

General Principles

Epidemiology

- Of the millions of patients undergoing noncardiac surgery annually, 1%–6% (depending on the population studied) will suffer a major cardiac event.
- Of those who have a perioperative MI, the risk of in-hospital mortality is estimated at 15%–25%.

Pathophysiology

- The exact mechanism of perioperative myocardial infarctions is not clear.
- Based on autopsy studies and angiographic evidence, it is likely that plaque rupture plays an integral role in a large number of these events, just as in nonperioperative infarcts.
- However, an undetermined number may be due to supply/demand mismatch engendered by the stresses of surgery.

Diagnosis

History

- The focus of the history is to identify factors/comorbid conditions that will affect perioperative risk.
- Different classification schema have identified somewhat different risk factors.
- The **American College of Cardiology (ACC)/American Heart Association (AHA) guidelines**[6] identify three classes of risk factors with gradations of risk:
  - Major
    - Unstable coronary syndromes
    - Decompensated congestive heart failure (CHF)
    - Uncontrolled/unstable arrhythmias
    - Severe/high-grade valvular lesions
  - Intermediate
    - Mild/stable angina
    - Evidence of previous MI
    - Compensated CHF
    - Diabetes mellitus
    - Renal insufficiency

- Minor
  - Advanced age
  - Abnormal ECG
  - Stable nonsinus rhythm
  - Poor functional capacity
  - Prior cerebrovascular accident (CVA)
  - Poorly controlled hypertension
- The **Revised Cardiac Risk Index**[7] is a validated risk-stratification tool that utilizes a smaller set of equally weighted variables:
  - High-risk surgery
  - Ischemic heart disease
  - History of CHF
  - Renal insufficiency
  - Diabetes mellitus requiring insulin therapy
  - History of cerebrovascular disease
- The **Eagle Criteria**[8] were developed for patients undergoing vascular surgery:
  - Q waves on the ECG
  - Angina
  - History of ventricular ectopy requiring therapy
  - Diabetes mellitus requiring medical therapy
  - Age >70 years
- An estimation of a patient's **functional status** should be made. A reliable assessment of functional status can usually be accomplished via history. In general, if patients cannot perform up to four metabolic equivalents (METs) of activity, they have poor functional status.
- Examples of activities that generally require more than four METs are[6]:
  - Able to climb one or more flights of stairs without severe fatigue
  - Able to walk a block at a brisk pace (>4 mph)
  - Able to run for a short distance
  - Able to perform heavy work around the home (mow the lawn, scrub the floors, etc.)
  - Able to participate in sporting activities

Physical Examination
- A complete physical exam is essential.
- Specific attention should be paid to:
  - Vital signs, particularly blood pressure. Though poorly controlled hypertension is only a minor criterion by the ACC/AHA guidelines, **a systolic >180 or diastolic >110 generally is a contraindication to elective surgery**, and therefore must be treated before proceeding.
  - Murmurs suggestive of significant valvular lesions, particularly aortic stenosis (see Valvular Heart Disease)
  - Evidence of congestive heart failure (jugular vein distension [JVD], crackles, S3, etc.)

Classification
- The most widely used algorithm for the preoperative assessment of cardiac risk for noncardiac surgery is the **2002 ACC/AHA guideline**. Since its publication, significant new information has been published, and new guidelines can be expected soon. Two similar algorithms are presented by the guideline to assist in the decision to pursue further cardiac testing prior to surgery. The "shortcut" method is presented here.
  - Consideration is given to the presence of major clinical risk predictors. If any of the major risk factors delineated above exist, the patient most likely would benefit from treatment of these issues prior to surgery.
  - If the patient has *undergone coronary revascularization within the prior 5 years* or has *undergone a cardiac evaluation by stress or angiography within the prior 2 years*, no further evaluation is necessary as long as no new symptoms have developed. The adequacy of this approach has since been questioned.[9]
  - Next, three factors have to be defined:
    1. Does the patient have any intermediate risk factors? These are detailed above.

   2. Is the surgery high risk?
   * The following stratifies surgeries by level of risk[6]:
      – **High risk** (cardiac risk >5%): major vascular surgery, prolonged surgery with marked volume shifts, emergency surgery
      – **Intermediate risk:** carotid endarterectomy, intraperitoneal/intrathoracic surgery, most orthopedic surgery, head and neck surgery
      – **Low risk** (cardiac risk <1%): superficial and endoscopic procedures, cataract surgery, breast surgery
   3. Does the patient have a poor functional status (maximum performance <four METs)?
   ▨ If *any two of these three risk factors* are present, then preoperative stress testing is recommended.
   ▨ It should be noted, however, that the full ACC/AHA algorithm does not recommend further testing prior to low risk procedures if no major clinical predictors.
   ▨ If high-risk results are obtained on the stress evaluation, then consideration should be given to proceeding to a cardiac catheterization preoperatively.
- Alternative strategies for assessing surgical risk are provided by the Revised Cardiac Risk Index and the Eagle Criteria.
- The **Revised Cardiac Risk Index** utilizes the six risk factors listed above. A major advantage of this methodology is the ability to identify patients at low risk of adverse cardiac outcomes despite a poor functional capacity.
   ▨ If one or none of the six risk factors is present, the patient is considered low risk (<1%) and no further testing is necessary.
   ▨ If two or more risk factors are present, further evaluation—likely by stress testing—will be necessary to determine the level of risk.
- The **Eagle Criteria** were developed in a cohort undergoing vascular surgery. The applicability of this method outside of that venue is unclear.
   ▨ If patients have none of the five clinical predictors of risk outlined above, they are considered low risk, and no further testing is necessary.
   ▨ If patients have one or two of the listed factors, then their risk assessment hinges on the results of nuclear perfusion stress results:
      * Patients with no redistribution (negative) perfusion imaging studies are low risk.
      * Patients with redistribution on their studies are high risk.
   ▨ Patients with three or more risk factors are high risk regardless of imaging results and risk reduction strategies would need to be implemented.

Objective Studies
- 12-lead electrocardiogram
   ▨ This is recommended for men aged >40 years and women aged >50 years undergoing intermediate or high-risk procedures.[10]
   ▨ Any patient in whom underlying cardiac disease is a concern because of risk factors (e.g., diabetes) should have an ECG.
   ▨ ECGs need not be routinely obtained in patients undergoing low-risk procedures unless otherwise clinically indicated.
- Resting echocardiogram
   ▨ In general, the indications for echocardiographic evaluation in the preoperative setting are no different than in the nonoperative setting. An echo is not routinely necessary.
   ▨ Murmurs found on physical exam suggestive of significant underlying valvular disease should be evaluated by echo.
   ▨ An assessment of left ventricular function should be considered when there is clinical concern for underlying CHF not previously diagnosed or if there is concern for deterioration since the last exam.
- Stress evaluation
   ▨ The decision to pursue a stress evaluation should be guided by an assessment of preoperative risk as detailed above. **Routine stress evaluation of all patients undergoing surgery is not warranted.**

- Exercise testing
  - If the patient is able to exercise adequately, exercise testing is the first choice. An inability to exercise adequately is itself a risk factor for poor outcomes.
  - Patients must be able to exercise to 85% of their predicted maximal heart rate.
  - The **presence of a left bundle branch block decreases the accuracy of exercise testing.** Vasodilator nuclear imaging is preferred in this instance.
  - Testing modalities
    - **Exercise ECG stress**
      - In general, this is considered the first choice among stress modalities.
      - Patients **must have no baseline ECG abnormalities that preclude interpretation of the test** (e.g., left ventricular [LV] strain).
    - **Exercise-echo** and **exercise-nuclear perfusion** stress testing
      - Neither is clearly superior to the other.
      - Patient comorbidities (e.g., obesity impeding echo windows) and additional questions to be answered (e.g., valvular disease making an echo more useful) should be considered in selecting the modality.
  - Pharmacologic stress testing
    - **Vasodilator-nuclear perfusion imaging** and **dobutamine-echocardiography** are the generally available options.
    - As with exercise testing, neither is clearly superior to the other for risk stratification.
    - Consideration must be given to patient comorbidities that make utilization of a modality's pharmacologic agent undesirable (e.g., supraventricular arrhythmias with dobutamine and bronchospasm with adenosine).
- **Coronary angiography**
  - Some patients will have a clear indication for angiography on clinical grounds apart from preoperative risk stratification (e.g., unstable coronary syndromes). Standard guidelines for the nonperioperative setting should guide the management of these patients.
  - Indications for preoperative coronary angiography in the majority of patients are in flux because of concerns that revascularization of lesions identified at angiography may not improve outcomes (see Revascularization).
  - At present, it is reasonable to pursue angiography in patients with high-risk results on noninvasive testing to further define their level of perioperative risk and to determine if they have disease that would generally mandate consideration of revascularization (e.g., left main disease).
  - The routine use of coronary angiography as a method of risk stratification cannot be recommended.

Treatment

Revascularization

- The best available data on preoperative revascularization comes from a prospective study of patients scheduled to undergo vascular surgery.[11] The group studied all had angiographically significant coronary artery disease and were randomized to revascularization (coronary artery bypass grafting [CABG] in 41% and percutaneous intervention in 59%) versus no revascularization. No difference between the groups in the occurrence of postoperative myocardial infarctions or long-term survival was demonstrated.
- Notable exclusions from the study population were patients found to have significant left main disease, severe LV dysfunction, severe aortic stenosis, and the presence of severe coexisting illnesses.
- Based on these results, **a strategy of routinely pursuing coronary revascularization as a method of decreasing perioperative cardiac risk cannot be recommended.**
- However, careful screening of patients is still essential to **identify those high-risk subsets excluded from study consideration (e.g., aortic stenosis, left main coronary artery disease)** and to identify patients who may obtain a survival benefit from revascularization **independent of their need for noncardiac surgery** (i.e., in accordance with standard guidelines for the performance of percutaneous coronary intervention [PCI] and/or CABG).

- Additional considerations in patients who do undergo **PCI** apply:
  - If an intracoronary stent is utilized, the risk of adverse cardiac outcomes perioperatively is greatly increased in the weeks following the PCI.[12,13] This is thought largely to be due to the occurrence of in-stent restenosis.
  - Any subsequent **surgery needs to be delayed for a minimum of 2 weeks**, though 6 weeks is preferred.
  - Whether this period may need to be lengthened for drug-eluting stents remains to be seen.
  - For angioplasty alone, a 1- to 2-week delay is recommended, though the event rates appear to be considerably lower regardless.[14]

Medical Therapy
- Beta-blockers
  - Evidence
    - There have been numerous studies of the cardioprotective benefit of beta-blockers in the perioperative setting. The use of β_1-selective antagonists appears to be associated with a substantial reduction in cardiac events.
    - Two studies provide the strongest evidence for perioperative beta-blockade:
      - In a study of patients undergoing noncardiac surgery either with coronary artery disease (CAD) or considered to be at risk for CAD (defined as the presence of two or more of the following: age >65, hypertension, current smoking, hypercholesterolemia, and diabetes); atenolol (5–10 mg IV 30 minutes prior to and again immediately after surgery, followed by 50–100 mg PO daily for up to 7 days postoperatively) produced a 15% absolute reduction versus placebo in the combined end point of MI, unstable angina, CHF, myocardial revascularization, or death at 6 months. In addition, atenolol reduced overall mortality at 6 months and 2 years.[15]
      - In a study of patients scheduled to undergo vascular surgery found to have evidence for ischemia on dobutamine echocardiography, bisoprolol was given beginning at least 7 days preoperatively and continuing for 30 days postoperatively. The bisoprolol group showed a 90% reduction in the occurrence of perioperative MI or cardiac death.[16]
      - It should be noted that both of the above studies targeted a reduction in the resting heart rate to <60–65.
    - More recent studies have, however, questioned the efficacy of perioperative beta-blockade, particularly in lower-risk patients.[16a,16b]
    - Recommendations
      - The body of evidence on perioperative beta-blocker use has led the ACC/AHA to issue the following recommendations[17]:
        - Patients with a pre-existing indication for beta-blocker use that are currently receiving them should be continued on therapy.
        - Patients undergoing vascular surgery with evidence of ischemia on preoperative testing should be treated.
        - Patients undergoing high- or intermediate-risk surgery (see Classification) that are found to have CAD or multiple clinical risk factors for CAD should also probably receive beta-blocker therapy.
        - Perioperative beta-blocker use should be considered in patients undergoing high- or intermediate-risk surgery if they have intermediate risk for CAD as defined by the presence of a single risk factor.
        - Because of the increased cardiovascular risk with major vascular surgery, perioperative beta-blocker use can also be considered in patients undergoing vascular surgery who otherwise would be considered to be at low risk for perioperative events.
      - Dosing should be sufficient to reduce the resting heart rate to a goal range of 50–60 so long as the systolic blood pressure remains above 100. Ideally, the heart rate should be kept below 80 intra- and postoperatively.
      - The selection of β_1-selective beta-blockers is recommended. However, it is not necessary to switch a patient previously effectively treated with a nonselective beta-blocker to a cardioselective beta-blocker.

- Attention should be paid to the presence of contraindications to beta-blocker use.
- α_2-**Agonists**
  - Evidence
    - Multiple studies of the perioperative cardiovascular benefit of α_2-agonists have been performed. These included a variety of agents. As clonidine is the α_2-agonist of choice in the United States, it will be the focus here.
    - A meta-analysis of the perioperative use of clonidine concluded that clonidine was able to decrease the incidence of perioperative ischemia in both cardiac and noncardiac surgeries.[18] The study was not able to address the effect on perioperative infarctions or mortality.
    - A subsequent trial of perioperative clonidine use was also able to show a decrement in the incidence of perioperative ischemia, but also showed improvements in both 30-day and 2-year mortality.[19] Whether this was due solely to fewer cardiac events was not clear.
  - Recommendations
    - It appears clonidine does have cardioprotective benefits, but the evidence is not as strong as that for beta-blockers.
    - The use of α_2-agonists as a risk-reduction strategy in patients at risk for adverse cardiac outcomes when beta-blockers are contraindicated appears a reasonable consideration.
    - If given, no particular administration protocol is clearly superior. That used in the study cited above consisted of clonidine 0.2 mg orally on the evening prior with the concurrent placement of a 0.2-mg/d clonidine patch (one time only). An additional 0.2-mg dose of clonidine was given on the morning of surgery due to the expected lag in onset of action of the transdermal preparation. Hemodynamics need to be monitored closely.
- **Statins**
  - Evidence
    - It had been previously recommended to hold statins (HMG-CoA reductase inhibitors) perioperatively because of concerns of increased risk of rhabdomyolysis. It appears now that this is unfounded.[20]
    - Moreover, recent studies suggest there is likely a benefit to the perioperative use of statins:
      - A reduction in in-hospital mortality associated with statin use was demonstrated by two retrospective studies. One was a case-control study of patients undergoing major vascular surgery.[21] The other was a retrospective cohort study of patients undergoing a variety of major noncardiac surgeries.[22]
      - The only (to date) published prospective study of perioperative statin use involved the administration of atorvastatin to patients scheduled to undergo vascular surgery. The atorvastatin group demonstrated an 18% absolute reduction versus placebo in the occurrence at 6 months of the composite end point of cardiac death, nonfatal MI, stroke, and unstable angina.[23]
  - Recommendations
    - Based on the available evidence, a cautious recommendation for the use of statins perioperatively can be made while awaiting the outcomes of larger studies.
    - Targets for statin therapy would appear to be chiefly patients who would otherwise benefit from aggressive lipid lowering such as diabetics.
    - Others would include patients undergoing vascular surgery and patients at high risk for adverse cardiac outcomes such as those with three or more risk factors according to the Revised Cardiac Risk Index (see Classification).
- **Aspirin**
  - Evidence
    - Controversy exists over the use of aspirin in the perioperative period.
    - Traditionally, aspirin is withheld for approximately 1 week prior to invasive procedures to minimize bleeding risk.
    - However, some evidence suggests that withdrawal of aspirin may be associated with an increased risk of cardiac events.[24]

- Also, early use of aspirin postoperatively appears to improve outcomes in coronary artery bypass surgery.[25]
- Recommendations
  - For planned surgeries where increased bleeding could result in significant morbidity (e.g., neurosurgery), aspirin should be held approximately 1 week prior to surgery.
  - For other surgeries, a risk–benefit assessment will need to be undertaken. Regardless, the period during which patients with substantial cardiac risk will be off of aspirin should be minimized.
  - For patients undergoing CABG, holding aspirin preoperatively with early resumption 6 hours postoperatively (if there are no bleeding complications) is recommended.[26]

Follow-Up
- **Postoperative surveillance**
  - Most perioperative events are thought to occur within 72 hours of surgery.
  - A substantial number of these will be asymptomatic, probably as the result of intraoperative occurrence or because of the influence of postoperative analgesics.
    - Therefore, in patients felt to be at intermediate or high risk for perioperative cardiac events, routine surveillance is recommended by the ACC/AHA guideline.
    - No specific protocol is clearly superior, but with what is known about the timing of events, surveillance that captures the 72-hour window when events are likely to occur seems reasonable.
  - The ACC and AHA recommend that ECGs be obtained immediately postoperatively and again on postoperative days 1 and 2. In addition, measurement of cardiac troponins 24 hours postoperatively and again on postoperative day 4 (or the day of discharge, whichever is first) is recommended.
  - Patients felt to be at low risk for perioperative events do not require routine surveillance. Evaluation should be based on clinical necessity.
  - Similarly, there is no need to perform MI surveillance in patients undergoing low-risk procedures.
- **Perioperative infarction**
  - Recent evidence suggests that even slight elevations in cardiac biomarkers are associated with substantial cardiac risk.[27]
  - Aggressive risk reduction in patients with even minor elevations is, therefore, recommended.
  - A full discussion of the management of acute coronary syndromes is detailed elsewhere (see Chapter 5, Ischemic Heart Disease).

SPECIFIC PERIOPERATIVE CARDIOVASCULAR CONDITIONS

Hypertension

General Principles
- Severe hypertension (BP >180/110) preoperatively often results in wider fluctuations in intraoperative BP and has been associated with an increased rate of perioperative cardiac events (see Preoperative Cardiac Evaluation).
- Antihypertensive agents patients are taking prior to admission for surgery may have an impact on the perioperative period:
  - When the patient is receiving beta-blockers or clonidine chronically, withdrawal of these medications may result in tachycardia and rebound hypertension, respectively.
  - Evidence suggests that holding angiotensin-converting enzyme inhibitors and angiotensin II–receptor blockers on the day of surgery may reduce perioperative hypotension. This is believed to be due to the effect of this class of medication in blunting the compensatory activation of the renin-angiotensin system perioperatively.

Treatment
- Hypertension in the postoperative period is a common problem with multiple possible causes.
  - All **remediable causes of hypertension,** such as pain, agitation, hypercarbia, hypoxia, hypervolemia, and bladder distention, should be excluded or treated.
  - Poor control of essential hypertension secondary to discontinuation in the immediate postoperative period of medications the patient was previously taking is not uncommon. Reviewing the patient's home medication list is recommended.
  - A rare cause of perioperative hypertension is **pheochromocytoma,** particularly if its presence was unrecognized. Patients can develop an acute hypertensive crisis perioperatively. Treatment with **phentolamine** or **nitroprusside** is recommended in this situation. Preoperative treatment when the diagnosis is suspected to minimize this risk is recommended. This is classically accomplished by titration of **phenoxybenzamine** preoperatively.
- Many parenteral antihypertensive medications are available for patients who are unable to take medications orally. Transdermal clonidine is also an option, but the onset of action is delayed.
- For further discussion of the management of hypertension, see Chapter 4, Hypertension.

Valvular Heart Disease

General Principles
- Symptomatic **stenotic lesions** such as mitral stenosis and aortic stenosis are associated with perioperative CHF and shock, and preoperative valvotomy or replacement is often needed.
- Severe aortic stenosis is associated with a very high incidence of perioperative MI and mortality.[28]
- Symptomatic **regurgitant lesions** are generally better tolerated perioperatively and can generally be managed medically so long as the patient is well compensated preoperatively.

Treatment
- If surgery is emergent, elective valvular repair will need to be deferred to a later time.
- If surgery can only be delayed for a short period, preoperative valvotomy can be considered.
- The need for **endocarditis prophylaxis** should be considered (see Chapter 13, Treatment of Infectious Diseases).
- Cardiology consultation should be considered when severe disease is present, especially with stenotic lesions.

Pacemakers and Implantable Cardioverter Defibrillators (ICDs)

General Principles
- The use of electrocautery intraoperatively can have adverse effects on the function of implanted cardiac devices.
- A variety of errors can occur from resetting of the device to inadvertent discharge of an ICD.

Treatment
- The following recommendations are adapted from the 2002 ACC/AHA guidelines:
  - Optimally, the device should be interrogated pre- and postoperatively to ensure it is functioning properly.
  - Rate-responsive pacemakers should have this mode deactivated intraoperatively.
  - ICDs should be deactivated immediately preoperatively and reactivated postoperatively to avoid accidental discharge.

PREOPERATIVE PULMONARY EVALUATION

General Principles

Epidemiology

- Clinically significant postoperative *pulmonary complications are probably more common* than cardiac complications,[29] and the occurrence of one probably increases the chances of the other occurring.[30]
- The most common complications include *pneumonia, respiratory failure, bronchospasm, atelectasis,* and *exacerbation* of underlying chronic lung disease.[31]

Etiology

- Much as with cardiovascular complications, both patient-dependent risk factors and surgery-specific risk factors combine to produce the level of risk. These are reviewed in detail in the 2006 guideline from the American College of Physicians.[32]
- Procedure-related risk factors
  - The **surgical site** is generally considered the greatest determinant of risk, with *upper abdominal* and *thoracic* surgeries imparting the greatest risk.[31] Repair of abdominal aortic aneurysms appears to have the single greatest surgical risk. Though not necessarily involving the trunk, head and neck and neurosurgical procedures also have a somewhat increased risk.[33]
  - The **surgery duration** also imparts risk, with prolonged procedures increasing the risk of pulmonary complications.[34]
  - The **type of anesthesia** utilized probably affects risk as well. Though controversial, neuraxial anesthesia is thought to carry less risk than general anesthesia.[35]
- Patient-dependent risk factors
  - **Chronic lung disease,** particularly COPD, has reliably been found to be a risk factor for postoperative pulmonary complications. How much the degree of lung dysfunction increases risk is not clear. Even patients with advanced lung disease can safely undergo surgery if it is deemed necessary.[36] Thus, there is no identified level of lung disease that precludes surgery.
  - **Advanced age** has also been identified as a predictor of postoperative pulmonary complications. The degree to which medical comorbidities confound this information is unclear, but multiple studies have found a significant association and it is included as a factor in risk prediction models, particularly age >60 years.[33,37]
  - **Smoking** is a risk factor for pulmonary complications. The degree of tobacco abuse correlates with the degree of risk as well.[38]
  - **Poor general health status** is, unsurprisingly, associated with increased perioperative pulmonary risk. Multiple measures of general health status have been correlated with poor pulmonary outcomes, including advancing ASA class,[39] higher scores on the Goldman cardiac risk index,[40] and functionally dependent status.[33]
  - **Congestive heart failure** also predicts, as would be expected, pulmonary complications postoperatively.[32]

Diagnosis

History

- The preoperative pulmonary evaluation should focus on evaluating the presence of and severity of patient-dependent risk factors.
  - Any history of chronic lung disease should be detailed. An effort should be made to determine the patient's baseline and whether there has been any recent deterioration, such as increased cough or sputum production.
  - Any symptoms of a current upper respiratory infection should be ascertained. Though not an absolute contraindication to surgery, it seems prudent to postpone purely elective procedures until such infections have resolved.
  - A full smoking history should be obtained.

- As noted, comorbid conditions impact the likelihood of pulmonary complications. Therefore, a complete medical history is necessary.

Physical Examination
- A complete physical examination should be part of any preoperative evaluation.
- Attention should be paid to evidence of chronic lung disease such as increased antero-posterior (AP) dimensions of the chest and the presence of adventitious lung sounds, particularly wheezing.
- The maximum laryngeal height should be determined. A value of <4 cm has been associated with pulmonary complications. Persistent coughing after a voluntary cough is also an indicator of increased risk.[38]

Laboratory Studies
- Pulmonary function tests (PFTs)
  - The value of preoperative PFTs is unclear and controversial outside of lung resection surgery, where their role is better defined.
  - Though PFTs can clearly be used to define lung disease, in the setting of nonpulmonary surgery there is concern that they add little beyond what can be gathered clinically.[41]
  - Firm recommendations for or against PFTs cannot be made.
  - However, in patients with unexplained pulmonary symptoms and patients with lung disease and an unclear baseline, PFTs should be considered.
- Arterial blood gas (ABG) analysis
  - It is unclear that ABG results add to the estimate of preoperative pulmonary risk beyond other clinically derived variables.
  - In general, an ABG is not an integral part of the preoperative pulmonary evaluation.[31]
  - An ABG should be obtained *when otherwise clinically necessary,* such as to determine if a patient's lung disease is compensated.
- Chest radiography
  - The value of a routine chest radiograph is variable.
  - Many findings deemed abnormal are chronic and do not affect management.[41]
  - However, as patients age, the value of a screening chest radiograph increases.
  - Though the yield of films that will alter management remains low, the minority of patients that will benefit probably justifies screening in the subset of patients *>50 years of age* or those with *known or suspected cardiopulmonary disease.*[10]
  - Chest radiography should not be used routinely to evaluate perioperative pulmonary risk.[32]
- Serum albumin
  - A decreased serum albumin level is a potent predictor of pulmonary risk.[42]
  - Though studies vary in definition, a level <3.5 mg/dL appears to be indicative of increased risk.
  - Despite the evidence identifying a decreased albumin level as a strong predictor of perioperative risk, there is at present no conclusive evidence that enteral or parenteral **nutritional supplementation** decreases risk.[43]

Classification
- Unlike the situation for preoperative cardiac risk stratification, relatively few tools for estimating preoperative pulmonary risk are available.
- Risk indexes for predicting postoperative respiratory failure[33] and postoperative pneumonia[37] have been developed.
- Though somewhat cumbersome, these represent the best available risk prediction tools.

Treatment
- Modifiable patient-related risk factors
  - Benefit from **smoking cessation** has been shown if patients stop smoking at least 8 weeks before surgery. All patients should be counseled to stop smoking even if

<8 weeks from surgery, however. Previous concerns about a paradoxical increase in complications appear unwarranted.[44]

■ **COPD therapy** should be optimized. Symptoms should be aggressively treated preoperatively. Although not all patients with COPD respond to corticosteroid therapy, a preoperative course of **steroids** is reasonable for symptomatic patients already receiving **maximal bronchodilator therapy** who are not at their best personal baseline level as determined by examination, chest radiography, and spirometry. Patients *with recent sputum changes* may benefit from a preoperative course of **antibiotics**.

■ Modifiable procedure-related risk factors
  ■ Consideration of alternative procedures with the lowest possible pulmonary risk should be undertaken for high-risk patients. **Laparoscopic procedures** may be associated with a lower risk of postoperative pulmonary complications.[45] Whether the complications that are prevented are clinically relevant is not clear.[43]
  ■ Though the choice of anesthesia is the province of the anesthesiologist, where possible, use of **neuraxial/regional** anesthetic methods should be considered.

■ Postoperative interventions
  ■ **Lung expansion maneuvers**, such as *incentive spirometry* or *deep breathing exercises*, should be employed.
  ■ **Continuous positive airway pressure (CPAP)** can be considered for patients unable to participate in other lung expansion maneuvers. A recent study utilizing a novel delivery device in patients with postoperative hypoxemia showed benefit, but whether the same would be seen with a conventional face or nasal mask is uncertain.[46] Because of the potential complications of its use, patients being treated with CPAP should be monitored closely.
  ■ **Appropriate analgesia** is essential to prevent splinting, but oversedation needs to be carefully avoided. The use of postoperative **epidural analgesia** has been shown to reduce the incidence of pulmonary complications, and its use should be considered.[31]
  ■ A strategy of **selective nasogastric tube placement** rather than routine use has also been shown to decrease the risk of pulmonary complications.[43]
  ■ Appropriate **DVT prophylaxis** is strongly encouraged (see Venous Thromboembolism Prophylaxis).

TRANSFUSION ISSUES IN SURGERY

General Principles

■ Transfusion of blood products is associated with substantial risks including transmission of bloodborne infections, transfusion reactions, and possibly immunomodulatory effects.
■ The threshold at which a red cell transfusion should be administered is unclear.
  ■ A study of intensive care unit (ICU) patients suggested that the classic transfusion threshold of a hemoglobin of 10 g/dL was too liberal, as patients treated with a more "restrictive" strategy (with a trigger of 7 g/dL) had outcomes that were at least equivalent and in some cases better.[47]
  ■ There is concern that the elderly may not tolerate such a conservative strategy as well. Perioperative myocardial ischemia may be more common in this population when the hematocrit drops below 28%.[48]

Treatment

■ It is generally agreed that **transfusion is not required when the hemoglobin exceeds 10 g/dL**.
■ Likewise, it is generally agreed that **a hemoglobin <7 g/dL necessitates transfusion**. Data from perioperative patients who refused transfusion on religious grounds provide a basis for this, showing a marked increase in mortality as hemoglobin levels dropped below 7 g/dL.[49]
■ The best strategy for patients with hemoglobin between 7 and 10 g/dL is unclear.
  ■ Physiologic markers of intolerance to anemia (e.g., tachycardia) should be considered.

■ Patients with **significant cardiopulmonary disease** and the **elderly (age >65)** will likely tolerate significant anemia less well. A reasonable transfusion threshold in this subset is a **hemoglobin <8 g/dL**.[50]

Special Considerations

■ Measures to *reduce the need for allogeneic blood* should be utilized where feasible.
  ■ Preoperative **autologous blood donation** should be considered for elective procedures where the anticipated need for transfusion is high.
  ■ **Preoperative erythropoietin** can be considered in patients with a decreased hemoglobin concentration.[51] Patients need to have adequate iron stores when this is utilized; supplemental iron therapy may be required.
  ■ **Intraoperative measures** include *normovolemic hemodilution* for elective surgery, *intraoperative blood salvage and autotransfusion*, and *positional blood pooling*.
■ Patients with **sickle cell anemia** require transfusion to a hemoglobin of 10 g/dL preoperatively to decrease the incidence of complications.

SURGERY IN THE PATIENT WITH LIVER DISEASE

General Principles

■ Patients with hepatic dysfunction suffer from an increased risk of morbid outcomes when undergoing surgery.
■ Probably because of decreased hepatic perfusion during anesthesia, patients with underlying liver disease are at substantial risk for acute hepatic decompensation postoperatively.[52]
■ The myriad systemic effects of liver dysfunction result in an increased frequency of other complications as well, such as bleeding.

Diagnosis

History and Physical Examination

■ As part of the preoperative history and physical, evidence of liver disease should be sought.
  ■ Historical details suggesting a risk for hepatic disease such as alcohol or drug abuse and prior blood transfusion should be sought.
  ■ Physical examination evidence of liver dysfunction should be noted. Some should be obvious, such as icterus and abdominal distension with ascites, but other abnormalities such as spider nevi, palmar erythema, and testicular atrophy may be more subtle.
■ Other indicators of a risk for liver disease may be noted in the preoperative evaluation (e.g., family history of hemochromatosis).

Laboratory Studies

■ Because of the low prevalence and because significant disease is usually clinically suspected, *routine laboratory screening for hepatic dysfunction in patients presenting for surgery who are without clinically suspected or known liver disease is not recommended*.[53]
■ Patients with known or suspected liver disease should undergo a thorough evaluation of liver function including **hepatic enzyme levels**, **albumin** and **bilirubin** measurements, and **evaluation for coagulopathy**.
■ **Renal function**, including electrolytes, blood urea nitrogen (BUN), and creatinine measurements, should also be evaluated.

Classification

■ The best validated measure of perioperative risk in patients *with cirrhosis* is the **Child-Pugh score**, reflecting increased risk with greater degrees of hepatic dysfunction.

- In a study of patients undergoing abdominal surgery (both elective and emergent), perioperative mortality was 10% for Child's class A, 30% for Child's class B, and 82% for Child's class C.[54]
- This is remarkably similar to data obtained in the prior decade.[55]
- The **MELD score** may also be a reliable indicator of postoperative mortality in cirrhotics, particularly a score ≥ 8.[56]

Treatment

- Patients with **acute viral or alcoholic hepatitis** tolerate surgery poorly, and *delaying surgery until recovery is recommended* if possible.
- Patients with **chronic hepatitis** without evidence of hepatic decompensation generally tolerate surgery well.
- Based on the high perioperative mortality rates in patients with **advanced cirrhosis,** nonoperative alternatives should be strongly considered.
- For patients who do require surgery, steps should be taken to optimize the preoperative status.
  - **Coagulopathy** should be corrected.
    - Vitamin K should be administered if the international normalized ratio (INR) is elevated. As the coagulopathy may well be refractory to this measure in the setting of liver disease, fresh frozen plasma and cryoprecipitate may be required.
    - **Thrombocytopenia** is a common occurrence and should generally be corrected if severe. The general recommendation for most surgical procedures is a minimum platelet count of 50,000. However, in the setting of liver disease, the coexistence of platelet dysfunction should be considered, particularly if there is clinical bleeding with an otherwise adequate platelet count.
  - **Renal and electrolyte abnormalities** should be addressed.
    - Careful attention should be paid to **volume status.**
    - Nephrotoxic substances, such as NSAIDs and aminoglycosides, should be avoided.
    - Patients with cirrhosis often have **hypokalemia** and **alkalosis.** These conditions should be corrected preoperatively to minimize the risks of cardiac arrhythmias and to limit encephalopathy.
    - If **hyponatremia** occurs, free water restriction may be required.
  - **Ascites** should be treated.
    - The presence of ascites may influence respiratory mechanics and increase the risk of abdominal wound dehiscence.
    - If time permits, **diuretic therapy** should be instituted.
    - **Paracentesis** should be considered preoperatively if diuretics are ineffective or if time constraints prevent their use.
  - **Encephalopathy** should be treated.
    - **Lactulose** titrated to two to three soft bowel movements per day should be started in patients with encephalopathy.
    - Protein restriction has been recommended for individuals who respond poorly to lactulose but should be done cautiously, because excessive restriction may actually contribute to malnutrition.
    - **Sedatives and other narcotics** can precipitate or worsen encephalopathy. They should be used only cautiously and dose reductions should be considered.
    - **Hypokalemia** should be avoided.
  - Adequate **nutrition** should be provided.

PERIOPERATIVE DIABETES MANAGEMENT

General Principles

- Hospitalized patients with diabetes and hyperglycemia are at increased risk for poor outcomes.[57]

- Improving glucose control in patients requiring critical care postoperatively appears to decrease mortality.[58]
- Poor glucose control is associated with an increased risk of postoperative infections.[59]
- It is unclear if improving glucose control in the non-ICU setting improves mortality, but given the association between hyperglycemia and poor outcomes in the general inpatient setting, this is suggested.
- Diabetics are at increased risk for cardiovascular disease. Appropriate *risk stratification for cardiac complications* of surgery is vital to the perioperative evaluation of these patients.

Diagnosis

Classification

- Establishing the etiology of hyperglycemia has important implications for subsequent patient care.
  - **Stress hyperglycemia** can occur in the perioperative setting because of the body's response to surgery with the release of counterregulatory hormones and cytokines that impede glucose metabolism. These patients need adequate glucose control during the perioperative period, but are unlikely to require such treatment later.
  - Type 2 diabetes is notoriously underdiagnosed, however, and the notation of perioperative hyperglycemia may be the first indication of its presence.
- It is also *essential to distinguish between type 1 and type 2 diabetes mellitus.*
  - **Type 1 diabetics** will require a continuous supply of insulin regardless of glucose level and oral intake.
  - The insulin requirement, if any, of **type 2 diabetics** during the perioperative period will vary.

Laboratory Studies

- Most patients should have a **hemoglobin A_{1c}** obtained.
  - This can assist in differentiating perioperative stress hyperglycemia from undiagnosed diabetes.
  - Knowledge of recent glycemic control in known diabetics is also helpful in determining what therapy is required.
- Evaluating **renal function** is also recommended given the increased prevalence of renal disease in diabetics.
- Cardiovascular risk stratification may require other evaluations (see Preoperative Cardiovascular Evaluation).

Treatment

- Elective surgery in patients with uncontrolled diabetes mellitus should preferably be scheduled after acceptable glycemic control has been achieved.
- If possible, the operation should be scheduled for early morning to minimize prolonged fasting.
- Frequent monitoring of blood glucose levels is required in all situations.
- **Type 1 diabetes**
  - Some form of **basal insulin is required at all times.**
  - On the evening prior to surgery, the regularly scheduled basal insulin should be continued. If taken in the morning, it is still recommended to give the regularly scheduled basal insulin without dose adjustment.[60]
  - **Glucose infusions** (e.g., D_5-containing fluids) can be administered to avoid hypoglycemia while the patient is NPO and until tolerance of oral intake postoperatively is established.
  - For complex procedures and procedures requiring a prolonged NPO status, a **continuous insulin infusion** will likely be necessary.
  - Caution should be exercised with the use of subcutaneous insulin in the intraoperative and critical care settings, as alterations in tissue perfusion may result in variable absorption.

- Type 2 diabetes
  - Treatment of type 2 diabetics varies according to their preoperative requirements and the complexity of the planned procedure.[61]
  - Consideration should be given to the efficacy of the patients' current regimen. If they are not well controlled at baseline, then an escalation in therapy may be required.
  - **Diet-controlled type 2 diabetes**
    - This can generally be managed without insulin therapy.
    - Glucose values should be checked regularly and elevated levels (>180 mg/dL) can be treated with intermittent doses of short-acting insulin.
  - **Type 2 diabetes managed with oral therapy**
    - **Short-acting sulfonylureas** and **other oral agents** should be withheld on the operative day.
    - **Metformin** and **long-acting sulfonylureas** (e.g., chlorpropamide) should be withheld 1 day before planned surgical procedures. Metformin is generally held for 48 hours postoperatively. Renal function should be normal prior to resuming treatment. Other oral agents can be resumed when patients are tolerating their preprocedure diet.
    - Most patients can be managed without an insulin infusion.
    - Glucose values should be checked regularly and elevated levels (>180 mg/dL) can be treated with intermittent doses of short-acting insulin.
  - **Type 2 diabetes managed with insulin**
    - If it is anticipated the patient will be able to eat postoperatively, basal insulin is still given on the morning of surgery.
      - If given as long-acting insulin (e.g., glargine insulin) and the patient usually takes the dose in the morning, 50%–100% of the usual dose can be given.[60]
      - If the patient utilizes intermediate-acting insulin (e.g., NPH), one-half to two thirds of the usual morning dose is given to avoid periprocedural hyperglycemia.
    - Dextrose-containing IV fluids may be required to avoid hypoglycemia.
    - Patients undergoing major procedures will typically require an insulin drip perioperatively.
      - Glucose and potassium will need to be administered concomitantly to avoid hypoglycemia and hypokalemia, respectively.
      - The presence of renal dysfunction may contraindicate the use of potassium, however.
      - The usual starting dose for an insulin infusion is 0.2 units/kg/hr.
    - The usual insulin treatment can be resumed once oral intake is established postoperatively.
- Target glucose levels
  - There are no generally agreed upon target glucose levels applicable to the entire postsurgical population.
    - The best data are available for critically ill postoperative patients, where a glucose target of 80–110 was shown to reduce mortality.[58]
    - There is also evidence that perioperative insulin infusion with a target glucose level of 100–150 in patients undergoing CABG improves mortality.[62]
    - In a general medical-surgical population, recurring glucose values >200 mg/dL were associated with a poor outcome.[57]
  - Based on this data, the American College of Endocrinology recommends a **target glucose of <110 mg/dL in patients requiring ICU care and <180 mg/dL in all other inpatients.**[63]

PERIOPERATIVE CORTICOSTEROID MANAGEMENT

General Principles

- Surgery is a potent activator of the hypothalamic-pituitary axis.
- Patients with adrenal insufficiency may lack the ability to respond appropriately to surgical stress.

- Further, patients receiving corticosteroids as medical therapy for indications other than adrenal dysfunction may develop adrenal insufficiency.
- How to best identify and treat these patients has undergone considerable change since the case reports of postoperative crises in the 1950s.

Pathophysiology
- The subtype of adrenal insufficiency has implications on management.
  - **Tertiary adrenal insufficiency** due to exogenous corticosteroid administration is the most common adrenal problem encountered. These patients should have intact mineralocorticoid function and therefore require only glucocorticoid supplementation.[64]
  - Likewise, **secondary adrenal insufficiency** should not result in mineralocorticoid deficiency. The possibility of deficits in other hormones due to pituitary disease should be considered.
  - **Primary adrenal insufficiency** requires replacement of both mineralocorticoids and glucocorticoids.
- The dose and duration of exogenous corticosteroids required to produce clinically significant tertiary adrenal insufficiency is highly variable, but general principles can be outlined.[61]
  - Daily therapy with **5 mg or less of prednisone (or its equivalent), alternate-day corticosteroid therapy,** and **any dose given for** <3 weeks *should not result in clinically significant adrenal suppression.*
  - Patients receiving **>20 mg/d of prednisone (or equivalent) for** >3 **weeks** and patients that are clinically **cushingoid in appearance** can be expected to have *significant suppression of adrenal responsiveness.*
  - The function of the hypothalamic-pituitary axis *cannot be readily predicted* in **patients receiving doses of prednisone 5–20 mg for** >3 **weeks and patients receiving doses >5 mg for** >3 **weeks within the prior year.**

Diagnosis

History and Physical Examination
- The dose and duration of prior corticosteroid therapy should be clarified.
- The coexistence of diseases that suggest the possibility of primary adrenal insufficiency should be sought (e.g., autoimmune thyroid disease, malignant tumors that metastasize to the adrenal such as lung cancer, etc.).
- Physical exam findings suggestive of adrenal hypofunction such as hyperpigmentation should be noted. As above, inspection for features of a cushingoid appearance should be performed.

Laboratory Studies
- For patients in whom clinical prediction of adrenal function is difficult, a **cosyntropin stimulation test** can be performed.
- **Electrolyte abnormalities** should be sought in patients with *primary adrenal insufficiency.* Patients with *other forms of adrenal insufficiency are unlikely to manifest the classic hyperkalemia and hyponatremia* due to intact mineralocorticoid function.

Treatment

- **Patients expected to have an intact adrenal function** (as outlined above) should take their regularly scheduled dose of corticosteroid. No further treatment is required.
- Some literature has suggested that patients with proven adrenal hyporesponsiveness may safely undergo surgery without glucocorticoid supplementation, but at present this has not been widely adopted.[65]
- At present, it is generally agreed that **patients with known or expected adrenal insufficiency** should be treated with perioperative glucocorticoids.
- In **patients whose hypothalamic-pituitary axis status is uncertain** and there is inadequate time to perform a cosyntropin stimulation test, corticosteroids can be administered preoperatively.

■ These guidelines are based on extrapolation from small studies in the literature, expert opinion, and clinical experience.[66]

　■ **Minor surgical stress** (e.g., colonoscopy, cataract surgery): Administer 25 mg hydrocortisone or 5 mg methylprednisolone IV on the day of the procedure only.

　■ **Moderate surgical stress** (e.g., cholecystectomy, hemicolectomy): Administer 50–75 mg hydrocortisone or 10–15 mg methylprednisolone IV on the day of the procedure and taper quickly over 1–2 days to the usual dose.

　■ **Major surgical stress** (e.g., major cardiothoracic surgery, Whipple procedure): Administer 100–150 mg hydrocortisone or 20–30 mg methylprednisolone IV on the day of the procedure and taper to the usual dose over the next 1–2 days.

　■ **Critically ill patients undergoing emergent surgery** (e.g., sepsis, hypotension): Administer 50–100 mg hydrocortisone IV every 6–8 hours or 0.18 mg/kg/hr as a continuous infusion plus 50 mcg/d of fludrocortisone until the shock has resolved. Then gradually taper the dose, monitoring vital signs and serum sodium closely.

■ Additional **mineralocorticoid supplementation** for patients with primary adrenal insufficiency may or may not be necessary, depending on the dose and mineralocorticoid potency of the corticosteroid given.

PERIOPERATIVE CARE OF KIDNEY DISEASE

Chronic Renal Insufficiency and End-Stage Renal Disease

General Principles
■ **Chronic renal insufficiency (CRI)** is an independent risk factor for **perioperative cardiac complications,** so all patients with renal disease need appropriate cardiac risk stratification.[7]
■ **Patients with end-stage renal disease (ESRD)** have a substantial mortality risk when undergoing surgery.[67]

Treatment
■ **Volume status**
　■ Every effort should be made to **achieve euvolemia** preoperatively to reduce the incidence of volume-related complications intra- and postoperatively.[68]
　■ Though this typically entails removing volume, some patients will be hypovolemic and require hydration.
　■ Patients with chronic renal insufficiency not receiving hemodialysis may require treatment with loop diuretics.
　■ Patients being treated with **hemodialysis** should undergo dialysis preoperatively.
　　• This is commonly performed on the day prior to surgery.
　　• Hemodialysis can be performed on the day of surgery as well. The possibility that transient electrolyte abnormalities and hemodynamic changes postdialysis can occur should be considered.
■ **Electrolyte abnormalities**
　■ **Hyperkalemia** in the preoperative setting should be treated, particularly as tissue breakdown associated with surgery may elevate the potassium level further postoperatively.
　　• For patients on dialysis, preoperative dialysis should be utilized.
　　• For patients with chronic renal insufficiency not undergoing dialysis, alternative methods of potassium excretion will be necessary.
　■ **Loop diuretics** can be utilized, particularly if the patient is also hypervolemic.
　■ **Sodium polystyrene sulfonate (SPS) resins** can also be utilized. The possibility that *intestinal necrosis* with SPS resins occurs more frequently in the perioperative setting has been suggested.[69]
　■ Although chronic **metabolic acidosis** has not been associated with elevated perioperative risk, some local anesthetics have reduced efficacy in acidotic patients.

Preoperative metabolic acidosis should be corrected with sodium bicarbonate infusions or dialysis.
- Bleeding diathesis
  - **Platelet dysfunction** has long been associated with uremia.
    - The value of a preoperative bleeding time in predicting postoperative bleeding has been questioned.[70] A preoperative bleeding time is, therefore, not recommended.
    - Patients that evidence perioperative bleeding should, however, be treated.
      - **Dialysis** for patients with ESRD will improve platelet function.
      - **Desmopressin** (0.3 mcg/kg IV or intranasally) can be utilized.
      - **Cryoprecipitate,** 10 U over 30 minutes IV, is an additional option.
      - In patients with coexisting anemia, **red blood cell transfusions** can improve uremic bleeding.
      - For patients **with a history of prior uremic bleeding,** preoperative desmopressin or **conjugated estrogens** (0.6 mg/kg/d IV or PO for 5 days) should be considered.
  - **Heparin** given with dialysis can increase bleeding risk. *Heparin-free dialysis* should be discussed with the patient's nephrologist when surgery is planned.
- Antibiotic prophylaxis
  - Patients with renal disease should be treated with surgery-appropriate prophylactic antibiotics to prevent surgical-site infections. Renal dosing may be necessary.
  - At present it is not clear that prophylactic antibiotics (as for endocarditis prophylaxis) are necessary in patients with surgically created dialysis access sites.[71]

Acute Renal Failure

General Principles
- Surgery has been associated with an increased risk of **acute renal failure (ARF).**[68]
- Patients with **chronic renal insufficiency (CRI)** are at increased risk of acute renal failure.
- The approach to acute renal failure in the perioperative setting is not substantially different from in the nonoperative setting.
- However, certain additional factors have to be considered when evaluating the cause in the perioperative setting:
  - **Intraoperative hemodynamic changes,** particularly hypotension, should be considered. A careful review of the operative record is advised.
  - Certain procedures can have an adverse effect on renal function (e.g., aortic clamping procedures). Therefore, careful attention to the details of the procedure is necessary.
  - The possibility that bleeding is responsible for a prerenal state deserves special attention.
- For further management, see Chapter 11, Renal Diseases.

References
1. Geerts WH, Pineo GF, Heit JA, et al. Prevention of venous thromboembolism: the Seventh ACCP Conference on Antithrombotic and Thrombolytic Therapy. *Chest* 2004;126:338S–400S.
2. Treatment of Pressure Ulcers Guideline Panel. Treatment of Pressure Ulcers. Clinical Practice Guideline, Number 15. AHCPR Publication No. 92-0652. Rockville, MD: Agency for Health Care Policy and Research, Public Health Service, U.S. Department of Health and Human Services. December 1994.
3. Lyder CH. Pressure ulcer prevention and management. *JAMA* 2003;289:223–226.
4. Bennett JS, Daugherty A, Herrington D, et al. The use of nonsteroidal anti-inflammatory drugs (NSAIDs): a science advisory from the American Heart Association. *Circulation* 2005;111:1713–1716.
5. Bertagnolli MM, Eagle CJ, Zauber AG, et al. Celecoxib for the prevention of sporadic colorectal adenomas. *N Engl J Med* 2006; 355:873–884.

6. Eagle KA, Berger PB, Calkins H, et al. American College of Cardiology. American Heart Association. ACC/AHA guideline update for perioperative cardiovascular evaluation for noncardiac surgery—executive summary: a report of the American College of Cardiology/American Heart Association Task Force on Practice Guidelines (Committee to Update the 1996 Guidelines on Perioperative Cardiovascular Evaluation for Noncardiac Surgery). *J Am Coll Cardiol* 2002;39:542–553.

7. Lee TH, Marcantonio ER, Mangione CM, et al. Derivation and prospective validation of a simple index for prediction of cardiac risk of major noncardiac surgery. *Circulation* 1999;100:1043–1049.

8. Eagle KA, Coley CM, Newell JB, et al. Combining clinical and thallium data optimizes preoperative assessment of cardiac risk before major vascular surgery. *Ann Int Med* 1989;110:859–866.

9. Bursi F, Babuin L, Barbieri A, et al. Vascular surgery patients: perioperative and long-term risk according to the ACC/AHA guidelines, the additive role of postoperative troponin elevation. *Eur Heart J* 2005;26:2448–2456.

10. Smetana GW, Macpherson DS. The case against routine preoperative laboratory testing. *Med Clin N Am* 2003;87:7–40.

11. McFalls EO, Ward HB, Moritz TE, et al. Coronary-artery revascularization before elective major vascular surgery. *N Engl J Med* 2004;351:2795–2804.

12. Kaluza GL, Joseph J, Lee Jr, et al. Catastrophic outcomes of noncardiac surgery soon after coronary stenting. *J Am Coll Cardiol* 2000;35:1288–1294.

13. Wilson SH, Fasseas P, Orford JL, et al. Clinical outcome of patients undergoing noncardiac surgery in the two months following coronary stenting. *J Am Coll Cardiol* 2003;42:234–240.

14. Brilakis ES, Orford JL, Fasseas P, et al. Outcome of patients undergoing balloon angioplasty in the two months prior to noncardiac surgery. *Am J Cardiol* 2005;96:512–514.

15. Mangano DT, Layug EL, Wallace A, et al. Effect of atenolol on mortality and cardiovascular morbidity after noncardiac surgery. *N Engl J Med* 1996;335:1713–1720.

16. Poldermans D, Boersma E, Bax JJ, et al. The effect of bisoprolol on perioperative mortality and myocardial infarction in high-risk patients undergoing vascular surgery. *N Engl J Med* 1999;341:1789–1794.

16a. Lindenauer PK, Pekow P, Wang K, et al. Perioperative beta-blocker therapy and mortality after major noncardiac surgery. *N Engl J Med* 2005;353:412–414.

16b. Juul AB, Wetterslev J, Gluud C, et al. Effect of perioperative beta blockade in patients with diabetes undergoing major non-cardiac surgery: randomised placebo controlled, blinded multicentre trial. *BMJ* 2006;332:1482.

17. Fleisher LA, Beckman JA, Brown KA, et al. ACC/AHA 2006 Guideline Update on Perioperative Cardiovascular Evaluation for Noncardiac Surgery: Focused Update on Perioperative Beta-Blocker Therapy. *A Report of the American College of Cardiology/American Heart Association Task Force on Practice Guidelines (Writing Committee to Update the 2002 Guidelines on Perioperative Cardiovascular Evaluation for Noncardiac Surgery).* J Am Coll Cardiol 2006;47:2343–2355.

18. Nishina K, Mikawa K, Uesugi T, et al. Efficacy of clonidine for prevention of perioperative myocardial ischemia: a critical appraisal and meta-analysis of the literature. *Anesthesiology* 2002;96:323–329.

19. Wallace AW, Galindez D, Salahieh A, et al. Effect of clonidine on cardiovascular morbidity and mortality after noncardiac surgery. *Anesthesiology* 2004;101:284–293.

20. Schouten O, Kertai MD, Bax JJ, et al. Safety of perioperative statin use in high-risk patients undergoing major vascular surgery. *Am J Cardiol* 2005;95:658–660.

21. Poldermans D, Bax JJ, Kertai MD, et al. Statins are associated with a reduced incidence of perioperative mortality in patients undergoing major noncardiac vascular surgery. *Circulation* 2003;107:1848–1851.

22. Lindenauer PK, Pekow P, Wang K, et al. Lipid-lowering therapy and in-hospital mortality following major noncardiac surgery. *JAMA* 2004;291:2092–2099.

23. Durazzo AE, Machado FS, Ikeoka DT, et al. Reduction in cardiovascular events after vascular surgery with atorvastatin: a randomized trial. *J Vasc Surg* 2004;39:967–976.

24. Ferrari E, Benhamou M, Cerboni P, et al. Coronary syndromes following aspirin withdrawal: a special risk for late stent thrombosis. *J Am Coll Cardiol* 2005;45:456–459.

25. Mangano DT. Aspirin and mortality from coronary bypass surgery. *N Engl J Med* 2002;347:1309–1317.

26. Stein PD, Schunemann HJ, Dalen JE, et al. Antithrombotic therapy in patients with saphenous vein and internal mammary artery bypass grafts: the Seventh ACCP Conference on Antithrombotic and Thrombolytic Therapy. *Chest* 2004;126(S):600S–608S.

27. Landesberg G, Shatz V, Akopnik I, et al. Association of cardiac troponin, CK-MB, and postoperative myocardial ischemia with long-term survival after major vascular surgery. *J Am Coll Cardiol* 2003;42:1547–1554.

28. Kertai MD, Bountioukos M, Boersma E, et al. Aortic stenosis: an underestimated risk factor for perioperative complications in patients undergoing noncardiac surgery. *Am J Med* 2004;116:8–13.

29. McAlister FA, Bertsch K, Man J, et al. Incidence of and risk factors for pulmonary complications after nonthoracic surgery. *Am J Respir Crit Care Med* 2005;171:514–517.

30. Fleischmann KE, Goldman L, Young B, et al. Association between cardiac and noncardiac complications in patients undergoing noncardiac surgery: outcomes and effects on length of stay. *Am J Med* 2003;115:515–520.

31. Smetana GW. Preoperative pulmonary evaluation. *N Engl J Med* 1999;340:937–944.

32. Qaseem A, Snow V, Fitterman N, et al. Risk assessment for and strategies to reduce perioperative pulmonary complications for patients undergoing noncardiothoracic surgery: a guideline from the American College of Physicians. *Ann Int Med* 2006;144:575–580.

33. Arozullah AM, Daley J, Henderson WG, et al. Multifactorial risk index for predicting postoperative respiratory failure in men after major noncardiac surgery. *Ann Surg* 2000;232:242–253.

34. Kroenke K, Lawrence VA, Theroux JF, et al. Operative risk in patients with severe obstructive pulmonary disease. *Arch Int Med* 1992;152:967–971.

35. Rodgers A, Walker N, Schug S, et al. Reduction of postoperative mortality and morbidity with epidural or spinal anaesthesia: results from overview of randomised trials. *BMJ* 2000;321:1493–1497.

36. Milledge JS, Nunn JF. Criteria of fitness for anaesthesia in patients with chronic obstructive lung disease. *Br Med J* 1975;3:670–673.

37. Arozullah AM, Khuri SF, Henderson WG, et al. Development and validation of a multifactorial risk index for predicting postoperative pneumonia after major noncardiac surgery. *Ann Int Med* 2001;135:847–857.

38. McAlister FA, Khan NA, Straus SE, et al. Accuracy of the preoperative assessment in predicting pulmonary risk after nonthoracic surgery. *Am J Respir Crit Care Med* 2003;167:741–744.

39. Hall JC, Tarala RA, Hall JL, et al. A multivariate analysis of the risk of pulmonary complications after laparotomy. *Chest* 1991;99:923–927.

40. Lawrence VA, Dhanda R, Hilsenbeck SG, et al. Risk of pulmonary complications after elective abdominal surgery. *Chest* 1996;110:744–750.

40a. De Nino LA, Lawrence VA, Averyt EC, et al. Preoperative spirometry and laparotomy: blowing away dollars. *Chest* 1997;111:1536–1534.

41. Joo HS, Wong J, Naik VN, et al. The value of screening preoperative chest x-rays: a systematic review. *Can J Anesth* 2005;52:568–574.

42. Smetana GW, Lawrence VA, Cornell JE. Preoperative pulmonary risk stratification for noncardiothoracic surgery: systematic review for the American College of Physicians. *Ann Int Med* 2006;144:581–595.

43. Lawrence VA, Cornell JE, Smetana GW. Strategies to reduce postoperative pulmonary

complications after noncardiothoracic surgery: systematic review for the American College of Physicians. *Ann Int Med* 2006;144:596–608.

44. Barrera R, Shi W, Amar D, et al. Smoking and timing of cessation: impact on pulmonary complications after thoracotomy. *Chest* 2005;127:1977–1983.

45. Torrington KG, Bilello JF, Hopkins TK, et al. Postoperative pulmonary changes after laparoscopic cholecystectomy. *South Med J* 1996;89:675–678.

46. Squadrone V, Coha M, Cerutti E, et al. Continuous positive airway pressure for treatment of postoperative hypoxemia: a randomized controlled trial. *JAMA* 2005;293: 589–595.

47. Hebert PC, Wells G, Blajchman MA, et al. A multicenter, randomized, controlled clinical trial of transfusion requirements in critical care. *N Engl J Med* 1999;340:409–417.

48. Goodnough LT, Brecher ME, Kanter MH, et al. Transfusion medicine. First of two parts—blood transfusion. *N Engl J Med* 1999;340:438–447.

49. Carson JL, Noveck H, Berlin JA, et al. Mortality and morbidity in patients with very low postoperative Hb levels who decline blood transfusion. *Transfusion* 2002;42:812–818.

50. Murphy MF, Wallington TB, Kelsey P, et al. Guidelines for the clinical use of red cell transfusions. *Br J Haematol* 2001;113:24–31.

51. Goodnough LT, Monk TG, Andriole GL. Erythropoietin therapy. *N Engl J Med* 1997;336:933–938.

52. Wiklund RA. Preoperative preparation of patients with advanced liver disease. *Crit Care Med* 2004;32(S):S106–115.

53. Rizvon MK, Chou CL. Surgery in the patient with liver disease. *Med Clin N Am* 2003;87:211–227.

54. Mansour A, Watson W, Shayani V, et al. Abdominal operations in patients with cirrhosis: still a major surgical challenge. *Surgery* 1997;122:730–735.

55. Garrison RN, Cryer HM, Howard DA, et al. Clarification of risk factors for abdominal operations in patients with hepatic cirrhosis. *Ann Surg* 1984;199:648–655.

56. Perkins L, Jeffries M, Patel T. Utility of preoperative scores for predicting morbidity after cholecystectomy in patients with cirrhosis. *Clin Gastroenterol Hepatol* 2004;2:1123–1128.

57. Umpierrez GE, Isaacs SD, Bazargan N, et al. Hyperglycemia: an independent marker of in-hospital mortality in patients with undiagnosed diabetes. *J Clin Endocrinol Metab* 2002;87:978–982.

58. van den Berghe G, Wouters P, Weekers F, et al. Intensive insulin therapy in the critically ill patients. *N Engl J Med* 2001;345:1359–1367.

59. Pomposelli JJ, Baxter JK 3rd, Babineau TJ, et al. Early postoperative glucose control predicts nosocomial infection rate in diabetic patients. *JPEN J Parenter Enteral Nutr* 1998;22:77–81.

60. Clement S, Braithwaite SS, Magee MF, et al. Management of diabetes and hyperglycemia in hospitals. *Diabetes Care* 2004;27:553–591.

61. Schiff RL, Welsh GA. Perioperative evaluation and management of the patient with endocrine dysfunction. *Med Clin N Am* 2003;87:175–192.

62. Furnary AP, Gao G, Grunkemeier GL, et al. Continuous insulin infusion reduces mortality in patients with diabetes undergoing coronary artery bypass grafting. *J Thorac Cardiovasc Surg* 2003;125:1007–1021.

63. Garber AJ, Moghissi ES, Bransome ED Jr, et al. American College of Endocrinology position statement on inpatient diabetes and metabolic control. *Endocr Pract* 2004;10:77–82.

64. Cooper MS, Stewart PM. Corticosteroid insufficiency in acutely ill patients. *N Engl J Med* 2003;348:727–734.

65. Glowniak JV, Loriaux DL. A double-blind study of perioperative steroid requirements in secondary adrenal insufficiency. *Surgery* 1997;121:123–129.

66. Coursin DB, Wood KE. Corticosteroid supplementation for adrenal insufficiency. *JAMA* 2002;287:236–240.

67. Kellerman PS. Perioperative care of the renal patient. *Arch Intern Med* 1994;154:1674–1688.

68. Joseph AJ, Cohn SL. Perioperative care of the patient with renal failure. *Med Clin N Am* 2003;87:193–210.

69. Gerstman BB, Kirkman R, Platt R. Intestinal necrosis associated with postoperative orally administered sodium polystyrene sulfonate in sorbitol. *Am J Kidney Dis* 1992;20:159–161.

70. Lind SE. The bleeding time does not predict surgical bleeding. *Blood* 1991;77:2547–2552.

71. Baddour LM, Bettmann MA, Bolger AF, et al. Nonvalvular cardiovascular device-related infections. *Circulation* 2003;108:2015–2031.

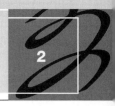
NUTRIENT REQUIREMENTS

General Principles

Energy

- **Total daily energy expenditure** (TEE) can be divided into resting energy expenditure (normally ~70% of TEE), thermic effect of food (normally ~10% of TEE), and energy expenditure of physical activity (normally ~20% of TEE).
- **Malnutrition** and **hypocaloric feeding** decrease resting energy expenditure to values 15%–20% below those expected for actual body size, whereas metabolic stressors, such as inflammatory diseases or trauma, often increase energy requirements. However, it is rare for illnesses or injury to increase resting energy expenditure by more than 50% of pre-illness values.
- It is impossible to determine **daily energy requirements** precisely with predictive equations because of the complexity of factors that affect metabolic rate. However, judicious use of predictive equations provides a reasonable estimate that should be modified as needed based on the patient's clinical course.
- Energy requirements per kilogram of body weight are inversely related to body mass index (BMI) (Table 2-1). The lower range within each category should be considered in insulin-resistant, critically ill patients, unless they are depleted in body fat.
- The **Harris-Benedict equation** provides a reasonable estimate of resting energy expenditure (in kcal/d) in healthy adults. The equation takes into account the effect of body size and lean tissue mass (which is influenced by gender and age) on energy requirements and can be used to estimate total daily energy needs in hospitalized patients:

$$\text{Men} = 66 + (13.7 \times \text{W}) + (5 \times \text{H}) - (6.8 \times \text{A})$$
$$\text{Women} = 665 + (9.6 \times \text{W}) + (1.8 \times \text{H}) - (4.7 \times \text{A})$$

- An **adjusted body weight** rather than actual body weight should be used in obese patients (BMI $\geq$30 kg/m^2) to avoid overfeeding:

$$\text{Adjusted body weight} = \text{ideal body weight} + [(\text{actual body weight} - \text{ideal body weight}) \times (0.25)].$$

- **Ideal body weight** can be estimated based on height. For men, 106 lb is allotted for the first 5 ft, then 6 lb is added for each inch above 5 ft; for women, 100 lb is given for the first 5 ft, with 5 lb added for each additional inch.
- Providing total daily energy equal to the Harris-Benedict calculation should be considered in obese and critically ill patients. Providing total daily energy equal to the Harris-Benedict calculation plus an additional 20% is a reasonable goal for nonobese, non–critically ill patients who have increased metabolic demands. An additional 300–500 kcal should be added to Harris-Benedict estimates in patients who are **underweight** (BMI <18.5 kg/m^2) or **pregnant**.

Protein

- Protein intake of 0.8 g/kg/d meets the requirements of 97% of the adult population.
- Individual protein requirements are affected by several factors, such as the amount of nonprotein calories provided, overall energy requirements, protein quality, and the

TABLE 2-1	Estimated Energy Requirements for Hospitalized Patients Based on Body Mass Index (BMI)

BMI (kg/m²)	Energy requirements (kcal/kg/d)
<15	35–40
15–19	30–35
20–24	20–25
25–29	15–20
≥30	<15

Note: These values are recommended for critically ill patients and all obese patients; add 20% of total calories in estimating energy requirements in non–critically ill patients.

patient's nutritional status. Protein requirements increase when nonprotein calorie intake is inadequate.

■ Inadequate amounts of any of the essential amino acids result in inefficient utilization.

■ Illness increases the efflux of amino acids from skeletal muscle; however, increasing protein intake to >1.2 g/kg/d of prehospitalization body weight in critically ill patients may not reduce the impact of illness on loss of lean body mass.[1]

■ Table 2-2 gives approximate protein requirements during different clinical conditions.

Essential Fatty Acids

■ The liver can synthesize most fatty acids, but humans lack the desaturase enzyme needed to produce the n-3 and n-6 fatty acid series. Therefore, linoleic acid should constitute at least 2% and linolenic acid at least 0.5% of the daily caloric intake to prevent the occurrence of essential fatty acid deficiency.

■ The plasma pattern of increased triene–tetraene ratio (>0.4) can be used to detect essential fatty acid deficiency, even before the presence of clinical manifestations (dermatitis, coarse hair, alopecia, poor wound healing).

■ Patients who are unable to receive intravenous or oral lipid solutions may receive a daily topical application of 1 tablespoon of safflower oil to provide essential fatty acids.

Carbohydrates

■ Certain tissues, such as bone marrow, erythrocytes, leukocytes, renal medulla, eye tissues, and peripheral nerves, cannot metabolize fatty acids and *require* glucose (~40 g/d) as a fuel, whereas other tissues, such as the brain, *prefer* glucose (~120 g/d).

TABLE 2-2	Recommended Daily Protein Intake

Clinical condition	Protein requirements (g/kg IBW/d)[a]
Normal	0.8
Metabolic "stress" (illness/injury)	1.0–1.5
Acute renal failure (undialyzed)	0.8–1.0
Hemodialysis	1.2–1.4
Peritoneal dialysis	1.3–1.5

IBW ideal body weight.
[a]Additional protein intake may be needed to compensate for excess protein loss in specific patient populations, such as those with burn injury, open wounds, and protein-losing enteropathy or nephropathy. Lower protein intake may be necessary in patients with chronic renal insufficiency who are not treated by dialysis and certain patients with hepatic encephalopathy.

Major Minerals

- Major minerals are important for ionic equilibrium, water balance, and normal cell function. The following are the daily recommended intakes (enteral and parenteral values, respectively):
  - Sodium, 0.5–5.0 g and 60–150 mEq
  - Potassium, 2–5 g and 60–100 mEq
  - Magnesium, 300–400 mg and 8–24 mEq
  - Calcium, 800–1200 mg and 5–15 mEq
  - Phosphorus, 800–1200 mg and 12–24 mEq

Micronutrients (Trace Elements and Vitamins)

- Trace elements and vitamins are essential constituents of enzyme complexes.
- The recommended dietary intake for trace elements, fat-soluble vitamins, and water-soluble vitamins (Table 2-3) is set at two standard deviations above the estimated mean so that it will cover the needs of 97% of the healthy population.
- The recommended dietary intake exceeds the micronutrient requirements of most persons.

Special Considerations

- Both the amount and location of gut resection influence mineral and vitamin needs.
- Patients who have an inadequate length of functional small bowel ($<\sim150$ cm of small bowel) because of intestinal resection or intestinal disease require additional vitamins and minerals if they are not receiving parenteral nutrition. Table 2-4 provides guidelines for supplementation in these patients.
- Resection of distal ileum may cause rapid development of B12 deficiency due to loss of enterohepatic recirculation. Proximal gut resection (i.e., stomach, duodenum) may increase the risk for iron, calcium and copper deficiency.
- Patients with excessive gastrointestinal (GI) tract losses require additional fluids and electrolytes. An assessment of fluid losses through diarrhea, ostomy output, and fistula volume should be made to help determine fluid requirements. Knowledge of fluid losses is also useful in calculating intestinal mineral losses by multiplying the volume of fluid loss by an estimate of intestinal fluid electrolyte concentration (Table 2-5).

ASSESSMENT OF NUTRITIONAL STATUS

General Principles

- The **assessment** of nutritional status can be divided into techniques that identify specific nutrient deficiencies and those used to assess protein-energy malnutrition.
- The best overall approach involves a careful clinical **evaluation,** which includes a nutritional history and physical examination in conjunction with appropriate laboratory studies to evaluate further the abnormal findings obtained during clinical examination.
- A careful history and physical examination, routine blood tests, and selected laboratory tests should be used to diagnose **specific** macronutrient, major mineral, vitamin, and trace mineral **deficiencies** (Table 2-3).
- Commonly used indicators of **protein-energy malnutrition** (i.e., plasma albumin and prealbumin concentration) correlate with clinical outcome. However, all these indicators are influenced by illness or injury, making it difficult to separate the contribution of malnutrition from the severity of illness itself on outcome.

Approach to the Patient

History

- Presence of mild ($<5\%$), moderate (5%–10%), or severe ($>10\%$) unintentional **body weight** loss in the last 6 months. In general, a 10% or greater unintentional loss in body weight in the last 6 months is associated with a poor clinical outcome.[2]

	TABLE 2-3	Trace Mineral, Fat-Soluble Vitamin, and Water-Soluble Vitamin Requirements and Assessment of Deficiency

Nutrient	Recommended daily enteral intake in normal adults	Recommended daily parenteral intake in normal adults	Symptoms or signs of deficiency	Laboratory evaluation
Chromium	30–200 mcg	10–20 mcg	Glucose intolerance, peripheral neuropathy, encephalopathy	Serum chromium
Copper	2 mg	0.3 mg	Anemia, neutropenia, osteoporosis, diarrhea	Serum copper, plasma ceruloplasmin
Iodine	150 mcg	70–140 mcg	Hypothyroidism, goiter	Urine iodine, thyroid-stimulating hormone
Iron	10–15 mg	1.0–1.5 mg	Microcytic hypochromic anemia	Serum iron and total iron-binding capacity, serum ferritin
Manganese	1.5 mg	0.2–0.8 mg	Hypercholesterolemia, dementia, dermatitis	Serum manganese
Selenium	50–200 mcg	20–40 mcg	Cardiomyopathy, muscle weakness	Serum selenium, blood glutathione peroxidase activity
Zinc	15 mg	2.5–4.0 mg	Growth retardation, delayed sexual maturation, hypogonadism, alopecia, acro-orificial skin lesion, diarrhea, mental status changes	Plasma zinc
Vitamin K (phylloquinone)	50–100 mcg	100 mcg	Easy bruising/bleeding	Prothrombin time
Vitamin A (retinol)	5000 International Units	3300 International Units	Night blindness, Bitot's spots, keratomalacia, follicular hyperkeratosis, xerosis	Serum retinol
Vitamin D (ergocalciferol)	400 International Units	200 International Units	Rickets, osteomalacia, osteoporosis, bone pain, muscle weakness, tetany	Serum 25-hydoxyvitamin D

Vitamin	10–15 International Units	10 International Units	Signs/Symptoms	Laboratory Test
Vitamin E (alpha tocopherol)			Hemolysia, retinopathy, neuropathy, abnormal clotting	Serum tocopherol: total lipid (triglyceride and cholesterol) ratio
Vitamin B$_1$ (thiamine)	1.0–1.5 mg	3 mg	Beriberi, cardiac failure, Wernicke's encephalopathy, peripheral neuropathy, fatigue, ophthalmoplegia	RBC transketolase activity
Vitamin B$_2$ (riboflavin)	1.1–1.8 mg	3.6 mg	Cheilosis, sore tongue and mouth, eye irritation, seborrheic dermatitis	RBC glutathione reductase activity
Vitamin B$_3$ (niacin)	12–20 mg	40 mg	Pellagra (dermatitis, diarrhea, dementia), sore mouth and tongue	Urinary N-methyl-nicotinamide
Vitamin B$_5$ (pantothenic acid)	5–10 mg	10 mg	Fatigue, weakness, paresthesias, tenderness of heels and feet	Urinary pantothenic acid
Vitamin B$_6$ (pyridoxine)	12 mg	4 mg	Seborrheic dermatitis, cheilosis, glossitis, peripheral neuritis, convulsions, hypochromic anemia	Plasma pyridoxal phosphate
Vitamin B$_7$ (biotin)	100–200 mcg	60 mcg	Seborrheic dermatitis, alopecia, mental status change, seizures, myalgia, hyperesthesia	Plasma biotin
Vitamin B$_9$ (folic acid)	400 mcg	400 mcg	Megaloblastic anemia, glossitis, diarrhea	Serum folic acid, RBC folic acid
Vitamin B$_{12}$ (cobalamin)	5 mcg	5 mcg	Megaloblastic anemia, paresthesias, decreased vibratory or position sense, ataxia, mental status changes, diarrhea	Serum cobalamin, serum methylmalonic acid
Vitamin C (ascorbic acid)	100 mg	100 mg	Scurvy, petechia, purpura, gingival inflammation, and bleeding, weakness, depression	Plasma ascorbic acid, leukocyte ascorbic acid

TABLE 2-4 Guidelines for Vitamin and Mineral Supplementation in Patients with Severe Malabsorption

Supplement	Dose	Route
Prenatal multivitamin with minerals[a]	1 tablet daily	PO
Vitamin D[a]	50,000 units 2–3 times/wk	PO
Calcium[a]	500 mg elemental calcium tid–qid	PO
Vitamin B$_{12}$[b]	1 mg daily	PO
	100–500 mcg q1–2 mo	SC
Vitamin A[b]	10,000–50,000 units daily	PO
Vitamin K[b]	5 mg/d	PO
	5–10 mg/wk	SC
Vitamin E[b]	30 units per day	PO
Magnesium gluconate[b]	108–169 mg elemental magnesium qid	PO
Magnesium sulfate[b]	290 mg elemental magnesium 1–3 times/wk	IM/IV
Zinc gluconate or zinc sulfate[b]	25 mg elemental zinc daily plus 100 mg elemental zinc/L intestinal output	PO
Ferrous sulfate[b]	60 mg elemental iron tid	PO
Iron dextran[b]	Daily dose based on formula or table	IV

[a]Recommended routinely for all patients.
[b]Recommended for patients with documented nutrient deficiency or malabsorption.

- Change in habitual **diet pattern** (number, size, and contents of meals). If present, the reason for altered food intake (e.g., change in appetite, mental status or mood, ability to prepare meals, ability to chew or swallow, GI symptoms) should be investigated.
- Evidence of **malabsorption**.
- Specific **nutrient deficiencies** (Table 2-3).
- Level of **metabolic stress**.
- **Functional status** (e.g., bedridden, suboptimally active, change from baseline).

Physical Examination

- **BMI,** defined as weight (in kilograms) divided by [height (meters)]^2 or weight (in pounds) times 704 divided by [height (inches)]^2. Patients can be classified by BMI as underweight (<18.5 kg/m^2), normal weight (18.5–24.9 kg/m^2), overweight (25.0–29.9 kg/m^2), class I obesity (30.0–34.9 kg/m^2), class II obesity (35.0–39.9 kg/m^2), or class III obesity (≥40.0 kg/m^2).[3] Patients who are **extremely underweight** (BMI <14 kg/m^2) have a

TABLE 2-5 Electrolyte Concentrations in Gastrointestinal Fluids

Location	Na (mEq/L)	K (mEq/L)	Cl (mEq/L)	HCO$_3$ (mEq/L)
Stomach	65	10	100	—
Bile	150	4	100	35
Pancreas	150	7	80	75
Duodenum	90	15	90	15
Mid–small bowel	140	6	100	20
Terminal ileum	140	8	60	70
Rectum	40	90	15	30

high risk of death and should be considered for admission to the hospital for nutritional support.

- **Tissue depletion** (loss of body fat and skeletal muscle wasting).
- **Muscle function** (strength testing of individual muscle groups).
- **Fluid status** [signs and symptoms of either dehydration (hypotension, tachycardia, postural changes, mucosal xerosis, decreased axillary sweat, or dry skin) or excess body fluid (i.e., edema or ascites)].
- Potential sources of **protein or nutrient losses**; large wounds or burns, nephrotic syndrome, drainage from surgical drains (e.g., chest tube, abdominal drains), chylothorax. These may be assessed by quantifying the volume of drainage and the concentration of protein or fat content.

Laboratory Studies

- Perform **laboratory studies** to determine specific nutrient deficiencies when clinically indicated (Table 2-3).
- Most hospitalized patients are vitamin D deficient, and caregivers should have a low threshold for checking plasma **25-OH vitamin D levels.**[4]
- The concentrations of several **plasma proteins** (e.g., albumin, prealbumin, retinol-binding protein, and transferrin) have been shown to correlate with clinical outcome.[5] However, illness or injury, not malnutrition, is responsible for hypoalbuminemia in sick patients.[6] Inflammation and injury decrease albumin synthesis, increase albumin degradation, and increase albumin transcapillary losses from the plasma compartment. In addition, certain GI, renal, and cardiac diseases can increase albumin losses through the GI tract and kidney, and albumin can be lost through surface tissues that have been damaged by wounds, burns, and peritonitis. **Plasma albumin and prealbumin concentration should not be used to assess patients for existing protein-caloric malnutrition or to monitor the adequacy of nutrition support.**

ENTERAL NUTRITION

General Principles

- Whenever possible, **oral/enteral** rather than parenteral **feeding** should be used in patients who need nutritional support.
- **Oral/enteral nutrition** helps to maintain the structural and functional integrity of the GI tract in different ways:
  - Prevents atrophy of the intestinal mucosa and pancreas
  - Preserves mucosal digestive and pancreatic secretory enzyme activity
  - Maintains GI immunoglobulin A (IgA) secretion
  - Prevents cholelithiasis
- Oral/enteral nutrition is usually **less expensive** than parenteral nutrition.

Contraindications

- The **intestinal tract cannot be used** effectively in some patients due to:
  - Persistent nausea or vomiting
  - Intolerable postprandial abdominal pain or diarrhea
  - Mechanical obstruction or severe hypomotility
  - Severe malabsorption
  - Presence of high-output fistulas that do not permit feedings proximal or distal to the fistula

Types of Feedings

- **Hospital diets** include a regular diet and diets modified in either nutrient content (amount of fiber, fat, protein, or sodium) or consistency (liquid, puréed, soft). There are ways that food intake can often be increased:
  - Encourage patients to eat

- Provide assistance at mealtime.
- Avoid unpalatable diets.
- Allow some food to be supplied by relatives and friends.
- Limit missed meals for medical tests and procedures.
- Milk-based formulas (e.g., Carnation Instant Breakfast) contain milk as a source of protein and fat and tend to be more palatable than other defined formula diets; milk-based formulas can be problematic for some lactose-intolerant patients but are often tolerated when infused continuously because this approach decreases the rate of lactose delivered to the intestine.
- Use of calorically dense supplements, e.g., Ensure or Boost.
- **Defined liquid formulas**
    - Elemental monomeric formulas (e.g., Vivonex, Glutasorb) contain nitrogen in the form of free amino acids and small amounts of fat ($<5\%$ of total calories) and are hyperosmolar (550–650 mOsm/kg). These formulas are not palatable and require either tube feeding or mixing with other foods or flavorings for oral ingestion. Absorption of monomeric formulas is not clinically superior to that of oligomeric or polymeric formulas in patients with adequate pancreatic digestive function. These formulas may exacerbate osmotic diarrhea in patients with short gut.
    - **Semielemental (oligomeric) formulas** (e.g., Propeptide, Peptamen) contain hydrolyzed protein in the form of small peptides and sometimes free amino acids.
    - **Polymeric formulas** are appropriate for most patients. They contain nitrogen in the form of whole proteins and include blenderized food, milk-based, and lactose-free formulas. Lactose-free formulas (e.g., Osmolite, Ensure) are the most commonly used polymeric formulas in hospitalized patients. These formulas are available as standard iso-osmolar solutions, containing approximately 1 kcal/ml, 16% calories as protein, 55% calories as carbohydrate, and 30% calories as fat. Most patients can be fed with standard iso-osmolar lactose-free formulas. Predigested (elemental and semielemental) formulas are more expensive than standard formulas and do not usually provide additional clinical benefits, even in patients with limited digestive and absorptive function, such as those with pancreatic insufficiency treated with enzyme replacement and those with short-bowel syndrome. Other formulas are also available that have modified nutrient content, such as high-nitrogen (e.g., Promote, Perative) or high-calorie (e.g., Two Cal HN) formulas for patients who require fluid restriction, fiber-enriched formulas (e.g., Jevity) for individuals with constipation or loose stools or those receiving long-term enteral tube feeding, and reduced protein, fluid, phosphorus, potassium, and magnesium for patients with renal insufficiency (e.g., Nepro).
- **Oral rehydration solutions** stimulate sodium and water absorption by taking advantage of the sodium-glucose cotransporter present in the brush border of intestinal epithelium. Oral rehydration therapy can be useful in patients with severe GI fluid and mineral losses, such as those with short-bowel syndrome[7] and HIV infection.[8] In patients with short-bowel syndrome, it is particularly important that the sodium concentration of the solution be between 90 and 120 mEq/L to avoid intestinal sodium secretion and negative sodium and water balance. The characteristics of several oral rehydration solutions are listed in Table 2-6.

Tube Feeding

- Tube feeding is useful in patients who have a **functional GI tract** but who cannot or will not ingest adequate nutrients.
- The type of tube-feeding approach selected (nasogastric, nasoduodenal, nasojejunal, gastrostomy, jejunostomy, pharyngostomy, and esophagostomy tubes) depends on physician experience, clinical prognosis, gut patency and motility, risk of aspirating gastric contents, patient preference, and anticipated duration of feeding.
- Short-term (<6 weeks) tube feeding can be achieved by placement of a soft, small-bore nasogastric or nasoenteric feeding tube. These tubes are made of silicone or polyurethane and do not cause the tissue irritation and necrosis associated with larger polyvinylchloride tubes. Tube feeding can be used to supplement oral intake. Although nasogastric

| **TABLE 2-6** | Characteristics of Selected Oral Rehydration Solutions |

Product	Na (mEq/L)	K (mEq/L)	Cl (mEq/L)	Citrate (mEq/L)	kcal/L	CHO (g/L)	mOsm
Equalyte	78	22	68	30	100	25	305
CeraLyte 70	70	20	98	30	165	40	235
CeraLyte 90	90	20	98	30	165	40	260
Pedialyte	45	20	35	30	100	20	300
Rehydralyte	74	19	64	30	100	25	305
Gatorade	20	3	NA	NA	210	45	330
WHO[a]	90	20	80	30	80	20	200
Washington University[b]	105	0	100	10	85	20	250

NA, not applicable; WHO, World Health Organization.
Note: Mix formulas with sugar-free flavorings as needed for palatability.
[a]WHO formula: Mix $^3/_4$ tsp sodium chloride, $^1/_2$ tsp sodium citrate, $^1/_4$ tsp potassium chloride, and 4 tsp glucose (dextrose) in 1 L (4$^1/_4$ cups) distilled water.
[b]Washington University formula: Mix $^3/_4$ tsp sodium chloride, $^1/_2$ tsp sodium citrate, and 3 tbsp + 1 tsp Polycose powder in 1 L (4$^1/_4$ cups) distilled water.

feeding is usually the most appropriate route, orogastric feeding in patients with nasal injury or gross nasal deformity and nasoduodenal or nasojejunal feeding in patients with gastroparesis can also be used. Nasoduodenal and nasojejunal feeding tubes can be placed at the bedside with a success rate approaching 90% when inserted by experienced personnel.[9]

- Long-term (>6 weeks) tube feeding usually requires a gastrostomy or jejunostomy tube that can be placed endoscopically, radiologically, or surgically, depending on the clinical situation and local expertise.
  - **Percutaneous endoscopic gastrostomy** can be performed within 30 minutes and is successfully completed in >90% of attempts.[10] Gastrostomy tubes can be placed percutaneously without endoscopy by inserting the catheter directly into the stomach via a peel-away sheath introduced over a previously placed J-wire guide.[11] Jejunal tube placement can be achieved by threading a tube through an existing gastrostomy or by direct percutaneous endoscopic jejunostomy in patients with previous partial or total gastrectomy.[12]
  - **Surgical gastrostomy and jejunostomy** can be performed by open and laparoscopic techniques and are particularly useful when endoscopic and radiologic approaches are technically impossible or cannot be performed safely because of prior abdominal surgeries or overlying bowel.
- **Feeding schedules.** Patients who have feeding tubes in the stomach can often tolerate intermittent bolus or gravity feedings, in which the total amount of daily formula is divided into four to six equal portions.
  - **Bolus feedings** are given by syringe as rapidly as tolerated.
  - **Gravity feedings** are infused over 30–60 minutes.
  - The patient's upper body should be elevated by 30–45 degrees during and for at least 2 hours after feeding. Tubes should be flushed with water after each feeding. Intermittent feedings are useful for patients who cannot be positioned with continuous head-of-the-bed elevation or who require greater freedom from feeding. However, patients who experience nausea and early satiety with bolus gravity feedings may require continuous infusion at a slower rate.
  - **Continuous feeding** can often be started at 20–30 mL/hr and advanced by 10 mL/hr every 6 hours until the feeding goal is reached. Patients who have gastroparesis often tolerate gastric tube feedings when they are started at a slow rate (e.g., 10 mL/hr) and advanced by small increments (e.g., 10 mL/hr every 8–12 hours). However, patients

with severe gastroparesis require passage of the feeding tube tip past the ligament of Treitz. Continuous feeding should always be used when feeding directly into the duodenum or jejunum to avoid distention, abdominal pain, and dumping syndrome.
- **Jejunal feeding** may be possible in patients with mild to moderate **acute pancreatitis** who are closely monitored.[13]

Complications
- Mechanical complications
  - **Nasogastric feeding tube misplacement** occurs more commonly in unconscious than in conscious patients. Intubation of the tracheobronchial tree has been reported in up to 15% of patients. Intracranial placement can occur in patients with skull fractures.
  - **Erosive tissue damage** can lead to nasopharyngeal erosions, pharyngitis, sinusitis, otitis media, pneumothorax, and GI tract perforation.
  - **Tube occlusion** is often caused by inspissated feedings or pulverized medications given through small-diameter (<No. 10 French) tubes. Frequent flushing of the tube with 30–60 mL of water and avoiding administration of pill fragments or "thick" medications help to prevent occlusion. Techniques used to unclog tubes include the use of a small-volume syringe (10 mL) to flush warm water or pancreatic enzymes (Viokase dissolved in water) through the tube. Commercially made products can be obtained that either dissolve or mechanically remove the obstruction.
- Hyperglycemia
  - Achieving tight control of blood glucose (<110 mg/dL) in critically ill patients appears to improve outcomes.[14]
  - Subcutaneously administered insulin can usually maintain good glycemic control. Intravenous (IV) insulin drip protocols may be used to control blood glucose in critically ill patients with anasarca or hemodynamic instability to ensure adequate insulin absorption.
  - Intermediate-duration insulin can often be used safely once tube feedings reach 1,000 kcal/d.
  - Patients who are receiving bolus feeds should receive short-acting insulin at the time of the feed.
  - Patients who are being given continuous (24 hours/d) feeding should receive intermediate or long-duration insulin every 12–24 hours.
- Pulmonary aspiration
  - The etiology of **pulmonary aspiration** can be difficult to determine in tube-fed patients because aspiration can occur from refluxed tube feedings or oropharyngeal secretions that are unrelated to feedings.
  - Addition of food coloring to tube feeds is not recommended for the diagnosis of aspiration. This method is insensitive for the diagnosis of aspiration. Several case reports suggest that food coloring can be absorbed by the GI tract in critically ill patients, which can lead to serious complications (i.e., refractory hypotension, metabolic acidosis) and death.[15]
  - Prevention of reflux
    - Decrease gastric acid secretion
    - Keep the patient sitting up or place in Trendelenburg position to achieve elevation of the head of the bed during feeds.
    - Gastric residuals are poorly predictive of aspiration risk.
    - Avoid gastric feeding in high-risk patients (e.g., those with gastroparesis, gastric outlet obstruction, or frequent vomiting; dysphagia is not a contraindication for gastric tube feeding)
- GI complications
  - Nausea
  - Vomiting
  - Abdominal pain
  - **Diarrhea** is often associated with antibiotic therapy[16] and the use of liquid medications that contain nonabsorbable carbohydrates, such as sorbitol.[17] If diarrhea from tube feeding persists after proper evaluation of possible causes, a trial of antidiarrheal

agents or fiber is justified. Diarrhea is common in patients who receive tube feeding and occurs in up to 50% of critically ill patients.
- Diarrhea in patients with short gut, who do not have other causes such as *Clostridium difficile* infection, may be minimized by use of small, frequent meals that do not contain concentrated sweets (e.g., soda). Intestinal transit time should be maximized to allow nutrient absorption using tincture of opium, loperamide, or diphenoxylate. Low-dose clonidine (0.025–0.05 mg orally twice a day in patients who are hemodynamically stable) may be used to reduce diarrhea in patients with short bowel by increasing enteral sodium absorption.[18]
- Intestinal ischemia/necrosis has been reported in a number of case reports. These cases have occurred predominantly in critically ill patients receiving vasopressors for blood pressure support in conjunction with enteral feeding. There are no reliable clinical signs for diagnosis, and the mortality rate is high. Caution should be used if enterally feeding critically ill patients requiring pressors.

PARENTERAL NUTRITION

General Principles

- Patients who are unable to consume "adequate" nutrients for a "prolonged" period of time by oral or enteral routes require parenteral nutritional therapy to prevent the adverse effects of malnutrition.
- The decision to use parenteral nutrition can be difficult because the precise definition of "adequate" and "prolonged" is not clear and depends on the patient's amount of body fat and lean tissue mass, the presence of preexisting medical illnesses, and the level of metabolic stress.
- In general, parenteral nutrition should be considered if energy intake has been, or is anticipated to be, inadequate (<50% of daily requirements) for more than 7 days and enteral feeding is not feasible. However, the efficacy of this approach has not been tested in clinical trials.
- Routine use of immediate postoperative total parenteral nutrition (TPN) does not appear to improve outcomes in unselected patients.[19]

Recommendations

Central Parenteral Nutrition (CPN)

- The infusion of hyperosmolar (usually >1,500 mOsm/L) nutrient solutions requires a large-bore, high-flow vessel to minimize vessel irritation and damage.
- Percutaneous subclavian vein catheterization with advancement of the catheter tip to the junction of the superior vena cava and right atrium is the most commonly used technique for CPN access. The internal jugular, saphenous, and femoral veins are also used. Although these sites either decrease or eliminate the risk of pneumothorax, they are less desirable because of decreased patient comfort and difficulty in maintaining sterility. Catheters that are tunneled under the skin prior to entering the vascular tree are preferred in patients who are likely to receive >~8 weeks of TPN to reduce the risk of mechanical failure.
- Peripherally inserted central venous catheters, which also eliminate the risk of pneumothorax, can be used to provide CPN in patients with adequate antecubital vein access.
- Macronutrient solutions
  - Crystalline amino acid solutions containing 40%–50% essential and 50%–60% nonessential amino acids (usually with little or no glutamine, glutamate, aspartate, asparagine, tyrosine, and cysteine) are used to provide protein needs (Table 2-2). Infused amino acids are oxidized and should be included in the estimate of energy provided as part of the parenteral formulation. Some amino acid solutions have been modified for specific disease states, such as those enriched in branched-chain amino acids for use in patients who have hepatic encephalopathy and solutions that contain mostly essential amino acids for use in patients with renal insufficiency.

- **Glucose** (dextrose) in IV solutions is hydrated; each gram of dextrose monohydrate provides 3.4 kcal. At least 150 g glucose/d is needed to maximize protein balance and provide energy to tissues that require and prefer glucose as a fuel.
- **Lipid emulsions** are available as a 10% (1.1 kcal/mL) or 20% (2.0 kcal/mL) solution and provide energy as well as a source of essential fatty acids. Emulsion particles are similar in size and structure to chylomicrons and are metabolized like nascent chylomicrons after acquiring apoproteins from contact with circulating endogenous high-density lipoprotein particles. Lipid emulsions are as effective as glucose in conserving body nitrogen economy once absolute tissue requirements for glucose are met. The optimal percentage of calories that should be infused as fat is not known, but 20%–30% of total calories is reasonable for most patients. The rate of infusion should not exceed 1.0 kcal/kg/hr (0.11 g/kg/hr) because most complications associated with lipid infusions have been reported when providing more than this amount.[20] A rate of 0.03–0.05 g/kg/hr is adequate for most patients who are receiving continuous CPN. Lipid emulsions should not be given to patients who have triglyceride concentrations of >400 mg/dL. Moreover, patients at risk for hypertriglyceridemia should have serum triglyceride concentrations checked at least once during lipid emulsion infusion to ensure adequate clearance. Underfeeding obese patients by the amount of lipid calories that would normally be given (e.g., 20%–30% of calories) facilitates mobilization of endogenous fat stores for fuel and may improve insulin sensitivity and glucose control; however intravenous lipids should be administered twice per week to provide essential fatty acids.

Complications

- **Mechanical complications** may occur during central line insertion:
  - Pneumothorax
  - Brachial plexus injury
  - Subclavian and carotid artery puncture
  - Hemothorax
  - Thoracic duct injury
  - Chylothorax
- Even when the subclavian vein is cannulated successfully, other mechanical complications can still occur:
  - Catheter can be advanced upward into the internal jugular vein.
  - The tip can be sheared off completely if it is withdrawn back through an introducing needle.
  - Air embolism can occur during insertion or whenever the connection between the catheter and IV tubing is disrupted.
- **Metabolic complications** are usually caused by overzealous or inadequate nutrient administration:
  - Fluid overload
  - Hypertriglyceridemia
  - Hypercalcemia
  - Specific nutrient deficiencies
  - Hypoglycemia
  - **Hyperglycemia** should be avoided because it is associated with leukocyte and complement dysfunction and increases the risk of infection:
    - Blood glucose goals for closely monitored intensive care unit (ICU) patients are ideally 80–120 mg/dL.
    - Blood glucose should be kept below 120 mg/dL in pregnant patients to avoid complications of gestational diabetes and large-for-gestational-age births.
  - Management of patients with hyperglycemia or diabetes[21]:
    - If blood glucose is >200 mg/dL or the patient has diabetes, consider obtaining better control of blood glucose before starting CPN.
    - If CPN is started, (1) limit dextrose to <200 g/d, (2) add 0.1 units of regular insulin for each gram of dextrose in CPN solution (e.g., 15 units for 150 g), (3) discontinue other sources of IV dextrose, and (4) order sliding-scale SC regular insulin

with blood glucose monitoring by fingerstick every 4–6 hours or sliding-scale IV regular insulin infusion with blood glucose monitoring by fingerstick every 1–2 hours.

- Supplemental corrective doses of insulin should be used to control hyperglycemia. In outpatients who use insulin, an estimate of the reduction in blood sugar that will be caused by the administration of 1 unit of insulin may be calculated by dividing 1,500 by the total daily insulin dose (e.g., for a patient receiving 50 units of insulin as an outpatient, 1 unit of insulin may be predicted to reduce plasma glucose concentration by 1,500/50 = 30 mg/dL).
- If blood glucose remains >200 mg/dL and the patient has been receiving SC insulin, add 50% of the supplemental short-acting insulin given in the last 24 hours to the next day's CPN solution and double the amount of SC insulin sliding-scale dose for blood glucose values >200 mg/dL.
- The insulin-to-dextrose ratio in the CPN formulation should be maintained while the CPN dextrose content is changed.

- Thrombosis and pulmonary embolus
  - Radiologically evident subclavian vein thrombosis occurs commonly (25%–50% of patients), but clinically significant manifestations, such as upper-extremity edema, superior vena cava syndrome, or pulmonary embolism, are rare.
  - Patients with hypercoagulable conditions are at increased risk of catheter-induced central vein thrombosis. Prophylactic use of low-dose warfarin (1–2 mg/d), which rarely increases the International Normalized Ratio, should be considered in these patients, and the dose of warfarin should be increased to full therapeutic anticoagulation if central vein thrombosis or pulmonary embolism occurs.
  - Fatal microvascular pulmonary emboli caused by nonvisible precipitate, containing calcium and phosphorus, in total nutrient admixtures underscore the importance of maintaining strict pharmacy standards regarding physical-chemical compatibility.
  - Inline filters should be used with all parenteral nutrient solutions. The smallest pulmonary capillaries are 5 m in diameter, and the size limit for visual detection of microprecipitates is 50–100 m.
- Infectious complications
  - Catheter-related sepsis is the most common life-threatening complication in patients who receive CPN and is most commonly caused by *Staphylococcus epidermidis* and *Staphylococcus aureus*.
  - In **immunocompromised patients** (e.g., those with AIDS, immunosuppressive therapy, chemotherapy, or absolute neutrophil count <200) and those with long-term (>2 weeks) CPN, *Enterococcus*, *Candida* species, *Escherichia coli*, *Pseudomonas*, *Klebsiella*, *Enterobacter*, *Acinetobacter*, *Proteus*, and *Xanthomonas* should be considered.
  - The principles of **evaluation and management** of suspected catheter-related infection are outlined in Chapter 13.
  - Although antibiotics are often infused through the central line, the **antibiotic lock technique** has been used successfully to treat and prevent central catheter-related infections.[22,23]
    - This technique involves injecting an antibiotic solution (e.g., vancomycin, 2 mg/mL) into the central catheter lumen and allowing the antibiotic to sit in the line for at least 12 hours.
    - The catheter can be used to infuse fluids or parenteral nutritional solutions during the remaining 12 hours of the day.
    - The catheter is periodically reinjected for a 14-day course. This approach is less expensive, delivers a higher antibiotic concentration into the catheter lumen, and has fewer side effects than systemic antibiotics.
- **Hepatobiliary complications.**[24] Although these abnormalities are usually benign and transient, more serious and progressive disease may develop in a small subset of patients, usually after 16 weeks of CPN therapy.
  - Biochemical
    - Elevated serum aminotransferase
    - Alkaline phosphatase

- Histologic alterations
  - Steatosis
  - Steatohepatitis
  - Lipidosis and phospholipidosis
  - Cholestasis
  - Fibrosis
  - Cirrhosis
- Biliary complications usually occur in patients who receive CPN for >3 weeks.
  - Acalculous cholecystitis
  - Gallbladder sludge
  - Cholelithiasis
  - Routine efforts to prevent hepatobiliary complications in all patients receiving long-term CPN include providing a portion (20%–40%) of calories as fat, cycling CPN so that the glucose infusion is stopped for at least 8–10 hours/d, encouraging enteral intake to stimulate gallbladder contraction and maintain mucosal integrity, and avoiding excessive calories.
  - If abnormal liver biochemistries or other evidence of liver damage occurs, an evaluation for other possible causes of liver disease should be performed.
  - Parenteral nutrition does not need to be discontinued, but the same principles used in preventing hepatic complications can be applied therapeutically.
  - When cholestasis is present, copper and manganese should be deleted from the CPN formula to prevent accumulation in the liver and basal ganglia. A 4-week trial of metronidazole or ursodeoxycholic acid has been reported to be helpful in some patients.
- Metabolic bone disease
  - Metabolic bone disease has been observed in patients receiving long-term (>3 months) CPN.
  - The clinical manifestations of bone disease are seen in asymptomatic patients who have radiologic evidence of demineralization, those who have bone pain, and those who experience bone fracture.[25]
  - Histologic examination has found osteomalacia, osteopenia, or both.
  - The precise causes of metabolic bone disease are not known, but several mechanisms have been proposed, including aluminum toxicity, vitamin D toxicity, and negative calcium balance.
  - Several therapeutic options should be considered in patients who have evidence of bone abnormalities.
    - Remove vitamin D from the CPN formulation if the parathyroid hormone and 1,25-hydroxy vitamin D levels are low
    - Reduce protein to <1.5 g/kg/d because amino acids cause hypercalciuria
    - Maintain normal magnesium status because magnesium is necessary for normal parathormone action and renal conservation of calcium
    - Provide oral calcium supplements of 1–2 g/d
    - Consider bisphosphonate therapy to decrease bone resorption.

Peripheral Parenteral Nutrition
- Peripheral parenteral nutrition is often considered to have limited usefulness because of the high risk of thrombophlebitis.
- Appropriate adjustments in the management of peripheral parenteral nutrition can increase the life of a single infusion site to >10 days.
- The following guidelines are recommended:
  - Provide at least 50% of total energy as a lipid emulsion piggy-backed with the dextrose–amino acid solution
  - Add 500–1000 U heparin and 5 mg hydrocortisone/L (to decrease phlebitis)
  - Place a fine-bore 22- or 23-gauge polyvinylpyrrolidone-coated polyurethane catheter in as large a vein as possible in the proximal forearm using sterile technique
  - Place a 5-mg glycerol trinitrate ointment patch (or 1/4 in. of 2% nitroglycerin ointment) over the infusion site
  - Infuse the solution with a volumetric pump

■ Keep the total infused volume <3,500 mL/d
■ Filter the solution with an inline 1.2-m filter.[26]

Long-Term Home Parenteral Nutrition

■ Long-term home parenteral nutrition is usually given through a **tunneled catheter** or an implantable subcutaneous port inserted in the subclavian vein and exiting the anterior chest.
■ **Nutrient formulations** can be infused overnight to permit daytime activities in patients who are able to tolerate the fluid load. IV lipids may not be necessary in patients who are able to ingest and absorb adequate amounts of fat.

Monitoring Nutrition Support

■ Adjustment of the nutrient formulation is often needed as medical therapy or clinical status changes.
■ When nutrition support is initiated, other sources of **glucose** (e.g., peripheral IV dextrose infusions) should be stopped and the volume of other IV fluids adjusted to account for CPN.
■ Vital signs should be checked every 8 hours.
■ In certain patients, body weight, fluid intake, and fluid output should be followed daily.
■ Serum electrolytes (including phosphorus) should be measured every 1 or 2 days after CPN is started until values are stable and then rechecked weekly.
■ Serum glucose should be checked up to every 4–6 hours by fingerstick until blood glucose concentrations are stable and then rechecked weekly.
■ If lipid emulsions are being given, **serum triglycerides** should be measured during lipid infusion in patients at risk for hypertriglyceridemia to demonstrate adequate clearance (triglyceride concentrations <400 mg/dL).
■ Careful attention to the catheter and catheter site can help to prevent **catheter-related infections**.
  ■ Gauze dressings should be changed every 48–72 hours or when contaminated or wet, but transparent dressings can be changed weekly.
  ■ Tubing that connects the parenteral solutions with the catheter should be changed every 24 hours.
  ■ A 0.22-m filter should be inserted between the IV tubing and the catheter when **lipid-free CPN** is infused and should be changed with the tubing.
  ■ A 1.2-m filter should be used when a total nutrient admixture containing a **lipid emulsion** is infused.
  ■ When a **single-lumen** catheter is used to deliver CPN, the catheter should not be used to infuse other solutions or medications, with the exception of compatible antibiotics, and it should not be used to monitor central venous pressure.
  ■ When a **triple-lumen** catheter is used, the distal port should be reserved solely for the administration of CPN.

REFEEDING THE SEVERELY MALNOURISHED PATIENT

Treatment

Complications

■ Initiating nutritional therapy in patients who are severely malnourished and have had minimal nutrient intake can have adverse clinical consequences and the **refeeding syndrome**.
  ■ **Hypophosphatemia, hypokalemia, and hypomagnesemia.** Rapid and marked decreases in these electrolytes occur during initial refeeding because of insulin-stimulated increases in cellular mineral uptake from extracellular fluid. For example, plasma phosphorus concentration can fall below 1 mg/dL and cause death within hours of initiating nutritional therapy if adequate phosphate is not given.[27]
  ■ **Fluid overload** and **congestive heart failure** are associated with decreased cardiac function and insulin-induced increased sodium and water reabsorption in

conjunction with nutritional therapy containing water, glucose, and sodium. Renal mass may be reduced, and thus may limit the ability to excrete salt or water loads.

- **Cardiac arrhythmias.** Patients who are severely malnourished often have bradycardia. Sudden death from ventricular tachyarrhythmias can occur during the first week of refeeding in severely malnourished patients and may be associated with a prolonged QT interval[28] or plasma electrolyte abnormalities.
- **Glucose intolerance.** Starvation causes insulin resistance, so that refeeding with high-carbohydrate meals or large amounts of parenteral glucose can cause marked elevations in blood glucose concentration, glucosuria, dehydration, and hyperosmolar coma. In addition, carbohydrate refeeding in patients who are depleted in thiamine can precipitate Wernicke's encephalopathy.

Recommendations

- Careful **evaluation** of cardiovascular function and plasma electrolytes (history, physical examination, electrocardiogram, and blood tests) and correction of abnormal plasma electrolytes are **important before initiation of feeding**.
- Refeeding by the oral or enteral route involves the frequent or continuous administration of small amounts of food or an isotonic liquid formula.
- Parenteral supplementation or complete parenteral nutrition may be necessary if the intestine cannot tolerate feeding.
- During initial refeeding, fluid intake should be limited to approximately 800 mL/d plus insensible losses. However, adjustments in fluid and sodium intake are needed in patients who have evidence of fluid overload or dehydration.
- Changes in body weight provide a useful guide for evaluating the efficacy of fluid administration. Weight gain greater than 0.25 kg/d or 1.5 kg/wk probably represents fluid accumulation in excess of tissue repletion. Initially, approximately 15 kcal/kg, containing approximately 100 g carbohydrate and 1.5 g protein/kg actual body weight, should be given daily.
- The rate at which the caloric intake can be increased depends on the severity of the malnutrition and the tolerance to feeding; however, in general, increases of 2–4 kcal/kg every 24 to 48 hours are appropriate.
- Sodium should be restricted to approximately 60 mEq or 1.5 g/d, but liberal amounts of phosphorus, potassium, and magnesium should be given to patients who have normal renal function.
- All other nutrients should be given in amounts needed to meet the recommended dietary intake (Table 2-3).
- Body weight, fluid intake, urine output, and plasma glucose and electrolyte values should be **monitored daily** during early refeeding (first 3–7 days) so that nutritional therapy can be appropriately modified when necessary.

References

1. Ishibashi N, Plank LD, Sando K, et al. Optimal protein requirements during the first 2 weeks after the onset of critical illness. *Crit Care Med* 1998;26(9):1529–1535.
2. Dewys WD, Begg C, Lavin PT, et al. Prognostic effect of weight loss prior to chemotherapy in cancer patients. Eastern Cooperative Oncology Group. *Am J Med* 1980;69:491–497.
3. NIH/NHLBl. Clinical guidelines on the identification, evaluation, and treatment of overweight and obesity in adults—the evidence report. *Obes Res* 1998;6(Suppl 2): S53–S54.
4. Thomas MK, Lloyd-Jones DM, Thadhani Rl, et al. Hypovitaminosis D in medical inpatients. *N Engl J Med* 1998:338:777–783.
5. Apelgren KN, Rombeau JL, Twomey PL, et al. Comparison of nutritional indices and outcome in critically ill patients. *Crit Care Med* 1982;10:305–307.
6. Klein S. The myth of serum albumin as a measure of nutritional status. *Gastroenterology* 1990;99:1845–1851.
7. Lennard-Jones JE. Oral rehydration solutions in short bowel syndrome. *Clin Ther* 1990;12(Suppl A):129–137.

8. Winick M. National Task Force on Nutrition in AIDS. Guidelines on nutritional support in AIDS. *Nutrition* 1989;5:390–394.

9. Taylor B, Schallom L. Bedside small bowel feeding tube placement in critically ill patients utilizing a dietician/nurse team approach. *Nutr Clin Pract* 2001;16:258–262.

10. Ponsky JL, Gauderer MW, Stellato TA, et al. Percutaneous approaches to enteral alimentation. *Am J Surg* 1985;149:102–105.

11. Russell TR, Brotman M, Norris F. Percutaneous gastrostomy. A new simplified and cost-effective technique. *Am J Surg* 1984;184:132–137.

12. Shike M, Schroy P, Ritchie MA, et al. Percutaneous endoscopic jejunostomy in cancer patients with previous gastric resection. *Gastrointest Endosc* 1987;33:372–374.

13. Simpson WG, Marsano L, Gates L. Enteral nutritional support in acute alcoholic pancreatitis. *J Am Coll Nutrition* 1995;14(6):662–665.

14. Van den Berghe G, Wouters P, Weekers F, et al. Intensive insulin therapy in the critically ill patients. *N Engl J Med* 2001;345:1359–1367.

15. Maloney J, Halbower A, Fouty R, et al. Systemic absorption of food dye in patients with sepsis. *N Engl J Med* 2000;343:1047–1048.

16. Mascidi EA, Randall S, Porter KA, et al. Thermogenesis from intravenous medium-chain triglycerides. *JPEN* 1991;15:27–31.

17. Edes TE, Walk BE, Austin JL. Diarrhea in tube-fed patients: feeding formula not necessarily the cause. *Am J Med* 1990;88:91–93.

18. McDoniel K, Taylor B, Huey W, et al. Use of clonidine to decrease intestinal fluid losses in patients with high-output short-bowel syndrome. *JPEN* 2004;28(4):265–268.

19. Sandström R, Drott C, Hyltander A, et al. The effect of postoperative intravenous feeding (TPN) on outcome following major surgery evaluated in a randomized study. *Ann Surg* 1993;217(2):185–195.

20. Miles JM. Intravenous fat emulsions in nutritional support. *Curr Opin Gastroenterol* 1991;7:306–311.

21. McMahon MM, Rizza RA. Nutrition support in hospitalized patients with diabetes mellitus. *Mayo Clin Proc* 1996;71:587–594.

22. Messing B. Catheter sepsis during home parenteral nutrition: use of the antibiotic-lock technique. *Nutrition* 1998;14:466–468.

23. Carratalà J, Niubó J, Fernández-Sevilla A, et al. Randomized, double-blind trial of an antibiotic-lock technique for prevention of gram-positive central venous catheter-related infection in neutropenic patients with cancer. *Antimicrob Agents Chemother* 1999;43:2200–2204.

24. Schiff L, Schiff ER (eds.), *Diseases of the Liver*, 7th ed. Philadelphia: JB Lippincott 1993:1505–1516.

25. Klein GL, Coburn JW. Parenteral nutrition: effect on bone and mineral homeostasis. *Annu Rev Nutr* 1991;11:93–119.

26. Everitt NJ, McMahon MJ. Peripheral intravenous nutrition. *Nutrition* 1994;10:49–57.

27. Weinsier RL, Krumdieck CL, Death resulting from overzealous total parenteral nutrition: the refeeding syndrome revisited. *Am J Clin Nutr* 1981;34:393–399.

28. Isner J, Roberts W, Heymsfield S, et al. Anorexia nervosa and sudden death. *Ann intern Med* 1985;102:49–52.

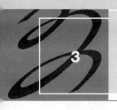

FLUID AND ELECTROLYTE MANAGEMENT
Kamalanathan Sambandam and Anitha Vijayan

FLUID MANAGEMENT AND PERTURBATIONS IN VOLUME STATUS

GENERAL PRINCIPLES

- **Total body water** (TBW). Water comprises approximately 60% of lean body weight in men and 50% in women. TBW is distributed in two major compartments: two-thirds is **intracellular fluid** (ICF) and one-third is **extracellular fluid** (ECF). The latter is further subdivided into intravascular and interstitial spaces in a ratio of 1:4. A 70-kg man, for example, would consist of 42 L of water (0.6 × lean weight), 28 L of which would be ICF (0.66 × TBW) and 14 L of which would be ECF (0.33 × TBW). The intravascular compartment would contain 3.5 L (0.25 × ECF) of water (i.e., the plasma volume; not including the water content of the cellular elements in blood, which, by definition, would be ICF) and the interstitial compartment 10.5 L (0.75 × ECF). Disturbances in TBW would manifest primarily as changes in the **osmolality** (see Disorders of Sodium Concentration, General Principles) of the fluid compartments.
- **Total body Na^+**. Eighty-five to ninety percent of **total body Na^+** is extracellular. Because most of the body's Na^+ is in the ECF, alterations in Na^+ content are manifest clinically as ECF volume depletion (hypotension, tachycardia) or ECF volume overload (peripheral and/or pulmonary edema). Na^+ *concentration* is distinct from Na^+ *content*, since one can have reduced serum $[Na^+]$ but increased total body Na^+ as occurs in heart failure.

THE EUVOLEMIC PATIENT

Treatment

- Maintenance fluid therapy can be provided enterally or, for patients who are unable to take food or liquid by mouth, intravenously. The patient who can be allowed free access to food and drink should be allowed this rather than providing parenteral therapy.
- Weighing the patient daily is the best means of assessing net gain or loss of total body fluid, because gastrointestinal (GI), renal, and insensible fluid losses are unpredictable and difficult to quantify accurately.
- A decision to provide intravenous maintenance fluid therapy should be an active one rather than by rote. There are indications/contraindications and adverse effects of intravenous fluids just as for any medication. Intravenous fluid (IVF) therapy should therefore be reassessed *at least* daily just as the inpatient medication list is reviewed at least daily.
- Consider the **water** and **electrolyte** needs of the patient separately when prescribing IVF therapy.
  - Minimum **water** requirements for daily fluid balance can be approximated from the sum of the minimum urine output necessary to excrete the daily solute load (~500–675 mL/d, which assumes an average solute load of 600–800 mOsm/d and a maximum urine concentrating capacity in healthy kidneys of 1,200 mOsm/L: 600 mOsm/d ÷ 1, 200 mOsm/L = 0.5 L/d), the water lost in stool (~200 mL/d),

and the **insensible water losses** from the skin and respiratory tract (each ~400–500 mL/d). The volume of water produced from endogenous metabolism (~250–350 mL/d) should be subtracted from this total. This comes to a minimum of about **1,400 mL/d** or **60 mL/hr** of water needed for maintenance. If the patient has any drains in place, these losses must be factored in the total water requirement. It must be kept in mind also that **insensible water losses** depend on respiratory rate, ambient temperature, humidity, and body temperature. Water losses increase by 100–150 mL/d for each degree of body temperature over 37°C. Fluid losses from sweating can vary enormously (100–2,000 mL/hr). It is not uncommon to administer 2–3 L of water per day to produce a urine volume >1,000–1,500 mL/d since there is no advantage to minimizing urine output.

■ The **electrolytes** that are usually administered during maintenance fluid therapy are Na^+ and K^+ salts. Requirements depend on minimum obligatory and ongoing losses. The kidneys are normally capable of compensating for wide fluctuations in dietary Na^+ intake; renal Na^+ excretion can fall to <5 mEq/d in the absence of Na^+ intake. It is customary to provide **75–175 mEq Na^+/d** as NaCl. (For comparison, a 2-g Na^+ diet provides 86 mEq Na^+/d.) Generally, **20–60 mEq K^+/d** is included if renal function is normal. Carbohydrate in the form of **dextrose, 100–150 g/d**, is given to minimize protein catabolism and prevent starvation ketoacidosis. The electrolyte losses from **insensible losses** may be disregarded since these fluids are quite **hypotonic** (see Disorders of Sodium Concentration, General Principles) and may be regarded simply as free water. If the patient has ongoing GI or renal losses from surgical drains or disease states such as diarrhea or salt-wasting nephropathy, these electrolyte losses should be accounted for and added to the total daily requirements. Gastrointestinal losses vary in composition and volume depending on their sources (see Chapter 2, Nutritional Therapy), and predictions of daily requirements based on this information may be made. Alternatively, laboratory measurement of the electrolyte composition of these GI losses can be performed to increase the accuracy of replacement. *(Note: Special considerations apply to hyperchloremic losses such as emesis and are described below* [see The Hypovolemic Patient, Treatment]).

■ Using these guidelines one can derive a **typical maintenance fluid regimen** for a patient: Dissolving 150 mEq Na^+, 40 mEq K^+, and 100 g dextrose in 2 L of water to be given over a day (these values were chosen arbitrarily, but are within the ranges of daily **water** and **electrolyte** requirements described above) would give a final solution consisting of 75 mEq/L Na^+, 20 mEq/L K^+, and 50 g/L dextrose. Using Table 3-1 which lists commonly used IV fluid preparations, one can see that this typical water and electrolyte requirement can be satisfied by a solution of D_5 0.45% NaCl with 20 mEq/L KCl additive running at 85 mL/hr (2,000 mL ÷ 24 hours). The more complicated scenarios with other ongoing gastrointestinal or renal losses can be approached in a similar way by determining the total water and total electrolyte losses separately and choosing the appropriate fluid to match both of those losses. (An example of this is provided below in Fluid Management and Perturbations in Volume Status, The Hypovolemic Patient, Treatment.) Calcium, magnesium, phosphorus, vitamins, and protein replacement are necessary after 1 week of parenteral therapy without PO intake (see Chapter 2, Nutritional Therapy).

THE HYPOVOLEMIC PATIENT

General Principles

Etiology
■ Volume depletion as we perceive it clinically generally results from a deficit in **total body Na^+** content as a result of **renal** or **extrarenal losses** that exceed Na^+ intake. Larger amounts of **water** alone must be lost to manifest as volume depletion since most of the loss (two thirds of it) occurs from the significantly larger ICF compartment, which is not easily accessible to clinical and laboratory examination.

TABLE 3-1	Commonly Used Parenteral Solutions

IV solution	Osmolality (mOsm/L)	[Glucose] (g/L)	[Na$^+$] (mEq/L)	[Cl$^-$] (mEq/L)	HCO$_3^-$ equivalents (mEq/L)
D$_5$W	278	50	0	0	0
D$_{10}$W	556	100	0	0	0
D$_{50}$W	2778	500	0	0	0
0.225% NaCl^a	77	—^{b}	38.5	38.5	0
0.45% NaCl^a	154	—^{b}	77	77	0
0.9% NaCl^a	308	—^{b}	154	154	0
3% NaCl	1026	—	513	513	0
D$_5$W with two ampules of NaHCO$_3$^{c}	478	50	100	0	100
Lactated Ringer's^d	274	—^{b}	130	109	28

D$_5$W, 5% dextrose in water; D$_{10}$W, 10% dextrose in water; D$_{50}$W, 50% dextrose in water.
^{a}NaCl 0.225%, 0.45%, and 0.9% are quarter-normal, half-normal, and normal saline, respectively.
^{b}Also available with 5% dextrose.
^{c}One 50 mL ampule of 8.4% NaHCO$_3$ contains 50 mEq each of Na$^+$ and HCO$_3^-$.
^{d}Also contains 4 mEq/L K$^+$, 1.5 mEq/L Ca^{++}, and 28 mEq/L lactate.

- **Renal losses** may be secondary to diuretics (pharmacologic or osmotic), salt-losing nephritis (medullary cystic disease, chronic interstitial nephritis, polycystic kidney disease), mineralocorticoid deficiency, or the tubular dysfunction and osmotic diuresis from resolving acute tubular necrosis (ATN) or the relief of bilateral urinary tract obstruction.
- **Extrarenal losses** include fluid loss from the GI tract (vomiting, nasogastric suction, fistula drainage, diarrhea), respiratory losses, skin losses (especially with burns), and hemorrhage. Another major consideration should be third-space accumulations as occur with peritonitis, pancreatitis, portal vein thrombosis, ileus or intestinal obstruction, bacterial enteritis or colitis, crush injuries and rhabdomyolysis, and during the postoperative period.

Diagnosis

Clinical Presentation
- A thorough history and physical examination are generally sufficient to determine the presence and cause of volume depletion.
- **Symptoms** are usually nonspecific and secondary to accompanying electrolyte imbalances and tissue hypoperfusion. These include complaints of thirst, fatigue, weakness, muscle cramps, and postural dizziness. Sometimes syncope and coma can result with more severe volume depletion.
- **Signs** of hypovolemia include low jugular venous pressure, postural hypotension, postural tachycardia, and the absence of axillary sweat. Diminished skin turgor and dry mucous membranes are poor markers of decreased interstitial fluid. Mild degrees of volume depletion are often not clinically detectable. Larger fluid losses often present as hypovolemic shock, heralded by hypotension, tachycardia, and signs of hypoperfusion such as cyanosis, cool extremities, oliguria, and altered mental status.

Laboratory Studies
- Laboratory studies corroborate the clinical suspicion. High urine osmolality, low urine Na$^+$, and contraction alkalosis may be present but cannot be relied upon. These data would be affected by the acid-base characteristics of the lost fluid and by the renal disease that may be causing the volume depletion in the first place.

- Serum [Na^+] does not reflect **total body Na^+ content** and therefore is not helpful in diagnosing Na^+ depletion. However, since it is intimately related to **osmolality**, [Na^+] does predict alterations in **TBW** (see Disorders of Sodium Concentration, General Principles). A high serum [Na^+] suggests the presence of a **water** deficit, which should be replaced as well (see Disorders of Sodium Concentration, Hypernatremia, Treatment).
- There may be a relative elevation in the hematocrit and serum [albumin] from hemoconcentration.

Treatment

- It is often difficult to estimate the **volume deficit** present. Weight loss can help in estimating the *total* volume deficit. The *ECF* deficit can be estimated from the formula, $ECF_{def} = 0.2 \times Lean\ Wt\ (kg) \times ([Hct \div Hct_{usu}] - 1)$, where Hct_{usu} corresponds to the patient's usual hematocrit when he or she is euvolemic. Unfortunately, the patient's euvolemic weight and hematocrit are not often known. Therapy is thus largely empiric and requires frequent reassessment of volume status through attention to the **signs** noted above while resuscitation is under way.
- Mild volume contraction can usually be corrected via the oral route. More severe cases of hypovolemia require IV therapy. The therapeutic goal is to first replenish **intravascular volume** with isotonic fluid and then restore the **total body volume deficit** as well as ongoing losses with fluid similar in composition to that being lost. The latter is done in a manner similar to that described above for calculation of maintenance fluids where the water and electrolyte losses are accounted for separately (see Fluid Management and Perturbations in Volume Status, The Euvolemic Patient, Treatment).
  - Normal saline (0.9% NaCl) is the initial fluid of choice for replenishing **intravascular volume**, especially in patients with hypotension or shock. Only approximately one third to one fourth of the administered volume of an isotonic fluid will remain in the intravascular space; the rest will leak into the interstitium. This is explained by the fact that the ECF is divided into intravascular space and interstitial space in a ratio of 1:4 (see Fluid Management and Perturbations in Volume Status, General Principles). Again, frequent reassessment should occur during resuscitation. Patients with significant hemorrhage or anemia may require blood transfusions.
    - One safe strategy for **intravascular volume** repletion would be to administer a bolus of isotonic fluid (either normal saline or Ringer's solution; hypo-osmolar solutions should never be used when bolusing to avoid the possibility of causing intravascular hemolysis) in a volume of 1–2 L, depending on the fluid deficit. After completion of the bolus, one should examine the patient for signs of improved hemodynamics (e.g., improved heart rate, blood pressure, and/or urine output) and for clinical evidence of impending volume overload with particular attention directed to the neck vein and pulmonary exams. If the patient still appears to be **intravascularly** volume depleted, then another iteration of the cycle of bolus followed by reassessment should be undertaken, and so on. Modifications to this strategy for poor cardiac reserve should be made through decreasing the size of the fluid bolus (even to as small as 250 mL) rather than decreasing the bolus infusion rate for all but the most profound states of heart failure.
  - **An example.** You estimate a patient who has been vomiting for 2 days has a **total volume deficit** of approximately 8 L. After iteratively bolusing a total 3 L of normal saline, you feel the patient is **intravascularly** replete. The patient continues to have 250 mL of emesis every 8 hours. A goal of repletion of the total body deficit in 24 hours is reasonable. The patient had 1,400 mL/d × 2 days = 2,800 mL of obligate water loss (for a derivation of daily obligate water loss see Fluid Management and Perturbations in Volume Status, The Euvolemic Patient, Treatment) and will lose an additional 1,400 mL during the next 24 hours of therapy. Therefore, fluid loss in emesis totals 5,200 mL (8,000 mL – 2,800 mL), plus an additional 750 mL over the next 24 hours to total 5,950 mL. The Na^+ and K^+ deficits can be estimated with a knowledge of the typical components of stomach fluid (see Chapter 2, Nutrition Support) or by laboratory analysis of the emesis and are 595 mEq (5.95 L × 100 mEq Cl^-/L) and 59.5 mEq (5.95 L × 10 mEq K^+/L), respectively. *(Note: When*

*dealing with significantly hyperchloremic fluid losses such as emesis where [Cl⁻] >>
[Na⁺], use [Cl⁻] in place of [Na⁺] when estimating the Na⁺ deficit since using [Na⁺]
will result in an underestimation. This underestimation occurs because the metabolic
alkalosis that results from GI Cl⁻ loss causes bicarbonaturia, which necessitates more
urinary cation loss, mostly Na⁺.)* Since 462 mEq Na⁺ (3 L × 154 mEq/L [see Table
3-1]) has already been given during the initial resuscitation, this leaves 133 mEq Na⁺
and 59.5 mEq K⁺ in a total volume of 7,150 mL (8,000 mL – 3,000 mL + 1,400 mL
[ongoing obligate water loss] + 750 mL [ongoing emesis]) left to replenish over the
next 24 hours. A routinely available solution (see Table 3-1) that would most closely
approximate these needs would be quarter normal saline with 10 mEq/L KCl running
at 300 mL/hr (7,150 mL ÷ 24 hours). Though a Na⁺ excess would be provided with
this volume of quarter normal saline (7.15 L × 38.5 mEq/L = 275 mEq Na⁺ vs. the
133 mEq required), this excess is within the capacity for renal excretion. This is a
rough estimate and the patient should frequently be reassessed throughout the day
by repeat physical examination and obtaining repeat labs.

THE HYPERVOLEMIC PATIENT

General Principles

Etiology

- Hypervolemia as perceived clinically results from a surplus in **total body Na⁺** as a result
  of salt intake that exceeds renal Na⁺ excretion, usually because of relative renal Na⁺
  retention. Na⁺ retention can be caused by a primary renal disorder such as renal failure
  or the nephrotic syndrome. Alternatively, it may be secondary to decreased **effective circulating volume** that results from heart failure, cirrhosis, or profound hypoalbuminemia.
- Hypervolemia can also occur with normal renal Na⁺ excretion during volume resuscitation with fluids with significant Na⁺ content.

Diagnosis

Clinical Presentation

- Volume overload is most apparent in the ECF compartment, again because this compartment is most accessible to clinical and laboratory evaluation.
- **Signs** of ECF volume excess result from expansion of the **interstitial compartment**, which
  presents as edema and effusions. Incipient edema may be detected only by the occurrence
  of weight gain, whereas overt edema is apparent only after 3–4 L of fluid has accumulated. Expansion of the **intravascular compartment** of the ECF results in pulmonary
  rales, elevated jugular venous pressure, hepatojugular reflux, an S₃ gallop, and sometimes hypertension.
- **Symptoms** may include dyspnea or complaints of peripheral or abdominal swelling.

Laboratory Studies

- Laboratory studies are generally not needed and hypervolemia is primarily a bedside
  diagnosis.
- Serum [Na⁺] does not reflect **total body Na⁺** and therefore is not helpful in establishing
  the presence of a Na⁺ surplus.
- The urine [Na⁺] may be low (<15 mEq/L) in states of decreased **effective circulating
  volume** reflecting renal sodium retention.
- A chest radiograph may show pulmonary edema or pleural effusions, but clear lung
  fields do not exclude volume overload.

Treatment

- Treatment must address not only the ECF volume excess, but also the underlying pathologic process. The main arms of therapy are limiting Na⁺ intake and promoting salt
  wasting through the use of diuretics. Treatment of the nephrotic syndrome and the

volume overload associated with renal failure is discussed in Chapter 11, Renal Diseases. Treatment of heart failure and cirrhosis is discussed in Chapter 6, Heart Failure, Cardiomyopathy, and Valvular Heart Disease, and Chapter 17, Liver Diseases, respectively.

DISORDERS OF SODIUM CONCENTRATION

GENERAL PRINCIPLES

- **Osmolality** is the solute or particle concentration of a fluid. Solutes that are restricted to the ECF (Na^+ and its accompanying anions) or the ICF (K^+ salts and organic phosphate esters) determine the **effective osmolality** or **tonicity** of each of those compartments. The osmolality of the ICF and ECF compartments is always equal because water diffuses rapidly across cell membranes in order to achieve **osmotic equilibrium**. Because of osmotic equilibrium, changes in the water content of one compartment affect *both* the ECF and ICF (as opposed to changes in Na^+ content, which affects primarily the ECF to which it is restricted). Also because of osmotic equilibrium, we can estimate the osmolality of TBW through the following relation: TBW osmolality = ECF osmolality = Plasma osmolality = $2 \times [Na^+] + ([BUN \text{ (blood urea nitrogen)}] \div 2.8) + ([glucose] \div 18)$. Since urea readily crosses plasma membranes, it is an **ineffective osmole**, and the contribution of glucose to osmolality in euglycemic individuals is small ($\sim$5 mOsm/L). Therefore, *effective* $TBW_{osm} = 2 \times [Na^+]$. It is thus obvious that $[Na^+]$ is intimately related to osmolality.
- Because of their relation to osmolality, **hypernatremia** and **hyponatremia** are primarily disorders of *water balance* or *water distribution* across the fluid compartments. Though alterations in Na^+ content change $[Na^+]$ transiently, there is a resulting perturbation in osmolality by the relation above which is met by compensatory changes in water balance. Regulation of water balance occurs primarily through **antidiuretic hormone** (ADH; vasopressin) and the **thirst control centers** of the hypothalamus, which return $[Na^+]$ to normal. A persistent abnormality in $[Na^+]$ would thus require an alteration in the action of ADH or the thirst response.

HYPONATREMIA

General Principles

Definition
- Hyponatremia is defined as a plasma $[Na^+]$ <135 mEq/L.

Etiology
- To maintain a normal plasma $[Na^+]$, the ingestion of solute-free water must eventually lead to the loss of the same volume of electrolyte-free water. Three steps are required for the kidney to excrete a water load: (a) glomerular filtration and delivery of fluid to the diluting sites of the nephron, (b) active reabsorption of Na^+ and Cl^- without water at those diluting segments (i.e., the distal convoluted tubule and the thick ascending limb of the loop of Henle), and (c) maintenance of a dilute urine due to impermeability of the collecting duct to water in the absence of **vasopressin**. Abnormalities of any of these steps can result in impaired free water excretion and eventual hyponatremia.
- **Hypo-osmolar hyponatremia.** Most causes of hyponatremia are associated with a low plasma osmolality. The ECF volume, reflecting **total body Na^+** content, may be decreased (**hypovolemic**), normal (**euvolemic**), or increased (**hypervolemic**) in hyponatremia.
    - **Hypovolemic hyponatremia** may result from **renal** or **nonrenal** causes of net Na^+ loss (see Fluid Management and Perturbations in Volume Status, The Hypovolemic

Patient, General Principles, Etiology). A decreased **effective circulating volume** stimulates the **hypothalamic thirst centers** and **vasopressin** release from the posterior pituitary gland, which both cause hyponatremia from free water accumulation.

- **Thiazide** use is a classic and very common cause of hyponatremia. Its use results in impaired water excretion by inducing a decreased effective circulating volume and impairing the action of the diluting segment of the nephron. Furthermore, thiazides may also be associated with a large K^+ deficit, resulting in *intracellular* hypo-osmolality (as noted in Disorders of Sodium Concentration, General Principles, K^+ is one of the major intracellular osmoles). Because of osmotic equilibrium, water shifts out of cells and hyponatremia worsens. This latter sodium-lowering effect can occur with any source of K^+ wasting, such as with vomiting.
- **Cerebral salt wasting** is a poorly understood entity that has been associated with neurosurgery and central nervous system (CNS) trauma, especially subarachnoid hemorrhage. It is characterized by excessive renal Na^+ excretion and its resulting ECF volume depletion after a CNS injury. The hyponatremia, however, does not always correct with volume resuscitation perhaps as a result of concomitant ADH release from the damaged brain. The disorder may be indistinguishable from the **syndrome of inappropriate antidiuretic hormone secretion (SIADH; see below)** by laboratory data.

■ **Hypervolemic hyponatremia** occurs in edematous states such as congestive heart failure (CHF), hepatic cirrhosis, and severe nephrotic syndrome as a result of a decrease in **effective circulating volume**, leading to increased **thirst** and **vasopressin** levels. The increase in **total body Na^+** is exceeded by the rise in **total body water**. The degree of hyponatremia often correlates with the severity of the underlying condition and is therefore an important prognostic factor. Oliguric renal failure may also be associated with hypervolemic hyponatremia if free water intake exceeds the kidney's limited ability to excrete an equivalent volume of free water.

■ **Euvolemic hyponatremia**

- **SIADH** is the most common cause of normovolemic hyponatremia. This disorder is caused by the nonphysiologic release of vasopressin from the posterior pituitary or an ectopic source. Common causes of SIADH include neuropsychiatric disorders (e.g., meningitis, encephalitis, acute psychosis, cerebrovascular accident, head trauma), pulmonary diseases (e.g., pneumonia, tuberculosis, positive pressure ventilation, acute respiratory failure), and malignant tumors (most commonly small cell lung cancer). **SIADH** is diagnosed by confirming (a) a hypo-osmotic hyponatremia, (b) an inappropriately concentrated urine (urine osmolality >100 mOsm/L), (c) euvolemia, and (d) an absence of adrenal, and thyroid dysfunction or other conditions associated with increased ADH action, which include the following:
  - **Pharmacologic agents** may cause hyponatremia by one of at least three mechanisms: (a) stimulation of vasopressin release (e.g., nicotine, carbamazepine, antidepressants, narcotics, antipsychotic agents, antineoplastic drugs); (b) potentiation of the antidiuretic action of vasopressin (e.g., chlorpropamide, methylxanthines, nonsteroidal anti-inflammatory drugs [NSAIDs]); or (c) vasopressin analogs (e.g., oxytocin, desmopressin acetate [dDAVP]).
  - **Physical/emotional stress and pain** are often associated with vasopressin release, possibly secondary to hypotension associated with stress-induced vasovagal reactions and/or coincident nausea.
  - Acute hypoxemia or hypercapnia also stimulates vasopressin secretion.
- **Hypothyroidism.** The mechanisms by which hypothyroidism leads to hyponatremia include decreased cardiac output and glomerular filtration rate (GFR) and increased vasopressin secretion in response to hemodynamic stimuli.
- **Glucocorticoid deficiency.** Although decreased *minleralo*corticoids may contribute to the hypovolemic hyponatremia of Addison disease, *gluco*corticoid deficiency alone as occurs in secondary adrenal insufficiency may lead to hypersecretion of ADH directly (ADH is cosecreted with corticotropin-releasing factor and cortisol provides negative feedback to the release of both) and indirectly (secondary to volume depletion from nausea/vomiting).

- **Psychogenic polydipsia** refers to a condition of compulsive fluid consumption that may overwhelm the large maximal renal excretory capacity of water of ∼12 L/d. These patients often have psychiatric illnesses and may be taking medications, such as phenothiazines, that enhance the sensation of thirst by causing a dry mouth.
- **Beer potomania** is similar to psychogenic polydipsia but is associated with a lower maximal renal excretory capacity of water. This results from the low protein and low solute diet seen with alcoholism, which generates a solute load of only 200–250 mOsm/d (600–800 mOsm/d is normal). Because urine can only be maximally diluted to 50 mOsm/L, a maximum of 4–5 L/d of urine can be generated. Beer drinking in excess of this capacity results in hyponatremia. A similar state, often referred to as the **tea-and-toast diet,** has been observed in malnourished elderly patients who maintain fluid intake without an adequate diet.
- **Reset osmostat** is a phenomenon in which the setpoint for plasma osmolality is reduced and ADH and thirst responses, though functional, maintain plasma osmolality at this new level. Thus, [Na^+] remains stable but below normal (usually 125–130 mEq/L). This phenomenon occurs in almost all pregnant women (perhaps in response to changes in the hormonal milieu), sometimes in states of chronic decreased effective circulating volume such as CHF, and rarely in severe malnutrition. The volume status of the patient can be quite variable. Distinction from SIADH is impossible but for the mildness of the hyponatremia and its stability over time.
- Hyponatremia with normal or high plasma osmolality
  - **Pseudohyponatremia** occurs as a result of a decrease in the aqueous portion of plasma. Plasma is 93% water, with the remaining 7% consisting of plasma proteins and lipids. Because Na^+ ions are dissolved in plasma water, increasing the nonaqueous component, as may occur in severe hyperlipidemia and paraproteinemias, artificially lowers the [Na^+] measured per liter of plasma (except when Na^+-sensitive electrodes are used for measurement). The plasma osmolality remains normal since its method of measurement is affected only by changes in the plasma water.
  - **Hyperosmolar hyponatremia** is usually caused by an increase in the concentration of a solute that is largely restricted to the ECF compartment. The resulting osmotic gradient causes water to shift from the ICF to the ECF, and dilutional hyponatremia ensues. Hyperosmolar hyponatremia is usually caused by hyperglycemia or, occasionally, the IV administration of mannitol. Quantitatively, the plasma [Na^+] falls by 2.4 mEq/L for every 100 mg/dL rise in the plasma [glucose]. (This was shown to be more accurate than the traditional 1.6 per 100 correction factor).[1]
  - **Posttransurethral resection of the prostate (post-TURP) syndrome.** Iso-osmolar or slightly hypo-osmolar hyponatremia can complicate transurethral resection of the prostate or bladder as a result of absorption of water and nonionic solute (either glycine, mannitol, or sorbitol) from the flushing solutions used during these procedures. Prompt renal excretion of the absorbed fluid and solute usually corrects the hyponatremia rapidly (glycine and sorbitol are also quickly metabolized by the tissues). Occasionally symptomatic hyponatremia results, especially in the setting of renal insufficiency.

Diagnosis

Clinical Presentation

- The clinical features of hyponatremia are related to osmotic intracellular water shift leading to cerebral edema. Therefore, the symptoms are primarily neurologic, and their severity is dependent on both the magnitude of the fall in plasma [Na^+] and the rapidity of the decrease. In **acute hyponatremia** (i.e., developing in <2 days), patients may complain of nausea and malaise with [Na^+] ∼125 mEq/L. As the plasma [Na^+] falls further, symptoms may progress to include headache, lethargy, confusion, and obtundation. Stupor, seizures, and coma do not usually occur unless the plasma [Na^+] falls acutely below 115 mEq/L.[2,3] In **chronic hyponatremia** (>3 days' duration), adaptive mechanisms designed to defend cell volume occur and tend to minimize the increase in ICF volume and its symptoms.

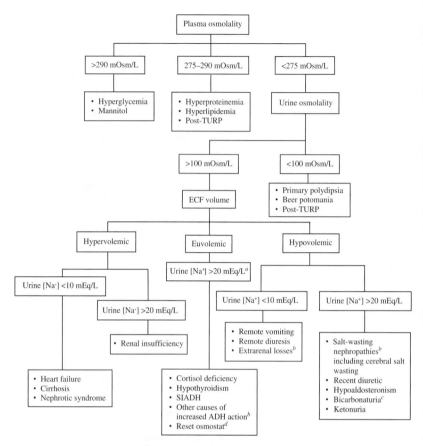

Figure 3-1. Algorithm depicting the diagnostic approach to hyponatremia. ECF, extracellular fluid; SIADH, syndrome of inappropriate antidiuretic hormone; post-TURP, posttransurethral resection of the prostate syndrome.
[a]Urine [Na+] may be <20 mEq/L with low Na+ intake.
[b]See text for details.
[c]From vomiting-induced contraction alkalosis or proximal renal tubular acidosis.
[d]Urine osmolality may be <100 mOsm/L after a water load.

- The underlying cause of hyponatremia can often be ascertained from an accurate history and physical examination, including an assessment of **ECF volume status** and the **effective circulating volume.**

Laboratory Studies
- Three laboratory analyses, when used with a clinical assessment of volume status, can narrow the differential diagnosis of hyponatremia: (a) the **plasma osmolality,** (b) the **urine osmolality,** and (c) the **urine [Na+]** (Fig. 3-1).
  - **Plasma osmolality.** Most patients with hyponatremia have a low plasma osmolality (<275 mOsm/L). If the plasma osmolality is not low, **pseudohyponatremia** and **hyperosmolar hyponatremia** must be ruled out.
  - **Urine osmolality.** The appropriate renal response to hypo-osmolality is to excrete a maximally dilute urine (urine osmolality <100 mOsm/L and specific gravity of

<1.003). This occurs in patients with primary polydipsia. If this is not the case, it suggests impaired free water excretion due to the action of vasopressin on the kidney. The secretion of vasopressin may be a physiologic response to decreased effective circulating volume, or it may be inappropriate in the presence of hyponatremia and euvolemia.

- **Urine [Na^+]** adds laboratory corroboration to the bedside assessment of effective circulating volume and is also used to discriminate between **extrarenal** and **renal losses** of Na^+ once it is established that hypovolemic hyponatremia is present. The appropriate response to decreased effective circulating volume in patients with normal renal electrolyte handling is to enhance tubular Na^+ reabsorption such that urine [Na^+] is <10 mEq/L. This is found with extrarenal volume losses and CHF. A urine [Na^+] of >20 mEq/L implies either euvolemia as in SIADH or hypovolemic hyponatremia as a result of renal Na^+ wasting. The latter can occur from dysfunctional tubular transport from diuretics, hypoaldosteronism, or intrinsic renal disease. Renal Na^+ loss can also be obligated by the urinary loss of anion in order to maintain tubular fluid electroneutrality, as occurs with ketonuria and the bicarbonaturia of contraction alkalosis.

Treatment

- The steps in therapy are to (a) **determine the required rate of correction,** (b) **correct the hypo-osmolality** at the rate desired, and (c) **correct the underlying disorder.** It is the hypo-osmolality, not the hyponatremia per se, that causes neuronal swelling and its symptoms, and therefore this is the target of treatment rather than simply the [Na^+]. The hyponatremia in hyperosmolar or iso-osmolar states is often a lab phenomenon and of little clinical significance by itself. Likewise, mild asymptomatic hyponatremia as is often seen with disorders such as reset osmostat usually have no adverse effect and do not require treatment.
- **The rate of correction** of hyponatremia depends on the acuity of its development and whether associated neurologic dysfunction is present. Regardless of the presence of symptoms, when hyponatremia is significant, therapy *must* be followed with frequent follow-up labs, beginning 2–3 hours into therapy.
  - **Symptomatic hyponatremia.** The risks of correcting hyponatremia too rapidly are volume overload and the development of **central pontine myelinolysis** (CPM). CPM is thought to result from the shrinkage of neurons away from their myelin sheaths due to the osmotic shift of water out of cells. In its most overt form, it is characterized by flaccid paralysis, dysarthria, and dysphagia, and in more subtle presentations it can be confirmed by computed tomography (CT) scan or magnetic resonance imaging (MRI) of the brain. The risk of precipitating CPM is increased with correction of the [Na^+] by >12 mEq/L in a 24-hour period.[4] The absolute magnitude of correction in 24 hours appears to be more important than the rate, such that an initially rapid rate of correction tapering off after several hours incurs less risk than a slow, steady correction that exceeds 12 mEq/L in one day. In addition to overaggressive correction, other risk factors for developing CPM include pre-existing hypokalemia, malnutrition, and alcoholism. Despite these concerns, in cases of severe neurologic signs such as obtundation or seizures, a rapid correction of the **hypo-osmolality** is required to reduce cerebral swelling, which poses a greater risk to the patient than of possibly causing CPM. Severe neurologic dysfunction should generally be treated with hypertonic saline; however, any saline solution that is hypertonic to the urine (if the urine osmolality is known at the start of therapy) can increase the [Na^+] when oral water intake is restricted. As an example of the converse, the administration of normal saline may actually *lower* the [Na^+] in a patient with a [Na^+] = 108 mEq/L and urine osmolality persistently >500 mOsm/L from SIADH. The 308 mOsm contained in 1 L of normal saline (see Table 3-1) will be excreted in 0.6 L of additional urine output (308 mOsm ÷ 500 mOsm/L), and 0.4 L of free water (1 L − 0.6 L) will be left to worsen the hyponatremia. The simultaneous administration of an IV loop diuretic to promote further water excretion can ameliorate this seemingly paradoxical effect.

- The change in $[Na^+]$ in mEq/L from the infusion of 1 L of a fluid can be estimated from $\triangle[Na^+] = \{[Na^+_i] + [K^+_i] - [Na^+_s]\} \div \{(Lean\ Wt \times 0.6) + 1\}$ where $[Na^+_i]$ and $[K^+_i]$ are the sodium and potassium concentrations in the infused fluid and $[Na^+_s]$ is the starting serum sodium.[5] The denominator must be modified to $\{(LeanWt \times 0.5) + 1\}$ in females. This formula does not account for ongoing electrolyte or water losses and is only a rough guide. **A goal increase of 1.5–2 mEq/L/hr for 3–4 hours until symptoms resolve but not to exceed 10 mEq/L in the first 24 hours** (which allows a margin of error from 12 mEq/L) **and <18 mEq/L over the first 48 hours appears to be safe.**[6] The slower rate of correction is much less critical in **acute** (<2 days in development) **symptomatic hyponatremia,** though immediate attainment of normonatremia is not suggested.
  - **An example.** If one wanted to correct a $[Na^+] = 108$ mEq/L in a 70-kg man who is seizing with hypertonic saline, one can determine that the $\triangle[Na^+]$ with 1 L of this fluid would be +9.4 mEq/L ($\{513$ [see Table 3-1] $- 108\} \div \{70 \times 0.6 + 1\}$). One could therefore estimate that 200 mL/hr ([2 mEq/L/hr] ÷ [9.4 mEq/L per 1,000 mL of saline]) of hypertonic saline should be given until symptoms improve but not to exceed 1,000 mL ([10 mEq/L] ÷ [9.4 mEq/L per 1,000 mL of saline]) in 24 hours. Frequent labs should be drawn to monitor therapy.
- **Chronic asymptomatic hyponatremia.** The plasma $[Na^+]$ should be raised significantly slower than 12 mEq/L/d (5–8 mEq/L/d would be reasonable) to avoid CPM in a patient without current symptoms and therefore with low risk for neurologic injury from the hypo-osmolality itself. The risk of treatment-related complication is increased due to the cerebral adaptation to the chronic hypo-osmolar state. It must be kept in mind that simple water restriction in primary polydipsia or saline resuscitation in hypovolemic patients may lead to overly rapid correction of hyponatremia, the latter as a result of ADH suppression and a resultant brisk water diuresis. This can be prevented by the administration of water or the use of the vasopressin analog, dDAVP, to slow down the rate of free water excretion.
- Specific therapies for the underlying disorder
  - **Hypovolemic hyponatremia.** First correct hemodynamic instability with enough **isotonic** saline to restore tissue perfusion. Using more normal saline than is required to restore stability may result in overcorrection of the hyponatremia. Further ECF volume repletion can be undertaken with fluid that is isotonic to the patient to avoid rapid changes in neuronal cell volume. Correcting any K^+ deficit, as occurs not uncommonly in this type of hyponatremia, will further increase the $[Na^+]$.
  - **Hypervolemic hyponatremia.** The hyponatremia in CHF and cirrhosis tends to reflect the severity of the underlying disease and is usually asymptomatic. Treatment should include restriction of Na^+ and water intake, correction of hypokalemia, and promotion of water loss in excess of Na^+. The latter may require the use of loop diuretics with replacement of a proportion of the urinary Na^+ loss. Dietary water restriction should be to a quantity that is less than the urine output.
  - **SIADH** can be treated by either limiting the intake of water or promoting its excretion, or both. The standard first-line therapy is water restriction and correction of any contributing factors (such as treating pain, and stopping drugs that may mimic SIADH). If this fails or if the patient is symptomatic, agents that enhance water excretion can be tried. Loop diuretics impair the ability to excrete concentrated urine and, when combined with Na^+ replacement in the form of salt tablets or saline, can enhance free water excretion. Another means to increase free water excretion is to increase the daily solute load. Because the urine osmolality is relatively fixed in SIADH, the urine output is a direct function of the solute excretion requirement. Thus, a high-salt, high-protein diet or administering oral urea (30–60 g) may increase renal water excretion and improve the hyponatremia. Drugs that interfere with the collecting tubule's ability to respond to ADH include lithium and demeclocycline. These agents are rarely used because of significant side effects and should only be considered in severe hyponatremia that is unresponsive to more conservative measures. ADH receptor antagonists are currently under development, but until oral formulations are available (conivaptan is the only one available in the United States, but is an intravenous medication), they add little extra to management of SIADH.

HYPERNATREMIA

General Principles

Definition
- Hypernatremia is defined as a plasma $[Na^+]$ >145 **mEq/L** and represents a state of **hyperosmolality** (see Disorders of Sodium Concentration, General Principles).

Etiology
- Hypernatremia may be caused by a primary Na^+ **gain** or a **water deficit**, the latter being much more common. In order for hypernatremia to persist, these must occur in the setting of a disturbance in the appropriate response to hyperosmolality: increased water intake stimulated by **thirst** and the excretion of a maximally concentrated urine from increased **vasopressin** effect.
- **Impaired thirst response.** If obligate water loss (see Fluid Management and Perturbations in Volume Status, The Euvolemic Patient, Treatment) is not met with an adequate free water consumption, hypernatremia will result. This may occur in situations where access to water is limited such as with infants, the physically handicapped, patients with impaired mental status, individuals in the postoperative state, and intubated patients in the intensive care unit. Rarely, hypernatremia may be caused by **primary hypodipsia** as a result of damage to the thirst-controlling hypothalamic osmoreceptors from a variety of pathologic changes, including granulomatous disease, vascular occlusion, and tumors. Often an impaired thirst response is a component of a multifactorial hypernatremia. Without this impairment, the disease states listed below would be met with a compensatory increase in water intake, allowing the $[Na^+]$ to change very little. Thus, *significant hypernatremia almost always requires an impaired thirst mechanism.*
- **Hypernatremia due to water loss.** The loss of water must occur in excess of electrolyte losses in order to raise $[Na^+]$ and can occur via the kidneys or from extrarenal sites.
  - **Nonrenal water loss** may be due to evaporation from the skin and respiratory tract (insensible losses) or loss from the GI tract. Insensible losses are increased with fever, exercise, heat exposure, and severe burns, and in mechanically ventilated patients. Diarrhea is the most common GI cause of hypernatremia. Osmotic diarrheas (induced by lactulose, sorbitol, or malabsorption of carbohydrate) and viral gastroenteritides in particular result in water loss exceeding that of Na^+ and K^+.
  - **Renal water loss** results from either **osmotic diuresis** or **diabetes insipidus.**
    - The most frequent cause of an **osmotic diuresis** is the glucosuria that occurs in poorly controlled diabetes mellitus. IV administration of mannitol, increased urea levels out of proportion to the decrease in GFR (as can occur in the catabolic ICU patient with moderate renal insufficiency on high-protein feeds and stress dose steroids), or large solute loads with high osmolar feeds can also result in an osmotic diuresis.
    - Hypernatremia secondary to nonosmotic urinary water loss is usually caused by (a) **central diabetes insipidus** (CDI) characterized by impaired vasopressin secretion or (b) **nephrogenic diabetes insipidus** (NDI), which results from resistance to the actions of vasopressin. Partial defects in both types of DI occur more frequently than complete defects. The most common cause of CDI is destruction of the neurohypophysis as a result of trauma, neurosurgery, granulomatous disease, neoplasms, vascular accidents, or infection. In many cases, CDI is idiopathic and may occasionally be hereditary. NDI may either be inherited or acquired. The latter can be further subdivided into disorders associated with intrinsic renal diseases (e.g., sickle cell nephropathy, polycystic kidney disease, obstructive nephropathy, Sjogren's), drugs (e.g., lithium, demeclocycline, amphotericin, glyburide), electrolyte disorders (hypercalcemia and hypokalemia), and conditions that impair medullary hypertonicity (e.g., osmotic diuresis, excessive water intake, and use of loop diuretics).
- **Hypernatremia due to primary Na^+ gain** occurs infrequently due to the kidney's capacity to excrete the extra Na^+, prompted by the hypervolemia that results. This may occur, however, in situations of significant **hypertonic saline** administration such as the

patient who receives several ampules of $NaHCO_3$ (which are hypertonic to plasma) during cardiopulmonary resuscitation. A variant of this hypervolemic hypernatremia occurs in states of chronic **mineralocorticoid excess**. With a normal functioning ADH axis, the increased Na^+ reabsorption would raise the serum $[Na^+]$, which would activate hypothalamic osmoreceptors, leading to ADH release and thus water retention. The $[Na^+]$ would therefore not rise significantly. However, the chronic moderate hypervolemia that results actually decreases the threshold for ADH release in an attempt to temporize the volume overload. The result is a reset osmostat of sorts in which a new mildly elevated $[Na^+]$ ($\sim$145 mEq/L) setpoint is defended.

- **Transcellular water shift** from ECF to ICF occurs in rare circumstances of transient intracellular hyperosmolality such as in some patients with seizures or rhabdomyolysis. Hypernatremia results as water moves intracellularly and **osmotic equilibrium** is reestablished.

Diagnosis

Clinical Presentation

- The maintenance of **osmotic equilibrium** in hypernatremia results in ICF volume contraction and cerebral cell shrinkage. Thus, the most severe symptoms of hypernatremia are neurologic and include altered mental status, weakness, neuromuscular irritability, focal neurologic deficits, and occasionally coma or seizures. As with hyponatremia, the severity of the clinical manifestations is related to the *acuity* and *magnitude* of the rise in plasma $[Na^+]$. **Chronic hypernatremia** is generally less symptomatic as a result of adaptive mechanisms designed to defend cell volume. Severe neurologic compromise tends to occur with acute rises in $[Na^+]$ to >158 mEq/L[7] but chronic elevations to as high as 170–180 mEq/L may be only mildly symptomatic.[8]
- **CDI** and **NDI** generally present with complaints of polyuria and thirst. For unknown reasons, patients with polydipsia from CDI tend to prefer ice-cold water. Signs of volume depletion or neurologic dysfunction are generally absent unless the patient has an associated thirst abnormality.
- Attention to the patient's volume status is helpful in determining the etiology of the derangement. The signs and symptoms of **hypovolemia** (see Fluid Management and Perturbations in Volume Status, The Hypovolemic Patient, Diagnosis, Clinical Presentation) are often present in patients with a history of excessive sweating, diarrhea, or an osmotic diuresis. Signs of **hypervolemia** (see Fluid Management and Perturbations in Volume Status, The Hypervolemic Patient, Diagnosis, Clinical Presentation) may be present with primary Na^+ gain.
- The history must include a list of current and recent medications, which may provide clues as to the etiology.

Laboratory Studies

- When used with a clinical assessment of volume status, the **urine output** and the **urine osmolality** with its **response to dDAVP** can help narrow the differential diagnosis for hypernatremia (see Fig. 3-2). The appropriate renal response to hypernatremia is excretion of a small volume (<800 mL/d) of concentrated (urine osmolality >800 mOsm/L) urine. This response suggests extrarenal or remote renal water loss.
  - Submaximal **urine osmolality** (<800 mOsm/L) suggests the presence of a defect in vasopressin action as occurs in CDI and NDI. A urine osmolality <300 mOsm in the setting of hypernatremia suggests a severe defect in vasopressin action as occurs in the complete forms of CDI and NDI (complete NDI is usually either congenital or from lithium toxicity). Most often, however, the defect is partial (300–800 mOsm/L).
  - **Urine output.** Polyuria can result from either an osmotic diuresis or diabetes insipidus. An osmotic diuresis will typically also have a urine osmolality of 300–800 mOsm/L. The two can be differentiated by quantifying the daily solute excretion (estimated by the urine osmolality × urine volume in 24 hours). A daily solute excretion >900 mOsm defines an osmotic diuresis. The osmotically active species can then be determined by measuring the urine [glucose] or [urea nitrogen].

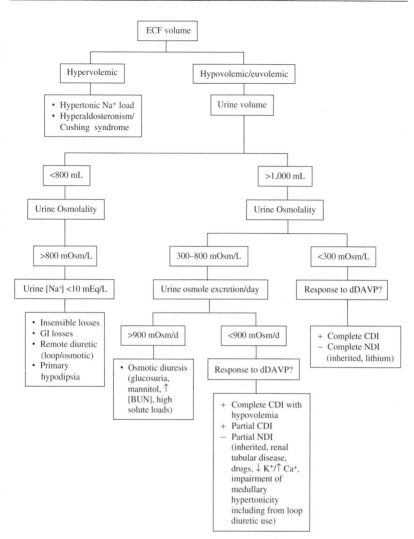

Figure 3-2. Algorithm depicting the diagnostic approach to hypernatremia. BUN, blood urea nitrogen; CDI, central diabetes insipidus; dDAVP, desmopressin acetate; ECF, extracellular fluid; GI, gastrointestinal; NDI, nephrogenic diabetes insipidus; $\downarrow K^+$, hypokalemia; $\uparrow Ca^+$, hypercalcemia; $(+)$, conditions with increase in urine osmolality in response to desmopressin acetate; $(-)$, conditions with little increase in urine osmolality in response to desmopressin acetate.

- **Response to dDAVP.** Complete CDI and NDI can be distinguished by administering the vasopressin analog dDAVP (10 mcg intranasally) after careful water restriction. The urine osmolality should increase by at least 50% in complete CDI and does not change in NDI. The diagnosis is sometimes difficult when partial defects are present.
- A primary Na^+ excess can be confirmed by the presence of ECF volume expansion and a urine $[Na^+]$ usually >100 mEq/L. A urine $[Na^+]$ <10 mEq/L is found in the hypovolemic hypernatremia caused by extrarenal losses. Thus, the urine $[Na^+]$ adds

little to the diagnosis of hypernatremic conditions other than to confirm the bedside volume assessment.

Treatment

- The therapeutic goals are to (a) **determine the rate of correction,** (b) **correct the water deficit** and hypovolemia at the rate desired, and (c) **correct the underlying disorder,** thereby reducing ongoing water loss.
- **The rate of correction** of hypernatremia depends on the acuity of its development and whether associated neurologic dysfunction is present. Regardless of the presence of symptoms, when hypernatremia is significant, therapy *must* be followed with frequent follow-up labs, beginning 2–3 hours into therapy.
  - **Symptomatic hypernatremia.** As in hyponatremia, aggressive correction of hypernatremia is potentially dangerous. The rapid shift of water into brain cells increases the risk of seizures or permanent neurologic damage. Therefore, the water deficit should be corrected slowly. A **goal decrease in $[Na^+]$ of 0.4–0.5 mEq/L/hr, or 10 mEq/L/d** (which allows for a margin for error from the observed safe rate of correction of 12 mEq/L/d[9]) is desired, similar to the treatment of hyponatremia. The safest route of administration of water is by mouth or via a nasogastric tube. Alternatively, D_5W or quarter normal saline can be given IV—the former is more appropriate in situations of pure water loss as in insensible losses or diabetes insipidus, the latter in situations of concurrent electrolyte loss as in GI and diuretic-induced losses. The change in $[Na^+]$ from the administration of these fluids can again be estimated by a simple formula: $\triangle[Na^+] = \{[Na^+_i] + [K^+_i] - [Na^+_s]\} \div \{(Lean\ Wt \times 0.6) + 1\}$[5] (see Disorders of Sodium Concentration, Hyponatremia, Treatment). Again, the denominator must be modified to $\{(Lean\ Wt \times 0.5) + 1\}$ in females. When calculating the rate of water replacement, ongoing losses of water and electrolytes, which may be widely variable in disease states, should be taken into account (see Fluid Management and Perturbations in Volume Status, The Euvolemic Patient, Treatment). The slower rate of correction is much less critical in **acute** (<2 days in development) **symptomatic hypernatremia,** though immediate attainment of normonatremia is not suggested.
    - **An example.** A 70-kg woman with diarrhea (2 L/d) from laxative abuse presents with obtundation and $[Na^+] = 168$ mEq/L, $[K^+] = 3.0$. A replacement fluid of quarter normal saline with 20 mEq KCl/L (to replace the diarrhea-induced hypokalemia) is chosen. The $\triangle[Na^+]$ with 1 L of this fluid would be −3 mEq/L ($\{38.5$ [see Table 3-1] $+ 20 - 168\} \div \{(70 \times 0.5) + 1\}$). Thus, one can predict that at least 3,300 mL ([10 mEq/L] ÷ [3 mEq/L per 1,000 mL of saline]) of this fluid will be required to correct the patient's $[Na^+]$ by 10 mEq/d. Since 1,400 mL/d of ongoing obligate water loss (see Fluid Management and Perturbations in Volume Status, The Euvolemic Patient, Treatment) and ongoing diarrhea of 2 L/d must also be accounted for, 6.7 L of this fluid should be given over the next 24 hours, or 275 mL/hr.
  - **Chronic asymptomatic hypernatremia.** The plasma $[Na^+]$ should be lowered significantly slower than 12 mEq/L/d (5–8 mEq/L/d would be reasonable) in a patient without current symptoms and therefore with low risk for neurologic injury from the hypernatremia itself. The risk of treatment-related complication is increased due to the cerebral adaptation to the chronic hyperosmolar state.
- **Specific therapies for the underlying cause**
  - **Hypovolemic hypernatremia.** First correct significant hemodynamic instability with enough **isotonic** saline to restore tissue perfusion before correcting the hyperosmolality. Using more normal saline than is required to restore stability may result in worsening hypernatremia. Therapy next involves the administration of hypotonic fluids as the cause of the water deficit is corrected (e.g., reducing the solute load in the patient on hyperosmolar feeds or administering dDAVP for DI as below).
  - **Hypernatremia from primary Na^+ gain.** Administration of free water alone may exacerbate the hypervolemic state. This can be prevented by administering a diuretic and infusing free water in the form of D5W or PO intake to match the urine output.

Attempting diuresis alone without water replacement may worsen the hypernatremia as hypo-osmolar urine is generated by loop diuretics.

■ **Diabetes insipidus without hypernatremia.** With an intact thirst mechanism, DI does not result in hypernatremia and therefore therapy, if required at all, is for the relief of symptomatic polyuria. Since therapy carries a risk of causing hyponatremia, transient, correctable DI is best treated by removing the underlying cause and waiting for improvements in symptoms to occur.

  • **CDI.** The appropriate treatment consists of administering dDAVP. Therapies used for NDI may be used in combination with desmopressin to increase response.

  • **NDI.** A low-Na^+ diet combined with *thiazide* diuretics will decrease polyuria through inducing mild volume depletion. This enhances proximal reabsorption of salt and water, decreasing excess water loss. Decreasing protein intake will further decrease urine output by minimizing the solute load that must be excreted. NSAIDs can potentiate vasopressin action, increasing urine osmolality.

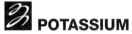 **POTASSIUM**

GENERAL PRINCIPLES

■ Potassium is the major intracellular cation. The normal plasma $[K^+]$ is 3.5–5.0 mEq/L, whereas that inside cells is approximately 150 mEq/L. The total body K^+ content in a normal adult is approximately **3,000–4,000 mEq**, 98% of which is in the cells. Thus, the ECF compartment from which we measure K^+ levels contains only 2% of the total body K^+ pool. The **Na^+/K^+-adenosine triphosphatase pump** actively transports Na^+ out of the cell and K^+ into the cell in a 3:2 ratio to maintain this difference in K^+ content between the ECF and ICF.

■ The K^+ intake of individuals on an average Western diet is approximately 1 mEq/kg/d, 90% of which is absorbed by the GI tract. Maintenance of the steady state necessitates matching K^+ excretion with ingestion.

  ■ **Renal excretion** is the major route of elimination of excess K^+. Ninety percent of filtered K^+ is reabsorbed by the proximal tubule and loop of Henle. Net distal K^+ secretion or reabsorption occurs in the setting of K^+ excess or depletion, respectively. The **principal cell** is responsible for K^+ secretion in the distal convoluted tubule and cortical collecting duct (CCD) and virtually all of the regulation of renal K^+ excretion occurs here. The driving force for K^+ secretion is a **lumen-negative transepithelial potential difference,** which depends on the relative rates of reabsorption of Na^+ and its accompanying anion (primarily Cl^-). In addition to variations in the K^+ secretion at the CCD, renal K^+ loss depends on the **distal urine flow rate,** a function of the daily solute load. Because K^+ excretion is equal to the product of concentration and flow, increased distal flow rate can significantly enhance urinary K^+ output.

  ■ Potassium secretion is regulated by two physiologic stimuli, **aldosterone** and the **potassium concentration.** Aldosterone is secreted in response to high angiotensin II or hyperkalemia. The plasma $[K^+]$ can also directly affect K^+ secretion independent of aldosterone.

HYPOKALEMIA

General Principles

Definition
■ Hypokalemia is defined as a plasma $[K^+]$ <3.5 mEq/L.

Etiology
■ **Spurious hypokalemia** may be seen in situations in which high numbers of metabolically active cells in drawn blood (as may occur in leukemia) uptake potassium when the tube is allowed to sit for some time prior to analysis.

- True hypokalemia may result from one or more of the following: (a) **decreased net intake,** (b) **shift into cells,** or (c) **increased net loss.**
- **Diminished intake** is seldom the sole cause of K^+ depletion because urinary excretion can be effectively decreased to <15 mEq/d. However, dietary K^+ restriction may exacerbate the hypokalemia from GI or renal loss.
- **Transcellular shift.** Movement of K^+ into cells may transiently decrease the plasma $[K^+]$ without altering total body K^+ content. The magnitude of the change is relatively small, often <1 mEq/L, but transcellular shift may amplify the hypokalemia due to other causes.
    - **Alkalemia** (see Acid-Base Disturbances, General Principles, Definitions), whether metabolic or respiratory, can shift K^+ into cells. Metabolic alkalosis may additionally result in excessive renal K^+ loss (see below), further lowering the $[K^+]$.
    - **Insulin therapy,** especially in the treatment of diabetic ketoacidosis (DKA), may lead to hypokalemia. The uncontrolled hyperglycemia and ketonuria contribute through promoting renal K^+ loss (see below).
    - Stress-induced **catecholamine** release and administration of β_2-adrenergic agonists directly induce the cellular uptake of K^+ and exert further effect by promoting insulin secretion by the pancreas.
    - **Anabolic states** can potentially result in K^+ shift into cells. This may occur after rapid cell growth, seen in patients with pernicious anemia treated with vitamin B_{12} or neutropenia treated with granulocyte-macrophage colony-stimulating factor. It can also be seen in patients receiving total parenteral nutrition (i.e., the refeeding syndrome).
    - A rare condition of episodic muscle weakness called **periodic paralysis** may be associated with transient hypokalemia or hyperkalemia from cellular shifts.
- **Nonrenal K^+ loss.** Hypokalemia from increased lower GI loss can occur in patients with enteritis, villous adenomas, vasoactive intestinal polypeptide (VIP)-omas, or laxative abuse. Integumentary K^+ loss can also be significant enough with excessive sweating to cause hypokalemia. Though stomach fluid has relatively high $[K^+]$, the profound hypokalemia seen in upper GI loss is more a result of renal K^+ wasting (see below).
- **Renal K^+ loss** accounts for most cases of chronic hypokalemia. This may be caused by factors that **increase CCD luminal K^+ concentration** or by factors that **augment distal tubular flow rate.**
    - **Augmented distal flow** occurs with diuretic use, osmotic diuresis (e.g., glucosuria), primary polydipsia/diabetes insipidus, and the recovery phase of ATN. The defects in the diuretic-responsive transporters in Bartter's and Gitelman's syndromes mimic diuretic use.
    - **Increased CCD luminal $[K^+]$**
        - **Primary mineralocorticoid excess** results in increased distal tubular K^+ secretion.
            - Primary hyperaldosteronism can be caused by an adrenal adenoma, a carcinoma, or adrenocortical hyperplasia.
            - Excess nonaldosterone mineralocorticoids may be found in congenital adrenal hyperplasia.
            - The presentation of Cushing's syndrome can include hypokalemia through cortisol's ability to also stimulate the aldosterone receptor. The syndrome of apparent mineralocorticoid excess reflects a type of local hypercortisolism due to 11-β-hydroxysteroid dehydrogenase deficiency. This enzyme normally converts cortisol to the less active cortisone. Ingestion of certain licorice, some chewing tobacco, or carbenoxolone can cause suppression of this enzyme with a similar clinical picture.
        - **Secondary hyperaldosteronism** from hyperreninism is seen in renovascular and malignant hypertension but occurs more commonly in any situation with decreased effective circulating volume. Hypovolemia stimulates aldosterone release, which augments K^+ secretion by the principal cells. The moderate to severe K^+ depletion often associated with vomiting or nasogastric suction is partly due to increased renal K^+ excretion through this mechanism. The metabolic alkalosis that is present in this setting promotes further kaliuresis (see below) as well as transcellular shift (see above).

- **Other mechanisms** of increased luminal [K^+]
  - Amphotericin B causes increased luminal [K^+] as a result of increased distal nephron permeability. It can also result in a distal (type 1) renal tubular acidosis (RTA; see Acid-Base Disturbances, Metabolic Acidosis, General Principles, Etiology), which itself is associated with impaired K^+ reabsorption and hypokalemia.
  - Hypomagnesemia appears to decrease K reabsorption in the loop of Henle and the collecting duct.
  - Increased distal delivery of Na^+ with a nonreabsorbable anion (i.e., not Cl^-) enhances the lumen-negative electrochemical force that drives K^+ secretion. This is seen with the bicarbonaturia of vomiting-induced metabolic alkalosis and proximal (type 2) RTA (see Acid-Base Disturbances, Metabolic Acidosis, General Principles, Etiology), the ketonuria of DKA, toluene abuse, and high doses of penicillin derivatives.
  - Liddle syndrome is a rare disorder that results from the constitutive activation of the renal epithelial sodium channel and is associated with low plasma renin and aldosterone and a hypokalemic metabolic alkalosis.

Diagnosis

Clinical Presentation

- The clinical features of K^+ depletion vary greatly, and their severity depends in part on the degree of hypokalemia. Symptoms seldom occur unless the plasma [K^+] is <3.0 mEq/L.
- Fatigue, myalgias, and muscular weakness or cramps of the lower extremities are common. Smooth muscle function may also be affected and may manifest with complaints of constipation or frank paralytic ileus. More severe hypokalemia may lead to complete paralysis, hypoventilation, or rhabdomyolysis.
- K^+ depletion is associated with an increased risk of arrhythmias (especially in the setting of digitalis use) which may present as complaints of palpitations or syncope.
- Polydipsia and polyuria may result from hypokalemia-induced NDI (see Disorders of Sodium Concentration, Hypernatremia, General Principles, Etiology).
- Diuretic and laxative abuse as well as surreptitious vomiting may be difficult to identify but should be excluded.
- Possible causes of transcellular shift should be sought, such as the use of bronchodilators in a patient with a chronic obstructive pulmonary disorder (COPD) exacerbation.
- Signs of mild hypervolemia and hypertension (see Fluid Management and Perturbations in Volume Status, The Hypervolemic Patient, Diagnosis, Clinical Presentation) or hypovolemia (see Fluid Management and Perturbations in Volume Status, The Hypovolemic Patient, Diagnosis, Clinical Presentation) may be apparent and would provide clues to the etiology.

Laboratory Studies

- Most commonly, the cause of hypokalemia will be obvious from the clinical context in which it occurs. However, when the etiology is not immediately apparent, a clinical assessment of ECF volume and blood pressure together with (a) **renal K^+ excretion,** (b) **acid-base status,** and (c) **urine [Cl^-]** can help narrow the differential diagnosis (Fig. 3-3).
  - **Renal K^+ excretion.** After eliminating spurious hypokalemia and intracellular shift as potential causes, examination of the renal K^+ excretion can help to clarify the source of K^+ loss. The appropriate response to K^+ depletion is to excrete <25 mEq/d of K^+ in the urine. This can be estimated by multiplying a spot urine [K^+] by the daily urine output. Hypokalemia with minimal renal K^+ excretion suggests extrarenal loss of K^+ or remote renal loss that has resolved. A spot urine [K^+] alone may be used to estimate renal K^+ avidity (urine [K^+] <20 mEq/L suggests appropriate K^+ reabsorption during extrarenal loss) but is less accurate in situations of either polyuria or oliguria.

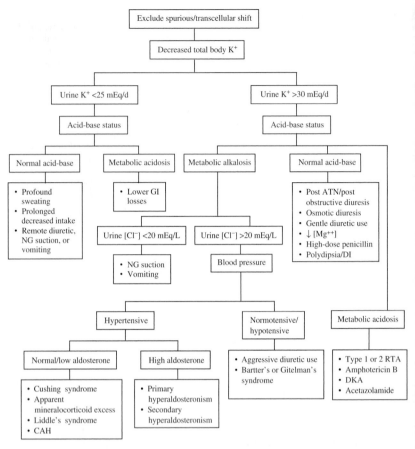

Figure 3-3. Algorithm depicting the diagnostic approach to hypokalemia. ATN, acute tubular necrosis; CAH, congenital adrenal hyperplasia; DI, diabetes insipidus; DKA, diabetic ketoacidosis; GI, gastrointestinal; NG, nasogastric; RTA, renal tubular acidosis.

- ▨ **Acid-base status.** Hypokalemia is frequently associated with derangements in acid-base status, a finding that is not surprising given the fact that aldosterone is important in regulating H^+ balance as well. States of hyperaldosteronism, either primary or secondary, cause metabolic alkalosis. In addition, K^+ depletion results in enhanced proximal HCO_3^- reabsorption, renal ammoniagenesis, and distal H^+ secretion, all of which tend to perpetuate the metabolic alkalosis that is frequently present in hypokalemic patients. Thus, the presence of a metabolic acidosis narrows the differential significantly, implying lower GI loss, RTA (including the "acquired proximal RTA" of acetazolamide use), or DKA.
- ▨ The **urine** $[Cl^-]$ serves as a surrogate for the urine $[Na^+]$ in the setting of urinary anion excretion, as occurs in the bicarbonaturia of a metabolic alkalosis. Excretion of anion obligates the excretion of cation, often causing inappropriate Na^+ wasting in states of hypovolemia and alkalosis such as refractory vomiting. The urine $[Cl^-]$, however, will remain <20 mEq/L unless diuretics have been recently administered.
- ■ Plasma renin and aldosterone levels are often helpful in differentiating the various causes of hyperaldosteronism.

- The **electrocardiogram (ECG)** changes of hypokalemia do not correlate well with the plasma [K$^+$]. Early changes may include flattening or inversion of the T wave, a prominent U wave, ST-segment depression, and a prolonged QU interval. Severe K$^+$ depletion may result in a prolonged PR interval, decreased voltage, and widening of the QRS complex.

Treatment

- **The therapeutic goals** are to (a) prevent life-threatening complications (arrhythmias, respiratory failure), (b) correct the K$^+$ deficit, and (c) minimize ongoing losses through treatment of the underlying cause.
- Hypomagnesemia should be sought in all hypokalemic patients and corrected (see Magnesium, Hypomagnesemia, Treatment) to allow effective K$^+$ repletion.
- **Oral therapy.** It is generally safer to correct hypokalemia via the oral route, and larger doses than can be given IV can be administered orally. Though the degree of K$^+$ depletion does not correlate well with the plasma [K$^+$], a decrement of 1 mEq/L may represent a total body K$^+$ deficit of 200–400 mEq. Factors that promote K$^+$ shift out of cells (see Potassium, Hyperkalemia, General Principles, Etiology) may result in an underestimation of the K$^+$ deficit. Therefore, the plasma [K$^+$] should be monitored frequently during therapy. KCl is usually the preparation of choice and promotes more rapid correction of hypokalemia and metabolic alkalosis than the other preparations. Potassium bicarbonate and citrate tend to alkalinize the blood and may be useful in correcting hypokalemia associated with chronic diarrhea or RTA.
- **IV therapy.** Patients with imminently life-threatening hypokalemia and those who are unable to take anything by mouth require IV replacement therapy with KCl. The maximum concentration of administered K$^+$ should be no more than 40 mEq/L via a peripheral vein or 100 mEq/L via a central vein. The rate of infusion should not exceed 20 mEq/hr unless paralysis or malignant ventricular arrhythmias are present. Ideally, KCl should be mixed in normal saline because dextrose solutions may initially exacerbate hypokalemia as a result of insulin-mediated movement of K$^+$ into cells. Rapid IV administration of K$^+$ should be used judiciously and requires close observation for the clinical manifestations of hyperkalemia (see Potassium, Hyperkalemia, Diagnosis, Clinical Manifestations).

HYPERKALEMIA

General Principles

Definition
- Hyperkalemia is defined as a plasma [K$^+$] >5.0 mEq/L.

Etiology
- **Pseudohyperkalemia** represents an artificially elevated plasma [K$^+$] due to K$^+$ movement out of cells immediately before or following venipuncture. Contributing factors include repeated fist clenching, hemolysis, and marked leukocytosis or thrombocytosis. Pseudohyperkalemia should be suspected in an otherwise asymptomatic patient with no obvious underlying cause.
- True hyperkalemia occurs as a result of (a) **transcellular shift,** (b) **increased K$^+$ intake,** and most commonly, (c) **decreased renal K$^+$ excretion.** Combinations of these mechanisms often underlie cases of hyperkalemia in clinical practice, and decreased renal excretion is nearly always some component of the pathophysiology.
- **Transcellular shift.** The ICF compartment buffers the addition of K$^+$ through the actions of catecholamines at the β-2 receptor, insulin, and the hyperkalemia itself.
  - The **insulin deficiency** and **hyperosmolality** that occurs in DKA promotes K$^+$ shift from the ICF to the ECF, resulting in hyperkalemia despite total body K$^+$ depletion.
  - Treatment with **nonselective beta-blockers** may contribute to an elevation in plasma [K$^+$] as well. **Digitalis** overdose can lead to hyperkalemia through inhibition of the Na$^+$/K$^+$-ATPase pump.

- **Metabolic acidoses,** with the exception of those due to the accumulation of organic anions, can be associated with mild hyperkalemia resulting from intracellular buffering of H^+.
- **Cell lysis** as occurs in the tumor lysis syndrome, GI bleeding, and rhabdomyolysis lead to K^+ release to the ECF.
- **Exercise-induced** hyperkalemia is due to release of K^+ from muscles. It is usually rapidly reversible and often associated with rebound hypokalemia. The mild hyperkalemia that occurs with depolarizing muscle relaxants such as succinylcholine represents this same phenomenon, but it can be significantly accentuated in patients with massive trauma, burns, or neuromuscular disease.
- **Hyperkalemic periodic paralysis** is a rare cause of hyperkalemia.
- **Increased K^+ intake** is rarely the sole cause of hyperkalemia though iatrogenic hyperkalemia may result from overzealous K^+ replacement. Increased intake more commonly becomes significant in situations of impaired renal excretion (see below).
  - Foods with a high content of K^+ include salt substitutes, dried fruits, nuts, tomatoes, potatoes, spinach, bananas, and oranges. Juices derived from these foods may be especially rich sources.
- **Decreased renal K^+ excretion.** The appropriate renal response to hyperkalemia is the excretion of at least 200 mEq K^+/d. Less excretion can occur through primarily three mechanisms: (a) **insufficient number of functioning nephrons,** (b) **diminished distal solute delivery,** or (c) inappropriately **low CCD luminal $[K^+]$** from reduced principal cell K^+ secretion.
  - **Insufficient functional renal mass.** The diseased kidney responds to progressive renal insufficiency with increased K^+ excretion per functional nephron. This adaptation is usually able to maintain normal K^+ levels, if a low-K^+ diet is followed, until the GFR falls to the point of oliguria. When hyperkalemia develops in a nonoliguric patient there is usually a superimposed factor, such as excessive K^+ intake.
  - **Diminished distal solute delivery.** Salt and water must be present in the distal tubule to allow for K^+ secretion to occur in exchange for Na^+ absorption. In states of decreased effective circulating volume, avid proximal tubular absorption leaves little solute in the distal tubule, thus retarding effective K^+ secretion. This is seldom the only cause of hyperkalemia but it occurs not uncommonly in concert with other mechanisms.
  - **Inappropriately low luminal $[K^+]$** occurs primarily from inappropriate hypoaldosteronism or hyporesponsiveness to the hormone's effect.
    - **Hypoaldosteronism**
      - Decreased aldosterone synthesis may be due to Addison's disease or congenital adrenal enzyme deficiency.
      - Hyporeninemic hypoaldosteronism occurs commonly in diabetics with moderate renal insufficiency and is commonly associated with a distal (type 4) RTA (see Acid-Base Disturbances, Metabolic Acidosis, General Principles, Etiology).
      - Drugs. Most of these drugs have only a modest effect on aldosterone and therefore require other causes of impaired K^+ excretion to manifest hyperkalemia. Heparin and ketoconazole directly decrease aldosterone production. Angiotensin-converting enzyme (ACE) inhibitors block the conversion of angiotensin I to angiotensin II, resulting in impaired aldosterone release, as do angiotensin II receptor antagonists. NSAIDs inhibit renin secretion, thereby preventing angiotensin I conversion as well. NSAIDs also decrease filtration at the glomerulus through the inhibition of vasodilatory renal prostaglandins and thus reduce distal solute delivery (see above). Cyclosporine may both lower renin and aldosterone levels and attenuate aldosterone's effect (see below).
    - **Aldosterone hyporesponsiveness**
      - Chronic tubulointerstitial disease from sickle cell disease or chronic obstruction may cause hyporesponsiveness to aldosterone often with an associated distal (type 1) RTA (see Acid-Base Disturbances, Metabolic Acidosis, General Principles, Etiology).
      - Pseudohypoaldosteronism is a rare disorder characterized by hyperkalemia, high aldosterone levels, and hypertension. Sodium is effectively reabsorbed,

contributing to the hypertension, but there is also abnormally enhanced distal Cl^- reabsorption. This eliminates the lumen-negative potential needed for effective K^+ secretion.

- Drugs. The kaliuretic response to aldosterone is impaired by K^+-sparing diuretics, trimethoprim, and pentamidine, which all block Na^+ reabsorption in exchange for K^+ secretion by the principal cell. Spironolactone is a competitive mineralocorticoid antagonist. A similar mechanism to that in pseudohypoaldosteronism may be partially responsible for the hyperkalemia associated with cyclosporine.

Diagnosis

Clinical Presentation

- The most serious effect of hyperkalemia is cardiac arrhythmogenesis secondary to potassium's pivotal role in determining the resting membrane potential and depolarization/repolarization events. Patients may present with palpitations, syncope, or sudden cardiac death.
- Severe hyperkalemia causes partial depolarization of the skeletal muscle cell membrane as well and may manifest as weakness that may progress to flaccid paralysis and hypoventilation if the respiratory muscles are involved.
- The history should focus on medications that impair K^+ handling and potential sources of K^+ intake.
- Evaluation of the ECF volume, effective circulating volume, and urine output are essential components of the physical examination. The presence of oliguria implies severe renal insufficiency.

Laboratory Studies

- If the etiology is not readily apparent and the patient is asymptomatic, **pseudohyperkalemia** should be excluded by drawing blood without fist clenching.
- Most commonly, the cause of hyperkalemia will be obvious from the context in which it occurs. However, when the etiology is not immediately apparent, a clinical assessment of the effective circulating volume together with laboratory assessment of the **CCD luminal** $[K^+]$ and **renin-angiotensin-aldosterone axis** can help narrow the differential diagnosis (Fig. 3-4).
  - Assessment of the **CCD luminal** $[K^+]$: the **transtubular potassium gradient (TTKG)**
    - The TTKG is a rapid and simple test that provides a means to represent the CCD luminal $[K^+]$ in comparison to the plasma $[K^+]$. TTKG = $([K^+_u] \div [K^+_p]) \div (Osm_u \div Osm_p)$, where $[K^+_u]$ = urine K^+ concentration, $[K^+_p]$ = plasma K^+ concentration, Osm_u = urine osmolality, and Osm_p = plasma osmolality. Dividing by the ratios of osmolality corrects for luminal water reabsorption, which will increase luminal $[K^+]$ without there being an actual increase in K^+ secretion. The formula assumes no further reabsorption or secretion of K^+ in the more distal collecting duct as occurs in profound K^+ depletion or excess and that vasopressin is present and active, ensured by confirming $Osm_u > Osm_p$.[10]
    - A TTKG <10 implies impaired K^+ secretion caused by either hypoaldosteronism or resistance to the renal effects of mineralocorticoid. A TTKG >10 occurs in situations when luminal K^+ is appropriately high as with excessive K^+ intake or with diminished distal flow (but urine $[Na^+]$ >15 mEq/L).
  - Assessment of the **renin-angiotensin-aldosterone axis and adrenal function.** Once a low TTKG reveals an inappropriately low luminal $[K^+]$, the precise etiology of the disturbance can be determined through measurement of the plasma renin, aldosterone, and cortisol levels. These should be measured in a morning specimen while the patient is on a low-salt diet and after the administration of a loop diuretic the night before to induce mild volume contraction.
    - High aldosterone levels can be found in states of aldosterone hyporesponsiveness (see above).

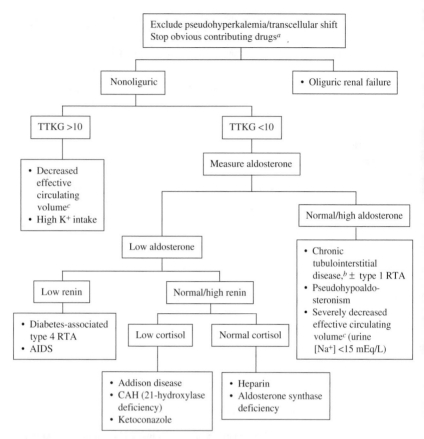

Figure 3-4. Algorithm depicting the diagnostic approach to hyperkalemia. AIDS, acquired immune deficiency syndrome; CAH, congenital adrenal hyperplasia; RTA, renal tubular acidosis; TTKG, transtubular K^+ gradient.
[a]See text for drugs commonly associated with hyperkalemia.
[b]Causes include sickle cell anemia, chronic obstruction, renal transplant rejection, and lupus.
[c]Causes include true hypovolemia, heart failure, cirrhosis, and nephrotic syndrome.

- The conditions with low aldosterone levels (see above) can be distinguished based on whether the decreased mineralocorticoid activity is from low renin or from adrenal insufficiency, the latter suggested by a low cortisol.
- Most of the conditions characterized by low aldosterone levels will respond with an increase in the TTKG after the administration fludrocortisone, 50–200 mcg PO.
- Because hyperkalemia inhibits renal ammoniagenesis and reabsorption of NH_4^+ in the loop of Henle, net acid excretion is impaired and there is a tendency toward a **metabolic acidosis.** Hypoaldosteronism also impairs H^+ secretion. Thus, a metabolic acidosis is not uncommon in the setting of hyperkalemic conditions.
- The **ECG** does not correlate well with the plasma $[K^+]$. The earliest ECG changes include increased T-wave amplitude, or peaked T waves. More severe degrees of hyperkalemia result in a prolonged PR interval and QRS duration, atrioventricular conduction delay, and loss of P waves. Progressive widening of the QRS complex and its merging with the T wave produce a sine wave pattern. The terminal event is usually ventricular fibrillation or asystole.

Treatment

- The approach to therapy depends on **changes in the ECG** and the **degree of hyperkalemia.**
- **Severe hyperkalemia with ECG changes** is a medical emergency and requires treatment directed at minimizing membrane depolarization over a few minutes, shifting K^+ into cells over the next 30–90 minutes, and the initiation of **longer-term** measures that promote K^+ loss. Exogenous K^+ intake and antikaliuretic drugs should be discontinued. **Acute therapy** may consist of some or all of the following (the hypokalemic effect is additive):
    - **Administration of calcium gluconate** decreases membrane excitability but does not lower $[K^+]$. The usual dose is 10 mL of a 10% solution infused over 2–3 minutes. The effect begins within minutes but is short lived (30–60 minutes), and the dose can be repeated if no improvement in the ECG is seen after 5–10 minutes.
    - **Insulin** causes K^+ to shift into cells and temporarily lowers the plasma $[K^+]$. Although glucose alone stimulates insulin release, a more rapid response generally occurs when exogenous insulin is administered (with glucose to prevent hypoglycemia). A commonly used combination is 10–20 units of regular insulin and 25–50 g glucose administered intravenously. If effective, the plasma $[K^+]$ will fall by 0.5–1.5 mEq/L in 15–30 minutes, and the effect will last for several hours. Hyperglycemic patients should not be given glucose, and simply lowering a significant plasma hyperosmolality with insulin has an even greater hypokalemic effect.
    - **Alkali therapy with IV $NaHCO_3$** can also shift K^+ into cells. This is safest when administered as an isotonic solution of three ampules of $NaHCO_3$ (150 mEq) added to 1 L of 5% dextrose and should be reserved for hyperkalemia associated with metabolic acidosis. Be aware that patients with end-stage renal disease may not tolerate the Na^+ load and resultant volume expansion.
    - **β_2-Adrenergic agonists** promote cellular uptake of K^+. The onset of action is 30 minutes, lowering the plasma $[K^+]$ by 0.5–1.5 mEq/L, and the effect lasts for 2–4 hours. Albuterol can be administered in a dose of 10–20 mg as a continuous nebulized treatment over 30–60 minutes.
- **Longer-term** means for $[K^+]$ removal
    - **Loop and thiazide diuretics,** often in combination, may enhance K^+ excretion if renal function is adequate. For states of decreased effective circulation volume, saline resuscitation or other therapies that improve renal perfusion should be given to improve distal tubular flow.
    - **Cation exchange resins,** such as sodium polystyrene sulfonate (Kayexalate), promote the exchange of Na^+ for K^+ in the GI tract. When given by mouth, the usual dose is 25–50 g mixed with 100 mL 20% sorbitol to prevent constipation. This generally lowers the plasma $[K^+]$ by 0.5–1.0 mEq/L within 1–2 hours and lasts for 4–6 hours. Sodium polystyrene sulfonate can also be administered as a retention enema consisting of 50 g resin in 150 mL tap water. Enemas should be avoided in postoperative patients because of the increased incidence of colonic necrosis, especially following renal transplantation.
    - **Dialysis** should be reserved for patients with renal failure and those with severe life-threatening hyperkalemia that is unresponsive to more conservative measures. Peritoneal dialysis removes K^+ but is significantly slower than hemodialysis.
- **Chronic therapy** may involve dietary modifications to avoid high K^+ foods (see Potassium, Hyperkalemia, General Principles, Etiology), correction of metabolic acidosis with oral alkali, promoting kaliuresis with diuretics, and/or administration of exogenous mineralocorticoid in states of hypoaldosteronism.

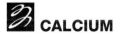 **CALCIUM**

GENERAL PRINCIPLES

- Calcium is essential for bone formation and neuromuscular function.
- Approximately 99% of body calcium is in bone; most of the remaining 1% is in the ECF. Nearly 50% of serum calcium is ionized (free), whereas the remainder is complexed to

albumin (40%) and anions such as phosphate (10%). Changes in serum albumin, especially hypoalbuminemia, and serum anions alter total serum calcium concentration without affecting the clinically relevant ionized calcium level. The ionized calcium concentration, which must lie within a narrow range (4.6–5.1 mg/dL) for optimal neuromuscular function, is normally precisely controlled by **parathyroid hormone.**

- **Calcium balance** is regulated by **parathyroid hormone** (PTH) and **calcitriol.**
    - **PTH** increases serum calcium by stimulating bone resorption, increasing calcium reclamation in the kidney, and promoting renal conversion of vitamin D to calcitriol. PTH also increases renal phosphate excretion. Serum calcium regulates PTH secretion by a negative feedback mechanism: hypocalcemia stimulates and hypercalcemia suppresses PTH release. Calcitriol also tends to feed back negatively on PTH release.
    - **Calcitriol** (1,25-dihydroxycholecalciferol, 1,25-dihydroxyvitamin D_3, or $1,25(OH)_2D_3$) is the most active metabolite of vitamin D in calcium homeostasis. Vitamin D is absorbed from food and synthesized in skin after exposure to sunlight. The liver converts it to 25-hydroxyvitamin D_3 ($25(OH)D_3$), which in turn is converted by **1-α-hydroxylase** in the kidney to $1,25(OH)_2D_3$. Calcitriol increases serum calcium by promoting intestinal calcium absorption and by playing a modest permissive role in the actions of PTH on the bone and kidney. It also enhances phosphate absorption by the intestine. Synthesis of $1,25(OH)_2D_3$ is stimulated by PTH and hypophosphatemia and is inhibited by hyperphosphatemia.

HYPERCALCEMIA

General Principles

Definition
- A serum calcium >**10.3 mg/dL** with a normal serum albumin or an ionized calcium >**5.2 mg/dL** defines hypercalcemia.

Etiology
- Clinically significant hypercalcemia is usually caused by both an increase in entry of calcium into the ECF from bone resorption or intestinal absorption and a decrease in renal calcium clearance (often volume depletion contributes to the latter). More than 90% of cases are due to **primary hyperparathyroidism** or **malignancy.**
- **Primary hyperparathyroidism** causes most cases of hypercalcemia in *ambulatory* patients. It is a common disorder, especially in elderly women, in whom the annual incidence is approximately 2 in 1,000. Nearly 85% of cases are due to an **adenoma** of a single gland, 15% to **hyperplasia** of all four glands, and 1% to **parathyroid carcinoma.**
- **Malignancy** is responsible for most cases of hypercalcemia among *hospitalized* patients. Patients usually have advanced, clinically obvious disease. There are three mechanisms of malignant hypercalcemia:
    - In **osteolytic hypercalcemia,** tumor cell products, often cytokines such as interleukin-1, act locally to stimulate osteoclast bone resorption. This form of malignant hypercalcemia occurs only with extensive bone involvement by tumor, most often due to breast carcinoma, non–small-cell lung cancer, myeloma, and lymphoma.
    - In **humoral hypercalcemia of malignancy,** tumor products act systemically to stimulate bone resorption and, in many cases, to decrease calcium excretion. **PTH-related peptide** (PTHrP), which acts via PTH receptors but is not detected by PTH immunoassays, is an important mediator of this syndrome; tumor-derived cytokines may also play a role. Humoral hypercalcemia of malignancy is caused most often by squamous carcinoma of the lung, head and neck, or esophagus, or by renal, bladder, or ovarian carcinoma.
    - **Tumoral calcitriol production** may occur in Hodgkin's and non-Hodgkin's lymphomas.

- Less common causes account for about 10% of cases of hypercalcemia:
  - **Increased vitamin D activity** occurs with exogenous overdosing of vitamin D analogs and from endogenous overproduction from certain malignancies (see above) and chronic granulomatous diseases (e.g., sarcoidosis, tuberculosis).
  - **Drugs.** The **milk-alkali syndrome** describes the acute or chronic development of hypercalcemia, alkalosis, and renal failure that may result from the ingestion of large quantities of calcium and base (e.g., $CaCO_3$). Both the alkalosis and the renal failure contribute to the decreased calcium excretion seen in this setting. Lithium increases the calcium concentration setpoint for PTH regulation. Vitamin A toxicity may cause hypercalcemia through increased stimulation of bone turnover. Finally, thiazide diuretics may elevate plasma calcium levels in combination with other hypercalcemic mechanisms (e.g., mild primary hyperparathyroidism) through their interference with renal calcium excretion.
  - **Other.** Hyperthyroidism, adrenal insufficiency, pheochromocytoma, and acromegaly may be associated with hypercalcemia. **Tertiary hyperparathyroidism** is characterized by excessive PTH production by autonomous parathyroid tissue resulting from long-standing secondary hyperparathyroidism. **Familial hypocalciuric hypercalcemia** is a rare, autosomal-dominant disorder characterized by asymptomatic hypercalcemia from childhood and a family history of hypercalcemia. Immobilization and Paget's disease cause increased bone resorption.

Diagnosis

Clinical Presentation

- Clinical manifestations generally are present only if serum calcium exceeds 12 mg/dL and tend to be more severe if hypercalcemia develops rapidly. Most patients with **primary hyperparathyroidism** have asymptomatic hypercalcemia that is found incidentally.
  - Renal manifestations include polyuria and nephrolithiasis. If serum calcium rises above 13 mg/dL, renal failure with nephrocalcinosis and ectopic soft tissue calcification are possible.
  - GI symptoms include anorexia, vomiting, constipation, and, rarely, signs of pancreatitis.
  - Neurologic findings include weakness, fatigue, confusion, stupor, and coma.
  - Osteopenia can result in fractures with little trauma. Rarely, when hyperparathyroidism is profound and prolonged, **osteitis fibrosa cystica** with "brown tumors" and marrow replacement can be found.
  - Polyuria and vomiting can cause signs of marked hypovolemia, resulting in impaired calcium excretion and rapidly worsening hypercalcemia.
- The history and physical examination should focus on (a) the duration of symptoms of hypercalcemia, (b) clinical evidence of any of the unusual causes of hypercalcemia, and (c) symptoms and signs of malignancy (which almost always precede **malignant hypercalcemia**). If hypercalcemia has been present for more than 6 months without an obvious etiology, primary hyperparathyroidism is almost certainly the cause.

Laboratory Studies

- In most patients, the diagnosis can be made with the history and physical and a limited laboratory workup.
  - The **serum calcium** should be interpreted with knowledge of the serum albumin, or an ionized calcium should be measured. Corrected $[Ca^{++}] = [Ca^{++}] + \{0.8 \times (4.0 - [Albumin])\}$. Many patients with primary hyperparathyroidism will have only a chronically high-normal calcium. A corrected $[Ca^{++}] > 13$ mg/dL that develops acutely is more suggestive of malignancy.
  - The **serum phosphorus** may be low in settings with high PTH or PTHrP activity (e.g., humoral hypercalcemia of malignancy, lithium). Phosphorus may be high when hypercalcemia is due primarily to increased vitamin D activity or increased bone resorption without hyperparathyroidism (e.g., Paget's disease).

- The **serum PTH** level should be measured. Assays measuring intact PTH should be used, as these are independent of renal function. In primary hyperparathyroidism, intact PTH levels are elevated or inappropriately normal in the setting of hypercalcemia. The PTH is almost always suppressed in patients with hypercalcemia due to other causes, except familial hypocalciuric hypercalcemia, tertiary hyperparathyroidism, and lithium use.
- When the intact PTH is suppressed:
  - **PTHrP** can be measured to confirm the diagnosis of humoral hypercalcemia of malignancy. It is rare that the presence of cancer is not clinically obvious prior to finding an elevated PTHrP.
  - **$1,25(OH)_2D_3$** levels are elevated in granulomatous disorders, primary hyperparathyroidism, calcitriol overdose, and acromegaly. **$25(OH)D_3$** levels are elevated with noncalcitriol vitamin D intoxication.
- If the family history and clinical picture is suggestive, patients with **familial hypocalciuric hypercalcemia** can be distinguished from primary hyperparathyroidism by documenting a low calcium clearance by 24-hour urine collection (<200 mg calcium/d) or fractional excretion of calcium (<1%) (the latter is calculated in a similar fashion to the fractional excretion of Na^+, as described in Chapter 11, Renal Disease). Primary hyperparathyroidism with coincident vitamin D deficiency must be ruled out.
- The **ECG** may reveal a shortened QT interval and, with very severe hypercalcemia, variable degrees of atrioventricular block.
- Hypernatremia from NDI (see Disorders of Sodium Concentration, Hypernatremia, General Principles, Etiology), distal (type 1) RTA (see Acid-Base Disturbances, Metabolic Acidosis, General Principles, Etiology), or renal insufficiency may be apparent. The latter may result from NDI-induced hypovolemia, nephrocalcinosis, or the intrarenal vasoconstriction caused by the hypercalcemia itself.

Treatment

- **Acute management** of hypercalcemia is warranted if severe symptoms are present or with serum calcium >12 mg/dL. Therapy includes measures that *increase calcium excretion* and *decrease resorption of calcium from bone*. The following regimen is presented in the order that therapy should be given.
  - **Correct hypovolemia** with 0.9% saline fluid boluses (for a typical strategy for **intravascular** volume resuscitation, see Fluid Management and Perturbations in Volume Status, The Hypovolemic Patient, Treatment). Severely hypercalcemic patients are volume depleted, which prevents effective calciuresis. The goal is restoration of normal GFR and this often requires at least 3–4 L in the first 24 hours. Continuing maintenance IVFs with hypotonic solutions after achieving euvolemia promotes further calcium excretion, with a reasonable goal being to achieve a urine output of 100–150 mL/hr. The patient should be monitored closely for signs of volume overload. Loop diuretics add little to the calciuretic effect of saline diuresis and may prevent adequate restoration of ECF volume. They are useful, however, if evidence of hypervolemia develops.
  - **IV bisphosphonate** inhibits bone resorption and should be administered early since its effect is delayed. Pamidronate 60 mg is infused over 2–4 hours; for severe hypercalcemia (>13.5 mg/dL), 90 mg can be given over the same duration. A hypocalcemic response is seen within 2 days, peaks at 7 days, and may persist for 2 weeks or longer. Treatment can be repeated after 7 days if hypercalcemia recurs. Zoledronate is a newer, more potent bisphosphonate that is given as a 4-mg dose infused over at least 15 minutes. During treatment with bisphosphonates, acute tubular necrosis can occur. Hydration should precede their use and renal insufficiency is a relative contraindication (the zoledronate dose, if given, should be lowered in renal insufficiency).
  - Other options
    - **Calcitonin** inhibits bone resorption and increases renal calcium excretion. Salmon calcitonin, 4–8 International Units/kg IM or SC q6–12h, lowers serum calcium

1–2 mg/dL within several hours in 60%–70% of patients. The hypocalcemic effect wanes after several days because of tachyphylaxis. Calcitonin is less potent than other inhibitors of bone resorption but has no serious toxicity, is safe in renal failure, and may have an analgesic effect in patients with skeletal metastases. It can be used early in the treatment of severe hypercalcemia to achieve a rapid response. Side effects include flushing, nausea, and, rarely, allergic reactions.

- **Glucocorticoids** lower serum calcium by inhibiting cytokine release, by direct cytolytic effects on some tumor cells, by inhibiting intestinal calcium absorption, and by increasing urinary calcium excretion. They are effective in hypercalcemia due to hematologic malignancies including myeloma, tumoral or granulomatous production of calcitriol, and vitamin D and A intoxication. The initial dose is 20–60 mg/d of prednisone or its equivalent. Serum calcium may take 5–10 days to fall. After serum calcium stabilizes, the dose should be gradually reduced to the minimum needed to control symptoms of hypercalcemia. Toxicity (see Chapter 23, Arthritis and Rheumatologic Diseases) limits the usefulness of glucocorticoids for long-term therapy.

- **Gallium nitrate** inhibits bone resorption as effectively as the IV bisphosphonates and has a similar delayed onset of 2 days. It is given as a 100–200-mg/m^2/d continuous infusion for up to 5 days, unless normocalcemia is achieved sooner. There is, however, a significant risk of nephrotoxicity and it is contraindicated if the serum creatinine is >2.5 mg/dL.

- **Dialysis.** Hemodialysis and peritoneal dialysis using dialysate with low calcium are very effective means of treating hypercalcemia. This therapy is particularly helpful for patients with very severe hypercalcemia (>16 mg/dL) and CHF or renal insufficiency prohibiting aggressive hydration.

- **Chronic management** of hypercalcemia
  - **Primary hyperparathyroidism.** The natural history of mild asymptomatic hyperparathyroidism is not fully known, but in many patients the disorder has a benign course, with little change in clinical findings or serum calcium concentration. The possibility of progressive loss of bone mass and increased risk of fracture are the main concerns, but the likelihood of these outcomes appears to be low. Deterioration of renal function is unlikely in the absence of nephrolithiasis.
    - Indications for **parathyroidectomy** include (a) corrected serum calcium >1 mg/dL over the upper limit of normal, (b) calciuria >400 mg/d, (c) renal insufficiency, (d) reduced bone mass (T score ≤2.5 by dual-energy absorptiometry), (e) age <50 years, and (f) unfeasibility of long-term follow-up.[11] Nephrolithiasis may also lean management toward surgery. Surgery is a reasonable choice in healthy patients even if they do not meet these criteria because it has a high success rate (95%), with low morbidity and mortality. Often a brief, 1- to 2-day period of mild, asymptomatic hypocalcemia ensues. In rare patients with overt bone disease, hypocalcemia may be severe and prolonged in the **hungry bone syndrome** (see Calcium, Hypocalcemia, General Principles, Etiology).
    - **Medical therapy** may be a reasonable option in asymptomatic patients who can be followed for evidence of any of the above criteria for surgery developing, and in patients who are not surgical candidates. Management consists of liberal oral hydration with a high-salt diet, daily physical activity to lessen bone resorption, and avoidance of thiazide diuretics and extremes of calcium intake (neither too high nor too restrictive). Drugs that are useful in lessening bone loss in this setting include estrogen replacement therapy or raloxifene in postmenopausal women, vitamin D if 25(OH)D$_3$ levels are low, and oral bisphosphonates. Cinacalcet is a new medication that is a calcimimetic, a noncalcium activator of the calcium receptor. Though it is not yet approved for use in primary hyperparathyroidism, preliminary data show that it is very effective for reducing PTH and calcium levels in this setting.
  - **Malignant hypercalcemia.** Because patients usually have extensive, unresectable disease, with a median survival of <3 months, the initial decision should be whether therapy is warranted at all. Repeated doses of IV bisphosphonate can be given. Prednisone usually controls hypercalcemia in multiple myeloma and other hematologic

malignancies. A calcium-restricted diet (<400 mg/d) and oral phosphate, which inhibits intestinal calcium absorption, can be tried if the serum phosphorus level is <3 mg/dL and renal function is normal, thus minimizing the risk of metastatic calcification. Doses of 0.5–1.0 g elemental phosphorus PO tid can be used, but the dose should be reduced if serum phosphorus exceeds 4.5 mg/dL or if the product of the serum calcium and phosphorus (measured in mg/dL) exceeds 60. Side effects include diarrhea and nausea. These maneuvers may control symptoms until antineoplastic therapy takes effect, but they rarely succeed for a long period of time unless the cancer responds to treatment.

HYPOCALCEMIA

General Principles

Definition

- A serum calcium <8.4 mg/dL with a normal serum albumin or an ionized calcium <4.2 mg/dL defines hypocalcemia.

Etiology

- **Pseudohypocalcemia** describes the situation in which the total calcium is reduced due to hypoalbuminemia but the **corrected [Ca^{++}]** (see Calcium, Hypercalcemia, Diagnosis, Laboratory Studies) and ionized calcium remain within the normal ranges.
- **Effective hypoparathyroidism.** The effect of decreased PTH activity is to lower serum calcium through three mechanisms: (a) decreased release of calcium to the circulation from bone, (b) reduced renal calcium reclamation, and (c) less calcitriol-induced intestinal calcium absorption. Reduced PTH activity can result from several etiologies:
  - Reduced PTH release can result from autoimmune (e.g., polyglandular autoimmune syndrome I), infiltrative (e.g., hemochromatosis, Wilson's disease, or malignant replacement), or iatrogenic (e.g., postthyroidectomy) destruction of parathyroid tissue. In rare patients the hypoparathyroidism is congenital, as in DiGeorge's syndrome or **familial hypocalcemia.** The latter results from an activating mutation in the calcium-sensing receptor, which decreases PTH release despite hypocalcemia.
  - **Pseudohypoparathyroidism** (types 1a, 1b and 2) represents PTH resistance from derangements in second messenger processes downstream of the PTH receptor.
  - **Hypomagnesemia** causes resistance to the effects of PTH, and when severe (<1 mg/dL) may decrease PTH release as well. Severe **hypermagnesemia** (>6 mg/dL) may also decrease PTH release.
- **Low vitamin D** results in a lowering of total body calcium stores, often with a preserved serum calcium from secondary hyperparathyroidism unless the vitamin D deficiency is severe.
  - Low vitamin D intake with limited sun exposure often occurs in the elderly. Malabsorption can also contribute in other populations.
  - Advanced chronic renal insufficiency leads to decreased 1-α-hydroxylase production of calcitriol, both from the decrease in functional renal mass and from the hyperphosphatemia (see Calcium, General Principles).
  - Severe chronic liver disease may result in decreased 25(OH)D$_3$, the precursor for calcitriol. Severe nephrotic syndrome can also lower 25(OH)D$_3$ levels through urinary wasting of the hormone with its vitamin D–binding protein.
  - P450-inducing medications (e.g., many anticonvulsants, isoniazid, or rifampin) may increase the metabolism of vitamin D.
  - **Vitamin D–dependent rickets** (types 1 and 2) results from inherited defects in 1-α-hydroxylase activity.
- **Extravascular deposition** of calcium occurs when tissue substances that can form complexes with calcium become accessible to the ECF. This occurs with the phosphate released in rhabdomyolysis and tumor lysis and with the fatty acids released with acute

pancreatitis. The **hungry-bone syndrome** represents a variant of this phenomenon in which bone that has been depleted of calcium from longstanding hyperthyroidism, hyperparathyroidism, or acidosis becomes very avid for calcium once the demineralizing stimulus is removed. Partial parathyroidectomy for severe primary hyperparathyroidism can thus result in prolonged (up to 3 months), profound hypocalcemia, as well as hypophosphatemia.

■ **Intravascular chelation** may result from the presence of substances in the circulation, which can complex with ionized calcium. Examples include IV foscarnet, hyperphosphatemia from any cause, and the administration of multiple units of citrate-containing blood products. The hypocalcemia from alkalemia is a variation of this in which the decrease in $[H^+]$ leaves negatively charged binding sites on albumin available to bind ionized calcium.

■ **Other.** A low serum free calcium level is common in critically ill patients perhaps due to a cytokine-mediated decrease in PTH and calcitriol release with target organ resistance to their effects. All of the agents used to treat hypercalcemia (see above) may precipitate hypocalcemia as well.

Diagnosis

Clinical Presentation

■ Clinical manifestations vary with the *degree of hypocalcemia* and *rate of onset.*
  ▪ Chronic hypocalcemia may be asymptomatic but may be associated with cataracts and calcification of the basal ganglia.
  ▪ Acute, moderate hypocalcemia may cause increased excitability of nerves and muscles leading to circumoral or distal paresthesias and tetany, including carpopedal spasms.
    • **Trousseau's sign** is the development of carpal spasm when a blood pressure cuff is inflated above systolic pressure for 3 minutes. **Chvostek's sign** refers to twitching of the facial muscles when the facial nerve is tapped anterior to the ear. The presence of these signs is known as **latent tetany.**
  ▪ Acute, severe hypocalcemia may cause laryngospasm, confusion, seizures, or vascular collapse with bradycardia and decompensated heart failure.
■ Clues to the diagnosis may be provided by a bedside evaluation for evidence of (a) previous neck surgery (as hypoparathyroidism may develop immediately or gradually over years), (b) disorders associated with the polyglandular autoimmune syndrome (e.g., hypothyroidism, adrenal failure, or candidiasis), (c) family history of hypocalcemia (which may be present in cases of familial hypocalcemia, hypoparathyroidism, or pseudohypoparathyroidism), (d) drugs that cause hypocalcemia or hypomagnesemia, (e) conditions associated with vitamin D deficiency (e.g., uremia or chronic diarrhea), and (f) findings of pseudohypoparathyroidism (short stature, short metacarpals).

Laboratory Studies

■ The cause of hypocalcemia will often be apparent with a history and physical and the results of only a few basic labs including serum albumin, phosphorus, magnesium, and creatinine. Measuring intact PTH and vitamin D levels may be all that is needed additionally if the diagnosis still remains elusive.
  ▪ **Magnesium** deficiency or excess should be ruled out since abnormal concentrations of this electrolyte are common and cause unpredictable alterations in many of the other labs via variable effects on PTH (e.g., PTH may be high, normal, or low with magnesium deficiency).
  ▪ **Serum phosphorus** will be low in conditions associated with **low vitamin D** activity (see above), except for renal failure where there is decreased clearance of phosphorus as well. Often the hypophosphatemia in these conditions will be more profound than the hypocalcemia due to the phosphaturia induced by secondary

hyperparathyroidism. The serum phosphorus will be increased in conditions with **effective hypoparathyroidism** (see above) and in rhabdomyolysis or tumor lysis.

- **Serum PTH** that is low or inappropriately normal in the setting of hypocalcemia is indicative of hypoparathyroidism. A high PTH is often found with vitamin D deficiency states and pseudohypoparathyroidism.
- **Vitamin D** stores are usually assessed by measuring only $25(OH)D_3$ since calcitriol $(1,25(OH)_2D_3)$ levels can be normal in vitamin D deficiency from the secondary rise in PTH. However, the isolated calcitriol deficiency of advanced renal insufficiency, or rarely, in type 2 vitamin D–dependent rickets, may have a normal $25(OH)D_3$ level.
- The ECG may show a prolonged QT interval and bradycardia.

Treatment

- **Acute management of symptomatic hypocalcemia** should be prompt and aggressive. **Hypomagnesemia**, if present, must be treated first in order to effectively correct the hypocalcemia. Two grams of magnesium sulfate can be given IV over 15 minutes followed by an infusion (see Magnesium, Hypomagnesemia, Treatment) and may even be given empirically if renal failure is not present. Next, 2 g of **calcium gluconate** (equal to 20 mL or two ampules of 10% calcium gluconate; 1 g = 93 mg elemental calcium) should be mixed in 50–100 mL of D_5W or saline and administered over 10–15 minutes. The effect is only transient and this must be followed by a continuous infusion most easily prepared by mixing 6 g of calcium gluconate (alternatively 2 g, 20 mL, or two ampules of 10% **calcium chloride**; 1 g = 272 mg elemental calcium) in 500 mL of D_5W or saline. This infusion should be administered to provide 0.5–1.5 mg/kg/hr of *elemental* calcium, adjusted to maintain a corrected calcium between 8 and 9 mg/dL. The serum calcium should be followed every 6 hours. Phosphate- or bicarbonate-containing solutions, if required, must be given through a separate vein because of their propensity to precipitate with calcium. The underlying cause should be treated or **chronic therapy** started (see below), and the IV infusion should be gradually tapered as oral therapy takes effect.
  - *Parenteral calcium is only necessary if the patient is symptomatic or has a significantly prolonged QT interval, especially if the patient is hyperphosphatemic or the underlying cause is rhabdomyolysis or tumor lysis. Aggressive repletion of calcium in these settings can lead to metastatic calcification and later rebound hypercalcemia as these calcium deposits are mobilized.*
- **Chronic management.** Treatment requires calcium supplements and vitamin D or its active metabolite to increase intestinal calcium absorption. Because PTH cannot limit urinary calcium excretion in **hypoparathyroidism** and **pseudohypoparathyroidism**, hypercalciuria and nephrolithiasis are potential side effects of therapy in these diseases. Maintaining serum calcium levels at slightly below the normal range (8.0–8.5 mg/dL) minimizes hypercalciuria. While the dose of vitamin D is being titrated, serum calcium should be measured twice a week. When a maintenance dose is achieved, serum and 24-hour urinary calcium levels should be monitored every 3–6 months. If urine calcium exceeds 250 mg/d, the dose of vitamin D should be reduced. If hypercalciuria develops at serum calcium levels of <8.5 mg/dL, salt restriction and hydrochlorothiazide can be used to reduce urinary calcium excretion. In the near future a synthetic PTH analog, teriparatide, may be approved for use in **hypoparathyroidism**, making hypercalciuria much less likely.
  - **Oral calcium supplements.** Calcium carbonate (Os-Cal, 250 or 500 mg elemental calcium per tablet; Tums Calcium for Life Bone Health, 500 mg elemental calcium per tablet; or various generic formulations) is the least expensive compound. The initial dosage is 1–2 g of *elemental* calcium PO tid during the transition from IV to oral therapy. For long-term therapy, the typical dosage is 0.5–1.0 g PO tid. Side effects include dyspepsia and constipation.
  - **Vitamin D.** Simple dietary deficiency can be corrected by the use of ergocalciferol 400–1,000 International Units/d, but treatment of other hypocalcemic disorders, especially those with hypoparathyroidism, requires much larger doses of ergocalciferol or the

use of an active metabolite. Ergocalciferol requires weeks to achieve its full effect and the initial dosage may be 50,000 International Units PO daily, with usual maintenance dosages of 25,000–100,000 International Units PO daily. The dose can be titrated at 4- to 6-week intervals. In comparison, calcitriol has a much more rapid onset of action. The initial dosage is 0.25 mcmg PO daily, and most patients are maintained on 0.5–2.0 mcmg PO daily. The dose can be increased at 2- to 4-week intervals. Calcitriol is much more expensive than ergocalciferol, but its lower risk of toxicity makes it the best choice for most patients. In expectation of the increase in intestinal phosphorus absorption with vitamin D, the serum phosphorus should be lowered to <6.5 mg/dL with oral phosphate binders (see Phosphorus, Hyperphosphatemia, Treatment) prior to starting vitamin D therapy.

■ **Development of hypercalcemia.** In the event that hypercalcemia develops, vitamin D and calcium supplements should be stopped until serum calcium falls to normal, then both should be restarted at lower doses. Hypercalcemia due to calcitriol usually resolves within 1 week. Hypercalcemia due to ergocalciferol may require >2 months to resolve. Symptomatic vitamin D–induced hypercalcemia should be treated with steroids (see Calcium, Hypercalcemia, Treatment).

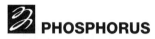 PHOSPHORUS

GENERAL PRINCIPLES

■ Phosphorus is critical for bone formation and cellular energy metabolism.
■ Approximately 85% of **total body phosphorus** is in bone, and most of the remainder is within cells. In fact, phosphate is the major intracellular anion. Only 1% of total body phosphorus is in the ECF. Thus, serum phosphorus levels may not reflect total body phosphorus stores.
■ Phosphorus exists in the body as **phosphate,** but the serum concentration is expressed as mass of phosphorus per volume (1 mg/dL phosphorus = 0.32 mM phosphate). The normal range is 3.0–4.5 mg/dL, with somewhat higher values in children and post-menopausal women. Serum phosphate is best measured in the fasting state because there is diurnal variation with a morning nadir.
■ **Phosphorus balance** is determined primarily by four factors:
  ▪ **PTH** lowers serum phosphate by decreasing proximal tubular reabsorption of phosphate, causing urinary wasting.
  ▪ The **phosphate concentration** itself further regulates renal excretion with hyperphosphatemia also decreasing proximal reabsorption in the nephron.
  ▪ **Insulin** lowers serum levels by shifting phosphate into cells.
  ▪ **Calcitriol** $(1,25[OH]_2D_3)$ increases serum phosphate by enhancing intestinal phosphorus absorption.

HYPERPHOSPHATEMIA

General Principles

Definition
■ A serum phosphate >4.5 mg/dL defines hyperphosphatemia.

Etiology
■ **Hyperphosphatemia** is caused by (a) **transcellular shift,** (b) **increased intake,** and most commonly (c) **decreased renal excretion.** Often combinations of these mechanisms underlie cases of hyperphosphatemia in clinical practice and renal insufficiency is usually the main predisposing factor.
  ▪ **Transcellular shift** with release of intracellular phosphate to the ECF occurs in rhabdomyolysis, tumor lysis syndrome, and massive hemolysis. Metabolic acidosis and

hypoinsulinemia each tend to prevent phosphorus shift into cells and account for the hyperphosphatemia that is not uncommonly found in DKA.

■ **Increased intake** leading to hyperphosphatemia usually occurs in the setting of renal insufficiency, either with patient dietary indiscretion in chronic kidney disease or as an iatrogenic complication. The most common example of the latter is when phosphosoda enemas (e.g., Fleets) are given to patients with renal insufficiency. Also, vitamin D intoxication can increase intestinal phosphorus absorption to the point of hyperphosphatemia, exacerbated by concomitant hypercalcemia-induced renal insufficiency (see Calcium, Hypercalcemia, Diagnosis, Laboratory Studies).

■ **Decreased renal excretion** occurs with renal failure, hypoparathyroidism, and pseudohypoparathyroidism (see Calcium, Hypocalcemia, General Principles, Etiology). Bisphosphonates can increase proximal tubular reabsorption of phosphate, but the decrease in bone resorption that occurs with these drugs tends to lessen the elevation in serum phosphorus. Rarely, acromegaly or familial tumoral calcinosis may be the cause of hyperphosphatemia through increased proximal tubular transport as well.

Diagnosis

Clinical Presentation

■ Symptoms and signs are those attributable to hypocalcemia (see Calcium, Hypocalcemia, Diagnosis, Clinical Presentation) and metastatic calcification of soft tissues, including blood vessels, cornea, skin, kidney, and periarticular tissue. **Calciphylaxis** describes the tissue ischemia that may result from the calcification of smaller blood vessels and their subsequent thrombosis.

■ Chronic hyperphosphatemia contributes to renal osteodystrophy (see Chapter 11, Renal Diseases).

Laboratory Studies

■ Hypocalcemia resulting from **intravascular chelation** or **extravascular deposition** with phosphate may result (see Calcium, Hypocalcemia, General Principles, Etiology).

Treatment

■ **Acute hyperphosphatemia** is treated by increasing renal excretion of phosphorus and, as such, is limited when renal insufficiency is present.
  ■ **Correcting renal insufficiency and removal of the underlying cause,** to the degree that these goals are achievable, will often correct the hyperphosphatemia in the patient within 12 hours. Saline and/or acetazolamide (15 mg/kg q4h) can be given to further encourage phosphaturia, if needed.
  ■ **Hemodialysis** may be required, especially if irreversible renal insufficiency or symptomatic hypocalcemia is present. The clearance of phosphate is quite limited, however, by the fact that most of it is intracellular and therefore not accessible to dialysis.

■ **Chronic hyperphosphatemia** is almost always associated with chronic renal insufficiency. Its management consists of reducing phosphorus intake through dietary modification and the use of phosphate binders. This is discussed more fully in Chapter 11, Renal Diseases.

HYPOPHOSPHATEMIA

General Principles

Definitions

■ A serum phosphate <2.8 mg/dL defines hypophosphatemia.

Etiology

■ Hypophosphatemia may be caused by (a) **impaired intestinal absorption,** (b) **increased renal excretion,** or (c) **transcellular shift** into cells. Often there are several of these mechanisms that work in concert to lower serum phosphate as in the severe hypophosphatemia of *chronic alcoholism* or *DKA*.

■ **Impaired intestinal absorption** occurs with the malabsorption syndromes, the use of oral phosphate binders, or vitamin D deficiency from any cause (see Calcium, Hypocalcemia, General Principles, Etiology). The secondary hyperparathyroidism that results from vitamin D deficiency contributes further to hypophosphatemia by increasing renal phosphate excretion. *Chronic alcoholism* is often associated with poor intake of both phosphate and vitamin D resulting in total body phosphorus depletion.

■ **Increased renal excretion** occurs with hyperparathyroidism, post renal transplantation (from residual secondary hyperparathyroidism), osmotic diuresis (as with the uncontrolled hyperglycemia of *DKA* or the diuretic phase of ATN), and intravascular volume expansion. A proximal tubular transport defect occurs frequently with *chronic alcoholism* and can further decrease total body phosphorus in addition to the mechanisms above. Rarely, urinary phosphate wasting occurs in the context of familial X-linked hypophosphatemic rickets, Fanconi syndrome, or oncogenic osteomalacia (a paraneoplastic production of a phosphaturic hormone by rare tumors).

■ **Transcellular shift** into cells is prompted by the administration of insulin or the endogenous rise in insulin provoked by IV dextrose infusions. This phenomenon further lowers the already low serum phosphorus when treatment for *DKA* is initiated or when an *alcoholic* is given glucose-containing maintenance fluids. The treatment of malnutrition from any cause, especially with hyperalimentation (the refeeding syndrome), and the hungry-bone syndrome (see Calcium, Hypocalcemia, General Principles, Etiology) also pull phosphorus out of the serum. Respiratory alkalosis may be the most common cause of *severe* hypophosphatemia in inpatients, through the stimulation of glycolysis by the rise in intracellular pH and the subsequent phosphorylation of the various intermediates in the pathway.

Diagnosis

Clinical Presentation
■ Signs and symptoms typically occur only if total body phosphate depletion is present and the serum phosphorus level is <1 mg/dL. These end-organ effects are due to the inability to form ATP and the impaired tissue oxygen delivery that occurs with a decrease in red blood cell 2,3-diphosphoglycerate.
  ■ Muscular abnormalities include weakness, rhabdomyolysis, impaired diaphragmatic function, and heart failure.
  ■ Neurologic abnormalities include paresthesias, dysarthria, confusion, stupor, seizures, and coma.
  ■ Hematologic manifestations are rare but may include hemolysis and platelet dysfunction with bleeding.
  ■ Chronic hypophosphatemia causes **rickets** in children and **osteomalacia** in adults.
■ The family history helps distinguish some of the causes of renal phosphate wasting.

Laboratory Studies
■ The cause is usually apparent from the clinical situation in which the hypophosphatemia occurs. If not, measurement of **urine phosphorus excretion** helps define the mechanism.
  ■ Renal excretion of >100 mg by 24-hour urine collection or a fractional excretion of phosphate >5% (this is calculated similarly to the fractional excretion of Na^+ [see Chapter 11, Renal Diseases]) during hypophosphatemia indicates excessive renal loss. Values less than these can be found with impaired intestinal absorption, unless there is associated vitamin D deficiency, which would cause phosphaturia from secondary hyperparathyroidism.
■ Low serum $25(OH)D_3$ suggests dietary vitamin D deficiency or malabsorption and an elevated **intact PTH** may occur in primary or secondary hyperparathyroidism.

- Hypercalciuria commonly occurs with prolonged hypophosphatemia by an unknown mechanism. Fanconi's syndrome would be associated with uricosuria, glucosuria, and amino aciduria as well.

Treatment

- **Acute moderate hypophosphatemia** (1.0–2.5 mg/dL) is common in the hospitalized patient and is often due simply to **transcellular shifts,** requiring no treatment if asymptomatic except correction of the underlying cause. In DKA, aggressive treatment of asymptomatic hypophosphatemia has not improved outcomes[12] and may even be associated with increased morbidity, primarily through the precipitation of hypocalcemia.[13]
- **Acute severe hypophosphatemia** (<1.0 mg/dL) may require IV phosphate therapy when associated with serious clinical manifestations. IV preparations include potassium phosphate (1.5 mEq potassium/mmol phosphate) and sodium phosphate (1.3 mEq sodium/mmol phosphate).
  - An infusion of phosphate, 0.08–0.16 mmol/kg in 500 mL 0.45% saline, is given intravenously over 6 hours (1 mmol phosphate = 31 mg phosphorus). If hypotension occurs, acute hypocalcemia should be suspected and the infusion should be stopped or slowed. Further doses should be based on symptoms and on the serum calcium, phosphorus, and potassium levels, which should be measured every 8 hours.
  - IV repletion should be stopped when the serum phosphorus level is >1.5 mg/dL and when oral therapy (see below) is possible. Because of the need to replenish intracellular stores, 24–36 hours of phosphate administration may be required.
  - Extreme care must be used to avoid hyperphosphatemia, which may cause hypocalcemia, ectopic soft tissue calcification, and renal failure. In renal insufficiency, IV phosphate should be given only if absolutely necessary.
- **Chronic hypophosphatemia.** Vitamin D deficiency, if present, should be treated first (see Calcium, Hypocalcemia, Treatment). Oral phosphate supplements, in a dose of 0.5–1.0 g elemental phosphorus PO bid–tid, can then be given. Preparations include Neutra-Phos (250 mg elemental phosphorus and 7 mEq each of Na^+ and K^+ per capsule) and Neutra-Phos K (250 mg elemental phosphorus and 14 mEq K^+ per capsule). The contents of the capsules should be dissolved in water. Fleet Phospho-soda (815 mg phosphorus and 33 mEq sodium per 5 mL) is an alternative oral agent. For patients who require long-term therapy, bulk powder is more economical; a 64-g bottle of Neutra-Phos dissolved in 1 gallon of water provides 250 mg of elemental phosphorus per 75 mL. Serum phosphorus, calcium, and creatinine should be measured daily as the dose is adjusted. Side effects include diarrhea, which is often dose limiting, and nausea. Hypocalcemia and ectopic calcification are rare unless hyperphosphatemia occurs.

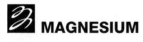 **MAGNESIUM**

GENERAL PRINCIPLES

- **Magnesium** plays an important role in neuromuscular function.
- Approximately 60% of body magnesium is in bone, and most of the remainder is within cells. Only 1% is in the ECF. Magnesium is not exchanged easily between these three pools and therefore there is little buffering of fluctuations in the serum magnesium concentration. Also as a result of this sluggish exchange, the serum magnesium is a poor predictor of intracellular and total body stores.
- Unlike the electrolytes discussed to this point, there are no hormones specifically delegated to the regulation of magnesium balance. The main determinant of magnesium balance is the **magnesium concentration** itself, which directly influences renal excretion. Hypomagnesemia stimulates tubular reabsorption of magnesium, whereas hypermagnesemia inhibits this.

HYPERMAGNESEMIA

General Principles

Definition
- A serum magnesium >2.2 mEq/L defines hypermagnesemia.

Etiology
- Most cases of clinically significant hypermagnesemia are **iatrogenic,** occurring with large doses of magnesium-containing antacids or laxatives and during treatment of pre-eclampsia with IV magnesium. Since renal excretion is the only means of lowering serum magnesium levels, the presence of significant renal insufficiency can lead to magnesium toxicity with even therapeutic doses of these antacids and laxatives.
- Mild, insignificant elevations in magnesium can occur in end-stage renal disease patients, theophylline intoxication, DKA, and the tumor lysis syndrome.

Diagnosis

Clinical Presentation
- Signs and symptoms are seen only if the serum magnesium level is >4 mEq/L.
  - Neuromuscular abnormalities usually include hyporeflexia (usually the first sign of magnesium toxicity), lethargy, and weakness that can progress to somnolence and paralysis. With diaphragmatic involvement this can lead to respiratory failure.
  - Cardiac findings include hypotension, bradycardia, and cardiac arrest.

Laboratory Studies
- Hypocalcemia may occur from diminished PTH release (see Calcium, Hypocalcemia, General Principles, Etiology).
- The ECG may reveal bradycardia and prolonged PR, QRS, and QT intervals with magnesium levels of 5–10 mEq/L. Complete heart block or asystole may eventually ensue with levels >15 mEq/L.

Treatment

- **Prevention.** In the setting of significant renal insufficiency, the inadvertent administration of magnesium-containing medications (e.g., Maalox, magnesium citrate), such as with inpatient PRN orders, should be avoided.
- **Asymptomatic hypermagnesemia.** In the setting of normal renal function, normal magnesium levels will quickly be attained with removal of the magnesium load.
- **Symptomatic hypermagnesemia**
  - Prompt supportive therapy is critical, including mechanical ventilation for respiratory failure and a temporary pacemaker for significant bradyarrhythmias.
  - The effects of hypermagnesemia can be antagonized quickly by the administration of 10% calcium gluconate, 10–20 mL IV (1–2 g) over 10 minutes. If renal function is normal, removal of the magnesium load will allow prompt improvement in the hypermagnesemia. Renal excretion can be encouraged with saline administration.
  - With significant renal insufficiency, hemodialysis is required for definitive therapy.

HYPOMAGNESEMIA

General Principles

Definition
- A serum magnesium <1.3 mEq/L defines hypomagnesemia.

Etiology
- Hypomagnesemia may be caused by (a) **impaired intestinal absorption,** (b) **increased renal excretion,** or, rarely, (c) **chelation from the serum.**

- **Decreased intestinal absorption** occurs in malnutrition, as is common in chronic alcoholics or any malabsorption syndrome. GI losses contain secreted magnesium, and prolonged diarrhea, nasogastric aspiration, or gastrointestinal tract drainage can cause negative magnesium balance.
- **Increased renal excretion** of magnesium occurs in a number of settings:
  - Calcium competes with magnesium at its major site of reabsorption in the thick ascending limb and thus hypercalcemia may cause magnesium wasting.
  - Increased tubular flow as occurs in an osmotic diuresis (as with uncontrolled diabetes) or volume expansion reduces magnesium reabsorption.
  - Tubular transport defects that occur with resolving ATN, chronic alcoholism, Bartter's or Gitelman's syndromes, and interstitial renal diseases can contribute.
  - **Drugs.** Several medications similarly induce defects in tubular magnesium transport including loop and thiazide diuretics, aminoglycosides, amphotericin B, cisplatin, pentamidine, and cyclosporine.
- **Chelation from circulation** can occur in many of the same settings as occurs with calcium, a cation with similar size and valence (see Calcium, Hypocalcemia, General Principles, Etiology). Hypomagnesemia can be seen with pancreatitis, the hungry-bone syndrome, citrate administration, and cardiopulmonary bypass.

Diagnosis

Clinical Presentation
- Neurologic manifestations include lethargy, confusion, tremor, fasciculations, ataxia, nystagmus, tetany, and seizures.
- Atrial and ventricular arrhythmias may occur, especially in patients treated with digoxin.
- Symptoms and signs associated with secondary **hypokalemia** (see Potassium, Hypokalemia, Diagnosis, Clinical Presentation) and **hypocalcemia** (see Calcium, Hypocalcemia, Diagnosis, Clinical Presentation) may contribute to the clinical picture.

Laboratory Studies
- In context of the clinical situations described above, **hypomagnesemia** is sufficient to establish the diagnosis of **magnesium deficiency**. However, routine measurement of serum magnesium without clinical suspicion of magnesium deficiency has little diagnostic value. Furthermore, due to the slow exchange of magnesium between the various pools (see Magnesium, General Principles), a normal serum level does not exclude total body **magnesium deficiency**.
- The etiology of hypomagnesemia usually is evident from the clinical context, but if there is uncertainty, measurement of **urine magnesium excretion** defines the mechanism. A 24-hour urine magnesium of >2 mEq (or >24 mg) or a fractional excretion of magnesium of $>2\%$ during hypomagnesemia suggests a cause that is characterized by **increased renal excretion** (see above). Calculating the fractional excretion of magnesium is done similarly to that of Na^+ (see Chapter 11, Renal Diseases), except that the serum magnesium concentration must be multiplied by 0.7 since only 70% is unbound and freely filtered across the glomerulus.
- Hypocalcemia (see Calcium, Hypocalcemia, General Principles, Etiology) and/or hypokalemia (see Potassium, Hypokalemia, General Principles, Etiology) can often be found as a result of hypomagnesemia-induced derangements in the handling of these electrolytes.
- **ECG** abnormalities may include a prolonged PR and QT interval with a widened QRS. **Torsades de pointes** is the classically associated arrhythmia.

Treatment

- In patients with normal renal function, excess magnesium is readily excreted, and there is little risk of causing hypermagnesemia with recommended doses. However, *magnesium must be given with extreme care in the presence of renal insufficiency*.

- The route of administration depends on whether clinical manifestations from magnesium deficiency are present.
  - **Asymptomatic hypomagnesemia** without ECG abnormalities can be treated orally, even if the deficiency is severe, if malabsorption is not present. Up to ~720 mg of oral elemental magnesium per day in divided doses can be given for severe deficiency and ~240 mg/d for mild deficiency. Numerous preparations exist including Mag-Ox 400 (240 mg elemental magnesium per 400-mg tablet), Uro-Mag (84 mg per 140-mg tablet), and sustained-release Slow-Mag (64 mg per tablet). The major side effect is diarrhea. Potassium-sparing diuretics such as amiloride can be administered to reduce inappropriate renal magnesium wasting, if present.
  - **Severe symptomatic hypomagnesemia** should be treated with 1–2 g magnesium sulfate (1 g magnesium sulfate = 96 mg elemental magnesium = 8 mEq magnesium) IV over 15 minutes, followed by an infusion of 6 g magnesium sulfate in 1 L or more of IV fluid over 24 hours. Because of the need to replenish intracellular stores, the infusion can be continued for 3–7 days. Serum magnesium should be measured q24h and the infusion rate adjusted to maintain a serum magnesium level of <2.5 mEq/L. Tendon reflexes should be tested frequently, as hyporeflexia suggests hypermagnesemia. Reduced doses and more frequent monitoring must be used even in mild renal insufficiency.

ACID-BASE DISTURBANCES

GENERAL PRINCIPLES

- The normal ECF **pH is 7.40** $\pm$ 0.03 ($[H^+]$ = 40 nmol/L $\pm$ 3 nmol/L) and it is maintained within a narrow range. Perturbations in pH occur with changes in the ratio of $[HCO_3^-]$ to pCO_2 (the partial pressure of carbon dioxide) as described by the **Henderson-Hasselbalch equation:** pH = 6.1 + log{$[HCO_3^-] \div (pCO_2 \times 0.3)$}.
- Acid-base homeostasis is essential for normal cellular function and consists of three integral components:
  - **Chemical buffering** minimizes variations in pH and is mediated by HCO_3^- in the ECF and by the much larger pool of proteins and phosphate buffers in the ICF.
  - **Alveolar ventilation** determines the pCO_2. The normal pCO_2 is 40 $\pm$ 5 mm Hg.
  - **Changes in renal H^+ excretion** alter the ECF $[HCO_3^-]$. Renal H^+ handling is determined by proximal tubular HCO_3^- reabsorption and distal tubular modifications in titratable acid (e.g., $H_2PO_4^-$) and NH_4^+ excretion. The normal $[HCO_3^-]$ is 24 $\pm$ 2 mEq/L.
    - Individuals who consume a typical Western diet generate approximately 1 mEq/kg/d of H^+ from the metabolism of sulfur-containing (cysteine and methionine) and cationic (arginine and lysine) amino acids. To achieve H^+ balance, the dietary acid load must be excreted (and HCO_3^- regenerated). The major adaptive response to an acid load is to stimulate ammoniagenesis and distal H^+ secretion, thereby increasing NH_4^+ excretion.

Definitions

- **Acidemia** and **alkalemia** refer to the final pH regardless of the mechanism or combination of mechanisms at play. An acidemia is present when the pH is <7.37 and alkalemia when the pH is >7.43. The underlying mechanisms consist of the following:
  - **Metabolic acidosis** is present when there is a primary decrease in the plasma $[HCO_3^-]$ due to either HCO_3^- loss or the accumulation of acid.
  - **Metabolic alkalosis** is characterized by a primary increase in the plasma $[HCO_3^-]$ due to either H^+ loss or HCO_3^- gain.
  - **Respiratory acidosis** is defined as a primary increase in pCO_2 resulting from alveolar hypoventilation.

▨ **Respiratory alkalosis** is present when hyperventilation leads to a primary decrease in pCO_2.

Diagnosis

Differential Diagnosis

■ After the physician is alerted to the possibility of an acid-base disorder, the analysis should be systematic so that accurate conclusions are drawn and appropriate therapy initiated. Once the underlying mechanisms for the disorder are discovered (i.e., metabolic acidosis, respiratory alkalosis, etc.), further diagnostic studies may be undertaken to determine the precise etiologies at play. The steps to dissecting an acid-base disorder, including mixed disorders, into its mechanisms are:

  ▨ **Step 1.** Predict what underlying mechanisms might be present based on the clinical scenario.
  ▨ **Step 2.** Verify that the arterial blood gas (ABG) values are internally accurate.
  ▨ **Step 3.** Tentatively establish the primary disturbance by determining whether the change in $[HCO_3^-]$ or pCO_2 can account for the observed deflection in pH.
  ▨ **Step 4.** Determine whether a mixed disorder is present. This is done by
  • noting whether metabolic or respiratory **compensation** is appropriate
  • calculating the **anion gap** (AG) to reveal a possible elevated AG metabolic acidosis
  • calculating the **corrected** $[HCO_3^-]$ if an elevated anion gap is found to determine if a second metabolic derangement is present.

■ **Step 1.** Predict what underlying mechanisms might be present based on the clinical scenario.

  ▨ This is done with a knowledge of some of the common causes of acid-base disorders (Table 3-2). This is especially helpful in interpreting mixed disorders, allowing one to discover mechanisms that may not be immediately obvious from the ABG.

■ **Step 2.** Verify that the ABG values are internally accurate.

  ▨ An ABG that is reported falsely will obviously not allow an accurate diagnosis to be made. The accuracy of the values can be established by confirming that they satisfy a simplified form of the Henderson-Hasselbalch equation: $[H^+](nmol/L) = 24 \times pCO_2(mm\ Hg) \div [HCO_3^-](mEq/L)$.
  • $[H^+] = 10\ exp(-pH)$. Within the pH range of 7.26–7.45, the $[H^+]$ in nmol/L = 80 – the decimal of the pH (e.g., for pH = 7.28, $[H^+]$ = 80 – 28 = 52 nmol/L).

■ **Step 3.** Tentatively establish the primary disturbance by determining whether the change in $[HCO_3^-]$ or pCO_2 can account for the observed deflection in pH.

  ▨ Increases in $[HCO_3^-]$ and decreases in pCO_2 tend toward alkalemia. Decreases in $[HCO_3^-]$ and increases in pCO_2 can cause acidemia. The change in $[HCO_3^-]$ or pCO_2 that can cause the observed change in pH indicates what the primary disturbance is.
  • An ABG with pH = 7.49, pCO_2 = 44, and $[HCO_3^-]$ = 32 suggests that the primary disturbance is a metabolic alkalosis since the elevated $[HCO_3^-]$ can cause the observed alkalemia but the elevated pCO_2 cannot.
  ▨ If both the pCO_2 and $[HCO_3^-]$ can cause the observed deflection in pH, then a combined disorder is present.
  ▨ If the pH is normal but the pCO_2 and $[HCO_3^-]$ are abnormal then a combined disorder is present.

■ **Step 4.** Determine whether a mixed disorder is present.

  ▨ Is the respiratory or metabolic compensation appropriate?
  • The kidney's response to a primary respiratory acid-base disorder is to vary its H^+ secretion, thus either raising or lowering the $[HCO_3^-]$. On the other hand, a primary metabolic derangement is met with a compensatory change in alveolar ventilation, thus modifying the pCO_2. The pH tends toward, but does not achieve, a normal value with these compensatory responses.
  • The expected compensations for the various primary acid-base derangements are given in Table 3-3.

TABLE 3-2 The Four Primary Acid-Base Disorders and Their Etiologies

Metabolic acidosis	Metabolic alkalosis	Respiratory acidosis	Respiratory alkalosis
High anion gap	*Chloride responsive[c]*	*Respiratory center depression*	*Central nervous system stimulation*
• Ketoacidosis—diabetic, alcoholic, starvation	• Upper GI losses (e.g., vomiting, NG suction)	• Sedative medications	• Pain
		• Brainstem lesions	• Meningoencephalitis
• Lactic acidosis—type A (when oxygen delivery to tissues is insufficient, e.g., shock, CO poisoning, seizures); type B (when cells cannot use the oxygen delivered, e.g., some HAART medications, CN poisoning); impaired clearance (e.g., D-lactate production, cirrhosis); metformin in renal insufficiency	• Previous diuretic use (except acetazolamide)	• Other (central sleep apnea, myxedema)	• Subarachnoid hemorrhage
	• Recovery from chronic hypercapnia	*Neuromuscular failure*	• Hepatic encephalopathy
		• Myopathic and motor end plate dysfunction (e.g., polymyositis, severe hypokalemia, organophosphate poisoning)	*Hypoxemia*
	Chloride unresponsive[d]		• Moderate asthma exacerbation
	• Effective mineralocorticoid excess (e.g., Conn's syndrome, CAH, Liddle's syndrome, some licorice, Cushing's syndrome, bilateral renal artery stenosis)	• Neuropathic (e.g., Guillain-Barré, amyotrophic lateral sclerosis, status epilepticus)	• Acute pulmonary edema
			• Pulmonary embolus
			• High altitude
			• Pneumonia
• Intoxications (e.g., ethylene glycol, methanol, salicylate)	• Current diuretic use (except acetazolamide)	*Decreased compliance*	*Drugs*
• Advanced renal failure	• Bartter's and Gitelman's syndromes	• Parenchymal (e.g., pulmonary fibrosis, ARDS)	• Progesterone
• Severe rhabdomyolysis	• Severe hypokalemia		• Salicylate poisoning
	• Excessive alkali administration (e.g., milk alkali syndrome, massive citrate infusion with blood products)	• Extraparenchymal (e.g., abdominal distention, severe kyphoscoliosis)	• Xanthines
Normal anion gap		*Increased airway resistance*	*Miscellaneous*
• GI HCO_3^- losses (e.g., lower GI fistulas, diarrhea, ureterosigmoidostomy)[a]		• Chronic obstructive pulmonary disease, emphysema, severe asthma	• Sepsis
• Renal tubular acidoses[b]		• Obstructive sleep apnea	• Mechanical hyperventilation
• Moderate renal insufficiency[b]		*Increased dead space*	• Pregnancy
• Acetazolamide use[b]		• Large pulmonary embolus	
• Large-volume saline resuscitation		• Emphysema	

CO, carbon monoxide; HAART, highly active antiretroviral therapy; CN^-, cyanide; NG, nasogastric; CAH, congenital adrenal hyperplasia; ARDS, acute respiratory distress syndrome.
[a]Disorders associated with a negative urine anion gap.
[b]Disorders associated with a positive urine anion gap though a type 2 RTA may have a variable gap.
[c]Disorders in which urine $[Cl^-] <20$ mEq/L.
[d]Disorders in which urine $[Cl^-] >20$ mEq/L.

TABLE 3-3	Expected Compensatory Responses to Primary Acid-Base Disorders

Disorder	Primary change	Compensatory response
Metabolic acidosis	↓ [HCO_3^-]	↓ pCO_2 1.2 mm Hg for every 1 mEq/L ↓ [HCO_3^-] OR pCO_2 = last two digits of pH
Metabolic alkalosis	↑ [HCO_3^-]	↑ pCO_2 0.7 mm Hg for every 1 mEq/L ↑ [HCO_3^-]
Respiratory acidosis	↑ pCO_2	
Acute		↑ [HCO_3^-] 1.0 mEq/L for every 10 mm Hg ↑ pCO_2
Chronic		↑ [HCO_3^-] 3.5 mEq/L for every 10 mm Hg ↑ pCO_2
Respiratory alkalosis	↓ pCO_2	
Acute		↓ [HCO_3^-] 2.0 mEq/L for every 10 mm Hg ↓ pCO_2
Chronic		↓ [HCO_3^-] 5.0 mEq/L for every 10 mm Hg ↓ pCO_2

- • An inappropriate compensatory response suggests the presence of a combined disorder.
- ■ Is an elevated anion gap present?
  - • AG = [Na^+] – [Cl^-] – [HCO_3^-]. The normal AG is 10 ± 2 mEq/L.
  - • In the normal individual, the anion gap is determined primarily by the [albumin], which is negatively charged. The AG should therefore be adjusted for changes in the albumin concentration: $AG_{correct}$ = AG + {(4 – [albumin]) × 2.5}.
  - • A significantly elevated AG suggests the presence of a metabolic acidosis with a circulating anion (see Table 3-2), irrespective of the final pH. If the presence of the metabolic acidosis was not suggested by Step 3, this can be a clue to a mixed disorder.
- ■ If an elevated anion gap is present, does the corrected [HCO_3^-] suggest the presence of a second metabolic derangement?
  - • [HCO_3^-]$_{correct}$ = [HCO_3^-] + ($AG_{correct}$ – 10).
  - • This formula can be conceptualized to describe how for every mEq of acidic anion in circulation, 1 mEq of HCO_3^- will be consumed by its disassociated proton. Therefore, the [HCO_3^-] prior to the addition of that strong acid can be predicted by adding the change in AG (i.e., $AG_{correct}$ – 10) to the [HCO_3^-].
  - • If an elevated anion gap metabolic acidosis exists without the presence of another metabolic derangement, then the [HCO_3^-]$_{correct}$ will equal a normally **compensated** [HCO_3^-] (i.e., the [HCO_3^-]$_{correct}$ may not be equal to 24 mEq/L if a concomitant respiratory derangement requiring metabolic compensation is present). If the [HCO_3^-]$_{correct}$ does not normalize, then a mixed metabolic disorder is present.
- ■ **An example.** A patient with a severe postoperative ileus requires the insertion of a nasogastric (NG) tube for decompression. After several days on the floor, he develops a line infection and is moved to the ICU once he becomes pressor dependent. The patient's ABG reveals a pH = 7.44, pCO_2 = 12, and [HCO_3^-] = 8. The [Na^+] = 145 with [Cl^-] = 102.
  - ■ **Step 1.** With knowledge of the common clinical scenarios leading to acid-base disturbances (see Table 3-2), this patient is at risk for developing a metabolic alkalosis from NG suction and a metabolic acidosis and respiratory alkalosis from sepsis.
  - ■ **Step 2.** [H^+] = 80 – 44 = 36. Does 36 = 24 × 12 ÷ 8? It does.
  - ■ **Step 3.** The patient is mildly alkalemic, which can be explained by the low pCO_2 but not by the low [HCO_3^-], suggesting that a respiratory alkalosis may be the primary derangement.

- ▪ Step 4
  - **a.** The drop in [HCO_3^-] might be an appropriate compensation for a chronic respiratory alkalosis (see Table 3-3). However, $24 - [(40 - 12) \div 10 \times 5] = 14$, which is not close to the observed [HCO_3^-] of 8. A mixed disorder is implied.
  - **b.** $AG = 145 - 102 - 8 = 35$. There is an elevated AG, which suggests a concomitant metabolic acidosis.
  - **c.** [HCO_3^-]$_{correct} = 8 + (35 - 10) = 33$. Therefore, if one were to be able to subtract out the effect of the elevated gap metabolic acidosis, an underlying metabolic alkalosis would also be revealed.
  - **a.** Since we now know that the patient has a metabolic acidosis and metabolic alkalosis, we must return to whether the patient in fact has a respiratory alkalosis or whether the observed fall the pCO_2 is compensatory. Using the expected compensation for a metabolic acidosis since the [HCO_3^-] is low, $40 - [(8 - 8) \times 1.2] = 21$ mm Hg. The observed pCO_2 is much lower than this so there is also a respiratory alkalosis.
  - ▪ This has proven to be a triple acid-base disorder with an elevated anion gap acidosis, a metabolic alkalosis, and a respiratory alkalosis, as was alluded to in Step 1.
- ■ Once the underlying mechanisms for the acid-base disturbance have been discovered, further evaluations can determine what specific disease processes are causing these derangements and therapy can then be offered. These diagnostic tests and therapies are discussed below.

METABOLIC ACIDOSIS

General Principles

Etiology

- ■ The causes of a metabolic acidosis can be divided into those that cause an **elevated anion gap** and those with a **normal anion gap.** Many of the causes seen in clinical practice can be found in Table 3-2.
- ■ The RTAs (**renal tubular acidoses**). This group of disorders consists of disease states in which there is a defect in the renal excretion of acid or in the reclamation of HCO_3^-. They result in a **normal anion gap acidosis** (see Table 3-2).
  - ▪ **Proximal (type 2) RTA** is due to impaired proximal tubular HCO_3^- reabsorption. A proximal RTA may be isolated or can occur in association with other transport defects in Fanconi's syndrome. Causes include inherited disorders (cystinosis, galactosemia, Wilson's disease), toxins (heavy metals, outdated tetracycline, ifosfamide), multiple myeloma, autoimmune diseases (Sjögren's syndrome), amyloidosis, and acetazolamide use. Osteomalacia or osteopenia is commonly associated with type 2 RTA due to the associated phosphaturia and calcitriol deficiency (calcitriol is made by the normal proximal tubule, which is dysfunctional in this disorder).
  - ▪ **Distal (type 1) RTA** results from impaired distal H^+ secretion (urine pH >5.5). Several unique mechanisms characteristic of various disease states can result in the low distal H^+ secretion seen:
    - • **Low H^+/adenosine triphosphatase pump activity** may be associated with inherited disorders (Ehlers-Danlos, Wilson's disease), autoimmune disease (Sjögren's syndrome, lupus, rheumatoid arthritis, or any form of chronic active hepatitis), medullary interstitial disease (medullar sponge kidney or nephrocalcinosis, light chain nephropathy), or drugs and toxins (lithium, toluene).
    - • **Back-leak of H^+** due to increased membrane permeability (e.g., amphotericin B)
    - • **Impairment in distal Na^+ reabsorption** resulting in reduced voltage augmentation of H^+ secretion. This can be seen with marked volume depletion, urinary tract obstruction, sickle cell nephropathy, and amiloride or triamterene use.
  - ▪ **Hypoaldosteronism-associated (type 4) RTA** may result from either low aldosterone levels or from resistance to its effect. The result is a decline in mineralocorticoid-stimulated H^+ and K^+ secretion. The resulting hyperkalemia further decreases acid

excretion through an inhibition of NH_4^+ recycling in the nephron. Hyporeninemic hypoaldosteronism can be found with diabetes and certain drugs (NSAIDs, beta-blockers, cyclosporine). Hyperreninemic hypoaldosteronism is seen with ACE inhibitor/angiotensin receptor blocker use, heparin, ketoconazole, and Addison's disease. Aldosterone resistance can be seen with spironolactone use.

■ **RTA of renal insufficiency** occurs when the GFR falls to 15–30 mL/min and there is insufficient renal mass to produce enough NH_4 to excrete the daily acid load.

Diagnosis

Laboratory Studies

■ The first step in narrowing the differential diagnosis for a metabolic acidosis is to calculate the **anion gap**, corrected for any change in the serum albumin (see Acid-Base Disturbances, Diagnosis, Differential Diagnosis).

  ■ If an **elevated anion gap** is present, the differential diagnosis is narrowed somewhat (see Table 3-2). Further laboratory studies that may be useful to arrive at a specific etiology include measuring lactate, creatinine, ketones (however, since the nitroprusside ketone reaction (Acetest) detects only acetoacetate and acetone, a significant ketoacidosis can still exist with a negative serum ketones if β-hydroxybutyrate is the major ketone present), and the **plasma osmolal gap.**

    • The plasma osmolal gap is the difference between the measured and the calculated plasma osmolality: $[Osm]_{meas} - [Osm]_{calc} = [Osm]_{meas} - \{([Na^+] \times 2) + ([glucose] \div 18) + ([BUN] \div 2.8)\}$. A high plasma osmolal gap reflects the presence of an unmeasured nonionized compound, usually an alcohol such as methanol, ethanol, isopropanol, or ethylene glycol.

  ■ If a **normal anion gap** is present, the differential is primarily limited to GI HCO_3^- losses, RTAs, or large-volume saline resuscitation (see Table 3-2). A **urine anion gap** (UAG) can help differentiate between GI HCO_3^- losses and RTAs.

    • The UAG is the difference between the major measured anions and cations in urine: $[Na^+]_u + [K^+]_u - [Cl^-]_u$. Because NH_4^+ is the major unmeasured urinary cation, a negative UAG reflects high NH_4^+ excretion. This would be the appropriate response to a metabolic acidosis with normal renal H^+ handling (i.e., with GI HCO_3^- losses). Conversely, a positive UAG signifies low NH_4^+ excretion, which, in the face of a metabolic acidosis, is inappropriate. This would be consistent with an RTA.

    • The various types of RTA can be differentiated with a knowledge of the typically associated conditions, by measuring various serum and urine studies, and by assessing the response to exogenous alkali administration (Table 3-4).

Treatment

■ **Ketoacidosis** attributable to ethanol abuse and starvation can be corrected with the resumption of caloric intake through PO intake or dextrose-containing fluids, and by correction of any volume depletion that may be present. The treatment of diabetic ketoacidosis is described in Chapter 21, Diabetes Mellitus and Related Disorders.

■ **Lactic acidosis** is corrected by treating the underlying cause for impaired oxygen delivery or its use by the tissues. Often this involves aggressive therapeutic maneuvers for the treatment of shock as described in Chapter 8, Critical Care. Of note, there is no clear benefit in terms of patient outcomes and improvements in physiologic parameters with using HCO_3^--containing fluids to correct an acidemia purely ascribable to a lactic acidosis, regardless of its severity.[14] Carnitine, thiamine, riboflavin, and coenzyme Q, which are involved in mitochondrial respiration, have all been used as therapies for drug-induced lactic acidosis, but their efficacy has not been established in randomized controlled trials.

TABLE 3-4 Differentiating the Various Renal Tubular Acidoses

	Type 1 RTA	Type 2 RTA	Type 4 RTA	RTA of renal insufficiency
Untreated urine pH	>5.5 (exclude UTI with urea-splitting organism)	<5.5	<5.5	<5.5
Untreated plasma [HCO$_3^-$]	May be <10 mEq/L	Usually 15–20 mEq/L	Usually 16–22 mEq/L	Usually 15–20 mEq/L
Untreated plasma [K$^+$]	Usually normal or ↓; if distal Na$^+$ reabsorption defect may be ↑	Normal or ↓	↑	Normal or ↑
Fractional excretion[a] of HCO$_3^-$ when [HCO$_3^-$] >20 mEq/L[b]	<3%	>15%	<3%	<3%
Other labs		May have glucosuria, phosphaturia, uricosuria, and amino aciduria	Serum aldosterone usually low, renin variable,[c] TTKG[d] <10 during hyperkalemia	TTKG[d] >10 during hyperkalemia
Associated complications	Nephrocalcinosis, nephrolithiasis	Osteomalacia, osteopenia	Often associated with moderate chronic renal insufficiency and volume overload when related to diabetes	Anemia, secondary hyperparathyroidism, volume overload

UTI, urinary tract infection; TTKG, transtubular potassium gradient.
[a]Fractional excretion of HCO$_3^-$ = ([HCO$_3^-$]$_{urine}$ × [Cr]$_{serum}$) ÷ ([HCO$_3^-$]$_{serum}$ × [Cr]$_{urine}$).
[b]Achieved with bicarbonate infusion of 0.5–1 mEq HCO$_3$/kg/hr.
[c]For conditions associated with hyperreninemia and hyporeninemia, see Acid-Base Disturbances, Metabolic Acidosis, General Principles, Etiology.
[d]See Potassium, Hyperkalemia, Diagnosis, Laboratory Studies.

97

- **Intoxication** therapy is described in Chapter 25, Medical Emergencies.
- **Normal AG metabolic acidosis.** Treatment with $NaHCO_3$ is appropriate for patients with a normal AG metabolic acidosis. Calculation of the HCO_3^- deficit in mEq ($0.5 \times$ Lean Wt $\times [24 - (HCO_3^-)]$) assumes a volume of distribution of 50% of total body weight. The HCO_3^- distribution space increases with the severity of the acidosis and may exceed 100% of total body weight in very severe acidosis. Parenteral $NaHCO_3$ should always be prescribed with caution because of the potential adverse effects, including pulmonary edema, hypokalemia, and hypocalcemia. Realize, however, that PO $NaHCO_3$ provides only 7 mEq of HCO_3^- per 650 mg pill versus the 50 mEq provided by 1 ampoule of IV $NaHCO_3$.
  - **Treatment of the RTAs.** Correction of the chronic acidemia associated with these disorders is warranted in order to prevent its catabolic effect on bone and muscle.
    - *Distal (type 1) RTA* therapy should be directed at reversing the underlying disorder. Correction of the metabolic acidosis consists of oral HCO_3^- replacement on the order of 1–2 mEq/kg/d with $NaHCO_3$ or sodium citrate. Potassium citrate replacement may be necessary for patients with hypokalemia, nephrolithiasis, or nephrocalcinosis.
    - *Proximal (type 2) RTA* therapy should also attempt to correct the underlying cause. Large amounts of alkali (10–15 mEq/kg/d) are required to reverse the acidosis. Citrate may cause fewer GI side effects than HCO_3^-. Administration of potassium salts minimizes the degree of hypokalemia associated with alkali therapy. Thiazide diuretics can be used to promote proximal tubule HCO_3^- reabsorption by inducing mild ECF volume depletion.
    - *Type 4 RTA* treatment is primarily concerned with correction of the hyperkalemia, which alone may correct the mild acidemia as well by improving NH_4^+ recycling in the tubule. This consists of dietary K^+ restriction (40–60 mEq/d) and possibly a loop diuretic with or without oral $NaHCO_3$ (0.5–1 mEq/kg/d). Chronic sodium polystyrene sulfonate therapy may also be necessary. Mineralocorticoid administration (fludrocortisone, 50–200 mcmg PO daily) should be used in patients with primary adrenal insufficiency and may be considered in other causes of hypoaldosteronism.
    - Therapy for *RTA of renal insufficiency* is described in Chapter 11, Renal Diseases.

METABOLIC ALKALOSIS

General Principles

Etiology

- A primary increase in the plasma $[HCO_3^-]$ may be due to either HCO_3^- **gain** or **excessive H^+ loss.** The latter mechanism is much more common and, by some schools of thought, is mechanistically more appropriately described as loss of Cl^- in excess of Na^+ and K^+. [A good review of this approach is cited below.[15]] Regardless, loss of excess Cl^- is equivalent to loss of H^+ and the two may be conceptually linked via aldosterone: Cl^- (with some Na^+) loss causes volume depletion, which results in secondary hyperaldosteronism and increased renal H^+ secretion. (There are other means by which hypochloremia increases H^+ loss but a description of these is beyond the scope of this text.) Thus, the causes of a metabolic alkalosis can be broken down into **chloride responsive** and **chloride unresponsive** (see Table 3-2).
- Since the kidney has a large capacity to excrete HCO_3^-, impaired renal HCO_3^- excretion is required to maintain the metabolic alkalosis induced by the causes in Table 3-2. This occurs as a result of a **decreased GFR** or enhanced tubular HCO_3^- reabsorption from **effective circulating volume depletion, hypokalemia,** and/or **hyperaldosteronism.**

Diagnosis

Clinical Presentation

- The history should focus on eating habits (vomiting) and drug use (diuretics).
- The physical examination should include an assessment of BP and ECF volume status. The two most common causes of metabolic alkalosis, vomiting and diuretic use, are both

associated with ECF volume contraction. In contrast, patients with mineralocorticoid excess tend to have a normal or expanded ECF compartment and are often hypertensive.

Laboratory Studies
- Urine electrolytes are generally useful in identifying the etiology of a metabolic alkalosis when the history and physical is unrevealing.
  - A **urine** [Cl^-] <20 mEq/L is consistent with a chloride-responsive metabolic alkalosis and usually indicates volume depletion. A urine [Cl^-] >20 mEq/L indicates a chloride-unresponsive cause (see Table 3-2).
  - Urine [Na^+] is not reliable in predicting the effective circulating volume in these conditions, since the bicarbonaturia that is present with alkalosis will obligate renal Na^+ wasting even in volume-depleted states.
- Hypokalemia is very common in metabolic alkalosis both as a contributor to the alkalosis and as a result of it. Hypokalemia contributes to alkalosis by increasing tubular H^+ secretion and Cl^- wasting through several mechanisms. Hypokalemia is also a result of alkalosis in that shift of K^+ into cells occurs in exchange for alkalosis-induced H^+ exit.

Treatment
- Hypokalemia, whenever present, should be corrected, and this alone will significantly improve the alkalemia in many cases.
- **Chloride-responsive** metabolic alkaloses are most effectively treated with saline resuscitation until euvolemia is achieved (for an example of a typical treatment strategy for emesis-induced hypovolemia, see Perturbations in Volume Status, The Hypovolemic Patient, Treatment). Untreated hypokalemia will lessen the effectiveness of this therapy, again stressing the importance of K^+ repletion.
- **Chloride-unresponsive** metabolic alkaloses are, as their name implies, saline resistant. These conditions are often associated with a normal or expanded ECF volume, and NaCl administration may be hazardous in this setting.
  - Mineralocorticoid excess states can be managed with a K^+-sparing diuretic (amiloride or spironolactone) and repletion of the K^+ deficit.
  - The alkalosis from excessive alkali administration will quickly resolve once the HCO_3^- load is withdrawn, assuming normal renal function.
- Acetazolamide may be useful in states of ECF overload with concurrent decreased effective circulating volume if further diuresis is still desired. This therapy promotes bicarbonaturia, but renal K^+ loss is enhanced as well.
- Severe alkalemia (pH >7.70) with ECF volume excess and/or renal failure can be treated with isotonic (150 mEq/L) HCl administered via a central vein.
- Metabolic alkalosis associated with renal failure can be corrected with hemodialysis against a bath with a low [HCO_3^-].

RESPIRATORY ACIDOSIS

General Principles
Etiology
- The causes of respiratory acidosis can be divided into hypoventilation from (a) **respiratory center depression**, (b) **neuromuscular failure**, (c) **decreased respiratory system compliance**, (d) **increased airway resistance**, and (e) **increased dead space** (see Table 3-2).

Diagnosis
Clinical Presentation
- The symptoms of respiratory acidosis result from the pH change in the cerebrospinal fluid (CSF) and not the elevated pCO_2 itself. A very severe hypercapnia may be well tolerated

if it is accompanied by renal compensation and a relatively normal pH. Conversely, a modest rise in pCO_2 can be very symptomatic if acute.

- The initial symptoms and signs may include headache and restlessness, which may progress to generalized hyperreflexia/asterixis and coma.

Treatment

- Treatment is directed at correcting the underlying disorder and improving ventilation (see Chapter 9, Pulmonary Diseases).
- Administration of $NaHCO_3$ in order to improve the acidemia may paradoxically worsen the pH in situations of limiting ventilation. The administered HCO_3^- will combine with H^+ in the tissues and form pCO_2 and water. If ventilation is fixed, this extra CO_2 generated cannot be blown off and worsening hypercapnia will result. Therefore, HCO_3^- should, in general, be avoided in *pure* respiratory acidoses.

RESPIRATORY ALKALOSIS

General Principles

Etiology

- The common causes of hyperventilation resulting in respiratory alkalosis are given in Table 3-2.

Diagnosis

Clinical Presentation

- The rise in CSF pH that occurs with **acute respiratory alkalosis** is associated with a significant reduction in cerebral blood flow that may lead to lightheadedness and impaired consciousness. Generalized membrane excitability can result in seizures and arrhythmias. Symptoms and signs of acute hypocalcemia (see Calcium, Hypocalcemia, Diagnosis, Clinical Presentation) may be evident from the abrupt fall in ionized calcium that can occur.
- **Chronic respiratory alkalosis** is usually asymptomatic since a normal pH is well defended by compensation.

Laboratory Studies

- The rise in pH from **acute respiratory alkalosis** can cause a reduced ionized calcium (see Calcium, Hypocalcemia, General Principles, Etiology), a profound hypophosphatemia (see Phosphorus, Hypophosphatemia, General Principles, Etiology), and hypokalemia (see Potassium, Hypokalemia, General Principles, Etiology).

Treatment

- Treatment of respiratory alkalosis should focus on identifying and treating the underlying disease.
- In ICU patients this may involve changing the ventilator settings to decrease ventilation (see Chapter 8, Critical Care).

References

1. Hillier T, Abbot R, Barett E. Hyponatremia: evaluating the correction factor for hyperglycemia. *Am J Med* 1999;106:399.
2. Ashraf N, Locksley R, Arieff A. Thiazide-induced hyponatremia associated with death or neurologic damage in outpatients. *Am J Med* 1981;70:1163.
3. Arieff A. Hyponatremia, convulsions, respiratory arrest, and permanent brain damage after selective surgery in healthy women. *N Engl J Med* 1986;314:1529.

4. Sterns R, Riggs J, Schochet S. Osmotic demyelination syndrome following correction of hyponatremia. *N Engl J Med* 1986;314:1525.
5. Adrogue H, Madias N. Aiding fluid prescription for the dysnatremias. *Intensive Care Med* 1997;23:309.
6. Sterns R, Cappuccio J, Silver S, et al. Neurologic sequelae after treatment of severe hyponatremia: a multicenter perspective. *J Am Soc Nephrol* 1994;4:1522.
7. Morris-Jones P, Houston I, Lord M, et al. Prognosis of the neurologic complications of acute hypernatremia. *Lancet* 1967;2:1385.
8. Kastin A, Lipsett M, Ommaya A, et al. Asymptomatic hypernatremia. *Am J Med* 1965;38:306.
9. Blum D, Brasseur D, Kahn A, et al. Safe oral rehydration of hypertonic dehydration. *J Pediatr Gastroenterol Nutr* 1986;5:232.
10. West M, Marsden P, Richardson R, et al. New clinical approach to evaluating disorders of potassium excretion. *Mineral Electrolye Metabol* 1986;12:234.
11. Bilezikian J, Potts J, Fuleihan G, et al. Summary statement from a workshop on asymptomatic primary hyperparathyroidism: a perspective for the 21st century. *J Bone Miner Res* 2002;17(Suppl 2):N2.
12. Wilson H, Keuer S, Lea A, et al. Phosphate therapy in diabetic ketoacidosis. *Arch Intern Med* 1982;142:517.
13. Zipf W, Bacon G, Spencer M, et al. Hypocalcemia, hypomagnesemia, and transient hypoparathyroidism during therapy with potassium phosphate in diabetic ketoacidosis. *Diabetes Care* 1979;2:265.
14. Forsyth S, Schmidt G. Sodium bicarbonate for the treatment of lactic acidosis. *Chest* 2000;117:260.
15. Kellum J. Determinants of blood pH in health and disease. *Crit Care* 2000;4:6.

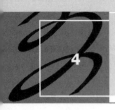

HYPERTENSION
Aubrey Morrison and Anitha Vijayan

GENERAL PRINCIPLES

Definition

- **Hypertension** is defined as the presence of a blood pressure (BP) elevation to a level that places patients at increased risk for target organ damage in several vascular beds, including the retina, brain, heart, kidneys, and large conduit arteries (Table 4-1).

Classification

- **Normal BP** is defined as <120/80; pharmacologic intervention is not indicated.
- **Prehypertension** is defined as a BP of 120–139/80–89. In these patients with no more than one cardiovascular risk factor, excluding diabetes mellitus, and no target organ damage, BP can be followed for up to 6 months with nonpharmacologic therapy. If treatment is ineffective or the patient has evidence of end-organ damage or diabetes, or both, pharmacologic therapy should be initiated. Lifestyle modifications should be encouraged.
- In stages **1** (140–159/90–99) and **2** (>160/>100) **hypertension,** pharmacologic therapy should be initiated in addition to lifestyle modification. Patients with BP levels >180/110 mm Hg often require more than one medication and frequent intervals of follow-up before adequate control is achieved. Patients with an average BP of 200/120 or greater require immediate therapy and, if symptomatic end-organ damage is present, hospitalization.
- **Hypertensive crisis** includes hypertensive emergencies and urgencies. It usually develops in patients with a previous history of elevated BP but may arise in those who were previously normotensive. The severity of a hypertensive crisis correlates not only with the absolute level of BP elevation, but also with the rapidity of development, because autoregulatory mechanisms have not had sufficient time to adapt.
- **Hypertensive urgencies** are defined as a substantial increase in BP, usually with a diastolic BP of 120–130 mm Hg, and occur in approximately 1% of hypertensive patients. Hypertensive urgencies (i.e., upper levels of stage 2 hypertension, hypertension with optic disk edema, progressive end-organ complications rather than damage, and severe perioperative hypertension) warrant BP reduction within several hours.[1]
- **Hypertensive emergencies** include **accelerated hypertension,** defined as a systolic BP typically exceeding 210 and diastolic BP >130 presenting with headaches, blurred vision, or focal neurologic symptoms, and **malignant hypertension,** which requires the presence of papilledema. Hypertensive emergencies require immediate BP reduction by 20%–25% to prevent or minimize end-organ damage [i.e., hypertensive encephalopathy, intracranial hemorrhage, unstable angina pectoris, acute myocardial infarction (MI), acute left ventricular failure with pulmonary edema, dissecting aortic aneurysm, progressive renal failure, or eclampsia].
- **Isolated systolic hypertension.** Isolated systolic hypertension—defined as a systolic BP >140 mm Hg—occurs frequently in the elderly (beginning after the fifth decade and increasing with age). Nonpharmacologic therapy should be attempted initially. If it fails,

TABLE 4-1	Manifestations of Target Organ Disease

Organ system	Manifestations
Large vessels	Aneurysmal dilation Accelerated atherosclerosis Aortic dissection
Cardiac	
Acute	Pulmonary edema, myocardial infarction
Chronic	Clinical or ECG evidence of CAD; LVH by ECG or echocardiogram
Cerebrovascular	
Acute	Intracerebral bleeding, coma, seizures, mental status changes, TIA, stroke
Chronic	TIA, stroke
Renal	
Acute	Hematuria, azotemia
Chronic	Serum creatinine >1.5 mg/dL, proteinuria >1+ on dipstick
Retinopathy	
Acute	Papilledema, hemorrhages
Chronic	Hemorrhages, exudates, arterial nicking

CAD, coronary artery disease; ECG, electrocardiogram; LVH, left ventricular hypertrophy; TIA, transient ischemic attack.

medication should be used to lower systolic BP to <140 mm Hg. Patient tolerance of antihypertensive therapy should be assessed frequently.

Epidemiology

- The public health burden of hypertension is enormous, affecting an estimated 50 million Americans. Indeed, for individuals aged 55–65 years of age, the lifetime probability of development of hypertension is 90%.
- Data derived from the Framingham study have shown that hypertensive patients have a fourfold increase in cerebrovascular accidents, as well as a sixfold increase in congestive heart failure (CHF) when compared to normotensive control subjects.
- Disease-associated morbidity and mortality, including atherosclerotic cardiovascular disease, stroke, heart failure (HF), and renal insufficiency, increase with higher levels of systolic and diastolic BP.

Etiology

- Of all hypertensive patients, 90% have essential hypertension; the remainder have hypertension secondary to causes such as renal parenchymal disease, renovascular disease, pheochromocytoma, Cushing syndrome, primary hyperaldosteronism, coarctation of the aorta, and uncommon autosomal-dominant or -recessive diseases of the adrenal–renal axis that result in salt retention.

DIAGNOSIS

Clinical Presentation

- Blood pressure elevation usually is discovered in asymptomatic individuals during screening.
- Optimal detection and evaluation of hypertension require accurate noninvasive BP measurement, which should be obtained in a seated patient with the arm level with the heart.

A calibrated, appropriately fitting BP cuff should be used because falsely high readings can be obtained if the cuff is too small.

■ Two readings should be taken, separated by 2 minutes. Systolic BP should be noted with the appearance of Korotkoff sounds (phase I) and diastolic BP with the disappearance of sounds (phase V).

■ In certain patients, the Korotkoff sounds do not disappear but are present to 0 mm Hg. In this case, the initial muffling of Korotkoff sounds (phase IV) should be taken as the diastolic BP. One should be careful to avoid spuriously low BP readings due to an auscultatory gap, which is caused by the disappearance and reappearance of Korotkoff sounds in hypertensive patients and may account for up to a 25-mm Hg gap between true and measured BP. Hypertension should be confirmed in both arms, and the higher reading should be used.

History

■ The history should seek to discover secondary causes of hypertension and note the presence of medications that can affect BP (e.g., decongestants, oral contraceptives, appetite suppressants, nonsteroidal anti-inflammatory agents, exogenous thyroid hormone, recent alcohol consumption, and illicit stimulants such as cocaine).

■ A diagnosis of secondary hypertension should be considered in the following situations:
   ■ Age at onset younger than 30 or older than 60 years
   ■ Hypertension that is difficult to control after therapy has been initiated
   ■ Stable hypertension that becomes difficult to control
   ■ Clinical occurrence of a hypertensive crisis
   ■ The presence of signs or symptoms of a secondary cause such as hypokalemia or metabolic alkalosis that is not explained by diuretic therapy

■ In patients who present with significant hypertension at a young age, a careful family history may give clues to forms of hypertension that follow simple mendelian inheritance.

Physical Examination

■ The physical examination should include investigation for target organ damage or a secondary cause of hypertension by noting the presence of carotid bruits, an S_3 or S_4, cardiac murmurs, neurologic deficits, elevated jugular venous pressure, rales, retinopathy, unequal pulses, enlarged or small kidneys, cushingoid features, and abdominal bruits.

Laboratory Studies

■ Tests are needed to help identify patients with possible target organ damage and provide a baseline for assessing adverse effects of therapy.
   ■ Urinalysis
   ■ Hematocrit
   ■ Plasma glucose
   ■ Serum potassium
   ■ Serum creatinine
   ■ Calcium
   ■ Uric acid
   ■ Chest radiography
   ■ Electrocardiogram (ECG)
   ■ Fasting serum cholesterol and triglyceride levels should be obtained to screen for hyperlipidemia.

■ Assessment of cardiac function or detection of left ventricular hypertrophy (LVH) by echocardiography may be of value for certain patients.

Monitoring

- BP measurements should be performed on multiple occasions under nonstressful circumstances (e.g., rest, sitting, empty bladder, comfortable temperature) to obtain an accurate assessment of BP in a given patient.
- Hypertension should not be diagnosed on the basis of one measurement alone, unless it is >210/120 mm Hg or accompanied by target organ damage. Two or more abnormal readings should be obtained, preferably over a period of several weeks, before therapy is considered.
- Care should also be used to exclude pseudohypertension, which usually occurs in elderly individuals with stiff, noncompressible vessels. A palpable artery that persists after cuff inflation (Osler sign) should alert the physician to this possibility.
- Home and ambulatory BP monitoring can be used to assess a patient's true average BP, which correlates better with target organ damage. Circumstances in which ambulatory BP monitoring might be of value include:
    - Suspected "white-coat hypertension" (increases in BP associated with the stress of physician office visits)
    - Prehypertension (120–139 mm Hg systolic, 80–89 mm Hg diastolic)
    - Evaluation of possible "drug resistance"
    - Episodic hypertension where hypertension is present if a patient's *average* BP is >140 mm Hg systolic or >90 mm Hg diastolic (Table 4-2)

Differential Diagnosis

- **Hypertension associated with withdrawal syndromes.** Hypertension may be part of several important syndromes of withdrawal from drugs, including alcohol, cocaine, and opioid analgesics. Rebound increases in BP also may be seen in patients who abruptly discontinue antihypertensive therapy (see Complications).
- **Cocaine and other sympathomimetic drugs** (e.g., amphetamines, phencyclidine hydrochloride) can produce hypertension in the setting of acute intoxication and when the agents are discontinued abruptly after chronic use. Hypertension often is complicated by other end-organ insults, such as ischemic heart disease, stroke, and seizures. Phentolamine is effective in acute management, and sodium nitroprusside or nitroglycerin can be used as an alternative (Table 4-3). β-Adrenergic antagonists should be avoided due to the risk of unopposed α-adrenergic activity, which can exacerbate hypertension.

TABLE 4-2	**Classification of Blood Pressure for Adults Aged 18 Years and Older**[a]	

Category	Systolic pressure (mm Hg)	Diastolic pressure (mm Hg)
Normal[b]	<120	<80
Prehypertension	120–139	80–89
Hypertension[c]		
Stage 1	140–159	90–99
Stage 2	>160	>100

[a]Not taking antihypertensive drugs and not acutely ill. When systolic and diastolic pressures fall into different categories, the higher category should be selected to classify the individual's blood pressure (BP) status. Isolated systolic hypertension is defined as a systolic BP of 140 mm Hg or more and a diastolic BP of <90 mm Hg and staged appropriately (e.g., 170/85 mm Hg is defined as stage 2 isolated systolic hypertension). In addition to classifying stages of hypertension on the basis of average BP levels, the clinician should specify the presence or absence of target organ disease and additional risk factors. This specificity is important for risk classification and management.
[b]Optimal BP with respect to cardiovascular risk is <120 mm Hg systolic and <80 mm Hg diastolic. However, unusually low readings should be evaluated for clinical significance.
[c]Based on the average of two or more readings taken at each of two or more visits after an initial screening.
Source: Seventh Report of the Joint National Committee on Detection, Evaluation, and Treatment of High Blood Pressure.[1]

TABLE 4-3 Commonly Used Antihypertensive Agents by Functional Class

Drugs by class	Properties	Initial dose	Usual dosage range (mg)
β-Adrenergic antagonists			
Atenolol[a,b]	Selective	50 mg PO daily	25–100
Betaxolol	Selective	10 mg PO daily	5–40
Bisoprolol[a]	Selective	5 mg PO daily	2.5–20
Metoprolol	Selective	50 mg PO bid	50–450
Metoprolol XL	Selective	50–100 mg PO daily	50–400
Nadolol[a]	Nonselective	40 mg PO daily	20–240
Propranolol[b]	Nonselective	40 mg PO bid	40–240
Propranolol LA	Nonselective	80 mg PO daily	60–240
Timolol[b]	Nonselective	10 mg PO bid	20–40
Carteolol[a]	ISA	2.5 mg PO daily	2.5–10
Penbutolol	ISA	20 mg PO daily	20–80
Pindolol	ISA	5 mg PO daily	10–60
Labetalol	α- and β-antagonist properties	100 mg PO bid	200–1,200
Carvedilol	α- and β-antagonist properties	6.25 mg PO bid	12.5–50
Acebutolol[a]	ISA, selective	200 mg PO bid, 400 mg PO daily	200–1,200
Calcium channel antagonists			
Amlodipine	DHP	5 mg PO daily	2.5–10
Diltiazem		30 mg PO qid	90–360
Diltiazem SR		60–120 mg PO bid	120–360
Diltiazem CD		180 mg PO bid	180–360
Diltiazem XR		80 mg daily	180–480
Isradipine	DHP	2.5 mg PO bid	2.5–10
Nicardipine[b]	DHP	20 mg PO tid	60–120
Nicardipine SR	DHP	30 mg PO bid	60–120
Nifedipine	DHP	10 mg PO tid	30–120
Nifedipine XL (or CC)	DHP	30 mg PO daily	30–90
Nisoldipine	DHP	20 mg PO daily	20–40
Verapamil[b]		80 mg PO tid	80–480
Verapamil COER		80 mg PO daily	180–480
Verapamil SR		120–140 mg PO daily	120–480
Angiotensin-converting enzyme inhibitors			
Benazepril[a]		10 mg PO bid	10–40
Captopril[a]		25 mg PO bid–tid	50–450
Enalapril[a]		5 mg PO daily	2.5–40
Fosinopril		10 mg PO daily	10–40
Lisinopril[a]		10 mg PO daily	5–40
Moexipril		7.5 mg PO daily	7.5–30
Quinapril[a]		10 mg PO daily	5–80
Ramipril[a]		2.5 mg PO daily	1.25–20
Trandolapril		1–2 mg PO daily	1–4
Angiotensin II receptor blocker			
Candesartan		8 mg PO daily	8–32
Irbesartan		150 mg PO daily	150–300
Losartan		25 mg PO daily	25–100
Telmisartan		20 mg PO daily	20–80
Valsartan		80 mg PO daily	80–320

TABLE 4-3   Commonly Used Antihypertensive Agents by Functional Class (continued)

Drugs by class	Properties	Initial dose	Usual dosage range (mg)
Diuretics			
Bendroflumethiazide	Thiazide diuretic	5 mg PO daily	2.5–15
Benzthiazide	Thiazide diuretic	25 mg PO bid	50–100
Chlorothiazide	Thiazide diuretic	500 mg PO daily (or IV)	125–1,000
Chlorthalidone	Thiazide diuretic	25 mg PO daily	12.5–50
Hydrochlorothiazide	Thiazide diuretic	25 mg PO daily	12.5–50
Hydroflumethiazide	Thiazide diuretic	50 mg PO daily	50–100
Indapamide	Thiazide diuretic	1.25 mg PO daily	2.5–5.0
Methyclothiazide	Thiazide diuretic	2.5 mg PO daily	2.5–5.0
Metolazone	Thiazide diuretic	2.5 mg PO daily	1.25–5
Polythiazide	Thiazide diuretic	2.0 mg PO daily	1–4
Quinethazone	Thiazide diuretic	50 mg PO daily	25–100
Trichlormethiazide	Thiazide diuretic	2.0 mg PO daily	1–4
Bumetanide	Loop diuretic	0.5 mg PO daily (or IV)	0.5–5
Ethacrynic acid	Loop diuretic	50 mg PO daily (or IV)	25–100
Furosemide	Loop diuretic	20 mg PO daily (or IV)	20–320
Torsemide	Loop diuretic	5 mg PO daily (or IV)	5–10
Amiloride	Potassium-sparing diuretic	5 mg PO daily	5–10
Triamterene	Potassium-sparing diuretic	50 mg PO bid	50–200
Eplerenone	Aldosterone antagonist	25 mg PO daily	25–100
Spironolactone	Aldosterone antagonist	50 mg PO daily	25–100
α-Adrenergic antagonists			
Doxazosin		1 mg PO daily	1–16
Prazosin		1 mg PO bid–tid	1–20
Terazosin		1 mg PO at bedtime	1–20
Centrally acting adrenergic agents			
Clonidine[b]		0.1 mg PO bid	0.1–1.2
Clonidine patch		TTS 1/wk (equivalent to 0.1 mg/d release)	0.1–0.3
Guanfacine		1 mg PO daily	1–3
Guanabenz		4 mg PO bid	4–64
Methyldopa[b]		250 mg PO bid–tid	250–2,000
Direct-acting vasodilators			
Hydralazine		10 mg PO qid	50–300
Minoxidil		5 mg PO daily	2.5–100
Miscellaneous			
Reserpine[b]		0.5 mg PO daily	0.01–0.25

DHP, dihydropyridine; ISA, intrinsic sympathomimetic activity; TTS, transdermal therapeutic system.
[a] Adjusted in renal failure.
[b] Available in generic form.

TREATMENT

Behavioral

- **Nonpharmacologic therapy.** Lifestyle modifications should be encouraged in all hypertensive patients regardless of whether they require medication. These changes may have beneficial effects on other cardiovascular risk factors. Some of these lifestyle modifications include cessation of smoking, reduction in body weight if the patient is overweight, judicious consumption of alcohol, and adequate nutritional intake of minerals and vitamins.

Medications

- **Initial drug therapy.** Data from the ALLHAT trial have shown decreased cardiovascular and cerebrovascular morbidity and mortality with the use of thiazide diuretics; thus, this class of drugs is favored as first-line agents in the absence of a contraindication to their use or if characteristics of a patient's profile (concomitant disease, age, race) mandate institution of a different agent. Calcium channel antagonists and angiotensin-converting enzyme (ACE) inhibitors have been shown to decrease BP to degrees similar to those observed with diuretics and β-adrenergic antagonists and also are reasonable initial agents because of their low side effect profile; however, it may be justifiable to choose agents that are off-patent to allow for cost containment. Initial drug choice may be affected by coexistent factors, such as age, race, angina, HF, renal insufficiency, LVH, obesity, hyperlipidemia, gout, and bronchospasm. Cost and drug interactions also should be considered. The BP response usually is consistent within a given class of agents; therefore, if a drug fails to control BP, another agent from the same class is unlikely to be effective. At times, however, a change within drug class may be useful in reducing adverse effects. The lowest possible effective dosage should be used to control BP, adjusted every 1–3 months as needed. The majority of patients with stage 1 hypertension can attain adequate BP control with single-drug therapy.
- **Additional therapy.** When a second drug is needed, it can generally be chosen from among the other first-line agents. A diuretic should be added first, as doing so may enhance effectiveness of the first drug, yielding more than a simple additive effect.
- **Adjustments of a therapeutic regimen.** In considering a modification of therapy because of inadequate response to the current regimen, the physician should investigate other possible contributing factors. Poor patient compliance, use of antagonistic drugs (i.e., sympathomimetics, antidepressants, steroids, nonsteroidal anti-inflammatory drugs, cyclosporine, caffeine, thyroid hormones, cocaine, erythropoietin), inappropriately high sodium intake, or increased alcohol consumption should be considered before antihypertensive drug therapy is modified. Secondary causes of hypertension must be considered when a previously effective regimen becomes inadequate and other confounding factors are absent.
- **Diuretics** (Table 4-3) are effective agents in the therapy of hypertension, and data have accumulated to demonstrate their safety and benefit in reducing the incidence of stroke and cardiovascular events. Chlorthalidone, a thiazide diuretic, may be more effective than α-adrenergic antagonists (doxazosin) in the treatment of hypertension and may also lessen the risk of cardiovascular disease and stroke in patients with hypertension and at least one risk factor for coronary heart disease.[2]
  - **Several classes of diuretics** are available, generally categorized by their site of action in the kidney. Thiazide and thiazidelike diuretics (e.g., hydrochlorothiazide, chlorthalidone) block sodium reabsorption predominantly in the distal convoluted tubule by inhibition of the thiazide-sensitive Na/Cl cotransporter. Loop diuretics (e.g., furosemide, bumetanide, ethacrynic acid, and torsemide) block sodium reabsorption in the thick ascending loop of Henle through inhibition of the Na/K/2Cl cotransporter and are the most effective agents in patients with renal insufficiency (creatinine >2.5 mg/dL). Spironolactone, a potassium-sparing agent, acts by competitively inhibiting the actions of aldosterone on the kidney. Triamterene and amiloride are potassium-sparing drugs that inhibit the epithelial Na^+ channel in the distal nephron to inhibit

reabsorption of Na^+ and secretion of potassium ions. Potassium-sparing diuretics are weak agents when used alone; thus, they are often combined with a thiazide for added potency. Aldosterone antagonists may have an additional benefit in improving myocardial function in HF; this effect may be independent of its effect on renal transport mechanisms.

■ **Side effects** of diuretics vary by class. Thiazide diuretics can produce weakness, muscle cramps, and impotence. Metabolic side effects include hypokalemia, hypomagnesemia, hyperlipidemia (with increases in low-density lipoproteins and triglyceride levels), hypercalcemia, hyperglycemia, hyperuricemia, hyponatremia, and, rarely, azotemia. Thiazide-induced pancreatitis also has been reported. Metabolic side effects may be limited when thiazides are used in low doses (e.g., hydrochlorothiazide, 12.5–25.0 mg/d). Loop diuretics can cause electrolyte abnormalities, such as hypomagnesemia, hypocalcemia, and hypokalemia, and also can produce irreversible ototoxicity (usually dose related and more common with parenteral therapy). Spironolactone can produce hyperkalemia; gynecomastia may occur in men, and breast tenderness has been noted in women. Triamterene (usually in combination with hydrochlorothiazide) can cause renal tubular damage and renal calculi. Unlike thiazides, potassium-sparing and loop diuretics do not cause adverse lipid effects.

■ **β-Adrenergic antagonists** (Table 4-3) are effective antihypertensive agents and are part of medical regimens that have been proven to decrease the incidence of stroke, MI, and HF.

■ The **mechanism of action** of β-adrenergic antagonists is competitive inhibition of the effects of catecholamines at β-adrenergic receptors, which decreases heart rate and cardiac output. These agents also decrease plasma renin and cause a resetting of baroreceptors to accept a lower level of BP. β-Adrenergic antagonists cause release of vasodilatory prostaglandins, decrease plasma volume, and also may have a central nervous system (CNS)-mediated antihypertensive effect.

■ **Classes of β-adrenergic antagonists** can be subdivided into those that are cardioselective, with primarily β_1-blocking effects, and those that are nonselective, with β_1- and β_2-blocking effects. At low doses, the cardioselective agents can be given with caution to patients with mild chronic obstructive pulmonary disease, diabetes mellitus, or peripheral vascular disease. At higher doses, these agents lose their β_1 selectivity and may cause unwanted effects in these patients. β-Adrenergic antagonists also can be categorized according to the presence or absence of partial agonist or intrinsic sympathomimetic activity (ISA). β-Adrenergic antagonists with ISA cause less bradycardia than do those without it.

■ **Side effects** include high-degree atrioventricular block, HF, Raynaud phenomenon, and impotence. Lipophilic β-adrenergic antagonists, such as propranolol, have a higher incidence of CNS side effects, such as insomnia and depression, than do the more hydrophilic agents. Propranolol also can cause nasal congestion. β-Adrenergic antagonists can cause adverse effects on the lipid profile; increased triglyceride and decreased high-density lipoprotein (HDL) levels occur mainly with nonselective β-adrenergic antagonists but generally do not occur when β-adrenergic antagonists with ISA are used. Pindolol, a selective β-adrenergic antagonist with ISA, may actually increase HDL and nominally increase triglycerides. Because β-receptor density is increased with chronic antagonism, abrupt withdrawal of these agents can precipitate angina pectoris, increases in BP, and other effects attributable to an increase in adrenergic tone.

■ **Selective α-adrenergic antagonists,** such as prazosin, terazosin, and doxazosin, have replaced nonselective α-adrenergic antagonists, such as phenoxybenzamine (Table 4-3), in the treatment of essential hypertension. However, based on the ALLHAT trial, they appear to be less efficacious than diuretics, calcium channel blockers, and ACE inhibitors in reducing primary end points of cardiovascular disease when used as monotherapy.[3]

■ **Side effects** of these agents include a "first-dose effect," which results from a greater decrease in BP with the first dose than with subsequent doses. Selective α_1-adrenergic antagonists can cause syncope, orthostatic hypotension, dizziness, headache, and drowsiness. In most cases, side effects are self-limited and do not recur with continued therapy. Selective α_1-adrenergic antagonists may improve lipid profiles by decreasing total cholesterol and triglyceride levels and increasing HDL levels. Additionally, these agents can improve the negative effects on lipids induced by thiazide diuretics and β-adrenergic antagonists. However, doxazosin specifically may be less effective in lowering systolic BP than thiazide diuretics and may additionally be associated with a higher risk of cardiovascular disease, particularly HF, and stroke in patients with hypertension and at least one additional risk factor for coronary heart disease.[2]

- **Agents with mixed properties** (labetalol, carvedilol) have α- and β-adrenergic antagonist actions (Table 4-3). In addition, carvedilol may have antioxidant properties. These agents are effective in white and in black hypertensive patients.
- **Side effects** of labetalol include hepatocellular damage, postural hypotension, a positive antinuclear antibody test (ANA), a lupuslike syndrome, tremors, and potential hypotension in the setting of halothane anesthesia. Labetalol has negligible effects on lipids. Carvedilol appears to have a similar side effect profile to other β-adrenergic antagonists. Rarely, reflex tachycardia may occur because of the initial vasodilatory effect of labetalol and carvedilol.
- **Centrally acting adrenergic agents** (Table 4-3) are potent antihypertensive agents. In addition to its oral dosage forms, clonidine is available as a transdermal patch that is applied weekly.
  - **Side effects** may include bradycardia, drowsiness, dry mouth, orthostatic hypotension, galactorrhea, and sexual dysfunction. Transdermal clonidine causes a rash in up to 20% of patients. These agents can precipitate HF in patients with decreased left ventricular function, and abrupt cessation can precipitate an acute withdrawal syndrome (AWS) of elevated BP, tachycardia, and diaphoresis (see Complications). Methyldopa produces a positive direct antibody (Coombs) test in up to 25% of patients, but significant hemolytic anemia is much less common. If hemolytic anemia develops secondary to methyldopa, the drug should be withdrawn. Severe cases of hemolytic anemia may require treatment with glucocorticoids. Methyldopa also causes positive ANA test results in approximately 10% of patients and can cause an inflammatory reaction in the liver that is indistinguishable from viral hepatitis; fatal hepatitis has been reported. Guanabenz and guanfacine decrease total cholesterol levels, and guanfacine also can decrease serum triglyceride levels.
- **Reserpine, guanethidine, and guanadrel** (Table 4-3) were among the first effective antihypertensive agents available. Currently, these drugs are not regarded as first- or second-line therapy because of their significant side effects.
  - **Side effects** of reserpine include severe depression in approximately 2% of patients. Sedation and nasal stuffiness also are potential side effects. Guanethidine can cause severe postural hypotension by effecting a decrease in cardiac output, a decrease in peripheral resistance, and venous pooling in the extremities. Patients who are receiving guanethidine with orthostatic hypotension should be cautioned to arise slowly and to wear support hose. Guanethidine also can cause ejaculatory failure and diarrhea.
- **Calcium channel antagonists** (Table 4-3) are effective agents in the treatment of hypertension. Generally, they have no significant CNS side effects and can be used to treat diseases, such as angina pectoris, that can coexist with hypertension. Concern has arisen that the use of short-acting dihydropyridine calcium channel antagonists may increase the number of ischemic cardiac events;[4] however, long-acting agents are safe in the management of hypertension.[5]
  - **Classes of calcium channel antagonists** include diphenylalkylamines (e.g., verapamil), benzothiazepines (e.g., diltiazem), and dihydropyridines (e.g., nifedipine). The dihydropyridines include many newer second-generation drugs (e.g., amlodipine, felodipine, isradipine, and nicardipine), which are more vasoselective and have longer plasma half-lives than nifedipine. Verapamil and diltiazem have negative cardiac inotropic and chronotropic effects. Nifedipine also has a negative inotropic effect, but, in clinical use, it is much less pronounced than that of verapamil or diltiazem because of peripheral vasodilation and reflex tachycardia. Less negative inotropic effects have been observed with the second-generation dihydropyridines. All calcium channel antagonists are metabolized in the liver; thus, in patients with cirrhosis, the

dosing interval should be adjusted accordingly. Some of these drugs also inhibit the metabolism of other hepatically cleared medications (e.g., cyclosporine). Verapamil and diltiazem should be used with caution in patients with cardiac conduction abnormalities and can cause or worsen HF in patients with decreased left ventricular function.

■ **Side effects** of verapamil include constipation, nausea, headache, and orthostatic hypotension. Diltiazem can cause nausea, headache, and rash. Dihydropyridines can cause lower extremity edema, flushing, headache, and rash. Calcium channel antagonists have no significant effects on glucose tolerance, electrolytes, or lipid profiles. In general, calcium channel antagonists should not be initiated in patients immediately after MI because of increased mortality in all but the most stable patients without evidence of HF (see Chapter 5, Ischemic Heart Disease). Additionally, in patients with hypertension and non–insulin-dependent diabetes mellitus, nisoldipine may be associated with a higher incidence of fatal and nonfatal MIs (Appropriate Blood Pressure Control in Diabetes [ABCD] trial),[6] although amlodipine appears to be safe and effective in this population.

■ **Inhibitors of the renin-angiotensin system** (Table 4-3) are effective antihypertensive agents in a broad array of patients.

  ■ **ACE inhibitors** may have beneficial effects in patients with concomitant HF or kidney disease. One study has also suggested that ACE inhibitors (ramipril) may significantly reduce the rate of death, MI, and stroke in patients without HF or low ejection fraction.[7] Additionally, they can reduce hypokalemia, hypercholesterolemia, hyperglycemia, and hyperuricemia caused by diuretic therapy and are particularly effective in states of hypertension associated with a high renin state (e.g., scleroderma renal crisis).

  ■ **Side effects** associated with the use of ACE inhibitors are infrequent. They can cause a dry cough (up to 20% of patients), angioneurotic edema, and hypotension, but they do not cause levels of lipids, glucose, or uric acid to increase. ACE inhibitors that contain a sulfhydryl group (e.g., captopril) may cause taste disturbance, leukopenia, and a glomerulopathy with proteinuria. Because ACE inhibitors cause preferential vasodilation of the efferent arteriole in the kidney, worsening of renal function may occur in patients who have decreased renal perfusion or who have preexisting severe renal insufficiency. ACE inhibitors can cause hyperkalemia and should be used with caution in patients with a decreased glomerular filtration rate who are taking potassium supplements or who are receiving potassium-sparing diuretics.

■ **Angiotensin-receptor blockers (ARBs)** are a class of antihypertensive drugs that are effective in diverse patient populations.[8] Several of these agents are now approved for the management of mild to moderate hypertension (Table 4-3). Additionally, ARBs may be useful alternatives in patients with HF who are unable to tolerate ACE inhibitors.[9]

  ■ **Side effects** of ARBs occur rarely but include angioedema, allergic reaction, and rash.

■ **Direct-acting vasodilators** are potent antihypertensive agents (Table 4-3) now reserved for refractory hypertension or specific circumstances, such as the use of hydralazine in pregnancy. Hydralazine in combination with nitrates is useful in treating patients with hypertension and HF (see Chapter 6, Heart Failure, Cardiomyopathy, and Valvular Heart Disease).

  ■ **Side effects** of hydralazine therapy may include headache, nausea, emesis, tachycardia, and postural hypotension. Asymptomatic patients may have a positive ANA test result, and a hydralazine-induced systemic lupuslike syndrome may develop in approximately 10% of patients. Patients who may be at increased risk for this latter complication include (1) those treated with excessive doses (e.g., >400 mg/d), (2) those with impaired renal or cardiac function, and (3) those with the slow acetylation phenotype. Hydralazine should be discontinued if clinical evidence of a lupuslike syndrome develops and a positive ANA test result is present. The syndrome usually resolves with discontinuation of the drug, leaving no adverse long-term effects. Side effects of minoxidil include weight gain, hypertrichosis, hirsutism, ECG abnormalities, and pericardial effusions.

■ **Parenteral antihypertensive agents** are indicated for the immediate reduction of BP in patients with hypertensive emergencies. Judicious administration of these agents (Table 4-4) may also be appropriate in patients with hypertension complicated by HF or MI. These drugs are also indicated for individuals who have perioperative hypertensive urgency or are in need of emergency surgery. If possible, an accurate baseline BP should be determined before the initiation of therapy. In the setting of hypertensive emergency, the patient should be admitted to an intensive care unit (ICU) for close monitoring, and an intra-arterial monitor should be used when available. Although parenteral agents are indicated as a first line in hypertensive emergencies, oral agents may also be effective in this group; the choice of drug and route of administration must be individualized. If parenteral agents are used initially, oral medications should be administered shortly thereafter to facilitate rapid weaning from parenteral therapy.

  ■ **Sodium nitroprusside,** a direct-acting arterial and venous vasodilator, is the drug of choice for most hypertensive emergencies (Table 4-4). It reduces BP rapidly and is easily titratable, and its action is short lived when discontinued. Patients should be monitored very closely to avoid an exaggerated hypotensive response. Therapy for more than 48–72 hours with a high cumulative dose or renal insufficiency may cause accumulation of thiocyanate, a toxic metabolite. Thiocyanate toxicity may cause paresthesias, tinnitus, blurred vision, delirium, or seizures. Serum thiocyanate levels should be kept at <10 mg/dL. Patients on high doses (>2–3 mg/kg/min) or those with renal dysfunction should have serum levels of thiocyanate drawn after 48–72 hours of therapy. In patients with normal renal function or those receiving lower doses, levels can be drawn after 5–7 days. Hepatic dysfunction may result in accumulation of cyanide, which can cause metabolic acidosis, dyspnea, vomiting, dizziness, ataxia, and syncope. Hemodialysis should be considered for thiocyanate poisoning. Nitrites and thiosulfate can be administered intravenously for cyanide poisoning.

  ■ **Nitroglycerin** given as a continuous IV infusion (Table 4-4) may be appropriate in situations in which sodium nitroprusside is relatively contraindicated, such as in patients with severe coronary insufficiency or advanced renal or hepatic disease. It is the preferred agent for patients with moderate hypertension in the setting of acute coronary ischemia or after coronary artery bypass surgery because of its more favorable effects on pulmonary gas exchange and collateral coronary blood flow. In patients with severely elevated BP, sodium nitroprusside remains the agent of choice. Nitroglycerin reduces preload more than afterload and should be used with caution or avoided in patients who have inferior MI with right ventricular infarction and are dependent on preload to maintain cardiac output.

  ■ **Labetalol** can be administered parenterally (Table 4-4) in hypertensive crisis, even in patients in the early phase of an acute MI, and is the drug of choice in hypertensive emergencies that occur during pregnancy. When given intravenously, the β-adrenergic antagonist effect is greater than is the α-adrenergic antagonist effect. Nevertheless, symptomatic postural hypotension may occur with IV use; thus, patients should be treated in a supine position. Labetalol may be particularly beneficial during adrenergic excess (e.g., clonidine withdrawal, pheochromocytoma, postcoronary bypass grafting). As the half-life of labetalol is 5–8 hours, intermittent IV bolus dosing may be preferable to IV infusion. IV infusion can be discontinued before oral labetalol is begun. When the supine diastolic BP begins to rise, oral dosing can be initiated at 200 mg PO, followed in 6–12 hours by 200–400 mg PO, depending on the BP response.

  ■ **Esmolol** is a parenteral, short-acting, cardioselective β-adrenergic antagonist (Table 4-4) that can be used in the treatment of hypertensive emergencies in patients in whom beta-blocker intolerance is a concern. Esmolol is also useful for the treatment of aortic dissection. β-Adrenergic antagonists may be ineffective when used as monotherapy in the treatment of severe hypertension and frequently are combined with other agents (e.g., with sodium nitroprusside in the treatment of aortic dissection).

  ■ **Nicardipine** is an effective IV calcium antagonist preparation (Table 4-4) approved for use in postoperative hypertension. Side effects include headache, flushing, reflex tachycardia, and venous irritation. Nicardipine should be administered via a central venous line. If it is given peripherally, the IV site should be changed q12h. Fifty

TABLE 4-4 **IV Antihypertensive Drug Preparations**

Drug	Administration	Onset	Duration of action	Dosage	Adverse effects and comments
Fenoldopam	IV Infusion	<5 min	30 min	0.1–0.3 mcg/kg/min	Tachycardia, nausea, vomiting
Sodium nitroprusside	IV infusion	Immediate	2–3 min	0.5–10 mcg/kg/min (initial dose, 0.25 mcg/kg/min for eclampsia and renal insufficiency)	Hypotension, nausea, vomiting, apprehension. Risk of thiocyanate and cyanide toxicity increased in renal and hepatic insufficiency, respectively; levels should be monitored. Must shield from light.
Diazoxide	IV bolus	15 min	6–12 hr	50–100 mg q5–10 min, up to 600 mg	Hypotension, tachycardia, nausea, vomiting, fluid retention, hyperglycemia. May exacerbate myocardial ischemia, heart failure, or aortic dissection.
Labetalol	IV bolus	5–10 min	3–6 hr	20–80 mg q5–10 min, up to 300 mg	Hypotension, heart block, heart failure, bronchospasm, nausea, vomiting, scalp tingling, paradoxical pressor response. May not be effective in patients receiving α or β antagonists.
Nitroglycerin	IV infusion IV infusion	1–2 min	3–5 min	0.5–2 mg/min 5–250 mcg/min	Headache, nausea, vomiting. Tolerance may develop with prolonged use.
Esmolol	IV bolus IV infusion	1–5 min	10 min	500 mcg/kg/min for first 1 min 50–300 mcg/kg/min	Hypotension, heart block, heart failure, bronchospasm
Phentolamine	IV bolus	1–2 min	3–10 min	5–10 mg q5–15 min	Hypotension, tachycardia, headache, angina, paradoxical pressor response
Hydralazine (for treatment of eclampsia)	IV bolus	10–20 min	3–6 hr	10–20 mg q20 min (if no effect after 20 mg, try another agent)	Hypotension, fetal distress, tachycardia, headache, nausea, vomiting, local thrombophlebitis. Infusion site should be changed after 12 hours.
Methyldopate (for treatment of eclampsia)	IV bolus	30–60 min	10–16 hr	250–500 mg	Hypotension
Nicardipine	IV infusion	1–5 min	3–6 hr	5 mg/hr, increased by 1.0–2.5 mg/hr q15 min, up to 15 mg/hr	Hypotension, headache, tachycardia, nausea, vomiting
Enalaprilat	IV bolus	5–15 min	1–6 hr	0.6255 mg q6h	Hypotension

percent of the peak effect is seen within the first 30 minutes, but the full peak effect is not achieved until after 48 hours of administration.

■ **Enalaprilat** is the active de-esterified form of enalapril (Table 4-4) that results from hepatic conversion after an oral dose. Enalaprilat (as well as other ACE inhibitors) has been used effectively in cases of severe and malignant hypertension. However, variable and unpredictable results also have been reported. ACE inhibition can cause rapid BP reduction in hypertensive patients with high renin states, such as renovascular hypertension, concomitant use of vasodilators, and scleroderma renal crisis, but should be used cautiously to avoid precipitating hypotension. Therapy can be changed to an oral preparation when IV therapy is no longer necessary.

■ **Diazoxide and hydralazine** now are used rarely in hypertensive crises and offer little or no advantage to the agents discussed previously. It should be noted, however, that hydralazine is a useful agent in pregnancy-related hypertensive emergencies because of its established safety profile.

■ **Fenoldopam** is a selective agonist to peripheral dopamine-1 receptors, which produce vasodilation, increase renal perfusion, and enhance natriuresis. Fenoldopam has a short duration of action; the elimination half-life is <10 minutes. The drug has important application as parental therapy for high-risk hypertensive surgical patients and the perioperative management of patients undergoing organ transplantation.

■ **Oral loading of antihypertensive agents** has been used successfully in patients with hypertensive crisis when urgent but not immediate reduction of BP is indicated.

■ **Oral clonidine loading** is achieved by using an initial dose of 0.2 mg PO followed by 0.1 mg PO q1h to a total dose of 0.7 mg or a reduction in diastolic pressure of 20 mm Hg or more. BP should be checked at 15-minute intervals over the first hour, 30-minute intervals over the second hour, and then hourly. After 6 hours, a diuretic can be added, and an 8-hour clonidine dosing interval can be begun. Sedative side effects are significant.

■ **Sublingual nifedipine** has an onset of action within 30 minutes but can produce wide fluctuations and excessive reductions in BP. **Because of the potential for adverse cardiovascular events (stroke/MI), sublingual nifedipine should be avoided in the acute management of elevated BP.** Side effects include facial flushing and postural hypotension.

Protocol

■ **Hypertensive crisis.** In hypertensive emergency, control of acute or ongoing end-organ damage is more important than the absolute level of BP. BP control with a rapidly acting parenteral agent should be accomplished as soon as possible (within 1 hour) to reduce the chance of permanent organ dysfunction and death. A reasonable goal is a 20%–25% reduction of mean arterial pressure or a reduction of the diastolic pressure to 100–110 mm Hg over a period of minutes to hours. A precipitous fall in BP may occur in patients who are elderly, volume depleted, or receiving other antihypertensive agents, and caution should be used to avoid cerebral hypoperfusion. BP control in hypertensive urgencies can be accomplished more slowly. The initial goal of therapy in urgency should be to achieve a diastolic BP of 100–110 mm Hg. Excessive or rapid decreases in BP should be avoided to minimize the risk of cerebral hypoperfusion or coronary insufficiency. Normal BP can be attained gradually over several days as tolerated by the individual patient.

Risk Management

■ **General considerations and goals.** The goal of treatment for hypertension is to prevent long-term sequelae (i.e., target organ damage). Barring an overt need for immediate pharmacologic therapy, most patients should be given the opportunity to achieve a reduction in BP over an interval of 3–6 months by applying nonpharmacologic modifications. The primary goal is to reduce BP to <140/90 mm Hg while concurrently controlling other modifiable cardiovascular risk factors. As isolated systolic hypertension is also associated with increased cerebrovascular and cardiac events, the therapeutic goal in this subset of patients should be to lower BP to <140 mm Hg systolic. Treatment should be more aggressive, with a goal BP of <130/80 in patients with chronic kidney disease or diabetes. Discretion is warranted in prescribing medication to lower BP that may affect cardiovascular risk adversely in other ways (e.g., glucose control, lipid metabolism, uric acid levels). In the absence of hypertensive crisis, BP should be reduced gradually to avoid end-organ (e.g., cerebral) ischemia.

Patient Education

- Patient education is an essential component of the treatment plan and promotes patient compliance. Physicians should emphasize that:
    - Lifelong treatment usually is required.
    - Symptoms are an unreliable gauge of severity of hypertension.
    - Prognosis improves with proper management.

Complications

- **Withdrawal syndrome associated with discontinuation of antihypertensive therapy.** In substituting therapy in patients with moderate to severe hypertension, it is reasonable to increase doses of the new medication in small increments while tapering the previous medication to avoid excessive BP fluctuations. On occasion, an AWS develops, usually within the first 24–72 hours. Occasionally, BP rises to levels that are much higher than those of baseline values. The most severe complications of AWS include encephalopathy, stroke, MI, and sudden death. The AWS is associated most commonly with centrally acting adrenergic agents (particularly clonidine) and β-adrenergic antagonists but has been reported with other agents as well, including diuretics. Rarely should BP medications be withdrawn, but, in discontinuing therapy, these drugs should be tapered over several days to weeks unless other medications are used to substitute in the interim. Discontinuation of antihypertensive medications should be done with caution in patients with preexisting cerebrovascular or cardiac disease. Management of AWS by reinstitution of the previously administered drug generally is effective. Sodium nitroprusside (Table 4-3) is the treatment of choice when parenteral administration of an antihypertensive agent is required or when the identity of the previously administered agent is unknown. In the AWS caused by clonidine, β-adrenergic antagonists should not be used because unopposed α-adrenergic activity will be augmented and may exacerbate hypertension. However, labetalol (Table 4-3) may be useful in this situation.

SPECIAL CONSIDERATIONS

Aortic Dissection

- Acute, proximal aortic dissection (type A) is a surgical emergency, whereas uncomplicated, distal dissection (type B) can be treated successfully with medical therapy alone. All patients, including those treated surgically, require acute and chronic antihypertensive therapy to provide initial stabilization and to prevent complications (e.g., aortic rupture, continued dissection). Medical therapy of chronic stable aortic dissection should seek to maintain systolic BP at or below 130–140 mm Hg if tolerated. Antihypertensive agents with negative inotropic properties, including calcium channel antagonists, β-adrenergic antagonists, methyldopa, clonidine, and reserpine, are preferred for management in the postacute phase.
    - **Sodium nitroprusside** is considered the initial drug of choice because of the predictability of response and absence of tachyphylaxis. The dose should be titrated to achieve a systolic BP of 100–120 mm Hg or the lowest possible BP that permits adequate organ perfusion. Nitroprusside alone causes an increase in left ventricular contractility and subsequent arterial shearing forces, which contribute to ongoing intimal dissection. Thus, when using sodium nitroprusside, adequate simultaneous β-adrenergic antagonist therapy is essential, regardless of whether systolic hypertension is present. Traditionally, propranolol has been recommended. **Esmolol, a**

cardioselective IV β-adrenergic antagonist with a very short duration of action, may be preferable, especially in patients with relative contraindications to β antagonists. If esmolol is tolerated, a longer-acting β-adrenergic antagonist should be used.

■ **IV labetalol** has been used successfully as a single agent in the treatment of acute aortic dissection. Labetalol produces a dose-related decrease in BP and lowers contractility. It has the advantage of allowing for oral administration after the acute stage of dissection has been managed successfully.

■ **Trimethaphan camsylate,** a ganglionic blocking agent, can be used as a single IV agent if sodium nitroprusside or β-adrenergic antagonists cannot be tolerated. Unlike sodium nitroprusside, trimethaphan reduces left ventricular contractility. Because trimethaphan is associated with rapid tachyphylaxis and sympathalgia (e.g., orthostatic hypotension, blurred vision, and urinary retention), other drugs are preferable.

Individual Patient Considerations

■ Cultural and other individual differences among patients must be considered in planning a therapeutic regimen. Although classification of adult BP is somewhat arbitrary, it may nevertheless be useful in making clinical decisions (Table 4-2).

■ **The elderly hypertensive patient** (older than 60 years) generally is characterized by increased vascular resistance, decreased plasma renin activity, and greater LVH than in younger patients. Often, elderly hypertensive patients have coexisting medical problems that must be considered in initiating antihypertensive therapy. Drug doses should be increased slowly to avoid adverse effects and hypotension. Diuretics as initial therapy have been shown to decrease the incidence of stroke, fatal MI, and overall mortality in this age group.[10] Calcium channel antagonists decrease vascular resistance, have no adverse effects on lipid levels, and also are good choices for elderly patients. Even though elderly patients tend to have low plasma renin activity, ACE inhibitors and ARBs may be effective agents in this population.

■ **Black hypertensive patients** generally have a lower plasma renin level, higher plasma volume, and higher vascular resistance than do white patients. Thus, black patients respond well to diuretics, alone or in combination with calcium channel antagonists. ACE inhibitors, ARBs, and labetalol (an α- and a β-adrenergic antagonist) are also effective agents in this population.

■ **The obese hypertensive patient** is characterized by more modest elevations in vascular resistance, higher cardiac output, expanded intravascular volume, and lower plasma renin activity at any given level of arterial pressure. Weight reduction is the primary goal of therapy and is effective in reducing BP and causing regression of LVH.

■ **The diabetic patient** with nephropathy may have significant proteinuria and renal insufficiency, which can complicate management (see Chapter 11, Renal Diseases). Control of BP is the most important intervention shown to slow loss of renal function. ACE inhibitors should be used as first-line therapy, as they have been shown to decrease proteinuria and to slow progressive loss of renal function independent of their antihypertensive effects.[11] ACE inhibitors also may be beneficial in reducing the rates of death, MI, and stroke in diabetics who have cardiovascular risk factors but lack left ventricular dysfunction. Furthermore, patients receiving ACE inhibitors may have a lower incidence of MI than those receiving the dihydropyridine class of calcium channel antagonists, although this observation was not evident in the ALLHAT trial. Hyperkalemia is a common side effect in diabetic patients treated with ACE inhibitors, especially in those with moderate to severe impairment of their glomerular filtration rate. ARBs also are effective antihypertensive agents and have been shown to slow the rate of progression to end-stage renal disease, thus supporting a renal protective effect [Reduction of Endpoints in Non–Insulin-Dependent Diabetes Mellitus with the Angiotensin II Antagonist Losartan (RENAAL) and irbesartan trials].

■ **The hypertensive patient with chronic renal insufficiency** has hypertension that usually is partially volume dependent. Retention of sodium and water exacerbates the existing hypertensive state, and diuretics are important in the management of this problem. With a serum creatinine >2.5 mg/dL, loop diuretics are the most effective class.

- **The hypertensive patient with LVH** is at increased risk for sudden death, MI, and all-cause mortality. Although there is no direct evidence, regression of LVH could be expected to reduce the risk for subsequent complications. ACE inhibitors appear to have the greatest effect on regression.

- **The hypertensive patient with coronary artery disease** is at increased risk for unstable angina and MI. β-Adrenergic antagonists can be used as first-line agents in these patients, as they can decrease cardiac mortality and subsequent reinfarction in the setting of acute MI and can decrease progression to MI in those who present with unstable angina. β-Adrenergic antagonists also have a role in secondary prevention of cardiac events and in increasing long-term survival after MI. Care should be exercised in those with cardiac conduction system disease. Calcium channel antagonists should be used with caution in the setting of acute MI, as studies have shown conflicting results from their use. ACE inhibitors are also useful in patients with coronary artery disease and decrease mortality in individuals who present with acute MI, especially those with left ventricular dysfunction, and more recently have been shown to decrease mortality in patients without left ventricular dysfunction.

- **The hypertensive patient with HF** is at risk for progressive left ventricular dilatation and sudden death. In this population, ACE inhibitors decrease mortality,[12] and in the setting of acute MI, they decrease the risk of recurrent MI, hospitalization for HF, and mortality.[13] ARBs have similar beneficial effects, and they appear to be an effective alternative in patients who are unable to tolerate an ACE inhibitor.[9] Nitrates and hydralazine also decrease mortality in patients with HF irrespective of hypertension, but hydralazine can cause reflex tachycardia and worsening ischemia in patients with unstable coronary syndromes and should be used with caution. Calcium channel antagonists should generally be avoided in patients in whom negative inotropic effects would affect their status adversely.

Pregnancy and Hypertension

- Hypertension in the setting of pregnancy is a special situation because of the potential for maternal and fetal morbidity and mortality associated with elevated BP and the clinical syndromes of preeclampsia and eclampsia. The possibility of teratogenic or other adverse effects of antihypertensive medications on fetal development also should be considered.

- **Classification of hypertension** during pregnancy has been proposed by the American College of Obstetrics and Gynecology.[14]
  - **Preeclampsia or eclampsia.** Preeclampsia is a condition defined by pregnancy, hypertension, proteinuria, generalized edema, and, occasionally, coagulation and liver function abnormalities after 20 weeks' gestation. Eclampsia encompasses those physical signs in addition to generalized seizures.
  - **Chronic hypertension.** This disorder is defined by a BP >140/90 mm Hg before the 20th week of pregnancy.
  - **Chronic hypertension with superimposed preeclampsia or eclampsia**
  - **Transient hypertension.** This condition results in increases in BP without associated proteinuria or CNS manifestations. BP returns to normal within 10 days of delivery.

- **Therapy.** Treatment of hypertension in pregnancy should begin if the diastolic BP is >100 mm Hg.
  - Nonpharmacologic therapy, such as weight reduction and vigorous exercise, is not recommended during pregnancy.
  - Alcohol and tobacco use should be discouraged strongly.
  - Pharmacologic intervention with methyldopa is recommended as first-line therapy because of its proven safety. Hydralazine and labetalol are also safe and can be used as alternative agents; both can be used parenterally.
  - Other antihypertensives have theoretical disadvantages, but none except the ACE inhibitors have been proven to increase fetal morbidity or mortality.
  - If a patient is suspected of having preeclampsia or eclampsia, urgent referral to an obstetrician who specializes in high-risk pregnancy is recommended.

Monoamine Oxidase Inhibitors (MAOIs)

■ MAOIs used in association with certain drugs or foods can produce a catecholamine excess state and accelerated hypertension. Interactions are common with tricyclic antidepressants, meperidine, methyldopa, levodopa, sympathomimetic agents, and antihistamines. Tyramine-containing foods that can lead to this syndrome include certain cheeses, red wine, beer, chocolate, chicken liver, processed meat, herring, broad beans, canned figs, and yeast. Nitroprusside, labetalol, and phentolamine have been used effectively in the treatment of accelerated hypertension associated with monoamine oxidase inhibitor use (Table 4-4).

References
1. Chobanian AV, Bakris GL, Black HR, et al. National High Blood Pressure Education Program Coordinating Committee. The Seventh Report of the Joint National Committee on Prevention, Detection, Evaluation, and Treatment of High Blood Pressure. The JNC 7 Report. *JAMA* 2003;289:2560–2572.
2. The ALLHAT Officers and Co-ordinators for the ALLHAT Collaborative Research Group. Major cardiovascular events in hypertensive patients randomly assigned to doxazosin vs chlorthalidone: the antihypertensive and lipid lowering treatment to prevent heart attack trial (ALLHAT). *JAMA* 2002;283:1967–1975.
3. The ALLHAT Officers and Coordinators for the ALLHAT Collaborative Research Group. Major outcomes in high-risk hypertensive patients randomized to angiotensin-converting enzyme inhibitor or calcium channel blocker vs diuretic: the Antihypertensive and Lipid-Lowering Treatment to Prevent Heart Attack Trial (ALLHAT). *JAMA* 2002;288:2981–2997.
4. Psaty BM, Heckbert SR, Koepsell TD, et al. The risk of myocardial infarction associated with antihypertensive drug therapies. *JAMA* 1995;274:620–625.
5. Kaplan NM. Do calcium antagonists cause myocardial infarction? *Am J Cardiol* 1996;77:81–82.
6. Estacio RO, Jeffers BW, Hiatt WE, et al. The effect of nisoldipine as compared with enalapril on cardiovascular outcomes in patients with non-insulin-dependent diabetes and hypertension. *N Engl J Med* 1998;338:645–652.
7. Yusuf S, Sleight P, Pogue J, et al. Effects of an angiotensin-converting enzyme inhibitor, ramipril, on cardiovascular events in high-risk patients. The Heart Outcomes Prevention Evaluation Study Investigators. *N Engl J Med* 2000;342:145–153.
8. Goodfriend TL, Elliott ME, Catt KJ. Angiotensin receptors and their antagonists. *N Engl J Med* 1996;334:1649–1654.
9. Cohn JN, Tognoni G. Valsartan Heart Failure Trial Investigators. A randomized trial of the angiotensin-receptor blocker valsartan in chronic heart failure. *N Engl J Med* 2001;345:1667–1675.
10. SHEP Cooperative Research Group. Prevention of stroke by antihypertensive drug treatment in older persons with isolated systolic hypertension: final results of the Systolic Hypertension in the Elderly Program (SHEP). *JAMA* 1991;265:3255–3264.
11. Lewis EJ, Hunsicker LG, Bain RP et al., for the Collaborative Study Group. The effect of angiotensin-converting-enzyme inhibition on diabetic nephropathy. *N Engl J Med* 1993;329:1456–1462.
12. The SOLVD Investigators. Effect of enalapril on mortality and the development of heart failure in asymptomatic patients with reduced left ventricular ejection fractions. *N Engl J Med* 1992;327:685–691.
13. Pfeffer MA, Braunwald E, Moyé LA et al., on behalf of the SAVE Investigators. Effect of captopril on mortality and morbidity in patients with left ventricular dysfunction after myocardial infarction: results of the survival and ventricular enlargement trial. *N Engl J Med* 1992;327:669–677.
14. Sibai BM. Treatment of hypertension in pregnant women. *N Engl J Med* 1996;335:257–265.

ISCHEMIC HEART DISEASE
Andrew Kates, Alan Zajarias, and Anne Goldberg

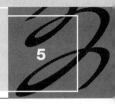

 # CORONARY ARTERY DISEASE

GENERAL PRINCIPLES

Definition
- Coronary artery disease (CAD) is typically defined as a >50% stenosis of any epicardial coronary artery.
- It is most commonly due to obstruction by atheromatous plaque.

Epidemiology
- CAD is the leading cause of morbidity and mortality in Western society and caused one of every five deaths in the United States in 2002.
- The morbidity associated with CAD is considerable: More than 1 million patients have a myocardial infarction (MI) annually. Many more are hospitalized for unstable angina and evaluation and treatment of stable chest pain syndromes.
- About 90% of patients with CAD have prior exposure to at least one major risk factor (see Risk Factors).

Pathophysiology
- The manifestations of CAD include stable angina, acute coronary syndromes (ACS), congestive heart failure, sudden cardiac death, and silent ischemia.
- ACS encompasses a spectrum of clinical conditions from unstable angina to ST-elevation MI.
- Stable angina most often results from fixed coronary lesions that produce a mismatch of myocardial supply and demand with increasing cardiac workload.
- The presence of ischemic heart disease can predispose patients to additional problems, including heart failure, cardiac arrhythmias, and sudden cardiac death.

Mechanisms of Injury
- The acute event usually represents rupture of a vulnerable atherosclerotic plaque, exposing a thrombogenic surface within the vessel.
  - Platelet aggregation of varying degrees ensues, limiting blood flow to the myocardium distal to the lesion.
  - The resulting myocardial oxygen supply–demand mismatch can result in tissue ischemia (unstable angina) or necrosis (MI).

DIAGNOSIS

Clinical Presentation

- A careful history and physical examination are usually sufficient to provide information to establish an appropriate pretest probability of coronary disease.
- Characteristics of angina
  - Angina is usually described as a chest discomfort or heaviness that may radiate to the neck, jaw, or arm(s) and can be further defined as follows:
    - Typical angina (definite) is (a) substernal chest discomfort with a characteristic quality and duration that is (b) precipitated by stress and (c) relieved by rest or nitroglycerin (NTG).
    - Atypical angina (probable) meets two of these characteristics.
    - Noncardiac chest pain meets one or none of these characteristics.
- Grading of angina
  - Grading of angina is based on the Canadian Cardiovascular Society (CCS) Classification System.
    - Class I: Angina occurs only with strenuous activity.
    - Class II: Angina occurs with moderate activity like walking more than two blocks or climbing more than one flight of stairs.
    - Class III: Angina occurs with mild activity like climbing a flight of stairs or walking less than two blocks.
    - Class IV: Angina occurs with any activity and may occur at rest.
- Associated symptoms may include dyspnea, diaphoresis, nausea, vomiting, dizziness, or palpitations. The patient's complaints may also be atypical in nature, such as epigastric discomfort.

Risk Factors

- Tobacco abuse is associated with a marked increased risk of CAD and has a synergistic effect with other risk factors. Environmental exposure to smoke (second-hand smoke) may also increase the risk of heart disease. Successful smoking cessation restores the risk of CAD to that of a nonsmoker within approximately 15 years.
- Hypertension is associated with increased cardiovascular risk. Lifestyle modification and pharmacologic therapy (if needed) should be used to achieve a goal of <140/90 mm Hg. More stringent control (<130/80 mm Hg) is appropriate if comorbid disease, including renal insufficiency, diabetes, or heart failure, is present (see Chapter 4, Hypertension).
- Diabetes mellitus. CAD is the primary cause of death in people with diabetes. In addition, most hospitalizations resulting from diabetes-associated complications are a consequence of CAD. Incidence of CAD disease is two- to fourfold higher in individuals with diabetes than without the disease. Moreover, increased insulin resistance, such as that seen with the metabolic syndrome, is associated with increased risk of CAD.
- Dyslipidemia. High low-density lipoprotein (LDL), low high-density lipoprotein (HDL), and elevated triglycerides are independent risk factors for CAD.
- Family history is appropriately defined as premature CAD in a first-degree relative (male relative <55; female relative <65).
- Obesity increases the risk of CAD and is associated with additional cardiac risk factors, including hypertension, diabetes, and lipid abnormalities. A body mass index of >25 kg/m^2 is considered overweight and >30 kg/m^2 is obese.

Physical Examination

- The clinical examination should include blood pressure, heart rate, and arterial pulses as well as an evaluation for the presence of heart failure (e.g., pulmonary rales, peripheral edema) or cardiac dysfunction (e.g., abnormal heart sounds, murmurs, or cardiac impulse).

- Complete exam should also include evaluation for evidence of significant dyslipidemia such as corneal arcus and xanthelasmas.

Diagnostic Evaluation

- **Electrocardiogram (ECG).** A baseline ECG should be recorded in all patients with suspected CAD. A normal tracing does not exclude the presence of disease, and an abnormal ECG does not indicate with certainty the presence of disease. Findings of significant Q waves or ST-T–wave abnormalities are consistent with (but not diagnostic of) underlying CAD. In addition to the baseline tracing, an ECG should be obtained if the patient is having anginal symptoms to assess for labile changes consistent with underlying ischemic disease.
- **Biochemical markers** including complete blood count (CBC), fasting glucose, troponin, and lipid profile should be obtained in all patients with suspected CAD or ACS. Additionally, elevated high-sensitivity C-reactive protein (CRP), lipoprotein (a), and homocysteine levels are associated with increased risk of CAD.
- **Chest radiograph** should be obtained if there is evidence of congestive heart failure (CHF), valvular disease, or aortic disease.

Exercise Stress Testing

- **Exercise treadmill testing** (ETT) is the test of choice for most patients. Patients can be exercised on a treadmill following a prescribed protocol.
  - The **Bruce protocol** is most commonly used, consisting of 3-minute stages of increasing treadmill speed and incline. The patient is monitored for an appropriate physiologic response to exercise with blood pressure (BP) and heart rate measurements during the walk and into the recovery period. The patient should be questioned for the presence of anginal symptoms. The patient's ECG is monitored throughout the study to evaluate for ischemic changes.
  - In properly selected patients the exercise stress test has a sensitivity and specificity of 70%–80% to detect disease if the patient has a normal resting ECG and if a target heart rate of 85% of the maximum heart rate for age is achieved.
  - Prior to obtaining a stress test, it is important to consider the likelihood of CAD in the patient who is being evaluated (Table 5-1). This pretest probability correlates with the positive and negative predictive values of an abnormal stress test.
  - Prognostic information can be quantified by the **Duke treadmill score,** which incorporates the duration of exercise on the Bruce protocol, maximal ST-segment deviation on the ECG, and anginal symptoms (Duke score = minutes exercise – [5 × mm ST-segment deviation] – [4 × anginal score]). Scores of >5, –10 to +4, and ≤11 are associated with low, moderate, and high risks, respectively, of subsequent cardiovascular events.
  - A positive study is present if new ST-segment depressions (>1 mm in multiple leads), a hypotensive response, new heart failure, or sustained ventricular arrhythmias develop.

TABLE 5-1   Pretest Likelihood of Coronary Artery Disease

Age (years)	Nonanginal chest pain		Atypical angina		Typical angina	
	Men	Women	Men	Women	Men	Women
30–39	4	2	34	12	76	26
40–49	13	3	51	22	87	55
50–59	20	7	65	31	93	73
60–69	27	14	72	51	94	86

Stress Testing in Specific Populations

- Patients **without known coronary disease**
    - **Low-risk** patients. In general, a "screening" exercise test is not warranted in asymptomatic patients at low risk for CAD.
    - **Intermediate-risk** patients can be considered for testing if their occupation is such that impairment might have an impact on public safety (e.g., airline pilot) or they plan to begin a vigorous exercise program.
    - **High-risk** patients for CAD due to other diseases, such as diabetes and peripheral vascular disease, can also be considered for testing.
- Patients **with known coronary disease**
    - **Stress testing after MI** provides useful prognostic information in patients who remain symptom free after their infarction and have not undergone coronary angiography.
        - A submaximal study performed 4–7 days after acute MI or a maximal exercise stress test 4–6 weeks after MI aids in determining the patient's ischemic burden, which, if significant, should prompt consideration for cardiac catheterization to define the coronary anatomy.
        - A treadmill stress test after acute MI, either with or without revascularization, helps guide recommendations for a cardiac rehabilitation program.
    - Risk assessment may be appropriate in **asymptomatic patients** with known disease who are scheduled to **undergo elective surgical procedure** (see Chapter 1, Patient Care in Internal Medicine).
    - The routine use of stress testing in **asymptomatic patients** after **percutaneous or surgical revascularization** remains controversial. If testing is done, it should be performed in conjunction with an imaging modality (nuclear or echocardiographic) to increase the sensitivity of the test and to localize area(s) of ischemia that may exist.
- **Women.** The use of exercise testing in women presents difficulties that are not experienced in men. These difficulties reflect the differences between men and women regarding the prevalence of CAD and the sensitivity and specificity of exercise testing. To compensate for the limitations of the test in women, some investigators have developed predictive models that incorporate more information from the test than simply the amount and type of ST-segment change. Although this approach is attractive, its clinical application remains limited.
- **The elderly.** Performance of exercise testing poses additional problems in the elderly as functional capacity is often compromised from muscle weakness and deconditioning.

Cardiac Stress Testing with Imaging

- Patients who are good candidates for cardiac stress testing with imaging (as opposed to exercise ECG alone) include those in the following categories:
    - Evidence of pre-excitation [Wolf-Parkinson-White (WPW) syndrome]
    - Left ventricular hypertrophy (LVH)
    - Left bundle branch block (LBBB) or significant intraventricular conduction delay (IVCD)
    - Digoxin effects
    - Paced rhythm
    - Resting ST- and T-wave changes
- **Myocardial perfusion imaging.** The radioactive tracers thallium-201 and technetium-99m are commonly used in conjunction with exercise or pharmacologic stress testing. Stress perfusion imaging allows the diagnosis and localization of areas of ischemia, allows determination of ejection fraction, and permits a determination of myocardial viability. Although false-positive and false-negative studies occur, the addition of nuclear imaging to an exercise stress test increases the sensitivity and specificity of the study to approximately 80%–90% in properly selected patients.
- **Echocardiographic imaging.** Exercise or dobutamine stress testing can be performed with echocardiography to aid in the diagnosis of CAD. As with nuclear imaging, echocardiography adds to the sensitivity and specificity of the test by translating myocardial ischemia into areas with wall motion abnormalities.

- **Adenosine magnetic resonance imaging** with contrast enhancement may be used to demonstrate myocardial ischemia and viability without requiring radiation exposure.

Pharmacologic Stress Testing

- **Exercise stress testing** (generally with a treadmill) is preferable to pharmacologic stress. However, when the patient cannot exercise to the necessary level or in other specified circumstances (see above), pharmacologic stress testing may be preferable.
- Three drugs are commonly used as substitutes for exercise stress testing: **dipyridamole, adenosine,** and **dobutamine.**
  - Dipyridamole and adenosine are **vasodilators** that are commonly used in conjunction with myocardial perfusion **scintigraphy.**
    - Dipyridamole or adenosine is the pharmacologic agent of choice in the patient with LBBB or paced rhythm on ECG.
  - Dobutamine is a **positive inotropic** (and chronotropic) agent commonly used with echocardiography.

Contraindications to Stress Testing

- Exercise stress testing is contraindicated in patients with the following:
  - Acute MI within 2 days
  - Unstable angina not previously stabilized by medical therapy
  - Cardiac arrhythmias causing symptoms or hemodynamic compromise
  - Symptomatic severe aortic stenosis
  - Symptomatic heart failure
  - Acute pulmonary embolus, myocarditis, pericarditis, aortic dissection

Diagnostic Procedures

- **Coronary angiography** is the **gold standard** for evaluating the coronary anatomy of the left and right coronary arterial systems. The presence and severity of atherosclerotic lesions can be directly identified. The rate of coronary flow down the epicardial vessels may be of prognostic value in patients who present with acute ischemic syndromes or after percutaneous revascularization. Coronary angiography may also be of benefit in defining aberrant anatomy or vasospasm.
  - **Intravascular ultrasound** (IVUS) can be used in selected patients to assess plaque burden, providing more definitive assessment of the coronary vasculature at the time of the cardiac catheterization.
  - **Doppler flow** can be used to determine the functional significance of a coronary lesion by measuring fractional flow reserve across the stenosis.
  - **Left ventricular (LV) catheterization** allows measurement of LV filling pressure, the gradient across the aortic valve, as well as the presence of regional wall motion abnormalities by **contrast ventriculography.**
  - **Pulmonary arterial catheterization** is typically reserved for patients with MI complicated by refractory hypotension, progressive renal dysfunction, or congestive heart failure. Measurement of cardiac filling pressures, pulmonary arterial pressures, and cardiac function (cardiac output) with a pulmonary arterial catheter may aid in establishing a diagnosis and guide the therapeutic intervention.
- **Electron beam computed tomography** (EBCT). Coronary calcification is often present in the advanced stages of atherosclerotic lesion formation. EBCT has a high sensitivity but a much lower specificity for the detection of functionally significant CAD. Given this fact and the potential for unnecessary additional testing in patients with false-positive results, current American Heart Association (AHA)/American College of Cardiology (ACC) guidelines do not recommend EBCT for diagnosing obstructive CAD.
- **Multiple-slice CT angiography** (MSCTA) is being studied to assess coronary anatomy and determine the presence of coronary artery stenosis and calcification. It provides a solely anatomic description of the coronary anatomy.

- **Magnetic resonance angiography** (MRA) is capable of examining the proximal portions of the coronary vasculature.
  - Both MRA and MSCTA have shown promise in the noninvasive evaluation of CAD. Further trials comparing these two methods with traditional coronary angiography are required before the clinical utility can be defined. The use of these modalities outside clinical protocols should be discouraged.

Differential Diagnosis

- Cardiovascular-related symptoms that are not due to atherosclerotic disease of the epicardial vessels may be due to **aortic dissection, coronary spasm,** or **pericarditis.**
- Other clinical conditions may also lead to a supply–demand mismatch, including **aortic stenosis, thyrotoxicosis,** and profound **anemia.**
- **Syndrome X** refers to ischemic chest pain in the presence of normal coronary arteries. The etiology of the ischemia is not fully understood but may represent microvascular disease in the heart. Compared with patients with classic coronary disease, those with syndrome X have a good prognosis.
- **Noncardiac causes** of angina-like symptoms include **esophageal disease** (gastroesophageal reflux and motility disorders), **biliary colic, musculoskeletal pain,** and **cervical radiculitis.** Pulmonary disease should also be considered, including **pulmonary embolism,** severe **pulmonary hypertension,** or **pneumonia** (Table 5-2).
- This list is not all-inclusive. The need to pursue a workup of nonischemic causes of angina should be individualized to each patient depending on the patient's physical examination, clinical course, and results of laboratory studies and diagnostic testing.

Primary Prevention of CAD

- According to a study of 52 countries (**INTERHEART**), nine easily measured and potentially modifiable risk factors account for over 90% of the risk of an initial acute MI.
  - These nine risk factors include **cigarette smoking,** abnormal blood **lipid levels, hypertension, diabetes,** abdominal **obesity,** a lack of **physical activity, low daily fruit and vegetable consumption,** alcohol overconsumption, and **psychosocial index.**
  - Institution of lifestyle changes that lower rates of smoking, promote physical activity, and lower trends in obesity all have a positive impact on chronic medical conditions,

| **TABLE 5-2** | **Selected Differential Diagnosis of Myocardial Infarction** |

Diagnosis	ECG findings	Diagnostic evaluation
Pericarditis	PR depression, diffuse or focal ST elevation	Echocardiography (to exclude wall motion abnormalities)
Myocarditis	ST elevation, Q waves	Cardiac enzymes (e.g., troponin), echo
Acute aortic dissection	ST elevation or depression, nonspecific ST- and T-wave changes	Transesophageal echocardiography, chest CT, MRI, or aortography
Pneumothorax	New poor R-wave progression in precordial leads, acute QRS-axis shift	Chest radiography
Pulmonary embolism	Inferior ST elevation, ST shifts in leads V_1–V_3	Ventilation-perfusion scan, D-dimer, or spiral CT scan
Acute cholecystitis	Inferior ST elevation	Gallbladder ultrasound or radio isotope scan

CT, computed tomography; ECG, electrocardiogram; MRI, magnetic resonance imaging.

including hypertension, diabetes, and hyperlipidemic syndromes, each of which contributes to increased cardiovascular risk.
- Risk factor screening in adults should begin at age 20 years and be re-evaluated every 5 years, or sooner if changes in clinical status warrant.
- Cardiovascular risk can be performed through various algorithms. One of the most common is the **Framingham Risk Score,** which provides an estimate of cardiovascular risk over a 10-year period.
- **Physical activity** for at least 30 minutes a day is recommended. Activity should be of moderate intensity. If the patient has coexisting medical conditions or is middle aged or older and sedentary, consultation with a physician is appropriate before an exercise program is initiated.
- **Hormone replacement therapy** (HRT) is not indicated in postmenopausal women for the prevention of CAD.
- The benefits of **folate** supplementation in primary prevention are unknown.
- **Aspirin** use should be considered in persons at higher risk of cardiovascular events (>10% risk of stroke or MI over 10 years), providing that the patient is not aspirin intolerant. Low-dose aspirin (75–160 mg/d) is as effective as higher doses at lowering cardiovascular risk.
- Patients at high risk for CAD based on presence of diabetes mellitus (DM), peripheral vascular disease, hypertension with multiple risk factors, or 10-year Framingham Risk Score >20% should be considered for **statin** therapy regardless of their baseline LDL.
- The use of **antioxidants** such as vitamin E does not appear to be helpful in the prevention of CAD.

 # CHRONIC STABLE ANGINA

GENERAL PRINCIPLES

Definition

Chronic stable angina is the manifestation of ischemic heart disease in approximately half of patients with CAD.

- **Typical angina pectoris** is described as (a) retrosternal pressure, pain, discomfort, or heaviness that (b) radiates to the neck, jaw, left arm, or shoulder, (c) precipitated by exertion and relieved by rest or nitroglycerin, lasting <10 minutes.
- **Associated symptoms** include dyspnea, diaphoresis, palpitations, nausea, vomiting, or lightheadedness.
- Women (more than men) may complain of **epigastric discomfort** that otherwise presents like typical angina.
- **Diabetic** patients may experience **anginal equivalent** symptoms (e.g., fatigue, epigastric distress) that are suspicious for underlying ischemia.

Pathophysiology

Angina is most commonly due to a **mismatch** between myocardial oxygen supply and demand.

- A fixed stenosis of an epicardial coronary artery, usually >70% of the original luminal diameter of the vessel, is sufficient to limit blood flow distal to the lesion. When myocardial workload (oxygen demand) exceeds the capacity of myocardial blood supply (oxygen delivery), angina may ensue.
- In addition to coronary atherosclerotic lesions, myocardial supply–demand mismatch may result from:
  - Disease of the coronary microvasculature (syndrome X)
  - Hypertrophic heart disease
  - Coronary spasm (Prinzmetal angina)

- Uncontrolled hypertension
- Valvular heart disease (e.g., aortic stenosis)

DIAGNOSIS

Clinical Presentation

- A detailed review of the patient's symptoms and focused physical examination are often helpful at directing further diagnostic testing.
    - Patients with typical angina often have CAD of one or more epicardial arteries.
    - Cardiac risk factors, including smoking, diabetes, hypertension, and family history, should be reviewed.
    - A history of peripheral or cerebrovascular disease increases the likelihood that CAD will be present.
- Patients can be characterized as being at low, intermediate, and high probability of significant angina based on their symptoms and cardiac risk profile (Table 5-1).
    - In men and older women the presence of typical angina in association with other cardiac risk factors suggests a 90% probability of CAD. In such patients, the role of cardiac tests is to assess the severity of CAD, guide treatment, and quantify the risk for MI.
    - In patients who experience noncardiac chest pain and lack cardiovascular risk factors, the prevalence of ischemic heart disease is low (<25%), and cardiac evaluation may identify people with CAD.
    - **Noninvasive cardiac imaging** is particularly useful in patients with **intermediate risk** of CAD.

Diagnostic Evaluation

- Laboratory studies in the initial evaluation of a patient with suspected stable angina should include laboratory testing for hemoglobin, fasting glucose, and fasting lipid profile.
    - Recent data suggest that **high-sensitivity CRP** is also of benefit in determining a patient's cardiovascular risk, although its role in secondary prevention remains unclear.
- **Electrocardiogram.** A resting ECG should be obtained during pain and when the patient is pain free. ECG will be without abnormality in <50% of patients with chronic stable angina.
    - *A normal rest ECG does not exclude the presence of severe CAD.*
    - ECG abnormalities including (a) pathologic Q waves (>0.4 seconds) consistent with a prior MI, (b) resting ST-segment depression, (c) T-wave inversion, or (d) LV hypertrophy increase the likelihood that the chest pain is cardiac in origin.
- **Echocardiography** measuring global LV systolic and diastolic function (e.g., ejection fraction) may be important in choosing appropriate medical or surgical therapy and making recommendations about activity level, rehabilitation, and work status.
    - Similarly, cardiac imaging may be helpful in establishing pathophysiologic mechanisms and guiding therapy in patients who have clinical signs or symptoms of heart failure in addition to chronic stable angina.
- **Exercise stress testing** provides functional information and allows risk stratification in patients with known angina.
    - **Beta-blockers, nodal blocking agents,** and **nitrates** should be discontinued in patients prior to performing stress tests.
    - Medications may be continued if the stress test is performed to optimize medical therapy.
    - A **positive stress test** indicative of severe CAD is defined with the presence of any of the following:
        - New ST-segment depression at the start of exercise
        - New ST-segment depression >2 mm in multiple leads
        - Inability to exercise for >2 minutes

- Decreased systolic blood pressure with exercise
- Development of heart failure or sustained ventricular arrhythmias
- Prolonged interval after exercise cessation (>5 minutes) before ischemic ST changes return to baseline

■ Patients with a markedly positive stress test should undergo cardiac catheterization to be evaluated for **coronary revascularization.**

■ **Cardiac stress testing with imaging**
  ■ **Stress echocardiography** or myocardial **perfusion imaging** with [201]thallium or [99m]technetium-sestamibi increase diagnostic sensitivity. Due to their increased costs, they should be used in specific indications (inability to exercise or evaluating for the presence of instant restenosis).
  ■ A markedly positive stress test demonstrating multiple areas of ischemia, transient LV cavity dilation, or uptake of radiotracer in the lungs should prompt referral for coronary angiography.

■ **Invasive diagnosis of CAD**
  ■ **Coronary angiography** is considered the gold-standard technique for diagnosing CAD. As with noninvasive testing, angiography can be used to establish a diagnosis or to characterize the degree of atherosclerosis in patients with known disease.
  ■ Coronary angiography should be performed in patients with known or suspected angina with a **markedly positive** stress test or who have survived **sudden cardiac death.**
  ■ Invasive testing should be considered as well for patients with a high pretest probability of **left main or three-vessel CAD** or for those whose occupation requires a definitive diagnosis.
  ■ Angiography can also be considered for patients if a recent stress test is nondiagnostic and for individuals who are unable to undergo noninvasive testing.
  ■ In selected patients with recurrent hospitalizations for chest pain or those with an overriding desire for a definite diagnosis and an intermediate or high pretest probability of CAD, invasive testing can be used to document the presence or extent of disease and facilitate long-term management.
  ■ Coronary angiography may also be useful in patients with angina who are suspected of having a **nonatherosclerotic cause** of ischemia (e.g., coronary anomaly, coronary dissection, radiation vasculopathy).

Risk Stratification

■ Risk assessment of patients with stable angina should be used to help guide decisions on referral for noninvasive or invasive cardiac testing in patients with an intermediate or high probability of CAD.
  ■ The **Duke treadmill score** provides useful information on survival. Patients in the low-risk group (Duke score >5) have an annual mortality of 0.25% and can often be **managed medically.**
  ■ Those in the moderate-risk group (Duke score –10 to +4) have a mortality of 1.25% per year.
    • Management of a patient at intermediate risk should be **individualized,** taking into account the patient's **clinical history, lifestyle,** and **comorbid** conditions.
  ■ Patients in the high-risk group (Duke score ≤10) have an annual mortality exceeding 5%, and should be referred for **coronary angiography.**
    • The probability of a patient having severe (three-vessel or left main) CAD can be estimated by review of the clinical history, physical examination, and demographic characteristics.
    • Independent predictors of severe CAD include **age** (>65), **diabetes,** evidence of a **prior MI** by history and ECG, complaints of **typical angina,** and **male** sex. Absence of all of these predictors is associated with a probability of severe disease ranging from <5% (30-year-old patient) to 20% (80-year-old patient). The probability of severe disease increases with an increasing number of predictors. With all five predictors present, the probability of severe disease ranges from 40%–80%, depending on the age of the patient.

- In **clinically stable** patients, once risk is assessed and a plan for management is enacted (invasive testing or medical management), there is **no need for routine reassessment.** If the patient experiences a significant worsening of symptoms or a change in therapy is contemplated, repeat testing may be warranted.

TREATMENT

Rationale

- The major purposes of treatment of patients with stable angina are to **prevent MI** and death and to **reduce or relieve symptoms,** leading to an improved quality of life.
- The combination of lifestyle modifications and medical therapy should be considered.

Medical Treatment

Specific treatment is aimed at **reducing myocardial oxygen demand, improving myocardial oxygen supply,** treating **cardiac risk factors** (hypertension, diabetes, obesity), and **controlling exacerbating factors** (valvular stenosis, anemia) that may precipitate ischemia.

- One approach to guide the treatment of patients with ischemic heart disease is the "ABCDE" mnemonic (aspirin and antianginal therapy; β-adrenergic antagonists and blood pressure control; cholesterol-lowering agents and cigarette-smoking cessation; diet; and exercise).
- **Aspirin** use in patients with stable angina has been shown to reduce cardiovascular events by 33%. In asymptomatic patients in the **Physician's Health Study,** aspirin (325 mg, every other day) decreased the incidence of MI.
  - Aspirin desensitization may be performed in selected patients with aspirin allergy.
  - **Clopidogrel** (75 mg/d) can be used in patients who are allergic or intolerant of aspirin.
- **β-Adrenergic antagonists** (Table 5-3). All β-blockers appear to be effective in controlling angina by decreasing heart rate and BP.
  - The dosage can be adjusted to result in a resting heart rate of 50–60 bpm.
  - In patients with persistent angina, a target heart rate of <50 bpm is warranted providing that no symptoms are associated with the bradycardia and that heart block does not develop.
  - If stress testing is performed as part of the evaluation, beta-blocker therapy in patients with known heart disease should limit the heart rate response with exercise to <75% of the heart rate associated with the onset of ischemia.
  - Use of beta-blockers is contraindicated in patients with severe **bronchospasm,** significant **atrioventricular (AV) block,** marked resting **bradycardia,** or poorly compensated heart failure.

TABLE 5-3	**Beta-Blockers Commonly Used for Ischemic Heart Disease**

Drug	β-Receptor selectivity	Dose
Propranolol	None	20–80 mg bid
Metoprolol	β_1	50–200 mg bid
Atenolol	β_1	50–200 mg daily
Nadolol	None	40–80 mg daily
Timolol	None	10–30 mg tid
Acebutolol	β_1	200–600 mg bid
Bisoprolol	β_1	10–20 mg daily
Esmolol (IV)	β_1	50–300 mcg/kg/min
Labetalol	Combined α/β	200–600 mg bid
Pindolol	None	2.5–7.5 mg tid
Carvedilol	Combined α, β_1, β_2	3.125–25 mg bid

TABLE 5-4 **Calcium Channel Blockers Commonly Used for Ischemic Heart Disease**

Drug	Duration of action	Usual dosage
Dihydropyridines		
Nifedipine		
Slow release	Long	30–180 mg/d
Amlodipine	Long	5–10 mg/d
Felodipine (SR)	Long	5–10 mg/d
Isradipine (SR)	Medium	2.5–10 mg/d
Nicardipine	Short	20–40 mg tid
Nondihydropyridines		
Diltiazem		
Immediate release	Short	30–80 mg qid
Slow release	Long	120–360 mg/d
Verapamil		
Immediate release	Short	80–160 mg tid
Slow release	Long	120–480 mg/d

- ▪ If additional BP control is necessary after incorporation of beta-blocker and calcium antagonist therapy, supplemental agents can be used, as outlined in Chapter 4, Hypertension.
- ■ **Calcium channel blockers** can be used in lieu of a beta-blocker if beta-blockers are contraindicated or not tolerated due to significant adverse effects.
  - ▪ Calcium antagonists can also be used in conjunction with beta-blockers if the latter are not fully effective at relieving anginal symptoms (Table 5-4). **Long-acting dihydropyridines** and **nondihydropyridine** agents can be used.
  - ▪ Use of **short-acting dihydropyridines** (e.g., nifedipine) should be avoided due to the potential to increase the risk of adverse cardiac events.
- ■ **Nitrates,** either long-acting formulations for chronic use or sublingual preparations for acute anginal symptoms, can be used as adjuncts to baseline therapy with beta-blockers or calcium antagonists, or both (Table 5-5). The patient should take the medication while seated because of possible side effects of hypotension.
  - ▪ **Sublingual preparations** should be used at the **first indication of angina** or prophylactically before engaging in activities that are known to precipitate angina. Patients should seek prompt medical attention if angina occurs at rest or fails to respond to the third sublingual dose.

TABLE 5-5 **Nitrate Preparations Commonly Used for Ischemic Heart Disease**

Preparation	Dosage	Onset (min)	Duration
Sublingual nitroglycerin	0.3–0.6 mg PRN	2–5	10–30 min
Aerosol nitroglycerin	0.4 mg PRN	2–5	10–30 min
Oral isosorbide dinitrate	5–40 mg tid	30–60	4–6 hr
Oral isosorbide mononitrate	10–20 mg bid	30–60	6–8 hr
Oral isosorbide mononitrate SR	30–120 mg daily	30–60	12–18 hr
2% Nitroglycerin ointment	0.5–2.0 in. tid	20–60	3–8 hr
Transdermal nitroglycerin patches	5–15 mg daily	>60	12 hr
Intravenous nitroglycerin	10–200 mcg/min	<2	During infusion

- Nitrate **tolerance** resulting in reduced therapeutic response may occur with all nitrate preparations. The institution of a **nitrate-free period** of 10–12 hours can enhance treatment efficacy.
- **Angiotensin-converting enzyme** (ACE) inhibitors have been investigated for treatment of stable angina, but their efficacy has not been established.
  - A reduction of exercise-induced myocardial ischemia has been reported with the addition of an ACE inhibitor in patients with stable angina with optimal beta-blockade and normal LV function.
- A new agent, **ranolizine**, with mechanisms different from previous antianginals was recently approved for use in patients who remain symptomatic despite optimal medical therapy.
- The use of **antibiotics** to prevent CAD is not recommended.

Revascularization

Medical therapy with at least two, and preferably three, classes of antianginal agents should be attempted before treatment is considered a failure.

- Patients who are **refractory** to medical therapy should be assessed with coronary angiography, if the anatomy has not already been defined.
- Revascularization with **percutaneous coronary intervention** (PCI) or coronary artery bypass grafting (CABG) should be considered, as the clinical history and anatomy dictate and may be associated with lower rates of death, nonfatal MI, or recurrent hospitalization.
  - Current percutaneous techniques include **balloon angioplasty, atherectomy** devices, and **intracoronary stenting.**
  - In appropriately selected cases, a clinical success rate of >90% can be expected.
  - The rate of coronary **restenosis** is related to the revascularization technique used; the nature of the lesion; and the presence of comorbid risks, such as diabetes and continued tobacco abuse.
  - Recently developed **drug-eluting stents** are associated with significantly lower rates of restenosis and failure compared to standard bare-metal stents.
- CABG is optimal for patients at high risk for cardiac mortality, including those with (a) left main disease, (b) two-vessel or three-vessel disease involving the proximal left anterior descending artery and LV dysfunction, or (c) diabetes and multivessel coronary disease with left ventricular dysfunction.
  - The **risk of surgery** includes 1%–3% mortality, a 5%–10% incidence of perioperative MI, a small risk of perioperative stroke or cognitive dysfunction, and a 10%–20% risk of vein graft failure in the first year. Approximately 75% of patients remain free of recurrent angina or adverse cardiac events at 5 years of follow-up. The risks of elective PCI include <1% mortality, a 2%–5% rate of nonfatal MI, and <1% need for emergent CABG for an unsuccessful procedure.
  - The use of **internal mammary artery grafts** is associated with 90% graft patency at 10 years, compared with 40%–50% for saphenous vein grafts. The long-term patency of **radial artery grafts** is currently under review. After 10 years of follow-up, 50% of patients develop recurrent angina or other adverse cardiac events related to late vein graft failure or progression of native CAD.
- Use of PCI is associated with a shorter hospital stay and faster recovery time, but has a higher rate of future reintervention when compared to CABG.

Alternate Therapies

Alternate therapies are available for patients with chronic stable angina who are refractory to medical management and who are not candidates for percutaneous or surgical revascularization.

- Transmyocardial **laser revascularization** has been delivered by percutaneous technique (YAG [yttrium-aluminum-garnet] laser) and by epicardial surgical techniques (CO_2 or YAG laser).

- The percutaneous approach has not been approved by the U.S. Food and Drug Administration and should therefore be considered **experimental** therapy.
- The goal in either approach is to create a series of **transmural endomyocardial channels.**
- Surgical transmyocardial laser revascularization has been shown to improve symptoms in patients with stable angina, although the mechanism that is responsible is controversial.
  - The data on whether exercise capacity is improved are conflicting, and no benefit has been demonstrated in terms of increasing myocardial perfusion or mortality.
- **Enhanced external counterpulsation** (EECP) is a nonpharmacologic technique for which 35 hours a week of treatment in patients with chronic stable angina and a positive stress test were shown to decrease the frequency of angina and increase the time to exercise-induced ischemia.
  - The treatment improved anginal symptoms in approximately 75%–80% of patients; however, additional clinical trial data are required before enhanced external counterpulsation can be definitively recommended.
- **Chelation** therapy and **acupuncture** have not been found to be effective to relieve symptoms and are not recommended for treatment of chronic stable angina.

Follow-Up

- **Patient follow-up** is discussed in detail in "Secondary Prevention."
- Minor changes in the patient's anginal complaints can be treated with titration or adjustment of the antianginal regimen.
- If the patient has a significant change in anginal complaints (frequency, severity, or time to onset with activity), a reassessment with a stress test (likely in conjunction with an imaging modality) or a cardiac catheterization is warranted.
- If the anatomy is amenable to revascularization (either percutaneous or surgical), this approach should be considered.

 # ACUTE CORONARY SYNDROME

UNSTABLE ANGINA/NON–ST-SEGMENT ELEVATION MYOCARDIAL INFARCTION

General Principles

Definition

- Acute coronary syndrome refers to any constellation of clinical symptoms that are compatible with acute myocardial ischemia and encompasses acute myocardial infarction [ST-segment elevation myocardial infarction (STEMI) and non–ST-segment elevation myocardial infarction (NSTEMI)] as well as unstable angina (UA).
- UA and NSTEMI are considered to be closely related conditions whose pathogenesis and clinical presentations are similar but differ in severity.
- These patients can be difficult to distinguish from one another solely on the basis of clinical symptoms and ECG findings.
  - Approximately three-fourths of patients will have an abnormal ECG, more often seen as labile ST-segment depression or T-wave inversions, or less frequently transient ST-segment elevations.
- NSTEMI is defined by an elevation of cardiac isoenzymes [creatine kinase MB (CK-MB) or troponin] and the absence of persistent ST-segment elevation.

Epidemiology

- Among patients with ACS, approximately 60% have UA and 40% have MI.
  - Of the patients with MI, two-thirds have NSTEMI and the remaining one-third present with acute ST-segment elevation MI.

Pathophysiology
- Thrombus formation, which may be episodic in nature, is the mechanism underlying the compromise in coronary blood flow.
- UA/NSTEMI most often represents acute atherosclerotic plaque rupture with exposure of a thrombogenic subendothelial matrix, but may also be due to progressive mechanical obstruction from advancing atherosclerotic disease or restenosis after percutaneous intervention.
- Causes other than plaque rupture include dynamic obstruction of the coronary artery due to vasospasm (Prinzmetal angina) and cardiac inflammation or infection.

Diagnosis
Immediate assessment of UA/NSTEMI includes the clinical presentation (history and physical examination), 12-lead ECG recording, and measurement of cardiac-specific marker (troponin or CK-MB).

History and Physical Examination
- The three principal presentations for UA are **rest angina** (angina occurring at rest and prolonged usually >20 minutes), **new-onset angina** (of at least CCS class III severity), and **increasing angina** (previously diagnosed angina that has become distinctly more frequent, longer in duration, or lower in threshold [i.e., increased by ≥1 CCS class to at least CCS class III severity]).
- Evaluation and management should be individualized to the patient's clinical presentation with a focused exam for evidence of heart failure, peripheral hypoperfusion, heart murmur, elevated jugular venous pulsation, pulmonary edema, and peripheral edema.
- The presence of severe underlying coronary disease is suggested in patients with clinical evidence of LV dysfunction, congestive heart failure, or transient ischemic ECG changes.

Electrocardiogram
- A 12-lead ECG should be obtained immediately in patients with ongoing chest discomfort and as rapidly as possible in patients who have a history of chest discomfort consistent with ACS but whose discomfort has resolved by the time of evaluation.

Measurement of Cardiac-Specific Markers
- Biomarkers of cardiac injury should be measured in all patients who present with chest discomfort consistent with UA/NSTEMI.
- In patients with negative cardiac markers within 6 hours of the onset of pain, another sample should be drawn within 6–12 hours.
- A cardiac-specific troponin is the preferred marker, and if available, it should be measured in all patients.
  - Troponin T or I levels increase 3–12 hours after the onset of MI and peak at 24–48 hours, then return to baseline over 5–14 days.
  - The risk of subsequent cardiac death is directly proportional to the increase in cardiac-specific troponin.
- CK-MB is also acceptable but its use is limited due to lack of specificity.
- Myoglobin is not cardiac specific but is released more rapidly from infarcted myocardium than CK-MB or the troponins.
  - It may be detected as early as 2 hours after the onset of myocardial necrosis.
  - The diagnosis of MI is limited by the brief duration of its elevation (<24 hours) and by its lack of cardiac specificity.
- C-reactive protein levels may aid in initial risk assessment in ACS patients. Elevated CRP levels may reflect inflammation of noncardiovascular origin (infections).

Classification and Risk Stratification
- The diagnosis of UA confers a 10%–20% risk of progression to acute MI in the untreated patient. Medical treatment reduces the risk of progression to 5%–7%.
- The choice of clinical testing and pharmacologic treatment, and the timing of possible invasive therapy, can be guided, in part, by the severity of the patient's risk. The higher the risk, the more aggressive the approach to care should be (Table 5-6).

TABLE 5-6	Risk Assessment in Patients Presenting with Acute Coronary Syndrome		
Feature	High risk (at least one of the following)	Intermediate risk (no high-risk features, but at least one of the following)	Low risk (no high- or intermediate-risk features but may have any of the following)
Clinical history	—	Prior MI, peripheral or cerebrovascular disease, CABG, or prior aspirin use	—
Characteristic of pain	Prolonged ongoing (<30 min) rest pain	Prolonged (>20 min) rest angina, now resolved, with moderate or high likelihood of CAD; rest angina (<20 min) or relieved with rest or SL-TNG	New-onset or progressive angina in the past 2 wk with moderate or high likelihood of CAD
Clinical findings	Pulmonary edema; new or worsening MR murmur; S$_3$, or new or worsening rales; hypotension, bradycardia, or tachycardia; age >75 yr	Age >70 yr	—
ECG	Angina at rest with transient ST changes >0.05 mV; new (or presumed new) bundle branch block; sustained ventricular tachycardia	T-wave inversions >0.02 mV; pathologic Q waves	Normal or unchanged ECG during an episode of angina
Biochemical cardiac markers	Elevated (troponin or CK-MB)	Borderline elevated (troponin or CK-MB)	Normal

CABG, coronary artery bypass graft; CAD, coronary artery disease; CK-MB, creatine kinase MB; ECG, electrocardiogram; MI, myocardial infarction; MR, magnetic resonance; SL-TNG, sublingual nitroglycerin. *Source:* Adapted with permission from Braunwald E, Antman EM, Beasley JW, et al. ACC/AHA guidelines for the management of patients with unstable angina and nonST-segment elevation myocardial infarction: executive summary and recommendations. A report of the American College of Cardiology/American Heart Association task force on practice guidelines (committee on the management of patients with unstable angina). *Circulation* 2000;102:1193.

- Patients at highest risk for progression include those with:
    - Rest angina
    - Associated labile ischemic ECG changes (ST-segment deviations or T-wave inversions)
    - Continued symptoms despite initiation of medical therapy
    - Thrombolysis in Myocardial Infarction (TIMI) risk score >6
- The TIMI risk score can be used to determine the patient's short-term risk of death or nonfatal MI. Antman et al. developed the seven-point TIMI risk score. Patients can be classified as low, intermediate, or high risk on the basis of their clinical profile (Fig. 5-1).
    - Low-risk patients may be initially observed in a facility with cardiac monitoring (chest pain or observation unit).
        - If the patient remains pain free and a subsequent ECG cardiac marker at 6–12 hours is normal, a stress test to provoke ischemia can be performed.
        - Low-risk patients with a negative stress test can be managed as outpatients.

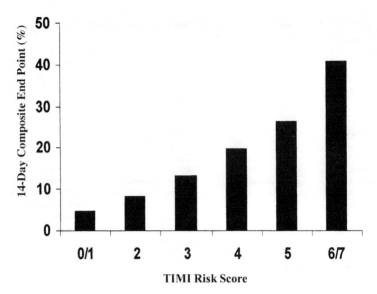

Figure 5-1. Effect of Thrombolysis in Myocardial Infarction (TIMI) risk score on cardiovascular events. Rate of death, myocardial infarction, or urgent revascularization after presentation with acute coronary syndromes. TIMI risk factors include (a) age >65 years, (b) three coronary artery disease (CAD) risk factors, (c) known CAD, (d) ST-segment deviation, (e) severe angina, (f) acetylsalicylic acid (ASA) use in the past, and (f) positive cardiac enzyme. (Adapted with permission from Antman EM, Cohen M, Bernink PJ, et al. The TIMI risk score for unstable angina/non-ST elevation MI: a method for prognostication and therapeutic decision making. *JAMA* 2000;284:835–842. Copyrighted 2000, American Medical Association.)

- Low-risk patients with a positive stress test should have management with medication and invasive testing individualized based on clinical status and the severity of the ischemic burden.
- Intermediate- and high-risk patients should be admitted to the hospital for observation and management. The choice between admission to the intensive care unit or a high-risk cardiac ward depends on the patient's clinical course. If the patient is rendered pain free with pharmacotherapy, he or she does not necessarily need intensive care unit (ICU) monitoring and the decision to proceed with noninvasive versus invasive testing must be made (see "Treatment").
- Patients with ongoing symptoms should be admitted to the ICU for more aggressive intervention and should be treated with anti-ischemic therapies and, if necessary, urgent cardiac catheterization with the goal of reperfusion of the culprit coronary lesion(s).

Treatment

Goals of Therapy
The primary goals of therapy for UA/NSTEMI are the prevention of thrombus, restoration of coronary flow, and reduction in myocardial oxygen demand.

Early Conservative Versus Invasive Strategies
Two different strategies have evolved for patients with UA/NSTEMI.

- **Early conservative strategy.** The patient is treated with medical therapy at maximally tolerated doses and coronary angiography is reserved for patients with evidence of recurrent ischemia or a strongly positive stress test, despite medical therapy. Although the choice should always be individualized to a particular patient, in general an early conservative approach can be used in low-risk patients and selected intermediate-risk patients without adverse effects on clinical outcomes.

■ **Early invasive strategy.** Patients are routinely recommended for coronary angiography and subsequent revascularization, as warranted. High-risk patients, including those with recurrent ischemia on medical therapy, evidence of congestive heart failure, LV dysfunction, sustained ventricular tachycardia (VT), or prior coronary revascularization (PCI within 6 months or CABG), are best assessed with an early invasive approach. Angiography in these individuals defines the anatomy and directs the choice of revascularization options, if appropriate.

   ▪ An early invasive strategy is also warranted in low- or intermediate-risk patients with repeated ACS presentations despite therapy. Cardiac catheterization of these patients provides a convenient approach to distinguish between those with no significant coronary disease and those with anatomy that is amenable to revascularization.

Medications

The goal of pharmacologic treatment is to provide relief of ischemia and prevent serious adverse outcomes (death or MI).

■ This approach should include anti-ischemia, antiplatelet, and anticoagulant (antithrombotic) therapies.

■ As with patients with ST-elevation MI, those with an UA/NSTEMI should be restricted to bedrest and be provided with supplemental oxygen and morphine (for adequate control of pain and anxiety).

Antiplatelet Therapy

■ All patients should receive **aspirin** unless a contraindication exists. Aspirin reduces subsequent MI and cardiac death in patients with unstable angina. Although doses as low as 75 mg/d have been used, the current AHA/ACC recommendation is 160–325 mg/d starting at the time of presentation and continued indefinitely.

■ **Clopidogrel** (75 mg/d) can be used in patients who are intolerant or allergic to aspirin.

   ▪ Clopidogrel (300-mg loading dose, then 75 mg/d) in addition to aspirin decreases the composite end point of cardiovascular death, MI, or stroke from 11.5%–9.3%.

   ▪ The optimal time to initiate clopidogrel therapy should factor in the risk of surgical disease as use of clopidogrel may result in delay or complications with CABG if urgent surgical intervention was required.

   ▪ A minimum of 1 month of therapy should be given if medical or percutaneous treatment is expected and can be continued for up to one year or longer.

■ The use of a **glycoprotein (GP) IIb/IIIa antagonist** (e.g., abciximab, eptifibatide, or tirofiban) should also be considered for high-risk patients (Table 5-7).

   ▪ If early catheterization and PCI are planned, any of the agents can be used.

   ▪ If the plan for management does not involve an early invasive strategy, one of the small-molecule GP IIb/IIIa antagonists (eptifibatide or tirofiban) should be used.

   ▪ GP IIb/IIIa antagonists should be used in conjunction with therapeutically dosed heparin, either unfractionated heparin (UFH) or enoxaparin.

Anticoagulant Therapy

■ Anticoagulant therapy is a key component of the antithrombotic management of patients with ACS. Treatment with heparin has been shown to reduce the early rate of death or MI by up to 60%.

■ **Enoxaparin** [low molecular weight heparin (LMWH), 1 mg/kg bid SC] or **intravenous UFH** (loading dose of 60 units/kg followed by a maintenance infusion of 12 units/kg/hr with a maximum of 5,000 units/hr and 1,000 units/hr, respectively) can be used.

   ▪ The activated partial thromboplastin time (aPTT) should be adjusted to maintain a value of 1.5–2.0 times control (50–70 seconds) for UFH therapy.

TABLE 5-7	Platelet Glycoprotein IIb/IIIa Receptor Inhibitors in Acute Coronary Syndromes		
	Abciximab	**Eptifibatide**	**Tirofiban**
Drug type	Monoclonal antibody	Cyclic heptapeptide	Nonpeptide small molecule
Dosage	0.25-mg/kg IV bolus, then 0.125 mcg/kg/min (max 10 mcg/min) · 12 hr (for ACS and planned PCI)	180-mcg/kg bolus, then 2 mcg/kg/min · 24–48 hr	0.4 mcg/kg/min for 30 min, then 0.1 mcg/kg/min × 24–48 hr
Metabolism/ excretion	Cellular catabolism	Renal excretion (dosage should be adjusted for patients with a serum creatinine >2.0)	Renal excretion (dosage should be adjusted for patients with a serum creatinine clearance <30 mL/min)
Recovery of platelet inhibition	48–96 hr	4–6 hr	4–6 hr
Reversibility	Platelet transfusion	None	None

ACS, acute coronary syndrome; PCI, percutaneous coronary intervention.
Note: Contraindications to glycoprotein IIb/IIIa receptor inhibition include a history of bleeding diathesis or active bleeding within the previous 30 days (2 years for abciximab), major surgery within the previous 6 weeks, a history of stroke, severe hypertension, platelet count <100,000, or international normalized ratio >1.2. All patients should be monitored for thrombocytopenia every 68 hours while receiving a glycoprotein IIb/IIIa inhibitor. All patients should receive weight-adjusted heparin therapy (unfractionated or low molecular weight [enoxaparin]).

- LMWH is easier to dose and does not require monitoring for clinical effect. However, if cardiac catheterization is planned, then the dose should be withheld on the morning of procedure.
- Thus far, enoxaparin is the only LMWH that has been shown to confer greater cardiac benefit than UFH in the ACS patient.
- **Heparin-induced thrombocytopenia** (HIT) develops in approximately 1%–3% of patients receiving heparin. Platelet counts usually drop after 5–7 days of therapy. If this occurs, the heparin should be discontinued, and if additional anticoagulation is needed, **lepirudin** can be used and is administered as a 0.4-mg/kg bolus IV (maximum, 44 mg) and then continuously infused at 0.15 mg/kg/hr. A dose reduction is required in renal impairment.

Anti-Ischemic Therapy
- **Nitroglycerin** reduces myocardial oxygen demand while enhancing myocardial oxygen delivery. The choice of preparation depends on the acuity of the patient's symptoms.
  - Nitroglycerin use is contraindicated in the presence of hypotension or if the patient has used a phosphodiesterase inhibitor [e.g., sildenafil (Viagra)] within the previous 24 hours.
  - Treatment can be initiated at the time of presentation with sublingual nitroglycerin (spray or tablets, 0.4 mg every 5 minutes for a total of three doses).
  - If the patient is clinically stable, topical or oral preparations can be used (Table 5-4).
  - Less stable patients, or those who require additional agents to control significant hypertension, should be treated with intravenous nitroglycerin (10 mcg/min, titrated up by 10–20 g/min every 3–5 minutes until pain relief, hypertension control, or both are achieved).
  - Significant antianginal effects are not seen above 200 mcg/min, but doses of up to 400 mcg/min can be used, if necessary, for BP control.

- β-**Adrenergic blockers** should be started early in the absence of contraindications. In high-risk patients, intravenous, followed by oral, preparations can be used (Table 5-2). Treatment with only an oral preparation is acceptable in intermediate- and low-risk patients.
  - The initial choice of agents includes metoprolol, atenolol, and propranolol. Esmolol can be used if a short-acting agent is required.
  - After the patient has stabilized and proved an ability to tolerate beta-blocker therapy, conversion to a long-acting agent can be considered.
- **Calcium channel antagonists** vary in the degree to which they produce decreased myocardial contractility, peripheral vasodilation, atrioventricular (AV) block, and a slowing of sinus node activity.
  - Nifedipine, diltiazem, verapamil, and amlodipine appear to have similar coronary dilatory properties.
  - Calcium antagonists can be used to control ongoing or recurrent ischemia if patients are either intolerant of or inadequately managed by beta-blocker therapy.
    - Short-acting nifedipine preparations must be avoided in the absence of adequate concurrent beta-blockade because of increased adverse outcomes with this medication.
    - Verapamil and diltiazem should be avoided in patients with evidence of severe LV dysfunction or pulmonary congestion (Table 5-3).
- **ACE inhibitors** are effective antihypertensive agents. Ischemia relief may be facilitated by this mechanism if hypotension or concerns of renal dysfunction do not preclude the use of these agents.
  - ACE inhibitors have been shown to reduce mortality in patients with MI and LV systolic dysfunction, particularly the diabetic population. These agents may also have mortality benefit in high-risk patients with normal systolic function.
- **Thrombolytic therapy** is not indicated in UA/NSTEMI.

Revascularization
In general, the indications for PCI and CABG in patients with UA/NSTEMI are similar to those for individuals with stable angina.

- Patients who are optimally managed with CABG include those with:
  - Significant left main CAD
  - Three-vessel disease and abnormal LV function (ejection fraction <50%)
  - Two-vessel disease with a significant proximal left anterior descending artery stenosis and abnormal LV function on noninvasive testing
  - Diabetes and multivessel disease
- The remaining patients with coronary disease requiring revascularization can be treated with CABG or PCI. Patients who are treated with CABG tend to have a lower incidence of angina and less need for subsequent revascularization, but there is no difference in the rates of cardiac death or MI between the two treatment strategies.

Risk Factor Modification
- Risk factor modification is addressed in detail in the section on STEMI and should include attention to smoking cessation, weight loss, exercise, and control of hypertension, diabetes, and hyperlipidemia, as warranted.

Follow-Up
- It is incumbent on the entire hospital staff (physicians, nurses, dietitians, pharmacists, and rehabilitation specialists) to prepare the patient for hospital discharge. The patient should be discharged on a medical regimen, as tolerated, to take advantage of proven methods of secondary prevention. The patient should also be provided a sublingual or spray formulation of nitroglycerin and instructed on its appropriate use.
- Arrangements for follow-up care should also be established before hospital discharge.

Complications
- The highest rate of progression to MI or development of recurrent MI is in the first 2 months after presentation with the index episode. Beyond that time point, most patients have a clinical course similar to those with chronic stable angina.

ST-SEGMENT ELEVATION MYOCARDIAL INFARCTION

General Principles
- STEMI is a medical emergency caused by the formation of an occluding thrombus over a ruptured atherosclerotic plaque in the coronary circulation.
- Over the past four decades, there has been a dramatic improvement in short-term mortality to the current rate of 6%–10%.
- Half of these deaths occur within the first hour of symptom initiation and are due to ventricular fibrillation. They can be markedly reduced if patients are transported to the hospital expeditiously for prompt reperfusion therapy, arrhythmia detection, and treatment. Transport to the emergency room should be done preferentially by ambulance in order to expedite triage and facilitate treatment.

Diagnosis

Criteria
- STEMI requires the presence of at least two of the following criteria:
  - History of prolonged chest discomfort or anginal equivalent (30 minutes)
  - Presence of ≥ 1 mm ST-segment elevation in two consecutive ECG leads
  - Presence of elevated cardiac biomarkers

History
- Chest pain from STEMI resembles angina, but lasts longer, is more intense, is not relieved by rest or sublingual nitroglycerin, and is accompanied by dyspnea, diaphoresis, palpitations, nausea, vomiting, fatigue, or syncope.
- STEMI may occur without chest discomfort in the elderly, hypertensive, diabetic, or postoperative patient. These patients may present with confusion, dyspnea, and exacerbation of congestive heart failure or unexplained hypotension.

Physical Examination
Physical examination should be directed at identifying hemodynamic instability and pulmonary congestion.

- The identification of a new systolic murmur may suggest the presence of ischemic mitral regurgitation or a ventricular septal defect.
- A limited neurologic exam to detect baseline cognitive and motor deficits and a vascular examination (lower extremity pulses and bruits) will aid in determining the candidacy for reperfusion treatment.
- Cardiogenic shock due to right ventricular myocardial infarction (RVMI) complicates inferior/posterior myocardial infarction and can be clinically suspected by the presence of hypotension, elevated jugular venous pressure, and absence of pulmonary congestion.

Clinical Stratification on Initial Presentation
- Patients with acute STEMI are stratified into low- or high-risk groups on the basis of their initial physical exam.
  - Those without pulmonary congestion or shock (Killip class I) have a mortality rate of <5%.
  - Patients with mild pulmonary congestion and/or the presence of S_3 (Killip class II) have a favorable prognosis.
  - Patients with pulmonary edema (Killip class III) often have extensive LV dysfunction and require aggressive management.

▨ Hypotensive patients with evidence of shock (Killip class IV) have a mortality that approaches 80% unless the cause of shock can be reversed.

Diagnostic Evaluation

ECG should be obtained promptly. If the diagnosis of STEMI is in doubt, serial ECG may elucidate the diagnosis.

- **T waves.** Peaked upright T waves may be the first ECG manifestation of myocardial ischemia.
- **ST-segment changes**
  - ▨ Convex ST-segment elevation ≥1 mm in two consecutive leads with peaked or inverted T waves usually is indicative of myocardial injury.
  - ▨ Posterior wall myocardial infarction is recognized by ST-segment depression in leads V_1–V_3 and is treated like a STEMI.
  - ▨ RVMI is diagnosed with ST-segment elevation in lead V_4R.
- **Q waves.** Development of new pathologic Q waves (>40 ms) is considered diagnostic for MI, but may occur in patients with prolonged ischemia.
- Infarction of the left circumflex territory may be electrocardiographically silent.
- **ECG changes that mimic MI.** ST-segment elevation and Q waves may result from pre-excitation, pericarditis, myocarditis, cardiomyopathy, COPD, pulmonary embolism, cholecystitis, and hyperkalemia.

Laboratory Studies

Blood samples should be sent for cardiac enzymes (troponin-I, CK-MB) complete blood count, coagulation studies [PTT, prothrombin time (PT), international normalized ratio (INR)], creatinine, electrolytes including magnesium, and type and screen. Fasting lipid profile should be obtained in all patients with STEMI for secondary prevention (see Dyslipidemia).

- **Cardiac-specific troponin I (cTnI) or troponin T (cTnT)** is the preferred biomarker for the diagnosis of STEMI.
  - ▨ In patients with acute ischemic syndromes, the risk of subsequent cardiac death is directly proportional to the increase in cardiac-specific troponins, even when CK-MB levels are not elevated.
  - ▨ Serum levels of cTnI and cTnT increase 3–12 hours after onset of MI, peak at 24–48 hours, and return to baseline over 5–14 days.
- **Creatinine kinase** (CK-MB) has >95% sensitivity and specificity for myocardial injury when measured 24–36 hours after the onset of chest pain.
  - ▨ In MI, levels increase within 3–12 hours of chest pain, peak at 24 hours, and return to baseline after 48–72 hours.
  - ▨ Increased CK-MB not caused by MI occurs infrequently as a result of release from noncardiac source, diminished clearance, or cross reactivity of some assays with CK-BB.
  - ▨ CK-MB is useful to detect small postprocedural infarctions.
- **Myoglobin** is not cardiac specific. It is the first protein to be detected in patients presenting with MI and can be detected as early as 2 hours. Myoglobin is invariably elevated in patients with end-stage renal disease and has a lower diagnostic yield in this population.
- **Use of cardiac enzymes.** Cardiac-specific troponins can be measured on admission and after 12 hours; if these are positive, CK-MB can be measured, if necessary, to confirm that the MI occurred within the previous 48 hours. Troponins should be measured daily until the peak level has been reached to determine the extent of myocardial damage. CK and CK-MB levels can be made on hospital admission, at 8–12 hours, and at 16–24 hours.
- **Routine use of cardiac noninvasive imaging** is not recommended for the initial diagnosis of STEMI. When the diagnosis is in question, a transthoracic echocardiogram can be performed to document regional wall motion abnormalities.
- A **portable chest radiograph** is useful to exclude other causes of chest pain, but it should not delay the initiation of reperfusion therapy.

Treatment

Acute Management

Since mortality and worsening LV function is directly related to the ischemic time, prompt treatment should be initiated as soon as the diagnosis is suspected.

- **Before presentation to the hospital.** The general public should be informed of the signs and symptoms consistent with an acute MI that should lead them to seek urgent medical care. Availability of "911" access and emergency medical services facilitates delivery of patients to emergency medical care.
- **Once in the emergency department,** care using an acute MI protocol should yield a targeted clinical examination and a 12-lead ECG within 10 minutes and an initial triage management plan shortly thereafter.
- **Immediate management.** The goal of immediate management in patients with STEMI is to identify candidates for reperfusion therapy.
  - Patients with ST elevation >1 mm in at least two contiguous leads or a new left bundle branch block that present within 12 hours of initiation of symptoms should be evaluated for PCI or fibrinolytic therapy.
    - The goal is a door-to-needle time of <30 minutes or door-to-balloon time of <90 minutes.
  - **Other priorities** include:
    - Relieve ischemic pain.
    - Provide supplemental oxygen.
    - Recognize and treat potential life-threatening complications like hypotension, pulmonary edema, and arrhythmia.
  - **General measures** include:
    - Continuous ECG, blood pressure, and pulse oximetry monitoring
      - Supplemental oxygen should be added if saturations are <90%. It is reasonable to administer supplemental oxygen for the first 6 hours of noncomplicated STEMI.
      - Institution of mechanical ventilation, when necessary, decreases the work of breathing and reduces myocardial oxygen demand.
    - Placement of two functioning IV lines while obtaining blood samples (see above) should follow.
    - Serial ECGs should be performed if the chest discomfort continues in patients who do not have ST-segment elevation on the initial ECG, as ST-segment elevation may develop.
    - Aggressive treatment of hypotension by volume expansion should be undertaken if necessary in volume depletion, RVMI, or cardiogenic shock.
  - **Coronary care unit (CCU)** use was the first major advance in the modern era of treatment of acute MI. The majority of patients benefit from the specialized training of the nursing and support staff in the CCU. Although there is a subset of patients with an uncomplicated MI who can be triaged initially to an intermediate level of care, most patients with acute MI should be observed for at least the first 12–24 hours in the CCU.

Medications

Antiplatelet Therapy

- **Aspirin** reduces mortality for all patients with MI. All patients who are not already receiving daily aspirin should be given 162–325 mg of non–enteric-coated aspirin, chewed in order to enhance absorption, and continued indefinitely on a daily basis (81–325 mg).
- **Clopidogrel** 75 mg/d can be substituted for true aspirin allergy.
- **GP IIb/IIIa inhibitors** are not indicated in the setting of STEMI unless they are used as an adjunctive to PCI.

Anticoagulation

- Anticoagulation should be started on all patients except those who receive nonselective fibrinolytic agents (see below) or those with a contraindication to heparin therapy.
- UFH should be initiated in all patients with MI who receive selective fibrinolytic agents (alteplase, reteplase, or tenecteplase) as an initial bolus of 60 units/kg (maximum of 5,000 units) followed by an infusion of 12 units/kg/hr (maximum of 1,000 units/hr) to keep a PTT of 1.5–2 times control.
- UFH should be given intravenously to patients treated with nonselective fibrinolytic agents (streptokinase, urokinase, anistreplase) who are at high risk for systemic embolization (atrial fibrillation, LV thrombus, large anterior MI), initiated 6 hours after the administration of the fibrinolytic.
- IV UFH or low molecular weight heparin (enoxaparin 1 mg/kg bid) can be used in patients who are committed to medical therapy or percutaneous revascularization.
  - After 48 hours the decision to continue anticoagulation will depend on individual patient's needs.

Antianginal Therapy

- Nitrates
  - Nitroglycerin should be administered to most patients with ischemic chest pain. Administration of nitroglycerin should be avoided in patients with the following:
    - Hypotension (systolic blood pressure <90 mm Hg)
    - Right ventricular MI
    - Tachycardia (>100 bpm) or bradycardia (<50 bpm)
    - Documented use of phosphodiesterase inhibitors (e.g., sildenafil)
  - Sublingual nitroglycerin 0.4 mg can be given every 5 minutes for a total of three doses in the absence of hypotension.
  - If the angina is not controlled, IV nitroglycerin drip at 10 mcg/min should be initiated. Dose titration may be performed in increments of 10 mcg/min every 5 minutes until chest pain resolves or the heart rate increases or BP decreases more than 10% from baseline.
- β-adrenergic blockade
  - β-adrenergic blockers reduce myocardial ischemia and may limit infarct size.
  - Therapy can be initiated with IV metoprolol (5 mg), which can be repeated every 5 minutes for three doses. Patients who tolerate this therapy can then be started on an oral agent (metoprolol 25–50 mg q6–12h).
  - Administration of beta-blockers should be avoided in patients with the following:
    - Clinical evidence of heart failure
    - Hypotension with a systolic blood pressure <90 mm Hg
    - Heart rate <60 bpm
    - Marked first-degree AV block (PR interval >250 ms)
    - Advanced heart block
    - Significant bronchospastic lung disease
  - Although no data have demonstrated the mortality benefit of esmolol, its short half-life (9 minutes) makes this agent useful in patients at high risk for beta-blocker therapy. If treatment with esmolol is successful, continued therapy with an oral agent is also likely tolerated.
- Atropine
  - Atropine (0.5 mg IV) can be used to treat symptomatic sinus bradycardia, or if the bradycardia is associated with low cardiac output, peripheral hypoperfusion, or AV block at or above the level of the AV node.
- Morphine sulfate
  - Adequate analgesia decreases levels of circulating catecholamines and reduces myocardial oxygen consumption. Morphine sulfate causes venodilation, which decreases preload and arterial vasodilation and has a vagotonic effect that decreases heart rate.

- It is given at a dose of 2–4 mg IV and may be repeated every 5 minutes until pain disappears or side effects ensue.
- **Other**
  - Nausea and vomiting can be treated with an antiemetic agent.
  - Magnesium and calcium channel blockers are not currently recommended in the setting of acute MI.

ACUTE CORONARY REPERFUSION

- Approximately 90% of patients with an acute MI and ST-segment elevation have a thrombotic occlusion of the infarct-related coronary artery. Early restoration of flow down the vessel limits infarct size, preserves LV function, and reduces mortality.
  - Unless spontaneous resolution of the infarction occurs (as determined by dissipation of angina and normalization of the ischemic changes on the ECG), the choices of reperfusion strategies include (a) thrombolytic therapy, (b) primary PCI, or (c) emergent CABG.
  - The choice of therapy is influenced by the duration of symptoms, the anatomic localization of the infarct, the presence of comorbid illnesses, and the rapid availability of a cardiac catheterization laboratory with qualified staff.
- **Thrombolytic therapy** (Table 5-8) offers the advantages of availability and rapid administration. The primary disadvantage of thrombolytic therapy is the risk of intracranial hemorrhage (0.7%–0.9%) and the uncertainty of whether normal coronary flow has been restored to the infarct-related artery.
  - Thrombolytic therapy should be considered in patients with ST-segment elevation in two or more contiguous ECG leads.
  - It is most effective if given within 12 hours of the onset of symptoms but can be administered for up to, but not beyond, 24 hours.
  - Thrombolytic therapy is ***not indicated*** if the symptoms have resolved or for patients with ST-segment depression on the presenting ECG.
  - **Contraindications** to thrombolytic therapy may be relative or absolute (Table 5-9). The risk of intracranial hemorrhage is increased twofold in the elderly (>75 years old), in those who weigh <70 kg, and in those with severe hypertension.
    - In patients with a relative contraindication to thrombolytic therapy, the decision to treat should be individualized, assessing the risk of bleeding with the risk of MI complications.
  - *Streptokinase* is a nonselective agent that induces a generalized fibrinolytic state characterized by extensive fibrinogen degradation. It is administered as an IV infusion of 1.5 million units over 60 minutes.
    - Allergic reactions (skin rashes and fever) may be seen in 1%–2% of patients.
    - Hypotension occurs in 10% of patients and usually responds to volume expansion.

TABLE 5-8	**Doses of Thrombolytic Agents for Myocardial Infarction**

Agents with fibrin specificity

Alteplase (rt-PA): IV bolus of 15 mg, followed by 0.75 mg/kg (up to 50 mg) by IV infusion over 30 min, then 0.5 mg/kg (up to 35 mg) by IV infusion over 60 min; maximum dose: 100 mg IV over 90 min

Reteplase (r-PA): IV bolus of 10 mg over 2 min, followed by another IV bolus of 10 units after 30 min

Tenecteplase (TNK-tPA): IV bolus of 0.5 mg/kg; ≤60 kg = 30 mg; 61–70 kg = 35 mg; 71–80 kg = 40 mg; 81–90 kg = 45 mg; ≥90 kg = 50 mg

Agents without fibrin specificity

Streptokinase (SK): IV infusion of 1.5 million units over 60 min

TABLE 5-9   **Contraindications to Thrombolytic Therapy**

Absolute contraindications	Relative contraindications
History of intracranial hemorrhage	Allergy or previous use (>5 d ago) of
Known structural cerebrovascular lesion (AVMs,	streptokinase or anistreplase
aneurysms)	Active peptic ulcer disease
Known intracranial tumor	Noncompressible vascular punctures
Ischemic stroke <3 mo	Internal bleeding (2–4 wk)
Aortic dissection	Prior ischemic stroke >3 mo
Trauma within 3 months	Prolonged/traumatic CPR >10 min
Severe uncontrolled hypertension (SBP	Major surgery <3 wk
>180 mm Hg, DBP >110 mm Hg)	Severe menstrual bleeding
Bleeding diathesis	History of intraocular bleeding
Acute pericarditis	
Aortic dissection	
History of hemorrhagic stroke	
Pregnancy	

AVM, arteriovenous malformation; CPR, cardiopulmonary resuscitation; DBP, diastolic blood pressure; SBP, systolic blood pressure.

- Allergic reactions and severe hypotension are treated as anaphylactic reactions, with IV antihistamines and steroids.
- Because of the development of antibodies, patients who were previously treated with streptokinase should be given an alternate thrombolytic agent if such treatment is warranted.
- ■ *Selective fibrinolytic agents*
  - **Recombinant tissue-plasminogen activator** (rt-PA) is more clot selective than streptokinase and does not cause allergic reactions or hypotension. rt-PA is administered as an IV bolus of 15 mg followed by an IV infusion of 0.75 mg/kg (up to 50 mg) over 30 minutes, then 0.5 mg/kg (up to 35 mg) by IV infusion over 60 minutes.
  - **Reteplase** (r-PA) has reduced fibrin specificity but a longer half-life than does rt-PA, permitting bolus administration. r-PA resulted in a similar decrease in mortality when compared to streptokinase and rt-PA in randomized trials. The initial dose is 10 units by IV bolus, with a second 10-unit bolus administered 30 minutes later.
  - **Tenecteplase** (TNK-tPA) is a genetically engineered variant of rt-PA with slower plasma clearance, better fibrin specificity, and high resistance to plasminogen-activator inhibitor-1, allowing single-bolus administration. When compared to rt-PA, TNK-tPA had a similar decrease in mortality in randomized trials. However, the incidence of mild to moderate bleeding was less in patients who received TNK-tPA. Dosing is approximately 0.5 mg/kg IV, with minimum and maximum doses of 30 and 50 mg, respectively.
  - **Heparin** is used as adjunctive therapy for all of the selective fibrinolytic agents.
  - The **choice of thrombolytic agent** is guided by considerations of cost, efficacy, and ease of administration.
    - rt-PA, r-PA, and TNK-tPA are more expensive than streptokinase. Compared with streptokinase, rt-PA is associated with a slightly greater risk of intracranial hemorrhage but offers the net clinical benefit of an additional 10 lives saved per 1,000 patients treated.
- ■ The **therapeutic efficacy** of thrombolytic treatment can be monitored by clinical response (resolution of chest pain), by improvement in ST-segment elevation, or by the presence of accelerated idioventricular rhythm on the ECG.

■ Individuals with persistent angina or persistent ischemic changes on the ECG (<50% reduction in ST-segment elevation) at 60–90 minutes after the initiation of fibrinolytic therapy should be considered for urgent coronary angiography and rescue PCI.

■ **Bleeding complications** are the most common adverse effect of thrombolytic therapy.
  • Venipuncture should be limited and arterial puncture avoided in patients treated with thrombolytic therapy for 24 hours after the initiation of treatment.
  • Major bleeding complications that require blood transfusion occur in approximately 10% of patients.
  • **Intracranial hemorrhage** is the most dreaded complication and generally results in death or permanent disability. In patients who experience a sudden change in neurologic status, anticoagulant and thrombolytic therapies should be terminated and evaluation with an urgent head CT scan should be undertaken. In patients who hemorrhage, fresh frozen plasma can be given to reverse the lytic state. Cryoprecipitate can also be used to replenish fibrinogen and factor VIII levels. Because platelet dysfunction often accompanies the lytic state, platelet transfusions may be useful in patients with markedly prolonged bleeding times. Neurologic and neurosurgical consultation should be obtained in a timely manner.

■ **Primary PCI** is an alternative to thrombolytic therapy in patients with acute MI and ST-segment elevation or new (or presumed new) LBBB.
  ■ Primary PCI results in mechanical reperfusion of a thrombosed coronary vessel with normal arterial flow (TIMI 3) in >95% of patients with ST-segment elevation MI.
  ■ Other advantages of primary PCI are immediate assessment of LV function and identification of other diseased vessels.
  ■ Primary PCI should be considered when a catheterization facility with experienced staff can anticipate providing a door-to-balloon time of <90 minutes.
  ■ Treatment is optimal when the angioplasty is performed within 12 hours of symptom onset but is effective beyond that point if symptoms persist.
  ■ PCI should be considered in patients with contraindications to thrombolytic therapy or those in whom cardiogenic shock develops within 36 hours of presentation with acute MI.
  ■ If the patient has **multivessel coronary disease,** the decision to revascularize the non-infarct-related arteries can be made after he or she has been stabilized.
    • In general, the approach to this question can be similar to that of patients with stable coronary disease. The functional significance of the lesion can be assessed by noninvasive testing and the vessel treated, if appropriate. Alternatively, the lesion can be treated empirically (without a prior noninvasive evaluation) if this is warranted in the judgment of the interventional cardiologist.

■ The **choice of therapy** between thrombolysis and PCI should almost be considered of secondary importance to the imperative of the overall goal of achieving reperfusion in a timely fashion with pharmacologic or mechanical intervention. The morbidity and mortality associated with an acute MI is linearly related to the time to treatment.
  ■ In general, primary PCI has been shown to result in improved outcomes compared with thrombolytic therapy, regardless of the anatomic distribution of the infarction or the age of the patient.
  ■ Preliminary data indicate that the added benefit of PCI is also present in patients who can be transferred emergently from a community hospital to a tertiary care center with catheterization facilities.
  ■ Facilitated PCI, a strategy of reduced dose of thrombolytic agent combined with PCI, is not currently recommended.
  ■ PCI is preferred over thrombolysis in patients who:
    • Are <75 years of age and present with cardiogenic shock within 36 hours of MI and PCI can be performed within 18 hours of shock
    • Have a contraindication to fibrinolytic therapy
    • Are at high risk of death or development of CHF
    • Underwent recent PCI or are post-CABG
  ■ **Thrombolysis** may be preferred if patients are presenting to the hospital within the first 2 hours of symptom onset.

- **Emergency CABG** is a high-risk procedure that should be considered only if the patient has refractory ischemia or cardiogenic shock and the coronary vasculature is not amenable to PCI or the procedure has failed.
- Emergency surgery should also be considered for patients with acute mechanical complications of MI, including papillary muscle rupture, ventricular septal defect (VSD), ventricular aneurysm formation in the setting of intractable ventricular arrhythmias or pump failure, or ventricular free wall rupture.

Special Clinical Situations

- **Intra-aortic balloon counterpulsation** should be considered in patients who are experiencing cardiogenic shock or hemodynamic instability.
    - It can be used as a stabilizing measure before cardiac catheterization and presumed revascularization, or in patients who have experienced a mechanical complication of MI, such as a VSD or acute mitral regurgitation due to papillary muscle rupture, before definitive surgical repair.
    - It is contraindicated in patients with peripheral vascular disease and aortic insufficiency.
    - Daily evaluation of lower extremities for ischemic/embolic complications and determination of platelet counts and serum creatinine should be obtained while the balloon pump is in place.
- **STEMI** in the setting of recent **cocaine use** presents a unique and challenging management situation. ST elevation can result from myocardial ischemia due to increased heart rate, blood pressure and oxygen demand, coronary vasospasm, in situ thrombus formation, or a combination of these factors.
    - Oxygen and aspirin should be administered to all patients with cocaine-associated STEMI.
    - Nitrates should be used preferentially to treat vasospasm. Additionally, benzodiazepines may confer additional relief by decreasing sympathetic tone.
        - β-Adrenergic blockers are contraindicated in these patients due to the potential for unopposed α-adrenergic activity.
    - **Phentolamine**, an α-adrenergic antagonist, may reverse coronary vasospasm and is recommended as a second-line agent.
    - The use of and choice of reperfusion therapy is controversial and should be reserved for those patients whose symptoms persist despite initial medical therapy.
        - Thrombolysis should be avoided unless its perceived benefits far outweigh the risks. Close attention should be paid to contraindications (both relative and absolute) in this population.
        - Primary angioplasty appears preferable for the patient with persistent symptoms and ECG changes, although the significant risk of coronary vasospasm makes its use somewhat less attractive as well.

Peri-Infarct Management

- **Bedrest** is appropriate intermediate care for the first 24 hours after presentation with an acute MI.
    - Bedside commode privileges are acceptable in hemodynamically stable patients if they are free of anginal symptoms.
    - Patients should be cautioned to avoid the Valsalva maneuver, which may predispose to ventricular arrhythmias. Stool softeners decrease the prevalence of unnecessary Valsalva maneuvers.
    - After 24 hours, clinically stable patients can progressively advance their activity with sitting, assisted bathing, standing, and finally walking, as tolerated.
- **Pain relief** and treatment of **anxiety** should be provided, as required.
- **Hemodynamic monitoring** may be useful to assess ambiguous clinical data or optimize medical therapy.
- **Cardiac pacing** may be required in the setting of an acute MI. Rhythm disturbance may be transient in nature, in which case temporary pacing is sufficient until a stable rhythm returns.

- **Transcutaneous patches** can be used if the need for pacing is anticipated but not required. The transcutaneous system may be associated with significant pain and appropriate analgesia should be administered.
- Patients at high risk or who have proven to have a need for pacing should receive a **temporary transvenous pacemaker.**
- Permanent pacing may be required in some patients if the arrhythmia persists beyond the acute time period of the MI (see Chapter 7, Arrhythmias).

Adjunctive Medical Treatment

- **Aspirin** is the preferred antiplatelet agent after MI and should be used indefinitely. Doses of 75–325 mg/d have been shown to reduce the chances of recurrent MI, stroke, and cardiac death.
- **Clopidogrel** (75 mg/d) can be used in patients with known allergic reaction to aspirin therapy.
- **Beta-blockers** confer a 23% mortality benefit in the first 30 days after an acute MI. Treatment should begin as soon as possible (preferably within the first 24 hours) and continued indefinitely.
- **Calcium channel blockers** (other than short-acting nifedipine) can be used in patients with normal ventricular function and no evidence of heart failure or AV block if beta-blocker therapy is contraindicated or ineffective for relief of ongoing ischemia or for arrhythmia management.
  - **Diltiazem should not be used** in patients with ventricular dysfunction because it has been shown to increase mortality in this patient population.
- **ACE inhibitors** provide a reduction in short-term mortality and incidence of congestive heart failure and recurrent MI when initiated within the first 24 hours of an acute MI.
  - Benefit is seen in asymptomatic patients with LV dysfunction (ejection fraction <40%) but is greatest in high-risk patients, including those with anterior infarctions and heart failure.
  - Therapy can be initiated with captopril, ramipril, trandolapril, or enalapril and titrated as BP permits.
  - ACE inhibitors should be used with caution in patients with renal insufficiency and are contraindicated in individuals with hypotension.
  - **IV enalaprilat should be avoided** as the initial therapeutic agent because of the possible increased mortality if BP is reduced excessively.
  - Patients with heart failure or asymptomatic LV dysfunction (ejection fraction <40%) should receive ACE inhibitors indefinitely.
- **Angiotensin II receptor blockers** can be used in patients who are intolerant of ACE inhibitors, although fewer data are available to demonstrate clear benefit.
  - Valsartan 160 mg bid and losartan 50 mg daily have been shown to be equivalent to captopril.
- **Anticoagulant therapy**
  - **IV heparin** should be given on initial presentation and continued for 48 hours, either as an adjunct to thrombolytic therapy or in association with cardiac catheterization. The role of LMWH (enoxaparin) in this setting has not been defined.
  - Beyond 48 hours, the use of anticoagulant therapy should be customized to the patient's needs. If the patient is not ambulatory, prophylactic dosing to prevent deep venous thrombosis is appropriate.
  - **Warfarin** should be used, absent contraindications, in patients with atrial fibrillation, a large anterior MI, or a documented LV thrombus. Heparin can be used until a therapeutic INR of 2–3 is achieved.
  - **Chronic anticoagulation** is appropriate for patients with LV dysfunction and a documented embolic event. Long-term use should also be considered in patients with severe LV dysfunction. In patients with an extensive anterior wall motion abnormality or a documented LV thrombus, warfarin can be used as prophylaxis against an embolic event and then discontinued after 3–6 months unless other indications warrant its continued use.

■ If **heparin-induced thrombocytopenia** (HIT) develops, heparin should be discontinued immediately and anticoagulation performed with thrombin inhibitors (lepirudin or argatroban)

■ **HMG-CoA reductase inhibitors** ("statins") should be started in all patients in the setting of ACS/STEMI in the absence of contraindications. Recent data suggest that aggressive treatment with a targeted LDL goal of <70 mg/dL results in additional benefit. Initial dose should target reduction in LDL of 30%–40%.

■ **Aldosterone blockade** with eplerenone 25 mg daily or spironolactone 25 mg daily should be started early in patients post-MI to decrease mortality if the ejection fraction is <40% in patients with symptomatic heart failure or diabetes, serum creatinine <2.0, serum potassium concentration <5.0 mEq/L, and are already receiving ACE inhibitors and beta-blockers.

■ Data on **HRT** and **antioxidant therapy** have *not* clearly demonstrated a benefit in secondary prevention after MI. Current recommendations allow for continued hormone replacement therapy (HRT) in women who are already taking the medication at the time of MI, but HRT should not be given de novo to postmenopausal women after a cardiac event.

Risk Assessment

After Medical Therapy (Including Thrombolysis)
■ Two possible strategies can be considered in the patient treated medically who has an uncomplicated post-MI course: noninvasive (stress test) evaluation and proceeding directly to catheterization.

■ **Stress testing** is done to determine prognosis or functional capacity.
   ▪ A submaximal stress test can be performed 4–6 days after the MI or a symptom-limited study at 10–14 days.
   ▪ The stress test can also be performed early after hospital discharge (2–3 weeks) or late after discharge (3–6 weeks) if the initial postinfarction stress test was submaximal.

■ With either approach, a **diagnostic cardiac catheterization** should be performed only if significant ischemic burden is identified.

■ **Catheterization without prior noninvasive assessment** is an alternative approach to the patient who was successfully managed medically at the time of initial presentation. At the time of catheterization, decisions on revascularization should be made based on the patient's anatomy, ventricular function, and clinical status.

■ Patients treated with initial medical management who experience any complications associated with the MI, including recurrent angina/ischemia, heart failure, a significant ventricular arrhythmia in the absence of ongoing ischemia, or a mechanical complication of the MI, should proceed directly to cardiac catheterization to assess the coronary anatomy and offer a revascularization strategy as the anatomy dictates.

Associated Conditions and Complications

Myocardial damage predisposes the patient to several potential adverse consequences or complications that should be considered if the patient presents after the original event with new clinical signs or symptoms.

■ **Recurrent chest pain** may be due to ischemia in the territory of the original infarction.
   ▪ The ischemia may result from incomplete revascularization, either by natural or pharmacologic fibrinolytic activity or by early restenosis at the site of a percutaneous intervention.
   ▪ Additional causes of chest pain to be considered include pericarditis, pulmonary embolism, and cardiac rupture.
   ▪ Evaluation of the patient may include:
      • Careful clinical examination for new murmurs or friction rubs
      • ECG to examine evidence of ischemic changes or findings consistent with pericarditis
      • Cardiac enzymes, which may help establish whether additional myocardial damage has occurred
      • Echocardiography or (repeat) angiography may also be indicated.

- **Ischemia** recurs in 20%–30% of patients after MI, with or without recent fibrinolytic therapy, and in up to 10% of patients in the early time period after percutaneous revascularization.
  - Patients should continue on heparin, nitrate, and β-adrenergic antagonist therapy.
  - If the ischemia is refractory to medical treatment, (repeat) angiography should be considered along with (repeat) dilation of the coronary lesion and stabilization with an intra-aortic balloon pump.
- **Extension or recurrence of infarction** occurs in up to 20% of patients after MI and is usually heralded by recurrent anginal symptoms.
  - Patients with recurrent chest pain should be evaluated for new ischemic ECG changes or a significant rise in cardiac enzyme levels.
  - Patients with recurrent ST elevation after fibrinolytic therapy should be considered for rescue angioplasty. If revascularization is not available on-site, or in a timely fashion with hospital transfer, patients can be treated 24 hours after the initial fibrinolytic therapy with additional doses of rt-PA or r-PA.
  - Because reinfarction increases the probability of death, heart failure, arrhythmias, and cardiac rupture, these patients should be monitored in-hospital for an extended period of time.
- **Acute pericarditis** occurs in approximately 15%–20% of patients with large MIs. Pericarditic pain is often pleuritic in nature and may be relieved in the upright position. A friction rub may be noted on clinical examination.
  - Symptoms may be mistaken for recurrent ischemia.
  - The ECG may show diffuse ST-segment elevation.
  - Treatment is directed at pain management.
  - Treatment consists of nonsteroidal anti-inflammatory drugs (NSAIDs) such as aspirin (650 mg PO qid) or indomethacin (25–50 mg qid).
  - Glucocorticoids (prednisone, 1 mg/kg daily) may be useful if symptoms are severe and refractory to initial therapy. Steroid use should be deferred until at least 4 weeks after acute MI due to their adverse impact on infarct healing and risk of ventricular rupture.
  - **Dressler syndrome** is thought to be an autoimmune process. It is characterized by malaise, fever, pericardial pain, leukocytosis, elevated sedimentation rate, and often a pericardial effusion occurring between the first and tenth week after acute MI.
- **Arrhythmias.** Cardiac rhythm abnormalities are common in patients with acute MI. Multiple factors may contribute to the rhythm disturbances.
  - Arrhythmias that result in hemodynamic compromise require prompt, aggressive intervention. If the arrhythmia precipitates refractory angina or heart failure, urgent therapy is also warranted. For all rhythm disturbances, even those that are not life threatening, exacerbating conditions should be addressed, including electrolyte imbalances, hypoxia, acidosis, and adverse drug effects.
  - **Intraventricular conduction disturbances.** One or more of the three fascicles of the His-Purkinje system may be affected in patients who present with acute MI. The left anterior fascicle is most commonly affected because of isolated coronary blood supply, compared with the left posterior and right fascicles, which receive dual coronary supply. Bifascicular or trifascicular block is associated with a high incidence of progression to complete heart block and other rhythm disturbances.
  - **Bradycardia.** Sinus bradycardia is common in patients with acute MI, particularly that involving the right coronary artery.
    - In the absence of hypotension or significant ventricular ectopy, observation alone is indicated.
    - If treatment is necessary, atropine (0.3–0.6 mg IV every 3–10 minutes; dose not to exceed 2 mg) can be used to achieve a rate of 60 bpm.
    - Temporary pacing may be required for more prolonged or refractory periods of bradycardia.
  - **First-degree AV block** usually does not require specific treatment. The conduction disturbance may be due to use of digoxin or other agents that slow AV conduction.
    - Beta-blocker therapy is contraindicated only if marked PR-interval prolongation or hemodynamic compromise from the loss of AV synchrony is noted.

- **Second-degree AV block**
    - Wenckebach (Mobitz I) occurs more often with inferior than anterior MI. The block is usually within the His bundle and does not require treatment unless symptomatic bradycardia is present.
    - Mobitz II second-degree AV block originates below the His bundle and is more commonly associated with anterior infarctions. Because of the significant risk of progression to complete heart block, Mobitz II block should be treated with temporary pacing, regardless of the patient's symptoms.
- **Third-degree AV block** may develop in up to 15% of patients with MI. Mortality in these individuals may approach 15% (or higher if right ventricular infarction is present).
    - In patients with anterior MI, third-degree heart block often occurs 12–24 hours after initial presentation and may appear suddenly.
    - Temporary pacing is recommended because of the risk of progression to ventricular asystole.
- **Asystole.** Complete loss of ventricular complexes may occur abruptly in patients with high-grade AV block or complex fascicular blocks. Temporary transvenous pacing is warranted in these patients.
- **Indications for pacing.** Conduction system disease at risk for progression to complete heart block or significant symptomatic bradycardia can be effectively treated with cardiac pacing. A transcutaneous pacing device can be used under emergent circumstances, and a temporary transvenous system can be used for longer-duration therapy (Table 5-10).
    - A temporary transvenous pacing system should be placed in patients with acute MI if they require transcutaneous pacing or have:
        - Asystole
        - Symptomatic bradycardia or Mobitz type I second-degree heart block that is unresponsive to atropine
        - Mobitz type II second-degree heart block
        - Recurrent sinus pauses
        - Incessant VT
        - New or age-indeterminate trifascicular block

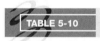

TABLE 5-10	Indications for Pacing in Acute Myocardial Infarction

Temporary transcutaneous pacing
Sinus bradycardia with hypotension unresponsive to drug therapy
Mobitz II heart block
Third-degree heart block
New bilateral bundle branch block
Newly acquired bundle branch or fascicular block
Left or right bundle branch block with first-degree atrioventricular (AV) block

Temporary transvenous pacing
Asystole
Symptomatic bradycardia and type 1 second-degree AV block
New bilateral bundle branch block
New bifascicular bundle branch block with first-degree AV block
Mobitz II second-degree AV block

Permanent pacing
Persistent second-degree AV block in the His-Purkinje system with bilateral bundle branch block or complete heart block
Transient second- or third-degree AV block associated with bundle branch block
Symptomatic AV block at any level
Persistent advanced (second- or third-degree) block at the AV node level

- Patients who are dependent on the atrial contribution to ventricular filling may benefit from atrial or AV sequential pacing.
- Temporary pacing can be considered in patients with a left bundle branch block if placement of a pulmonary arterial catheter is indicated, due to the risk of progression to complete heart block with catheter placement.
- Temporary AV sequential pacing may be helpful in patients with an inferior MI complicated by right ventricular infarction and complete heart block.
- If the rhythm abnormality presents or persists late in the post-MI course, the patient should be evaluated for permanent pacemaker implantation (see Chapter 7, Arrhythmias).

■ **Supraventricular tachycardias** (see Chapter 7, Arrhythmias).
  - **Sinus tachycardia** is common in patients with acute MI and is often due to enhanced sympathetic activity resulting from pain, anxiety, hypovolemia, anxiety, heart failure, or fever.
    - Treatment of the underlying contributing factors is indicated.
    - Persistent sinus tachycardia suggests poor underlying ventricular function and is associated with excess mortality.
    - Invasive monitoring of these patients may facilitate choices in volume management and pharmacologic therapy in these individuals.
  - **Paroxysmal supraventricular tachycardias** occurs infrequently in the setting of acute MI. Rate control and rhythm management with beta-blocker or calcium antagonist agents are effective at limiting myocardial oxygen demand in the postinfarction period.
  - **Atrial fibrillation** and **flutter** are observed in up to 20% of patients with acute MI, with atrial fibrillation occurring more commonly than flutter.
    - Adverse consequences of these rhythms include the loss of AV synchrony and the potential for a rapid ventricular response.
    - Treatment with beta-blockers or calcium antagonists is effective at rate and rhythm control. Because atrial fibrillation and atrial flutter are usually transient in the acute MI period, long-term anticoagulation is often not necessary after documentation of stable sinus rhythm.
  - **Accelerated junctional rhythm** occurs in conjunction with inferior MI. The rhythm is usually benign and warrants treatment only if hypotension is present. Digitalis intoxication should be considered in patients with accelerated junctional rhythm.

■ **Ventricular arrhythmias** (see Chapter 7, Arrhythmias)
  - Ventricular premature depolarizations (VPDs) are common in the course of an acute MI.
  - Beta-blocker therapy used for secondary prevention beginning in the early time period after presentation may reduce the frequency of VPDs and provide symptomatic relief for patients who are aware of the ectopic beats.
  - Prophylactic treatment with lidocaine or other antiarrhythmics has been associated with increased overall mortality and is **not recommended.**
  - **Accelerated idioventricular rhythm** is a ventricular rhythm at a rate between 60 and 125 bpm and may be seen in up to 20% of patients, often within the first 2 days of the acute MI.
    - It is commonly seen after successful reperfusion with thrombolytic therapy. This rhythm is not associated with an increased incidence of adverse outcomes.
    - Specific treatment is not warranted unless the loss of AV synchrony results in hemodynamic compromise. If needed, sinus activity may be restored with atropine or temporary atrial pacing.
  - **Nonsustained ventricular tachycardia** (NSVT), defined as three or more consecutive beats >100 bpm that last for <30 seconds, occur in the majority of patients in the first 24 hours after acute MI. The early appearance of this rhythm is not associated with an increase in mortality.
    - Hypokalemia may increase the risk of NSVT. Serum potassium and magnesium should be corrected, as necessary, to values >4.5 mEq/L and 2.0 mEq/L, respectively.
    - NSVT later in the post-MI course is associated with increased mortality.

- **Ventricular tachycardia.** Episodes of sustained VT during the first 48 hours after acute MI are associated with increased in-hospital mortality.
  - Synchronized cardioversion with 200 joules should be used for monomorphic VT.
  - Unsynchronized cardioversion should be used for polymorphic VT. The addition of prophylactic drug therapy is warranted for 24–48 hours (see Chapter 7, Arrhythmias).
  - Patients who experience VT after appropriate coronary revascularization or later in the post-MI course should be considered for long-term antiarrhythmic therapy or defibrillator placement.
  - Ventricular fibrillation. Primary VF occurs in up to 5% of patients in the early post-MI period. Treatment with immediate unsynchronized cardioversion is appropriate.
- **Hypertension.** Patients with hypertension in the setting of an acute MI should be treated initially with short-acting IV agents.
  - Bedrest, pain control, and sedation may facilitate hypertension management.
  - *β*-**Adrenergic antagonists.** Beta-blocker therapy is an effective antihypertensive agent that also decreases myocardial oxygen demand by reducing heart rate and contractility. Unless contraindications of hypotension or severe bradycardia exist, beta-blocker therapy should be initiated early in the post-MI course.
  - **ACE inhibitors.** As with beta-blocker therapy, ACE inhibitors can be used for hypertension management and for secondary prevention after MI.
    - Therapy should be initiated within the first 3 days after MI unless prohibited by contraindications of hypotension or renal dysfunction.
  - **Calcium channel blockers.** If beta-blocker or ACE inhibitor therapy is contraindicated or not sufficient to manage hypertension, calcium channel blockers can be used for antihypertensive and for antianginal effects.
    - Short-acting dihydropyridines (nifedipine) are associated with increased in-hospital mortality after acute MI and should be avoided.
    - Although diltiazem and verapamil have not been demonstrated to benefit infarct size or mortality after MI, these agents can be used for BP control and management of supraventricular arrhythmias.
  - **Nitroprusside.** Moderate to severe hypertension can be treated with intravenous nitroprusside (see Chapter 7, Hypertension).
  - **Nitroglycerin.** Predominately a venodilating agent, intravenous nitroglycerin may effectively decrease BP at high doses or in patients with elevated LV filling pressures. Nitroglycerin may also attenuate hypertension through its anti-ischemic effects.
- **Left ventricular failure.** Acute MI may be associated with systolic or diastolic dysfunction, or both. The degree of dysfunction is usually in proportion to the severity of the infarction. The approach to therapy must be individualized to the patient according to etiology, acuity, and extent of the compromise in function.
  - Normotensive patients with pulmonary congestion or a summation gallop on clinical examination can be treated empirically.
  - Cardiac function (ventricular and valvular) can be assessed by echocardiography or at the time of cardiac catheterization, if performed.
  - Diuretics should be administered to control the patient's volume, but care should be given to avoid intravascular volume depletion.
  - ACE inhibitors can favorably affect both morbidity and mortality after acute MI in patients with documented ventricular dysfunction but are also beneficial in the absence of ventricular dysfunction.
  - In the patient unable to take an ACE inhibitor, an angiotensin receptor blocking agent can be substituted; however, the efficacy is less well established.
  - *β*-Adrenergic antagonists confer additional benefits in the treatment of compensated heart failure after acute MI.
  - **Aldosterone blockade** with eplerenone 25 mg daily or Aldactone 25 mg daily should be started early in patients post-MI to decrease mortality if the ejection fraction is <40% in patients with symptomatic heart failure or diabetes, serum creatinine

<2.0, and serum potassium concentration <5.0 mEq/L and are already receiving ace inhibitors and beta-blockers.

■ **Digitalis** has not been clearly demonstrated to reduce mortality following infarction. Improved contractility may be achieved when it is used in patients with severe dysfunction.

- Digoxin can also be used for rate control in patients with atrial fibrillation in the setting of acute MI.
- Digitalis, especially in the setting of hypokalemia, may provoke arrhythmias within the first few hours after acute MI.

■ **Nitrates** may reduce pulmonary congestion. Intravenous nitroglycerin should be titrated to reduce BP by approximately 10%, but not below 90 mm Hg.

- Care should be given to avoid a reflex tachycardia.
- After stabilization, the patient can be converted to an oral preparation.

■ **Inotropes/vasoactive amines** (dopamine/dobutamine) may be used to improve blood pressure and enhance myocardial contractility. Their use increases myocardial oxygen consumption and may worsen ischemia.

■ **Right ventricular myocardial infarction** is seen in approximately 50% of patients with an acute inferior MI. Roughly half of these patients have hemodynamic compromise as a result of the right ventricular involvement.

- The LV filling pressures are normal or decreased, the right atrial pressures are elevated (>10 mm Hg), and the cardiac index is depressed. In some patients, elevated right atrial pressures may not be evident until IV fluids are administered.
- Clinical signs may include hypotension (possibly to the extent of cardiogenic shock), elevated jugular venous pulsation, a Kussmaul sign (an increase in jugular venous pressures with inspiration), and right-sided third or fourth heart sounds with clear lung fields.
- Right precordial ECG leads should be obtained and analyzed for ST elevation (V_4R is the most sensitive and specific lead and is transient).
- Initial therapy is intravenous fluids. If hypotension is excessive, inotropic support with dobutamine or an intra-aortic balloon pump may be necessary.
- In patients with heart block resulting in AV dyssynchrony, sequential AV pacing may have a marked beneficial effect.

■ **Cardiogenic shock** is defined as hypotension and cardiac function that is inadequate to meet the metabolic needs of the peripheral tissue. Organ hypoperfusion may be manifest as progressive renal failure or mental status changes. Hemodynamic monitoring reveals elevated filling pressures (wedge pressure >20 mm Hg) and a depressed cardiac index (<2.5 L/kg/min) in the setting of a systemic BP of <90 mm Hg.

- Patients with cardiogenic shock in the setting of an MI have a mortality well in excess of 50%. All patients should receive inotropic support.
- For patients younger than 75 years, an early revascularization strategy decreases 6-month mortality; however, patients older than 75 years benefit from initial medical stabilization.
- **Dopamine** is the preferred therapeutic agent in patients with a systolic BP of 70–90 mm Hg, but norepinephrine may be required in markedly hypotensive patients (systolic BP <70 mm Hg).
- In patients with a systolic BP near 90 mm Hg, inotropic support with dobutamine is often sufficient and does not adversely affect ventricular afterload.
- **Milrinone** should be added in patients who are either not responding to or are developing excessive tachycardia in response to dobutamine. It should not be used in patients with renal insufficiency.
- All patients in whom contraindications do not exist should be considered for insertion of an **intra-aortic balloon pump** and should be evaluated for surgically treatable mechanical complications of MI, such as VSD or severe mitral regurgitation (see below).

■ **Mechanical complications**

- **Aneurysm.** After an MI, the affected area of the myocardium may undergo infarct expansion and thinning, forming an aneurysm. The wall motion may become dyskinetic, and the endocardial surface is at risk for mural thrombus formation.

- LV aneurysm is suggested by persistent ST elevation on the ECG (>1 month from MI) and may be diagnosed by imaging studies, including ventriculography or echocardiography.
- Empiric anticoagulation (warfarin target INR, 2.0–3.0) is warranted to lower the risk of systemic embolization, especially if a mural thrombus is present.
- Surgical intervention may be appropriate if the aneurysm results in heart failure or ventricular arrhythmias that are not satisfactorily managed with medical therapy.
- Incomplete rupture of the myocardial free wall can result in formation of a ventricular pseudoaneurysm in which complete extravasation of blood is prevented by the visceral pericardium. Echocardiography is the preferred diagnostic test to assess for a pseudoaneurysm, often allowing differentiation from a true aneurysm.
- Prompt surgical intervention for pseudoaneurysms is advised because of the high incidence of myocardial rupture.

■ **Papillary muscle rupture** is a rare complication after MI and is associated with abrupt clinical deterioration. The posterior medial papillary muscle is most commonly affected due to its isolated vascular supply, but anterolateral and right ventricular papillary rupture have been reported.
- Papillary muscle rupture may be seen in the setting of a relatively small MI.
- The physical exam may not reveal an audible murmur in ~50% of patients.
- The diagnostic test of choice is echocardiography with Doppler imaging.
- Stabilization with afterload reduction using nitroprusside or nitroglycerin as well as inotropic support with dobutamine and intra-aortic balloon pump may be necessary for hemodynamically unstable patients until definitive therapy with surgical repair can be performed.

■ **Ventricular septal rupture** (or defect) formation is more commonly associated with anterior MI. The perforation may follow a direct course between the ventricles or a serpiginous route through the septal wall.
- Diagnosis can be made by echocardiography with Doppler imaging.
- A step-up in hemoglobin oxygen saturation >5% between the right atrium and right ventricle suggests a clinically significant shunt.
- Diagnosis should be suspected in the postinfarct patient who develops heart failure symptoms and a new holosystolic murmur.
- Stabilization with afterload reduction using nitroprusside or nitroglycerin as well as inotropic support with dobutamine and intra-aortic balloon pump may be necessary for hemodynamically unstable patients until definitive therapy with surgical repair can be performed.
- In hemodynamically stable patients, surgery is best deferred at least a week to improve patient outcome. Left untreated, mortality approaches 90%.

■ **Free wall rupture** represents a catastrophic complication of acute MI accounting for 10% of early deaths. This complication can occur after anterior or inferior MI but is more commonly seen in hypertensive women with a first large transmural MI, treated late with fibrinolytic therapy, and given NSAIDs or glucocorticoids.
- Rupture typically occurs within the first week after MI.
- The diagnosis should be suspected in patients who have experienced sudden hemodynamic collapse.
- Echocardiography may identify patients with particularly thinned ventricular walls at risk for rupture.
- Pericardiocentesis and intra-aortic balloon pump support may be necessary awaiting emergent surgical correction.
- Despite optimal intervention, mortality of free wall rupture remains greater than 90%.

Hemodynamic Monitoring

■ Hemodynamic monitoring with a pulmonary artery catheter should be considered in patients with acute MI if their course is complicated by:
  ▪ Hypotension not corrected by fluid administration
  ▪ Hypotension in the presence of congestive heart failure

- Cardiogenic shock
- Potential or confirmed mechanical complications
- Unexplained cyanosis or hypoxia
- Right ventricular MI

- Patients with MI requiring hemodynamic monitoring can be categorized into one of several groups that are useful for defining treatment strategies.
  - **Hypovolemic hypotension** is characterized by decreased LV filling pressures and systemic hypotension.
    - Volume resuscitation with normal saline to a pulmonary arterial wedge pressure of 15–20 mm Hg should be attempted when accompanied by decreased cardiac index (<2.5 L/min/m^2), oliguria, or persistent sinus tachycardia.
  - **Pulmonary congestion** is evident when the pulmonary arterial wedge pressure is elevated (>20 mm Hg) in the setting of a normal cardiac index. The condition may be due to volume overload or decreased cardiac compliance.
    - Treatment should consist of intravenous nitroglycerin to reduce preload and diuresis to accomplish more normal cardiac filling pressures.
  - **Peripheral hypoperfusion** is apparent when the BP is maintained but the LV filling pressure is elevated (wedge pressure >20 mm Hg) and the cardiac index is depressed (<2.5 L/kg/min). With sufficient BP, the treatment of choice is afterload reduction.
    - **Nitroglycerin** is preferred early after the onset of MI because it may also induce coronary vasodilation and increase myocardial blood flow to ischemic regions.
    - **Nitroprusside** has less favorable effects than nitroglycerin in terms of coronary blood flow, and its use should be reserved for patients with marked hypertension that is unresponsive to nitroglycerin. It should be used with caution in patients with renal insufficiency. Determination of thiocyanide levels should be determined daily to avoid cyanide toxicity.
    - The hemodynamic goal should be to reduce the systemic vascular resistance below 1,000 dynes/sec/cm^{-5}.
    - Patients who respond to intravenous therapy can be converted to an oral ACE inhibitor and weaned off the nitroglycerin or nitroprusside.
    - An inotropic agent such as dobutamine should be added if the BP falls or the cardiac index does not improve with vasodilator therapy.
  - Caution should be used placing a pulmonary artery catheter in patients with a left bundle branch block on ECG because of the risk of inducing complete heart block with the procedure.
  - Establishing trends is more important than single absolute values, and therapy must be based on individual responses to initial therapy.
  - All hemodynamic data should be evaluated in terms of the clinical response and viewed critically if they fail to correlate with other physiologic parameters such as urine output.
  - The duration of catheter use should be kept to a minimum.

Secondary Prevention

- The goal of secondary prevention is to produce a favorable impact on the morbidity and mortality associated with CAD.
  - The strategies outlined for primary prevention and the management of stable angina have also been shown to decrease the rates of repeat infarction, progression to congestive heart failure, and incidence of cardiovascular deaths in patients with known CAD.
  - Important in the goal of secondary prevention is appropriate short- and long-term follow-up with a cardiologist.
- **Antiplatelet agents**
  - Aspirin is the preferred antiplatelet agent after MI and should be used indefinitely. Doses of 75–325 mg/d have been shown to reduce the chances for recurrent MI, stroke, and death.
  - Clopidogrel (75 mg/d) or warfarin (target INR 2.0–3.0) can be used in patients with contraindications to aspirin therapy, including hypersensitivity reactions.

Allergy consultation should be obtained if necessary to determine if a true aspirin allergy exists.
- Clopidogrel (in addition to aspirin) is also recommended for a minimum of 4, 12, and 24 weeks after placement of a bare-metal, sirolimus-eluting, and paclitaxel-eluting coronary stents, respectively, to reduce the risk of in-stent thrombosis. When added to clopidogrel, 81 mg of aspirin has a lower risk of gastrointestinal bleeding.
- The combination of aspirin and low-dose warfarin is not superior to aspirin alone in reducing cardiac events.
- Warfarin should be used, often in addition to aspirin, in patients with atrial fibrillation or a large anterior MI and may be of benefit in patients with severe LV dysfunction. Patients with atrial fibrillation should be treated until at least 3–4 weeks after maintenance of sinus rhythm is ensured. Those with a large anterior MI, LV aneurysm, or documented mural thrombus should receive warfarin for 3–6 months.
- **ACE inhibitors/angiotensin receptor blockers/aldosterone blockers**
  - **ACE inhibitors** reduce mortality and the incidence of congestive heart failure and recurrent MI.
    - Benefit is seen in asymptomatic patients with LV dysfunction (ejection fraction <40%) and all patients after MI.
    - Therapy should be titrated to the maximally tolerated dose and continued treatment indefinitely.
    - Although fewer data are available to demonstrate clear benefit, angiotensin receptor blockers can be used in patients who are intolerant to ACE inhibitors.
  - **Aldosterone blockade** is beneficial in patients with LV dysfunction (ejection fraction <40%) who are normokalemic, have preserved renal function, and are tolerating ACE inhibitors.
  - The combination of ACE inhibitors/angiotensin receptor blockers and aldosterone antagonists have a high risk of **hyperkalemia.** Serum potassium determinations should be taken frequently while initiating or modifying therapy.
- **β-Adrenergic blockers**
  - β-Adrenergic blockers reduce cardiac events after MI and should be continued indefinitely after MI.
  - Treatment with β_1-selective or nonselective agents is effective (e.g., metoprolol, 100 mg bid; atenolol, 100 mg daily; timolol, 10 mg bid; propranolol, 80 mg tid).
  - Dosing should be adjusted as necessary if issues of hypotension, bradycardia, or bronchospasm arise. Additional care should be given when using these agents in symptomatic heart failure.
  - In addition to their role in secondary prevention, beta-blocker agents may also be effective in the treatment of hypertension, angina, and rhythm abnormalities.
- **Cholesterol treatment**
  - Cholesterol-lowering agents should be used to lower cardiovascular event rates after MI (discussed in detail in Hyperlipidemia in Patients with Ischemic Heart Disease).
  - Treatment with a statin is preferred with a target LDL <100 mg/dL for all patients with CAD and <70 mg/dL in those at very high risk, including those patients with an acute coronary syndrome or STEMI.
  - Recent data indicate that all patients with CAD benefit from statins, regardless of baseline LDL.
- **Calcium channel blockers**
  - The combination of calcium channel blockers and nitrates reduces angina but has not been shown to reduce mortality.
- **Tobacco cessation**
  - Continued smoking after MI significantly increases the incidence of recurrent ischemic events. Patients should be clearly instructed to quit smoking and attempt to avoid second-hand smoke.
  - Counseling and support group interventions should be used, in addition to pharmacologic therapy.
    - Bupropion (150 mg bid) treatment is needed for a minimum of 7 weeks to be effective, although some patients require up to a year of therapy. After treatment, patients should be slowly tapered off bupropion to reduce the chance of relapse

and the risk of seizures. Bupropion is contraindicated in patients with a known seizure disorder or in those taking monoamine oxidase inhibitors.
- Nicotine patches and gums can be used in conjunction with a supervised smoking cessation program but should be avoided until after the acute hospitalization.
- Diet
  - Patients should be counseled about the National Cholesterol Education Program Therapeutic Lifestyle Changes (NCEP-TLC) Diet for reducing cholesterol and achieving optimal body weight.
  - A body mass index of <25 kg/m^2 is desirable. When body mass index is >25 kg/m^2, a goal for waist circumference of <40 in. in men and <35 in. in women should be pursued.
- Diabetes
  - Although no clear data currently link tight glycemic control with reduced progression of atherosclerotic disease or cardiac events, current recommendations favor appropriate hypoglycemic therapy to achieve near-normal fasting plasma glucose levels and a target hemoglobin A1c of $<7\%$.
  - The diabetic with CAD should be considered at very high risk for recurrent cardiovascular event.
- Exercise
  - In patients who are physically capable, an exercise stress test can be used for prognostic assessment and to determine functional capacity. A submaximal study can be performed 4–6 days after MI, or symptom-limited study can be performed at 10–14 days.
  - Alternatively, a maximal stress test can be administered 3–6 weeks after MI. With an appreciation of the patient's functional exercise capacity, a program of activity can be formulated.
  - The goal is a minimum of 3–4 days per week of 30–60 minutes of activity.

Follow-Up Care

Routine office visits every 4–12 months are suggested for the first year after presentation with an index ischemic event, and annual visits thereafter.
- Our practice has been to maintain cardiology follow-up indefinitely once the diagnosis of CAD has been made.
- Five specific questions should be answered during the visits:
  - Has the patient decreased his or her level of physical activity since the last visit?
  - Has the patient's pattern of angina (frequency, severity, or level of activity to provoke) changed since the last visit?
  - How is the patient tolerating therapy?
  - Has the patient attempted to address risk factor modification?
  - What is the status of known or new comorbid illnesses that may affect the patient's ischemic heart disease?
- Patients should be instructed to seek more frequent or urgent follow-up evaluation if they experience any noticeable change in their clinical status.
- Specific plans for a patient's long-term follow-up should be individualized and are affected by their clinical status, anatomy, prior interventions, and any changes in symptoms.
- Routine testing is not warranted in patients with no change in clinical status or in those with an estimated annual mortality (by prior risk assessment) of $<1\%$.
- Patients with evidence of new congestive heart failure should be evaluated with a chest radiograph and echocardiogram to assess for changes in ventricular function, for new wall motion abnormalities, and for new or worsening valvular disease.
- A stress imaging study is appropriate for patients who have a significant change in clinical status (either heart failure or angina).
- Coronary angiography should be considered for patients with significant ischemic burden on stress testing that is potentially amenable to revascularization or those with marked limitations of ordinary activity despite maximal medical therapy.

- If new or recurrent coronary disease is identified, options of (repeat) revascularization or other treatments (e.g., CABG, transmyocardial laser revascularization, or cardiac transplantation) should be considered.

DYSLIPIDEMIA

General Principles

- Lowering cholesterol levels has been shown to decrease the risk of recurrent coronary events and procedures in patients with coronary artery disease as well as to prevent coronary artery disease in people with hypercholesterolemia.
- Several studies have shown evidence of regression of atherosclerotic lesions in patients whose lipid levels are lowered.
  - Randomized placebo-controlled event trials such as the **Scandinavian Simvastatin Survival Study** showed a decrease in total as well as cardiovascular mortality in patients with coronary artery disease who had their cholesterol levels lowered with diet and drug therapy.[1]
  - In the **Cholesterol and Recurrent Events** (CARE) Study, patients with a history of myocardial infarction and baseline LDL cholesterol (LDL-C) levels of 115–175 mg/dL had a decrease in event rate when treated with cholesterol-lowering medication.[2]
  - The **West of Scotland** Study confirmed a decrease in risk of coronary events in men with elevated cholesterol levels and no previous history of myocardial infarction.[3]
  - The Air Force/Texas Coronary Atherosclerosis Prevention Study (**AFCAPS**)[4] showed the benefits of LDL lowering for primary prevention in both men and women with HDL cholesterol (HDL-C) levels <50 mg/dL. In addition, another secondary prevention trial, the Long-Term Intervention with Pravastatin in Ischemic Disease (**LIPID**)[5] study, showed decreased coronary events in patients with previous heart disease and a wide range of baseline cholesterol levels.
- More recently, studies such as the **Heart Protection Study**[6] and Pravastatin or Atorvastatin Evaluation and Infection Therapy (**PROVE-IT**)[7] study indicates that statin use at lower baseline levels of LDL or to achieve LDL levels lower than NCEP targets may be beneficial in decreasing risk in high-risk patients.

Screening and Diagnosis

- All patients with evidence of coronary disease should have lipid profiles performed. For primary prevention of cardiovascular disease, all adults over 20 should have a fasting lipoprotein profile and evaluation of cardiovascular risk factors every 5 years (Table 5-11).

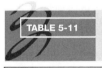

TABLE 5-11	National Cholesterol Education Program Adult Treatment Panel III Guidelines: Major Risk Factors (Exclusive of Low Density Lipoprotein Cholesterol) That Modify Low Density Lipoprotein Cholesterol Goals

Cigarette smoking
Hypertension (blood pressure ≥140/90 mm Hg or on antihypertensive medication)
Family history of premature CHD (CHD in male first-degree relative <55 years; CHD in female first-degree relative <65 years)
Low HDL cholesterol (<40 mg/dL)[a]
Age: men ≥45 years
women ≥55 years

CHD, coronary heart disease; HDL, high-density lipoprotein.
[a]If HDL cholesterol level is ≥60 mg/dL (1.55 mmol/L), subtract one risk factor.

- The **NCEP** has published guidelines for the diagnosis, evaluation, and treatment of high blood cholesterol levels in adults.[8] A recent review of clinical trials available since the Adult Treatment Panel III report was published in July 2004.[9] The paper provides updated rationale and goals for treatment of high-risk patients.
  - Lipoprotein analysis should be performed on serum obtained after a **12-hour fast.** Total cholesterol, triglycerides, and HDL-C are measured, and LDL-C is calculated using the **Friedewald formula:**

    $$\text{LDL-C} = \text{total cholesterol} - \text{HDL-C} - (\text{triglycerides}/5)$$

    where triglyceride/5 represents the cholesterol contained in very-low-density lipoprotein (VLDL). This formula is not valid when triglyceride levels are >400 mg/dL. In such patients, the most reliable way to ascertain LDL-C is to measure it directly using ultracentrifugation. An immunoassay for measuring direct LDL is now widely available and can be useful in assessing LDL levels in patients with very high triglyceride levels. In patients who have had an acute MI, lipoprotein levels measured within the first 24 hours provide an approximation of their usual levels; otherwise, levels may not be stable for up to 6 weeks.
  - **Risk assessment** is the first step in the evaluation of patients. Risk is determined based on the lipoprotein profile, the presence or absence of CHD, and other major risk factors (Table 5-12).
  - **Initial classification** is based on LDL-C level, which is the primary target of therapy.
    - Optimal LDL-C is <100 mg/dL.
    - Near or above optimal LDL-C is 100–129 mg/dL.
    - Borderline-high LDL-C is 130–159 mg/dL.
    - High LDL-C is 160–189 mg/dL.
    - Very-high LDL-C is ≥190 mg/dL.
  - **Total cholesterol** and **HDL-C** classification
    - Desirable total cholesterol is <200 mg/dL.
    - Borderline-high blood cholesterol is 200–239 mg/dL.
    - High blood cholesterol is ≥240 mg/dL.
    - Low HDL-C is <40 mg/dL and is counted as a risk factor.
    - High HDL-C is ≥60 mg/dL and is a negative risk factor; its presence removes one risk factor from the total count.

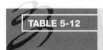

TABLE 5-12 National Cholesterol Education Program Adult Treatment Panel III Guidelines: Treatment Decisions Based on LDL Cholesterol[a]

Risk category	LDL goal	LDL level at which to initiate therapeutic lifestyle changes (TLCs)	LDL level at which to consider drug therapy
CHD or CHD risk equivalents (10-yr risk >20%)	<100 mg/dL	≥100 mg/dL	≥130 mg/dL (100–129 mg/dL: drug optional)
2+ Risk factors (10-yr risk ≤20%)	<130 mg/dL	≥130 mg/dL	10-yr risk 10%–20%: ≥130 mg/dL 10-yr risk <10%: ≥160 mg/dL
0–1 Risk factor	<160 mg/dL	≥160 mg/dL	≥190 mg/dL (160–189 mg/dL: LDL-lowering drug optional)

CHD, coronary heart disease; LDL, low-density lipoprotein.
[a]Very-high-risk patients have an optional LDL goal of <70 mg/dL.

■ **Risk categories** modify LDL-C goals. Patients in the category of **highest risk** are those with CAD and CAD risk equivalents. **CAD risk equivalents** include clinical CAD, carotid artery disease, peripheral vascular disease, and abdominal aortic aneurysm. Other CAD risk equivalents include diabetes mellitus and the presence of multiple risk factors that confer a 10-year risk for CAD >20% (Table 5-12).

- **Very high risk** is defined as established vascular disease and additional conditions including multiple risk factors (especially diabetes), severe and poorly controlled risk factors (e.g., cigarette smoking), metabolic syndrome (high TG, low HDL-C), and acute coronary syndromes. These patients have an optimal LDL **goal of <70 mg/dL.** Patients with CAD and CAD risk equivalents who do not fall into the very-high-risk group have an LDL **goal of <100 mg/dL.**
- The next category consists of patients with two or more risk factors (Table 5-11). Goal LDL for these patients is <130 mg/dL.
- The third category consists of people with one or zero risk factors. The goal LDL for this group is <160 mg/dL.

■ **The estimation of 10-year risk of CAD** is performed in patients with two or more risk factors using Framingham scoring.[8]

- A 10-year risk of >20% is considered a CAD risk equivalent, and the goal LDL is <100 mg/dL.
- A 10-year risk of 10%–20% qualifies the patient for a more aggressive approach than a 10-year risk of <10% even though the goal LDL is <130 mg/dL for both groups.
- A 10-year risk of <10% usually corresponds to fewer than two risk factors.

■ **Classification** of patients with CAD. Patients with CAD or CAD equivalents need aggressive therapy to lower LDL-C.

- Optimal LDL-C is ≤100 mg/dL. These patients should have instruction on diet and physical activity. Other lipid and nonlipid risk factors should be treated. If patients have vascular disease and other conditions putting them into the very-high-risk category, consideration should be given to lipid-lowering therapy with a reduction in LDL-C to <70 mg/dL.
- Higher than optimal LDL-C is above 130 mg/dL. Patients with baseline LDL above 130 mg/dL require intensive lifestyle therapy and maximal control of other risk factors. Drug therapy can be started simultaneously with lifestyle therapy. The goal of therapy is <100 mg/dL unless the patients are in the very-high-risk category. Patients with LDL-C levels between 100 and 129 mg/dL should have lifestyle therapy started or intensified and should be considered for initial or intensified drug therapy. The Heart Protection Study included patients with vascular disease and low LDL levels, with benefits from drug therapy shown even in patients whose baseline LDL-C levels were below 115 mg/dL.[6] When LDL-lowering medication is used, a decrease of at least 30% should be obtained.

■ **Elevated serum triglyceride levels** are an independent risk factor for atherosclerotic disease. They may be associated with increased concentrations of atherogenic particles such as chylomicron remnants, VLDL remnants, and small, dense LDL particles. Patients with hypertriglyceridemia frequently have low levels of HDL-C.

- Normal triglycerides are <150 mg/dL.
- Borderline-high hypertriglyceridemia levels are between 150 and 199 mg/dL. Nonpharmacologic therapy, including diet, exercise, and weight loss, is the initial form of treatment in these patients. Drug therapy is considered for those who are not at goal level of LDL, which is the first target of therapy in this group of patients.
- High triglycerides are defined as triglyceride levels between 200 and 499 mg/dL. Nonpharmacologic treatment with diet, exercise, and weight loss is initial therapy. LDL-C remains the primary target of therapy, but non-HDL-C is a secondary target. Non-HDL-C is equal to total cholesterol minus HDL. Table 5-13 shows non-HDL cholesterol goals.
- Very high triglycerides are >500 mg/dL. These patients are at increased risk for **pancreatitis.** Nonpharmacologic measures and a search for secondary causes are needed. These patients must be treated aggressively and often require drug therapy.

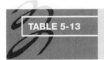

	National Cholesterol Treatment Program Adult Treatment Panel III Guidelines: Comparison of Low-Density Lipoprotein (LDL) Cholesterol and Non–High-Density Lipoprotein (HDL) Cholesterol Goals for Three Risk Categories

Risk category	LDL goal (mg/dL) [mmol/L]	Non-HDL goal (mg/dL) [mmol/L]
CHD and CHD risk equivalent	<100 [2.56]	<130 [3.36]
Multiple (2+ risk factors)	<130 [3.36]	<160 [4.13]
0–1 Risk factor	<160 [4.13]	<190 [4.9]

CHD, coronary heart disease.

Once triglyceride levels are lowered to <500 mg/dL, LDL is again the primary target of therapy.

Specific Disorders

- **Familial hypercholesterolemia** (FH) is an autosomal-dominant disorder involving the LDL receptor.
  - **Heterozygotes** for FH have 50% of the normal number of LDL receptors, elevated LDL-C levels, and cholesterol levels of 250–500 mg/dL. The incidence is approximately 1 in 500 persons. Affected patients often have premature vascular disease and may have tendon xanthomas.
    - Treatment usually requires drug as well as diet therapy. More severe cases may require the combination of two or more medications, typically a hydroxymethylglutaryl-coenzyme A (HMG-CoA) reductase inhibitor and a bile acid sequestrant resin or cholesterol absorption inhibitor.
    - Patients with insufficient response to tolerated doses of lipid-lowering medications may be candidates for LDL apheresis.
  - **Homozygotes** for FH have few or no LDL receptors and thus have markedly elevated LDL-C levels and blood cholesterol levels of 600–1,000 mg/dL. The incidence is 1 in 1 million. Heart disease often begins in early childhood, and many patients die of heart disease in their 20s and 30s.
    - Affected children may have planar and tuberous as well as tendon xanthomas.
    - They respond poorly to both diet and drug therapy although there may be some response to higher doses of potent statins. LDL apheresis is the preferred therapy. Liver transplantation has been performed in a few patients.
- **Familial defective apolipoprotein B-100** is an autosomal dominant disorder caused by an abnormality in the LDL receptor–binding region of apolipoprotein B-100, the major protein on the surface of LDL particles. It appears to have frequency, clinical features, and lipoprotein levels similar to those of heterozygous FH.
- **Familial combined hyperlipidemia** (FCHL) is associated with an increased risk of vascular disease. Patients may have elevated cholesterol, triglycerides, or both. The molecular basis of this disorder is unknown; many patients overproduce VLDL. FCHL appears to be an autosomal-dominant disorder and occurs in 1%–2% of the population. The diagnosis is made by the presence of multiple lipoprotein phenotypes within one family.
  - Family members may have elevated VLDL, elevated LDL-C, or increased levels of both VLDL and LDL-C. HDL is often low. Many patients will have increased levels of small, dense LDLs, particles that are atherogenic.
  - Apolipoprotein B levels are frequently elevated.
  - Diet therapy, weight loss, and exercise are useful initial therapies, but many patients will require drug therapy aimed at correcting specific lipoprotein abnormalities.
- **Severe polygenic hypercholesterolemia** is found in adults whose LDL-C is above 220 mg/dL and who do not clearly demonstrate a monogenic inheritance of hypercholesterolemia. These patients are usually at increased risk for premature CHD. Many will require medication to achieve LDL-C goals.

- **Hypertriglyceridemia** may be secondary to diet, obesity, excess alcohol intake, diabetes mellitus, hypothyroidism, uremia, dysproteinemias, β-adrenergic antagonists, estrogen, oral contraceptive drugs, retinoids, antiretroviral medications, tacrolimus, and sirolimus.
  - Triglyceride levels >400 mg/dL are often associated with an underlying primary disorder. Primary hypertriglyceridemia can be due to FCHL or familial hypertriglyceridemia (FHTG).
  - Families with familial hypertriglyceridemia have multiple members with elevated triglyceride levels due to increased VLDL levels. FHTG appears to be an autosomal dominant disorder without a clearly defined molecular basis. Families may show less pronounced risk of CHD than those with FCHL.
- **Dysbetalipoproteinemia** (type III hyperlipoproteinemia) is a rare (approximately 1 in 5,000) disorder caused by an abnormality of apoprotein E, a protein on the surface of VLDL and other lipoproteins, which is important in the uptake of remnant particles by cell surface receptors. Cholesterol-enriched VLDL (β-VLDL), an atherogenic particle, accumulates.
  - Both cholesterol and triglycerides are elevated.
  - Isoelectric focusing, which shows an abnormal apoprotein E pattern, can be confirmed by specific genotyping. Patients may have palmar or tuberoeruptive xanthomas, and there is increased risk of vascular disease. Patients with this disorder may respond well to diet and weight loss.
- **Hyperchylomicronemia** is diagnosed by the presence of a chylomicron layer when plasma is centrifuged or when chylomicrons float to the top of plasma that has been refrigerated overnight.
  - Chylomicrons can be seen when triglyceride levels are in excess of 1,000 mg/dL. The patient may have rare syndromes involving absence of lipoprotein lipase activity or absent apoprotein CII (a cofactor of lipoprotein lipase). Chylomicrons alone may be increased, as in lipoprotein lipase deficiency, or both VLDL and chylomicrons may be elevated.
  - Total cholesterol levels are often markedly elevated because of the presence of large numbers of VLDL particles that contain cholesterol as well as triglycerides. Patients with primary hypertriglyceridemia, FCHL, or dysbetalipoproteinemia may develop hyperchylomicronemia in the presence of excessive dietary fat intake, uncontrolled diabetes, alcohol excess, obesity, or other secondary causes of hyperlipidemia.
  - The chylomicronemia syndrome may include abdominal pain, hepatomegaly, splenomegaly, eruptive xanthomas, lipemia retinalis, and pancreatitis. Memory loss, paresthesias, and peripheral neuropathy can also occur.
- **Family members** of patients with hyperlipidemia should be screened to facilitate diagnosis of primary hyperlipidemias as well as to identify other patients in need of treatment.
- **Secondary causes of hyperlipidemia** include diet, hypothyroidism, diabetes mellitus, nephrotic syndrome, chronic renal failure, and dysproteinemia. Certain drugs can have effects on lipids. Thiazide diuretics, β-adrenergic antagonists (particularly less selective ones), glucocorticoids, estrogens, progestins, retinoids, anabolic steroids, protease inhibitors, and alcohol have variable effects on cholesterol, triglycerides, and HDL cholesterol. Treatment of diabetes mellitus with good control of blood sugars is particularly important if reasonable control of hypertriglyceridemia is to be achieved.
- **Low HDL-C levels** (<40 mg/dL) may be due to a genetic disorder or to secondary causes.
  - *Primary disorders* include familial hypoalphalipoproteinemia, primary hypertriglyceridemias, and rare disorders such as fish-eye disease, Tangier disease, and lecithin-cholesterol-acyl transferase (LCAT) deficiency.
  - *Secondary causes* of low HDL-C levels include cigarette smoking, obesity, lack of exercise, androgens, some progestational agents, anabolic steroids, β-adrenergic antagonists, and hypertriglyceridemia.
- **The metabolic syndrome** is a secondary target of risk reduction therapy. It is a constellation of factors including abdominal obesity, insulin resistance or diabetes, hypertension, and atherogenic lipid profile (elevated triglyceride levels; small, dense LDL; low HDL).

- Patients are considered to have the metabolic syndrome if they have three of the following:
  - Abdominal obesity: waist circumference >102 cm in men and 88 cm in women
  - Triglycerides ≥150 mg/dL
  - HDL-C <40 mg/dL in men and 50 mg/dL in women
  - Blood pressure ≥130/85 mm Hg
  - Fasting glucose ≥100 mg/dL
- **Elevated levels of lipoprotein (a) above 30 mg/dL** are associated with increased risk of atherosclerotic cardiovascular disease. Measurement of lipoprotein (a) may be useful in assessing risk in patients with few risk factors but with a strong family history of premature atherosclerosis. Lipoprotein (a) responds poorly to both nonpharmacologic and drug therapy. There can be modest reductions with niacin. The primary approach to therapy is reduction of LDL-C.

Treatment

- Patients who have **coronary disease** should have LDL-C levels reduced to 100 mg/dL or less (<70 mg/dL in very-high-risk patients).
  - Therapy should begin during hospitalization for an acute coronary event if patients are not already being treated.
  - Patients with coronary disease should be treated with the NCEP-TLC diet, which restricts saturated fat to 7% of total calories and daily cholesterol intake to <200 mg. Patients should see a dietitian for assistance in making diet changes. Patients with elevated triglycerides need to restrict simple sugars and alcohol as well.
- **LDL-C** can be lowered with the HMG-CoA reductase inhibitors (statins): lovastatin, pravastatin, simvastatin, fluvastatin, atorvastatin, and rosuvastatin; the bile acid sequestrant drugs cholestyramine, colestipol, and colesevelam; the cholesterol absorption inhibitor ezetimibe; and nicotinic acid (niacin).
  - The **HMG-CoA reductase inhibitors** lower LDL cholesterol well in most patients. These are the drugs of choice for lowering LDL for secondary prevention. LDL cholesterol can drop by 20%–60% depending on the drug and dosage. HDL may increase by up to 15% and triglycerides decrease by up to 30%.
    - All the statins are similar in mechanism of actions and side effects.
    - Atorvastatin and rosuvastatin have half-lives of approximately 13 hours and 20 hours, respectively. The other reductase inhibitors have half-lives of approximately 2–3 hours. Extended-release formulations of lovastatin and fluvastatin have longer half-lives than their counterparts. Lovastatin is best given with food, usually with evening meal; pravastatin, simvastatin, and fluvastatin can be administered without food, preferably in the evening.
    - Side effects occur infrequently (approximately 5%–10% of patients) and most commonly include mild gastrointestinal discomfort and myalgias.
    - **Liver function tests** should be monitored every 6–12 weeks initially and then every 6–12 months (or according to package inserts). About 1% of patients will have transaminase elevations to greater than three times the upper limit of normal; the transaminase elevation will often decrease while the patient continues on the statin. A common cause of this problem is fatty liver, which responds to small amounts of weight loss. If transaminases continue to be elevated, changing to a different statin may be helpful. Other drugs or conditions may contribute to elevated transaminases, such as increased alcohol intake.
    - **Myopathy** may occur in up to 10% of patients. Patients may have complaints of muscle cramps, aching, or weakness. Myopathy has been reported more often when the reductase inhibitors are combined with fibric acid derivatives, cyclosporine, niacin, and erythromycin. Patients with myalgias due to statins may have normal or elevated CK levels. Symptoms usually improve within a few days after the drug is discontinued. Some patients who have myalgias with one statin may be able to tolerate another statin. The myalgias may also be dose related in some patients.

- **Rhabdomyolysis** is a rare complication of statin use. It is more likely to occur in elderly or debilitated patients, individuals with renal or congestive heart failure, or patients on medications that affect the metabolism of the statins, including fibric acid derivatives (especially gemfibrozil), cyclosporine, macrolide antibiotics, or drugs with significant cytochrome P-450 metabolism such as itraconazole.[10]

- **Bile acid sequestrant resins** lower LDL by 15%–30%. Because the resins can raise triglycerides, they should not be used as monotherapy in patients with triglycerides above 250 mg/dL. Usual dosages are 4–20 g/d of cholestyramine or colestipol. Up to 24 g of cholestyramine or 30 g of colestipol may be used.
  - **Cholestyramine** and **colestipol** are available in powder form, in bulk, or in single-dose packets. Colestipol is also available in 1-g tablets. Once- or twice-daily dosing close to meals is desirable. A single daily dose of up to 8–12 g may be useful to fit the resin into a medication schedule. Resins can be combined with nicotinic acid or reductase inhibitors to treat patients with severe elevations of LDL cholesterol where greater reductions of LDL are required.
  - **Colesevelam** is another bile acid–binding drug. It is available in 625-mg tablets with a recommended dose of six tablets per day and a maximum dose of seven tablets per day. LDL cholesterol reduction is 15%–18%. Interactions with other drugs and gastrointestinal side effects may be less frequent than with the older resins. The addition of bile acid–binding drugs to statins can produce additional reduction of LDL levels that are needed to get to goal in some patients.
  - The most common side effects of the resins are bloating, hard stools, and constipation. Initiation of therapy with low doses, patient education, and use of stool softeners or psyllium can increase compliance. Many patients like the idea of taking a medication that is not absorbed. Patients with severe constipation and very complicated drug regimens are not usually good candidates for resin therapy. Side effects are generally less with colesevelam than with the older resins. Other medications must be taken 1 hour before or 4 hours after the cholestyramine or colestipol.

- **Ezetimibe** is a cholesterol absorption inhibitor. It blocks the absorption of cholesterol at the level of the enterocyte. LDL cholesterol levels can decrease by about 20%. The dose is 10 mg daily, and it is not affected by food. Ezetimibe can be used alone or in combination with statins.
  - The addition of ezetimibe to a given dose of a statin may produce additional lowering of LDL by 20% or more.
  - Side effects include diarrhea and myalgias.
  - Liver enzyme elevations can occur with the combination of ezetimibe and statins, and transaminases should be monitored with the combination as they would be with the statins.
  - Fixed-dose simvastatin/ezetimibe combination tablets are available and can be considered in patients who are using this combination.

- **Nicotinic acid** or **niacin** can lower triglycerides, raise HDL, and lower LDL in higher doses. It is particularly useful in combined hyperlipidemia and in patients with low levels of HDL. Niacin requires extensive patient education because of the flushing and other side effects that can occur.
  - To initiate therapy with nicotinic acid, patients should begin taking 100 mg/d for 2–3 days, then increase to 100 mg tid for 1 week, then 200 mg tid the second week, and 300 mg tid the third week, and repeat lipids; serum chemistries should be obtained after another 3 weeks while patients remain on 300 mg tid. The dose can gradually be increased to the highest dose the patient can tolerate that produces desired results, up to 3,000 mg/d. Patients should report any nausea or increased fatigue as these may be signs of toxicity; liver function tests should be measured and the dose decreased if these are elevated. For patients on higher doses, 500-mg non–time-release tablets are available from several manufacturers. A prescription-only, extended-release formulation can be given once a day at bedtime; significant liver toxicity was not reported at doses up to 2,000 mg/d in clinical trials. Thus, the maximum dose is 2,000 mg/d. The initial dose is 500 mg at bedtime. The dose can be increased by 500 mg at 4-week intervals up to the

maximum dose. The entire dose should be given at bedtime, and this preparation should not be combined with any other niacin preparations.

- **Adverse effects.** Some over-the-counter sustained-release preparations have been associated with severe liver toxicity; crystalline or non–time-release preparations should be used. Flushing can be decreased by starting with low doses, use of aspirin before each dose, and having the patient take nicotinic acid with meals. Uric acid, blood glucose, and serum transaminases should be monitored every 6–8 weeks during the titration phase. Nicotinic acid should be avoided in patients with a history of gout, active peptic ulcer disease, and liver disease. Diabetic patients should only use niacin if they have hemoglobin A_{1c} levels of approximately 7% or less and should monitor blood sugars closely.

- **Hypertriglyceridemia** usually responds to a combined approach using nonpharmacologic and drug therapy.
  - Patients should be instructed to decrease their intake of alcohol and simple sugars and to exercise regularly. Some patients who markedly increase their carbohydrate intake will have increases in triglyceride levels. Hypertriglyceridemic patients should generally not be on diets with fat content <25% of calories, except for patients with the chylomicronemia syndrome. The response to very-low-fat diets (i.e., 10% of calories from fat) may be disappointing in patients with impaired glucose tolerance unless the diet is sufficiently hypocaloric. Very-high-carbohydrate diets that are isocaloric may lead to poor glycemic control and increased triglyceride levels. A particular problem is a high intake of nonfat desserts leading to increased calories in an otherwise low-fat diet. Modest amounts of weight loss can be extremely helpful. In addition, patients with diabetes, especially those with very high triglyceride levels, should have good glycemic control.
    - Omega-3 fatty acids, found in fish oils, can help reduce triglyceride levels. Fish oil capsules containing the long-chain fatty acids eicosapentaenoic acid (EPA) and docosahexaenoic acid (DHA) can be used as an adjunct to other therapies in patients with hypertriglyceridemia. At doses of 3–6 g/d of eicosapentaenoic acid and docosahexaenoic acid, triglycerides may decrease by up to 30%. The major drawbacks to high doses of these fatty acids are large numbers of pills to be taken, eructation, and occasional diarrhea. They have a mild antiplatelet effect, which may be of concern in patients who are receiving warfarin or antiplatelet drugs. A prescription-only omega-3 preparation is available. Four tablets contain about 3.6 g of omega-3 acid ethyl esters and can lower triglycerides by 20%–30%.
  - **Drug therapy**
    - Patients with triglycerides of 400 mg/dL or less and elevated LDL cholesterol levels may respond adequately to a statin added to nonpharmacologic measures.
    - If the triglycerides are above 400 mg/dL despite adequate dietary modifications and exercise, the choice of medication could include a statin at higher doses, gemfibrozil, fenofibrate, niacin, or omega-3 fatty acids.
    - For patients with triglycerides over 1,000 mg/dL, fibrates and niacin are the drugs of choice. If LDL cholesterol levels remain high after the triglycerides are lowered, combination therapy can be considered.
    - Combination therapy of niacin and a statin or fibrate and a statin may increase the risk of **myopathy** including **rhabdomyolysis.** The risk is less with a statin–niacin combination. The combination of a fibrate and statin should be avoided in patients with renal insufficiency, congestive heart failure, severe debility, or other conditions, which may affect the metabolism of medications. Patients whose triglycerides remain above 200 mg/dL should have non-HDL cholesterol evaluated as a secondary goal of therapy. If non-HDL cholesterol is not at goal, therapeutic lifestyle changes should be emphasized. The dose of statin can be increased or a second medication such as ezetimibe can be added. Gemfibrozil and fenofibrate are the fibric acid derivatives that are available in the United States.
    - The usual dose of **gemfibrozil** is 600 mg bid before meals. Triglyceride levels are usually reduced by 30%–50%. The drug should not be used in patients with very low creatinine clearances. Abdominal pain and nausea are the most common side effects. The incidence of gallstones is increased in patients who are receiving

the fibric acid derivatives due to increased cholesterol content of bile. Patients on warfarin need to have their INR monitored closely after they start taking gemfibrozil.

- The use of **fenofibrate** is similar to that of gemfibrozil. Fenofibrate is available in several different strengths, including 48- and 145-mg tablets; 54- and 160-mg tablets; 67-, 134-, and 200-mg capsules; and 43-, 87-, and 130-mg capsules. Fenofibrate can be given once a day with a meal. Although the starting dosages are the lower strengths, many patients require the full dose of 145 or 160 mg/d. However, a lower dose should be used in patients with renal insufficiency. It can be given once a day with a meal. Side effects, which occur in 5%–10% of patients, are primarily mild gastrointestinal discomfort and, less frequently, rash and pruritus. Increased transaminases occur in about 5% of patients and return to normal when the drug is discontinued. Infrequently, myalgias and increased CPK have been reported. In addition to its use for lowering triglycerides, fenofibrate may also be useful in some patients with combined hyperlipidemia who have moderately elevated LDL cholesterol levels and high triglycerides.

- Drugs such as **estrogen, retinoids,** and **thiazides** may contribute to hypertriglyceridemia. The use of transdermal estrogen instead of oral estrogen preparations can lead to significant decreases in triglyceride levels in women who are receiving postmenopausal HRT. Oral estrogen preparations should be avoided in women with triglyceride levels above 500 mg/dL.

- The **chylomicronemia syndrome** requires a diet that is very low in total fat. Patients with triglycerides above 2,000 mg/dL should initiate a diet with <10% of total calories as fat. It may be possible to gradually increase the fat content as the triglyceride level falls to <500 mg/dL. Primary lipoprotein lipase deficiency is treated with fat restriction and does not respond to drug therapy.

- The **metabolic syndrome** is a secondary target of risk reduction therapy. Weight control and increased physical activity are important in the treatment of the metabolic syndrome. Other risk factors such as hypertension should also be treated. Elevated triglycerides or low HDL, or both, should be treated once the LDL goal has been reached.

- **Low HDL cholesterol** levels are associated with an increased risk of cardiovascular disease. Attention should be given to factors that lower HDL, such as cigarette smoking and certain medications such as β-adrenergic–blocking agents, androgenic compounds, and progestins. Nonpharmacologic therapy such as exercise, weight loss, and smoking cessation should be stressed. Niacin is the most effective agent for increasing HDL. Some increase (approximately 10%–20%) can occur with fibrates, but generally only in patients with elevated triglycerides. Once patients have reached LDL cholesterol goals, the addition of niacin may be useful to raise HDL cholesterol levels in suitable patients.

References

1. Randomised trial of cholesterol lowering in 4444 patients with coronary heart disease: the Scandinavian Simvastatin Survival Study (4S). *Lancet* 1994;344:1383–1389.
2. Sacks FM, Pfeffer MA, Moye LA, et al. The effect of pravastatin on coronary events after myocardial infarction in patients with average cholesterol levels. Cholesterol and Recurrent Events Trial Investigators. *N Engl J Med* 1996;335:1001–1009.
3. Shepherd J, Cobbe SM, Ford I, et al. Prevention of coronary heart disease with pravastatin in men with hypercholesterolemia. West of Scotland Coronary Prevention Study Group. *N Engl J Med* 1995;333:1301–1307.
4. Downs JR, Clearfield M, Weis S, et al. Primary prevention of acute coronary events with lovastatin in men and women with average cholesterol levels: results of AF-CAPS/TexCAPS. Air Force/Texas Coronary Atherosclerosis Prevention Study. *JAMA* 1998;279:1615–1622.
5. The Long-Term Intervention with Pravastatin in Ischemic Disease (LIPID) Study Group. Prevention of cardiovascular events and death with pravastatin in patients with coronary heart disease and a broad range of initial cholesterol levels. *N Engl J Med* 1998;339:1349–1357.

6. Heart Protection Study Collaborative Group. MRC/BHF Heart Protection Study of cholesterol lowering with simvastatin in 20,536 high-risk individuals: a randomised placebo-controlled trial. *Lancet* 2002;360:7–22.

7. Cannon CP, Braunwald E, McCabe CH, et al. Intensive versus moderate lipid lowering with statins after acute coronary syndromes. *N Engl J Med* 2004;350:1495–1504.

8. Executive Summary of The Third Report of The National Cholesterol Education Program (NCEP) Expert Panel on Detection, Evaluation, and Treatment of High Blood Cholesterol in Adults (Adult Treatment Panel III). Expert Panel on Detection, Evaluation, and Treatment of High Blood Cholesterol in Adults. *JAMA* 2001;285:2486–2497.

9. Grundy SM, Cleeman JI, Merz CN, et al. Implications of recent clinical trials for the National Cholesterol Education Program Adult Treatment Panel III guidelines. *Circulation* 2004;110:227–239.

10. Pasternak RC, Smith SC Jr, Bairey-Merz CN, et al. ACC/AHA/NHLBI Clinical Advisory on the Use and Safety of Statins. *Circulation* 2002;106:1024–1028.

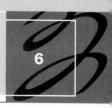

HEART FAILURE

GENERAL PRINCIPLES

Definition

- Heart failure (HF) is the inability of the heart to maintain an output adequate to meet the metabolic demands of the body. It is an increasingly common condition that affects approximately 5 million Americans and is associated with extremely high morbidity and mortality. It is a syndrome and not a disease.

Epidemiology

- About 5 million cases of heart failure are prevalent in the United States.
- Incidence is estimated at 550,000 cases per year.
- The 5-year mortality rate following diagnosis with heart failure is approximately 50%.

Classification

- HF may be secondary to abnormalities in myocardial contraction (systolic dysfunction), ventricular relaxation and filling (diastolic dysfunction), or both.
- Severity can be classified according to New York Heart Association (NYHA) status, ACC/AHA stage (Table 6-1) or metabolic capacity.

Pathophysiology

- HF is manifested as organ hypoperfusion and inadequate tissue oxygen delivery due to a low cardiac output and decreased cardiac reserve, as well as pulmonary and systemic venous congestion.
- A variety of "compensatory adaptations" occur, including (a) increased left ventricular (LV) volume (dilation) and mass (hypertrophy), (b) increased systemic vascular resistance (SVR) secondary to enhanced activity of the sympathetic nervous system and elevated levels of circulating catecholamines, and (c) activation of the renin-angiotensin-aldosterone and vasopressin (antidiuretic hormone) systems. These secondary mechanisms, in conjunction with pump failure, play an important role in the pathophysiology of HF.

Etiology

- Hypertension (HTN) and coronary artery disease are the most frequent causes of HF in the United States.
- Other causes include valvular heart disease, toxic or metabolic disease, infiltrative disease, infections, and drugs.

TABLE 6-1 American College of Cardiology/American Heart Association Guidelines of Evaluation and Management of Chronic Heart Failure in Adults

Stage	Description	Treatment
A	No structural heart disease and no symptoms but risk factors: CAD, HTN, DM, cardiotoxins, familial cardiomyopathy	Lifestyle modification—diet, exercise, smoking cessation; treat hyperlipidemia and use ACEI for HTN
B	Abnormal LV systolic function, MI, valvular heart disease but no HF symptoms	Lifestyle modifications, ACEI, β-adrenergic blockers
C	Structural heart disease and HF symptoms	Lifestyle modifications, ACEI, β-adrenergic blockers, diuretics, digoxin
D	Refractory HF symptoms to maximal medical management	Therapy listed under A, B, C and mechanical assist device, heart transplantation, continuous IV inotropic infusion, hospice care in selected patients

ACEI, angiotensin-converting enzyme inhibitor; CAD, coronary artery disease; DM, diabetes mellitus; HF, heart failure; HTN, hypertension; LV, left ventricular; MI, myocardial infarction.
Source: Adapted from SA Hunt, DW Baker, MH Chin, et al. ACC/AHA guidelines for the evaluation and management of chronic heart failure in the adult: executive summary. *J Am Coll Cardiol* 2005;46:1116–1143.

■ Precipitants of HF include myocardial ischemia, HTN, arrhythmias, infection, thyroid disease, volume overload, alcohol/toxins, drugs (nonsteroidal anti-inflammatory drugs [NSAIDs], calcium channel antagonists, doxorubicin), pulmonary embolism, and dietary or medical noncompliance.

DIAGNOSIS

Clinical Presentation

■ Clinical manifestations of HF vary depending on the rapidity of cardiac decompensation, underlying etiology, age, and comorbidities of the patient.
■ Extreme deterioration in cardiac output and elevated SVR result in hypoperfusion of vital organs such as the kidney (decreased urine output) and brain (confusion and lethargy) and, ultimately, cardiogenic shock.

Symptoms

■ Fatigue
■ Exercise intolerance
■ Dyspnea with exertion
■ Orthopnea, paroxysmal nocturnal dyspnea
■ Presyncope, palpitations, and angina may be present in varying circumstances.

Physical Examination

■ Chronic pulmonary and systemic venous congestion results in pulmonary crackles, peripheral edema, elevated jugular venous pressure, pleural and pericardial effusions, hepatic congestion, and ascites.
■ Third or fourth heart sounds may be present.

Laboratory Studies

- B-type natriuretic peptide (BNP) is synthesized by right and left ventricular myocytes and released in response to stretch, volume overload, and elevated filling pressures. Serum levels of BNP are elevated in patients with asymptomatic LV dysfunction as well as symptomatic HF.
- A serum BNP of <100 pg/mL has a good negative predictive value and typically excludes HF as primary diagnosis in dyspneic patients.
- BNP levels correlate with the severity of HF and predict survival.[1]
- Associated laboratory abnormalities include elevated levels of blood urea nitrogen (BUN) and creatinine, hyponatremia, anemia, and elevated serum levels of hepatic enzymes.

Imaging

- Abnormalities in the electrocardiogram (ECG) are common and include supraventricular and ventricular arrhythmias, conduction delays, and nonspecific ST-T changes.
- Radiographic evidence of cardiomegaly and pulmonary vascular redistribution is common.
- Depressed ventricular function should be confirmed by echocardiography, radionuclide ventriculography, or cardiac catheterization with left ventriculography.

TREATMENT

Behavioral

- Exercise training is recommended in stable HF patients. Ideally, it should be started slowly in a monitored outpatient setting and reach a target of 20–45 minutes a day for 3–5 days a week for a total of 8–12 weeks. Short-term effects of exercise training in chronic stable HF patients are additive to pharmacologic treatment and are associated with a decrease in neurohormonal activation.
- Patients enrolled in exercise training programs notice increased exercise capacity, decreased symptoms, increased quality of life, and decreased hospitalization rate.
- The effects of long-term exercise training on survival are not defined.[2]
- Restriction of physical activity may be required in acute HF exacerbations to reduce myocardial workload and oxygen consumption.
- Weight loss and fluid restriction should be instituted when appropriate.
- Patients should be counseled about smoking cessation.

Medications

- The general principle of pharmacologic therapy involves the antagonism of neurohormones that are increased in patients with HF and have deleterious effects on the myocardium and the peripheral vasculature. Vasodilator therapy and β-adrenergic blockade are the cornerstone of therapy for patients with HF. Diuretics are reserved for relieving volume overload. Most patients require a multidrug regimen to control symptoms and prolong survival (Table 6-1).
- β-**Adrenergic receptor antagonists** (see Chapter 4, Hypertension, and Table 6-2) are critical components of HF pharmacotherapy that block the cardiac effects of chronic adrenergic stimulation, including myocyte toxicity.
  - Large randomized trials have documented the beneficial effects of β-adrenergic antagonists on functional status and survival in patients with NYHA class II–IV symptoms.
  - Improvement in ejection fraction (EF), exercise tolerance, and functional class are common after the institution of a β-adrenergic antagonist.
  - Typically, 2–3 months of therapy is required to observe significant effects on LV function, but reduction of cardiac arrhythmia and incidence of sudden cardiac death may occur much earlier.[3]
  - β-Adrenergic antagonists should be instituted at a low dose and titrated with careful attention to blood pressure (BP) and heart rate. Some patients experience volume

TABLE 6-2	Drugs Commonly Used for Treatment of Heart Failure	

Drug	Initial dose	Target
Angiotensin-converting enzyme inhibitors		
Captopril	6.25–12.5 mg q6–8h	50 mg tid
Enalapril	2.5 mg bid	10 mg bid
Fosinopril	5–10 mg daily; can use bid	20 mg daily
Lisinopril	2.5–5.0 mg daily; can use bid	10–20 mg bid
Quinapril	2.5–5.0 mg bid	10 mg bid
Ramipril	1.25–2.5 mg bid	5 mg bid
Trandolapril	0.5–1.0 mg daily	4 mg daily
Angiotensin receptor blockers		
Valsartan[a]	40 mg bid	160 mg bid
Losartan	25 mg daily; can use bid	25–100 mg daily
Irbesartan	75–150 mg daily	75–300 mg daily
Candesartan[a]	2–16 mg daily	2–32 mg daily
Olmesartan	20 mg daily	20–40 mg daily
Thiazide diuretics		
HCTZ	25–50 mg daily	25–50 mg daily
Metolazone	2.5–5.0 mg daily or bid	10–20 total mg daily
Loop diuretics		
Bumetanide	0.5–1.0 mg daily or bid	10 mg total daily (maximum)
Furosemide	20–40 mg daily or bid	400 total mg daily (maximum)
Torsemide	10–20 mg daily or bid	200 total mg daily (maximum)
Aldosterone antagonists		
Eplerenone	25 mg daily	50 mg daily
Spironolactone	12.5–25.0 mg daily	25 mg daily
Beta-blockers		
Bisoprolol	1.25 mg daily	10 mg daily
Carvedilol	3.125 mg q12h	25–50 mg q12h
Metoprolol succinate	12.5–25.0 mg daily	200 mg daily
Digoxin	0.125–0.25 mg daily	0.125–0.25 mg daily

HCTZ, hydrochlorothiazide.
[a]Valsartan and Candesartan are the only U.S. Food and Drug Administration–approved angiotensin II-receptor blockers in the treatment of heart failure.

retention and worsening HF symptoms that typically respond to transient increases in diuretic therapy. Individual β-adrenergic antagonists have unique properties (see Chapter 4, Hypertension), and the beneficial effect of β-adrenergic antagonists in HF may not be a class effect.[4]

- Therefore, β-adrenergic antagonists with proven effects on patient survival in large clinical trials (bisoprolol, metoprolol succinate, and carvedilol) should be used.
  - **Carvedilol** (Table 6-2) is the best studied β-adrenergic antagonist in heart failure. It has been shown to be superior to metoprolol tartrate for chronic treatment.[4,5]
  - **Bisoprolol** (Table 6-2)[6]
  - **Metoprolol succinate** (Table 6-2)[7]
- **Vasodilator therapy** is another mainstay of treatment in patients with HF. Arterial vasoconstriction (afterload) and venous vasoconstriction (preload) occur in patients with HF as a result of activation of the renin-angiotensin-aldosterone system and adrenergic nervous system, as well as increased secretion of arginine vasopressin. Agents with predominantly venodilatory properties decrease preload and ventricular filling pressures. In the absence of LV outflow tract obstruction, arterial vasodilators reduce

afterload by decreasing SVR, resulting in increased cardiac output, decreased ventricular filling pressure, and decreased myocardial wall stress. The efficacy and toxicity of vasodilator therapy depend on intravascular volume status and preload. Vasodilators should be used with caution in patients with a fixed cardiac output [e.g., aortic stenosis (AS) or hypertrophic cardiomyopathy (HCM)] or with predominantly diastolic dysfunction.

- Oral vasodilators should be the initial therapy in patients with symptomatic chronic HF and in patients in whom parenteral vasodilators are being discontinued. When treatment with oral vasodilators is being initiated in hypotensive patients, it is prudent to use agents with a short half-life.
  - **ACE inhibitors** (Table 6-2) attenuate vasoconstriction, vital organ hypoperfusion, hyponatremia, hypokalemia, and fluid retention attributable to compensatory activation of the renin-angiotensin system.
    - Treatment with ACE inhibitors decreases afterload while increasing cardiac output.
    - Large clinical trials have clearly demonstrated that ACE inhibitors improve symptoms and survival in patients with LV systolic dysfunction.
    - ACE inhibitors may also prevent the development of HF in patients with asymptomatic LV dysfunction and in those at high risk of developing structural heart disease or HF symptoms (coronary artery disease, diabetes mellitus, HTN). Currently, no consensus has been reached regarding the optimal dosing of ACE inhibitors in HF, although one study suggested that higher doses decrease morbidity without improving overall survival.[8]
    - Absence of an initial beneficial response to treatment with an ACE inhibitor does not preclude long-term benefit.
    - Most ACE inhibitors are excreted by the kidneys, necessitating careful dose titration in patients with renal insufficiency. Acute renal insufficiency may occur in patients with bilateral renal artery stenosis. Additional adverse effects include rash, angioedema, dysgeusia, increases in serum creatinine, proteinuria, hyperkalemia, leukopenia, and cough.
    - *ACE inhibitors are contraindicated in pregnancy.*
    - Oral potassium supplements, potassium salt substitutes, and potassium-sparing diuretics should be used with caution during treatment with an ACE inhibitor.
    - Agranulocytosis and angioedema are more common with captopril than with other ACE inhibitors, particularly in patients with associated collagen vascular disease or serum creatinine >1.5 mg/dL.
  - **Angiotensin II receptor blockers (ARBs)** (Table 6-2) inhibit the renin-angiotensin system via specific blockade of the angiotensin II receptor.
    - In contrast to ACE inhibitors, they do not increase bradykinin levels, which may be responsible for adverse effects such as cough.
    - ARBs reduce mortality and morbidity associated with HF in patients who are not receiving an ACE inhibitor.[9–11]
    - ARBs should be considered in patients who are intolerant to ACE inhibitors due to cough or angioedema.
    - Caution should be exercised when ARBs are used in patients with renal insufficiency and bilateral renal artery stenosis because hyperkalemia and acute renal failure can develop.
    - Renal function and potassium levels should be periodically monitored.
    - *ARBs are contraindicated in pregnancy.*
  - **Hydralazine** acts directly on arterial smooth muscle to produce vasodilation and to reduce afterload. In combination with nitrates, hydralazine improves survival in patients with HF.[12]
    - A **combination of hydralazine and isosorbide dinitrate** (starting dose: 37.5/20 mg three times daily) when added to standard therapy with beta-blockers and ACE inhibitors has been shown to reduce mortality in black patients.[13]
    - Reflex tachycardia and increased myocardial oxygen consumption may occur, requiring cautious use in patients with ischemic heart disease.

- **Nitrates** are predominantly venodilators and help relieve symptoms of venous and pulmonary congestion. They reduce myocardial ischemia by decreasing ventricular filling pressures and by directly dilating coronary arteries.
  - Nitrate therapy may precipitate hypotension in patients with reduced preload.
- **Parenteral vasodilators** should be reserved for patients with severe HF or those who are unable to take oral medications. IV vasodilator therapy may be guided by central hemodynamic monitoring (pulmonary artery catheterization) to assess efficacy and avoid hemodynamic instability. Parenteral agents should be started at low doses, titrated to the desired hemodynamic effect, and discontinued slowly to avoid rebound vasoconstriction.
  - **Nitroglycerin** is a potent vasodilator, with effects on venous and, to a lesser extent, arterial vascular beds. It relieves pulmonary and systemic venous congestion and is an effective coronary vasodilator.
    - Nitroglycerin is the preferred vasodilator for treatment of HF in the setting of *acute myocardial infarction* (MI) or *unstable angina*.
  - **Sodium nitroprusside** is a direct arterial vasodilator with less potent venodilatory properties. Its predominant effect is to reduce afterload, and it is particularly effective in patients with HF who are hypertensive or who have severe aortic or mitral valvular regurgitation.
    - Nitroprusside should be used cautiously in patients with myocardial ischemia because of a potential reduction in regional myocardial blood flow (*coronary steal*).
    - The initial dose of **0.25 mcg/kg/min** can be titrated (**maximum dose of 10 mcg/kg/min**) to the desired hemodynamic effect or until hypotension develops. The half-life of nitroprusside is 1–3 minutes, and its metabolism results in the release of cyanide, which is metabolized hepatically to thiocyanate and then is excreted renally.
    - *Toxic levels* of thiocyanate (>10 mg/dL) may develop in patients with renal insufficiency. Thiocyanate toxicity is manifested as nausea, paresthesias, mental status changes, abdominal pain, and seizures (see Chapter 4, Hypertension).
    - *Methemoglobinemia* is a rare complication of treatment with nitroprusside.
  - **Recombinant BNP (nesiritide)** is an arterial and venous vasodilator.
    - Intravenous infusion of nesiritide reduces right atrial and left ventricular end-diastolic pressures (LVEDP) and SVR and results in an increase in cardiac output.
    - It is administered as a 2-mcg/kg IV bolus followed by a continuous IV infusion starting of 0.01 mcg/kg/min. Nesiritide is approved for use in acute HF exacerbations and relieves HF symptoms early after its administration.[14] It should not be used to improve renal function or to enhance diuresis. *Nesiritide is not recommended for intermittent outpatient use.*
    - *Hypotension* is the most common side effect of nesiritide, and its use should be avoided in patients with systemic hypotension (systolic BP <90 mm Hg) or evidence of cardiogenic shock. Episodes of hypotension should be managed with discontinuation of nesiritide and cautious volume expansion or pressor support if necessary.
  - **Enalaprilat** is an active metabolite of the ACE inhibitor enalapril that is available for IV administration.
    - Its onset of action is more rapid and its pharmacologic half-life shorter than that of enalapril. The initial dosage is 1.25 mg IV q6h, which can be titrated to a maximum dosage of 5 mg IV q6h. Patients who take diuretics or those with impaired renal function (serum creatinine >3 mg/dL, creatinine clearance <30 mL/min) initially should receive 0.625 mg IV q6h. When dosing is being converted from IV to PO administration, enalaprilat, 0.625 mg IV q6h, is approximately equivalent to enalapril, 2.5 mg PO daily.
- **α-Adrenergic receptor antagonists**
  - These agents have not been shown to improve survival in HF, and hypertensive patients treated with doxazosin as first-line therapy had an increased risk of developing HF.[15]
- **Digitalis glycosides** increase myocardial contractility and may attenuate the neurohormonal activation associated with HF.

- Digoxin decreases the number of HF hospitalizations without altering overall mortality.[16]
- Discontinuation of digoxin in patients who are stable on a regimen of digoxin, diuretics, and an ACE inhibitor may result in clinical deterioration.[17]
- *The toxic–therapeutic ratio is narrow*, and serum levels should be followed closely, particularly in patients with unstable renal function.
- The usual daily dose is 0.125–0.25 mg and should be decreased in patients with renal insufficiency. Clinical benefits may not be related to the serum levels, and, although serum digoxin levels of 0.8–2.0 ng/mL are considered "therapeutic," toxicity can occur in this range.
- Observations suggest that women and patients with higher serum digoxin levels (1.2–2.0 ng/mL) have an increased mortality risk.[18,19]
- *Drug interactions with digoxin* are common. Oral antibiotics such as erythromycin and tetracycline may increase digoxin levels by 10%–40%. Quinidine, verapamil, flecainide, and amiodarone also increase digoxin levels significantly.
- *Digoxin toxicity* may be caused or exacerbated by drug interactions, electrolyte abnormalities (particularly hypokalemia), hypoxemia, hypothyroidism, renal insufficiency, and volume depletion.

- **Diuretic therapy** (Table 6-2), in conjunction with restriction of dietary sodium and fluids, often leads to clinical improvement in patients with symptomatic HF. Frequent assessment of the patient's weight along with careful observation of fluid intake and output is essential during initiation and maintenance of therapy. Frequent complications of therapy include hypokalemia, hyponatremia, hypomagnesemia, volume contraction alkalosis, intravascular volume depletion, and hypotension. Serum electrolytes, BUN, and creatinine levels should be followed after institution of diuretic therapy. Hypokalemia may be life threatening in patients who are receiving digoxin or in those who have severe LV dysfunction that predisposes them to ventricular arrhythmias. Potassium supplementation or a potassium-sparing diuretic should be considered in addition to careful monitoring of serum potassium levels.
  - **Thiazide diuretics** (hydrochlorothiazide, chlorthalidone) can be used as initial agents in patients with normal renal function in whom only a mild diuresis is desired. Metolazone, unlike other thiazides, exerts its action at the proximal as well as the distal tubule and may be useful in combination with a loop diuretic in patients with a low glomerular filtration rate.
  - **Loop diuretics** (furosemide, ethacrynic acid, bumetanide) should be used in patients who require significant diuresis and in those with markedly decreased renal function. Furosemide reduces preload acutely by causing direct venodilation when administered IV, making it useful for managing severe HF or acute pulmonary edema. Use of loop diuretics may be complicated by hyperuricemia, hypocalcemia, ototoxicity, rash, and vasculitis. Furosemide and bumetanide are sulfa derivatives and may cause drug reactions in sulfa-sensitive patients. Ethacrynic acid can generally be used safely in such patients.
- **Potassium-sparing diuretics** do not exert a potent diuretic effect when used alone.
  - **Spironolactone** (25 mg daily) is an aldosterone receptor antagonist that has been shown to improve survival and decrease hospitalizations in NYHA class III–IV patients.[20] The potential for development of life-threatening hyperkalemia exists with the use of these agents. Gynecomastia may develop in 10%–20% of men treated with spironolactone. Serum potassium must be monitored closely after initiation; concomitant use of ACE inhibitors and NSAIDs and the presence of renal insufficiency (creatinine >2.5 mg/dL) increase the risk of hyperkalemia.
  - **Eplerenone**, a selective aldosterone receptor antagonist without the hormonal side effects of spironolactone, is Food and Drug Administration (FDA) approved for treatment of HTN and HF and reduces mortality in patients with HF associated with acute MI.[21]
- **Inotropic agents**
  - **Sympathomimetic agents** are potent drugs that are primarily used to treat severe HF. Beneficial and adverse effects are mediated by stimulation of myocardial β-adrenergic

TABLE 6-3	Inotropic Agents		
Drug	**Dose**	**Mechanism**	**Effects/side effects**
Dopamine	1–3 mcg/kg/min	Dopaminergic receptors	Splanchnic vasodilation
	2–8 mcg/kg/min	β_1-Receptor agonist	+Inotropic
	7–10 mcg/kg/min	α-Receptor agonist	↑ SVR
Dobutamine	2.5–15.0 mcg/kg/min	β_1->β_2->α-receptor agonist	+Inotropic, ↓ SVR, tachycardia
Milrinone[a]	50-mcg/kg bolus IV over 10 min, 0.375–0.75 mcg/kg/min	↑ cAMP	↓ SVR, +inotropic; atrial and ventricular tachyarrhythmias

cAMP, cyclic adenosine monophosphate; SVR, systemic vascular resistance; ↑, increased; ↓, decreased.
[a]Needs dose adjustment for creatinine clearance.

receptors. The most important adverse effects are related to the arrhythmogenic nature of these agents and the potential for exacerbation of myocardial ischemia. Treatment should be guided by careful hemodynamic and ECG monitoring. Patients with refractory chronic HF may benefit symptomatically from continuous ambulatory administration of IV inotropes as palliative therapy or as a bridge to mechanical ventricular support or cardiac transplantation.[2] However, this strategy may increase the risk of life-threatening arrhythmias or indwelling catheter-related infections.
- **Dopamine** (Table 6-3) should be used primarily for stabilization of the hypotensive patient.
- **Dobutamine** (Table 6-3) is a synthetic analog of dopamine. Dobutamine tolerance has been described, and several studies have demonstrated increased mortality in patients treated with continuous dobutamine. Dobutamine has no significant role in the treatment of HF resulting from diastolic dysfunction or a high-output state.
- **Phosphodiesterase inhibitors** increase myocardial contractility and produce vasodilation by increasing intracellular cyclic adenosine monophosphate. Milrinone is currently available for clinical use and is indicated for treatment of refractory HF. Hypotension may develop in patients who receive vasodilator therapy or have intravascular volume contraction, or both. Milrinone may improve hemodynamics in patients who are treated concurrently with dobutamine or dopamine. Data suggest that in-hospital short-term milrinone administration in addition to standard medical therapy does not reduce the length of hospitalization or the 60-day death or rehospitalization rate when compared with placebo.[22]
- **Minimization of medications** with deleterious effects in HF should be attempted.
  - **Negative inotropes** (e.g., verapamil, diltiazem) should be avoided in patients with impaired ventricular contractility, as should over-the-counter β stimulants [e.g., compounds containing ephedra, pseudoephedrine hydrochloride (Sudafed)].
  - **NSAIDs,** which antagonize the effect of ACE inhibitors and diuretic therapy, should be avoided if possible.

Nonoperative Management

- **Coronary revascularization** reduces ischemia and may improve systolic function in some patients with coronary artery disease.
- **Cardiac resynchronization therapy** or **biventricular pacing** (see Chapter 7, Cardiac Arrhythmias) appears to be beneficial in patients with an ejection fraction of 35% or less, NYHA class III–IV HF, and conduction abnormalities (left bundle branch block and

atrioventricular delay). It has been demonstrated to improve quality of life and reduce the risk of death in carefully selected patients.[23]

- An **intra-aortic balloon pump** (IABP) can be considered for patients in whom other therapies have failed, have transient myocardial dysfunction, or are awaiting a definitive procedure such as transplantation.
  - The IABP is positioned in the aorta with its tip distal to the left subclavian artery.
  - Balloon inflation is synchronous with the cardiac cycle and results in significant preload and afterload reduction, with decreased myocardial oxygen demand and improved coronary blood flow, resulting in improved cardiac output.
  - **Severe aortoiliac atherosclerosis** and aortic valve insufficiency are contraindications to IABP placement.

Surgery

- **Ventricular assist devices** require surgical implantation and are indicated for patients with severe HF after cardiac surgery, for individuals with intractable cardiogenic shock after acute MI, and for patients whose conditions deteriorate while they await cardiac transplantation.
  - Currently available devices vary with regard to degree of mechanical hemolysis, intensity of anticoagulation required, and difficulty of implantation. The decision to institute ventricular assist device circulatory support must be made in consultation with a cardiac surgeon who has experience with this procedure.
  - Ventricular assist devices improve survival in patients with refractory HF who are not candidates for cardiac transplantation ("destination therapy").[24]
- **Cardiac transplantation** is an option for selected patients with severe end-stage HF that has become refractory to aggressive medical therapy and for whom no other conventional treatment options are available.
  - Candidates considered for transplantation should be younger than 65 years (although selected older patients may also benefit), have advanced HF (NYHA class III–IV), have a strong psychological support system, have exhausted all other therapeutic options, and be free of irreversible extracardiac organ dysfunction that would limit functional recovery or predispose them to posttransplantation complications.[25]
  - Survival rates of 90% at 1 year and 70% at 5 years have been reported since the introduction of cyclosporine-based immunosuppression.
  - In general, functional capacity and quality of life improve significantly after transplantation.
  - **Posttransplant complications** include acute and chronic rejection, typical and atypical infections, and adverse effects of immunosuppressive agents. Cardiac allograft vasculopathy (coronary artery disease/chronic rejection) and malignancy are the leading causes of death after the first posttransplant year.

SPECIAL CONSIDERATIONS

- **Fluid and free water restriction** (<1.5 L/d) is especially important in the setting of hyponatremia (serum sodium <130 mEq/L) and volume overload.
- **Administration of oxygen** may relieve dyspnea, improve oxygen delivery, reduce the work of breathing, and limit pulmonary vasoconstriction in patients with hypoxemia. Sleep apnea has prevalence as high as 37% in the HF population. Treatment with nocturnal positive airway pressure improves symptoms and LV EF.[26,27]
- **Dialysis** or **ultrafiltration** may be necessary in patients with severe HF and renal dysfunction who cannot respond adequately to fluid and sodium restriction and diuretics. Other mechanical methods of fluid removal such as therapeutic thoracentesis and paracentesis may provide temporary symptomatic relief of dyspnea. Care must be taken to avoid rapid fluid removal and hypotension.
- **End-of-life considerations** may be necessary in the patient with advanced HF that is refractory to therapy. Discussions regarding the disease course, treatment options, survival, functional status, and advance directives should be addressed early in the treatment of

the patient with HF. For those with end-stage disease (stage D, NYHA class IV) with multiple hospitalizations and severe decline in their functional status and quality of life, hospice and palliative care should be considered.

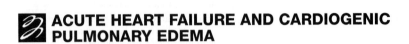

ACUTE HEART FAILURE AND CARDIOGENIC PULMONARY EDEMA

GENERAL PRINCIPLES

Pathophysiology

- Cardiogenic pulmonary edema (CPE) occurs when the pulmonary capillary pressure exceeds the forces that maintain fluid within the vascular space (serum oncotic pressure and interstitial hydrostatic pressure).
- Increased pulmonary capillary pressure may be caused by LV failure of any cause, obstruction to transmitral flow [e.g., mitral stenosis (MS), atrial myxoma], or, rarely, pulmonary veno-occlusive disease.
- Accumulation of fluid in the pulmonary interstitium is followed by alveolar flooding and impairment of gas exchange.

DIAGNOSIS

Clinical Presentation

- Clinical manifestations of CPE may occur rapidly and include dyspnea, anxiety, and restlessness.
- The patient may expectorate pink frothy fluid.
- Physical signs of decreased peripheral perfusion, pulmonary congestion, use of accessory respiratory muscles, and wheezing often are present.

Imaging and Diagnostic Studies

- Radiographic abnormalities include cardiomegaly, interstitial and perihilar vascular engorgement, Kerley B lines, and pleural effusions.
- The radiographic abnormalities may follow the development of symptoms by several hours, and their resolution may be out of phase with clinical improvement.

TREATMENT

Initial Management

- **Supplemental oxygen** should be administered initially to raise the arterial oxygen tension to >60 mm Hg.
    - Mechanical ventilation is indicated if oxygenation is inadequate by noninvasive means or if hypercapnia coexists.
    - Placing the patient in a sitting position improves pulmonary function.
    - Strict bedrest, pain control, and relief of anxiety can decrease cardiac workload.
- **Precipitating factors** should be identified and corrected.
    - Common precipitants of pulmonary edema include severe HTN, MI, or myocardial ischemia [particularly if associated with mitral regurgitation (MR)]; acute valvular regurgitation; new-onset tachyarrhythmias or bradyarrhythmias; and volume overload in the setting of severe LV dysfunction. Successful resolution of pulmonary edema can often be accomplished only by correction of the underlying process.

Medications

- **Morphine sulfate** reduces anxiety and dilates pulmonary and systemic veins.
  - Morphine, 2–5 mg IV, can be given over several minutes and can be repeated every 10–25 minutes until an effect is seen.
- **Furosemide** is a venodilator that decreases pulmonary congestion within minutes of IV administration, well before its diuretic action begins.
  - An initial dose of 20–80 mg IV should be given over several minutes and can be increased based on response, to a maximum of 200 mg in subsequent doses.
- **Nitroglycerin** is a venodilator that can potentiate the effect of furosemide.
  - IV administration is preferable to oral and transdermal forms as it can be rapidly titrated.
- **Nitroprusside** is an effective adjunct in the treatment of acute CPE.
  - It is useful in CPE that results from acute valvular regurgitation or HTN (see Valvular Heart Disease).
  - Pulmonary and systemic arterial catheterization should be considered to guide titration of nitroprusside therapy.
- **Inotropic agents** , such as dobutamine or phosphodiesterase inhibitors, may be helpful after initial treatment of CPE in patients with concomitant hypotension or shock.
- **Recombinant BNP (nesiritide)** is administered as an IV bolus followed by an IV infusion.
  - Nesiritide reduces intracardiac filling pressures by producing vasodilation and indirectly increases the cardiac output.
  - In conjunction with furosemide (Lasix), nesiritide produces natriuresis and diuresis.

SPECIAL CONSIDERATIONS

- **Right heart catheterization** (e.g., Swan-Ganz catheter) may be helpful in cases in which a prompt response to therapy does not occur.
  - The pulmonary artery catheter allows differentiation between cardiogenic and noncardiogenic causes of pulmonary edema via measurement of central hemodynamics and cardiac output and helps to guide subsequent therapy.
- **Acute hemodialysis and ultrafiltration** may be effective, especially in the patient with significant renal dysfunction and diuretic resistance.

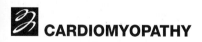 **CARDIOMYOPATHY**

DILATED CARDIOMYOPATHY

General Principles

Definition
- Dilated cardiomyopathy is a disease of heart muscle characterized by dilation of the cardiac chambers and reduction in ventricular contractile function.

Epidemiology
- Lifetime incidence of 36.5 cases per 100,000 persons
- Approximately 10,000 U.S. deaths annually[28]

Pathophysiology
- Dilated cardiomyopathy may be secondary to progression of any process that affects the myocardium and dilation is directly related to neurohormonal activation. The majority of cases are idiopathic.

- Dilation of the cardiac chambers and varying degrees of hypertrophy are anatomic hall-marks. Tricuspid and MR are common due to the effect of chamber dilation on the valvular apparatus.
- **Atrial and ventricular arrhythmias** are present in as many as one-half of these patients and probably are responsible for the high incidence of sudden death in this population.

Diagnosis

Clinical Presentation
- Symptomatic heart failure (dyspnea, volume overload) is often present.
- A portion of patients with preclinical disease may be asymptomatic.
- The ECG is usually abnormal, but changes are typically nonspecific.

Imaging and Diagnostic Studies
- The diagnosis of dilated cardiomyopathy can be confirmed with echocardiography or radionuclide ventriculography.
- Two-dimensional and Doppler echocardiography is helpful in differentiating this condition from hypertrophic or restrictive cardiomyopathy, pericardial disease, and valvular disorders.
- Endomyocardial biopsy provides little information that affects treatment of patients with dilated cardiomyopathies and is not routinely recommended.

Treatment

Medications
- The medical management of symptomatic patients is identical to that for HF from other causes.
- Therapeutic strategies include control of total body sodium and volume in addition to appropriate preload and afterload reduction using vasodilator therapy.
- β-Adrenergic antagonists should be used unless contraindicated.
- Immunizations against influenza and pneumococcal pneumonia are recommended.
- Chronic oral anticoagulation has not been shown to decrease the risk of thromboembolism in patients with LV dysfunction. Anticoagulation should be strongly considered in individuals with a history of thromboembolic events, atrial fibrillation, or evidence of an LV thrombus. The level of anticoagulation recommended varies but is generally an international normalized ratio of 2.0–3.0.
- Immunosuppressive therapy with agents such as prednisone, azathioprine, and cyclosporine for biopsy-proven myocarditis has been advocated by some, but efficacy has not been established.[29]

Nonoperative Management
- Dilated cardiomyopathy (of nonischemic origin) is associated with an increased incidence of **sudden cardiac death** (SCD) and **ventricular arrhythmia**. When compared to NYHA Class IV HF patients, who are more likely to die of progressive pump failure, sudden cardiac death is relatively more common in patients with mild to moderate symptoms.
- Suppression of asymptomatic ventricular premature beats or nonsustained ventricular tachycardia (NSVT) using antiarrhythmic drugs in patients with HF does **not improve survival and may increase mortality** as a result of the proarrhythmic effects of the drugs.[30,31]
- Primary prevention of SCD is recommended by implantation of an implantable cardioverter-defibrillator (ICD) in patients with dilated cardiomyopathy, an ejection fraction of 35% or less, and NYHA class II–III symptoms. Patients should receive aggressive medical treatment including neurohormonal blockade, correction of electrolyte imbalances, and discontinuation of proarrhythmic drugs. Medical therapy is recommended for 3 months following a new diagnosis of dilated cardiomyopathy (DCM) prior to ICD implantation for primary prevention.[32]
- Cardiac resynchronization therapy may be beneficial in selected patients with symptomatic HF.

Surgery

- Cardiac transplantation should be considered for selected patients with HF that is refractory to medical therapy.
- Intra-aortic balloon counterpulsation or placement of a ventricular assist device may be necessary for stabilization of patients in whom cardiac transplantation is an option or before other definitive surgical therapies.
- Mitral valve annuloplasty or replacement can be used for symptomatic relief in patients with severe MR.

DIASTOLIC DYSFUNCTION

General Principles

Definition
- **Diastolic dysfunction** refers to abnormality in the mechanical function of the heart during diastole. Usually, this involves elevated filling pressures and impairment of ventricular filling. A number of echocardiographic criteria are used to evaluate for the presence or absence of diastolic dysfunction.
- **Diastolic heart failure** refers to the syndrome of heart failure in the presence of preserved systolic function.

Epidemiology
- Twenty percent to 40% of patients admitted with a primary HF diagnosis have diastolic heart failure.

Etiology
- Causes include hypertension, ischemia, hypertrophic cardiomyopathy (HCM), restrictive cardiomyopathies, infiltrative disease (amyloidosis, sarcoidosis), and constrictive pericarditis.

Diagnosis

Imaging and Diagnostic Studies
- Differentiating between diastolic and systolic heart failure cannot be reliably accomplished without two-dimensional echocardiography.
- Diagnosis is based on echocardiographic criteria and Doppler findings of normal LV systolic function with impaired diastolic relaxation.

Treatment

- Treatment is directed toward improving the symptoms with diuretic therapy and correcting the precipitating factors (e.g., hypertension, coronary artery disease, tachycardia).

HYPERTROPHIC CARDIOMYOPATHY

General Principles

Definition
- **Hypertrophic cardiomyopathy (HCM)** is a myocardial disorder characterized by ventricular hypertrophy, diminished LV cavity dimensions, normal or enhanced contractile function, and impaired ventricular relaxation.
- The idiopathic form of HCM has an early onset (as early as the first decade of life) without associated HTN.
- An acquired form also occurs in elderly patients with chronic HTN.

Pathophysiology
- The pathophysiologic change in HCM is myocardial hypertrophy that is typically predominant in the ventricular septum (asymmetric hypertrophy) but may involve all ventricular segments equally.
- Many cases of HCM have a genetic component, with mutations in the myosin heavy-chain gene that follow an autosomal-dominant transmission with variable phenotypic expression and penetrance.
- HCM can be classified according to the presence or absence of LV outflow tract obstruction.
- LV outflow obstruction may occur at rest, but is enhanced by factors that increase LV contractility or decrease ventricular volume.
- Delayed ventricular diastolic relaxation and decreased compliance are common and may lead to pulmonary congestion.
- Myocardial ischemia is frequently secondary to a myocardial oxygen supply–demand mismatch.
- Systolic anterior motion of the anterior leaflet of the mitral valve often is associated with MR and may contribute to LV outflow tract obstruction.

Diagnosis

Clinical Presentation
- Presentation varies but may include dyspnea, angina, arrhythmias, syncope, cardiac failure, or sudden death.
- Sudden death is most common in children and young adults between the ages of 10 and 35 years and often occurs during periods of strenuous exertion.

History
- Family history of HCM is suggestive of the familial subtype.

Physical Examination
- Physical findings include bisferious carotid pulse (in the presence of obstruction).
- Forceful double or triple apical impulse and a coarse systolic outflow murmur localized along the left sternal border that is accentuated by maneuvers that decrease preload (e.g., standing, Valsalva maneuver) may also be found.

Imaging and Diagnostic Studies
- The ECG may show conduction system disease or low voltage, in contrast to the increased voltage seen with ventricular hypertrophy.
- Two-dimensional echocardiography and Doppler flow studies can establish the presence of a significant LV outflow gradient at rest or with provocation.
- Additional risk stratification should be pursued with 24- to 48-hour Holter monitoring and exercise testing.

Treatment

- Management is directed toward relief of symptoms and prevention of endocarditis, arrhythmias, and sudden death.
- Treatment in asymptomatic individuals is controversial, and no conclusive evidence has been found that medical therapy is beneficial.
- All individuals with HCM should avoid strenuous physical activity, including most competitive sports.

Medications
- β-Adrenergic antagonists may reduce symptoms of HCM by reducing myocardial contractility and heart rate. However, symptoms may recur during long-term therapy.
- Calcium channel antagonists, particularly verapamil and diltiazem, may improve the symptoms of HCM, primarily by augmentation of diastolic ventricular filling. Therapy should be initiated at low doses, with careful titration in patients with outflow obstruction. The dose should be increased gradually over several days to weeks if symptoms

persist. Dihydropyridines should be avoided in patients with LV outflow tract obstruction as a result of their vasodilatory properties.

- Diuretics may improve pulmonary congestive symptoms in patients with elevated pulmonary venous pressures. These agents should be used cautiously in patients with severe LV outflow obstruction because excessive preload reduction worsens the obstruction.
- Nitrates and vasodilators should be avoided because of the risk of increasing the LV outflow gradient.
- Atrial and ventricular arrhythmias occur commonly in patients with HCM. Supraventricular tachyarrhythmias are tolerated poorly and should be treated aggressively; cardioversion is indicated if hemodynamic compromise develops.
  - **Digoxin is relatively contraindicated** because of its positive inotropic properties and potential for exacerbating ventricular outflow obstruction.
  - Atrial fibrillation should be converted to sinus rhythm when possible, and anticoagulation is recommended if paroxysmal or chronic atrial fibrillation develops.
  - **Diltiazem, verapamil, or β-adrenergic antagonists** can be used to control the ventricular response before cardioversion. Procainamide, disopyramide, or amiodarone (see Chapter 7, Cardiac Arrhythmias) may be effective in the chronic suppression of atrial fibrillation.
  - Patients with NSVT detected on ambulatory monitoring are at increased risk for sudden death. However, the benefit of suppressing these arrhythmias with medical therapy has not been established, and the risk of a proarrhythmic effect of antiarrhythmic drugs exists.
  - ICD placement should be considered in high-risk patients: those with genetic mutations associated with SCD; prior SCD or sustained ventricular tachyarrhythmia; a history of syncope or near-syncope, recurrent or exertional, in young patients; multiple nonsustained episodes of VT on Holter recordings; hypotensive response to exercise; LV hypertrophy with a wall thickness >30 mm in young patients; and a history of sudden, premature death in close relatives.[33] There is very limited benefit for invasive electrophysiologic testing in the risk stratification of patients with HCM.
- Symptomatic ventricular arrhythmias should be treated as outlined in Chapter 7, Cardiac Arrhythmias.
- Dual-chamber pacing (see Chapter 7, Cardiac Arrhythmias) improves symptoms in some patients with HCM.[34] Alteration of the ventricular activation sequence via right ventricular (RV) pacing may minimize LV outflow tract obstruction secondary to asymmetric septal hypertrophy.
- Only 10% of the patients with HCM meet the criteria for pacemaker implantation, and the effect on decreasing the left ventricular outflow tract (LVOT) gradient is only 25%. Dual chamber pacing has not been demonstrated to decrease morbidity and mortality in patients with HCM.

Surgery
- Surgical therapy is useful in the treatment of symptoms but has not been shown to alter the natural history of HCM.
- The most frequently used operative procedure involves septal myotomy-myectomy with or without mitral valve replacement (MVR).
- Alcohol septal ablation, a catheter-based alternative to surgical myotomy-myectomy, seems to be equally effective at reducing obstruction and providing symptomatic relief when compared to the gold standard surgical procedure.[35]
- Cardiac transplantation should be reserved for patients with end-stage HCM with symptomatic HF.

Counseling
- Genetic counseling and family screening are recommended for first-degree relatives of patients at high risk for SCD, because the disease is transmitted as an autosomal-dominant trait.

RESTRICTIVE CARDIOMYOPATHY

General Principles

Definition
- Restrictive cardiomyopathy results from pathologic infiltration of the myocardium.
- Myocardial infiltration results in abnormal diastolic ventricular filling and varying degrees of systolic dysfunction.

Pathophysiology
- Restrictive cardiomyopathy is most commonly associated with amyloidosis or sarcoidosis.
- Less common causes include glycogen storage diseases, hemochromatosis, endomyocardial fibrosis, and hypereosinophilic syndromes.

Diagnosis

Imaging and Diagnostic Studies
- In restrictive cardiomyopathy, echocardiography with Doppler analysis may demonstrate thickened myocardium with normal or abnormal systolic function, abnormal diastolic filling patterns, and elevated intracardiac pressure.
- In restrictive cardiomyopathy, cardiac catheterization reveals elevated RV and LV filling pressures and a classic dip-and-plateau pattern in the RV and LV pressure tracing.
- RV endomyocardial biopsy may be diagnostic and should be considered in patients in whom a diagnosis is not established.
- It is often difficult to differentiate between restrictive cardiomyopathy and constrictive pericarditis because of similar clinical presentations and hemodynamics, but this distinction is critical as surgical therapy may be effective for constrictive pericarditis.

Treatment

- Specific therapy aimed at amelioration of the underlying cause should be initiated.
- Cardiac hemochromatosis may respond to reduction of total body iron stores via phlebotomy or chelation therapy with deferoxamine.
- Cardiac sarcoidosis may respond to glucocorticoid therapy, but prolongation of survival with this approach has not been established.
- No therapy is known to be effective in reversing the progression of cardiac amyloidosis.
- Digoxin should be avoided in patients with cardiac amyloidosis because of enhanced susceptibility to digoxin toxicity.

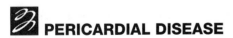 # PERICARDIAL DISEASE

CONSTRICTIVE PERICARDITIS

General Principles

- Constrictive pericarditis may develop as a late complication of pericardial inflammation.
- The noncompliant pericardium causes impairment of ventricular filling and progressive elevation of venous pressure.
- Most cases are idiopathic, but pericarditis after cardiac surgery and mediastinal irradiation are important identifiable causes.
- Tuberculous pericarditis is a leading cause of constrictive pericarditis in some underdeveloped countries.
- Constrictive pericarditis often is difficult to distinguish from restrictive cardiomyopathy.

Diagnosis

Clinical Presentation
- In contrast to cardiac tamponade, the clinical presentation of constrictive pericarditis is insidious, with gradual development of fatigue, exercise intolerance, and venous congestion.
- Physical findings include jugular venous distention with prominent X and Y descents, inspiratory elevation of the jugular venous pressure (Kussmaul sign), peripheral edema, ascites, and a pericardial knock during diastole.

Imaging and Diagnostic Studies
- Echocardiography may reveal pericardial thickening and diminished diastolic filling.
- Chest computed tomography (CT) scan or magnetic resonance imaging (MRI) demonstrates pericardial thickening.
- Cardiac catheterization is usually necessary to demonstrate elevated and equalized diastolic pressures in all four cardiac chambers.

Treatment

- Definitive treatment requires complete pericardiectomy, which is accompanied by significant perioperative mortality (5%–10%) but results in clinical improvement in 90% of patients.
- Patients who are minimally symptomatic can be managed with judicious sodium and fluid restriction and diuretic therapy but must be followed closely to detect hemodynamic deterioration.

CARDIAC TAMPONADE

General Principles

- Cardiac tamponade results from increased intrapericardial pressure secondary to fluid accumulation within the pericardial space.
- Pericarditis of any cause may lead to cardiac tamponade.
- Idiopathic (or viral) and neoplastic forms are the most frequent causes.

Diagnosis

Clinical Presentation
- The diagnosis of cardiac tamponade should be suspected in patients with elevated jugular venous pressure, hypotension, pulsus paradoxus, tachycardia, evidence of poor peripheral perfusion, and distant heart sounds.
- ECG often reveals a tachycardia with low voltage and electrical alternans.

Imaging and Diagnostic Studies
- Echocardiography can confirm the diagnosis of pericardial effusion and demonstrate hemodynamic significance by right atrial and RV diastolic collapse, increased right-sided flows during inspiration, and respiratory variation of the transmitral flow.
- Right heart catheterization is also helpful in determining the hemodynamic significance of a pericardial effusion, especially in patients with a subacute or chronic presentation.
- Hemodynamic findings of elevated, equalized diastolic pressures are present in the patient with cardiac tamponade.

Treatment

- Treatment for cardiac tamponade consists of drainage of the pericardial space via pericardiocentesis or surgical pericardiotomy. Urgent pericardiocentesis should be performed with echocardiographic guidance, if possible.

- If pericardial drainage cannot be performed, stabilization with parenteral inotropic support and aggressive administration of IV saline to maintain adequate ventricular filling are indicated.
- Diuretics, nitrates, and any other preload-reducing agents are absolutely contraindicated for cardiac tamponade.

VALVULAR HEART DISEASE

MITRAL STENOSIS

General Principles

- Mitral stenosis (MS) impedes blood flow from the lungs and left atrium into the left ventricle.
- Rheumatic heart disease is the most common etiology.
- MS may result from calcium deposition in the mitral annulus and leaflets, from congenital valvular malformation, or from connective tissue disorders.
- Left atrial myxoma or cor triatriatum may mimic MS.
- Prosthetic mitral valves (particularly bioprosthetic valves) may become stenotic late after implantation.

Pathophysiology

- Significant MS results in elevation of left atrial, pulmonary venous, and pulmonary capillary pressures, with consequent pulmonary congestion.
- The degree of pressure elevation depends on the severity of obstruction, flow across the valve, diastolic filling time, and presence of effective atrial contraction.
- Factors that normally augment flow across the mitral valve, such as tachycardia, exercise, fever, and pregnancy, result in a marked increase in left atrial pressure and may exacerbate HF symptoms.
- Left atrial enlargement and fibrillation may result in atrial thrombus formation, which contributes to the high incidence (20%) of systemic embolization in patients with MS who are not anticoagulated.

Diagnosis

Clinical Presentation

- Pulmonary congestion, such as dyspnea, cough, and occasionally hemoptysis are prominent.
- Physical signs of pulmonary venous congestion and right heart volume and pressure overload often are present.
- A loud S_1, early diastolic opening snap, and rumbling diastolic murmur are present on auscultation.

Imaging and Diagnostic Studies

- The diagnosis and severity of MS can be confirmed by two-dimensional and Doppler echocardiography.
- Transesophageal echocardiography (TEE) can also be used to confirm the diagnosis, define the anatomy more fully, and provide diagnostic information in patients in whom transthoracic echocardiography is suboptimal.
- Cardiac catheterization is indicated in patients in whom there is a likelihood of concomitant coronary artery disease and in whom echocardiographic studies are either technically suboptimal or nondiagnostic.

Treatment

Nonoperative Management

- Factors that increase left atrial pressure, including tachycardia and fever, should be identified and alleviated.
- Vigorous physical activity should be avoided in patients with moderate to severe MS.
- Diuretics are the mainstay of therapy for pulmonary congestion and edema.
- **Atrial fibrillation** may not be well tolerated.
    - Anticoagulant therapy is indicated for patients with MS and atrial fibrillation (because of the high thromboembolism risk), prior embolic event, or known atrial thrombi. Heparin therapy should be instituted at the onset of atrial fibrillation, followed by long-term warfarin therapy.
    - When the patient is hemodynamically stable, the ventricular response rate to atrial fibrillation can be controlled using digoxin, calcium channel antagonists, or β-adrenergic antagonists.
    - Synchronized direct current cardioversion should be performed if hemodynamic compromise (hypotension, pulmonary edema, and angina) occurs.
    - An attempt to restore and maintain sinus rhythm may be beneficial. It should be preceded by anticoagulation therapy for at least 3 weeks to minimize the risk of systemic embolization on resumption of normal sinus rhythm.
    - A TEE should be performed to evaluate the left atrium for presence of thrombi in patients who require cardioversion prior to completion of a full course of anticoagulation.
    - After conversion to sinus rhythm has been accomplished, antiarrhythmics may be beneficial to maintain sinus rhythm.
- Infective **endocarditis prophylaxis** is indicated.
- Continuous prophylaxis against recurrent rheumatic fever is indicated in young patients, patients at high risk for streptococcal infection (parents of young children, schoolteachers, medical and military personnel, and those in crowded living conditions), and those who have had acute rheumatic fever within the previous 10 years.

Surgery

- Patients with severe symptoms or pulmonary hypertension and significant MS (valve area <1 cm^2/m^2) should undergo commissurotomy or mitral valve replacement (MVR).
- Patients with mild to moderate symptoms may improve with diuretics and can be followed with clinical evaluations and serial echocardiograms.
- A single systemic thromboembolic event does not necessarily mandate MVR. However, the recurrence rate of systemic thromboembolism in patients with MS is high, even with systemic anticoagulation, and MVR should be strongly considered.
- Percutaneous balloon mitral valvuloplasty can reduce the mitral valve pressure gradient and improve cardiac output. This procedure is an alternative to surgery and carries acceptable morbidity and mortality in selected patients without severe MR or severe valvular calcification.

AORTIC STENOSIS

General Principles

- **Aortic stenosis** (AS) in the adult population may result from calcification and degeneration of a normal valve, calcification and fibrosis of a congenitally bicuspid aortic valve, or rheumatic valvular disease.

Pathophysiology

- AS produces a pressure gradient between the left ventricle and the aorta, causing pressure overload of the left ventricle that leads to concentric hypertrophy.
    - LV compliance is reduced, LVEDP rises, and myocardial oxygen demand is increased.
    - Elevated LVEDP decreases the perfusion pressure across the myocardium, leading to subendocardial ischemia.

Diagnosis

Clinical Presentation

■ Diagnosing significant AS may be difficult, as the condition may be asymptomatic for a number of years.
■ AS should be suspected clinically with the presence of one or more of the classic symptoms in the triad of angina, syncope, and HF.

Physical Examination

■ Physical findings include a slowly rising carotid pulse that is sustained (pulsus parvus et tardus) and a mid- to late-peaking harsh systolic murmur.
■ The pressure gradient across the stenotic aortic valve is directly related to the severity of obstruction and cardiac output.
  ■ The intensity of the systolic murmur may diminish as the cardiac output decreases with increasingly severe AS. In general, murmurs of long duration that peak late in systole indicate severe AS.

Imaging and Diagnostic Studies

■ Doppler echocardiography estimates the aortic valve gradient and valve area, which correlates well with the findings at cardiac catheterization.
■ TEE may be required in patients with suboptimal transthoracic echocardiograms.
■ Coronary arteriography should be performed in men older than 40 years and women older than 50 years, as well as in all patients with anginal symptoms.
  ■ Left ventriculography is indicated in patients with coexistent MR (although a high-quality transthoracic echocardiogram or a TEE may suffice).
  ■ Most adult patients being considered for aortic valve replacement (AVR) require preoperative cardiac catheterization to determine the extent of concomitant coronary artery disease.

Treatment

Nonoperative Management

■ Vigorous exercise and physical activity should be avoided in patients with moderate to severe AS.
■ Asymptomatic patients with mild to moderate AS can be followed closely with clinical assessment and Doppler echocardiography performed at 6- to 12-month intervals.
■ Infective **endocarditis prophylaxis** is indicated.
■ **Atrial (and ventricular) arrhythmias** are poorly tolerated and should be treated (see Chapter 7, Cardiac Arrhythmias).
■ **Digoxin** may be useful in patients with HF in the presence of LV dilation and impaired systolic function. In severe AS caused by the fixed obstruction of LV outflow, however, inotropic therapy is of little benefit.
■ **Diuretics** may be useful in treating congestive symptoms but must be used with extreme caution. Reduction of LV filling pressure in patients with AS may decrease cardiac output and systemic BP.
■ **Nitrates** and other vasodilators should be used with caution in patients with severe AS, as they may result in severe hypotension and hemodynamic collapse.
  ■ In patients with severe AS and new-onset angina, nitroglycerin should be initiated cautiously. If nitroglycerin results in hypotension that does not respond to aggressive volume expansion, parenteral inotropic agents (e.g., dobutamine) or vasopressors, or both, should be given.

Surgery

■ Symptomatic patients with severe AS (aortic valve area <1.0 cm^2) and patients with severe AS who are undergoing cardiac or aortic surgery should undergo AVR concurrently.
■ Asymptomatic patients with severe AS should be considered for AVR if LV dilation or decreased systolic function is present or if they have a hypotensive response to exercise.[36]

- Intra-aortic balloon counterpulsation may stabilize patients with critical AS and hemodynamic decompensation until AVR can be accomplished. An IABP should not be used when significant aortic insufficiency (AI) coexists.
- Percutaneous balloon aortic valvuloplasty can reduce the aortic valve gradient and improve symptoms and LV function with relatively low morbidity and mortality in selected patients.
- Restenosis occurs in approximately 50% of patients within 6 months.
- At present, this therapeutic modality is used primarily in patients who require noncardiac surgery before definitive AVR.

CHRONIC MITRAL REGURGITATION

General Principles

- **Chronic mitral regurgitation** (MR), as an isolated lesion, is most commonly caused by myxomatous degeneration of the mitral valve.
- Other etiologies include rheumatic heart disease, mitral valve annulus calcification, coronary artery disease with associated papillary muscle dysfunction, infective endocarditis, and connective tissue diseases (e.g., Marfan's syndrome, Ehlers-Danlos syndrome).
- MR may occur secondary to cardiomyopathy and LV dilation.

Pathophysiology

- Chronic MR imposes volume overload on the left ventricle as a result of regurgitation of a fraction of the LV blood flow into the left atrium.
- Early in the disease course, normal forward cardiac output is maintained.
- With progressive MR, compensatory mechanisms no longer accommodate increasing LV end-diastolic volume (LVEDV). Accordingly, the ejection fraction falls, and symptoms of right and left HF develop.

Diagnosis

Clinical Presentation

- MR is suggested by characteristic physical findings of well-preserved carotid pulsations, an enlarged point of LV impulse, and an apical holosystolic murmur.

Imaging and Diagnostic Studies

- Two-dimensional echocardiography with Doppler confirms the diagnosis, estimates the severity of MR, and provides clues to its etiology.
- TEE is particularly useful for the evaluation of the mitral valve and is commonly used to evaluate the patient with MR.

Treatment

Nonoperative Management

- **Infective endocarditis** prophylaxis should be given.
- **Anticoagulant therapy** should be considered, particularly in the presence of atrial fibrillation, an enlarged left atrium, or a previous embolic event.
- **Vasodilators** provide hemodynamic improvement in MR by reducing SVR, thus decreasing the regurgitant fraction and augmenting forward cardiac output.
  - Beneficial effects have been demonstrated with nitroprusside, captopril, enalapril, and hydralazine.
- **Digoxin** may be useful in the presence of impaired LV systolic function.
- **Diuretics** are useful for treating congestive symptoms.
- Nitrates can be used to reduce preload and ventricular size, and may decrease the severity of MR.

Surgery
- Patients with moderate to severe symptoms despite medical therapy should be considered for mitral valve repair or replacement if the LV EF is >40%.
- Mitral valve repair may improve symptoms and improve cardiac output in patients with severe MR secondary to LV dilation associated with depressed LV systolic function (EF <25%).[37]
- Patients with minimal or no symptoms should be followed closely with assessment of LV size and systolic function (by echocardiography or radionuclide ventriculography) every 6–12 months.
- Mitral valve repair (or replacement) should be considered when the echocardiogram demonstrates an LV end-systolic dimension of >45 mm or an LV EF of <60%, or both.[36]
- Generally, a decreased EF signifies that marked LV dysfunction has occurred and MVR with its attendant increase in LV afterload may be poorly tolerated or may fail to improve the patient's symptoms.

ACUTE MITRAL REGURGITATION

General Principles

- Acute MR can result from papillary muscle dysfunction or rupture caused by myocardial ischemia or infarction, infective endocarditis with flail or perforated leaflets, severe myxomatous disease with rupture of a chorda that results in a flail leaflet, or trauma.

Pathophysiology
- The pathophysiologic features of acute MR differ from those of chronic MR in that compensatory increases in left atrial and LV compliance do not occur.
- This results in a sudden increase in pulmonary venous pressure that leads to acute pulmonary edema, and frequently cardiogenic shock.

Treatment
Nonoperative Management
- Afterload reduction should be initiated urgently with sodium nitroprusside and should be guided by systemic BP and central hemodynamic monitoring. Approximately 50% of patients with acute MR can be stabilized in this manner, allowing MVR to proceed under more controlled conditions.
- Diuretics, with or without nitrates, can be used (as systemic BP tolerates) to relieve pulmonary congestion. However, the direct venodilatory effect of nitroprusside may render other preload-reducing maneuvers unnecessary.
- Intra-aortic balloon counterpulsation is indicated in cases of severe hemodynamic instability to reduce SVR and improve forward cardiac output.

Surgery
- Surgery is indicated urgently in patients with acute MR and hemodynamic compromise whose condition cannot be stabilized medically.
- In those with infective endocarditis who are hemodynamically stable, MVR should be delayed for several days while antibiotic therapy is initiated. If refractory hemodynamic deterioration develops, surgery should not be delayed.

MITRAL VALVE PROLAPSE

General Principles

- Mitral valve prolapse (MVP) is characterized by prolapse of one or both MV leaflets into the left atrium more than 2 mm in midsystole.

- MVP may be associated with supraventricular and ventricular tachyarrhythmias such as Wolff-Parkinson-White and long QT syndrome.
- MVP can be inherited as an autosomal-dominant trait with variable penetrance, or may be associated with connective tissue diseases, congenital heart disease, musculoskeletal deformities, MV surgery, or ischemia.

Diagnosis

Clinical Presentation
- Symptoms are nonspecific, varying from fatigue, anxiety, palpitations, lightheadedness, and chest pain to presyncopal and syncopal episodes. Most patients are asymptomatic.
- Examination reveals a midsystolic click, typically followed by an MR murmur.
- The early or late occurrence of the click in systole and the duration of the MR murmur are dependent on the LV loading conditions (high LV volume, LV pressures–late midsystolic click).

Treatment

Nonoperative Management
- If palpitations, near-syncope, or syncope is of concern, evaluation with Holter monitor and echocardiography is recommended. If there is evidence of NSVT or sustained VT on Holter monitoring, electrophysiologic evaluation is warranted, with possible implantation of a defibrillator if the patient has inducible sustained VT.
- Symptomatic isolated atrial premature complexes or ventricular premature complexes may respond to treatment with β-adrenergic blockers.
- Anticoagulation therapy is recommended in the presence of atrial fibrillation or previous embolic event.
- Subacute bacterial endocarditis (SBE) prophylaxis is indicated if MR is present or the MV leaflets are thickened, or both.
- Management of the MR associated with MVP may require treatment with afterload-reducing agents and possible surgical correction.

AORTIC INSUFFICIENCY

General Principles

- **Aortic insufficiency** may result from an abnormality of the aortic valve, the aortic root, or both.
- Causes of AI include rheumatic fever, endocarditis, trauma, connective tissue disorders, and congenital bicuspid aortic valve.
- Dilation or distortion of the aortic root may be due to systemic hypertension, ascending aortic dissection, syphilis, cystic medial necrosis, Marfan syndrome, or ankylosing spondylitis.

Pathophysiology
- The diastolic regurgitant flow from the aorta into the left ventricle causes increased LV end-diastolic volume and pressure. In turn, the LV becomes dilated and hypertrophied, which maintains stroke volume and prevents further increase in LVEDP.
- In acute AI, the chronic compensatory mechanisms are not active, and therefore, the increase in LVEDP is marked.
- In chronic AI, increases in peripheral resistance (e.g., HTN) lead to increased regurgitant flow and raise diastolic filling pressure and volume.

Diagnosis

Clinical Presentation
- Chronic AI typically presents insidiously, while acute AI may present with severe HF and cardiogenic shock.

- AI may be suspected on the basis of clinical findings, including a wide pulse pressure, bounding pulses, and an aortic diastolic murmur.

Imaging and Diagnostic Studies
- The diagnosis of AI can be confirmed by two-dimensional and Doppler echocardiography or cardiac catheterization with ascending aortography.

Treatment
Nonoperative Management
- Medical therapy is reserved for patients with chronic stable AI or for stabilization of patients with severe or acute AI prior to definitive surgical correction.
- Treatment of underlying or precipitating causes, such as endocarditis, syphilis, and connective tissue diseases, should occur concurrently with treatment of symptoms.
- Strenuous physical activity should be restricted in patients with AI and associated LV dysfunction. Activities that involve increases in isometric work (lifting heavy objects) are more detrimental than are activities such as walking or swimming.
- Patients should receive prophylaxis for endocarditis.
- Fluid and salt restriction, diuretics, digoxin, and vasodilators are the cornerstones of therapy for patients with chronic AI who have evidence of LV dysfunction. Nifedipine may reduce the need for AVR in patients with symptomatic AI and normal LV function.[38]
- Sodium nitroprusside or inotropes should be used in a patient with acute AI to stabilize his or her condition before AVR.

Surgery
- AVR and repair of associated aortic root abnormalities should be performed urgently in individuals with acute hemodynamic compromise, or both.
  - In patients with infective endocarditis who are hemodynamically stable with medical therapy, AVR can be deferred for several days while treatment with antibiotics is initiated.
- AVR should be recommended in patients with severe chronic AI in whom signs or symptoms of HF (NYHA class II–III) or LV dysfunction develop.
  - Echocardiography should be performed every 6–12 months and AVR considered when LV dilation (end-systolic dimension >55 mm or end-diastolic dimension >75 mm) or LV systolic dysfunction develops.
  - The clinical outcome and extent of reversibility of LV dysfunction after AVR depend on the duration of dysfunction, dilation of the left ventricle (end-systolic diameter and volume), and degree of systolic dysfunction.

References
1. Maisel AS, Krishnaswamy P, Nowak RM. Rapid measurement of B-type natriuretic peptide in the emergency diagnosis of heart failure. *N Engl J Med* 2002;347:161–167.
2. Hunt SA, Baker DW, Chin MH, et al. ACC/AHA guidelines for the evaluation and management of chronic heart failure in the adult: executive summary. A report of the American College of Cardiology/American Heart Association Task Force on Practice Guidelines (Committee to revise the 1995 Guidelines for the Evaluation and Management of Heart Failure). *J Am Coll Cardiol* 2001;38(7):2101–2113.
3. Krum H, Roecker EB, Mohacsi P, et al. Effects of initiating carvedilol in patients with severe chronic heart failure: results from the COPERNICUS Study. *JAMA* 2003;289(6):712–718.
4. Poole-Wilson PA, Swedberg K, Cleland JG, et al. Comparison of carvedilol and metoprolol on clinical outcomes in patients with chronic heart failure in the Carvedilol Or Metoprolol European Trial (COMET): randomised controlled trial. *Lancet* 2003;362:7–13.
5. Packer M, Coats A, Fowler MB, et al. Effect of Carvedilol on Survival in Severe Chronic Heart Failure. *N Engl J Med* 2001;344:1651–1658.
6. The Cardiac Insufficiency Bisoprolol Study II (CIBIS-II): a randomised trial. *Lancet* 1999;353:9–13.

7. Hjalmarson A, Goldstein S, Fagerberg B, et al. Effects of controlled-release metoprolol on total mortality, hospitalizations, and well-being in patients with heart failure: the Metoprolol CR/XL Randomized Intervention Trial in congestive heart failure (MERIT-HF). *JAMA* 2000;283:1295.

8. Packer M, Poole-Wilson PA, Armstrong PW, et al. Comparative Effects of Low and High Doses of the Angiotensin-Converting Enzyme Inhibitor, Lisinopril, on Morbidity and Mortality in Chronic Heart Failure. *Circulation* 1999;100:2312–2318.

9. Pitt B, Poole-Wilson PA, Segal R, et al. Effect of losartan compared with captopril on mortality in patients with symptomatic heart failure: randomised trial—the Losartan Heart Failure Survival Study ELITE II. *Lancet* 2000;355:1582–1587.

10. Cohn JN, Tognoni G, the Valsartan Heart Failure Trial Investigators. A Randomized Trial of the Angiotensin-Receptor Blocker Valsartan in Chronic Heart Failure. *N Engl J Med* 2001;345:1667–1675.

11. Yusuf S, Pfeffer MA, Swedberg K, et al. Effects of candesartan in patients with chronic heart failure and preserved left-ventricular ejection fraction: the CHARM-Preserved Trial. *Lancet* 2003;362:772–776.

12. Cohn JN, Archibald DG, Ziesche S, et al. Effect of vasodilator therapy on mortality in chronic congestive heart failure. Results of a Veterans Administration Cooperative Study. *N Engl J Med* 1986;314:1547–1552.

13. Taylor AL, Ziesche S, Yancy C, et al. Combination of Isosorbide Dinitrate and Hydralazine in Blacks with Heart Failure. *N Engl J Med* 2004;351:2049–2057.

14. Publication Committee for the VMAC Investigators. Intravenous nesiritide vs nitroglycerin for treatment of decompensated congestive heart failure: a randomized controlled trial. *JAMA* 2002;287:1531–1540.

15. ALLHAT Collaborative Research Group. Major cardiovascular events in hypertensive patients randomized to doxazosin vs chlorthalidone: the antihypertensive and lipid-lowering treatment to prevent heart attack trial (ALLHAT). *JAMA* 2000;283:1967–1975.

16. The Digitalis Investigation Group. The effect of digoxin on mortality and morbidity in patients with heart failure. *N Engl J Med* 1997;336:525–533.

17. Packer M, Gheorghiade M, Young JB, et al. Withdrawal of digoxin from patients with chronic heart failure treated with angiotensin-converting-enzyme inhibitors. *N Engl J Med* 1993;329:1–7.

18. Rathore SS, Wang Y, Krumholz HM. Sex-based differences in the effect of digoxin for the treatment of heart failure. *N Engl J Med* 2002;347:403–411.

19. Rathore SS, Curtis JP, Wang Y, et al. Association of serum digoxin concentration and outcomes in patients with heart failure. *JAMA* 2003;289:871–878.

20. Pitt B, Zannad F, Remme WJ, et al. The effect of spironolactone on morbidity and mortality in patients with severe heart failure. *N Engl J Med* 1999;341:709–717.

21. Pitt B, Remme W, Zannad F, et al. Eplerenone, a selective aldosterone blocker, in patients with left ventricular dysfunction after myocardial infarction. *N Engl J Med* 2003;348:1309–1321.

22. Cuffe MS, Califf RM, Adams KF Jr, et al. Short-term intravenous milrinone for acute exacerbation of chronic heart failure: a randomized controlled trial. *JAMA* 2002;287:1541–1547.

23. Cleland JG, Daubert JC, Erdmann E, et al. The effect of cardiac resynchronization on morbidity and mortality in heart failure. *N Engl J Med* 2005;352:1539–1549.

24. Rose EA, Gelijns AC, Moskowitz AJ, et al. Long-term mechanical left ventricular assistance for end-stage heart failure. *N Engl J Med* 2001;345:1435–1443.

25. Cardiac Transplantation, 24th Bethesda Conference. November 5-6, 1992. *J Am Coll Cardiol* 1993;22:1–64.

26. Leung RS, Bradley TD. Sleep Apnea and Cardiovascular Disease. *Am J Respir Crit Care Med* 2001;164:2147–2165.

27. Kaneko Y, Floras JS, Usui K, et al. Cardiovascular effects of continuous positive airway pressure in patients with heart failure and obstructive sleep apnea. *N Engl J Med* 2003;348:1233–1241.

28. Manolio TA, Baughman KL, Rodeheffer R, et al. Prevalence and etiology of idiopathic

dilated cardiomyopathy (Summary of a National Heart, Lung, and Blood Institute workshop). *Am J Cardiol* 1992;69:1458–1466.

29. Mason JW, O'Connell JB, Herskowitz A, et al. A clinical trial of immunosuppressive therapy for myocarditis. The Myocarditis Treatment Trial Investigators. *N Engl J Med* 1995;333:269–275.

30. The Cardiac Arrhythmia Suppression Trial (CAST) Investigators. Preliminary report: effect of encainide and flecainide on mortality in a randomized trial of arrhythmia suppression after myocardial infarction. *N Engl J Med* 1989;321:406–412.

31. Singh SN, Fletcher RD, Fisher SG, et al. Amiodarone in patients with congestive heart failure and asymptomatic ventricular arrhythmia. Survival Trial of Antiarrhythmic Therapy in Congestive Heart Failure. *N Engl J Med* 1995;333:77–82.

32. Bardy GH, Lee KL, Mark DB, et al. Amiodarone or an implantable cardioverter-defibrillator for congestive heart failure. *N Engl J Med* 2005;352:225–237.

33. Maron BJ, Shen WK, Link MS, et al. Efficacy of implantable cardioverter-defibrillators for the prevention of sudden death in patients with hypertrophic cardiomyopathy. *N Engl J Med* 2000;342:365–373

34. Fananapazir L, Cannon RO, Tripodi D, et al. Impact of dual-chamber permanent pacing in patients with obstructive hypertrophic cardiomyopathy with symptoms refractory to verapamil and beta-adrenergic blocker therapy. *Circulation* 1992;85:2149–2161.

35. Firoozi S, Elliott PM, Sharma S, et al. Septal myotomy-myectomy and transcoronary septal alcohol ablation in hypertrophic obstructive cardiomyopathy. A comparison of clinical, haemodynamic and exercise outcomes. *Eur Heart J* 2002;23:1617–1624.

36. ACC/AHA guidelines for the management of patients with valvular heart disease. *J Am Coll Cardiol* 1998;32:1486–1588.

37. Bach DS, Bolling SF. Early improvement in congestive heart failure after correction of secondary mitral regurgitation in end-stage cardiomyopathy. *Am Heart J* 1995;129:1165–1170.

38. Scognamiglio R, Rahimtoola SH, Fasoli G, et al. Nifedipine in asymptomatic patients with severe aortic regurgitation and normal left ventricular function. *N Engl J Med* 1994;331:689–694.

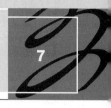

CARDIAC ARRHYTHMIAS

Daniel H. Cooper and Mitchell N. Faddis

7

 APPROACH TO TACHYARRHYTHMIAS

GENERAL PRINCIPLES

- Tachyarrhythmias are commonly encountered entities in the inpatient setting. Approaching these abnormal rhythms in a prompt, stepwise manner will facilitate early recognition of the likely arrhythmia mechanism for timely initiation of appropriate therapy.
- Tachyarrhythmias are defined as cardiac rhythms whose ventricular rate exceeds 100 bpm. Based on the QRS duration, they are typically divided into **narrow-complex** (QRS <120 ms) or **wide-complex** (QRS >120 ms) tachycardias.
- **Reentrant mechanisms** account for the majority of tachyarrhythmias. Re-entry refers to conduction of the electrical activation wavefront retrograde into a myocardial region that was initially refractory to antegrade conduction of the wavefront. Differential refractory periods of myocardial tissue are a necessary component to allow re-entry to occur. As a result of re-entry, propagation of the activation wavefront around a myocardial circuit sustains the arrhythmia. **Enhanced automaticity** and **triggered activity** are other, less common mechanisms of tachyarrhythmias.

DIAGNOSIS

History

- There is an array of **symptoms** that can be attributable to tachyarrhythmias. Important historical points to elicit include the presence or absence of palpitations, chest pain, lightheadedness, shortness of breath, and syncope. Also, symptoms that may reflect underlying left ventricular dysfunction should be addressed including poor or worsening exercise tolerance, dyspnea on exertion, orthopnea, paroxysmal nocturnal dyspnea, and lower extremity swelling.
- If **palpitations** are mentioned, one should inquire as to the nature of their onset and termination. A sudden onset and termination of the palpitations are highly suggestive of a tachyarrhythmia. Also, if symptoms abate with breath holding or Valsalva maneuver, the diagnosis of a supraventricular origin of the tachyarrhythmia is more likely. Specifically, it provides support that the atrioventricular (AV) node plays an integral role in the maintenance of the arrhythmia and can help further distinguish between atrial tachyarrhythmias and paroxysmal supraventricular tachycardia (SVT).
- A history of **organic heart disease** (i.e., ischemic, nonischemic, valvular cardiomyopathy) or **endocrinopathies** (i.e., thyroid disease, pheochromocytoma) should be sought. A history of **familial or congenital causes of arrhythmias** such as hypertrophic cardiomyopathy, congenital long-QT syndrome, or other congenital heart disease should be addressed as well.

- An accurate list of all **medications** taken, including all over-the-counter and herbal remedies, is critical to the workup of a tachyarrhythmia. Particular attention should be paid to those medicines that target the cardiac conduction system in addition to those that have known arrhythmogenic side effects.

Physical Examination

- The role of the physical examination in the workup of tachyarrhythmias is largely confined to helping the clinician to determine if there are underlying cardiovascular abnormalities that may make certain rhythms more or less likely.
  - The presence of physical examination findings consistent with **congestive heart failure,** including elevated jugular venous pressure (JVP), peripheral edema, and third heart sounds, make the diagnosis of malignant ventricular arrhythmias more likely.
  - **Mitral valve prolapse** is associated with a number of supraventricular and ventricular arrhythmias and often produces a midsystolic click audible on cardiac auscultation.
  - **Hypertrophic obstructive cardiomyopathy** produces a harsh systolic ejection murmur heard best along the left sternal border. The murmur is increased during Valsalva and reduced by squatting. This disorder is associated with atrial arrhythmias, principally atrial fibrillation, as well as malignant ventricular arrhythmias.
- Occasionally, the rhythm disturbance may be of sufficient duration and hemodynamic stability to allow for examination during the arrhythmia.
  - The pulse should be palpated and assessed for rate and regularity.
    - Rates of approximately 150 bpm should lead one to suspect underlying atrial flutter with 2:1 block, whereas rates exceeding 150 bpm are more commonly seen with atrioventricular nodal re-entrant tachycardia (AVNRT) or atrioventricular re-entrant tachycardia (AVRT). Rates of ventricular arrhythmias are more variable.
    - Pulse irregularity with no pattern suggests the presence of an irregularly irregular rhythm discussed below. Irregularity with a discernible pattern (i.e., "group beating") suggests the presence of second-degree heart block.
  - "Cannon" A waves may be seen upon inspection of the jugular venous pulsation as a result of atrial contraction against a closed tricuspid valve.
    - If they are seen irregularly, then it is suggestive of underlying AV dissociation as seen with ventricular tachycardia.
    - If they are seen regularly and in a 1:1 ratio with the peripheral pulse, this is suggestive of an underlying re-entrant tachyarrhythmia such as AVNRT and AVRT or a junctional tachycardia, all leading to retrograde atrial activation occurring simultaneously with ventricular contraction.

Diagnostic Tools and Laboratory Studies

- A **12-lead electrocardiogram** (ECG) at baseline is critical for the initial evaluation of any patient with a possible cardiac arrhythmia. The tracing should be examined for any evidence of conduction abnormalities, such as pre-excitation or bundle branch block, or signs of structural heart disease, such as a prior myocardial infarction (MI). If a patient presents with an arrhythmia and is hemodynamically stable, initial data should consist of a standard 12-lead ECG and a continuous rhythm strip with leads that best demonstrate atrial activation (e.g., V1, II, III, aVF). Comparison of a 12-lead ECG at baseline with that obtained during an arrhythmia can highlight subtle features of the QRS deflection that indicate the superposition of atrial and ventricular depolarization. A continuous rhythm strip is very useful to document the response to interventions (e.g., vagal maneuvers, antiarrhythmic drug therapy, electrical cardioversion).
- **Continuous ambulatory ECG monitoring** for 24–72 hours may be useful for documentation of symptomatic transient arrhythmias that occur with sufficient frequency. This recording mode is also useful for assessment of a patient's heart rate response to daily activities or response to an antiarrhythmic drug treatment. The correlation

between patient-reported symptoms in a time-marked diary and heart rhythm recordings is the most useful method to determine whether the symptoms are attributable to an arrhythmia.

- **Event recorders** can be kept by patients for a month or more and are more useful than 24- to 72-hour monitors for diagnosis of transient arrhythmias that occur infrequently. A "loop" recorder is worn by the patient and continuously records the ECG. When the patient is symptomatic, the monitor is triggered and the ECG recording is saved with the preceding time period. An "event monitor" is connected only when the patient experiences symptoms. The **implantable loop recorder** is placed surgically, to provide automated or patient-activated recording of significant arrhythmic events that occur infrequently over several months. These recorders are implanted subcutaneously for up to 1–2 years and are useful for patients with very infrequent symptoms or those who are unable to activate external recorders.
- **Exercise ECG** is useful for studying exercise-induced arrhythmias or to assess the sinus node response to exercise.
- **Electrophysiology study (EPS)** is an invasive, catheter based procedure that is used to study a patient's susceptibility to arrhythmias or to investigate the mechanism of a known arrhythmia. EPS is also combined with catheter ablation for curative treatment of many arrhythmia mechanisms. The efficacy of EPS to induce and study arrhythmias is highest for re-entrant mechanisms.
- **Serum electrolytes, complete blood count (CBC), thyroid function tests, and a toxicology screen** should be considered for all patients. **Chest radiography** and **transthoracic echocardiograms** can help provide evidence of structural heart disease that may make ventricular arrhythmias more likely. **Serum concentrations of digoxin** should be obtained where appropriate to help rule out toxicity.

APPROACH TO SUPRAVENTRICULAR TACHYCARDIAS

GENERAL PRINCIPLES

- The evaluation of SVT, when the QRS duration is <120 ms, should always begin with prompt assessment of hemodynamic stability and clinical "substrate." One must consider that a tachyarrhythmia in an otherwise healthy adult may be well tolerated, allowing more time for evaluation and diagnosis. However, the same arrhythmia may be poorly tolerated in a patient with left ventricular (LV) dysfunction, valvular heart disease, or other cardiopulmonary comorbidity.
- If the patient is deemed unstable by either the presence of hypotension, significant dyspnea, angina, or change in mental status, then one should immediately proceed to cardioversion per advanced cardiac life support (ACLS) guidelines (see Appendix G).
- If the patient is hemodynamically stable, a thorough evaluation of the rhythm can be performed by asking the following questions:
  - *Question 1: What are the odds?*
    - When approaching any diagnostic dilemma it is always helpful to have a rough idea of how commonly or rarely a particular diagnosis presents in your patient population.
    - **Atrial fibrillation (AF)** is the most common narrow-complex tachycardia seen in the inpatient setting. **Atrial flutter (AFl)** can often accompany AF and is diagnosed one-tenth as often as AF but is twice as prevalent as the paroxysmal SVTs. The other atrial tachyarrhythmias are far less common.
    - In one case series, AVNRT was reported as the most common diagnosis of the paroxysmal SVTs (60%) followed by AVRT (30%).[1] However, if your patient is younger than age 40, then AVRT, often in the context of Wolfe-Parkinson-White Syndrome, is more likely.

■ *Question 2: Is the rhythm regular or irregular?*
If regular, move on to Question 3.
OR
If irregularly irregular, the differential diagnosis includes:

- **AF** is the most common sustained tachyarrhythmia for which patients seek treatment and the most likely etiology for an irregularly irregular rhythm discovered on an inpatient ECG. AF is typically a disease of the elderly affecting more than 10% of those older than 75 years old. Disease processes that are often associated with AF include hypertension, valvular and ischemic heart disease, endocrinopathies (i.e., thyroid disorders, pheochromocytoma), pericarditis, acute alcohol ingestion, theophylline, or other stimulant toxicity. AF is a particularly common occurrence following cardiac surgery. An irregularly fluctuating baseline on ECG with an irregular, and often rapid, ventricular rate (>100 bpm) is typical of AF. Symptoms, which are usually secondary to the rapid ventricular response rather than the arrhythmia itself, can range from severe (acute pulmonary edema, palpitations, angina, syncope) to nonspecific (fatigue) to none at all. However, the loss of the contribution of atrial systole to LV filling can cause significant symptomatology in patients with significant ventricular dysfunction. Prolonged episodes of tachycardia due to AF may lead to a **tachycardia-induced cardiomyopathy.**

- **AFl with variable AV block.** Atrial flutter results from a single re-entrant circuit around functional or structural conduction barriers within the atria. The atrial rate in atrial flutter is 250–350 bpm with conduction to the ventricle that is usually not 1:1. Disease processes associated with AFL are similar to those seen with AF. Prior cardiac surgery that required an atriotomy incision can be associated with atrial flutter. In "typical" atrial flutter, flutter waves are best visualized as a "sawtooth" pattern in the inferior leads (II, III, and aVF) with positive deflections in V1 at an atrial rate of about 300 bpm. Although atrial flutter commonly conducts to the ventricle in a 2:1 pattern, a variable pattern of atrioventricular coupling (i.e., 2:1 to 4:1 to 3:1, etc.) is possible, producing an irregularly irregular rhythm. AFl and AF frequently occur in the same patient. In patients with pure AFl, stroke risks appear to be higher than previously thought. Therefore, recommendations for anticoagulation are the same for patients with AF and AFl.

- **Multifocal atrial tachycardia (MAT).** MAT is an irregular SVT that is distinguished by at least three distinct P-wave morphologies apparent on a 12-lead ECG. MAT is often associated with chronic obstructive pulmonary disease or heart failure. MAT may be potentiated by chronic theophylline treatment. Therapy for MAT is targeted at treatment of the underlying pathophysiologic process.

- **Sinus tachycardia with frequent premature atrial complexes (PACs).** Frequent atrial ectopy can lead to the appearance of an irregularly irregular rhythm on ECG in a patient with underlying sinus tachycardia. It is distinguished by the predominance of "sinus" beats intermixed with premature atrial beats that do not meet aforementioned criteria for MAT. Management of this rhythm is aimed at treatment of the underlying condition that is precipitating the tachycardia.

- **Ectopic atrial tachycardia (EAT) with variable block.** EAT with variable block is an uncommon arrhythmia that is distinguished from atrial flutter by an atrial rate that is usually in the range of 150–200 bpm. The combination of EAT with variable AV block is a well-known consequence of digoxin toxicity, although other mechanisms are possible. EAT is thought to be due to enhanced automaticity, although the combination of atrial pathology and antiarrhythmic drug treatment may produce atrial rates associated with intra-atrial re-entry that are in a similar range. When present, treatment of digoxin toxicity may terminate the arrhythmia.

■ *Question 3: Are there discernible P waves?*
If P waves are readily apparent, move on to Question 4.
OR
If P waves are not clearly present, consider performance of a "vagal" maneuver that will transiently enhance vagal tone or administration of intravenous adenosine to potentially slow or terminate the tachycardia.

- **Vagal maneuvers** should be performed with the patient lying down to avoid injury from prolonged heart block that may occur. Ideally, the patient should be on continuous ECG monitoring during any vagal maneuver including rhythm strips that emphasize atrial activity (i.e., V1, II) to enhance the diagnostic value of the maneuver. The **Valsalva maneuver is performed by** exhaling forcefully against a closed airway for several seconds followed by relaxation. The vagal stimulation that results from this maneuver occurs during the relaxation phase. Alternatively, **carotid sinus massage** may be performed. **Carotid massage should not be performed in patients with carotid bruits or a history of cerebrovascular disease (i.e., transient ischemic attack [TIA] or stroke).** Following careful auscultation of the carotids, the patient should be placed in a recumbent position with neck extended, head facing slightly away from side of stimulation. At first apply enough pressure to simply feel the carotid pulse with your index and middle fingers below the angle of the jaw, the approximate location of the carotid sinus. This slight pressure alone can have sufficient effect in some patients. If no effect, then use a rotating motion with enough pressure to cause mild discomfort for a period of 3–5 seconds. If no response occurs, then the opposite carotid sinus can be stimulated with a similar protocol. **Never massage both carotid sinuses simultaneously. Alternative vagal maneuvers that may also have value include gagging, deep breathing, and cold water stimulation of the face.**
- **Adenosine** is a short-acting agent with a serum half-life of approximately 4–8 seconds. The recommended initial dose is 6 mg given IV as a rapid bolus via an antecubital vein, followed by a 10- to 30-mL saline flush. If within 1–2 minutes SVT is not terminated and AV block is not seen, 12 mg followed by 18 mg can be given. A lower initial dose (3 mg) should be used if the drug is injected through a central venous line.
  - Toxicities of adenosine include precipitation of prolonged asystole in patients with sick sinus syndrome or second- or third-degree AV block.
  - Its effects are antagonized by methylxanthines (caffeine or theophylline) and larger doses may be required.
  - Effects are potentiated by dipyridamole and carbamazepine and in heart transplant recipients. In these situations, a smaller initial dosage should be used.
  - Common side effects, including facial flushing, dyspnea, and chest pressure, usually are of brief duration. Adenosine also rarely may exacerbate bronchoconstriction, and this effect may persist beyond the duration of the presence of adenosine. Because of this, patients with significant bronchospasm should not receive a bolus of intravenous adenosine.
- Many SVTs will terminate with adenosine such as AVNRT, AVRT, and many atrial tachycardias. Therefore, the diagnostic value of adenosine termination to distinguish tachycardia mechanisms is limited. However, in the case of atrial flutter, the appearance of the flutter waveform may be helpful.

■ *Question 4: What is the P wave morphology and its relationship to the QRS complex?*
- The atrial activity seen on ECG should be studied closely with respect to morphology and axis. These properties can indicate the regional origin of atrial activity. Negative P waves in the inferior leads (II, III, aVF) suggest an atrial origin near the AV node. A negative P wave in lead aV1 can indicate an origin in the left atrium. P waves that have morphology and axis similar to sinus beats (i.e., upright in I, II, aVF; biphasic in V1) suggest an origin near or within the sinus node complex. Alternatively, one may see the classic "sawtooth" appearance of atrial flutter waves in the inferior leads confirming the presence of typical, counterclockwise atrial flutter.
- A P:QRS relationship >1:1 excludes AVRT and most forms of AVNRT. In this case, EAT or atrial flutter is most likely.

■ *Question 5: What is the RP interval?*
- A differential diagnosis of tachycardia mechanisms can be generated on the basis of the **RP interval**, the time interval between the peak of an R wave and the subsequent P wave, during the tachyarrhythmia.

- **Short RP tachycardias** have an RP interval of <50% of the RR interval. These include:
  - **"Typical" AVNRT.** This re-entrant rhythm occurs in patients who have functional dissociation of their AV node into "slow" and "fast" pathways. In typical AVNRT, conduction proceeds antegrade down the slow pathway, with retrograde conduction up the fast pathway. Atrial and ventricular excitation occur concurrently with every tachycardia circuit. On a 12-lead ECG, the P waves are often hidden within the QRS complexes and are not visible (i.e., a "no RP" tachycardia) or they are buried at the end of the QRS complexes creating a pseudo-r' (V1) or pseudo-s' (II). These **retrograde P waves** may be distinguished only by a comparison of the QRS morphologies in tachycardia and in sinus rhythm. Epidemiologic studies have shown that the arrhythmia has a predilection for middle age and female gender, but AVNRT is common in all age groups.
  - **Orthodromic AVRT (O-AVRT)** is an accessory pathway–mediated re-entrant rhythm that occurs when anterograde conduction to the ventricle takes place through the AV node and retrograde conduction to the atrium occurs through an accessory atrioventricular "bypass" tract. Retrograde P waves on a 12-lead ECG are frequently seen shortly after each QRS complex and are usually distinguishable from the QRS (i.e., separated by >70 ms) in contrast to AVNRT. O-AVRT is the most common mechanism of SVT in patients with Wolfe-Parkinson-White (WPW) syndrome characterized by paroxysmal SVT in patients with pre-excitation (defined by a short PR and a delta wave on the upstroke of the QRS) present on a sinus rhythm 12-lead ECG. O-AVRT may also occur in patients without pre-excitation in which conduction through the bypass tract occurs only during tachycardia in a retrograde fashion; pathways with this property are referred to as "concealed."
  - **Sinus tachycardia or ectopic atrial tachycardia associated with first-degree AV block.** The two rhythms differ with respect to the P-wave axis and morphology. In these situations, the P wave after each QRS is actually conducting to the subsequent QRS complex with a prolonged PR interval.
  - **Junctional tachycardia** arises from automaticity within the AV junction and, in the absence of concomitant bundle branch block, is a narrow-complex tachycardia. In junctional tachycardia, the electrical impulses conduct to the ventricle and atrium simultaneously, similar to typical AVNRT, so that the retrograde P waves frequently record simultaneously with the QRS complex. Junctional tachycardia is common in young children but is rare in adults.
- **Long RP tachycardias** have an RP interval that is >50% of the RR interval. These include:
  - **Sinus tachycardia (ST)** is the most common mechanism of a long RP tachycardia. Most often, ST is a normal physiologic response to the hyperadrenergic states caused by exertion, emotional distress, acute illness, fever, pain, hypovolemia, hypoxia, anemia, and endocrinopathies. ST can also be induced by both illicit (cocaine, amphetamines, methamphetamine) and prescription drugs (theophylline, atropine, β-adrenergic agonists). Management should be directed at correcting the aforementioned influences on the sinus rate. ST is distinguished from inappropriate sinus tachycardia and sinoatrial re-entry by the absence of an identifiable stimulus of the sinus rate.
    - **Inappropriate sinus tachycardia** refers to a persistently elevated sinus rate in the absence of an identifiable physical, pathologic, or pharmacologic influence. Patients will often describe symptoms out of proportion to the physiologic impact of the tachycardia. In addition, sinus rates tend to normalize when the patient is asleep. Fluctuations in sinus rate are usually gradual.
    - **Sinus node re-entrant tachycardia** is caused by a re-entrant circuit localized at least partially within the sinoatrial (SA) node. This tachycardia typically has an abrupt onset, is triggered by a premature atrial complex, and has an equally abrupt termination. The P-wave morphology and axis are identical to the native sinus P-wave morphology during normal sinus rhythm.

- "Atypical" AVNRT. Less common than "typical" AVNRT, this arrhythmia mechanism occurs when anterograde conduction proceeds over the fast AV nodal pathway with retrograde conduction over the slow AV nodal pathway in patients with dual AV nodal physiology. Because retrograde conduction to the atrium is slow, the retrograde P wave is inscribed well after the QRS complex.
- **O-AVRT mediated by an accessory bypass tract with slow or decremental conduction properties.** In this less common form of O-AVRT, retrograde conduction over the accessory pathway to the atrium proceeds slowly enough for atrial activation to occur in the second half of the RR interval. Because the associated tachycardia is often incessant, this arrhythmia may cause a tachycardia-mediated cardiomyopathy.
- **EAT.** These rhythms are characterized by a regular atrial activation pattern with a P-wave morphology originating outside of the sinus node complex. Proposed mechanisms for EAT include enhanced automaticity, triggered activity, and, possibly, micro-re-entry.

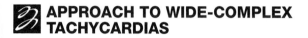

APPROACH TO WIDE-COMPLEX TACHYCARDIAS

GENERAL PRINCIPLES

- Wide-complex tachycardia (WCT) may be due to either SVT with aberrant conduction (presence of bundle branch block) or ventricular tachycardia (VT). The differentiation between these mechanisms is of the utmost importance. **The pharmacologic agents utilized in the management of SVT (i.e., beta blockers, calcium channel blockers) can cause severe hemodynamic instability if used erroneously in the setting of VT.** Therefore, all WCTs are considered to be ventricular in origin until clearly proven otherwise.
  - Ventricular arrhythmias are the major cause of **sudden cardiac death (SCD)**. SCD is defined as death that occurs within 1 hour of the onset of symptoms. In the United States, 350,000 cases of SCD occur annually. Among patients with aborted SCD, ischemic heart disease is the most common associated cardiac structural abnormality. Most cardiac arrest survivors do not evolve evidence of an acute MI; however, more than 75% have evidence of previous infarcts. A nonischemic cardiomyopathy is also associated with an elevated risk for SCD.
  - **Sustained monomorphic VT** is defined as tachycardia composed of ventricular complexes that last longer than 30 seconds (or 30 beats by some definitions), at a rate of 100–250 bpm with a single QRS morphology.
  - **Polymorphic VT** is characterized by an ever-changing QRS morphology and is often due to ischemia. **Torsades de pointes (TdP)** is a variant of polymorphic VT that is preceded by a prolonged QT interval in sinus rhythm. Polymorphic VT is usually associated with hemodynamic collapse or instability.
  - **Ventricular fibrillation (VF)** is associated with disorganized mechanical contraction, hemodynamic collapse, and sudden death. The ECG reveals irregular and rapid oscillations (250–400 bpm) of highly variable amplitude without uniquely identifiable QRS complexes or T waves.
- The evaluation of WCTs should always begin with prompt assessment of vital signs and clinical symptoms. If the arrhythmia is poorly tolerated, postpone further detailed evaluation and proceed to acute management per ACLS guidelines. If stable, there are several important questions to address that can guide one toward the most likely diagnosis. A common mistake is the assumption that hemodynamic stability supports the diagnosis of SVT over VT when VT can often be hemodynamically well tolerated.
- Other, less common mechanisms of WCT include **antidromic AVRT, hyperkalemia-induced arrhythmia, or pacemaker-induced tachycardia.**
- VT represents the vast majority of WCT seen in the inpatient setting with reported prevalence upwards of 80%. With that in mind, one can then proceed to elicit several historical points of emphasis and scrutinize electrocardiographic properties of the arrhythmia to

further delineate the mechanism of the underlying rhythm disturbance. Begin with the following questions:

■ *Does the patient have a history of structural heart disease?*
  • Patients with structural heart disease are much more likely to have VT than SVT as the etiology of a WCT. In one report, 97% of patients with WCT that had prior MI proved to have VT.[2]

■ *Does the patient have a pacemaker, implantable cardioverter defibrillator (ICD), or wide QRS at baseline (i.e., right bundle branch block [RBBB], left bundle branch block [LBBB], interventricular conduction delay [IVCD])?*
  • The presence of either a pacemaker or an ICD should raise suspicion for a device-mediated WCT.
    ◦ **Device-mediated WCT** can be due to ventricular pacing at a rapid rate either due to device tracking of an atrial tachyarrhythmia or an "endless loop tachycardia" created by tracking of the retrograde atrial impulses created by the preceding ventricular paced beat. In either case, the tachycardia rate is a clue to the mechanism as this is typically equal to the programmed upper rate limit (URL) of the device. A commonly programmed URL is 120 paces per minute (ppm). A tachycardia rate above the URL effectively excludes a device-mediated WCT.
  • History of device implantation can be confirmed by inspection of the chest wall (usually left chest for right-handed patients), chest radiograph, or the presence of pacing spikes seen on telemetry or ECG. Typically, the wide QRS induced by right ventricular pacing leads has an LBBB pattern and is preceded by a short pacing spike. Modern devices utilize bipolar pacing, in most cases, which is often difficult to recognize on the 12-lead ECG due to the small size of the electrical artifact. Therefore, one should not exclude the presence of a device-mediated tachycardia mechanism by the absence of visible pacing spikes during the tachycardia.
  • Patients with known RBBB, LBBB, or IVCD at baseline who present with WCT will have a QRS morphology identical to baseline in the presence of SVT. In addition, some patients with a narrow QRS at baseline will manifest a WCT due to SVT when a rate-related bundle branch block is present. This phenomenon is referred to as SVT with aberrancy and can be distinguished from VT reliably with the criteria described below.

■ *What medications is the patient taking?*
  • The medication list should be scanned for any medication with proarrhythmic side effects, especially those that can prolong the baseline QT interval and increase the risk for polymorphic VT or TdP. These medications include many of the class I and III antiarrhythmics, certain antibiotics, antipsychotics, and many more. The University of Arizona–sponsored website, www.qtdrugs.org, provides a comprehensive list of QT-prolonging agents.
  • Medications that can lead to electrolyte abnormalities such as loop and potassium-sparing diuretics, angiotensin-converting enzyme (ACE) inhibitors, and angiotensin receptor blockers (ARBs) should be ascertained. Also, digoxin toxicity is always an important consideration in the setting of any arrhythmia.

■ **Differentiation of SVT with aberrancy from VT** on the basis of analysis of the surface ECG is critical in the determination of appropriate acute and chronic therapy. For acute therapy of SVT, IV medications such as adenosine, calcium channel blockers, or beta-blockers are used. However, calcium channel blockers and beta-blockers can produce hemodynamic instability in patients with VT. Chronically, many SVTs are amenable to radiofrequency ablation, whereas most VTs are malignant and require an antiarrhythmic agent and/or ICD implantation.
  ■ Features that are diagnostic of VT are **AV dissociation, capture or fusion beats,** an absence of an RS morphology in the precordial leads (V1–V6), and an **LBBB morphology with right axis deviation.** In the absence of these features, examination of an RS complex in a precordial lead for an RS interval >100 ms is consistent with VT (Fig. 7-1). In addition, characteristic QRS morphologies that are suggestive of VT may be sought, as shown in Figure 7-2.
  ■ **Antidromic AVRT** is a re-entrant form of SVT that occurs when conduction to the ventricle is down an accessory bypass tract with retrograde conduction through the

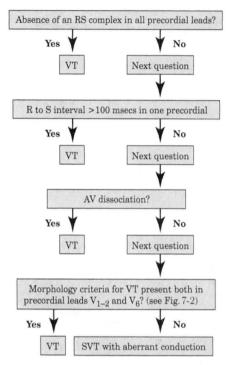

Figure 7-1. Overview of the Brugada criteria for the differentiation of VT from aberrantly conducted SVT.

AV node or a second bypass tract. The resulting QRS is consistent with VT originating from the base of the heart; however, the presence of pre-excitation on the baseline QRS should be diagnostic for WPW syndrome. Antidromic AVRT is seen in <5% of patients with WPW syndrome.

 # TREATMENT OF TACHYARRHYTHMIAS

- The acute treatment of symptomatic tachyarrhythmias should follow the protocols of advanced cardiac life support as outlined in Appendix I. Chronic treatment for tachyarrhythmias is aimed at either prevention of recurrence or prevention of the complications associated with the specific tachyarrhythmia.
  - **SVT.** Initial therapy of acute episodes of regular, narrow-complex tachycardias includes vagal maneuvers (e.g., carotid massage, Valsalva maneuver) and, if unsuccessful, bolus administration of short-acting agents that slow or block AV nodal conduction.
    - IV adenosine (administered as described above) is the most common agent utilized for acute treatment of SVT. Alternative agents include metoprolol (5 mg IV q5min), verapamil (dosed with IV boluses of 5–10 mg over 2–3 minutes that can be repeated after 15–30 minutes, if necessary), and diltiazem (given as an IV bolus of 0.25 mg/kg over 2 minutes, with a repeat bolus of 0.35 mg/kg if the desired effect is not obtained). After bolus administration of diltiazem, a continuous infusion can be initiated at 10 mg/hr, with the infusion rate titrated to the desired effect.

Configuration	SVT (n=22)	VT (n=60)	Favors	Sens.	Spec.
Taller left peak 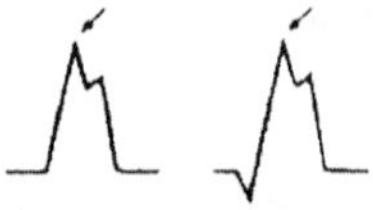	0	14	VT	23%	100%
Biphasic RS or QR 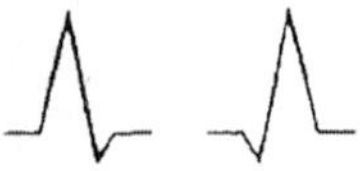	1	11	VT	18%	95%
Triphasic rsR' or rR' 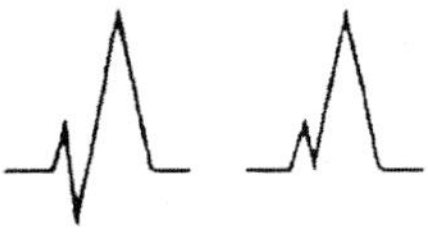	14	8	SVT	64%	87%

A

Configuration	SVT (n=13)	VT (n=38)	Favors	Sens.	Spec.
In V_1, V_2 any of: (a) r $\geq$0.04 sec (b) Notched S downstroke (c) Delayed S nadir >0.06 sec 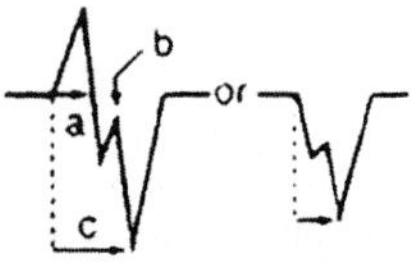	0	33	VT	87%	100%
In V_1, V_2 absence of: (a) r $\geq$0.04 sec (b) Notched S downstroke (c) Delayed S nadir >0.06 sec 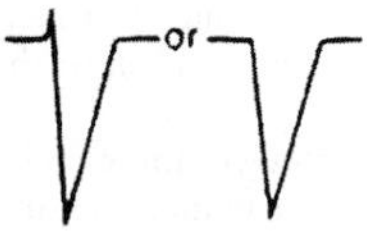	13	4	SVT	100%	89%

B

Figure 7-2. Brugada morphologic criteria. **A:** Lead V_1 criteria in right bundle-branch block (RBBB). R > R' and biphasic RS or QR favor VT, whereas triphasic rSR' or rR' favors SVT. **B:** Lead V_1 criteria in left bundle-branch block. r >40 msecs, a notched S, and delayed intrinsicoid deflection (onset of QRS to nadir of S) >60 msecs all favor VT. (*continued*)

Configuration	SVT (n = 35)	VT (n = 98)	Favors	Sens.	Spec.
Monophasic QS 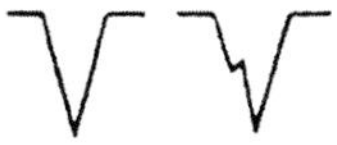	0	29	VT	30%	100%
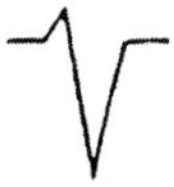 Biphasic rS (RBBB-type)	0	23	VT	38%	100%
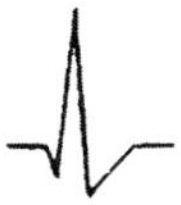 Triphasic qRs (RBBB-type)	8	3	SVT	36%	95%

C

Figure 7-2. (*continued*) **C:** Lead V_6 criteria. Monophasic QS or biphasic rS favors VT. Triphasic qRs favors SVT. (From *Circulation* 1991;83:1649)

- Many SVTs can be terminated by AV nodal–blocking agents or techniques, whereas AFl, AF, and some atrial tachycardias will persist with a slowing of the ventricular rate due to partial AV nodal blockade.
- Chronic pharmacologic therapy for SVT can include calcium channel antagonists (diltiazem sustained release at 120–360 mg PO daily or verapamil sustained release at 120–480 mg PO daily), β-adrenergic antagonists (metoprolol, 25–100 mg PO bid or sustained release with daily dosing, or atenolol, 25–100 mg PO daily), and digoxin (0.125–0.5 mg PO daily, depending on the renal function).
- **Correction of electrolyte abnormalities** may have some preventative value in patients with a history of tachyarrhythmias. Particular emphasis should be placed on correcting hypokalemia and hypomagnesemia.
- **Radiofrequency ablation** offers definitive cure for many SVTs, including AVNRT, accessory bypass tract–mediated tachycardias, focal atrial tachycardia, and AFl. Complication rates are usually <1% and include bleeding, groin hematomas, cardiac perforation or tamponade, strokes, and complete heart block requiring permanent pacemakers. Given the high success rate of ablation procedures, antiarrhythmic drugs are now rarely indicated for the treatment of SVT.

■ **AF.** The management of atrial fibrillation requires careful consideration of three issues: rate control, prevention of thromboembolism, and rhythm control. Recent studies have shown that there is no mortality advantage to a management strategy aimed at maintaining sinus rhythm. Therefore, the approach to atrial fibrillation has evolved to focus largely on anticoagulation and rate-controlling agents. Rhythm control is reserved for patients who remain symptomatic despite efforts to optimize ventricular response to AF.

- **Rate control** of AF can be achieved with agents that prolong conduction through the AV node. These include the nondihydropyridine calcium channel blockers (diltiazem, verapamil), β-adrenergic blockers, and digoxin. Refer to Table 7-1 for loading and dosing recommendations.
  - **Digoxin** is useful in controlling the resting ventricular rate in AF in the setting of LV dysfunction and congestive heart failure (CHF), and may be useful as adjunctive therapy in combination with calcium channel antagonists or β-adrenergic antagonists for optimum rate control of chronic AF. It is less useful for rate control during exertion.

TABLE 7-1 Pharmacologic Agents Used for Heart Rate Control in Atrial Fibrillation

Drug	Loading dose	Onset of action	Maintenance dose	Major side effects	Recommendation
Without evidence of accessory pathway:					
Esmolol[b]	IV: 0.5 mg/kg over 1 min	5 min[a]	0.06–0.2 mg/kg/min	↓ BP, ↓ HR, HB, HF, bronchospasm	I
Metoprolol[b]	IV: 2.5–5.0 mg bolus over 2 min (up to 3 doses)	5 min	NA	↓ BP, ↓ HR, HB, HF, Bronchospasm	I
	PO: Same as maintenance	4–6 h	25–100 mg bid		
Propranolol[b]	IV: 0.15 mg/kg	5 min	NA	↓ BP, ↓ HR, HB, HF, bronchospasm	I
	PO: Same as maintenance	60–90 min	80–240 mg daily in divided doses		
Diltiazem	IV: 0.25 mg/kg over 2 min	2–7 min	5–15 mg/hr	↓ BP, HB, HF	I
	PO: Same as maintenance	2–4 h	120–360 mg daily in divided doses; slow release available		
Verapamil	IV: 0.075–0.15 mg/kg over 2 min	3–5 min	NA	↓ BP, HB, HF	I
	PO: Same as maintenance	1–2 h	120–360 mg daily in divided doses; slow release available		
With evidence of accessory pathway[c]:					
Amiodarone	IV: 150 mg over 10 min	Days	1 mg/min × 6 hr, then 0.5 mg/min	See below	IIa
In patients with heart failure and without accessory pathway:					
Digoxin	IV: 0.25 mg q2h, up to 1.5 mg	60 min or more	0.125–0.375 mg daily IV or orally	Digoxin toxicity, HB, ↓ HR	I
	PO: 0.5 mg daily	2 days			
Amiodarone[d]	IV: 150 mg over 10 min	Days	1 mg/min × 6 hr, then 0.5 mg/min	↓ BP, HB, ↓ HR, warfarin interaction; see text for description of dermatologic, thyroid, pulmonary, corneal, and liver side effects	Acute setting:
	PO: 800 mg/d for 1 wk,	1–3 wks	100–400 mg PO daily		IIa (IV)
	600 mg/d for 1 wk,				Nonacute/chronic:
	400 mg/d for 1 wk,				IIb (PO)

↓ BP: hypotension; ↓ HB, heart block; HF, heart failure; HR, bradycardia; NA, not applicable.

[a]Onset is variable and some effects occur earlier.

[b]Only representative members of the type of beta-blockers are included in the table, but other similar agents could be used for this indication in appropriate doses.

[c]Conversion to sinus rhythm and catheter ablation of the accessory pathway are generally recommended; pharmacologic therapy for rate control may be appropriate therapy in certain patients. See text for discussion of atrial fibrillation (AF) in setting of pre-excitation/Wolf-Parkinson-White syndrome.

[d]Amiodarone can be useful to control the heart rate in patients with AF when other measures are unsuccessful or contraindicated.

Adapted from Fuster V, Ryden LE, Cannom DS, et al. ACC/AHA/ESC 2006 Guidelines for the Management of Patients With Atrial Fibrillation: A report of the American College of Cardiology/American Heart Association Task Force on Practice Guidelines and the European Society of Cardiology Committee for Practice Guidelines (Writing Committee to Revise the 2001 Guidelines for the Management of Patients With Atrial Fibrillation). *Circulation* 2006;114:e257–e354.

- **Digitalis toxicity** is usually diagnosed clinically with presenting symptoms including nausea, abdominal pain, vision changes, confusion, and delirium. It is often seen in patients with renal dysfunction or in those patients on agents known to increase digoxin levels (verapamil, diltiazem, erythromycin, cyclosporine, etc.). Paroxysmal atrial tachycardia with varying degrees of AV block and bidirectional VT are the most commonly seen arrhythmias in association with digitalis toxicity. Treatment is supportive, by withholding the drug, insertion of temporary pacemakers for AV block, and IV phenytoin for bidirectional VT.
  - **Nonpharmacologic therapies. Catheter ablation of the AV node with pacemaker implantation** can be performed for ventricular rate control when drug therapy is ineffective or if the patient cannot tolerate high doses of AV nodal–blocking agents secondary to hypotension or CHF. It is important to remember such therapy is for rate control only and the underlying atrial rhythm persists; therefore, these patients require anticoagulation for stroke prevention.
- **Prevention of thromboembolic complications** is a central tenet of AF management and should begin with individual risk assessment of each patient. Chronic warfarin anticoagulation is currently the most effective therapy for attenuating the risk of stroke associated with AF; however, its initiation requires careful risk–benefit analysis to identify the patients that are at sufficient risk for embolic cerebrovascular accident (CVA) to outweigh the increased risk of hemorrhagic complications.
  - The **CHADS$_2$ score** is a validated, risk stratification tool that can categorize nonvalvular AF patients as low, intermediate, or high risk for stroke based on the presence of these risk factors: CHF, Hypertension (HTN), Age >75, Diabetes mellitus, or prior Stroke/TIAs (Table 7-2).
  - In one study, high-risk patients have a 6%–7% per year stroke risk that can be reduced to 3.6% per year if placed on aspirin 325 mg/d or reduced further to 2.3% per year if placed on therapeutic doses of warfarin.[3] It is also of general consensus that patients younger than 65 years old without structural heart disease or hypertension (i.e. "lone AF") are at low risk (approximately 1% per year) and can be managed with daily aspirin (ASA) alone. The current American Heart Association (AHA)/American College of Cardiology (ACC)/European Society of Cardiology (ESC) recommendations for chronic antithrombotic therapy in AF are summarized in Table 7-3.
  - The role of antithrombotic therapy leading up to and after restoration of sinus rhythm is discussed below.
- **Restoration of sinus rhythm** can be achieved with electrical direct-current (DC) cardioversion or with antiarrhythmic agents (chemical cardioversion). With either method, one must consider the potential for a thromboembolic event.
  - AF with a rapid ventricular response in the setting of ongoing myocardial ischemia, MI, hypotension, or marked CHF should receive prompt cardioversion regardless of the anticoagulation status.
  - If the duration of AF is documented to be <48 hours, cardioversion may proceed without anticoagulation. If AF has persisted for >48 hours (or for an unknown duration), patients should be anticoagulated with warfarin, with an international normalized ratio (INR) of 2.0–3.0, for at least 3 weeks before cardioversion, and anticoagulation should be continued in the same therapeutic range following successful cardioversion.
  - An alternative to anticoagulation for 3 weeks before cardioversion is to perform a **transesophageal echocardiogram** to rule out left atrial appendage thrombus before cardioversion. This method is safe and has the advantage of shorter time to cardioversion than warfarin and therefore is indicated in patients who are not able to wait weeks before cardioversion. Therapeutic anticoagulation with warfarin is indicated after the cardioversion for a minimum of 4 weeks,[4] although the AFFIRM trial suggests that in patients with high-risk factors for strokes, warfarin should be continued indefinitely.

TABLE 7-2 Stroke Risk in Patients with Nonvalvular AF Not Treated with Anticoagulation According to the CHADS2 Index

CHADS2 risk	Score
Cardiac failure	1
Hypertension	1
Age >75 yr	1
Diabetes mellitus	1
Prior stroke or TIA	2

Patients (N = 1,733)[a]	Adjusted stroke rate (%/yr) (95% CI)	CHADS2 score	Risk category	Recommended antithrombotic therapy
120	1.9 (1.2–3.0)	0	Low	Aspirin 81–325 mg PO daily
463	2.8 (2.0–3.8)	1	Moderate	Aspirin or warfarin
523	4.0 (3.1–5.1)	2	Moderate	Previous CVA/TIA/embolism? – Yes = Warfarin – No = Aspirin or warfarin
337	5.9 (4.6–7.3)	3	High	
220	8.5 (6.3–11.1)	4	High	Warfarin (INR 2.0–3.0)
65	12.5 (8.2–17.5)	5	High	
5	18.2 (10.5–27.4)	6	High	

AF, atrial fibrillation; CHADS2, cardiac failure, hypertension, age, diabetes, and stroke (doubled); CI, confidence interval; CVA, cerebrovascular accident; INR, international normalized ratio; TIA, transient ischemic attack.

[a]The adjusted stroke rate was derived from multivariate analysis assuming no aspirin usage.

Adapted from Fuster V, Ryden LE, Cannom DS, et al. ACC/AHA/ESC 2006 Guidelines for the Management of Patients With Atrial Fibrillation: A Report of the American College of Cardiology/American Heart Association Task Force on Practice Guidelines and the European Society of Cardiology Committee for Practice Guidelines (Writing Committee to Revise the 2001 Guidelines for the Management of Patients With Atrial Fibrillation). *Circulation* 2006;114:e257–e354. Data from Gage BF, Waterman AD, Shannon W, et al. Validation of clinical classification schemes for predicting stroke: results from the National Registry of Atrial Fibrillation. *JAMA* 2001;285:2864–2870 (426).

TABLE 7-3	Appropriate Anticoagulation in Various AF Populations	

Patient features	Antithrombotic therapy	Class of recommendation
Age <60 yr, no heart disease (lone AF)	Aspirin (81–325 mg/d) or no therapy	I
Age <60 yr, heart disease but no RFs[a]	Aspirin (81–325 mg/d)	I
Age 60–74 yr, no RFs[a]	Aspirin (81–325 mg/d)	I
Age 65–74 yr with diabetes mellitus or CAD	Oral anticoagulation (INR 2.0–3.0)	I
Age 75 yr or older, women	Oral anticoagulation (INR 2.0–3.0)	I
Age 75 yr or older, men, no other RFs	Oral anticoagulation (INR 2.0–3.0) or aspirin (81–325 mg/d)	I
Age 65 or older, heart failure	Oral anticoagulation (INR 2.0–3.0)	I
LV ejection fraction <35% or fractional shortening <25%, and hypertension	Oral anticoagulation (INR 2.0–3.0)	I
Rheumatic heart disease (mitral stenosis)	Oral anticoagulation (INR 2.0–3.0)	I
Prosthetic heart valves; prior thromboembolism	Oral anticoagulation (INR 2.0–3.0 or higher)	I
Persistent atrial thrombus on TEE	Oral anticoagulation (INR 2.0–3.0 or higher)	IIa

AF, atrial fibrillation; CAD, coronary artery disease; INR, international normalized ratio; TEE, transesophageal echocardiography.
[a]Risk factors (RFs) for thromboembolism include heart failure (HF), left ventricular (LV) ejection fraction <35%, and history of hypertension.
Adapted from Fuster V, Ryden LE, Cannom DS, et al. ACC/AHA/ESC 2006 Guidelines for the Management of Patients With Atrial Fibrillation: A Report of the American College of Cardiology/American Heart Association Task Force on Practice Guidelines and the European Society of Cardiology Committee for Practice Guidelines (Writing Committee to Revise the 2001 Guidelines for the Management of Patients With Atrial Fibrillation). *Circulation* 2006;114:e257–e354.

- **DC cardioversion** is the safest and most effective method of acutely restoring sinus rhythm.
  - For cardioversion of atrial arrhythmias, the anterior patch electrode should be positioned just right of the sternum at the level of the third or fourth intercostal space, with the second electrode positioned just below the left scapula posteriorly. Care should be taken to position patch electrodes at least 6 cm from permanent pacemaker or defibrillator generators.
  - When practical, sedation should be accomplished with midazolam (1–2 mg IV q2min to a maximum of 5 mg), methohexital (25–75 mg IV), etomidate (0.2–0.6 mg/kg IV), or propofol (initial dose, 5 mg/kg/hr IV).
  - Proper synchronization to the QRS is critical to avoid induction of ventricular fibrillation by a cardioversion shock delivered during a vulnerable period. Synchronization of the external cardioverter defibrillator should be confirmed by noting the presence of a synchronization marker superimposed on the QRS complex.
  - If electrode paddles are being used, firm pressure and conductive gel should be applied to minimize contact impedance. Direct contact with the patient or the bed should be avoided.
  - Atropine (1 mg IV) should be readily available to treat prolonged pauses. Reports of serious arrhythmias, such as VT, VF, or asystole, are rare and

are more likely in the setting of improperly synchronized cardioversion, digitalis toxicity, or concomitant antiarrhythmic drug therapy.
- Cardioversion is ineffective in multifocal atrial tachycardia or other paroxysmal atrial arrhythmias.
- **Pharmacologic cardioversion** of AF to sinus rhythm requires similar considerations regarding anticoagulation as for electrical cardioversion. Although oral antiarrhythmics have low rates of conversion, conversions are possible, and patients should be adequately anticoagulated before oral agents are started.
  - **Ibutilide** is the only drug that is approved by the U.S. Food and Drug Administration for pharmacologic cardioversion. Clinical trials have shown a 45% conversion rate for AF and a 60% conversion rate for AFL. Ibutilide is associated with a 4%–8% risk for TdP, especially in the first 2–4 hours after administration of the drug. Because of this risk, patients must be monitored on telemetry with an external defibrillator immediately available during ibutilide infusion and for at least 4 hours after ibutilide infusion. The risk for TdP is higher in patients with cardiomyopathy and congestive heart failure. Ibutilide is given as an IV bolus, at a dosage of 1 mg (0.01 mg/kg if patient is <60 kg), **infused slowly over 10 minutes.**
  - Other antiarrhythmic agents that have proven efficacy for pharmacologic cardioversion of AF are available. The 2006 AHA/ACC/ESC guidelines made the following recommendations based on duration of AF:
    ○ If AF is ≤7 days in duration, dofetilide, **flecainide, ibutilide,** and **propafenone** are generally agreed to be useful and effective. To a lesser degree, **amiodarone** is considered effective.
    ○ If AF is ≥7 days in duration, **dofetilide** has shown efficacy with less convincing evidence for amiodarone and ibutilide.
- **Maintenance of normal sinus rhythm** generally requires an antiarrhythmic agent. Maintenance of sinus rhythm has not been shown to reduce mortality or stroke risks, and antiarrhythmic agents are associated with a small risk for life-threatening proarrhythmia. As a result, antiarrhythmic therapy should be reserved for patients who have highly symptomatic AF in spite of adequate rate control. Antiarrhythmic agents are grouped by the predominate mechanism of action according to the Vaughan-Williams classification. Class I agents inhibit the fast sodium channel, class II agents are β-adrenergic antagonists, class III agents primarily block potassium channels, and class IV agents are calcium channel antagonists. Commonly used antiarrhythmic agents, their major route of elimination, and dosing regimen are listed in Table 7-4.
  - **Class Ia** agents include quinidine, procainamide, and disopyramide. All may cause TdP as a result of QT prolongation. Quinidine and procainamide are rarely used for the treatment of AF because of a poor efficacy, numerous side effects, and inconvenient dosing regimen.
    - **Quinidine** is commonly associated with gastrointestinal side effects, including nausea, vomiting, diarrhea, abdominal pain, and anorexia.
    - Long-term use of **procainamide** may be associated with lupuslike reactions (fever, pleuropericarditis, hepatomegaly, arthralgias). In addition, procainamide has an active metabolite, N-acetylprocainamide, which exerts an action that is typical of class III agents and can prolong the QT interval. Combined procainamide and N-acetylprocainamide levels >30 mg/L are associated with increased toxicity.
    - **Disopyramide** may be an effective agent for the treatment of vagally mediated AF. Side effects include urinary retention, dry mouth, and exacerbation of glaucoma and are due to its potent anticholinergic properties. In addition, its negative inotropic effects may worsen congestive heart failure for patients with LV dysfunction.
  - **Class Ib** agents, including lidocaine, mexiletine, tocainide, and phenytoin, have very little effect on atrial tissues and are not used for AF.

TABLE 7-4 Commonly Used Antiarrhythmic Drugs

Class	Drug	Route of administration (elimination)[a]	Initial/loading dose	Maintenance dose	Major adverse effects[b]/comments
Ia	Procainamide	IV (R, H) PO (R, H)	15–18 mg/kg at 20 mg/min 50 mg/kg/24 hr, max: 5 g/24 hr	1–4 mg/min IR: 250–500 mg q3–6h; SR: 500 mg q6h; Procainbid: 1,000–2,500 mg q12h	GI, CNS, + ANA/SLE-like syndrome, fever, hematologic anticholinergic effects. Follow QTc, serum procainamide (4–8 mg/L), and NAPA levels (<20 mg/mL).
	Quinidine	PO (H)	Sulfate, 200–400 mg q6h; gluconate, 324–972 mg q8–12h	NA	↑ QT, TdP, ↓ BP, thrombocytopenia, cinchonism, GI upset
	Disopyramide	PO (H, R)	300–400 mg	IR: 100–200 mg q6h; SR: 200–400 mg q12h	Anticholinergic, HF
Ib	Lidocaine	IV (H)	1 mg/kg over 2 min (may repeat ×2 up to 3 mg/kg total)	1–4 mg/min	↓ HR, CNS, GI. Adjust dose in patients with hepatic failure, AMI, HF, or shock.
	Mexiletine	PO (H)	400 mg one-time dose	200–300 mg q8h	GI, CNS
Ic	Flecainide	PO (H, R)	50 mg q12h	Increase by 50–100 mg/d every 4 d to max 400 mg/d	HF, GI, CNS, blurred vision
	Propafenone	PO (H)	IR:150 mg q8h ER: 225 mg q12h	IR: Increase at 3- to 4-d intervals up to 300 mg q8h; ER: may increase in 5-day intervals, up to 425 mg q12h	GI, dizziness
III	Sotalol	PO (R)	80 mg q12h	May increase every 3 days up to 240–320 mg/d in 2–3 divided doses.	↓ HR, ↓ BP, CHF, CNS. Limit QTc prolongation to <550 ms
	Dofetilide	PO (R, H)	CrCl (mL/min): Dose (mcg bid): >60: 500 40–60: 250 20–39: 125 <20: Contraindicated	Dose adjusted based on QTc 2–3 hr after inpatient doses 1 through 5. Chronic therapy requires calculation of QTc and CrCl every 3 months with adjustment as necessary.	↑ QT, VT/TdP, HA, dizziness. See text for further details on initiating and monitoring treatment.
	Ibutilide	IV (H)	1 mg (0.01 mg/kg if patient <60 kg) over 10 min; can repeat if no response 10 min after initial infusion	NA	↑ QT, TdP, AV block, GI, HA
	Amiodarone	IV (H) PO (H)	IV: 150 mg over 10 min PO: 800 mg/d for 1 wk, then 600 mg/d for 1 wk, then 400 mg/d for 1 wk	1 mg/min ×6 hr, then 0.5mg/min. 100–400 mg PO daily	↓ BP, HB, ↓ HR, warfarin interaction. See text for description of dermatologic, thyroid, pulmonary, corneal, and liver effects.

AMI, acute myocardial infarction, ↓ BP, hypotension; ER, extended release H, hepatic; ↓ HA, headache; HB, heart block; HF, heart failure; HR, bradycardia; IR, immediate release; NA, not applicable; R, renal; TdP, torsades de pointes, VT, ventricular tachycardia;

[a] Please refer to Appendix E for dosing in setting of renal impairment.

[b] Either common or life-threatening adverse effects of these medications are listed. This is not a comprehensive list of all possible adverse effects.

- **Class Ic** agents flecainide and propafenone are more effective than class Ia agents in the management of AF.
    - Both agents may cause QRS widening, and the effects are more apparent at higher heart rates (use dependence). Therefore, monitoring for toxicity usually involves an exercise stress test, after a stable dose has been reached, to look for QRS widening at high heart rates.
    - Both agents are potent negative inotropes; therefore, their use is contraindicated in patients with a history of structural heart disease. Flecainide and propafenone should never be used in post-MI patients, as they are associated with increased mortality in this particular group.[5]
    - The dose should be reduced or the drug should be discontinued if the QRS duration exceeds 0.2 seconds. Flecainide and propafenone may also cause sinus node depression and AV conduction abnormalities. Both drugs may cause conversion of AF to AFL.
    - The slowing of atrial rate from AF to AFL may result in 1:1 conduction to the ventricle. Therefore, nodal blocking agents, such as beta-blockers or calcium channel blockers, should always be used in conjunction with class Ic agents.
- **Class III** agents prolong repolarization through potassium channel blockade, causing an increase in the QT interval. Ibutilide is a class III agent that is only available in IV form for the acute conversion of AF. Oral class III agents that are commonly used for treatment of AF are sotalol and dofetilide.
    - **Sotalol** is a mixture of stereoisomers (dl-); d-sotalol is a potassium channel blocker while l-sotalol is a β-antagonist. Side effects reflect both mechanisms of action. In addition to QT interval prolongation, dl-sotalol may result in sinus bradycardia or AV conduction abnormalities and should be avoided in patients with decompensated CHF due to the negative inotropic effect.
    - **Dofetilide** blocks the rapid component of the delayed rectifier potassium current, I_{Kr}. As a result, dofetilide increases the QT interval at clinically effective doses. QT prolongation is intensified by bradycardia, a characteristic known as reverse use dependence. The main risk of dofetilide is TdP.
        - Dofetilide is contraindicated in patients with a baseline corrected QT (QT_c) >440 ms, or 500 ms in patients with bundle branch block. Initial dosing of dofetilide is based on the creatinine clearance.
        - A 12-lead ECG should be obtained before the first dose of dofetilide and 1–2 hours after each dose. If the QT_c interval after the first dose prolongs by 15% of the baseline or exceeds 500 ms, a 50% dosage reduction is indicated. If the QT_c exceeds 500 ms after the second dose, dofetilide must be discontinued.
        - Several medications block the renal secretion of dofetilide (verapamil, cimetidine, prochlorperazine, trimethoprim, megestrol, ketoconazole) and are contraindicated with dofetilide.
        - In patients who previously received amiodarone, dofetilide can be started only after amiodarone has been discontinued for at least 3 months.
        - The advantages of dofetilide are that it is not associated with increased CHF or mortality in patients with LV dysfunction,[6] and dofetilide does not cause sinus node dysfunction or conduction abnormalities.
- **Class II and IV** are β-antagonists and calcium channel antagonists, respectively. Their use in the treatment of AF is for rate control by increasing the AV nodal refractory period. These agents are not effective in the conversion or maintenance of sinus rhythm.
- **Amiodarone** has the properties of class I, II, III, and IV drugs, and is arguably the most effective antiarrhythmic agent for maintenance of sinus rhythm. **Because of the extensive toxicity profile of amiodarone, it should not be considered as a first-line agent for rhythm control of atrial fibrillation in patients**

in whom an alternative antiarrhythmic can be safely used. Intravenous amiodarone has a low efficacy for acute conversion of AF, although conversion after several days of IV amiodarone has been observed. Given its common use and relative high incidence of side effects, a more detailed discussion of these effects is required.

- Adverse effects of oral amiodarone are partially dose dependent and may occur in up to 75% of patients treated at high doses for 5 years. At lower dosages (200–300 mg/d), adverse effects that require discontinuation occur in approximately 5%–10% of patients per year.
- **Pulmonary toxicity** occurs in 1%–15% of treated patients but appears less likely in those who receive <300 mg/d.[7] Patients characteristically have a dry cough and dyspnea associated with pulmonary infiltrates and rales. The process appears to be reversible if detected early, but undetected cases may result in a mortality of up to 10% of those affected. A chest radiograph and pulmonary function tests should be obtained at baseline and every 12 months or when patients complain of shortness of breath. The presence of interstitial infiltrates on the chest radiograph and a decreased diffusing capacity raise concern of amiodarone pulmonary toxicity.
- **Photosensitivity** is a common adverse reaction, and, in some patients, a violaceous skin discoloration develops in sun-exposed areas. The blue-gray discoloration may not resolve completely with discontinuation of therapy.
- **Thyroid dysfunction** is a common adverse effect. Hypothyroidism and hyperthyroidism have been reported, with an incidence of 2%–5% per year. Thyroid-stimulating hormone should be obtained at baseline and monitored every 6 months. If hypothyroidism develops, concurrent treatment with levothyroxine may allow continued amiodarone use.
- **Corneal microdeposits**, detectable on slit-lamp examination, develop in virtually all patients. These deposits rarely interfere with vision and are not an indication for discontinuation of the drug. Optic neuritis, leading to blindness, is rare but has been reported in association with amiodarone.
- The most common **ECG changes** are lengthened PR intervals and bradycardia; however, high-grade AV block may occur in patients who have pre-existing conduction abnormalities. Amiodarone may prolong QT intervals, although usually not extensively, and TdP is rare. Other agents that prolong the QT interval, however, should be avoided in patients who are taking amiodarone.
- **Liver dysfunction** usually manifests in an asymptomatic and transient rise in hepatic transaminases. If the increase exceeds three times normal or doubles in a patient with an elevated baseline level, amiodarone should be discontinued or the dose should be reduced. Aspartate transaminase (AST) and alanine transaminase (ALT) should be monitored every 6 months in patients who are receiving amiodarone.
- **Drug interactions.** Amiodarone may raise the blood levels of warfarin and digoxin; therefore, these drugs should be reduced routinely by one-half when amiodarone is started, and levels should be followed closely.
- **Choosing and monitoring antiarrhythmic agents.** In general, loading of antiarrhythmic drugs should be performed in an inpatient setting for four to five doses, with daily ECGs performed to check QT and QRS intervals, and continuous telemetry to monitor for the development of bradycardia and TdP. Renal function must be carefully assessed and followed for patients who are receiving renally cleared drugs. The loading of dofetilide requires a mandatory 3-day hospitalization for monitoring. Outpatient loading of antiarrhythmic drugs is acceptable in limited circumstances, generally for patients without any structural cardiac diseases or conduction abnormalities. Event monitors are recommended in these cases, as recordings can be sent by patients daily to monitor for bradyarrhythmias and QT/QRS intervals.

Nonpharmacologic methods of rhythm control
- The initiation and maintenance AF has been shown to arise from focal sites within the pulmonary veins[8] for many patients with atrial fibrillation. Catheter ablation

strategies that electrically isolate the pulmonary veins and left atrial periosteal tissue have been shown to be curative in the majority of patients who undergo these procedures. Complications associated with this procedure include stroke, perforation with tamponade, pulmonary vein stenosis, and atrial esophageal fistula formation. As a result, catheter ablation of atrial fibrillation should be reserved for symptomatic patients in whom no other therapeutic options are available.

- The **Maze procedure** is a cardiac surgery that utilizes multiple incisions in the right and left atrium to create narrow corridors of atrial tissue that do not support atrial fibrillatory waves. The procedure has been used successfully in conjunction with other heart operations, in particular mitral valve surgery. Cure rates associated with the Maze procedure are about 90%.

■ Special considerations: WPW and AF
- For hemodynamically stable pre-excited AF, IV procainamide or amiodarone can be used to slow conduction over the accessory pathway, but **AV nodal–blocking agents (adenosine, calcium channel antagonists, beta-blockers, or digoxin) must be avoided,** as they may facilitate conduction over the accessory pathway and increase the ventricular rate paradoxically, initiating VF.
- Hemodynamic compromise or clinical instability should be treated with prompt DC cardioversion.
- Because AF in these patients most commonly results from AVRT, the therapy of choice is ablation of the accessory pathway.
- Pharmacologic therapy for WPW patients is targeted at slowing conduction and prolonging refractoriness of the accessory bypass tract with an antiarrhythmic agent (class Ia, Ic, and III agents) and is reserved for those who are unable to undergo or who refuse an ablation procedure.

■ AFL differs from AF in that AFL results from a single macro–re-entrant circuit around the tricuspid valve in the right atrium. AFL is treated similarly to AF. Although data for thromboembolic risks in patients with AFL are not as extensive as those for AF, the risk of thromboembolus appears to be similar to AF.[9] As a result, the same guidelines for anticoagulation in AF should be followed for patients with AFL.
- Rate control of the ventricular response to AFL can be achieved with agents that reduce AV nodal conduction with the same agents discussed above for AF.
- Electrical or chemical cardioversion is appropriate for highly symptomatic patients in whom rhythm control is warranted. In patients with implanted pacemakers, cardioversion can be achieved in many by overdrive atrial pacing at an atrial rate faster than the atrial flutter rate. This should only be attempted by a cardiovascular disease specialist with specific training for management of pacemakers.
- Catheter ablation of atrial flutter is often preferable to antiarrhythmic drug therapy for maintenance of sinus rhythm in highly symptomatic patients.[10] Catheter ablation of typical right AFL is associated with a chronic success rate of about 90%. Complications are rare but can include complete heart block or injury to the right coronary artery with inferior MI. Ablation of atypical forms of AFL is associated with a lower rate of success.
  - **Similar considerations regarding anticoagulation for electrical or pharmacologic cardioversion should be observed** before an attempt is made at overdrive pace termination or catheter ablation of AFL.

■ VT and VF. Immediate unsynchronized DC cardioversion is the primary therapy for pulseless VT and VF. VF that is resistant to external defibrillation requires the addition of IV antiarrhythmic agents. Intravenous lidocaine is frequently used; however, IV amiodarone appears to be more effective in increasing survival of VF when used in conjunction with defibrillation.[11] After successful cardioversion, continuous IV infusion of effective antiarrhythmic therapy should be maintained until any reversible causes have been corrected.
- Chronic antiarrhythmic drug therapy is indicated for the treatment of recurrent symptomatic ventricular arrhythmias. In the setting of hemodynamically unstable ventricular arrhythmias treated with an ICD, antiarrhythmic drug therapy is often necessary to suppress frequent device discharges.

- **Class I** agents in general have not been shown to reduce mortality in patients with VT/VF. In fact, the class Ic agents **flecainide** and propafenone are associated with increased mortality in patients with ventricular arrhythmias.[12]
  - **Lidocaine** is a class Ib agent available only in IV form with efficacy in the management of sustained and recurrent VT/VF. The prophylactic use of lidocaine for suppression of premature ventricular contractions (PVCs) and nonsustained ventricular tachycardia (NSVT) in the otherwise uncomplicated post-MI setting is not indicated and may lead to an increase in mortality from bradyarrhythmias.[13] Toxicities of lidocaine include central nervous system (CNS) effects (convulsions, confusion, stupor, and, rarely, respiratory arrest), all of which resolve with discontinuation of therapy. Negative inotropic effects are seen only at high drug levels.
  - **Mexiletine** is similar to lidocaine but is available in oral form. Mexiletine is most often used in combination with either amiodarone or sotalol for chronic treatment of refractory ventricular arrhythmias. Mexiletine may have a limited role in the treatment of some patients with congenital long QT syndromes. CNS toxicity includes tremor, dizziness, and blurred vision. Higher levels may result in dysarthria, diplopia, nystagmus, and an impaired level of consciousness. Nausea and vomiting are common side effects.
  - **Phenytoin** is used primarily in the treatment of digitalis-induced ventricular arrhythmias. It may have a limited role in the treatment of ventricular arrhythmias associated with congenital long QT syndromes. The IV loading dose is 250 mg given over 10 minutes (maximum rate of 50 mg/min). Subsequent doses of 100 mg can be given q5min as necessary and as blood pressure (BP) tolerates, to a total of 1,000 mg. Frequent monitoring of the ECG, BP, and neurologic status is required. Continuous infusion is not recommended (see Chapter 24, Neurologic Disorders).
- **Class II** agents, the β-adrenergic antagonists, are the only class of antiarrhythmic agent to have consistently shown improved survival in post-MI patients. Beta-blockers reduce postinfarction total mortality by 25%–40% and SCD by 32%–50%.[14]
- Sotalol is the only **class III** agent indicated for the chronic treatment of VT/VF. **Sotalol** prevents the recurrence of sustained VT and VF in 70% of patients[15] but must be used with caution in individuals with congestive heart failure as noted above.
- **Class IV** agents have no role in the chronic management of VT. Intravenous calcium channel blockers should never be used in the acute management of VT, as they may cause hemodynamic collapse. Oral calcium channel blockers are not effective in the management of VT. Short-acting nifedipine is associated with a trend toward increasing mortality when used in the post-MI patient.[16]
- **Amiodarone** is safe and well tolerated for the acute management of ventricular arrhythmias. Amiodarone has complex pharmacokinetics and is associated with significant toxicities arising from chronic therapy.[17]
  - After oral loading, amiodarone prevents the recurrence of sustained VT or VF in up to 60% of patients. A therapeutic latency of more than 5 days exists before beneficial antiarrhythmic effects are observed with oral dosing, and full suppression of arrhythmias may not occur for 4–6 weeks after therapy is initiated.
  - Amiodarone has become the most studied antiarrhythmic agent in the treatment of SCD and the main drug against which ICDs are compared, in secondary and in primary prevention trials.
  - The balance of multiple prospective clinical trials does not support the prophylactic use of amiodarone for prevention of SCD in cardiomyopathy patients.
- Primary VF that occurs within the first 72 hours of an acute MI is not associated with an elevated risk of recurrence and does not require chronic antiarrhythmic therapy.

- In the case of **TdP associated with long QT syndrome,** acute therapy is immediate DC cardioversion. Bolus administration of magnesium sulfate in 1- to 2-g increments up to 4–6 g IV is highly effective. In cases of acquired long QT syndrome, identification and treatment of the underlying condition should be undertaken, if possible. Elimination of long–short triggering sequences and shortening of the QT interval can be achieved by increasing the heart rate to the range of 90–120 bpm by either IV isoproterenol infusion (initial rate at 1–2 mcg/min) or temporary transvenous pacing.
- **Nonpharmacologic therapy for VT/VF** includes automatic ICD and catheter ablation.
  - **ICDs** provide automatic recognition and treatment of ventricular arrhythmias. ICD implantation improves survival in patients resuscitated from ventricular arrhythmias (secondary prevention of SCD) and in individuals without prior symptoms who are at high risk for SCD (primary prevention of SCD).
  - **Secondary prevention of SCD** with ICD implantation is indicated for most patients who survive SCD outside of the peri-MI setting. The superiority of ICD therapy to chronic antiarrhythmic drug therapy has been demonstrated in multiple prospective clinical trials.[18]
  - **Primary prevention of SCD** with ICD implantation is indicated for patients who are at high risk of SCD. The efficacy of ICD implantation for primary prevention of SCD in the setting of cardiomyopathy has been established in multiple prospective clinical trials.[19–22] Most patients with a left ventricular ejection fraction of <35% for more than 3 months meet current indications for prophylactic ICD implantation.
  - **Other indications for ICD**
    - Phenotypes associated with **hypertrophic cardiomyopathy, arrhythmogenic right ventricular cardiomyopathy, congenital long QT syndrome, or Brugada syndrome have a high risk of SCD.** ICD implantation is indicated if patients with one of these syndromes have had a resuscitated cardiac arrest or documented ventricular arrhythmias. Prophylactic ICD implantation for asymptomatic patients is generally considered appropriate, particularly in patients who have had syncope or with a family history of sudden death.
    - Patients who are awaiting cardiac transplantation are at high risk for SCD, especially if they are receiving an intravenous inotrope. Prophylactic ICD implantation is reasonable to protect against SCD prior to transplantation.
    - ICDs are contraindicated in patients who have incessant VT, significant psychiatric illnesses, or life expectancy of <6 months.[23]
  - **Radiofrequency catheter ablation of VT** is most successfully performed in patients with hemodynamically stable forms of idiopathic VT that is not associated with structural heart disease. Long-term cure rates in these patients are similar to those achieved for catheter ablation of SVT. In the presence of structural heart disease, and particularly with hemodynamically unstable VT, catheter ablation is generally reserved for drug refractory VT due to a lower efficacy and a higher morbidity associated with the ablation procedure.
    - **Idiopathic VT is usually associated with a structurally normal heart, but an associated tachycardia-mediated cardiomyopathy has been described.**
      - **Right ventricular outflow tract VT (RVOT-VT)** often presents as repetitive, nonsustained bursts of VT that can be exercise induced. The ECG pattern is diagnostic with an LBBB morphology and an inferior axis. RVOT-VT is usually responsive to beta-blockers, diltiazem or verapamil, and adenosine.
      - **Idiopathic LV VT** has an RBBB morphology with a superior axis and is frequently responsive to verapamil.
      - Both forms of idiopathic VT are benign without an increased incidence of SCD. Therefore, ICD implantation is not appropriate. All forms of

idiopathic VT are amenable to treatment with radiofrequency ablation or drug therapy.

- **Bundle branch re-entry VT (BBRT)** is a form of VT that involves the His-Purkinje system in a re-entrant circuit. BBRT can be treated successfully by catheter ablation of the right bundle branch. Because BBRT usually occurs in patients with cardiomyopathy and an abnormal conduction system, an ICD is generally implanted in conjunction with ablation.
- **VT associated with ischemic heart disease** can also be treated by catheter ablation; however, success rates are significantly lower compared to idiopathic VT. The reasons for the lower success rate include the hemodynamic instability of VT and the multiple different VT circuits (due to multiple areas of scars from prior MIs) that are often present. Catheter ablation of ischemic VT in patients with antiarrhythmic drug-refractory VT and an implanted ICD has been successful in reducing frequent ICD shocks.[24]
- **Ablation of VT in nonischemic cardiomyopathy** is possible, but VT circuits may be intramyocardial or epicardial. As a result, success rates are typically lower than those associated with ischemic VT.

APPROACH TO BRADYARRHYTHMIAS

GENERAL PRINCIPLES

- **Bradyarrhythmias** are rhythms that result in a ventricular rate of <60 bpm.
- The conduction disturbances can be attributed to dysfunction somewhere within the native conduction system from the SA node through the AV node to the His-Purkinje network.
- One must consider both intrinsic conduction disease in patients with bradycardia and extrinsic influences on the conduction system.

Anatomy of Conduction System

- Under normal conditions, the **sinus node,** a collection of specialized pacemaker cells located in the high right atrium, initiates a wave of depolarization that spreads inferiorly and leftward via atrial myocardium and intranodal tracts, producing atrial systole.
  - The typical resting rate of the SA node is between 50 and 90 bpm, is inversely related to age, and is determined by the balance of sympathetic and parasympathetic input.
  - Arterial blood is supplied to the SA node via the sinus node artery, which has variable anatomic origins as follows: right coronary artery (RCA), 65%; circumflex, 25%; or dual (RCA and circumflex), 10%.
- The wave of depolarization then reaches the **AV node,** another grouping of special cells located in the right atrial side of the intraatrial septum. The AV node should serve as the only electrical connection between the atria and the ventricle.
  - Conduction through the AV node is decremental, produces a delay typically in the range of 55–110 ms, and accounts for the majority of the PR interval measured on ECG.
  - The primary blood supply to the AV node comes from the **AV nodal artery** that originates typically from the proximal posterior descending artery (PDA) (80%), but can also come from the circumflex (10%) or both (10%). In addition, it receives collateral flow from the left anterior descending (LAD) artery and is, therefore, relatively protected against vascular compromise.
  - The AV node is also innervated by the autonomic nervous system, which modulates the ventricular response to atrial depolarization.
- From the AV node, the wave of propagation travels down the **His bundle,** located in the membranous septum, into the **right and left bundle branches** before reaching the Purkinje fibers that depolarize the rest of the ventricular myocardium.

- The His and right bundle receive blood via the AV node artery and from septal perforators off the LAD.
- The left bundle divides further into the anterior and posterior fascicles, of which the former is supplied by septal perforators and the latter by branches off the PDA and septal perforators off the LAD.

Definitions

- **Sinus bradycardia** is defined as a sinus rate of <60 bpm with a normal P-wave configuration consistent with an origin in the sinus node area.
- **Sick sinus syndrome (SSS)** represents an array of rhythm disturbances that result from sinus node dysfunction. It is usually a disorder of the elderly and is presumed to arise from intrinsic disease of the sinoatrial node caused by aging, or in association with structural heart disease.
  - **Chronotropic incompetence** is the inability to increase the heart rate appropriately in response to metabolic need.
  - **Sinus pause or sinus arrest** occurs when the sinus node intermittently fails to produce an impulse or when sinus node inactivity is prolonged, respectively. Sinus pauses that result in ventricular asystole of >3 seconds in the awake patient are an indication for permanent pacemaker therapy in the absence of reversible causes.
  - **Tachy-brady syndrome** occurs when bradyarrhythmias alternate with tachyarrhythmias, especially AF. Sinus pauses occur after termination of AF as a result of suppression of sinus node function by the rapid atrial rate. Drugs used to treat the tachycardia frequently exacerbate underlying sinus node disease.
- **AV block** occurs when an atrial impulse is conducted with delay or fails to conduct to the ventricle at a time when the AV node should not be refractory.
  - **First-degree AV block** describes a conduction delay, usually within the AV node, that results in a prolonged PR interval on the surface ECG of >200 ms.
  - **Second-degree AV block** is present when some atrial impulses are not conducted to the ventricle. Distinctions between type I and type II second-degree AV block are important, as they carry different prognostic implications.
    - **Mobitz type I block (Wenckebach)** is a progressive delay in AV conduction with successive atrial impulses, as evidenced by progressive PR interval prolongation, before the block of an atrial impulse. The characteristic ECG pattern is of QRS complexes occurring in regular groupings (grouped beating) separated by the blocked beat. The RR interval progressively shortens before a blocked P wave, and the PR interval just after the block is shorter than the PR interval just before the block.
      - The site of conduction block is usually within the AV node. Mobitz type I block is benign and usually does not portend development of complete heart block.
      - Symptomatic type I AV block is managed initially with atropine, 0.5 mg IV every 2 minutes to a maximum of 0.04 mg/kg. For persistent symptoms without treatable causes, permanent pacemaker therapy is indicated.
    - **Mobitz type II block** is characterized by abrupt AV conduction block without evidence of progressive conduction delay. The ECG demonstrates no change in PR intervals preceding a nonconducted P wave.
      - The site of block is localized most often to the His-Purkinje system.
      - Etiologies include conduction system disease and myocardial ischemia (typically in an anterior distribution).
      - Type II block, especially in the setting of a bundle branch block, often antedates the development of complete heart block, and permanent pacemakers are indicated in symptomatic and in asymptomatic patients. Hemodynamically unstable patients should be treated initially with temporary transvenous pacemakers.
      - Atropine is usually not effective in the treatment of Mobitz type II block and may worsen the condition by accelerating the sinus rate, resulting in higher degrees of block.

- **AV 2:1 block** may be caused by either Mobitz type I or II mechanisms but differentiating between the two is difficult.
  - Mobitz type I 2:1 block often occurs concomitantly with first-degree AV block or AV Wenckebach with grouped beating, or both. An increase in the sinus rate from increased sympathetic input often results in resumption of 1:1 conduction if the mechanism is Mobitz type I.
  - The concomitant presence of bundle branch block or fascicular block suggests the presence of type II second-degree AV block. An increase in the sinus rate frequently worsens the block if Mobitz type II block is present (i.e., 2:1 block may progress to 3:1 or 4:1 block).
- **Third-degree (complete) AV block** is present when all atrial impulses fail to conduct to the ventricle and the prevailing ventricular escape rhythm is slower than the atrial rate.
  - This pattern is distinct from **AV dissociation**, which is present when the ventricular rate exceeds the atrial rate. The ventricular escape rate should be regular in complete heart block. The site of block may be the AV node (as occurs in congenital heart block) or within the His-Purkinje system (typical for acquired heart block).
  - Etiologies of acquired complete AV block include ischemia or infarction, drug toxicity, idiopathic degeneration of the conduction system, infiltrative diseases (amyloidosis, sarcoidosis, metastatic disease), rheumatologic disorders (polymyositis, scleroderma, rheumatoid nodules), infectious diseases (Chagas disease, Lyme disease), calcific aortic stenosis, and endocarditis.
  - **Isorhythmic AV dissociation** describes a condition in which a junctional rhythm is competing with underlying sinus bradycardia.

DIAGNOSIS

History and Physical Examination

- As seen in tachyarrhythmias, there is a broad range of presenting symptoms that can be attributed to an underlying bradyarrhythmia.
  - Those patients capable of augmenting stroke volume to compensate for bradycardia can tolerate very low heart rates without clinically significant consequences. Others, however, can present with symptoms ranging from the nonspecific (fatigue, lightheadedness, weakness, exercise intolerance) to the overt (syncope).
  - Ischemic heart disease, usually involving the right-sided circulation, can present with bradycardia and hypotension and, therefore, symptoms of acute coronary syndromes should always be ascertained.
- **Precipitating circumstances** surrounding symptomatic episodes may be helpful in the diagnosis of autonomically mediated bradyarrhythmias occurring as a component of a neurocardiogenic syndrome.
- **History of tachyarrhythmias** and inquiries regarding palpitations should also be made to search for the presence of underlying tachy-brady syndrome. In that syndrome, a significant pause often follows the termination of an episode of tachyarrhythmia.
- History of structural heart disease, collagen vascular disease, infiltrative diseases (amyloidosis, sarcoid, hemochromatosis), hypothyroidism, neuromuscular disorders, and prior cardiac surgery (valve replacement, congenital repair) should be sought.
- **Medications** that affect the SA and AV node should be sought with particular emphasis on common medications such as β-adrenergic antagonists, calcium channel blockers, digoxin, and clonidine.
- Physical examination findings consistent with the aforementioned comorbidities known to cause bradyarrhythmias should be sought.
- A regularly irregular rhythm (i.e., **"group beating"**) discovered on physical examination may indicate an underlying second-degree AV block.
- Emphasis should be placed on delineating **whether the presenting symptoms correlate directly with rhythm changes** discovered on the following diagnostic modalities.

Diagnostic Tools

- The **12-lead ECG** as described previously is essential to any diagnostic workup where arrhythmia is suspected. Rhythm strips from leads that provide the best illustration of atrial activity (II, III, aVf, or V1) should be utilized. Evidence of both old and acute manifestations of ischemic heart disease should be sought.
- Often episodes of bradycardia are transient and episodic; therefore, a baseline ECG may not be sufficient to record the bradycardia. Some form of continuous monitoring is often required.
  - In the inpatient setting, **continuous central telemetry monitoring** can be utilized.
  - If further workup is done as an outpatient, **24- to 72-hour Holter monitoring** can be used if the episodes occur somewhat frequently. If the episodes are infrequent, an **event recorder** or **implantable loop recorder** should be considered.
  - Again, it is vital to correlate symptoms with the rhythm disturbances discovered via continuous monitoring—a task easily accomplished during inpatient care but more difficult as an outpatient. Therefore, the importance of accurate symptom diaries in the ambulatory setting should be emphasized to patients.
- **Exercise ECG** is useful in assessing the sinus node's response to exertion.
- **EPS** can also be used to assess sinus node function and AV conduction, but it is rarely necessary if the rhythm is already discovered via noninvasive modalities.
- **Laboratory studies** should include thyroid function tests, serum electrolytes, and serum digoxin level (if appropriate).
- The role of **tilt-table testing** will be discussed below in the setting of a syncope evaluation.

TREATMENT

- Identification of reversible causes of symptomatic bradycardia should be undertaken immediately after diagnosis. Symptomatic sinus bradycardia, first-degree AV block, or Mobitz I second-degree AV block may respond acutely to atropine, 0.5–2.0 mg IV. For irreversible causes of symptomatic bradycardia, pacemaker therapy should be considered.
  - **Temporary pacemakers.** Temporary pacing is best achieved by insertion of a temporary transvenous pacemaker, although placement of an external transthoracic unit can be used.
    - Temporary pacing is indicated for **symptomatic second- or third-degree heart block caused by transient drug intoxication or electrolyte imbalance and complete heart block or Mobitz II second-degree AV block in the setting of an acute MI.**
    - Sinus bradycardia, AF with a slow ventricular response, or Mobitz I second-degree AV block should be treated with temporary pacemakers **only if symptoms or hemodynamic instability is present.**
  - **Permanent pacemaker implantation.** Contemporary pacemakers can maintain AV synchrony and adapt the rate of pacing to mimic the normal physiologic heart rate response to exertion. Before a pacemaker is implanted, the patient must be free of any active infections, and anticoagulation issues must be carefully considered. Hematomas over the pacemaker pocket are most often seen in patients who are receiving IV heparin or subcutaneous enoxaparin sodium (Lovenox) and may require surgical evacuation in severe cases.
    - **Class I indications** are conditions in which permanent pacing is considered to be acceptable and necessary for adequate treatment and are listed in Table 7-5. For a full discussion of current guidelines, refer to the joint AHA/ACC/NASPE report released in 2002.
    - **Pacing modalities.** A four-letter alphabetic code is used to identify pacing modalities. The first initial defines the chamber that is paced (Ventricle, Atrium, Dual chamber, O if neither), the second identifies the chamber that is sensed (Ventricle, Atrium, Dual chamber, O for neither), the third indicates the response to a sensed event (Inhibited, Triggered, Dual function, O for no response), and the fourth,

TABLE 7-5   **Class I Indications for Permanent Pacemakers**

Symptomatic sinus bradycardia or atrioventricular (AV) block
Sinus bradycardia as a result of necessary drug therapy
Symptomatic chronotropic incompetence
Advanced AV block with:
  Asystole ≥3 sec in the awake patient
  Escape rate <40 beats/min
  Catheter ablation of AV node
  Neuromuscular disease
  Postoperative AV block that is not expected to recover
Intermittent complete heart block
Intermittent type II second-degree block
Alternating bundle branch block
Recurrent syncope with carotid sinus massage causing asystole ≥3 sec

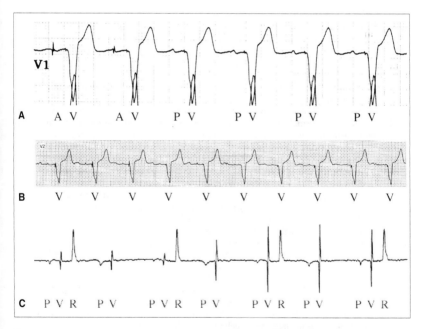

Figure 7-3. A: Normal dual-chamber (DDD) pacing. First two complexes are atrioventricular (AV) sequential pacing, followed by sinus with atrial sensing and ventricular pacing. **B:** Normal single-chamber (VVI) pacing. Underlying rhythm is atrial fibrillation (no distinct P waves), with ventricular pacing at 60 beats/minute. **C:** Pacemaker malfunction. The underlying rhythm is sinus (P) at 80 beats/minute with 2:1 heart block and first-degree AV block (long PR). Ventricular pacing spikes are seen (V) after each P wave, demonstrating appropriate sensing and tracking of the P waves; however, there is failure to capture. A, paced atrial events; V, paced ventricular events; P, sensed atrial events; R, sensed ventricular events.

when present, denotes Rate response mode. Some examples of normal and abnormal pacing functions are shown in Figure 7-3.

- The **VVI** and **DDD** modes are used most commonly. VVI units pace and sense in the ventricle; a sensed (native QRS) event inhibits the ventricular stimulus. DDD units pace and sense in both chambers. Events sensed in the atrium inhibit the atrial stimulus and trigger a ventricular response after an appointed interval (AV delay), whereas ventricle-sensed events inhibit ventricular stimulus.
- **Lower rate limit** is the intrinsic heart rate below which the pacemaker begins to pace.
- **Upper rate limit** is the maximum heart rate that the pacemaker paces. In patients with atrial arrhythmias (most commonly AF) and AV block, a DDD pacemaker may allow for tracking of AF, resulting in ventricular pacing at the upper rate limit.
- Pacemakers today have detection protocols that allow automatic switching of pacing modes to prevent rapid ventricular pacing in response to rapid atrial rates ("mode switch").
- **Application of a magnet to a pacemaker turns off the sensing modality**, thereby making a pacemaker asynchronous. For example, VVI mode becomes VOO (ventricular asynchronous pacing), and DDD mode becomes DOO (asynchronous AV pacing).

 # APPROACH TO SYNCOPE

GENERAL PRINCIPLES

- Syncope is defined as a **sudden, brief loss of consciousness and postural tone followed by rapid and complete recovery as a result of transient cerebral hypoperfusion.**
- Syncope is common in the general population. Of an unselected population, 40% report at least one lifetime syncopal event. Syncope accounts for approximately 6% of all hospital admissions.
- Because a syncopal event may herald an otherwise unsuspected, potentially lethal cardiac condition, a careful evaluation of the patient with syncope is warranted.
- In general, the **presence of known structural heart disease, symptoms suggestive of cardiac syncope, abnormal ECG, age older than 65 years, focal neurologic findings, and severe orthostatic hypotension suggest a potentially more ominous etiology. Therefore, these patients should be admitted** for their workup to avoid delay and adverse outcomes.
- The etiologies of syncope are myriad and can be divided into primary cardiac and noncardiac mechanisms.
  - **Primary cardiac syncope** is caused either by mechanical obstruction of cardiac output (e.g., hypertrophic cardiomyopathy, valvular stenosis, aortic dissection, myxomas, pulmonary embolism) or by a hemodynamically significant arrhythmia. Cardiac causes of syncope account for approximately 9.5% of all identified causes of syncope and are **associated with increased mortality.**
  - **Neurocardiogenic syncope** is the most commonly diagnosed cause of syncope (21%), particularly in those without underlying heart disease or other comorbidities. This form of syncope is generally associated with a benign prognosis.
    - The two components of neurocardiogenic syncope are described as **cardioinhibitory**, in which bradycardia or asystole results from increased vagal outflow to the heart, and **vasodepression**, where the peripheral vasodilation results from sympathetic withdrawal to peripheral arteries. Most patients have a combination of both components as the mechanism of their syncope.
    - Specific stimuli may evoke a neurocardiogenic mechanism, leading to a **situational syncope** (e.g., micturition, defecation, coughing, swallowing).
  - Other **noncardiac causes of syncope** include orthostatic hypotension, toxic or metabolic influences (e.g., drug toxicities, hypoglycemia, hypoxia, etc.), neurologic etiologies (e.g., seizures or cerebrovascular accidents), and psychiatric etiologies (e.g., conversion disorders and anxiety disorders).

History and Physical Examination

- The clinical history and physical examination have the highest utility for identification of a potential mechanism of a syncopal event. Special attention should be focused on the events or symptoms that precede and follow the syncopal event, the time course of loss and resumption of consciousness (abrupt vs. gradual), and any description of vital signs before, during, and after the event.
    - A characteristic prodrome of nausea, diaphoresis, or flushing preceding loss of consciousness suggests neurocardiogenic syncope, as does the identification of a particular emotional or situational trigger or a postsyncopal sensation of fatigue that lasts for many minutes to hours.
    - Alternatively, an unusual sensory prodrome, incontinence, or a decreased level of consciousness that gradually clears suggests a seizure as a likely diagnosis.
    - With transient ventricular arrhythmias, an abrupt loss of consciousness may occur, with a rapid recovery.
    - A clear history of palpitations preceding syncope is seldom elicited.
- Physical examination should include assessment of orthostatic vital signs and careful neurologic, pulmonary, and cardiovascular assessment.
    - Bedside manipulations may be useful, including Valsalva maneuvers and squatting, with attention to cardiac auscultatory findings to detect valvular and subvalvular lesions.

DIAGNOSIS

- The 12-lead ECG will be abnormal in 50% of the cases but, alone, will yield a diagnosis in only 5% of these patients.
- Following a thorough history, physical examination, and analysis of the baseline ECG, the etiology will be either diagnosed, suggested, or unexplained. At this point in the evaluation, 40% of diagnoses will be apparent or suggested.
    - If the diagnosis is apparent, then one should treat the condition accordingly.
    - If "suggestive," then further workup (i.e., electroencephalogram [EEG], head computed tomography [CT] scan, echocardiography, troponins, stress test, spiral chest CT, toxicology screening, etc.) should be tailored to the likely etiology.
    - If "unexplained," consider the following:
        - If the patient has known heart disease or baseline ECG abnormalities, a cardiac arrhythmia is most likely. In these patients, a transthoracic echocardiogram, noninvasive stress test, continuous ECG monitoring, cardiac consultation, and, ultimately, EPS are more likely to yield a diagnosis.
        - If the patient has no history of heart disease and a normal ECG, neurally mediated processes become more likely. In these patients, one could consider maneuvers to test for carotid sinus hypersensitivity or tilt-table testing if the symptoms are recurrent or if the patient has a higher-risk occupation (e.g., truck/taxi driver, construction, etc.).
- **Routine laboratory tests are typically unhelpful;** however, for patients with comorbid conditions or those who take electrophysiologically active drugs, such screening should be performed. Toxicology screening should be done for suspected illicit drug use or inadvertent drug exposure.

TREATMENT

- Appropriate therapy for patients with syncope is determined by the underlying etiology.
    - Syncope in the setting of ischemic or nonischemic cardiomyopathy carries a poor prognosis, and the implantation of ICDs is appropriate when no reversible causes are found. Syncope due to reversible causes, whether cardiac, neurologic, or medication related, should be appropriately treated.

■ When the clinical history or diagnostic testing is suggestive of a **neurocardiogenic mechanism,** initial treatment is targeted at counseling patients to take precautionary steps to avoid injury. Patients should be aware of their prodromal symptoms and maintain horizontal positions at those times, increase fluid uptake, keep their feet elevated, and use support stockings to minimize the impact of peripheral vasodilatation.

- Medical therapy begins with **β-adrenergic antagonists,** which block peripheral adrenergic-mediated vasodilation and decrease cardiac inotropy, or volume expansion with salt tablets or fludrocortisone, or both. Metoprolol and atenolol are commonly used beta-blockers. In patients with baseline sinus bradycardia, the use of beta-blockers with intrinsic sympathomimetic activities (pindolol, 5–10 mg bid, or acebutolol, 200–400 mg bid) may prevent worsening bradycardia.

- **Midodrine,** an α_1-adrenergic agonist that induces venous and arterial vasoconstriction, appears to be effective in patients with vasodepressor syncope.[25] Midodrine is given 5 mg PO tid and can be increased as needed to 15 mg tid. As with salt tablets and fludrocortisone, midodrine may cause hypertension.

- **Disopyramide** may have utility to prevent neurocardiogenic syncope, probably through its strong negative inotropic action in reducing stimulation of ventricular mechanoreceptors. However, given its antiarrhythmic properties and potential for causing malignant arrhythmias, it is rarely used to treat benign vasovagal syncope.

- Centrally acting agents such as **selective serotonin reuptake inhibitors** or **yohimbine** may be useful to attenuate central reflex centers involved in neurocardiogenic mechanisms.

- **Permanent dual-chamber pacemakers** with a hysteresis function (high-rate pacing in response to a detected sudden drop in heart rate) have been shown to be useful in highly selected patients with recurrent neurocardiogenic syncope with a prominent cardioinhibitory component.[26]

References

1. Trohman RG. Supraventricular tachycardia: implications for the intensivist. *Crit Care Med* 2000 Oct;28(10 Suppl):N129–135.
2. Tchou P, Young P, Mahmud R, et al. Useful clinical criteria for the diagnosis of ventricular tachycardia. *Am J Med* 1988 Jan;84(1):53–56.
3. Stroke Prevention in Atrial Fibrillation Investigators. Stroke prevention in atrial fibrillation study: final results. *Circulation* 1991;84:527–539.
4. Berger M, Schweitzer P. Timing of thromboembolic events after electrical cardioversion of atrial fibrillation or flutter: a retrospective analysis. *Am J Cardiol* 1998;82:1545–1547.
5. Cardiac Arrhythmia Suppression Trial. Preliminary report: effect of encainide and flecainide on mortality in a randomized trial of arrhythmia suppression after myocardial infarction. *N Engl J Med* 1989;321:406–412.
6. Torp-Pedersen C, Moller M, Bloch-Thomsen PE. Dofetilide in patients with congestive heart failure and left ventricular dysfunction. Danish Investigations of Arrhythmia and Mortality on Dofetilide Study Group. *N Engl J Med.* 1999;341:857–865.
7. Dusman RE, Stanton MS, Miles WM et al. Clinical features of amiodarone-induced pulmonary toxicity. *Circulation,* 1990;82:51–59.
8. Haissaguerre M, Jais P, Shah DC, et al. Spontaneous initiation of atrial fibrillation by ectopic beats originating in the pulmonary veins. *N Engl J Med.* 1998;339:659–666.
9. Seidl K, Hauer B, Schwick NG, Zellner D, Zahn R, Senges J. Risk of thromboembolic events in patients with atrial flutter. *Am J Cardiol.* 1998;82:580–583.
10. Feld GK, Fleck RP, Chen PS, et al. Radiofrequency catheter ablation for the treatment of human type 1 atrial flutter: Identification of a critical zone in the reentrant circuit by endocardial mapping techniques. *Circulation* 1992;86:1233–1240.
11. Dorian P, Cass D, Schwartz B, et al. Amiodarone as compared with lidocaine for shock-resistant ventricular fibrillation [Published erratum appears in N Engl J Med 2002;347:955]. *N Engl J Med* 2002;346:884–890.
12. Echt DS, Liebson PR, Mitchell LB, et al. Mortality and morbidity in patients receiving

encainide, flecainide, or placebo: the Cardiac Arrhythmia Suppression Trial. *N Engl J Med* 1991;324:781–788

13. Hine LK, Laird N, Hewitt P, et al. Meta-analytic evidence against prophylactic use of lidocaine in acute myocardial infarction. *Arch Intern Med.* 1989;149:2694–2698.

14. Hjalmarson A, Elmfeldt D, Herlitz J, et al. Effect on mortality of metoprolol in acute myocardial infarction. A double-blind randomised trial. *Lancet.* 1981;2:823–827.

15. Mason JW. A comparison of seven antiarrhythmic drugs in patients with ventricular tachyarrhythmias. Electrophysiologic Study versus Electrocardiographic Monitoring Investigators. *N Engl J Med* 1993;329:452–458.

16. Goldbourt U, Behar S, Reicher-Reiss H, et al. Early administration of nifedipine in suspected acute myorcardial infarction. The Secondary Prevention Reinfarction Israel Nifedipine Trial 2 Study. *Arch Intern Med* 1993;153:345–353.

17. Weinberg BA, Miles WM, Klein LS, et al. Five-year follow up of 589 patients treated with amiodarone. *Am Heart J.* 1993;125:109–120.

18. The Antiarrhythmics Versus Implantable Defibrillators (AVID) Investigators. A comparison of antiarrhythmic-drug therapy with implantable defibrillators in patients resuscitated from near-fatal ventricular arrhythmias. *N Engl J Med.* 1997;337:1576–1583.

19. Moss AJ, Zareba W, Hall WJ, et al, for the Multicenter Automatic Defibrillator Implantation Trial II Investigators. Prophylactic implantation of a defibrillator in patients with myocardial infarction and reduced ejection fraction. *N Engl J Med.* 2002;346:877–883.

20. Moss AJ, Hall WJ, Cannom DS, et al, for the Multicenter Automatic Defibrillator Implantation Trial Investigators. Improved survival with an implanted defibrillator in patients with coronary disease at high risk for ventricular arrhythmia. *N Engl J Med.* 1996;335:1933–1940.

21. Buxton AE, Lee KL, Fisher JD, et al. A randomized study of the prevention of sudden death in patients with coronary artery disease: Multicenter Unsustained Tachycardia Trial (MUSTT) Investigators. *N Engl J Med* 1999;341:1882–1890.

22. Bardy GH, Lee KL, Mark DB, et al. Amiodarone or an implantable cardioverter-defibrillator for congestive heart failure. *N Engl J Med* 2005;352:225–237.

23. Gregoratos G, Abrams J, Epstein AE, et al. ACC/AHA/NASPE 2002 guideline update for implantation of cardiac pacemakers and antiarrhythmia devices: summary article. *Circulation.* 2002;106:2145–2161.

24. Strickberger SA, Man KC, Daoud EG, et al. A prospective evaluation of catheter ablation of ventricular tachycardia as adjuvant therapy in patients with coronary artery disease and an implantable cardioverter-defibrillator. *Circulation* 1997;96:1525–1531.

25. Samniah N, Sakaguchi S, Lurie KG, et al. Efficacy and safety of midodrine hydrochloride in patients with refractory vasovagal syncope. *Am J Cardiol* 2001;88:80–83.

26. Pongiglione G, Fish F, Strasburger J, et al. Heart rate and blood pressure response to upright tilt in young patients with unexplained syncope. *J Am Coll Cardiol.* 1990;16:165–170.

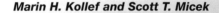

CRITICAL CARE
Marin H. Kollef and Scott T. Micek

8

The goals of critical care medicine are to save the lives of patients with life-threatening but reversible medical or surgical conditions and to offer the dying a peaceful and dignified death. Open discussions between physicians and patients and their family members ensure that critical care is provided in a manner that is most consistent with the patient's wishes.

RESPIRATORY FAILURE

General Considerations

- **Hypercapnic respiratory failure** occurs with acute carbon dioxide retention [arterial carbon dioxide tension ($PaCO_2$) >45–55 mm Hg], producing a respiratory acidosis (pH <7.35).
- **Hypoxic respiratory failure** occurs when normal gas exchange is seriously impaired, resulting in hypoxemia [arterial oxygen tension (PaO_2) <60 mm Hg or arterial oxygen saturation (SaO_2) <90%]. Usually, this type of respiratory failure is associated with tachypnea and hypocapnia; however, its progression can lead to hypercapnia as well. Hypoxic respiratory failure can result from a variety of insults, as shown in Table 8-1.
  - The **acute respiratory distress syndrome** (ARDS) is a form of hypoxic respiratory failure caused by acute lung injury. The common end result is disruption of the alveolar capillary membrane, leading to increased vascular permeability and accumulation of inflammatory cells and protein-rich edema fluid within the alveolar space.
  - The **American-European Consensus Conference** has defined ARDS as follows: (a) acute bilateral pulmonary infiltrates, (b) ratio of PaO_2 to inspired oxygen concentration (FIO_2) <200, and (c) no evidence for heart failure or volume overload as the principal cause of the pulmonary infiltrates.[1]

Pathophysiology

- **Hypoxic respiratory failure** usually is the result of the lung's reduced ability to deliver oxygen into the bloodstream, owing to one of the following six processes.
  - **Shunt.** This term refers to the fraction of mixed venous blood that passes into the systemic arterial circulation after bypassing functioning lung units. Congenital shunts are due to developmental anomalies of the heart and great vessels. Acquired shunts usually result from diseases that affect lung units, although acquired cardiac and peripheral vascular shunts also can occur. Table 8-1 lists some of the more common disease processes that produce clinically significant pulmonary shunts. Shunts are associated with a widened alveolar-arterial oxygen tension [$P(A-a)O_2$] gradient, and the resultant hypoxemia is resistant to correction with supplemental oxygen alone when the shunt fraction of the cardiac output (CO) is >30%.
  - **Ventilation–perfusion mismatch.** Diseases associated with airflow obstruction [e.g., chronic obstructive pulmonary disease (COPD), asthma], interstitial inflammation (e.g., pneumonia, sarcoidosis), or vascular obstruction (e.g., pulmonary embolism) often produce lung regions with abnormal ventilation-to-perfusion relationships. In

TABLE 8-1	Causes of Shunts and Hypoxic Respiratory Failure

Clinical presentation	Causes
Cardiogenic pulmonary edema (low permeability, high hydrostatic pressure)	Acute myocardial infarction Left ventricular failure Mitral regurgitation Mitral stenosis Diastolic dysfunction
Noncardiogenic pulmonary edema/ARDS (high permeability, low hydrostatic pressure)	Aspiration Sepsis Multiple trauma Pancreatitis Near-drowning Pneumonia Reperfusion injury Inhalational injury Drug reaction (aspirin, narcotics, interleukin-2)
Mixed pulmonary edema (high permeability, high hydrostatic pressure)	Myocardial ischemia or volume overload associated with sepsis, aspiration, etc. High-altitude exposure
Pulmonary edema of unclear etiology	Upper airway obstruction Neurogenic cause Lung re-expansion

ARDS, acute respiratory distress syndrome.

ventilation–perfusion mismatch, unlike shunt physiology, increases in FIO_2 result in increases in PaO_2.

■ **Low inspired oxygen.** Usually, FIO_2 is reduced at high altitudes or when toxic gases are inhaled. In patients with other cardiopulmonary disease processes, an inappropriately low FIO_2 can contribute to hypoxic respiratory failure.

■ **Hypoventilation.** This condition is associated with elevated $PaCO_2$ values, and the resultant hypoxemia is due to increased alveolar carbon dioxide, which displaces oxygen. Usually, oxygen therapy improves hypoxemia as a result of hypoventilation but may worsen the overall degree of hypoventilation, especially in patients with chronic airflow obstruction. Primary treatment is directed at correcting the cause of the hypoventilation.

■ **Diffusion impairment.** Hypoxemia due to diffusion impairments usually responds to supplemental oxygen therapy, as is seen in patients with interstitial lung diseases.

■ **Low mixed venous oxygenation.** Normally, the lungs fully oxygenate pulmonary arterial blood, and mixed venous oxygen tension ($P\bar{v}O_2$) does not affect PaO_2 significantly. However, a decreased $P\bar{v}O_2$ can lower the PaO_2 significantly when either intrapulmonary shunting or ventilation–perfusion mismatch is present. Factors that can contribute to low mixed venous oxygenation include anemia, hypoxemia, inadequate CO, and increased oxygen consumption. Improving oxygen delivery to tissues by increasing hemoglobin or CO usually decreases oxygen extraction and improves mixed venous oxygen saturation (SvO_2).

■ **Hypercapnic respiratory failure** usually involves some combination of the following three processes.

■ **Increased carbon dioxide production** (i.e., respiratory acidosis) can be precipitated by fever, sepsis, seizures, and excessive carbohydrate loads in patients with underlying lung disease. The oxidation of carbohydrate fuels is associated with more carbon dioxide production per molecule of oxygen consumed as compared to the oxidation of fat fuels.

- **Increased dead space** occurs when areas of the lung are ventilated but not perfused or when decreases in regional perfusion exceed decreases in ventilation. Examples include intrinsic lung diseases (e.g., COPD, asthma, cystic fibrosis, pulmonary fibrosis) and chest wall disorders associated with parenchymal abnormalities (e.g., scoliosis). Usually, these disorders are associated with widened $P(A-a)O_2$ gradients.

- **Decreased minute ventilation** can result from central nervous system (CNS) disorders (e.g., spinal cord lesions), peripheral nerve diseases (e.g., Guillain-Barré syndrome, botulism, myasthenia gravis, amyotrophic lateral sclerosis), muscle disorders (e.g., polymyositis, muscular dystrophy), chest wall abnormalities (e.g., thoracoplasty, scoliosis), drug overdoses, metabolic abnormalities (e.g., myxedema, hypokalemia), and upper airway obstruction. These disorders usually are associated with a normal $P(A-a)O_2$ gradient unless accompanying lung disease is also present.

- **Mixed respiratory failure** is seen most commonly after surgery, particularly in patients with underlying lung disease who are undergoing upper abdominal procedures. Abnormalities in oxygenation usually occur on the basis of atelectasis, which often is multifactorial in origin (decreased lung volumes and cough due to the effects of anesthesia, abnormal diaphragmatic function resulting from the surgery or associated pain, and interstitial edema causing small airways to close). Hypoventilation can also result from abnormal diaphragmatic function, particularly when complete paralysis occurs, as with phrenic nerve injury.

- **Blood Gas Analysis** (see Acid-Base Disturbances in Chapter 3, Fluid and Electrolyte Management)

OXYGEN THERAPY

The goal of oxygen administration is to facilitate adequate uptake of oxygen into the blood to meet the needs of peripheral tissues. When this goal cannot be accomplished with the methods detailed below, endotracheal intubation may be necessary.

- **Nasal prongs** allow patients to eat, drink, and speak during oxygen administration. Their disadvantage is that the exact FIO_2 delivered is not known, as it is influenced by the patient's peak inspiratory flow demand. As an approximation, the following guide can be used: 1 L/min of nasal prong oxygen flow is approximately equivalent to an FIO_2 of 24%, with each additional liter of flow increasing the FIO_2 by approximately 4%. Flow rates should be limited to <5 L/min.

- **Venturi masks** allow the precise administration of oxygen. Usual FIO_2 values delivered with these masks are 24%, 28%, 31%, 35%, 40%, and 50%. Often, Venturi masks are useful in patients with COPD and hypercapnia because one can titrate the PaO_2 to minimize carbon dioxide retention.

- **Nonrebreathing masks** achieve higher oxygen concentrations (approximately 80%–90%) than do partial rebreathing systems. A one-way valve prevents exhaled gases from entering the reservoir bag in a nonrebreathing system, thereby maximizing the FIO_2.

- A **continuous positive airway pressure (CPAP) mask** can be used if the PaO_2 is <60–65 mm Hg during use of a nonrebreathing mask and the patient is conscious and cooperative, able to protect the lower airway, and hemodynamically stable.[2] CPAP is delivered by a tight-fitting mask equipped with pressure-limiting valves. Many patients cannot tolerate a CPAP mask because of persistent hypoxemia, hemodynamic instability, or feelings of claustrophobia or aerophagia. In these patients, endotracheal intubation should be performed. Initially, 3–5 cm H_2O of CPAP should be applied while the PaO_2 or SaO_2 is monitored. If the PaO_2 is still <60 mm Hg (SaO_2 <90%), the level of CPAP should be increased in steps of 3–5 cm H_2O up to a level of 10–15 cm H_2O.

- **Bilevel positive airway pressure (BiPAP)** is a method of noninvasive ventilation whereby inspiratory and expiratory pressure can be applied by a mask during the patient's respiratory cycle. The inspiratory support decreases the patient's work of breathing. The expiratory support (CPAP) improves gas exchange by preventing alveolar collapse.

Noninvasive ventilation using face or nasal masks has been successfully performed in patients with neuromuscular disease, COPD, and postoperative respiratory insufficiency as a means of decreasing the need for endotracheal intubation and mechanical ventilation.[3] In using BiPAP, a pressure-support ventilation (PSV) level of 5–10 cm H_2O and a CPAP level of 3–5 cm H_2O are reasonable starting points. The PSV level can be increased in increments of 3–5 cm H_2O, using the patient's respiratory rate as a guide of effectiveness.

AIRWAY MANAGEMENT AND TRACHEAL INTUBATION

Establishment of a patent airway and ventilatory support are required by many intensive care unit (ICU) patients. Specific indications for airway support in the form of endotracheal intubation include (a) initiation of mechanical ventilation, (b) airway protection, (c) inadequate oxygenation using less invasive methods, (d) prevention of aspiration and allowing for the suctioning of pulmonary secretions, and (e) hyperventilation for the treatment of increased intracranial pressure. In an emergency situation, such simple maneuvers as a jaw thrust with mask-to-face ventilation may assist the patient in clearing an obstructed airway and in maintaining adequate ventilation until endotracheal intubation can be performed.

Airway Management

- **Head and jaw positioning.** The oropharynx should be inspected, and all foreign bodies should be removed. For patients with inadequate respirations, the jaw thrust or head tilt–chin lift maneuvers should be performed (see Acute Upper Airway Obstruction in Chapter 25, Medical Emergencies).
- **Oral and nasopharyngeal airways.** When head and jaw positioning fail to establish a patent airway or when more permanent airway maintenance is desired, an oral or nasopharyngeal airway can be used. Initially, oral airways are positioned with the concave curve of the airway facing up into the roof of the mouth. The oral airway then is turned 180 degrees so that the concave curve of the airway follows the natural curve of the tongue. A tongue depressor can also be used to displace the tongue inferiorly and laterally to allow direct positioning of the oral airway. Careful monitoring of airway patency is required, as malpositioning of oral airways can push the tongue posteriorly and can result in obstruction of the oropharynx. Nasopharyngeal airways are made of soft plastic. These airways are passed easily down one of the nasal passages to the posterior pharynx after topical nasal lubrication and anesthesia with viscous lidocaine jelly.
- **Laryngeal mask airway (LMA).** The LMA is an endotracheal tube with a small mask on one end that can be passed orally over the larynx to provide ventilatory assistance and prevent aspiration. Placement of the LMA is more easily performed than endotracheal intubation. However, it should be considered a temporary airway for patients who require prolonged ventilatory support.
- **Mask-to-face ventilation.** After an airway is established, respiratory efforts should be evaluated and monitored closely. Ineffective respiratory efforts can be augmented with simple mask-to-face ventilation. Proper fitting and positioning of the mask ensure a tight seal around the mouth and nose, optimizing ventilation. Additionally, proper head positioning and the use of airway adjuncts (e.g., oral or nasopharyngeal airways) optimize ventilation with a mask-to-face system.

Endotracheal Intubation[4]

- **Technique.** Depending on the skill of the operator and the urgency of the situation, one of several techniques can be selected for intubation of the trachea. Such techniques include (a) direct laryngoscopic orotracheal intubation, (b) blind nasotracheal intubation, and (c) flexible fiberoptically guided orotracheal or nasotracheal intubation. In emergency situations, the direct laryngoscopic technique allows for the most rapid intubation of the trachea with the largest endotracheal tube. Nasotracheal intubation often requires smaller endotracheal tubes that are more susceptible to kinking and obstruction and is associated with a higher incidence of otitis media and sinusitis. Before endotracheal intubation is attempted, a systematic evaluation of the patient's head and neck positioning must be performed. The oral, pharyngeal, and tracheal axes should be aligned before any intubation attempts. This "sniffing" position is achieved by flexing the patient's neck and extending the head. A small pillow or several towels placed under the occiput can assist in maintaining this position. Table 8-2 offers a step-by-step approach to performing successful orotracheal intubation. After successful intubation of the trachea, the tracheal tube cuff pressures should be monitored at regular intervals and should be maintained below capillary filling pressure (i.e., <25 mm Hg) to prevent ischemic mucosal injury.

- **Verification of correct endotracheal tube positioning.** Proper tube positioning must be ensured by (a) direct view of the endotracheal tube entering the trachea through the vocal cords, (b) fiberoptic inspection of the airways through the endotracheal tube, or (c) use of an end-tidal carbon dioxide monitor. Clinical evaluation of the patient (i.e., listening for bilateral breath sounds over the chest and the absence of ventilation over the stomach) and radiographic evaluation (e.g., standard portable chest radiograph) can be unreliable for establishing correct endotracheal tube positioning. If uncertainty exists regarding the positioning of the endotracheal tube, it should be withdrawn and the patient reintubated.

- **Complications.** Improper endotracheal tube positioning is the most important immediate complication to be recognized and corrected. Ideally, the tip of the endotracheal tube should be 3–5 cm above the carina, depending on head and neck positioning. Esophageal or right main-stem intubation should be suspected if hypoxemia,

---

TABLE 8-2 **Procedure for Direct Orotracheal Intubation**

Administer oxygen by face mask.

Ensure that basic equipment is present and easily accessible [oxygen source, bag-valve device, suctioning device, endotracheal (ET) tube, blunt stylet, laryngoscope, 20-mL syringe].

Place patient on nonmobile rigid surface.

If patient is in hospital bed, remove backboard and adjust bed height.

Depress patient's tongue with tongue depressor and administer topical anesthesia to patient's pharynx.

Position patient's head in sniffing position (see Airway Management and Tracheal Intubation).

Administer IV sedation and neuromuscular blocker if necessary.[a]

Have assistant apply Sellick maneuver (compressing cricothyroid cartilage posteriorly against vertebral bodies) to prevent regurgitation and aspiration of stomach contents from esophagus.

Grasp laryngoscope handle in left hand while opening patient's mouth with gloved right hand.

Insert laryngoscope blade on right side of patient's mouth and advance to base of tongue, displacing tongue to the left.

Lift laryngoscope away from patient at a 45-degree angle using arm and shoulder strength. Do not use patient's teeth as a fulcrum.

Suction oropharynx and hypopharynx if necessary.

Grasp ET tube with inserted stylet in right hand and insert it into right corner of patient's mouth, avoiding obscuration of epiglottis and vocal cords.

Advance ET tube through vocal cords until cuff is no longer visible and remove stylet.

Inflate cuff with enough air to prevent significant air leakage.

Verify correct ET tube positioning by auscultation of both lungs and the abdomen.

Obtain a chest radiograph or use end-tidal CO_2 monitor to verify correct position of the ET tube.

---

[a]Neuromuscular blockade can result in complete airway collapse and airway obstruction. Personnel who are skillful in establishment of an emergency surgical airway should be available if paralysis is used.

hypoventilation, barotrauma, or cardiac decompensation occurs. Abdominal distention, lack of breath sounds over the thorax, and regurgitation of stomach contents through the endotracheal tube indicate an esophageal intubation. Any uncertainty regarding the possibility of an esophageal intubation calls for immediate verification of tube positioning or reintubation of the patient, with direct confirmation of endotracheal tube positioning. Other complications associated with endotracheal intubation include dislodgment of teeth, trauma to the upper airway, and increased intracranial pressure.

Surgical Airways

- **Tracheostomy.** The main indications for surgical tracheostomy are (a) the need for prolonged respiratory support, (b) potentially life-threatening upper airway obstruction (due to epiglottitis, facial burns, or worsening laryngeal edema), (c) obstructive sleep apnea that is unresponsive to less invasive therapies, and (d) congenital abnormalities (e.g., Pierre-Robin syndrome). Tracheostomy sites usually require at least 72 hours to mature. Tube dislodgment before site maturation, followed by blind attempts at tube reinsertion, can lead to tube malpositioning within a false channel in the pretracheal space; this misplacement can result in complete loss of the airway followed by progressive hypoxemia and hypotension. If a tracheostomy tube cannot be reinserted easily, standard direct orotracheal intubation should be performed (Table 8-2). Optimal timing of surgical tracheostomy is controversial but should be considered after 7–14 days of mechanical ventilation if prolonged ventilation is anticipated.[5]
- **Cricothyrotomy.** This procedure is indicated for the establishment of an emergency airway when direct tracheal intubation cannot be performed owing to upper airway obstruction. A pillow or towel roll should be placed under the patient's shoulders to extend the neck. The thyroid cartilage superiorly and the cricoid cartilage inferiorly should be located where they border the cricothyroid membrane. The thumb and second finger of the surgeon's nondominant hand should grasp and stabilize the lateral aspects of the cricothyroid membrane. With a scalpel, a transverse skin incision is made over the entire distance of the membrane. The incision then is deepened to the cricothyroid membrane, avoiding injury to surrounding structures. Standard tracheostomy tubes or endotracheal tubes can be inserted into the stoma to ventilate the patient. Alternatively, prepackaged kits using the Seldinger technique with progressive dilation of the stoma can be used.
- **Cricothyroid needle cannulation.** In emergency settings when standard endotracheal intubation cannot be performed and placement of a surgical airway is not immediately possible, needle cannulation of the cricothyroid membrane can be performed as an intermediate procedure until a more definitive airway can be established. The ends of the cricothyroid membrane are grasped with the nondominant hand and a 22-gauge needle is inserted into the airway, aspirating air to confirm positioning. Lidocaine then is injected into the trachea to blunt the patient's cough reflex before the needle is withdrawn. By the same technique, a 14-gauge (or larger) needle-through-cannula device can be passed through the cricothyroid membrane at a 45-degree angle to the skin. When air is aspirated freely, the outer cannula is passed into the airway caudally, and the needle is removed. A 3-mL syringe barrel then can be attached to the catheter and a 7-mm inner-diameter endotracheal tube adapter attached to the syringe to allow bag-valve ventilation. Alternatively, the cannula can be attached directly to high-flow oxygen (i.e., 10–15 L/min).

MECHANICAL VENTILATION

Indications

- The decision to begin mechanical ventilation is a clinical judgment that should take into account the reversibility of the underlying disease process as well as the patient's overall medical condition. Usual indications include severely impaired gas exchange, rapid onset of respiratory failure, an inadequate response to less invasive medical treatments, and increased work of breathing with evidence of respiratory muscle fatigue. Parameters that can help to guide the decision as to whether mechanical ventilation is needed include respiratory rate (>35), inspiratory force (>25 cm H_2O), vital capacity (<10–15 mL/kg), PaO_2 (<60 mm Hg with FIO_2 $>60\%$), $PaCO_2$ (>50 mm Hg with pH <7.35), and an absent gag or cough reflex.

Initiation of Mechanical Ventilation

Certain variables should be considered when initiating mechanical ventilation.

- **Ventilator type.** Often, ventilator selection is dictated by what is available at a particular hospital. A volume-cycled ventilator is used in most clinical circumstances.
- **Mode of ventilation.** Several modes of mechanical ventilation are available. General guidelines for the use of the more commonly administered or referred to modes are provided.
  - **Assist-control ventilation (ACV)** should be the initial mode of ventilation used in most patients with respiratory failure. It produces a ventilator-delivered breath for every patient-initiated inspiratory effort. Controlled ventilator-initiated breaths are delivered automatically when the patient's spontaneous rate falls below the selected backup rate. Respiratory alkalosis is a potential concern when using ACV for patients with tachypnea.
  - **Intermittent mandatory ventilation (IMV)** allows patients to breathe at a spontaneous rate and tidal volume without triggering the ventilator, while the ventilator adds additional mechanical breaths at a preset rate and tidal volume.
  - **Synchronized intermittent mandatory ventilation (SIMV)** allows the ventilator to become sensitized to the patient's respiratory efforts at intervals determined by the frequency setting. This capability allows coordination of the delivery of the ventilator-driven breath with the respiratory cycle of the patient to prevent inadvertent stacking of a mechanical breath on top of a spontaneous inspiration. Potential advantages of SIMV include less respiratory alkalosis, fewer adverse cardiovascular effects due to lower intrathoracic pressures, less requirement for sedation and paralysis, maintenance of respiratory muscle function, and facilitation of long-term weaning. However, considerable patient-initiated respiratory muscle work may contribute to respiratory muscle fatigue and failure to wean from mechanical ventilation in some patients. This nonphysiologic work of spontaneous breathing can be alleviated by the addition of low levels of PSV (4–8 cm H_2O) or the addition of flow-by, or both.
  - **PSV** augments each patient-triggered respiratory effort by an operator-specified amount of pressure that is usually between 5 and 50 cm H_2O. PSV is used primarily to augment spontaneous respiratory efforts during IMV modes of ventilation or during weaning trials. PSV can also be used as a primary form of ventilation in patients who can trigger the ventilator spontaneously. Increased airway resistance, decreased lung compliance, and decreased patient effort result in diminished tidal volumes and, frequently, in decreased minute ventilation. PSV is not recommended as a primary ventilatory mode in patients in whom any of the aforementioned parameters are expected to fluctuate widely.
  - **Inverse ratio ventilation (IRV)** uses an inspiratory-to-expiratory ratio that is greater than the standard 1:2–1:3 ratio (i.e., $\geq$1:1) to stabilize terminal respiratory units (i.e., alveolar recruitment) and to improve gas exchange primarily for patients with ARDS.[6] The goals of IRV are to decrease peak airway pressures, to maintain adequate alveolar ventilation, and to improve oxygenation. The use of IRV can be considered in patients with a PaO_2 of <60 mm Hg despite an FIO_2 of $>60\%$, peak airway pressures >40–45 cm H_2O, or the need for positive end-expiratory pressure (PEEP) of >15 cm H_2O. However, lung strain may be greater in acute lung injury when IRV is employed.[7]
  - **Lung-protective, pressure-targeted ventilation** (i.e., permissive hypercapnia) is a method whereby controlled hypoventilation is allowed to occur with elevation of the $PaCO_2$ to minimize the detrimental effects of excessive airway pressures. This form

of ventilation has been used in patients with respiratory failure due to asthma and ARDS. In patients with ARDS the application of tidal volumes ≤ 6 mL/kg has been used as a lung-protective strategy and has been associated with improved outcomes.[8] The use of smaller tidal volumes is thought to prevent ventilator-induced lung injury. Additional methods for improving oxygenation while minimizing lung injury during mechanical ventilation in ARDS include prone positioning[9] and the administration of nitric oxide (NO), although these interventions have not been associated with a survival advantage. The administration of corticosteroids for established ARDS is still controversial despite one small randomized trial demonstrating improved survival.[10] For patients with asthma, the use of a helium–oxygen mixture may result in improved lung mechanics compared to the use of oxygen alone.[11]

- **Independent lung ventilation** uses two independent ventilators and a double-lumen endotracheal tube. Usually, this modality is reserved for severe unilateral lung disease, such as unilateral pneumonia, respiratory failure associated with hemoptysis, or a bronchopleural fistula.
- **High-frequency ventilation** uses rates that are substantially faster (60–300 breaths/min) than conventional ventilation with small tidal volumes (2–4 mL/kg). The use of high-frequency ventilation is controversial except during upper airway surgery.
- **Airway pressure release ventilation (APRV)** uses CPAP with an intermittent pressure release phase. APRV applies CPAP to maintain adequate lung volume and promote alveolar recruitment. A time-cycled release phase to a lower set pressure allows ventilation to occur. APRV allows spontaneous breathing to be integrated independent of the ventilator cycle, making mechanical ventilation more comfortable for some patients.[12]
- **Mechanical ventilation with inhaled NO** has been demonstrated to improve gas exchange in adults and children with respiratory failure, including patients with ARDS, primary pulmonary hypertension, or cor pulmonale secondary to congenital heart disease, and after cardiac surgery or heart or lung transplantation. Inhaled NO acts as a selective pulmonary artery (PA) vasodilator, decreasing PA pressures [without decreasing systemic blood pressure (BP) or CO] and improving oxygenation by reducing intrapulmonary shunt.[13] Generally, 5–20 ppm NO is administered, and the level of methemoglobin is monitored periodically.

- **Ventilator management**
  - **FIO_2.** Hypoxemia is more dangerous than brief exposure to high inspired levels of oxygen. The initial FIO_2 should be 100%. Adjustments in the FIO_2 can be made to achieve a PaO_2 of >60 mm Hg or an SaO_2 of >90%.
  - **Minute ventilation.** Minute ventilation is determined by the respiratory rate and the tidal volume. In general, a respiratory rate of 10–15 breaths/min is an appropriate rate with which to begin. Close monitoring of minute ventilation is especially important in ventilating patients with COPD and carbon dioxide retention. In these individuals, the minute ventilation should be adjusted to achieve the patient's baseline $PaCO_2$ and not necessarily a normal $PaCO_2$. Inadvertent hyperventilation with resultant metabolic alkalosis in these patients may be associated with serious serum electrolyte shifts and arrhythmias. Initial tidal volumes usually can be set at 10–12 mL/kg. Patients with decreased lung compliance (e.g., ARDS) often need smaller lung volumes (6–8 mL/kg) to minimize peak airway pressures and iatrogenic morbidity.
  - **PEEP** is defined as the maintenance of positive airway pressure at the end of expiration. It can be applied to the spontaneously breathing patient in the form of CPAP or to the patient who is receiving mechanical ventilation. The appropriate application of PEEP usually increases lung compliance and oxygenation while decreasing the shunt fraction and the work of breathing. PEEP increases peak and mean airway pressures, which can increase the likelihood of barotrauma and cardiovascular compromise. PEEP is used primarily in patients with hypoxic respiratory failure (e.g., ARDS, cardiogenic pulmonary edema). Low levels of PEEP (3–5 cm H_2O) may also be useful in patients with COPD, to prevent dynamic airway collapse from occurring during expiration. The main goal of PEEP is to achieve a PaO_2 of >55–60 mm Hg with an FIO_2 of $\leq 60\%$ while avoiding significant cardiovascular sequelae. Usually, PEEP is

applied in 3- to 5-cm H_2O increments during monitoring of oxygenation, organ perfusion, and hemodynamic parameters. Patients who receive significant levels of PEEP (i.e., >10 cm H_2O) should not have their PEEP removed abruptly, because removal can result in collapse of distal lung units, the worsening of shunt, and potentially life-threatening hypoxemia. PEEP should be weaned in 3- to 5-cm H_2O increments while oxygenation is monitored closely.

■ **Inspiratory flow rate.** Flow rates set inappropriately low can be associated with prolonged inspiratory times that can lead to the development of auto-PEEP. The resultant lung hyperinflation can affect patient hemodynamics adversely by impairing venous return to the heart. Patients with severe airflow obstruction are at the greatest risk for development of lung hyperinflation when improper flow rates are used. Increasing the inspiratory flow rate usually allows for longer expiratory times that help to reverse this process.

■ **Trigger sensitivity.** Most mechanical ventilators use pressure triggering either to initiate a machine-assisted breath or to permit spontaneous breathing between IMV breaths, or during trials of CPAP. The patient must generate a decrease in the airway circuit pressure equal to the selected pressure sensitivity. Most patients do not tolerate a trigger sensitivity of ≤1 or –2 cm H_2O because of autocycling of the ventilator. Alternatively, excessive trigger sensitivity can increase the patient's work of breathing, contributing to failure to wean from mechanical ventilation. In general, the smallest trigger sensitivity should be selected, allowing the patient to initiate mechanical or spontaneous breaths without causing the ventilator to autocycle.

■ **Flow-by.** To decrease the patient work of breathing, flow-by can be used as an adjunct to conventional modes of mechanical ventilation. Flow-by refers to triggering of the ventilator by changes in airflow as opposed to changes in airway pressures. A continuous base flow of gas is provided through the ventilator circuit at a preselected flow rate (5–20 L/min). A flow sensitivity (i.e., patient rate of inhaled flow that triggers the ventilator to switch from base flow to either a machine-delivered or a spontaneous breath) is selected (usually 2 L/min). Flow-triggered systems are more responsive than are pressure-triggered systems and result in a decreased work of breathing.

Management of Problems and Complications

■ **Airway malpositioning and occlusion** (see Airway Management and Tracheal Intubation)
■ **Worsening respiratory distress or arterial oxygen desaturation** may develop suddenly as a result of changes in the patient's cardiopulmonary status or secondary to a mechanical malfunction. The first priority is to ensure patency and correct positioning of the patient's airway so that adequate oxygenation and ventilation can be administered during the ensuing evaluation.

■ **Briefly note ventilator alarms, airway pressures, and tidal volume.** Low-pressure alarms with decreased exhaled tidal volumes may suggest a leak in the ventilator circuit.

■ **Disconnect the patient from the ventilator and manually ventilate with an anesthesia bag using 100% oxygen.** For patients receiving PEEP, manual ventilation with a PEEP valve should be used to prevent atelectasis and hypoxemia.

■ **If manual ventilation is difficult, check airway patency by passing a suction catheter through the endotracheal tube or tracheostomy.** Additionally, listen for prolonged expiration continuing up to the point of the next manual breath. This suggests the presence of gas trapping and auto-PEEP.

■ **Check vital signs and perform a rapid physical examination with attention to the patient's cardiopulmonary status.** Be attentive to asymmetry in breath sounds or tracheal deviation suggesting tension pneumothorax. Note other parameters, including cardiac rhythm and hemodynamics.

■ **Treat appropriately on the basis of the foregoing evaluation.** Treatment should be specific to the identified problems. If the presence of gas trapping and auto-PEEP is suspected, a reduction in the minute ventilation is appropriate. In some circumstances, periods of hypoventilation (4–6 breaths/min) or even apnea for 30–60 seconds may be necessary to reverse the hemodynamic sequelae of auto-PEEP (e.g., shock, electromechanical dissociation).

- **Return the patient to the ventilator only after checking its function.** Increase the level of support provided by the ventilator to the patient after an episode of respiratory distress or arterial oxygen desaturation. Usually, this adjustment means increasing the FIO_2 and the delivered minute ventilation unless significant auto-PEEP is present.

- An **acute increase in the peak airway pressure** usually implies either a decrease in lung compliance or an increase in airway resistance. At a minimum, considerations that should be entertained as causes of increased airway pressure include (a) pneumothorax, hemothorax, or hydropneumothorax; (b) occlusion of the patient's airway; (c) bronchospasm; (d) increased accumulation of condensate in the ventilator circuit tubing; (e) main-stem intubation; (f) worsening pulmonary edema; or (g) the development of gas trapping with auto-PEEP.

- **Loss of tidal volume,** as evidenced by a difference between the tidal volume setting and the delivered tidal volume, implies a leak in either the ventilator or the inspiratory limb of the circuit tubing. A difference between the delivered tidal volume and the expired tidal volume implies the presence of a leak at the patient's airway due either to cuff malfunction or to malpositioning of the airway (e.g., positioning of the cuff at or above the level of the glottis) or a leak within the patient (e.g., presence of a bronchopleural fistula in a patient with a chest tube).

- **Asynchronous breathing ("fighting" or "bucking" the ventilator)** occurs when a patient's breathing coordinates poorly with the ventilator. This difficulty may indicate unmet respiratory demands. A careful evaluation is mandated, with attention focused at the identification of leaks in the ventilator system or airway, inadequate FIO_2, or inadequate ventilatory support. The problem can be alleviated by adjustments in the mode of mechanical ventilation, rate, tidal volume, inspiratory flow rate, and level of PEEP. The identification of gas trapping with auto-PEEP may require changing multiple settings to allow adequate time for exhalation (e.g., decreasing rate and tidal volume, increasing inspiratory flow rate, switching from assist-control to SIMV in selected cases). Additionally, measures aimed at reducing the work of breathing with mechanical ventilation also may resolve the problem (addition of flow-by triggering or low levels of PSV to patients taking spontaneous breaths). If these adjustments are unsuccessful, sedation should be attempted. Muscle paralysis should be reserved for patients in whom effective gas exchange and ventilation cannot be achieved with other measures.

- **Organ hypoperfusion or hypotension** can occur. Positive-pressure ventilation can result in decreased CO and BP by decreasing venous return to the right ventricle, increasing pulmonary vascular resistance, and impairing diastolic filling of the left ventricle because of increased right-sided heart pressures. Increasing the preload to the left ventricle with fluid administration should increase stroke volume and CO in most cases. Occasionally, the administration of dobutamine (after appropriate preload replacement) or vasopressors becomes necessary. Under these circumstances, consideration should be given to reducing airway pressures (peak airway pressures <40 cm H_2O) at the expense of relative hypoventilation (i.e., pressure-targeted ventilation).

- **Auto-PEEP** is the development of end-expiratory pressure caused by airflow limitation in patients with airway disease (emphysema, asthma), excessive minute ventilation, or an inadequate expiratory time. Graphic tracings on modern ventilators can suggest the presence of gas trapping by demonstrating persistent airflow at end expiration. The level of auto-PEEP can be estimated in the spontaneously breathing patient by occluding the expiratory port of the ventilator briefly just before inspiration and measuring the end-expiratory pressure reading on the ventilator's manometer. The presence of auto-PEEP can increase the work of breathing, contribute to barotrauma, and result in organ hypoperfusion by impairing CO. Appropriate adjustments to the ventilator can reduce or eliminate the presence of auto-PEEP.

- **Barotrauma or volutrauma** in the form of subcutaneous emphysema, pneumoperitoneum, pneumomediastinum, pneumopericardium, air embolism, and pneumothorax is associated with high peak airway pressures, PEEP, and auto-PEEP. Subcutaneous emphysema, pneumomediastinum, and pneumoperitoneum seldom threaten the patient's well-being. However, the occurrence of these disorders usually indicates a need to reduce peak airway pressures and the total level of PEEP. The occurrence of a pneumothorax is a potentially life-threatening complication and should be considered whenever airway pressure rises acutely, breath sounds are diminished unilaterally, or BP falls abruptly (see Pneumothorax in Chapter 25, Medical Emergencies). In most cases, acute tension pneumothorax should be treated as an emergency by inserting a 14-gauge catheter-over-needle device into the pleural space at the xiphoid level in the midaxillary line or anteriorly into the second or third intercostal space in the midclavicular line. Chest tube insertion should follow.

- **Positive fluid balance and hyponatremia** in mechanically ventilated patients often develop from several factors, including applied PEEP, humidification of inspired gases, administration of hypotonic fluids and diuretics, and increased levels of circulating antidiuretic hormone.

- **Cardiac arrhythmias,** particularly multifocal atrial tachycardia and atrial fibrillation, are common in respiratory failure and should be treated as outlined in Chapter 7, Cardiac Arrhythmias.

- **Aspiration** commonly occurs despite the use of a cuffed endotracheal tube, especially in patients who are receiving enteral nutrition. Elevating the head of the bed and avoiding excessive gastric distention help to minimize the occurrence of aspiration. Additionally, pooling of secretions around the cuff of the endotracheal tube requires suctioning of these secretions before deflation or manipulation of the cuff.

- **Ventilator-associated pneumonia** is a frequent complication connected with increased patient morbidity and mortality. Prevention of ventilator-associated pneumonia is aimed at avoiding colonization in the patient of pathogenic bacteria and their subsequent aspiration into the lower airway.[14]

- **Upper gastrointestinal (GI) hemorrhage** may develop secondary to gastritis or ulceration. The prevention of stress bleeding requires ensuring hemodynamic stability and, in high-risk patients [e.g., those receiving prolonged mechanical ventilation (>48–72 hours) or with a coagulopathy], the administration of proton pump inhibitors, H_2-receptor antagonists, antacids, or sucralfate.

- **Thromboembolism** (deep venous thrombosis and pulmonary embolism) may complicate the clinical course of patients who require mechanical ventilation. This disorder can be prevented in most patients by the prophylactic administration of low-dose unfractionated heparin [e.g. heparin 5,000 units SC q8h] or low molecular weight heparin [e.g. enoxaparin 40 mg SC q24h], or the use of intermittent pneumatic compression devices (see Chapter 1, Patient Care in Internal Medicine).

- **Acid-base complications** are common in the critically ill patient (see also Chapter 3, Fluid and Electrolyte Management).
  - **Nonanion gap metabolic acidosis** may render weaning difficult, as minute ventilation must increase to normalize pH.
  - **Metabolic alkalosis** may compromise weaning by blunting ventilatory drive to maintain a normal pH. In patients with chronic ventilatory insufficiency (e.g., emphysema, cystic fibrosis), correction of metabolic alkalosis usually is inappropriate and can cause an unsustainable minute ventilation requirement. Under these circumstances, a patient should be allowed to slow minute ventilation gradually to a more appropriate level. This change may be facilitated by switching from ACV to SIMV or PSV.
  - **Respiratory alkalosis** may develop rapidly during mechanical ventilation. When severe, it can lead to arrhythmias, CNS disturbances (including seizures), and a decrease in CO. Changing the ventilator settings to reduce the minute ventilation or changing the mode of ventilation (ACV to SIMV) usually corrects the alkalosis. However, some patients (such as those with ARDS, interstitial lung disease, pulmonary embolism, asthma) are driven to high respiratory rates by local pulmonary stimuli. In such patients, sedation with or without paralysis may be indicated briefly during the acute phase of the respiratory compromise.

- **Oxygen toxicity** commonly is accepted to occur when an FIO_2 of >0.6 is administered, particularly for more than 48 hours. However, the highest FIO_2 necessary should be used initially to maintain the SaO_2 at more than 0.9. The application of PEEP or other maneuvers that increase mean airway pressure (e.g., IRV) can be used to reduce FIO_2

requirements. However, an FIO_2 of 0.6–0.8 should be accepted before a plateau pressure above 30 cm H_2O is accepted. This cautionary note is due to the greater risk of morbidity associated with plateau pressures above this level.[15]

Weaning From Mechanical Ventilation

Weaning is the gradual withdrawal of mechanical ventilatory support.[16] Successful weaning depends on the condition of the patient and on the status of the cardiovascular and respiratory systems. In patients who have had brief periods of mechanical ventilation, the manner in which ventilatory support is discontinued often is not crucial. In patients with marginal respiratory function, chronic underlying lung disease, or incompletely resolved respiratory impairment, the approach to weaning may be critical to obtaining a favorable outcome.

- **Weaning strategies.** In general, the level of supported ventilation (minute ventilation) is decreased gradually, and the patient assumes more of the work of ventilation with each of the techniques described. However, it is important during the weaning process not to fatigue the patient excessively, which can prolong the duration of mechanical ventilation.
- **IMV** allows a progressive change from mechanical ventilation to spontaneous breathing by decreasing the ventilator rate gradually. However, the weaning process may be prolonged if ventilator changes are not made often enough. Prolonged periods at low rates (<6 breaths/min) may promote a state of respiratory muscle fatigue because of the imposed work of breathing through a high-resistance ventilator circuit. The addition of PSV may alleviate this fatigue but can prolong the weaning process if not titrated appropriately. Very often, tachypnea that occurs during weaning of the IMV rate represents a problem related to the imposed work from the ventilator circuit and the endotracheal tube rather than a diagnosis of persistent respiratory failure. In circumstances in which this problem is suspected, a trial of extubation may be appropriate.
- **T-tube technique** intersperses periods of unassisted spontaneous breathing through a T tube (or other continuous-flow circuit) with periods of ventilator support.[17] Short daytime periods (5–15 minutes two to four times per day) are used initially and then are increased progressively in duration. Small amounts of CPAP (3–5 cm H_2O) during these periods may prevent distal airway closure and atelectasis, although the effects on weaning success appear to be negligible.[18] Similar to IMV weaning, small amounts of pressure support (4–8 cm H_2O) can be used to decrease inspiratory resistance imposed by the ventilator circuit and the endotracheal tube. Extubation may be appropriate when the patient can comfortably tolerate more than 30–90 minutes of T-tube ventilation. More prolonged periods of T-tube breathing may produce fatigue, especially when small endotracheal tubes (i.e., <8 mm internal diameter) are used.
- **PSV** is preferred by some practitioners when respiratory muscle weakness appears to be compromising weaning success.[19] PSV can reduce the patient's work of breathing through the endotracheal tube and the ventilator circuit. The optimal level of PSV is selected by increasing the PSV level from a baseline of 15–20 cm H_2O in increments of 3–5 cm H_2O. A decrease in respiratory rate with achieved tidal volumes of 10–12 mL/kg signals that the optimal PSV level has been reached. When the patient is ready to begin weaning, the level of PSV is reduced gradually by 3- to 5-cm H_2O increments. Once a PSV level of 5–8 cm H_2O is reached, the patient can be extubated without further decreases in PSV.
- **Protocol-guided weaning of mechanical ventilation** has been safely and successfully used by nonphysicians.[20] The use of protocols or guidelines can reduce the duration of mechanical ventilation by expediting the weaning process.

Failure to Wean

- Patients who do not wean from mechanical ventilation after 48–72 hours of the resolution of their underlying disease process need further investigation. Table 8-3 lists the factors that should be considered when weaning failure occurs. The acronym "WEANS NOW" has been developed to aid in addressing each of these factors. Commonly used parameters that can be assessed in predicting weaning success are listed in Table 8-4.

TABLE 8-3	Factors To Be Considered in the Weaning Process

Weaning parameters
  See Table 8-4.

Endotracheal tube
  Use largest tube possible.
  Consider use of supplemental pressure-support ventilation.
  Suction secretions.

Arterial blood gases
  Avoid or treat metabolic alkalosis.
  Maintain PaO_2 at 60–65 mm Hg to avoid blunting of respiratory drive.
  For patients with carbon dioxide retention, keep $PaCO_2$ at or above the baseline level.

Nutrition
  Ensure adequate nutritional support.
  Avoid electrolyte deficiencies.
  Avoid excessive calories.

Secretions
  Clear regularly.
  Avoid excessive dehydration.

Neuromuscular factors
  Avoid neuromuscular-depressing drugs.
  Avoid unnecessary corticosteroids.

Obstruction of airways
  Use bronchodilators when appropriate.
  Exclude foreign bodies within the airway.

Wakefulness
  Avoid oversedation.
  Wean in morning or when patient is most awake.

Extubation

- Usually, extubation should be performed early in the day, when full ancillary staff are available. The patient should be clearly educated about the procedure, the need to cough, and the possible need for reintubation. Elevation of the head and trunk to more than 30–45 degrees improves diaphragmatic function. Equipment for reintubation should be available, and a high-humidity, oxygen-enriched gas source with a higher-than-current FIO_2 setting should be available at the bedside. The patient's airway and the oropharynx above the cuff should be suctioned. The cuff of the endotracheal tube should be deflated partially, and airflow around the outside of the tube—indicating the absence of airway obstruction—should be detected. After the cuff is deflated completely, the patient should be extubated, and high-humidity oxygen should be administered by a face mask. Coughing and deep breathing should be encouraged while the examiner monitors the patient's vital signs and upper airway for stridor. Inspiratory stridor may result from glottic and subglottic edema. If clinical status permits, treatment with nebulized 2.5% racemic epinephrine (0.5 mL in 3 mL normal saline) should be administered. If upper airway obstruction persists or worsens, reintubation should be performed.
- Extubation should not be reattempted for 24–72 hours after reintubation for upper airway obstruction. Otolaryngology consultation may be beneficial to exclude other causes of upper airway obstruction and to perform tracheostomy if upper airway obstruction persists.

TABLE 8-4	Guidelines for Assessing Withdrawal of Mechanical Ventilation

Patient's mental status: awake, alert, cooperative
PaO_2 >60 mm Hg with an FIO_2 <50%
PEEP ≤5 cm H_2O
$PaCO_2$ and pH acceptable
Spontaneous tidal volume >5 mL/kg
Vital capacity >10 mL/kg
MV <10 L/min
Maximum voluntary ventilation double of MV
Maximum negative inspiratory pressure >25 cm H_2O
Respiratory rate <30 breaths/min
Static compliance >30 mL/cm H_2O
Rapid shallow breathing index (ratio of respiratory rate to tidal volume) <100 breaths/min/L
Stable vital signs after a 1- to 2-hr spontaneous breathing trial

FIO_2, inspired oxygen concentration; MV, minute ventilation; $PaCO_2$, arterial carbon dioxide tension; PaO_2, arterial oxygen tension; PEEP, positive end-expiratory pressure.
Source: From Yang KL, Tobin MJ. A prospective study of indexes predicting the outcome of trials of weaning from mechanical ventilation. *N Engl J Med* 1991;324:1445; and Ely EW, Baker AM, Dunagan DP, et al. Effect on the duration of mechanical ventilation of identifying patients capable of breathing spontaneously. *N Engl J Med* 1996;335:1864, with permission.

Medications

■ **Drugs** are commonly used in the ICU to facilitate tracheal intubation and mechanical ventilation (Table 8-5). Nondepolarizing muscle relaxants have been implicated in muscle dysfunction and prolonged weakness after their use in ICU patients.[21] Some reports suggest a drug interaction between muscle relaxants and glucocorticoids, potentiating this effect. To minimize the chances of this complication, the continuous use of muscle relaxants should be limited to as brief a period as possible. Peripheral nerve stimulators should be used to titrate the dose of the muscle relaxant to the lowest effective dose. Finally, glucocorticoids should be avoided in patients who are receiving muscle relaxants unless their use is clearly indicated (e.g., for status asthmaticus, anaphylactic shock).

Shock

Circulatory shock is a process in which blood flow and oxygen delivery to tissues are disturbed; this event leads to tissue hypoxia, with resultant compromise of cellular metabolic activity and organ function. Oliguria, decreased mental status, decreased peripheral pulses, and diaphoresis represent the major clinical manifestations of circulatory shock. Survival from shock is related to the adequacy of the initial resuscitation and the degree of subsequent organ system dysfunction. The main goal of therapy is rapid cardiovascular resuscitation with the re-establishment of tissue perfusion using fluid therapy and vasoactive drugs. The definitive treatment of shock requires reversal of the underlying etiologic process.

Resuscitative Principles

■ **Fluid resuscitation** is usually the first treatment used. All patients in shock should receive an initial IV fluid challenge. The amount of fluid necessary is unpredictable but should be based on changes in clinical parameters, including arterial BP, urine output, cardiac filling pressures, and CO. Crystalloid fluid solutions (0.9% sodium chloride or Ringer

TABLE 8-5 Intensive Care Unit Drugs to Facilitate Endotracheal Intubation and Mechanical Ventilation

Drug	Bolus dosages (IV)	Continuous-infusion dosages[a]	Onset	Duration after single dose
Succinylcholine[b]	0.3–1 mg/kg	—	45–60 sec	2–10 min
Pancuronium	0.05–0.1 mg/kg	1–2 mcg/kg/min	2–4 min	60–90 min
Vecuronium	0.08–0.1 mg/kg	0.3–1 mcg/kg/min	2–4 min	30–45 min
Atracurium	0.2–0.6 mg/kg	5–15 mcg/kg/min	2–4 min	20–35 min
Lorazepam	0.03–0.1 mg/kg	0.01–0.1 mg/kg/hr, titrate to effect	5–20 min	2–6 hr[c]
Midazolam	0.02–0.08 mg/kg	0.04–0.2 mg/kg/hr, titrate to effect	1–5 min	30–60 min[c]
Morphine	0.01–0.15 mg/kg	0.1–0.5 mg/kg/hr, titrate to effect	2–10 min	2–4 hr[c]
Fentanyl	0.35–1.5 mcg/kg	1–10 mcg/kg/hr, titrate to effect	30–60 sec	30–60 min[c]
Thiopental	50–100 mg; repeat up to 20 mg/kg	—	20 sec	10–20 min
Methohexital	1–1.5 mg/kg	—	15–45 sec	5–20 min
Etomidate[b]	0.3–0.4 mg/kg	—	10–20 sec	4–10 min
Propofol	0.25–0.5 mg/kg	25–80 mcg/kg/min	15–60 sec	3–10 min[c]
Dexmedetomidine	1 mcg/kg	0.2–0.7 mcg/kg/hr	10 min	30 min

[a] A continuous infusion should be started or titrated upward only after the desired level of sedation is achieved with bolus administration.
[b] Use only in the process of rapid sequence intubation.
[c] Duration is prolonged with continuous IV administration. Frequent titration to the minimum effective dose is required to prevent accumulation of drug.

lactate) usually are administered, owing to their lower cost and comparable efficacy compared to colloid solutions (5% and 25% albumin, 6% hetastarch, dextran 40, and dextran 70). Blood products should be administered to patients with significant anemia or active hemorrhage. Young, adequately resuscitated patients usually tolerate hematocrits of 20%–25%. In older patients, individuals with atherosclerosis, and patients who exhibit ongoing anaerobic metabolism, hematocrits of 30% or greater may be required to optimize oxygen transport to tissues.

- **Vasopressors and inotropes** play a crucial role in the management of shock states. Their use usually requires monitoring with intra-arterial and PA catheters.
  - **Dopamine** is capable of stimulating cardiac β_1-receptors, peripheral α-receptors, and dopaminergic receptors in renal, splanchnic, and other vascular beds. The effects of dopamine are dose dependent. At dosages of <5 mcg/kg/min, dopamine primarily acts as a vasodilator, increasing renal and splanchnic blood flow. At dosages of 5–10 mcg/kg/min, dopamine increases cardiac contractility and CO via the activation of cardiac β_1-receptors. At higher dosages (>10 mcg/kg/min), dopamine increases BP by activation of peripheral α-receptors.
  - **Dobutamine** is an inotropic agent that is generally considered a selective β_1-agonist. It exerts powerful inotropic effects, reduces afterload by indirect (reflex) peripheral vasodilation, and is a relatively weak chronotropic agent, accounting for its favorable hemodynamic response (increased stroke volume with modest increases in heart rate unless used in high dose or in the setting of hypovolemia).
  - **Epinephrine** has α_1- and nonselective β-adrenergic activity. It is the agent of choice for anaphylactic shock. Like dopamine, its relative effects are dose dependent.
  - **Norepinephrine** also has α_1- and β_1-adrenergic activity but primarily is a potent vasoconstricting agent.
  - **Vasopressin** is a vasoconstrictor mediated by three different G-peptide receptors called V_{1a}, V_{1b}, and V_2. The usual dose of vasopressin for hypotension is 0.01–0.04 U/min.[22]
  - **Milrinone** is a noncatecholamine inhibitor of phosphodiesterase III that acts as an inotrope and a direct peripheral vasodilator to increase CO.

Classification

- **Individual shock states** usually can be classified into four broad categories. These categories include hypovolemic shock (e.g., hemorrhage, dehydration), cardiogenic shock (e.g., acute myocardial infarction, cardiac tamponade), obstructive shock (e.g., acute pulmonary embolism), and distributive shock (septic shock and anaphylactic shock). Table 8-6 gives the main hemodynamic patterns seen with each of these shock states.
- **Hypovolemic shock** results from a decrease in effective intravascular volume that decreases venous return to the right ventricle. Significant hypovolemic shock (i.e., >40% loss of intravascular volume) that lasts for more than several hours is often associated with a fatal outcome despite resuscitative efforts. Therapy of hypovolemic shock usually is aimed at re-establishing the adequacy of the intravascular volume. At the same time, ongoing sources of volume loss, such as a bleeding vessel, may require surgical intervention. Crystalloid solutions are used initially for the resuscitation of patients in hypovolemic shock. Fluid resuscitation must be prompt and should be given through large-bore catheters placed in large peripheral veins. **Rapid infusers or pumps** are available to increase the rate of fluid resuscitation. In the absence of overt signs of congestive heart failure (CHF), the patient should receive a 500- to 1000-mL initial bolus of normal saline or Ringer lactate, with further infusions adjusted to achieve adequate BP and tissue perfusion. When shock is due to hemorrhage, packed red blood cells (RBCs) should be given as soon as feasible. When hemorrhage is massive, type-specific unmatched blood can be given safely. Rarely, type O-negative blood is needed.
- **Cardiogenic shock** is seen most commonly after acute myocardial infarction (see Chapter 5, Ischemic Heart Disease) and usually is the result of pump failure. Other causes of cardiogenic shock include septal wall rupture, acute mitral regurgitation, myocarditis, dilated cardiomyopathy, arrhythmias, pericardial tamponade, and right ventricular failure due to pulmonary embolism. Cardiogenic shock secondary to acute myocardial

TABLE 8-6	Hemodynamic Patterns Associated with Specific Shock States							
Type of shock	**CI**	**SVR**	**PVR**	**SvO$_2$**	**RAP**	**RVP**	**PAP**	**PAOP**
Cardiogenic (e.g., MI, cardiac tamponade[a])	↓	↑	N	↓	↑	↑	↑	↑
Hypovolemic (e.g., hemorrhage)	↓	↑	N	↓	↓	↓	↓	↓
Distributive (e.g., septic)	N–↑	↓	N	N–↑	N–↓	N–↓	N–↓	N–↓
Obstructive (e.g., massive pulmonary embolism)	↓	↑–N	↑	N–↓	↑	↑	↑	N–↓

CI, cardiac index; MI, myocardial infarction; N, normal; PAOP, pulmonary artery occlusion pressure; PAP, pulmonary artery pressure; PVR, pulmonary vascular resistance; RAP, right atrial pressure; RVP, right ventricular pressure; SvO$_2$, mixed venous oxygen saturation; SVR, systemic vascular resistance; ↑, increased; ↓, decreased.
[a]Equalization of RAP, PAOP, diastolic PAP, and diastolic RVP establishes a diagnosis of cardiac tamponade.

infarction usually is associated with hypotension (mean arterial BP <60 mm Hg), decreased cardiac index (<2.0 L/min/m^2), elevated intracardiac pressures [pulmonary artery occlusive pressure (PAOP) >18 mm Hg], increased peripheral vascular resistance, and organ hypoperfusion (e.g., decreased urine output, altered mentation) (Table 8-6).

■ Certain **general measures** should be undertaken. A PaO$_2$ of >60 mm Hg should be achieved, and the hematocrit should be maintained at equal to or >30%. Endotracheal intubation and mechanical ventilation should be considered to reduce the work of breathing (and therefore oxygen requirements) and to increase juxtacardiac pressures (P$_{JC}$), which may improve cardiac function. Noninvasive mechanical ventilation with BiPAP can be used to accomplish similar end points in patients who are able to sustain spontaneous breathing. Careful attention to fluid management is necessary to ensure that an adequate preload is present to optimize ventricular function (especially in the presence of right ventricular infarction) and to avoid excessive volume administration with resultant pulmonary edema.

■ **Pharmacologic treatment** usually involves two classes of drugs: inotropes and vasopressors. Vasodilators generally are not used in patients with cardiogenic shock due to severe hypotension. The use of vasodilators can be considered after the patient's hemodynamics have stabilized as a means of improving left ventricular function. **Dopamine** usually is administered first in patients with cardiogenic shock because it has inotropic and vasopressor properties. Typically, the dose is titrated to maintain a mean arterial BP of 60 mm Hg or greater. Subsequent guidance using a PA catheter helps to define what further measures are required, including inotropic support (dobutamine, milrinone), afterload reduction (nitroprusside), and changes in intravascular volume (fluid administration vs. diuresis).

■ **Mechanical circulatory assist devices** are required in patients who do not respond to medical therapy or who have specific conditions identified as the cause of shock (e.g., acute mitral valve insufficiency, ventricular septal defect). Intra-aortic balloon counterpulsation (see Chapter 5, Ischemic Heart Disease) usually is performed with the device inserted percutaneously. The balloon filling is controlled electronically so that it is synchronized with the patient's electrocardiogram (ECG). The balloon inflates during diastole and deflates during systole, thus reducing afterload and improving CO. Additionally, coronary artery blood flow is improved during diastolic inflation. Intra-aortic balloon pumps should be considered only as an interim step to more definitive therapy.

■ **Definitive treatment** must be considered for any patient with cardiogenic shock. This treatment can take the form of relatively noninvasive procedures (e.g., angioplasty) or more invasive surgical procedures (e.g., coronary artery bypass surgery, valve replacement, heart transplantation).

- **Obstructive shock** usually is caused by massive pulmonary embolism. Occasionally, air embolism, amniotic fluid embolism, or tumor embolism also may cause obstructive shock. When shock complicates pulmonary embolism, therapy is directed toward preserving peripheral organ perfusion and removing the vascular obstruction. Fluid administration and the use of vasoconstrictors (e.g., norepinephrine, dopamine) may preserve BP while more definitive measures, such as thrombolytic therapy (e.g., streptokinase, alteplase, reteplase) or surgical embolectomy, are considered.

- **Distributive shock** occurs primarily as septic shock or anaphylactic shock. These two forms are associated with significant decreases in vascular tone.

  - **Septic shock** is caused by the systemic release of mediators that usually are triggered by circulating bacteria or their products, although the systemic inflammatory response syndrome can be seen without evidence of infection (e.g., pancreatitis, crush injuries, and certain drug ingestions such as salicylates).[23] Septic shock is characterized primarily by hypotension due to decreased vascular tone. CO also is increased, owing to increased heart rate and end-diastolic volumes despite overall myocardial depression. The main goals of treatment of septic shock include initial fluid resuscitation, adequate treatment of the underlying infection, and interruption of the mediator-associated systemic inflammatory response. **Initial resuscitation** includes appropriate large-volume fluid administration to compensate for the decrease in vascular tone and dilated ventricular capacity.

    - Goal-directed fluid administration, using a targeted central venous pressure (CVP) of 8–12 cm H_2O, appears to be important in such patients to determine the adequacy of preload and the need for inotropic or vasoconstrictor agents.[24]
    - A new therapy for septic shock has been developed. **Drotrecogin alfa** (activated), or **recombinant human activated protein C**, has antithrombotic, anti-inflammatory, and profibrinolytic properties. It has been shown to reduce mortality significantly in patients with severe sepsis when the patient has two or more acute organ failures and/or an APACHE II score is 25 or greater.[25,26] The usual dosage of drotrecogin alfa is a continuous infusion of 24 mcg/kg body weight/hr for 96 hours. The main contraindication to its use is an increased risk of hemorrhage (e.g., recent invasive procedure, severe thrombocytopenia).
    - Septic shock can also be associated with relative adrenal insufficiency. Among patients with septic shock who were classified as nonresponders to a corticotropin test (i.e., an increase in the serum cortisol level of <9 mcg/dL), a 7-day course of hydrocortisone (50 mg q6h IV) and fludrocortisone (50 mcg once a day via enteral route) was associated with a significant 28-day survival advantage.[27]

  - **Anaphylactic shock** is discussed further in the section Anaphylaxis in Chapter 10, Allergy and Immunology.

HEMODYNAMIC MONITORING AND PULMONARY ARTERY CATHETERIZATION

Indications

- A PA catheter can be placed to differentiate between cardiogenic and noncardiogenic forms of pulmonary edema, to identify the etiology of shock (Table 8-6), for the evaluation of acute renal failure or unexplained acidosis, for the evaluation of cardiac disorders, or to monitor high-risk surgical patients in the perioperative setting.
- The PA catheter allows measurement of intravascular and intracardiac pressures, CO, and $P\bar{v}O_2$ and SvO_2.

Obtaining a PAOP "Wedge Pressure" Tracing

- The PA catheter is advanced through a central vein after the distal balloon is inflated. Bedside waveform analysis is used to determine successful passage of the catheter through the right atrium, right ventricle, and PA into a PAOP position. Fluoroscopy should be used when difficulty is encountered in positioning the PA catheter.

■ If, at any time after passage into the PA, the tracing is found to move off the scale of the graph, overwedging of the catheter has occurred. An overwedged catheter should be withdrawn immediately 2–3 cm **after balloon deflation**, and catheter positioning should then be rechecked with reinflation of the balloon. Overwedging of a PA catheter increases the likelihood of serious complications (e.g., PA rupture).

Acceptance of PAOP Readings

■ Respiratory variation on the waveform, atrial pressure characteristics (including *a* and *v* waves), mean value of the PAOP tracing obtained at end expiration at less than the mean value of the PA pressure measurement, and the aspiration of highly oxygenated blood with the catheter in the PAOP position all indicate an accurate reading.

Transmural Pressure

■ When PEEP is present (applied or auto-PEEP), the positive intra-alveolar pressure at end expiration is transmitted through the lung to the pleural space. In these circumstances, the measured PAOP reflects the sum of the hydrostatic pressure within the vessel and the P_{JC}. When significant levels of total PEEP are present (>10 cm H_2O), it is more appropriate to use the transmural pressure as a measure of left ventricular filling (transmural pressure = PAOP – P_{JC}). For patients with normal lung compliance, one half of the total PEEP can be used as an estimate of P_{JC}. When lung compliance is depressed significantly (e.g., in ARDS), one third of the total PEEP can be used as an estimate for P_{JC}.

Cardiac Output

■ PA catheters are equipped with a thermistor to measure CO. At least two measurements that differ by <10%–15% should be obtained. Injections should be synchronized with the respiratory cycle to minimize variability between results. Often, thermodilution measurements of CO are inaccurate at an extremely low CO (e.g., <1.5 L/min) or an extremely high CO (e.g., >7.0 L/min), in the presence of significant valvular disease (e.g., severe tricuspid insufficiency), and when large intracardiac shunts are present. Calculation of the CO using the Fick formula may be more accurate in these circumstances.

Interpretation of Hemodynamic Readings

PAOP can be used as an index of left ventricular filling (preload) and as an index of the patient's propensity for development of pulmonary edema.

■ **Optimizing cardiac function.** Improving cardiac function by optimizing preload is more efficient in terms of myocardial oxygen consumption than similar improvements in cardiac function by use of inotropes when preload is inadequate. As a general rule, preload should be optimized before inotropic agents (which can increase myocardial oxygen consumption) or vasodilators (which can cause hypotension when preload is inadequate) are used. Fluid boluses should be administered in patients who are suspected of having inadequate cardiac filling pressures (i.e., inadequate preload) and should be followed by repeat measurements of PAOP, CO, heart rate, and stroke volume. In low CO states, if the PAOP increases by <5 mm Hg without significant changes in heart rate, CO, and stroke volume, additional fluid boluses may have to be given. An increase in the PAOP by more than 5 mm Hg usually signals that adequate ventricular filling is being achieved. Once the patient's preload has been optimized, cardiac performance can be reassessed and, if necessary, further therapy with inotropes (e.g., dobutamine, amrinone) or with vasodilators (e.g., nitroprusside, hydralazine, angiotensin-converting enzyme inhibitors) can be initiated to achieve further improvements in cardiac performance and tissue perfusion.

■ **Reducing unnecessary lung water.** PAOP is a reflection of the lung's tendency to develop pulmonary edema. Decreased left ventricular compliance results in a "critical pressure" being reached sooner for similar volume changes as compared to a normally compliant left ventricle. This difference is due to the increased stiffness of the noncompliant ventricle that causes higher pressures to be achieved for similar changes in volume. To optimize cardiac performance and to minimize the tendency for pulmonary edema formation, PAOP should be kept at the lowest point at which cardiac performance is acceptable.

- **Differentiating hydrostatic from nonhydrostatic pulmonary edema.** The management of pulmonary edema depends in large part on whether the excessive accumulation of lung water is due to increased hydrostatic pressures (e.g., left ventricular failure, mitral stenosis, acute volume overload), increased permeability of the alveolocapillary barrier (e.g., ARDS due to sepsis, aspiration, or trauma), or a combination of these factors. Clinical and radiographic criteria alone often are insufficient to determine the underlying mechanisms of pulmonary edema. Therefore, less than optimal management of the patient's underlying disease process may occur. In general, a PAOP of <18 mm Hg suggests that the primary mechanism of pulmonary edema is nonhydrostatic. Values above 18 mm Hg support a hydrostatic cause for the increased lung water.

- **Adequacy of organ perfusion.** Oxygen delivery to tissues depends on (a) an intact respiratory system to provide oxygen for hemoglobin saturation, (b) the concentration of hemoglobin, (c) CO, (d) tissue microcirculation, and (e) the unloading of oxygen from hemoglobin for diffusion into the tissue beds. Oxygen delivery can be measured as the product of CO and arterial oxygen content (CaO_2). CaO_2 is the sum of hemoglobin-bound and dissolved oxygen. Inadequate organ perfusion generally is associated with elevated blood lactate levels and decreased SvO_2 (usually <0.6). Factors that contribute to a low SvO_2 include anemia, hypoxemia, inadequate CO, and increased oxygen consumption. Factors that may elevate measured SvO_2 despite tissue hypoxia include peripheral arteriovenous shunting, the blood flow maldistribution of sepsis or cirrhosis, and cellular poisoning, such as that associated with cyanide toxicity. In general, optimization of gas exchange and CO along with an adequate hemoglobin (usually $\geq$10 g/dL) results in improved oxygen delivery to tissues.

References

1. Ware LB, Matthay MA. The acute respiratory distress syndrome. *N Engl J Med* 2000;342:1334–1349.
2. Antonelli M, Conti G, Rocco M, et al. A comparison of noninvasive positive-pressure ventilation and conventional mechanical ventilation in patients with acute respiratory failure. *N Engl J Med* 1998;339:429–435.
3. Brochard L. Noninvasive ventilation for acute respiratory failure. *JAMA* 2002;288:932–935.
4. Hurford W. Orotracheal intubation outside the operating room: Anatomic considerations and techniques. *Respir Care* 1999;44:615–626.
5. Ahrens T, Kollef MH. Early tracheostomy—has its time arrived? *Crit Care Med* 2004;32:1796–1797.
6. Sessler CN. Mechanical ventilation of patients with acute lung injury. *Crit Care Clin* 1998;14:707–729.
7. Tobin MJ. Critical care medicine in AJRCCM 2003. *Am J Respir Crit Care Med* 2004;169:239–253.
8. Fessler HE, Brower RG. Protocols for lung protective ventilation. *Crit Care Med* 2005;33:S223–7.
9. Gattinoni L, Tognoni G, Pesenti A, et al. Effect of prone positioning on the survival of patients with acute respiratory failure. *N Engl J Med* 2001;345:568–573.
10. Thompson BT. Glucocorticoids and acute lung injury. *Crit Care Med* 2003;31:S253–57.
11. Kress JP, Noth I, Gehlbach BK, et al. The utility of albuterol nebulized with heliox during acute asthma exacerbations. *Am J Respir Crit Care Med* 2002;165:1317–1322.
12. Habashi NM. Other approaches to open-lung ventilation: airway pressure release ventilation. *Crit Care Med* 2005;33:S228–40.
13. Taylor RW, Zimmerman JL, Dellinger RP, et al. Low-dose inhaled nitric oxide in patients with acute lung injury: a randomized controlled trial. *JAMA* 2004;291:1603–1609.
14. Shaw MJ. Ventilator-associated pneumonia. *Curr Opin Pulm Med* 2005;11:236–241.

15. Amato MB, Barbas CS, Medeiros DM, et al. Effect of a protective-ventilation strategy on mortality in the acute respiratory distress syndrome. *N Engl J Med* 1998;338:347–354.
16. Simonds AK. Streamlining weaning: protocols and weaning units. *Thorax* 2005;60:175–182.
17. Esteban A, Frutos F, Tobin MJ, et al. A comparison of four methods of weaning patients from mechanical ventilation. Spanish Lung Failure Collaborative Group. *N Engl J Med* 1995;332:345–50.
18. Jones DP, Byrne P, Morgan C, et al. Positive end-expiratory pressure vs T-piece. Extubation after mechanical ventilation. *Chest* 1991;100:1655–1659.
19. Brochard L, Rauss A, Benito S, et al. Comparison of three methods of gradual withdrawal from ventilatory support during weaning from mechanical ventilation. *Am J Respir Crit Care Med* 1994;150:896–903.
20. Dries DJ, McGonigal MD, Malian MS, et al. Protocol-driven ventilator weaning reduces use of mechanical ventilation, rate of early reintubation, and ventilator-associated pneumonia. *J Trauma* 2004;56:943–951.
21. De Jonghe BA, Sharshar TB, Hopkinson NB, et al. Paresis following mechanical ventilation. *Curr Opin Crit Care* 2004;10:47–52.
22. Dellinger RP, Carlet JM, Masur H, et al. Surviving Sepsis Campaign guidelines for management of severe sepsis and septic shock. *Crit Care Med* 2004;32:858–873.
23. Matthay MA. Severe sepsis—a new treatment with both anticoagulant and antiinflammatory properties. *N Engl J Med* 2001;344:759–762.
24. Rivers E, Nguyen B, Havstad S, et al. Early Goal-Directed Therapy in the Treatment of Severe Sepsis and Septic Shock. *N Engl J Med* 2001;345:1368–1377.
25. Bernard GR, Vincent JL, Laterre PF, et al. Efficacy and safety of recombinant human activated protein C for severe sepsis. *N Engl J Med* 2001;344:699–709.
26. Abraham E, Laterre PF, Garg R, et al. Drotrecogin Alfa (Activated) for Adults with Severe Sepsis and a Low Risk of Death. *N Engl J Med* 2005;353:1332–1341.
27. Annane D, Sébille V, Charpentie C. Effect of Treatment With Low Doses of Hydrocortisone and Fludrocortisone on Mortality in Patients With Septic Shock. *JAMA* 2002;288:862–871.

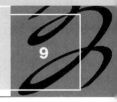

PULMONARY DISEASE

*Roger D. Yusen, Martin L. Mayse, Murali Chakinala,
Tonya Russell, and Daniel B. Rosenbluth*

9

 PULMONARY HYPERTENSION

GENERAL PRINCIPLES

Definition and Nomenclature

- Pulmonary hypertension (PH) is the sustained elevation of the mean pulmonary artery pressure ($\geq$25 mm Hg at rest or $\geq$30 mm Hg during exertion).
- PH is subcategorized into five major etiologic groups (Table 9-1)
    - Pulmonary arterial hypertension (PAH)
    - Pulmonary venous hypertension
    - Parenchymal lung disease and/or chronic hypoxemia
    - Chronic thrombotic and/or embolic disease
    - Miscellaneous
- PAH specifically represents a group of disorders with similar pathologies, clinical presentation, and propensity for right heart failure.

Epidemiology

- PH is most often due to left heart disease or parenchymal lung disease.
- Idiopathic pulmonary arterial hypertension (IPAH), formerly known as primary pulmonary hypertension (PPH), is a rare disorder (estimated incidence 1 in 500,000).
    - Historical median survival for IPAH prior to current medical therapy was 2.8 years.[1]
- PAH associated with progressive systemic sclerosis (PSS) or scleroderma represents the largest group within the PAH subcategory.
- Incidence of chronic thromboembolic pulmonary hypertension (CTEPH) may be as high as 4% among survivors of acute pulmonary embolism.[2]

Pathophysiology

- Central physiologic abnormality of PH is increased right ventricular (RV) afterload due to elevated pulmonary vascular resistance (PVR).
- The highest PVRs are encountered in PAH and CTEPH.
- Chronically elevated RV afterload affects RV contractility and overall cardiac output.
- Unlike the left ventricle, the RV has limited ability to overcome high afterload.
    - Initially, cardiac output is diminished during strenuous exercise. As the PH severity worsens, maximal cardiac output is achieved at progressively lower workloads; ultimately resting cardiac output is reduced.
- Death in PAH is most commonly due to right heart failure.
- In advanced stages, pulmonary artery pressures decline as the RV fails to generate enough blood flow to maintain high pressures.

TABLE 9-1	Clinical Classification of Pulmonary Hypertension: Venice 2003 Classification

1. Pulmonary arterial hypertension (PAH)
   a. Idiopathic pulmonary arterial hypertension (IPAH)
   b. Familial pulmonary arterial hypertension (FPAH)
   c. Associated pulmonary arterial hypertension (APAH)
       i. Collagen vascular disease
       ii. Congenital systemic-to-pulmonary shunts
       iii. Portal hypertension
       iv. HIV infection
       v. Drugs and toxins
       vi. Other (glycogen storing disease, Gaucher disease, hereditary hemorrhagic telangiectasia, hemoglobinopathies, myeloproliferative disorders, splenectomy)
   d. Associated with significant venous or capillary involvement
       i. Pulmonary veno-occlusive disease
       ii. Pulmonary capillary hemangiomatosis
2. Pulmonary venous hypertension
   a. Left-sided atrial or ventricular heart disease
   b. Left-sided valvular heart disease
3. Pulmonary hypertension associated with parenchymal lung disease and/or chronic hypoxemia
   a. Chronic obstructive lung disease
   b. Interstitial lung disease
   c. Sleep-disordered breathing
   d. Alveolar-hypoventilation disorders
   e. Chronic exposure to high-altitude
4. Pulmonary hypertension due to chronic thrombotic and/or embolic disease
   a. Thromboembolic obstruction of proximal pulmonary arteries
   b. Thromboembolic obstruction of distal pulmonary arteries
   c. Pulmonary embolism (tumor, parasites, foreign material)
5. Pulmonary hypertension due to miscellaneous conditions
   a. Sarcoidosis
   b. Pulmonary langerhans cell histiocytosis
   c. Lymphangiomatosis
6. Compression of pulmonary vessels (fibrosing mediastinitis, tumor, adenopathy)
From *JACC* 2004;43:5S–12S.[3]

- When PH is due to other conditions (i.e., non-PAH), pathophysiology is due to the underlying entity (e.g., chronic obstructive pulmonary disease [COPD]) and the associated pulmonary vascular abnormalities.

Clinical Presentation

- **Symptoms** include **dyspnea** (most common), exercise intolerance, fatigue, and palpitations.
- Symptoms of right heart failure include exertional dizziness, **syncope**, chest pain, lower extremity swelling, increased abdominal girth (ascites), and hoarseness (impingement of recurrent laryngeal nerve by enlarging pulmonary artery).
- Assess for exposure to **anorectic drugs** and symptoms of **underlying diseases** (e.g., connective tissue diseases, congestive heart failure [CHF], obstructive sleep apnea–hypopnea syndrome, and venous thromboembolism [VTE]).

- Ausculatory signs of PH include **prominent second heart sound** (loud S_2) and loud P_2, right ventricular S_3, and tricuspid regurgitation, and pulmonary insufficiency murmurs.
- Signs of right heart failure include elevated jugular venous pressure, hepatomegaly, pulsatile liver, pedal edema, and ascites.
- Physical examination should focus on identifying underlying conditions linked to PH: skin changes of scleroderma, stigmata of liver disease, clubbing (congenital heart disease), and abnormal breath sounds (parenchymal lung disease).

DIAGNOSIS

- Diagnostic testing should (a) **confirm clinical suspicion of PH,** (b) **determine etiology of PH,** (c) **gauge severity of condition,** and (d) **assist with treatment planning.**
- Acute illnesses (e.g., pulmonary edema, pulmonary embolism, adult respiratory distress syndrome) can cause *acute* PH that is *mild* (pulmonary artery systolic pressure [PASP] <50) or can worsen pre-existing PH. Evaluation of *chronic* PH becomes necessary if pulmonary artery pressures remain elevated after resolution of the acute process.
- If chronic PH is entertained based on clinical suspicion or during the evaluation of a vulnerable population (e.g., first-degree relative of IPAH patient, liver transplant candidate, or pre-existing scleroderma), transthoracic echocardiogram should be the initial test. Additional studies, as outlined below, should be completed if PAH is still under consideration after echocardiography.[4]
- **Transthoracic echocardiogram with Doppler and agitated saline injection**
  - Preferred test for initial evaluation of suspected PH.
  - **Estimate PASP** by Doppler interrogation of tricuspid valve regurgitant jet; absence of tricuspid regurgitation does not exclude elevated pulmonary artery pressure. Sensitivity for predicting PH is 80%–100% and correlation coefficient with invasive measurement is 0.6–0.9.[4] However, invasive measurement is recommended if suspicion of PH remains despite estimation by echocardiogram.
  - **Assess RV pressure overload and dysfunction** (e.g., hypertrophied RV free wall, dilated chamber, hypokinesis, displaced interventricular septum, paradoxical septal motion, compression of left ventricle, and pericardial effusion).
  - **Identify etiologies for PH** (e.g., left ventricular systolic or diastolic dysfunction, primary left-sided valvular disease, left atrial structural anomalies, and congenital systemic to pulmonary [left-to-right] shunts).
- **Pulmonary function testing**
  - Spirometry and lung volumes to assess for obstructive (e.g., **COPD**) or restrictive (e.g., interstitial lung disease) ventilatory abnormalities.
  - Diffusing capacity for carbon monoxide is usually reduced with parenchymal lung diseases, but isolated mild–moderate reduction is often encountered in PAH.
- **Arterial blood gas (ABG)**
  - Low PaO_2 may be indicative of parenchymal lung disease.
  - Elevated $PaCO_2$ is an important clue for a hypoventilation syndrome or parenchymal lung disease.
- **Six-minute walk (6MW) or simple exercise test**
  - Unexplained **exercise-induced desaturation** is suggestive of PH.
  - Distance covered helps **assign overall functional classification** (Table 9-2) and provides intermediate-term **prognostic information.**[5]
- **Nocturnal oximetry**
  - Screen for nocturnal desaturations and need for polysomnography (see Obstructive Sleep Apnea–Hypopnea Syndrome).
- **Laboratory tests**
  - **Evaluate for causative conditions and gauge degree of cardiac impairment.**
  - Tests include complete blood counts, electrolytes, blood urea nitrogen, serum creatinine, hepatic function tests, brain natriuretic peptide (BNP), coagulation studies, human immunodeficiency virus serology, thyroid-stimulating hormone (TSH), antinuclear antibody (ANA), antitopoisomerase and anticentromere antibodies, and antiphospholipid antibody.

TABLE 9-2	Functional Assessment for Patients with PH
Class I	No limitation of physical activity. Ordinary physical activity does not cause undue dyspnea or fatigue, chest pain, or near syncope.
Class II	Slight limitation of physical activity. Comfortable at rest. Ordinary physical activity causes undue dyspnea or fatigue, chest pain, or near syncope.
Class III	Marked limitation of physical activity. Comfortable at rest. Less than ordinary activity causes undue dyspnea or fatigue, chest pain, or near syncope.
Class IV	Unable to carry out any physical activity without symptoms. Dyspnea and/or fatigue may be present at rest. Discomfort is increased by any physical activity. Signs of right heart failure are present.

Source: Modified after the New York Heart Association Functional Classification; World Health Organization, 1999.

- Chest radiography
    - General findings of PH include enlarged central pulmonary arteries (diameter >17 mm in males and >15 mm in females), RV enlargement (opacification of retrosternal space on lateral view), and pulmonary artery calcification.
    - Clues to specific PH diagnosis include decreased peripheral vascular markings or pruning (PAH), very large pulmonary vasculature throughout lung fields (congenital-to-systemic shunt), regional oligemia of pulmonary vasculature (chronic thromboembolic disease), interstitial infiltrates (interstitial lung disease), and hyperinflated lungs (COPD).
- Electrocardiography
    - Signs of **right heart enlargement** include right ventricular hypertrophy, right atrial enlargement, right bundle branch block, and right ventricular strain pattern (S wave in lead I with Q wave and inverted T wave in lead III).
- Ventilation–perfusion (V/Q) lung scan
    - Evaluate for **chronic thromboembolic disease** (see the section Thromboembolic Disorders in Chapter 18, Disorders of Hemostasis).
    - **Heterogeneous perfusion** patterns are associated with PAH.
    - Presence of one or more segmental mismatches raises concern for chronic thromboembolic disease and should be investigated with computed tomography and pulmonary angiography.[6]
- Additional investigations. The following investigations should be conducted, if necessary, to elaborate results from the initial studies (as outlined above).
    - Chest computed tomography (CT) scan
        - **Evaluates lung parenchyma and mediastinum.**
        - **High-resolution images** assess for interstitial or bronchiolar disease.
        - CT angiogram can identify chronic thromboembolic changes.
    - Pulmonary arteriogram
        - Further **evaluates for chronic thromboembolic disease,** if suggested by V/Q scan or chest CT scan.
        - Provides a direct measurement of pulmonary artery and right atrial pressures.
        - **Inferior vena cava filter** can be deployed at time of angiography, if chronic thromboembolic disease is detected.
        - Angiography's risk in the setting of severe PH is minimized by using limited amounts of **nonionic contrast** with slow injection of contrast.
    - Radionuclide ventriculography
        - **Assesses right and left ventricular function.**
        - Quantification of ejection fraction can be confounded by tracer detection from overlapping adjacent structures (e.g., dilated atrium or ventricle).
        - Significant valvular regurgitation may exaggerate the calculated **ejection fraction.**

- Magnetic resonance imaging (MRI)
  - MRI investigates cardiac anomalies that lead to the development of PAH.
  - Provides anatomic and functional information on the RV, including contractility measures.
  - Role is not clearly defined but may be a useful modality for longitudinal assessment of RV.
- Transesophageal echocardiogram (TEE)
  - The TEE identifies intracardiac shunts suspected by transthoracic echocardiogram.
  - Because of the distance between probe and tricuspid valve regurgitant jet, **TEE estimation of PASP is less accurate than TTE.**
- Additional laboratory testing
  - If PAH is suspected, additional studies that may be indicated based on the initial evaluation include free thyroxine, hepatitis B and C serologies, hemoglobin electrophoresis, extractable nuclear antigen, and lupus anticoagulant.
- Polysomnogram
  - Evaluates for **sleep-disordered breathing** (SDB), which can cause mild PH or aggravate PH caused by other conditions (see Obstructive Sleep Apnea–Hypopnea Syndrome).
  - Titrate **supplemental oxygen** to correct nocturnal oxyhemoglobin desaturation.
  - **Hypercarbia** due to **hypoventilation** can cause significant PH and should be corrected with **noninvasive positive pressure ventilation** (NIPPV).
- Cardiopulmonary exercise test (CPET)
  - PH pattern of abnormalities include **reduced peak oxygen consumption,** early anaerobic threshold, **reduced oxygen-pulse,** oxyhemoglobin desaturation, and increased dead-space ventilation with exercise.
  - The CPET is infrequently needed and **should be performed with caution,** only by experienced personnel.
- Lung biopsy
  - Lung biopsy is rarely performed but useful if lung disease requires histologic confirmation (e.g., pulmonary **vasculitis** or **veno-occlusive disease**).
  - The risk of **surgery** is usually prohibitive in the setting of severe PH or RV dysfunction.
  - **Transbronchial biopsy** is contraindicated in the setting of severe PH.
- Right heart catheterization
  - **An essential investigation if PAH is suspected, whether present on echocardiography or not, and treatment is being considered.**
    - **Confirm noninvasive estimate of PASP,** as echocardiography can under- and overestimate pulmonary artery systolic pressure.[7]
    - **Measure cardiac output and mean right atrial pressure (RAP) to gauge severity of condition and predict future course;** increased RAP is an indicator of RV dysfunction and had the greatest odds ratio for predicting mortality in the IPAH Registry[1]. Since tricuspid regurgitation produces inaccurate thermodilution cardiac output data, use of the **Fick (estimated) method** is advised.
    - **Investigate etiologies of PH,** including left heart disease (by measuring pulmonary artery occlusion pressure [PAOP]) or missed systemic-to-pulmonary shunts (by noting "step-ups" in oxygen saturations).
  - **Acute vasodilator testing** is recommended if PAH is suspected (i.e., PH with normal PAOP).
    - Performed with a *short*-acting vasodilator, such as intravenous adenosine, intravenous epoprostenol (Flolan), or inhaled nitric oxide; *long*-acting **calcium channel blockers (CCBs) should not be used for initial vasodilator testing** due to risk of sustained systemic hypotension or drop in cardiac output.[8]
    - **Not recommended for patients in extreme right heart failure** (mean RAP >20).
    - Definition of a **responder** is decline in mean pulmonary artery pressure (mPAP) ≥ 10 mm Hg *and* concluding mPAP ≤ 40 mm Hg.[8]

- Responders should then undergo a CCB trial with pulmonary artery catheter in place. If similar vasoresponsiveness is documented, chronic CCB therapy can be prescribed (see Treatment).
- **Left heart catheterization** is only necessary to directly measure **left ventricular end-diastolic pressure** (LVEDP) if PAOP cannot reliably exclude left heart disease.

TREATMENT

- **Management of PH depends on the specific category of PH** (Table 9-1).
  - Patients with PH due to left heart disease or parenchymal lung diseases should receive appropriate therapy for underlying causative condition.
    - Chronic thromboembolic pulmonary hypertension may be treated by **pulmonary thromboendarterectomy** at specialized centers and requires careful screening to determine surgical resectability and expected hemodynamic response.[6]
    - PH resulting from congenital systemic-to-pulmonary shunts, in select cases, may be improved with **percutaneous or surgical correction** of the underlying defect.
  - PAH patients should be offered **vasomodulator/vasodilator** therapy.
- Regardless of PH diagnosis, normoxemia should be maintained to avoid hypoxic vasoconstriction and further aggravation of pulmonary artery pressures. **Supplemental oxygen** to maintain adequate arterial saturations (>89%) 24 hours a day is recommended. However, normoxemia may not be possible in the presence of a significant right-to-left shunt (e.g., patent foramen ovale).
- **In-line filters** should be used to prevent paradoxical air emboli from intravenous catheters in PH patients with significant right-to-left shunts.
- **Pneumovax and influenza vaccination** should be given to avoid respiratory tract infections.
- Patients with severe PH and RV dysfunction should minimize high-risk behaviors that can induce acute pulmonary hypertensive crisis and/or circulatory collapse:
  - **Valsalva** maneuvers can raise intrathoracic pressure and induce syncope through diminished central venous return (e.g., vigorous exercise, severe coughing paroxysms, straining during defecation or micturition)
  - **High altitudes** (>5,000 feet) due to low inspired concentration of oxygen
  - **Cigarette smoking,** because of nicotine's vasoactive effects
  - **Pregnancy,** due to hemodynamic alterations that further strain the heart
  - Systemic **sympathomimetic** agents, such as decongestants and cocaine

Medications

- **Modified New York Heart Association (NYHA) classification** defines clinical severity, based on functional limitations, and guides treatment (Table 9-2).
- Vasomodulator/vasodilator agents
  - **Calcium channel blockers (CCBs)** (nifedipine or diltiazem)
    - Mechanism: vasodilate pulmonary *and* systemic circulation
    - Indication: **responders** during acute vasodilator testing *and* after verification of vasodilatory response to CCB during a short-term CCB trial; **only a minority of IPAH patients (~8%) are proven long-term responders to CCB.**[9]
    - Dose variable, and based on tolerance (determined by symptoms and hemodynamics), but doses of oral nifedipine 240 mg/d or diltiazem 720 mg/d (in divided doses) may be needed.
    - Effects: improve symptoms, exercise tolerance, hemodynamics, and survival[10]
    - Hazards: **rebound pulmonary hypertension** with abrupt discontinuation; negative inotropic effects that can worsen right heart failure symptoms
  - **Endothelin receptor antagonist** (bosentan)
    - Mechanism: blocks **endothelin-1** at receptor level
    - Indication: functional class II–IV (Table 9-2)
    - Dose: 62.5 mg PO bid × 1 month, then increase dose to **125 mg PO bid,** as tolerated

- Effects: improves exercise capacity and delays time to clinical worsening[11]
- Hazards: **hepatotoxicity** (7% discontinuation rate); drug interaction with oral hypoglycemic agents and warfarin
- Specific monitoring: monthly liver function tests
▣ **Phosphodiesterase-5 inhibitor** (sildenafil)
  - Mechanism: smooth muscle cell relaxation by up-regulating **cyclic guanosine monophosphate (cGMP)** pathway
  - Indication: functional class II–IV
  - Dose: **20 mg PO tid** (anecdotal experiences with higher dosing)
  - Effects: improves exercise capacity and hemodynamics[12]
  - Hazards: **hypotension** (usually transient), drug interaction with nitrates, visual disturbances
▣ **Prostanoids** (epoprostenol)
  - Mechanism: **vasodilator, inotrope, inhibitor of platelet aggregation**
  - Indication: functional class III–IV
  - Dose: **gradually titrated and based on side effects and PH symptoms (range 2–50 ng/kg/min,** delivered **intravenously** as continuous infusion)
  - Effects: improved exercise capacity, hemodynamics, and **survival (in IPAH)**[13,14]
  - Hazards: frequent drug-related side effects (e.g., jaw pain, nausea, diarrhea, flushing, and headache), **catheter-related infections,** and acute deterioration from abrupt discontinuation from malfunction of delivery system
▣ **Alternative prostanoids** (treprostinil, iloprost)
  - Mechanism: same as epoprostenol
  - Indication: treprostinil—functional class II–IV; iloprost—functional class III–IV
  - Dose: **treprostinil** administered as **continuous infusion, SC or IV (based on side effects and residual PH symptoms, range 10–150 ng/kg/min); iloprost inhalational delivery** (2.5–5.0 μg q2–3h during awake period)
  - Effects: Both agents reduce symptoms and improve hemodynamics,[15,16] although long-term hemodynamic regression was not demonstrated with iloprost. Neither has been conclusively shown to improve survival.
  - Hazards: Treprostinil has similar drug-related side effects to epoprostenol and **pain at injection site** with subcutaneous delivery. Iloprost drug levels and hemodynamics fluctuate between doses.
■ **Inotropic agents** (dobutamine, milrinone, digoxin)
  ▣ Modestly improves right heart function, cardiac output, and symptoms.
  ▣ Dobutamine and milrinone are best suited for **short-term use** in extremely decompensated states.
  ▣ Digoxin's effects on right ventricular contractility are limited and use is somewhat controversial and quite variable.
■ **Anticoagulation** (warfarin)
  ▣ Chronic anticoagulation improves survival, based on limited data in IPAH patients.[10,17]
  ▣ Warfarin is dosed to **target international normalized ratio (INR) of 1.5–2.5** (see Anticoagulants, Chapter 18, Disorders of Hemostasis).[8]
  ▣ Anticoagulant therapy is not urgent and should be avoided in the setting of invasive procedures or active bleeding.
■ **Diuretic therapy** (loop diuretic often in conjunction with aldosterone antagonist)
  ▣ Alleviates **right heart failure** and improves symptoms.
  ▣ Overdiuresis or too rapid of a diuresis can be poorly tolerated due to **preload dependency** of the RV and limited ability of the cardiac output to compensate for systemic hypotension.
■ Because current therapies for PAH are only palliative and not curative, patients require close follow-up as deterioration may induce an alteration of medical therapy or surgical intervention in certain cases. While there is no consensus for follow-up strategy, periodic functional (e.g., 6-minute walk and World Health Organization [WHO] Functional Classification) and hemodynamic (e.g., echocardiography or right heart catheterization) assessments provide the most comprehensive assessment.

Surgery

- Lung transplantation or heart–lung transplantation
    - Reserved for suitable patients with PAH that **remain in advanced functional class (III–IV) despite maximal medical therapy.**
    - Because the RV recovers after **isolated lung transplantation,** heart transplantation is usually reserved for complex congenital heart defects that cannot be repaired.
    - A randomized trial of medical versus transplant therapy has not been conducted, but lung transplantation is thought to prolong survival in selected advanced cases that have poor intermediate-term prognosis with medical therapy.
    - Median survival after lung transplantation is ~5 years and **survival for IPAH patients at 5 years is ~50%.**[18]
- Atrial septostomy
    - Palliative procedure performed in cases of right heart failure (i.e., syncope, hepatic congestion, prerenal azotemia) refractory to medical therapy.
    - Percutaneous creation of a right-to-left shunt across the interatrial septum in patients whose right atrial pressures are greater than left atrial pressures.
    - Despite arterial oxyhemoglobin desaturation and hypoxemia, **oxygen delivery** increases from improved left ventricular filling and cardiac output.

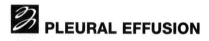

PLEURAL EFFUSION

GENERAL PRINCIPLES

Definition

- Pleural effusion is the accumulation of fluid in the pleural space.

Mechanisms of Injury

- Normally, the pleural space only contains a small amount of fluid that is not radiographically apparent.
- **Transudative pleural effusions** result from alteration of hydrostatic and oncotic factors that increase the formation or decrease the absorption of pleural fluid (e.g., increased mean capillary pressure [heart failure] or decreased oncotic pressure [cirrhosis or nephrotic syndrome]).
- **Exudative pleural effusions** occur when damage or disruption of the normal pleural membranes or vasculature (e.g., tumor involvement of the pleural space, infection, inflammatory conditions, or trauma) leads to increased capillary permeability or decreased lymphatic drainage.
- **Parapneumonic effusions** are exudates that develop secondary to pulmonary infections. Patients with pneumonia and a pleural effusion should undergo **rapid diagnostic testing** because an infected pleural space (empyema) needs to be **treated without delay.**
- **Malignant pleural effusions** arise from tumor involvement of the pleura or mediastinum. Patients with malignancy are also at increased risk for pleural effusions from postobstructive pneumonia, pulmonary emboli, chylothorax, and drug or radiation reactions.
- While pleural effusion occurs in a vast array of disease states, **90% of pleural effusions are the result of only five diseases.**[19]
    - Congestive heart failure (36%)
    - Pneumonia (22%)
    - Malignancy (14%)
    - Pulmonary embolism (11%)
    - Viral disease (7%)

DIAGNOSIS

Clinical Presentation

- The underlying cause of the effusion usually dictates the symptoms, although patients may be asymptomatic.
- Pleural inflammation, abnormal pulmonary mechanics, and worsened alveolar gas exchange produce **symptoms and signs** of disease.
    - Inflammation of the parietal pleura leads to pain in local (intercostal) involved areas or referred (phrenic) distributions (shoulder).
    - Dyspnea is frequent and may be present and out of proportion to the size of the effusion.
    - Cough can occur.
    - Chest examination is notable for dullness to percussion, decreased or absent tactile fremitus, and decreased breath sounds.
    - Tracheal shift to the contralateral side or an ipsilateral pleural rub may be present.

History and Physical Examination

- The clinical setting is crucial to establishing a proper diagnosis. A definitive diagnosis based solely upon pleural fluid analysis is possible in the minority of pleural effusions.
- History or physical examination findings suggestive of congestive heart failure, malignancy, pneumonia, pulmonary embolism, myocardial infarction, surgery, cirrhosis, or rheumatologic arthritis provide important clues to the underlying diagnosis.

Laboratory and Imaging Studies

- Pleural effusions are typically **detected by chest radiography** as blunting of the costophrenic angle or opacification of the base of the hemithorax without loss of volume of the hemithorax (which would suggest atelectasis), and may be accompanied by air bronchograms (which would suggest an alveolar filling process such as pneumonia).
- Prior to invasive diagnostic or therapeutic procedures, the patient should undergo imaging to confirm the presence and size of the effusion. Preferred modalities include:
    - **Decubitus chest radiography** showing layering fluid will confirm the presence of pleural effusion and demonstrates that at least a portion of the fluid is not loculated.
    - **Thoracic ultrasonography** is one of the best modalities to assess for pleural fluid loculations. Ultrasonography can also provide real-time guidance for pleural procedures and can reduce both the complication and failure rate of thoracentesis.
    - **Computed tomography of the chest** with contrast helps differentiate pleural fluid from lung masses and atelectatic lung, and helps define the extent of pleural thickening, pleural nodularity, and other associated findings.
- Pleural fluid analysis
    - Thoracentesis can be performed safely at the bedside, in the absence of disorders of hemostasis, on effusions that extend >10 mm from the inner chest wall on a lateral decubitus film. Loculated effusions can be localized with ultrasonography or CT scan. Proper technique and sonographic guidance minimize the risk of pneumothorax and other complications. **Repeat thoracentesis** increases the diagnostic yield.
        - Serum lactate dehydrogenase (LDH), protein, pH, glucose and albumin should be measured within hours of the thoracentesis to allow appropriate comparison.
    - Pleural fluid appearance
        - **Red-tinged pleural effusions** indicate the presence of blood.
        - In exudative pleural effusions, **serosanguineous** fluid is usually not helpful in narrowing the diagnosis. If the blood is due to thoracentesis, the degree of discoloration should clear during the aspiration.
        - **Bloody pleural fluid** usually indicates the presence of malignancy, pulmonary embolism (PE), or trauma.
        - The presence of gross blood should lead to the measurement of a pleural fluid hematocrit. **Hemothorax** is defined as a pleural fluid–to–blood hematocrit ratio of >0.5, and chest tube drainage should be considered.

■ The **transudate/exudate classification system** of pleural effusions narrows the **differential diagnosis.**

- **Transudative pleural effusions** have (a) a pleural fluid-to-serum **protein ratio** of ≤ 0.5, (b) a pleural fluid-to-serum **LDH ratio** of ≤ 0.6, **AND** (c) a pleural fluid **LDH** of less than or equal to two-thirds of the upper limit of normal for serum LDH.[20] Most **transudates** are clear, straw colored, nonviscid, and without odor. The white blood cell (WBC) count is usually $<100/mm^3$, and the red blood cell (RBC) count is generally $<10,000/mm^3$. The pleural fluid glucose level is usually similar to the serum level, and the pleural fluid pH is higher than the blood pH. Transudates should lead to further evaluation of the heart, liver, and kidneys, and therapy is directed accordingly.

- **Exudative pleural effusions** have high protein or LDH values. Specifically, they are pleural effusions that meet any of **Light's criteria** of (a) a pleural fluid-to-serum **protein ratio** of >0.5, (b) a pleural fluid-to-serum **LDH ratio** of >0.6, **OR** (c) a pleural fluid **LDH** of more than two-thirds of the upper limit of normal for serum LDH are exudates.

- In patients who have an exudative effusion according to Light's criteria but in whom clinical suspicion for heart, liver, or kidney disease is high, a serum-to-pleural fluid albumin gradient should be checked. A gradient of >1.2 g/dL suggests that the pleural fluid is likely due to congestive heart failure, liver disease, or kidney disease.

- Exudates have a broad differential diagnosis.

  • The **WBC differential** is often not diagnostic, although **neutrophilia** is suggestive of infection. **Eosinophilia** ($>10\%$ of total nucleated cell count) is suggestive of air or blood in the pleural space. If air or blood is not present in the pleural space, consideration should be given to fungal and parasitic infection, drug-induced disease, PE, asbestos-related disease, and Churg-Strauss syndrome. **Lymphocytosis** ($>50\%$ of the total nucleated cell count) is suggestive of malignancy or tuberculosis. The presence of **mesothelial cells** argues against the diagnosis of tuberculosis. Many **plasma cells** suggest a diagnosis of multiple myeloma.

  • Exudative effusions with **normal protein but high LDH** are likely to be parapneumonic or secondary to malignancy. LDH is an indicator of the degree of pleural inflammation.

  • A **glucose** concentration of <60 mg/dL is probably due to tuberculosis, malignancy, rheumatoid arthritis, or parapneumonic effusion. For parapneumonic pleural effusions with a glucose of <60 mg/dL, tube thoracostomy should be considered (Table 9-3).

TABLE 9-3	Indications for Tube Thoracostomy in Parapneumonic Effusions

Radiographic criteria
Pleural fluid loculations
Effusion filling more than half the hemithorax
Air–fluid level

Microbiologic criteria
Pus in the pleural space
Positive stain for microorganisms
Positive pleural fluid cultures

Chemical criteria
Pleural fluid pH <7.2
Pleural fluid glucose <60 mg/dL

From Colice GL, Curtis A, Deslauriers J, et al. Medical and Surgical Treatment of Parapneumonic Effusions. *Chest* 2000;118:1158–1171.[22]

- In addition to testing pleural fluid for LDH and protein, **other useful tests** of pleural fluid include pH, albumin, glucose, cell count and differential, microbiologic stains, cultures, cytology, triglycerides, and amylase.
  - **Pleural fluid with a low pH** usually has a low glucose and a high LDH; otherwise, the low pH may be due to poor sample collection technique. A pH of <7.3 is seen with empyema, tuberculosis, malignancy, collagen vascular disease, or esophageal rupture. For parapneumonic pleural effusions with a pH of <7.20, tube thoracostomy should be considered (Table 9-3). Pleural fluid for pH testing should be collected anaerobically in a heparinized syringe and placed on ice.
  - An elevation of **amylase** suggests that the patient has pancreatic disease, malignancy, or esophageal rupture. Malignancy and esophageal rupture have salivary amylase elevations and not pancreatic amylase elevations.
  - **Turbid or milky fluid** should be centrifuged. If the supernatant clears, the cloudiness is likely due to cells and debris. If the supernatant remains turbid, pleural lipids should be measured. Elevation of triglycerides (>110 mg/dL) suggests that a chylothorax is present, usually due to disruption of the thoracic duct from trauma, surgery, or malignancy (i.e., lymphoma).
  - **Cytology** is positive in approximately 60% of malignant effusions. Priming the fluid collection bag with unfractionated heparin (UFH; e.g., 1,000 International Units) may increase the yield. The volume of pleural fluid analyzed does not impact the yield of cytologic diagnosis.[21]
  - Pleural fluid LDH, protein, pH, and Gram stain/culture are used to define complicated parapneumonic effusions and to guide treatment (Table 9-3).[22]
- **Surgical diagnostic procedures**
  - **Closed pleural biopsy** adds little to the diagnostic yield of thoracentesis, except in the diagnosis of tuberculosis. For tuberculous effusions, pleural fluid cultures alone are positive in only 20%–25% of cases. However, the combination of pleural fluid studies and pleural biopsy (demonstrating granulomas or organisms) is 90% sensitive in establishing tuberculosis as the etiology of the effusion.
  - **Diagnostic thoracoscopy** has largely replaced closed pleural biopsy. Thoracoscopy allows directed biopsies that increase the diagnostic yield for malignancy while maintaining the high diagnostic yield of closed pleural biopsy for TB.
- **Other diagnostic procedures** that are useful in establishing the etiology of a pleural effusion when the aforementioned tests are nondiagnostic include evaluation of liver function and renal function, cardiac echo, biopsy of other abnormal sites (e.g., a mediastinal or lung mass), and evaluation of PE (see Thromboembolic Disorders in Chapter 18, Disorders of Hemostasis).

TREATMENT

- **Transudates** resolve with treatment of the underlying heart, kidney, or liver disease. Uncommonly, more aggressive approaches including pleurodesis and shunts are required.
- **Parapneumonic effusions and empyema** should be managed with **tube drainage** when indicated based on the size, gross appearance, or biochemical analysis of the pleural fluid or the presence of loculations (Table 9-3).[22] Multiple tubes are sometimes required to adequately drain the pleural space.
  - Failure to adequately and quickly drain a complicated parapneumonic effusion can lead to organization of the pleural fluid and formation of a thick pleural "rind," which may necessitate surgical removal known as **decortication**.
- **Malignant pleural effusions**[23]
  - **Observation** without invasive interventions may be appropriate for some patients with malignant pleural effusions.
  - **Therapeutic thoracentesis** may improve patient comfort and relieve dyspnea. The rapid removal of more than 1 L of pleural fluid may rarely result in re-expansion pulmonary edema, especially if the lung is unable to re-expand. The subjective response to drainage and the rate of fluid reaccumulation should be monitored.

Repeated thoracenteses are reasonable if they achieve symptomatic relief and if fluid reaccumulation is slow. Unfortunately, 95% of malignant effusions will recur with a median time to recurrence of less than a week. When frequent or repeated thoracentesis is required for effusions that reaccumulate, early consideration should be given to tube drainage with pleurodesis or placement of a chronic indwelling pleural catheter.

- **Chemical pleurodesis** is an effective therapy for recurrent effusions. This treatment is recommended in patients whose symptoms are relieved with initial drainage but who have rapid reaccumulation of fluid.
  - Talc pleurodesis is effective and inexpensive. Fever and hypoxia are common following instillation of talc into the pleural space, and respiratory failure has been described on occasion. Overall efficacy is similar for talc slurry delivered via chest tube versus dry talc insufflated during thoracoscopy. Insufflated dry talc has added benefit for patients with lung or breast cancer.[24]
  - Doxycycline or minocycline can also be instilled into the pleural space via a chest tube. Pain is more prevalent and severe following doxycycline and minocycline than following talc.
  - Bleomycin appears to be less effective and more expensive than other drugs.
  - Systemic analgesics and the administration of lidocaine in the sclerosing agent solution help to decrease the appreciable discomfort associated with the procedure.[25]
  - If the chest tube drainage remains high (>100 mL/d) more than 2 days after the initial pleurodesis, a second dose of the sclerosing agent can be administered.
- **Chronic indwelling pleural catheters** can provide good control of effusion-related symptoms via intermittent drainage. The Pleurx catheter is better at controlling symptoms than doxycycline administered via a chest tube.[26] Furthermore, repeated drainage via a Pleurx catheter leads to pleurodesis in roughly 50% of patients, allowing the catheter to be removed.
- **Pleurectomy or pleural abrasion** requires thoracic surgery and should be reserved for patients with a good prognosis who have had ineffective pleurodesis or inadequate response to chronic pleural drainage.
- **Chemotherapy and mediastinal radiotherapy** may control effusions in responsive tumors, such as lymphoma or small-cell bronchogenic carcinoma, although it has poor efficacy in metastatic carcinoma.

OBSTRUCTIVE SLEEP APNEA–HYPOPNEA SYNDROME

GENERAL PRINCIPLES

Definition

- Obstructive sleep apnea–hypopnea syndrome (OSAHS) is a disorder in which patients experience apneas (cessation of breathing) or hypopneas (shallow breathing) and is associated with excessive daytime somnolence.[27] OSAHS may be associated with consequences such as motor vehicle accidents.[28]

Epidemiology

- Patients with OSAHS have an increased risk of death,[29] mainly due to cardiovascular events.
- Of middle-aged adults, 2%–4% have OSAHS.[30]

Pathophysiology

- Sleep apnea may be **central, obstructive,** or a combination of both.
  - In **central** sleep apnea, the absent central drive to breathe results in no respiratory effort and no airflow, despite adequate airway patency. However, most cases of sleep

apnea are obstructive sleep apnea (OSA) and result from decreased or absent respiratory airflow due to narrowing or collapse of the upper airway. OSA with symptoms of excessive daytime sleepiness results in OSAHS.

DIAGNOSIS

History

- Lack of recognition and diagnosis of OSAHS is a significant problem.
- Habitual loud **snoring** is the most common symptom of OSAHS, although not all people who snore have this syndrome.
- Excessive daytime sleepiness (**daytime hypersomnolence**) is a classic symptom of OSAHS (Table 9-4). Patients may describe falling asleep while driving or having difficulty concentrating at work.
- Patients may also complain of personality changes, intellectual deterioration, morning headaches, automatic behavior, loss of libido, and chronic fatigue.
- Disorders commonly associated with OSA include obesity, nasal obstruction, adenoidal or tonsillar hypertrophy, micrognathia, retrognathia, macroglossia, acromegaly, hypothyroidism, vocal cord paralysis, and bulbar involvement from neuromuscular disease.[31]
- Patients with OSAHS often have **associated cardiovascular disease,** including systemic **hypertension**[32,33] and heart failure and stroke.[34]
  - Recent data have demonstrated an increased risk of **stroke** associated with obstructive sleep apnea.[35]
  - A small study has shown significantly higher glucose and insulin levels in obese OSA patients when compared to matched controls, suggesting a link between diabetes mellitus and OSA.[36]
- Subjective sleepiness can be assessed by a validated scale, such as the **Epworth Sleepiness Scale** (Table 9-5).[37]

Physical Examination

- All patients should have a thorough **nose and throat examination** to detect sources of upper airway obstruction that are surgically correctable (e.g., septal deviation, enlarged tonsils, enlarged uvula), especially if continuous positive airway pressure (CPAP; see nonoperative management) is poorly tolerated.
- The **Mallampati score** is used by anesthesiologists to assess the difficulty of intubation. A grade of I–IV (IV being most severe) is assigned based on the visibility of the tonsils, tonsillar pillars, soft palate, and uvula. Increased severity of obstructive sleep apnea has been associated with increased severity of Mallampati score.[38]

Diagnostic Testing

- The gold standard for the diagnosis of OSAHS is **overnight polysomnography** (PSG or "sleep study")[39] with direct observation by a qualified technician. Sleep studies are typically performed in the outpatient setting.

TABLE 9-4	**Symptoms Associated With Obstructive Sleep Apnea–Hypopnea Syndrome**
Excessive daytime sleepiness	Enuresis
Snoring	Awakening unrefreshed
Nocturnal arousals	Morning headaches
Apneas	Impaired memory and concentration
Nocturnal gasping, grunting, and choking	Irritability and depression
Nocturia	Impotence

TABLE 9-5	Epworth Sleepiness Scale

How likely are you to doze off or fall asleep in the following situations, in contrast to just feeling tired? This refers to your usual way of life in recent times. Even if you have not done some of these things recently, try to work out how they would have affected you. Use the following scale to choose the most appropriate number for each situation:

0 = would never doze   2 = moderate chance of dozing
1 = slight chance of dozing   3 = high chance of dozing

Situation
Sitting and reading
Watching TV
Sitting, inactive, in a public place
Sitting as a passenger in a car for an hour
Lying down in the afternoon
Sitting and talking to someone
Sitting quietly after a lunch without alcohol
Sitting in a car, while stopped for a few minutes in traffic

Note: The scores for each situation are summed to obtain the Epworth score. An Epworth score >10 suggests that significant daytime sleepiness is present.
Adapted from Johns MW. A new method for measuring daytime sleepiness: the Epworth sleepiness scale. *Sleep* 1991;14:541.[37]

- **Typical indications** for a sleep study include snoring with excessive daytime sleepiness, titration of optimal nasal CPAP therapy, and assessment of objective response to therapeutic interventions.
  - Other indications include unexplained pulmonary hypertension, polycythemia, daytime hypercapnia, and poorly controlled hypertension.
- PSG stages sleep using **electroencephalogram (EEG), electromyography,** and **electrooculography,** and assesses respiratory airflow and effort, oxyhemoglobin saturation, heart electrical activity (ECG), and body position.
- The sleep study is analyzed for **sleep staging** and for the frequency of respiratory events, and events are categorized as **obstructive** or **central.**
  - **Obstructive.** Airflow is absent or reduced despite continuous respiratory efforts.
  - **Central.** Airflow and respiratory effort are absent.
- The **apnea–hypopnea index** (AHI) is used to diagnose sleep-disordered breathing and to quantify its severity. All events must have a duration of at least 10 seconds to qualify.
  - **Apnea** is defined as a complete cessation of airflow.
  - **Hypopnea** is defined as a >30% reduction in baseline airflow that must be associated with a 4% decrease in oxygen saturation.[40]
  - The (AHI) is the sum of apneic and hypopneic episodes per hour of sleep. The **respiratory disturbance index** (RDI) may also be reported and can include events that do not qualify for the AHI, such as snore arousals or respiratory effort–related arousals.
  - OSA is present when a sleep study shows an AHI of at least five events per hour in a symptomatic patient.
    - Mild OSA has an AHI of 5–15, moderate OSA has an AHI of 16–30, and severe OSA has an AHI of more than 30.[27] The risk of death, hypertension, and poor neuropsychological functioning rises as the AHI increases.
  - Most sleep studies are performed as **"split studies,"** where the first few hours of the study are diagnostic and the later part of the study is used for CPAP titration if the AHI is moderate to severe. Because some patients only have significant events when lying in certain positions (usually supine) or during rapid eye movement (REM) sleep, these patients may require a complete overnight study for diagnosis and a full second overnight study for initiation of therapy.

Differential Diagnosis

- Patients should be assessed for hypothyroidism.
- In addition to OSA and sleep-related hypoventilation, the differential diagnosis for daytime sleepiness includes sleep deprivation, periodic limb movement disorder, nacrolepsy, and medication side effects.

TREATMENT

- The therapeutic approach to OSAHS depends on the severity of the disease, the underlying medical condition, the cardiopulmonary sequelae, and the expected degree of patient compliance. Treatment must be highly individualized, with special attention to correcting potentially reversible exacerbating factors.

Behavioral

- Weight reduction for the obese is recommended.[41]
- OSAHS patients should avoid use of alcohol, tobacco, and sedatives.

Medications

- Nasal saline and decongestants help with dryness and congestion.
- Modafinil may improve daytime sleepiness in patients with persistent symptoms despite adequate CPAP use.

Nonoperative Management

- **Oxygen supplementation** should be used when needed.
- **Positive airway pressure**
  - **CPAP** is used to deliver air via a nasal or oral mask. Nasal CPAP (nCPAP) is the current treatment of choice for most patients with OSAHS. nCPAP pneumatically splints open the upper airway and prevents collapse. The sleep study determines the positive pressure (cm H_2O) required to optimize airflow. The nCPAP pressure is gradually increased until obstructive events, snoring, and oxygen desaturations are minimized. Some patients, such as those with COPD, also require supplemental oxygen to maintain adequate oxygen saturations (SaO_2 90%). CPAP leads to consolidated sleep and decreased daytime hypersomnolence in almost all patients. Hypertensions, nocturia, peripheral edema, polycythemia, and pulmonary hypertension may improve.
    - Autotitrating or "smart" CPAP machines use flow and pressure transducers to sense airflow patterns and then automatically adjust the CPAP, but their effectiveness has not been well studied.
    - The **compliance rate** with nCPAP is approximately 50%. Compliance can be improved with education, instruction, follow-up, adjustment of the mask for fit and comfort, humidification of the air to decrease dryness, and treatment of nasal or sinus symptoms.
    - Use of a full face mask (oronasal) has not improved compliance compared to the use of nasal masks. However, full face masks are frequently used in patients requiring higher nCPAP pressures, due to air leak through the mouth.
  - **Bilevel positive airway pressure** (BiPAP) can be used to treat patients with OSAHS. BiPAP is more expensive than CPAP and does not improve patient compliance. Patients with intolerance of very high levels of CPAP, a poor response to CPAP, or concomitant alveolar hypoventilation may respond well to noninvasive mechanical ventilation with BiPAP or volume ventilation.
  - **Oral appliances** for mild OSAHS, such as the mandibular repositioning device, aim to increase airway size to improve airflow. The devices can be fixed or adjustable, and most require customized fitting. Many devices have not been well studied.
    - Contraindications: tempromandibular joint disease, bruxism, full dentures, inability to protrude mandible.

Surgery

- Tracheostomy
  - Tracheostomy has been consistently effective in OSAHS patients, but is rarely used since the advent of positive airway pressure therapy.
  - Tracheostomy should be reserved for patients with life-threatening disease (cor pulmonale, arrhythmias, or severe hypoxemia) or significant alveolar hypoventilation that cannot be controlled with other measures.
- Uvulopalatopharyngoplasty
  - Uvulopalatopharyngoplasty (UPPP) is the most common surgical treatment of mild to moderate OSAHS in patients who do not respond to medical therapy.
  - UPPP enlarges the airway by removing tissue from the tonsils, tonsillar pillars, uvula, and posterior palate. UPPP may be complicated by change in voice, nasopharyngeal stenosis, foreign body sensation, and velopharyngeal insufficiency with associated nasal regurgitation during swallowing, and CPAP tolerance problems.
  - The success rate of UPPP for treatment of OSAHS is only approximately 50%, when defined as a 50% reduction of the AHI, and improvements related to UPPP may diminish over time.[42] Thus, UPPP is considered a second-line treatment for patients with mild to moderate OSAHS who cannot successfully use CPAP and who have retropalatal obstruction.
- In experienced centers, other staged procedures for obstructive sleep apnea can be performed, including **genioglossus advancement, hyoid myotomy with suspension,** and **maxillomandibular advancement.**[43]

Special Therapy

- Concomitant conditions (e.g., COPD, hypertension, hypothyroidism) should be treated in the standard fashion.

Referrals

- Patients with risk factors and symptoms or sequelae of OSAHS should be referred to a sleep specialist and sleep laboratory for further evaluation.

Complications

- When OSAHS is associated with disorders such as obesity and chronic lung disease, patients may develop hypoxemia, hypercapnia, polycythemia, and cor pulmonale.[44]
- All noninvasive positive pressure or mechanical ventilation devices may induce dryness of the airway, nasal congestion, rhinorrhea, epistaxis, skin reactions to the mask, nasal bridge abrasions, and aerophagia.

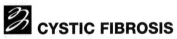 CYSTIC FIBROSIS

GENERAL PRINCIPLES

Definition

- **Cystic fibrosis (CF)** is an autosomal-recessive disorder caused by mutations of the cystic fibrosis transmembrane conductance regulator (**CFTR**), a gene located on chromosome 7.

Epidemiology

- CF is the most common lethal genetic disease in whites, with an incidence of 1 in 3,200 live births in the United States.[45] Although CF is less common in nonwhites, the diagnosis needs to be considered in patients of diverse backgrounds.
- The diagnosis of CF is typically made during childhood, but 8% of patients are diagnosed during adolescence or adulthood.[46]

- With improved therapy, the median survival has been extended to approximately 35 years.[47]
  - Predictors of increased mortality include age, female gender, low weight, low forced expiratory volume in 1 second (FEV$_1$), pancreatic insufficiency, diabetes mellitus, infection with *Burkholderia cepacia*, and the number of acute exacerbations.[48]

Pathophysiology

- CFTR normally regulates and participates in the transport of electrolytes across epithelial cell and intracellular membranes.[49] The primary pulmonary manifestations of disease are thought to be related to abnormal electrolyte transport in the airway, which results in desiccated airway secretions and impaired mucociliary clearance. Secretions become infected, and a vicious cycle of infection, inflammation, and chronic airway obstruction ensues, resulting in bronchiectasis, chronic infection, and ultimately premature death.[50]

DIAGNOSIS

- The diagnosis of CF is based on a compatible clinical and family history and persistently elevated concentrations of sweat chloride, two known disease-causing CF mutations, or nasal transepithelial potential difference measurements that are typical of CF. Atypical patients may lack classic symptoms and signs or have normal sweat tests. Although genotyping may assist in the diagnosis, it alone cannot establish or rule out the diagnosis of CF, and the initial test of choice remains the sweat test.

Clinical Presentation

- **Pulmonary symptoms** lead to consideration of the diagnosis of CF in 50% of cases.[46] In almost all patients, chronic (sino) pulmonary disease eventually develops, most notable for bronchiectasis and chronic airflow obstruction. Symptoms initially include cough and purulent sputum production. Dyspnea ensues as the disease progresses. Acute pulmonary disease exacerbations may lead to significant deterioration and subsequent hospitalization. Isolation of mucoid variants of *Pseudomonas aeruginosa* from the respiratory tract occurs frequently.
- **Extrapulmonary manifestations** of CF include pancreatic exocrine insufficiency, which is seen in 90% of patients and leads to fat malabsorption and malnutrition. Pancreatitis occasionally develops. Gastrointestinal (GI) complications include distal intestinal obstruction syndrome, volvulus, intussusception, and rectal prolapse. CF also affects the endocrine pancreatic (diabetes mellitus in approximately 20% of adults), the hepatobiliary system (fatty liver, cirrhosis, portal hypertension, cholelithiasis, and cholecystitis), the genitourinary (male infertility and epididymitis), and the skeletal (retardation of growth, osteoarthropathy, osteopenia) systems. Digital clubbing appears in childhood in virtually all symptomatic patients. Although fertility may be decreased in women with CF secondary to thickened cervical mucus, many women with CF have tolerated pregnancy well.[51]

Laboratory Studies

- **Skin sweat testing** with a standardized quantitative pilocarpine iontophoresis method remains the gold standard for the diagnosis of CF.
  - **A sweat chloride concentration of >60 mmol/L** is consistent with the diagnosis of CF. However, the diagnosis requires an elevated sweat chloride concentration on two separate occasions in a patient with a typical phenotype or with a history of CF in a sibling. Borderline sweat test results (40–60 mmol/L sweat chloride) or nondiagnostic results in the setting of high clinical suspicion should also lead to repeat sweat testing, nasal potential difference testing, or genetic testing. Sweat testing should be performed at a CF care center to ensure reliability of results. Abnormal sweat chloride concentrations are rarely detected in non-CF patients (e.g., Addison disease and untreated hypothyroidism).

- **Genetic tests** have detected more than 1,000 putative CF mutations.
  - Two recessive genes must be abnormal to cause CF. The most commonly encountered CF mutation is the $\Delta F508$ CFTR mutation, which is present in approximately 70% of alleles in affected individuals.
  - Commercially available probes identify more than 90% of the abnormal genes in a white Northern European population, although they test for only a minority of the known CF genes.
- **Sputum cultures** typically identify *P. aeruginosa* or *Staphylococcus aureus*, or both, and **sputum sensitivity testing** should direct therapy.
- **Testing for malabsorption due to pancreatic exocrine insufficiency** is often not formally performed, because clinical evidence (the presence of foul-smelling, bulky, and loose stools; **low fat-soluble vitamin levels [vitamins A, D, and E]**; and a **prolonged prothrombin time** [vitamin K dependent]) and a clear response to pancreatic enzyme treatment are usually considered sufficient for the diagnosis.
- Tests that identify chronic **sinusitis** or **infertility**, especially obstructive azoospermia in men, would also support the diagnosis of CF.
- Monitoring of electrolytes is indicated in patients with a history of electrolyte abnormalities or renal insufficiency.

Imaging and Diagnostic Testing

- Typically, **chest radiography** eventually shows enlarged lung volumes, with cystic lung disease and bronchiectasis, especially in the upper lobes.
- **Pulmonary function tests** eventually show expiratory airflow obstruction with increased residual volume and total lung capacity. Impairment of alveolar gas exchange may be present as well, progressing to oxyhemoglobin desaturation with exertion, hypoxemia, and hypercapnia.
- **High-resolution CT scan** may be helpful in evaluating patients with early or mild disease.

Pathologic Findings

- Respiratory tract disease is characterized by neutrophil-dominated airway inflammation with the development of bronchiectasis. Airway obstruction may lead to focal pneumonia and areas of cavitation within the lung.
- Interstitial fibrosis is seen with more advanced disease.

Differential Diagnosis

- **Primary ciliary dyskinesia** or **immunoglobulin deficiency** may lead to bronchiectasis, sinusitis, and infertility. However, limited GI symptoms and normal sweat electrolytes distinguish these diseases from CF.
- **Shwachman syndrome,** consisting of pancreatic insufficiency and cyclic neutropenia, may also lead to lung disease, but sweat chloride concentrations are normal and the neutropenia is distinguishing.
- Men with **Young syndrome** have bronchiectasis, sinusitis, and azoospermia, but this disorder only has mild respiratory symptoms, lacks GI symptoms, and has normal sweat chloride levels.

TREATMENT

- CF therapy aims to improve quality of life and functioning, decrease the number of exacerbations and hospitalizations, avoid complications associated with therapy, and decrease mortality. A comprehensive program addressing multiple organ/system derangements, as provided at CF care centers, is recommended. The greatest number of adults with CF have significant lung disease and a large portion of therapy is focused on clearing pulmonary secretions and controlling infection.[52]

Behavioral

- Avoidance of irritating inhaled fumes, dusts, or chemicals including second-hand smoke is recommended.

Medications

- **Inhaled bronchodilators** such as β-adrenergic agonists (albuterol metered-dose inhaler [MDI], two to four puffs bid–qid; salmeterol or formoterol, one dry powder inhalation bid) are used to treat the reversible components of airflow obstruction and facilitate mucus clearance (see Chronic Obstructive Pulmonary Disease). These agents are contraindicated in the rare patient with associated paradoxical deterioration of airflow after their use.
- **Airway clearance** for pulmonary disease may be accomplished by various airway clearance techniques, including postural drainage with chest percussion and vibration, with or without mechanical devices (flutter valves, high-frequency chest oscillation vests, low- and high-pressure positive expiratory pressure devices, etc.), and breathing and coughing exercises.
- **Recombinant human deoxyribonuclease (Dnase, dornase-α, Pulmozyme)** digests extracellular DNA, decreasing the viscoelasticity of the sputum. It improves pulmonary function and decreases the incidence of respiratory tract infections that require parenteral antibiotics.[53,54] The recommended dose is 2.5 mg (one ampule) per day inhaled using a jet nebulizer. Adverse effects may include pharyngitis, laryngitis, rash, chest pain, and conjunctivitis.
- **Hypertonic saline.** A recent study showed fewer exacerbations and possible improvement in lung function in patients treated with 4 mL of inhaled 7% saline twice daily. Inhaled bronchodilators should be administered prior to treatments to avoid treatment-induced bronchospasm.
- **Antibiotics.** *P. aeruginosa* is the most frequent pulmonary pathogen. A combination of an IV semisynthetic penicillin, a third- or fourth-generation cephalosporin, or a quinolone and an aminoglycoside is typically recommended during acute exacerbations. Sputum culture sensitivities should guide therapy.
  - The duration of antibiotic therapy is dictated by the clinical response. At least 14 days of antibiotics is typically given to treat an exacerbation. Home IV antibiotic therapy is common, but hospitalization may allow better access to comprehensive therapy and diagnostic testing. PO antibiotics are recommended only for mild exacerbations.
  - The use of chronic or intermittent prophylactic antibiotics can be considered, especially in patients with frequent recurrent exacerbations, but antimicrobial resistance may develop. Inhaled aerosolized tobramycin (300 mg nebulized bid, 28 days on alternating with 28 days off, using appropriate nebulizer and compressor) improves pulmonary function, decreases the density of *P. aeruginosa*, and decreases the risk of hospitalization.[55] Voice alteration (13%) and tinnitus (3%) are potential adverse events associated with long-term inhaled tobramycin.[55]
- Patients with CF have atypical **pharmacokinetics** and often require higher drug doses at more frequent intervals. In patients with CF, for example, cefepime is often dosed at 2 g IV q8h and gentamicin or tobramycin is often dosed at 3 mg/kg IV q8h (aiming for peak levels of 10 mg/mL and trough levels of <2 mg/mL). Once-daily aminoglycoside dosing should be guided by pharmacokinetic testing.
  - Monitoring levels (peaks and troughs) of drugs such as aminoglycosides helps to ensure therapeutic levels and decrease the risk of toxicity (see Antibacterial Agents, Chapter 12, Antimicrobials).
- **Anti-inflammatory therapy.** The anti-inflammatory effects of short courses of glucocorticoid therapy may be helpful to some patients, but long-term therapy should be avoided to minimize the side effects that include glucose intolerance, osteopenia, and growth retardation. High-dose ibuprofen has been used as a chronic anti-inflammatory in patients with mild impairment of lung function.
- **Azithromycin.** Recent studies have shown that chronic PO azithromycin (500 mg PO Mon, Wed, Fri) mildly improves lung function and reduces days in the hospital for

treatment of respiratory exacerbations in patients who are chronically infected with *P. aeruginosa.*[56]

- **Pulmonary rehabilitation** that includes exercise rehabilitation may improve functioning.
- **Oxygen therapy** is indicated based on standard recommendations (see Chronic Obstructive Pulmonary Disease). Rest and exercise oxygen assessments should be performed as clinically indicated.
- **Noninvasive ventilation** for chronic respiratory failure due to CF-related bronchiectasis has not been clearly demonstrated to provide a survival benefit, although it may provide symptomatic relief or it can be used as a bridge to transplantation.

Surgery

- **Lung transplantation**
  - The majority of patients with CF die from pulmonary disease. FEV_1 is a strong predictor of mortality[57] and has been helpful in deciding when to refer patients for lung transplantation. However, other factors such as marked alveolar gas exchange abnormalities (resting hypoxemia or hypercapnia), evidence of PH, or increased frequency or severity of pulmonary exacerbations should also be considered when deciding on referral for transplantation.
- **Massive hemoptysis** is usually controlled with bronchial artery embolization. Surgical lung resection is rarely needed.

Management of Extrapulmonary Disease

- Pancreatic insufficiency is managed with **pancreatic enzyme supplementation.**
  - Enzyme dose should be titrated to achieve one to two semisolid stools per day, and to maintain adequate growth and nutrition. Enzymes are taken immediately before meals and snacks. Dosing of pancreatic enzymes should be initiated at 500 Units lipase/kg/meal and should not exceed 2,500 Units lipase/kg/meal. High doses (6,000 Units lipase/kg/meal) have been associated with chronic intestinal strictures.[58] **Generic** enzyme substitutes may not provide adequate lipase needed for absorption. Gastric acid suppression may enhance enzyme activity.
- **Vitamin supplementation** is recommended in extrapulmonary disease, especially with fat-soluble vitamins that are not well absorbed in the setting of pancreatic insufficiency. Vitamins A, D, E, and K can all be taken orally on a regular basis (see Table 2-4 in Chapter 2). Iron-deficiency anemia requires iron supplementation.
- **Treatment of CF-related diabetes mellitus** is usually accomplished with **insulin** (see Chapter 21, Diabetes Mellitus and Related Disorders), but typical diabetic dietary restrictions are liberalized (high-calorie diet with unrestricted fat) to meet the increased energy requirements of patients with CF and to encourage appropriate growth and weight maintenance.
- **Osteopenia** screening should be routinely performed on patients with CF, and if present may be managed with calcium, vitamin D supplementation, and bisphosphonate therapy as clinically indicated.[59]
- **Sinusitis regimens** are used in the typical fashion for extrapulmonary disease. Many patients will benefit from chronic nasal steroid administration. Patients whose symptoms cannot be controlled with medical management may benefit from functional endoscopic sinus surgery and nasal polypectomy.

Risk Management

- **Yearly influenza vaccination** (0.5 mL IM) decreases the incidence of infection and subsequent deterioration.[60] Pneumovax (0.5 mL IM) may also provide benefit (see Appendix C, Immunizations and Postexposure Therapies).

Complications

- Other pulmonary complications of CF may include **allergic bronchopulmonary aspergillosis, massive hemoptysis,** and **pneumothorax.**

CHRONIC OBSTRUCTIVE PULMONARY DISEASE

GENERAL PRINCIPLES

Definition

- COPD is a mostly **preventable** and always **treatable** disease state characterized by expiratory airflow limitation that is not fully reversible. The airflow limitation is usually progressive and associated with an abnormal inflammatory response of the lungs to noxious particles or gases (e.g., cigarette smoking). COPD also causes adverse systemic consequences. Of note, this COPD definition does not specifically mention the terms **emphysema** and **chronic bronchitis,** though these diseases are typically used to help classify two types of patients that have COPD.
    - **Emphysema** is defined pathologically as enlargement of the distal airways with destruction of the acinus, without associated fibrosis.
    - **Chronic bronchitis** may be defined clinically as cough, productive of at least 2 tablespoons of sputum (not postnasal drip) on most days of 3 consecutive months in 2 consecutive years, in the absence of other lung diseases, such as bronchiectasis.
- Patients with (a) emphysema on CT scan and normal spirometry or (b) symptoms of chronic bronchitis and normal spirometry do not have COPD according to the current definition of COPD. Also, patients may have expiratory airflow obstruction due to conditions other than emphysema or chronic bronchitis, such as bronchiectasis or sarcoidosis.

Epidemiology

- Chronic respiratory diseases and allied conditions mainly due to COPD affect over 15 million people and are the fourth leading cause of death.
- In the year 2000, the number of women dying from COPD exceeded the number of men dying from COPD for the first time.
- The incidence of COPD is increasing.

Etiology

- Most cases of COPD are attributable to cigarette smoking, especially in developed countries. Though only a minority of cigarette smokers develop clinically significant COPD, a much higher proportion develop abnormal lung function.
- Environmental (e.g., wood-burning stove) and occupational dusts, fumes, gases, and chemicals are other known risk factors for COPD.

Pathophysiology

- In the setting of defective or overwhelmed normal protective and repair mechanisms of the lungs, exposure to inhaled noxious particles and gases may produce COPD.
- Processes important in the pathogenesis of COPD include inflammation, imbalance of proteinases and antiproteinases in the lung, apoptosis, and oxidative stress.
- Pathologic changes characteristic of COPD are found in the central airways, peripheral airways, lung parenchyma, and pulmonary vasculature.
- Dilation and destruction of the terminal airways, structural changes in the airway wall due to inflammation, airway edema, and mucus hypersecretion contribute to the development of COPD.
- Physiologic changes of the lungs characteristic of COPD include mucus hypersecretion, ciliary dysfunction, airflow limitation, pulmonary hyperinflation, alveolar gas exchange abnormalities, and pulmonary vascular disease.
- COPD has systemic consequences, such as skeletal muscle dysfunction, that may contribute to limitation of exercise capacity and decline of health status.

- COPD exacerbations lead to potentially reversible significant decrement in pulmonary function, especially alveolar gas exchange, that may progress to acute respiratory failure requiring mechanical ventilatory support.
  - The most common identifiable causes of acute COPD exacerbations are infections, typically due to viruses and less often due to bacteria.

DIAGNOSIS

Clinical Presentation and History

- Though most patients seek medical attention for the hallmark symptom of dyspnea, clinicians should also assess for the presence and severity of cough, sputum production, wheezing, and chest discomfort.
- Dyspnea on exertion gradually progresses over time.
- Significant nocturnal symptoms should lead to a search for comorbidities such as gastroesophageal reflux, congestive heart failure, or sleep-disordered breathing.
- Most patients with COPD have smoked cigarettes, and clinicians should quantify exposure to environmental and occupational risk factors.
- α_1-Antitrypsin deficiency should be considered in a patient with emphysema who has (a) a minimal smoking history, (b) early-onset COPD (e.g., younger than 45 years), (c) a family history of lung disease, or (d) a predominance of lower lobe emphysema.
- A variety of insults may provoke a COPD exacerbation, which consists of some combination of increased dyspnea, cough, sputum purulence, and sputum volume, often associated with wheezing.
- Weight loss occurs in patients with end-stage COPD, but other etiologies, such as malignancy, should be sought.

Physical Examination

- Until significant impairment of lung function occurs, physical signs of COPD have low sensitivity and specificity.
- Patients with severe or very severe COPD show prolonged exhalation, use of accessory muscles of respiration, chest hyperresonance to percussion, enlarged thoracic volume, and decreased breath sounds.
- Expiratory wheezing may or may not be present.
- Signs of cor pulmonale may accompany very severe disease (see Pulmonary Hypertension).
- Clubbing is not a feature of COPD, and its presence should prompt an evaluation for etiologies such as lung cancer.
- Marked tachypnea, cyanosis, and signs of increased work of breathing (e.g., paradoxical abdominal motion) may characterize a severe COPD exacerbation and may signify the need for assisted ventilation.

Laboratory Studies

- A baseline **ABG** is often recommended for assessing patients with severe or very severe COPD, and annual monitoring could be considered.
  - ABGs should be obtained during serious acute exacerbations of COPD because measurement of oxyhemoglobin saturation with a pulse oximeter neglects to provide information about alveolar ventilation (i.e., arterial carbon dioxide tension, or $PaCO_2$).
  - ABGs detect acute and chronic hypercapnia, and the development of acute respiratory acidosis may signal acute respiratory failure and the need for assisted ventilation.
  - An elevated venous HCO_3 may signify the presence of a chronic respiratory acidosis.
  - An elevated hemoglobin (i.e., polycythemia) may signify chronic hypoxemia and inadequate supplemental use.

Imaging

- **Chest radiographs** are not sensitive for the diagnosis of COPD, but they are useful for evaluating for alternative diagnoses.
  - With increasing disease severity, patients develop thoracic hyperinflation, with flattening of the diaphragm and increased retrosternal/retrocardiac air spaces, and hyperlucency with diminished vascular markings. Bullae may be visible.
  - Though emphysema is usually most prominent in the upper lung zones, patients with a_1-antitrypsin deficiency and emphysema typically shows a basilar predominance.
- Chest radiographs are valuable during an acute exacerbation to exclude such complications as pneumonia, pneumothorax, or congestive heart failure.
- Chest radiographs may detect other conditions associated with tobacco smoking and COPD, such as lung cancer.
- **Chest CT** is not routinely used for diagnosing COPD, though it may help evaluate for other diagnoses and it is used in the evaluation of patients for lung volume reduction surgery and lung transplantation.

Physiologic Testing

- **Pulmonary function testing,** especially spirometry, is the main method for diagnosing COPD, although it has limited utility during an acute illness in a patient already diagnosed with COPD.
- A diagnosis of COPD requires the presence of expiratory airflow obstruction, defined as a low 1-second forced expiratory volume/forced vital capacity ratio (FEV_1/FVC <0.7). The FEV_1 defines the severity of the expiratory airflow obstruction.
  - The decrement in the FEV_1 is often used to assess the clinical course and response to therapy, and it is an important predictor of prognosis and mortality in patients with COPD (Table 9-6). When the FEV_1 falls to <1 L, the 5-year survival is approximately 50%.

TABLE 9-6	**GOLD Classification of Severity of COPD**
Stage	**Characteristics**
0: At risk	Normal spirometry
	Chronic symptoms (cough, sputum production)
I: Mild COPD	FEV_1/FVC <70%
	FEV_1 ≥80% predicted
	With or without chronic symptoms (cough, sputum production)
II: Moderate COPD	FEV_1/FVC <70%
	50% ≤FEV_1 <80% predicted
	With or without chronic symptoms (cough, sputum production)
III: Severe COPD	FEV_1/FVC <70%
	30% ≤FEV_1 <50% predicted
	With or without chronic symptoms (cough, sputum production)
IV: Very severe COPD	FEV_1/FVC <70%
	FEV_1 <30% predicted or FEV_1 <50% predicted plus chronic respiratory failure[a]

Classification based on postbronchodilator FEV_1.
COPD, chronic obstructive pulmonary disease; FEV_1, forced expiratory volume in 1 second; FVC, forced vital capacity.
[a]Respiratory failure, arterial partial pressure of oxygen (PaO_2) <8.0 kPa (60 mm Hg) with or without arterial partial pressure of CO_2 ($PaCO_2$) >6.7 kPa (50 mm Hg) while breathing air at sea level.
Source: NIH/NHLBI. *Global initiative for chronic obstructive lung disease* ("GOLD"), April 2001, updated July 2003. NIH Publication 2701. Available at: www.goldcopd.com.

- Routine monitoring of spirometry provides clinical and prognostic information that may assist with evaluation for disability and referral for lung volume reduction surgery and lung transplantation.
- Spirometry may help assist in the evaluation of worsened symptoms of unclear etiology.
- Smoking cessation for more than a year leads to an improvement in lung function, and an FEV_1 decline similar to that of nonsmokers.[61]
- Total lung capacity (TLC), functional residual capacity (FRC), and residual volume (RV) increase to supranormal values in patients with COPD, indicating lung hyperinflation and air trapping.
- Emphysema and many other diseases produce a reduction in the diffusing capacity of the lung (D_{LCO}).

Differential Diagnosis

- Although emphysema and chronic bronchitis are the main diseases associated with COPD, asthma (see Chapter 10, Allergy and Immunology), bronchiectasis, obliterative bronchiolitis, airway tumors, sarcoidosis, tuberculosis, lung damage from previous infections, eosinophilic granuloma, and lymphangioleiomyomatosis may also produce expiratory airflow obstruction.
- Concomitant illnesses such as bronchogenic carcinoma, tuberculosis, and sleep-disordered breathing may also worsen symptoms and signs of COPD.

TREATMENT

- Treatment of COPD should include ongoing assessments, monitoring, education, and reduction of risk factors. Management of COPD should focus on both long-term goals and treatment of acute exacerbations.
- **Long-term management**[62] of patients with COPD should aim to improve quality of life (e.g., relieve symptoms, increase functioning), decrease the frequency and the severity of acute exacerbations, slow the progression of disease, prevent morbidity, and prolong survival.
    - Of all chronic medical therapies, smoking cessation and the correction of hypoxemia with supplemental oxygen produce the greatest survival benefit. Though medications have not been shown to modify the long-term decline in lung function, they may improve quality of life and decrease the frequency and the severity of acute exacerbations.

Medications

- **Inhaled bronchodilators** (Table 9-7)
    - Inhaled bronchodilators, the foundation of COPD pharmacotherapy, work by decreasing or preventing an increases in airway smooth muscle tone. The two main classes of inhaled bronchodilators consist of β-agonists and anticholinergics. Short-acting agents have a duration of action of 4–6 hours and long-acting β-agonists have a duration of action of 8–12 hours; long-acting anticholinergic therapy lasts more than 24 hours.
    - For patients with mild airflow obstruction and intermittent symptoms, a single short-acting or long-acting bronchodilator will likely provide adequate symptom relief, though short-acting agents should be used for acute symptom relief.
    - Patients with at least moderate airflow obstruction would likely derive benefit from long-acting bronchodilator therapy. A short-acting agent should also be used for acute symptom relief.
    - **Combination therapy** (β-agonist and anticholinergic) should be used in patients that did not achieve adequate relief with one class of drugs.
    - Use of an **MDI** with a **spacer device or reservoir** is as effective as delivery of the drug by a **nebulizer** in most patients.[63] To ensure effective bronchodilator delivery, health care providers should assess patient technique and provide instruction.

TABLE 9-7	Inhaled Drugs for the Treatment of Chronic Obstructive Pulmonary Disease	

Generic name	Brand name	Dose
Sympathomimetic bronchodilators [a]		
Albuterol		MDI: 90 mcg
		Nebulizer: 0.5% solution, 2.5–5.0 mg; (0.5–1.0 mL) diluted in 1.02.5 mL of NS
		Rotocaps inhalation powder: 200 mcg
Metaproterenol		MDI: 650 mcg
		5% solution, 0.2–0.3 mL diluted in 25 mL of NS
		MDI: 200 mcg
Pirbuterol acetate		Autohaler: 200 mcg
Bitolterol mesylate		MDI: 370 mcg
		Nebulizer: 0.2% solution
Formoterol fumarate[b]	Foradil	Inhalation powder: 1 cap = 12 mcg
Salmeterol xinafoate[b]	Serevent	Diskus: 50 mcg
Arformoterol tartrate[b]	Brorana	Nebulizer 15 mcg/2 mL
Combination drugs		
Ipratropium/albuterol	Combivent	MDI: ipratropium, 18 mcg/albuterol, 103 mcg/puff
	DuoNeb	Nebulizer: 0.5 mg ipratropium, 2.5 mg albuterol
Salmeterol/fluticasone[b]	Advair	Diskus (inhalation powder):
		Fluticasone, 100 mcg/salmeterol, 50 mcg/inhalation
		Fluticasone, 250 mcg/salmeterol, 50 mcg/inhalation
		Fluticasone, 500 mcg/salmeterol, 50 mcg/inhalation
Anticholinergic bronchodilators[a]		
Atropine	Atropine	Nebulizer: 0.025 mg/kg diluted to 35 mL with saline
Glycopyrrolate	Robinul	Nebulizer: 0.3–2.0 mg; 1.5–10.0 mL
Ipratropium bromide	Atrovent	MDI: 18 mcg
		Nebulizer: 0.02% solution 2.5 mL
Tiotropium bromide	Spiriva	HandiHaler: 18 mcg/capsule
Corticosteroids[c]		See Table 10-5

MDI, metered-dose inhaler.
[a]Usual dosing qid, although more frequent dosing can be used during acute exacerbations.
[b]Maximum frequency q12h.
[c]Once daily.

- β_2-Adrenergic agonists
  - **Short-acting inhaled β_2-adrenergic agonists** are used at two to four puffs bid–qid and PRN.
  - Long-acting β-agonists salmeterol, formoterol or arformoterol are dosed twice daily, and may limit the need for short-acting inhaler use.
  - β_2-Adrenergic agonists may cause tremor, nervousness, tachycardia, tachyarrhythmias, and hypokalemia.
- Anticholinergic agents
  - **Short-acting inhaled anticholinergic agents** are used at two to four puffs bid–qid and PRN. Ipratropium bromide and glycopyrrolate are available in solution for nebulization.
  - Long-acting anticholinergic tiotropium is dosed as one inhalation once daily. Short-acting anticholinergic therapy is usually discontinued with long-acting anticholinergic therapy, since minimal additional benefit is expected, side effects may increase, and use of two inhaled anticholinergic agents has not been well studied.
  - Anticholinergic agents often cause dry mouth and may result in bladder outlet obstruction or an exacerbation of acute angle glaucoma.

- Combination agents
  - Compared to short-acting β-agonist or anticholinergic therapy, combination short-acting therapy has equivalent or fewer side effects and greater and more sustained improvements in FEV_1.
  - Short-acting β-agonists and anticholinergic agents can be nebulized together or used together in an MDI (Combivent) for synergistic bronchodilation.[64]
  - The combination of the long-acting β-agonist salmeterol with fluticasone (Advair) performs better than either agent alone for chronic therapy.[65]
  - Short-term treatment with a combined inhaled glucocorticoid and a long-acting β-agonist produces greater control of lung function and symptoms than combined inhaled short-acting anticholinergic and β-agonist therapy.
- Methylxanthines
  - Patients not responding adequately to inhaled bronchodilator therapy may benefit from treatment with oral methylxanthines (theophylline), though inhaled bronchodilator therapy is preferred due to the potential toxicity of systemic methylxanthine therapy.
  - Sustained-release theophylline is dosed once or twice a day. Levels should be maintained below 20 mg/L (between 6 and 12 mg/L) to avoid toxicity.
  - Theophylline and a number of other drugs interact, which may increase or decrease the dosage requirements and the incidence of toxicity.
  - Continued inhalation of tobacco smoke lowers theophylline levels.
  - IV methylxanthines have a higher risk of acute side effects than the oral form.
  - Patients with severe COPD may experience significant clinical deterioration with discontinuation of theophylline.
  - If symptoms of **toxicity** develop, including anxiety, tremor, headache, insomnia, nausea, vomiting, dyspepsia, tachycardia, and tachyarrhythmias, the drug should be stopped and a level should be measured. Toxic levels may lead to seizures and death.
- Glucocorticoids
  - Inhaled steroids improve lung function in patients with COPD, though they have not been shown to decrease the rate of decline. Inhaled steroids also reduce the frequency of exacerbations and improve quality of life in patients with COPD who experience frequent exacerbations, especially patients with severe airflow obstruction.[66] Inhaled steroids are clearly indicated in patients with asthma combined with COPD, though their use in patients with COPD and bronchial hyperresponsiveness is less clear. Withdrawal of inhaled steroids in patients with COPD may lead to an exacerbation.
  - Systemic oral glucocorticoids are not recommended for the long-term management of COPD. However, oral steroids are sometimes used in patients with severe disease who are not responding to all other therapies. If used, chronic oral steroid therapy should be minimized to lessen the risk and severity of side effects.
- Vaccinations
  - Influenza and pneumococcal vaccinations reduce serious illness and mortality in patients with COPD.
- Intravenous α-1 antitrypsin (A1AT) augmentation therapy may benefit select patients with A1AT deficiency and COPD.
- For standard therapy of stable COPD, antibiotics, mucolytics, antioxidants, immunoregulators, antitussives, vasodilators, respiratory stimulants, narcotics, and leukotriene inhibitors have not shown significant benefit.

Additional Therapy

- **Supplemental oxygen therapy** has been shown to decrease mortality and improve physical and mental functioning in hypoxemic patients with COPD.
  - A **room air resting arterial blood gas** is the gold standard test for determining the need for supplemental oxygen. Pulse oximetry may be useful for routine checks after a baseline oxyhemoglobin saturation (SpO_2) is assessed and compared for accuracy with the measured arterial oxyhemoglobin saturation (SaO_2). Oxygen therapy is indicated for any patient with a PaO_2 of 55 mm Hg or less or an SaO_2 of 88% or less. If a patient has a PaO_2 of 59 mm Hg or less or an SaO_2 of 89% or less and

evidence of PH, polycythemia (hematocrit >55%), or heart failure, oxygen therapy is indicated.

- Supplemental oxygen requirements are typically greatest during exertion and least at rest while awake. Patients who require supplemental oxygen during exertion often need it during sleep. Although the exact amount of supplemental oxygen required during sleep might be measured with pulse oximetry, it is reasonable to initially estimate the amount needed during sleep by setting the oxygen flow rate at 1 L/min greater than that required during rest while awake.
- The **oxygen prescription** should state the delivery system required (compressed gas, liquid, or concentrator) and the required oxygen flow rates (L/min) for rest, sleep, and exercise.
- Stable patients receiving long-term oxygen therapy should undergo routine re-evaluation no less than once a year.[67]

- **Pulmonary rehabilitation** is defined by the American Thoracic Society as a multidisciplinary program of care for patients with chronic respiratory impairment that is individually tailored and designed to optimize physical and social performance and autonomy.[68]
  - Pulmonary rehabilitation improves exercise tolerance and dyspnea, and may improve quality of life and decrease the frequency of exacerbations in patients with COPD.
  - Patients with COPD who should be referred to a comprehensive rehabilitation program include those who have dyspnea have reduced exercise tolerance or poor functional status despite optimal medical management.
- **Chest physiotherapy** and mechanical clearance devices may improve clearance of secretions in patients with copious respiratory secretions (>50 mL/d), although they are not routinely recommended during acute COPD exacerbations.
  - Chest percussion or postural drainage may produce or worsen hypoxemia.
- **Psychoactive drugs**
  - Patients with COPD often suffer from **depression** and **anxiety**.
  - Low-dose benzodiazepines (e.g., alprazolam 0.25—0.5 mg PO tid) produce significant anxiety reduction.
  - Because of their respiratory depressant properties, benzodiazepines and narcotics should be used with caution in patients with COPD.
- **Smoking cessation.** In patients with COPD, abstinence from tobacco smoking produces a marked reduction in the rate of lung function decline and may improve survival.[61]
  - Tobacco dependence warrants repeated treatment until patients become abstinent.
  - Most smokers fail initial attempts at smoking cessation, and relapse reflects the chronic nature of the dependence and not the failure of the patient or the physician.
  - A multimodality approach is recommended to optimize quit rates. Standard interventions include (a) counseling (on the preventable health risks of smoking, providing advice to stop smoking, and encouraging patients to make further attempts to stop smoking even after previous failures), (b) providing smoking cessation materials to patients, and (c) pharmacotherapy.[69]
  - **Pharmacotherapy** doubles the quit rate. Pharmacotherapy is most effective when used in **conjunction with formal smoking cessation programs** or close medical follow-up.[70]
  - **Strategies to help the patient who is willing to quit smoking** include **asking** about tobacco use, **advising** quitting, **assessing** willingness to quit, **assisting** the patient in quitting, and **arranging** follow-up.[71]
  - Current U.S. Food and Drug Administration–approved medications for smoking cessation include nicotine replacement therapy, bupropion, and varenicline.
    - **Nicotine replacement.** Heavy smokers typically require **combination therapy** with the long-acting patch and a short-acting nicotine product to decrease cravings and improve efficacy. Nicotine products are typically for 12 weeks, followed by tapering over 6–12 weeks. **Contraindications** to nicotine use include significant vascular disease, pregnancy, breast-feeding, and allergy to the drug. Nicotine therapy **side effects** may include headache, insomnia, nightmares, nausea, dizziness, and blurred vision.

- Nicotine-containing chewing gum (2-mg or 4-mg pieces). One piece is chewed for a few minutes until a tingling sensation arises, and then it is "parked" between the cheek and the gums for 20–30 minutes until the craving returns, repeating the process, as needed, up to 60 mg/d.
- The **transdermal nicotine patch** regimen usually consists of 6 weeks of a high-dose patch (21 mg/d) followed by 2–4 weeks of an intermediate-dose patch (14 mg/d) and then 2–4 weeks of a low-dose patch (7 mg/d). Nonheavy smokers often do not require nicotine patch therapy during sleep. Patients should replace patches once a day, and they should rotate sites. Redness and pruritus at the patch site might develop.
- The **nicotine nasal spray** regimen consists of one (0.5 mg) spray to each nostril q1–2h PRN, not to exceed five doses per hour or 40 doses per day. Side effects may also include sneezing, excess lacrimation, and cough.
- The **nicotine inhaler** (10 mg/cartridge) is used over 20 minutes, 6–16 cartridges per day. Side effects may also include cough and irritation of the mouth.
- **Nicotine lozenges** (2 mg) are used q1–2h, not to exceed 20 lozenges over 24 hours, and weaned over many weeks. Patients who smoke their first cigarette within 30 minutes of waking should use the 4-mg strength.
- **Sublingual nicotine tablet** (2 mg) are used twice an hour, not to exceed 40 tabs per day.

■ **Nonnicotine pharmacotherapy. Bupropion hydrochloride SR** (Zyban) started 1 week before quitting smoking (150 mg PO daily for 3 days, then 150 mg PO bid for 7–12 weeks) increases the smoking cessation rate when used with a behavior modification program. Bupropion **combined** with nicotine replacement may improve efficacy.[72] Longer-duration (e.g., 6 months) use of bupropion has been recommended to improve long-term cessation rates. Bupropion should be avoided in patients taking monoamine oxidase inhibitors. **Side effects** may include dizziness, headache, insomnia, nausea, xerostomia, hypertension, and, uncommonly, seizures.

■ **Varenicline (Chantix),** started 1 week before quitting smoking (0.5 mg PO daily for 3 days, 0.5 mg PO bid for 4 days, and then 1 mg PO bid for 12 weeks), binds to nicotine receptors, blocks their activation by nicotine, and prevents smoking-induced reinforcement and reward. The most common side effects are nausea, vomiting, and insomnia.

Surgery

■ **Surgical treatment options** exist for carefully selected patients with COPD.
  ■ **Lung transplantation** is indicated in patients with very severe expiratory airflow obstruction and severe limitations in quality of life, especially individuals with hypercapnia, marked hypoxemia, or PH. Lung transplantation is typically not an option for elderly patients or those with significant comorbidities.[73]
  ■ **Giant bullectomy** is considered in patients with COPD and dyspnea in whom a bulla or bullae occupy approximately one-third to one-half of the hemithorax.
  ■ **Lung volume reduction surgery** may provide quality of life and survival benefits in highly selected patients with severe COPD due to emphysema.[74,75] Target areas for surgical resection consist of large peripheral focal areas of severe emphysema. Ideally, the areas of lung not targeted for resection are significantly spared from emphysema. Poor candidates for lung volume reduction surgery include patients with very poor lung function (i.e., PaO_2 <45 mm Hg, $PaCO_2$ >55 mm Hg, FEV_1 and DL_{CO} $\leq$20% of the predicted normal value, or very high supplemental oxygen requirements [>6 lpm] with exertion) or those with diffuse or homogeneous emphysema on chest CT scan.

Acute Exacerbation of COPD

■ Increased breathlessness, often accompanied by cough, sputum production, wheezing, chest tightness, or other symptoms (and signs) of acutely worsened respiratory status define a COPD exacerbation.

- Infection and air pollution cause most exacerbations.
- Though many COPD exacerbations have an unclear etiology, the differential diagnosis list for a decompensation includes pneumothorax, pneumonia, aspiration, CHF, volume overload, cardiac ischemia, and PE.
- In addition to a history and physical examination, patients with concerning symptoms should undergo chest radiograph, routine blood work, oxyhemoglobin saturation, and arterial blood gas testing. In patients that require hospitalization, sputum culture, nasal viral swab, etc., may be useful.
- Clinicians may best judge the severity of an exacerbation and need for hospitalization by the medical history, physical examination, and alveolar gas exchange abnormalities.
    - **Intensive care unit (ICU) admission** indications include severe dyspnea that does not adequately respond to therapy, mental status changes, and persistent or worsening hypoxemia, hypercapnia, or respiratory acidosis despite medical therapy.
- Patients with acute exacerbations of COPD require adjustments and additions to chronic therapy.
- Inhaled bronchodilators (Table 9-7)
    - **Short-acting inhaled β_2-adrenergic agonists** are the first-line therapy for COPD exacerbations. Inhaled β_2-adrenergic agonists, such as albuterol, have a reduced duration of action in acute exacerbations of COPD, allowing a treatment frequency of q30–60min as tolerated[76]; subsequent treatments can be decreased to two to four puffs q4h as the acute exacerbation of COPD starts resolving.
    - **Short-acting inhaled anticholinergic agents,** such as ipratropium bromide, have similar efficacy to short-acting β_2-adrenergic agonists in the treatment of acute exacerbations of COPD. However, anticholinergic agents have less tendency to produce hypoxemia and other side effects of β_2-adrenergic agents.[77] During acute exacerbations, the usual dose of ipratropium, two puffs qid, can be increased to four to six puffs q4–6h to produce maximal bronchodilation.
    - **Combination β_2-agonist and anticholinergic therapy** for acute exacerbations appears to be the most efficacious bronchodilator strategy.
- Methylxanthines
    - Due to the significant risk for serious side effects, clinicians typically avoid using methylxanthines as mainline therapy for acute exacerbations, though chronic use is not necessarily discouraged and sudden discontinuation during an exacerbation is discouraged due to the risk of decompensation.
- Antimicrobial therapy
    - Antimicrobial therapy is typically not recommended as chronic therapy for patients with COPD. Controversy surrounds the role of **antimicrobial therapy** for COPD exacerbations.
    - For routine exacerbations of COPD in the absence of pneumonia, current methods do not reliably differentiate exacerbations caused by bacteria versus those produced by other agents.
    - Antibiotic therapy most often benefits patients who have more severe underlying lung disease, severe exacerbations,[78] and two or three cardinal symptoms (increased dyspnea, sputum volume, and sputum purulence).
    - Mild exacerbations due to bacterial infection are most often caused by *Haemophilus influenzae, Streptococcus pneumoniae, and Moraxella catarrhalis*, whereas patients with moderate to severe exacerbations have a higher incidence of infection with Gram-negative rods.
    - Traditional first-line antibiotic regimens for acute bacterial exacerbations of chronic bronchitis (**AECB**) consist of a 7- to 10-day course of oral therapy (e.g., trimethoprim/sulfamethoxazole, 160 mg/800 mg [one double-strength tablet] PO bid; amoxicillin, 250 mg PO tid; doxycycline, 100 mg PO bid; or a PO cephalosporin).
    - For moderate to severe exacerbations, recommended antibiotics include azithromycin (500 mg PO on day 1 and 250 mg PO on days 2–5), or a 7- to 10-day course of clarithromycin (500 mg PO bid or extended-release, 1 g PO daily), amoxicillin/clavulanate (500 mg PO tid or 875 mg PO bid), a second- or third-generation cephalosporin, or quinolones with enhanced activity against penicillin-resistant

S. pneumoniae, such as levofloxacin (500 mg PO daily) or moxifloxacin (400 mg PO daily).

- Patients requiring mechanical ventilation should receive antibiotic therapy that also covers *P. aeruginosa* such as high-dose (750 mg per tube or 400 mg IV bid). Ciprofloxacin or a β-lactam with *P. aeruginosa* activity.
- **Glucocorticoids**
  - Inhaled steroids currently do not have an important role in the treatment of an acute COPD exacerbation. However, systemic steroids produce improvement in hospital length of stay, lung function, and the incidence of relapse compared with placebo for treatment of acute exacerbations of COPD.[79]
  - The role of systemic glucocorticoids for acute exacerbations in outpatients with COPD remains controversial, though practitioners frequently prescribe short oral steroid "bursts" or "tapers." In patients with moderate to severe COPD, short courses of PO steroids in combination with other medical therapy can improve outcomes of those with exacerbations who are discharged from the emergency department.[80]
  - For patients with a COPD exacerbation, prednisone PO 40–60 mg daily is a typical starting dose, and this could be tapered off over a week or two as tolerated. Patients who use long-term PO steroids or high-dose inhaled steroid therapy might require a longer tapering period.
  - For patients hospitalized for a severe COPD exacerbation, initial moderate to high doses of oral (e.g., prednisone 60 mg PO daily) or IV glucocorticoids (e.g., methylprednisolone 60 mg IV q6h) may be useful, although they increase the risk of hyperglycemia and other complications. High steroid doses should not be continued for prolonged periods, and gradual tapering over 1–2 weeks is generally recommended.
- **Supplemental oxygen**
  - Adequate oxygenation must be maintained, despite the presence of hypercapnia, though excessively unnecessary amounts should be avoided. Increasing requirements of supplemental oxygen suggest that a complicating condition exists (e.g., PE, pneumonia, pneumothorax, or right-to-left shunt).
  - After return to baseline from a COPD exacerbation, patients with increased supplemental oxygen requirements should undergo an oxygen reassessment to redefine the appropriate oxygen needs.
- **Mechanical ventilation**
  - **Indications for invasive mechanical ventilation** include severe dyspnea with increased work of breathing (e.g., marked tachypnea, use of accessory muscles, and paradoxical abdominal motion), life-threatening hypoxemia, severe respiratory acidosis, respiratory arrest, impaired mental status, cardiovascular complications, other major complicating conditions, and failure of noninvasive ventilation.
  - The use of noninvasive ventilation in end-stage COPD should depend on the reversibility of the precipitating event and patient preferences.
  - Risks of invasive ventilation include ventilator-associated pneumonia (see Chapter 8, Critical Care), barotrauma, and failure to wean.
- **Noninvasive ventilation,** typically consisting of positive pressure ventilation delivered via a nasal or face mask, provides an alternative to intubation in selected patients with acute exacerbation of COPD.[81] **Indications** are similar to those for invasive ventilation, except that **exclusion criteria for noninvasive positive pressure ventilation** include respiratory arrest, cardiovascular instability, impaired mental status, high aspiration risk, copious secretions, significant facial/gastroesophageal/craniofacial/nasopharyngeal disease, and extreme obesity.[82]
- **Discharge criteria** for patients with acute exacerbations of COPD include use of inhaled bronchodilators less frequently than every 4 hours; clinical and ABG stability for at least 12–24 hours; acceptable ability to eat, sleep, and ambulate; adequate patient understanding of home therapy; and adequate home arrangements.
  - Prior to discharge from the hospital, chronic therapy issues should be readdressed including vaccination updates, smoking cessation, education, assessment of inhaler technique, and pulmonary rehabilitation.

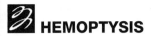 **HEMOPTYSIS**

GENERAL PRINCIPLES

- **Hemoptysis,** the expectoration of blood, is a nonspecific sign associated with many pulmonary diseases.
  - Infection (e.g., acute bronchitis, lung abscess, tuberculosis, aspergilloma, pneumonia, bronchiectasis)
  - Neoplasm
  - Cardiovascular disease (e.g., mitral stenosis, pulmonary embolus, pulmonary vascular malformations)
  - Trauma
  - Autoimmune disorders (e.g., Wegener granulomatosis, Goodpasture syndrome, systemic lupus erythematosus)
  - Drugs or toxins (e.g., cocaine, anticoagulants, thrombolytic agents, penicillamine, solvents)
- Often, the specific etiology of hemoptysis is never determined.

DIAGNOSIS

History and Physical Examination

- History and physical examination should confirm that the source of bleeding is located in the respiratory tract and not in the GI tract or nasopharynx.
- An attempt should be made to estimate the amount of bleeding.
- **Massive hemoptysis** is defined as more than 600 mL blood over 48 hours or quantities that are sufficient to impair alveolar gas exchange.
- The clinician should assess the patient for symptoms and signs of underlying diseases.

Laboratory Studies

- The following tests should be included in the evaluation of the patient with hemoptysis: Tests of hemostasis (INR and partial thromboplastin time), complete blood count to look for anemia and thrombocytopenia, liver function tests to evaluate for hepatic dysfunction if the platelet count is low or the INR is prolonged, serum creatinine to evaluate for renal dysfunction, sputum bacterial and mycobacterial (and sometimes fungal) stains and cultures, sputum cytology, urinalysis to evaluate for RBCs or RBC casts that may be associated with Wegener granulomatosis or Goodpasture syndrome, and arterial blood gas analysis.

Imaging

- **Chest radiography** should be performed to look for the cause of hemoptysis, such as pneumonia or lung cancer.
- Evaluation for PE (see Thromboembolic Disorders, Chapter 18, Disorders of Hemostasis) should be performed, if indicated, preferentially using CT scan over V/Q scanning because alternative etiologies are best detected with CT.
- Chest CT scan is also indicated if there is concern for underlying parenchymal disease.

Diagnostic Procedures

- **Bronchoscopy** is indicated in patients who have hemoptysis and a risk factor for carcinoma, even if the hemoptysis is minor and the radiograph is normal.

- Risk factors for carcinoma include (a) age older than 40 years, (b) significant smoking history, (c) hemoptysis of more than 1 week's duration, and (d) unexplained abnormality on chest radiograph.
- If bleeding is brisk, rigid bronchoscopy may be required.
- Bronchoalveolar lavage (BAL) fluid should be sent for cytology and culture (e.g., mycobacterial, fungal, bacterial). Alveolar hemorrhage can be detected on BAL, where the returned fluid becomes progressively bloody.

TREATMENT

- **Therapy is tailored to the severity of the episode and to the underlying cause.** The primary immediate goals of therapy are to maintain the airway, optimize oxygenation, stabilize the hemodynamic status, and cease the bleeding. Therapy for minor bleeding or blood-streaked sputum should be directed at the specific etiology.
- Causal laboratory abnormalities should be corrected: fresh frozen plasma for elevated INR or partial thromboplastin time, platelets for thrombocytopenia or platelet dysfunction (due to aspirin or other nonsteroidal anti-inflammatory drugs), and desmopressin acetate in the setting of uremia (see Chapter 18, Disorders of Hemostasis). Bedrest, mild cough suppression, and avoidance of excessive thoracic manipulation (e.g., chest percussion, incentive spirometry) are helpful.
- Patients should undergo pulse oximetry monitoring and should receive supplemental oxygen for oxyhemoglobin desaturation.
- For massive hemoptysis, while awaiting surgical consultation, clinically stable patients should be positioned with the bleeding side in a dependent position to reduce aspiration of blood into the contralateral lung.

Medications

- Sedatives aid patient cooperation, but excessive sedation may suppress airway protection and mask signs of respiratory decompensation.

Operative Management

- Once stabilization is accomplished, diagnostic and therapeutic interventions should be performed promptly, because recurrent bleeding occurs unpredictably.
  - **Early fiberoptic bronchoscopy,** especially during active bleeding, may localize the specific site and identify the cause of the bleeding. Immediate control of the airway can sometimes be obtained with endobronchial tamponade or unilateral intubation of the nonbleeding lung.
- **If bleeding continues** but the site of origin is uncertain, lung isolation or use of a double-lumen tube should be considered, provided that the staff is skilled in this procedure. If the bleeding cannot be localized because the rate of hemorrhage does not allow adequate visualization of the airway, emergency rigid bronchoscopy or arteriography and embolization are indicated.
- **Urgent surgical intervention** should be considered in operative candidates with unilateral bleeding when embolization is unavailable or unfeasible, when bleeding continues despite embolization, or when bleeding is associated with persistent hemodynamic and respiratory compromise. Contraindications to surgical treatment may include inoperable lung cancer and previous pulmonary function studies precluding pulmonary resection.

INTERSTITIAL LUNG DISEASE

GENERAL PRINCIPLES

- This section focuses mainly on subacute and chronic interstitial lung diseases (**ILDs**), and focuses on two of the classic ILDs: idiopathic pulmonary fibrosis and sarcoidosis.

Definition

- ILDs are a heterogeneous group of disorders, pathologically characterized by infiltration of the alveolar walls by cells, fluid, and connective tissue. Though a recent classification system prefers to use the words **diffuse parenchymal lung diseases (DPLDs)**, this chapter will refer to ILD and DPLD in the same manner.
- **Idiopathic pulmonary fibrosis (IPF)**, one of the idiopathic interstitial pneumonias (IIPs), is a relatively uncommon ILD in which lung inflammation and fibrosis occur.
- **Sarcoidosis**, one of the granulomatous ILDs, is a syndrome of unknown etiology, consisting of multiorgan involvement with noncaseating granulomas. A diagnosis of sarcoidosis usually requires the demonstration of lesions in more than one organ system of the body (e.g., lung and lymph nodes) and exclusion of other disorders known to cause granulomatous disease (e.g., mycobacterial or fungal infection, inhalation of metal dusts, fumes, and organic antigens).

Epidemiology

- **Idiopathic pulmonary fibrosis.** Approximately 30% of patients with chronic ILD have IPF, a primary lung disease of unclear etiology.
  - IPF occurs more frequently in men than in women, with onset typically occurring in middle age, and it may run in families.
  - IPF has a highly variable but progressive course. From the time of diagnosis, patients with IPF have a median survival of <5 years. Relatively good prognostic factors include (a) young age; (b) female gender; (c) recent onset of symptoms, less severe breathlessness, and relatively preserved lung function; (d) radiographic infiltrates at presentation; (e) predominantly cellular histology (as opposed to fibrosis); (f) increased proportion of lymphocytes in BAL; (g) stability or initial responsiveness after 3–6 months of glucocorticoid therapy; and (h) current cigarette smoking at time of diagnosis.[83,84]
  - Treatment responses are usually partial and transient, though treatment may slow the progression of disease. Spontaneous remissions are not expected.
- **Sarcoidosis.** Patients typically develop sarcoidosis before the age of 40 years.
  - Half of the patients present with asymptomatic abnormalities incidentally noted on chest radiographs.
  - Multiple system involvement is a hallmark of sarcoidosis.
    - The lungs and thoracic lymph nodes are involved in more than 90% of patients.
    - Cardiac involvement is clinically evident in only 5% of the patients, most of whom have extensive extracardiac disease. Cardiac disease is frequently unrecognized antemortem and is the most common cause of death attributed to sarcoidosis.[85]
    - Skin involvement occurs in approximately 25% of patients.
    - Eye involvement is variable in frequency and severity, and uveitis is the most common eye lesion.
    - **Lupus pernio** represents chronic sarcoidosis and consists of indurated skin plaques and discoloration of the nose, cheeks, lips, and ears.
    - **Erythema nodosum** is the hallmark of acute sarcoidosis, with erythematous painful bumps on the anterior legs, often associated with adjacent swollen painful joints.
    - **Löfgren's syndrome** consists of fever, bilateral hilar adenopathy, erythema nodosum, and arthralgia.
    - **Heerfordt's syndrome** consists of anterior uveitis, fever, parotid enlargement, and facial palsy.

Pathophysiology

- With ILDs, the decreased distensibility of the lung may produce a restrictive pulmonary function pattern and dyspnea. Some of the ILDs that have accompanying cystic lung disease (e.g., sarcoidosis, lymphangioleiomyomatosis [LAM], and eosinophilic granuloma [EG]), may produce an obstructive ventilatory pattern or a mixed restrictive-obstructive pattern.

■ With long-standing ILD, PH may develop late in the course, or PH may occur out of proportion to the restrictive ventilatory pattern or the imaging abnormalities.

Etiology

■ Clues about the ILD etiology come from assessment of **chronicity** of disease, **underlying systemic disease or exposure**, and **immune status**.
  ■ Inflammation (infectious or not), increased lung water, or infiltrative material causes ILD.
  ■ Infection and cardiogenic pulmonary edema most commonly cause acute ILD.

DIAGNOSIS

History

■ The history should focus on possible reversible causes of lung injury, especially **exposure** to infections, inhalants (i.e., dusts, fumes, chemicals, and fibers), and drugs with known pulmonary toxicity (e.g., amiodarone and nitrofurantoin). Clinicians should seek information regarding gastroesophageal reflux disease (GERD) and possible recurrent aspiration.
■ The past medical history may provide key information, such as a history of cancer (e.g., lymphangitic spread to the lung, radiation pneumonitis, or chemotherapy-induced ILD) or congestive heart failure.
■ The occupational, social, and family history provide useful information.
■ Patients with acute and chronic ILD typically present with dyspnea on exertion and cough. Chest pain, wheezing, and hemoptysis are less common.
■ Unlike IPF, sarcoidosis may involve multiple other organs, and patients may complain about adenopathy, skin rash, joint pains, and neurologic abnormalities.
■ *If the patient is known to be immunosuppressed and acutely ill, urgent evaluation is warranted.*

Physical Examination

■ The **physical examination** findings depend on the etiology of the ILD.
■ IPF often demonstrates bibasilar inspiratory crackles, which are less common with sarcoidosis.
■ Signs of PH and right heart failure may be present with any ILD.
■ Extrapulmonary findings may assist with the diagnosis. Though clubbing is associated with IPF, it may be associated with bronchogenic carcinoma. Clubbing rarely occurs with sarcoidosis. Erythema nodosum, adenopathy, and splenomegaly suggest the presence of sarcoidosis. Telangiectasias and sclerodactyly may accompany scleroderma.

Laboratory Studies

■ Routine blood testing is **rarely diagnostic,** although certain abnormalities may define the underlying disorder: eosinophilia due to eosinophilic pneumonia or drug reaction, thrombocytopenia due to collagen vascular disease, hypercalcemia due to sarcoidosis, and iron-deficiency anemia due to alveolar hemorrhage.
  ■ Rheumatoid arthritis (i.e., rheumatoid factor), systemic lupus erythematosus (i.e., antinuclear antibody), polymyositis (i.e., anti JO-1), and other connective tissue diseases may produce **elevated serologic test results,** and other diseases, such as IPF and silicosis, may cause nonspecific mild serology elevations.
  ■ The presence of cytoplasmic antineutrophil cytoplasmic antibody (c-ANCA) provides evidence for Wegener granulomatosis.
  ■ Serum precipitating antibody testing may support the presence of extrinsic allergic alveolitis related to farming or pigeon breeding.

- The angiotensin-converting enzyme level is neither sensitive nor specific for the diagnosis of sarcoidosis.

Pulmonary Function Tests and Arterial Blood Gas Analysis

- All stable patients who present with subacute or chronic ILD should undergo (a) **pulmonary function testing** (spirometry, lung volumes, and diffusing capacity); (b) resting ABG analysis; and (c) exercise assessment of arterial oxygenation (PaO_2 or SaO_2).
- Most patients with ILD have abnormal routine pulmonary function tests, although some are initially normal. As the lungs become stiffer, the vital capacity and total lung capacity decrease, producing a restrictive ventilatory pattern. The restriction is often accompanied by a decrease in D_{LCO}, a widening of the alveolar-arterial difference for oxygen at rest, and at times a dramatic fall in the SaO_2 with exercise.
- With advanced ILD that typically causes a restrictive ventilatory pattern, distortion of the airways and lung parenchyma may produce a concomitant obstructive ventilatory pattern. Some ILD may show an obstructive ventilatory pattern or a mixed restrictive–obstructive ventilatory pattern (e.g., sarcoid, eosinophilic granuloma, lymphangioleiomyomatosis, and IPF associated with severe cystic lung disease).
- Most patients with ILD present with a respiratory alkalosis. Hypoxemia develops as disease progresses. Carbon dioxide retention occurs only in very severe ILD. Marked oxyhemoglobin desaturation is common as disease progresses.

Imaging

- ILDs typically produce abnormal **imaging** test results (**chest radiograph or CT scan**), though some patients initially have normal tests. Imaging studies most often provide nonspecific but useful information (Table 9-8). All patients with ILD should undergo chest radiography. Further imaging is appropriate, especially when acute diseases (e.g., infection or pulmonary edema) are not suspected.
  - The **CT scan,** including **high-resolution CT** (HRCT), is more sensitive than chest radiography and occasionally provides specific diagnostic information that obviates the need for further testing (e.g., lymphangioleiomyomatosis).
  - Chest CT may also provide information regarding complication of the underlying ILD, such as aspergilloma, infection, or malignancy.
  - HRCT also detects associated findings such as mediastinal lymphadenopathy and provides guidance for surgical lung biopsy.
- For patients with IPF, typical radiologic studies show lower lobe–predominant patchy peripheral and subpleural basal reticular abnormalities, often with traction bronchiectasis and honeycombing. Though often present, ground-glass opacities are not a predominant feature of IPF and suggest the presence of other disorders such as nonspecific interstitial pneumonitis (NSIP).
- Sarcoidosis has five roentgenographic stages of intrathoracic disease.[86] Clinical and radiographic features have the highest diagnostic accuracy for the lower stages of disease. Five percent to 10% of patients have a normal chest radiograph (stage 0).
  - Stage 0: Normal
  - Stage I: Bilateral hilar adenopathy (BHL) without ILD
  - Stage II: BHL and ILD
  - Stage III: ILD without BHL
  - Stage IV: ILD with fibrosis

Surgical Diagnostic Procedures

- The clinician should exclude pulmonary edema as the cause of the ILD before embarking on invasive testing. To obtain biologic specimens for diagnostic purposes, clinicians should consider performing at least one of three types of tests.
- **Bronchoalveolar lavage (BAL)** obtains cells and material from the periphery of the airways during bronchoscopy. BAL provides the most useful information in patients with infections (i.e., positive stains and cultures), particularly in immunosuppressed patients,

TABLE 9-8 Chest Radiograph Patterns in Diffuse Interstitial Lung Disease

Category	Example
Lower lobe predominance	Idiopathic pulmonary fibrosis
	Collagen vascular disease (scleroderma)
	Asbestosis
	Hypersensitivity pneumonitis
Upper lobe predominance	Pneumoconiosis (silicosis)
	Ankylosing spondylitis
	Eosinophilic granuloma (EG; Langerhans cell granulomatosis)
	Sarcoid
Hilar adenopathy	Sarcoid
	Hypersensitivity pneumonitis, including some drugs (e.g., methotrexate)
Associated pneumothorax	EG
	Lymphangioleiomyomatosis (LAM)/tuberous sclerosis
Increased lung volumes	EG
	LAM
	Sarcoidosis
Eggshell calcification of lymph nodes	Silicosis
	Sarcoidosis
	Radiation

eosinophilic pneumonia (i.e., eosinophils of at least 25%), and alveolar hemorrhage (i.e., progressively bloody BAL return). BAL as the sole diagnostic tool in patients with other ILDs is so limited as to almost never be worthwhile.

- **Transbronchial lung biopsy (TBBx)** obtains small pieces of lung tissue close to the distal airways. It is most useful in diseases that follow an airway distribution (e.g., sarcoidosis and lymphangitic carcinoma). With the exception of infection, TBBx is much less useful and may be inadequate if a large amount of tissue is needed to make a specific diagnosis of other types of ILD.[87] The finding of inflammation or fibrosis is considered nondiagnostic on the small specimens obtained from TBBx.
  - A definitive diagnosis of IPF relies on obtaining adequate quantity and quality of lung tissue. Bronchoscopy with TBBx often does not obtain sufficient lung tissue to define the disease process adequately, and a diagnostic surgical biopsy should be considered in patients with an atypical presentation.
- In diseases with associated adenopathy (e.g., sarcoid), **transbronchial needle aspirate (TBNA)** of lymph nodes may provide diagnostic information.
- **Surgical lung biopsy (video-assisted thoracoscopic surgery or thoracotomy)** is the procedure of choice to obtain sufficient lung tissue for diagnosis. Pathologic classification of ILD aids in assessing prognosis and choosing therapy.[88] The surgeon should biopsy the most active sites of inflammation as determined by HRCT and should avoid biopsying only end-stage fibrotic areas or the easily accessible right middle lobe or lingula. Patients with rapidly advancing disease, suspicion of vasculitis, marked systemic symptoms, or atypical imaging findings should receive strong consideration for surgical biopsy. The risks of a biopsy may exceed the benefits in patients with advanced age, severe comorbidity, stable or very slowly progressive disease, known collagen vascular disease, and typical imaging and functional abnormalities.

Pathologic Findings

- The classic histologic appearance of IPF consists of usual interstitial pneumonitis (UIP), although other diseases (e.g., collagen vascular disease) may show similar biopsy findings.

- Sarcoidosis is most often diagnosed by demonstrating characteristic noncaseating granulomas in the affected organs and ruling out other etiologies of granulomatous disease such as infection with fungi or tuberculosis and cancer with granulomatous reactions in regional lymph nodes.

Differential Diagnosis

- The **differential diagnosis** of ILD is extensive (Table 9-9).
- A confident diagnosis of IPF can be made in the absence of a surgical lung biopsy specimen if the four major criteria and three of the four minor criteria are met,[89] as shown in Table 9-10.

TREATMENT

- Treatment of ILD varies depending on the underlying etiology. Before embarking on a course of treatment, the clinician likely needs to narrow down the differential diagnosis in an orderly fashion. Patients with more of an acute presentation should undergo assessment for infection and pulmonary edema, and should possibly receive empiric treatment. Based on test results and response to empiric therapy, lung fluid and tissue might be necessary to obtain an accurate diagnosis. Depending on the ILD etiology, treatment might include antibiotics, immunosuppression, or avoidance of exposures to offending agents.
- In many cases, particularly those of sarcoid, bronchiolitis obliterans organizing pneumonia, and chronic eosinophilic pneumonia, various regimens of corticosteroids produce dramatic improvements. Clinicians also need to watch for and potentially treat disease sequelae (e.g., PH and right heart failure associated with ILD; see Pulmonary Hypertension), side effects of medications, other conditions that accompany ILD, and concomitant disease (e.g., pulmonary embolism, congestive heart failure, infection).

Specific Clinical Situations

- **Idiopathic pulmonary fibrosis.** Treatment options for IPF include corticosteroids, immunosuppressive/cytotoxic agents, antifibrotic agents, and lung transplantation.
  - Small studies have suggested that the minority of patients experience modest and limited benefit from medical therapy. Few large clinical trials have been conducted.
  - Given the poor efficacy and the high risk of complications of treatment, the American Thoracic Society (ATS)[84] recommends a cautious undertaking of treatment in patients with advanced age, extreme obesity, severe comorbidity (e.g., diabetes mellitus, cardiac disease, osteoporosis), or end-stage honeycomb lung on HRCT examination.
  - For patients who are undergoing therapy, the ATS recommends combined therapy with corticosteroids and either azathioprine or cyclophosphamide. Contraindications and side effects of immunosuppressive agents are discussed in Chapter 23, Arthritis and Rheumatologic Diseases.
  - Clinicians should address the routine care of patients with chronic lung disease, and treatment options include supplemental oxygen, vaccinations, and pulmonary rehabilitation (see Chronic Obstructive Pulmonary Disease)
- **Sarcoidosis.** Patients with sarcoidosis undergo systemic immunosuppressive treatment mainly for progressive and severe disease, especially that which involves critical organs such as the brain, eye (not responding to topical therapy), heart, and kidney.
  - Since recurrences are common, patients responsive to therapy should typically continue it for a minimum of 1 year.
  - **Asymptomatic patients** (stages 0, I, and many with stage II pulmonary disease) without evidence of clinical or radiologic lung disease progression (and without other critical organ involvement) could be followed closely without treatment.
  - Fifty-five percent to 90% of patients with bilateral hilar lymphadenopathy (stage I) usually experience stability or resolution without therapy within a few years of diagnosis.

TABLE 9-9 Classification of Interstitial Lung Disease

Category	Examples
Granulomatous disease	Sarcoidosis
	Berylliosis
	Hypersensitivity pneumonitis
Connective tissue diseases	Scleroderma
	Rheumatoid arthritis
	Polymyositis-dermatomyositis
	Systemic lupus erythematosus
	Mixed connective tissue disease
	Ankylosing spondylitis
	Sjögren syndrome
	Psoriatic arthritis
	Behçet disease
	Relapsing polychondritis
Iatrogenic	Drug induced
	Antibiotics
	Nitrofurantoin
	Sulfasalazine
	Antiarrhythmics
	Amiodarone
	Chemotherapeutic immunosuppresive agents
	Bleomycin
	Methotrexate
	Azathioprine
	Illicit
	Crack cocaine (inhaled)
	Radiation
	Bone marrow transplantation
	Vitamins
	L-tryptophan
Familial	Tuberous sclerosis/neurofibromatosis
	Idiopathic pulmonary fibrosis
	Sarcoidosis
Occupational and environmental	Inorganic dusts
	Asbestos
	Hard metals
	Silicates
	Talc
	Organic dusts (hypersensitivity pneumonitis)
	Bird breeder's lung
	Farmer's lung
	Fumes
Idiopathic	Idiopathic pulmonary fibrosis
	Autoimmune-associated pulmonary fibrosis (see Connective Tissue Disease)
	Nonspecific interstitial pneumonitis
	Acute interstitial pneumonitis/Hamman-Rich syndrome
	Lymphocytic interstitial pneumonia
	Respiratory bronchiolitis

(continued)

TABLE 9-9   **Classification of Interstitial Lung Disease (*Continued*)**

Category	Examples
	Lymphangioleiomyomatosis
	Eosinophilic granuloma (EG)
	Chronic eosinophilic pneumonia
	Eosinophilic pneumonia
	Bronchiolitis obliterans and organizing pneumonia
	Pulmonary hemorrhage syndromes
	Amyloidosis
	Alveolar microlithiasis
	Metastatic calcification
	Acute respiratory distress syndrome
	Postinfectious
	Pulmonary alveolar proteinosis
Neoplasm	Lymphangitic carcinoma
	Bronchoalveolar carcinoma
	Lymphoma
Lung water	Pulmonary edema
	Cardiogenic
	Noncardiogenic
Infectious	Mycobacterial
	Fungal (including *Pneumocystis carinii/jiroveci*)
	Viral
	Parasitic
	Bacterial
Chemical	Aspiration
	Lipoid pneumonia

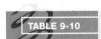

TABLE 9-10   **Major and Minor Criteria for the Diagnosis of Idiopathic Pulmonary Fibrosis**

Major criteria

Exclusion of other known causes of interstitial lung disease

Abnormal pulmonary function test results that include evidence of restriction and impaired gas exchange

Bibasilar reticular abnormalities with minimal ground-glass opacities seen on high-resolution computed tomography scan

Transbronchial lung biopsy or bronchoalveolar lavage fluid specimens without features to support an alternative diagnosis

Minor criteria

Age >50 years

Insidious onset of otherwise unexplained dyspnea on exertion

Duration of illness >3 months

Bibasilar, inspiratory "Velcro-like" crackles

- Forty percent to 70% of patients with stage II sarcoidosis have spontaneous resolution of their lung infiltrates and adenopathy.
- Though only 10%–20% of patients with stage III sarcoidosis have spontaneous remission, therapy for stage III is controversial, because about half of patients experience improvement without therapy within 2 years. Decisions regarding initiation of therapy should be individualized in patients with mild to moderate pulmonary function abnormalities.
- Patients with stage IV sarcoidosis do not experience remission, but they also may not benefit from immunosuppressive therapy, and referral for lung transplantation should be considered.

Medications

- Idiopathic pulmonary fibrosis
  - Corticosteroids (prednisone, 0.5–1.0 mg/kg PO daily) should be initiated *early* in the course of the illness. If an objective response occurs within 3 months, and side effects are tolerable, then therapy should be continued. The steroid dosage should be gradually decreased to 0.25–0.5 mg/kg PO daily over the next few months. Eventually, prednisone is tapered slowly to the minimal dosage that maintains clinical stability, such as 10–15 mg PO every other day. For patients with unequivocal responses to therapy, prolonged therapy is recommended.[84]
  - Azathioprine, 2–3 mg/kg PO daily, not to exceed 150 mg/d, or cyclophosphamide, 2 mg/kg (lean body weight) PO daily, not to exceed 150 mg/d, in combination with low-dose glucocorticoids was suggested as first-line therapy for willing patients with acceptable prognostic features.[84] Dosing of either can begin at 25–50 mg/d and increase by 25-mg increments every 1–2 weeks until the maximum dose is reached (as tolerated by WBC count, platelet count, etc.).
  - Other drug therapies, including colchicine, methotrexate, penicillamine, pirfenidone, interferon-γ, interferon-β, and thalidomide, have not clearly demonstrated efficacy. Interferon-γ-1b may improve lung function and oxygenation in patients with IPF who had no response to glucocorticoids alone.[90] Colchicine (0.6 mg PO daily or bid) might have similar efficacy to corticosteroids with fewer side effects.
  - Treatment should be continued for at least 6 months. Studies should be performed to evaluate response. If the patient's condition is improved or stable, therapy should generally be continued. If the patient's condition worsens, as is frequently the case, the drugs can be tapered and stopped or changed.
- Sarcoidosis
  - Corticosteroids are the mainstay of treatment for sarcoidosis in patients with progressive impairment of pulmonary function, vital organ dysfunction (eye, central nervous system [CNS], heart, kidney), or persistent hypercalcemia.
  - Lung involvement. Although there is still debate as to their long-term effectiveness, corticosteroids may reverse the early changes of pulmonary parenchymal involvement. Corticosteroid therapy is a long-term commitment, as the patient will likely require it for at least 1 year to prevent relapse. The lowest dose that will continue to suppress the patient's symptoms should be maintained, while monitoring for toxicity. The efficacy of other immunosuppressive agents in sarcoid has not been clearly defined, although they may allow treatment with a lower dose of steroids.
  - Other organ involvement. CNS and cardiac involvement respond poorly to therapy. Hypercalcemia due to sarcoid responds well to corticosteroids and avoidance of ultraviolet light exposure.

Risk Management

- *Pneumocystis jiroveci* (previously *Pneumocystis carinii*) pneumonia prophylaxis should be considered in patients receiving immunosuppressive therapy.

Follow-Up and Monitoring

■ **Monitoring** of the clinical course with clinical, radiographic, and physiologic parameters may be useful, especially if the patient is being treated. A battery of information should be obtained at baseline and at regular intervals to assess progression or remission. Typical tests include complete pulmonary function tests, arterial blood gas at rest while breathing room air, exercise test, and high-resolution chest CT without contrast. Follow-up should occur frequently within the first few years of presentation, and for patients with more severe disease.

■ **Bone density** assessment should be considered on an annual or twice-yearly basis for patients receiving chronic systemic steroid therapy, especially patients with additional risk factors, and aggressive prevention and treatment of osteoporosis (see Chapter 22, Endocrine Diseases) is recommended.

■ For patients on immunosuppressive therapy, WBC and platelet counts should be regularly monitored (see Rheumatologic Diseases, Chapter 23, Arthritis and Rheumatologic Diseases).

■ Patients receiving azathioprine should undergo monthly monitoring of **liver** function tests (see Rheumatologic Diseases, Chapter 23, Arthritis and Rheumatologic Diseases).

■ Patients receiving cyclophosphamide should undergo routine **urine** monitoring for hematuria (see Rheumatologic Diseases, Chapter 23, Arthritis and Rheumatologic Diseases).

■ Patients with a positive **PPD** should be considered for INH prophylaxis prior to the initiation of steroid and immunosuppressive therapy.

■ Because untreated uveitis can lead to blindness, all patients with sarcoid should regularly receive a detailed ophthalmologic evaluation.

■ Patients with ILD should be considered for intermittent echocardiographic monitoring for the development of PH.

References

1. Rich S, Dantzker DR, Ayres SM, et al. Primary pulmonary hypertension. A national prospective study. *Ann Intern Med* 1987;107:216–223.
2. Pengo V, Lensing AWA, Prins MH, et al. Incidence of chronic thromboembolic pulmonary hypertension after pulmonary embolism. *N Engl J Med* 2004;350:2257–2264.
3. Simonneau G, Galiè N, Rubin LJ, et al. Clinical classification of pulmonary hypertension. *J Am Coll Cardiol* 2004;43:5S–12S.
4. McGoon M, Gutterman D, Steen V, et al. Screening, Early Detection, and Diagnosis of Pulmonary Arterial Hypertension: ACCP Evidence-Based Clinical Practice Guidelines. *Chest* 2004;126:14S–34S.
5. Miyamoto S, Nagaya N, Satoh T, et al. Clinical correlates and prognostic significance of six-minute walk test in patients with primary pulmonary hypertension: comparison with cardiopulmonary exercise testing. *Am J Respir Crit Care Med* 2000;161:487–492.
6. Fedullo PF, Auger WR, Kerr KM, et al. Chronic thromboembolic pulmonary hypertension. *N Engl J Med* 2001;345:1465–1472.
7. Hinderliter AL, Willis PW, Barst RJ, et al. Effects of long-term infusion of prostacyclin (epoprostenol) on echocardiographic measures of right ventricular structure and function in primary pulmonary hypertension. *Circulation* 1997;95:1479–86.
8. Badesch DB, Abman SH, Ahearn GS, et al. Medical Therapy For Pulmonary Arterial Hypertension: ACCP Evidence-Based Clinical Practice Guidelines. *Chest* 2004;126:35S–62S.
9. Sitbon O, Humbert M, Jas X, et al. Long-Term Response to Calcium Channel Blockers in Idiopathic Pulmonary Arterial Hypertension. *Circulation* 2005;111:3105–3111.
10. Rich S, Kaufmann E, Levy PS. The effect of high doses of calcium-channel blockers on survival in primary pulmonary hypertension. *N Engl J Med* 1992;327:76–81.
11. Rubin LJ, Badesch DB, Barst RJ, et al. Bosentan therapy for pulmonary arterial hypertension. *N Engl J Med* 2002;346:896–903.
12. Galie N, Ghofrani HA, Torbicki A, et al. Sildenafil citrate therapy for pulmonary arterial hypertension. *N Engl J Med* 2005;353:2148–2157.
13. Barst RJ, Rubin LJ, Long WA, et al. A comparison of continuous intravenous

epoprostenol (prostacyclin) with conventional therapy for primary pulmonary hypertension. *N Engl J Med* 1996;334:296–302.

14. Sitbon O, Humbert M, Nunes H, et al. Long-term intravenous epoprostenol infusion in primary pulmonary hypertension: prognostic factors and survival. *J Am Coll Cardiol* 2002;40:780–788.

15. Simonneau G, Barst RJ, Galie N, et al. Continuous subcutaneous infusion of treprostinil, a prostacyclin analogue, in patients with pulmonary arterial hypertension: a double-blind, randomized, placebo-controlled trial. *Am J Respir Crit Care Med* 2002;165:800–804.

16. Olschewski H, Simonneau G, Galie N, et al. Inhaled iloprost for severe pulmonary hypertension. *N Engl J Med* 2002;347:322–329.

17. Fuster V, Steele PM, Edwards WD, et al. Primary pulmonary hypertension: natural history and the importance of thrombosis. *Circulation* 1984;70:580–587.

18. Trulock EP, Edwards LB, Taylor DO et al. Registry of the International Society for Heart and Lung Transplantation: Twenty-second official adult lung and heart-lung transplant report-2005. *J Heart Lung Transplant* 2005;24:956–967.

19. Light RW: Pleural Diseases. Fourth Edition. Lippincott, Williams and Wilkins, Baltimore, 2001.

20. Sallach SM, Sallach JA, Vasquez E, et al. Volume of Pleural Fluid Required for Diagnosis of Pleural Malignancy. *Chest* 2002;122:1913–1917.

21. Colice GL, Curtis A, Deslauriers J, et al. Medical and surgical treatment of parapneumonic effusions: An evidence-based guideline. *Chest* 2000;118:1158–1171.

22. Light RW, Macgregor MI, Luchsinger PC, et al. Pleural effusions: The diagnostic separation of transudates and exudates. *Ann Intern Med* 1972;77:507–513.

23. Sahn SA. Pleural effusion in lung cancer. *Clin Chest Med* 1993;14:189–200.

24. Dresler CM, Olak J, Herndon JE, et al. Phase III Intergroup Study of Talc Poudrage vs Talc Slurry Sclerosis for Malignant Pleural Effusion. *Chest* 2005;127:909–915.

25. Walker-Renard PB, Vaughan LM, Sahn SA. Chemical pleurodesis for malignant pleural effusions. *Ann Intern Med* 1994;120:56–64.

26. Putnam JB, Light RW, Rodriguez RM, et al. Randomized comparison of indwelling pleural catheter with doxycycline pleurodesis in the management of malignant pleural effusions. *Cancer* 1999;86:1992–1999.

27. Sleep-related breathing disorders in adults: Recommendations for syndrome definition and measurement techniques in clinical research. The Report of an American Academy of Sleep Medicine Task Force. *Sleep* 1999;22:667–689.

28. Young T, Blustein J, Finn L, et al. Sleep-disordered breathing and motor vehicle accidents in a population-based sample of employed adults. *Sleep* 1997;20:608–613.

29. Partinen M, Guilleminault C. Daytime sleepiness and vascular morbidity at seven-year follow-up in obstructive sleep apnea patients. *Chest* 1990;97:27–32.

30. Young T, Palta M, Dempsey J, et al. The occurrence of sleep-disordered breathing among middle-aged adults. *N Engl J Med* 1993;328:1230–1235.

31. Westbrook PR. Sleep disorders and upper airway obstruction in adults. *Otolaryngol Clin North Am* 1990;23:727–743.

32. Peppard PE, Young T, Palta M, et al. Prospective study of the association between sleep-disordered breathing and hypertension. *N Engl J Med* 2000;342:1378–1384.

33. Nieto FJ, Young TB, Lind BK, et al. Association of sleep-disordered breathing, sleep apnea, and hypertension in a large community-based study. Sleep Heart Health Study. *JAMA* 2000;283:1829–1836.

34. Naughton MT, Bradley TD. Sleep apnea in congestive heart failure. *Clin Chest Med* 1998;19:99–113.

35. Yaggi HK, Concato J, Kernan WN, et al. Obstructive sleep apnea as a risk factor for stroke and death. *N Engl J Med* 2005;353:2034–2041.

36. Vgontzas AN, Papanicolaou DA, Bixler EO, et al. Sleep apnea and daytime sleepiness and fatigue: relation to visceral obesity, insulin resistance, and hypercytokinemia. *J Clin Endocrinol Metab* 2000;85:1151–1158.

37. Johns MW. A new method for measuring daytime sleepiness: the Epworth sleepiness scale. *Sleep* 1991;14:540–545.

38. Liistro G, Rombaux P, Belge C, et al. High Mallampati score and nasal obstruction are associated risk factors for obstructive sleep apnoea. *Eur Respir J* 2003;21:248–252.
39. Indications and standards for cardiopulmonary sleep studies - Report of an ATS Consensus Conference. *Am Rev Respir Dis* 1989;139:559–568.
40. Meoli AL, Casey KR, Clark RW, et al. Hypopnea in sleep-disordered breathing in adults. *Sleep* 2001;24:469–470.
41. Suratt PM, McTier RF, Findley LJ, et al. Changes in breathing and the pharynx after weight loss in obstructive sleep apnea. *Chest* 1987;92:631–637.
42. Sher AE, Schechtman KB, Piccirillo JF. The efficacy of surgical modifications of the upper airway in adults with obstructive sleep apnea syndrome. *Sleep* 1996;19:156–177.
43. Li KK, Powell NB, Riley RW, et al. Long-term Results of Maxillomandibular Advancement Surgery. *Sleep and Breathing* 2000;4:137–139.
44. Kaplan J, Staats BA. Obstructive sleep apnea syndrome. *Mayo Clin Proc* 1990;65:1087–1094.
45. Hamosh A, FitzSimmons SC, Macek M, et al. Comparison of the clinical manifestations of cystic fibrosis in black and white patients. *J Pediatr* 1998;132:255–259.
46. FitzSimmons SC. The changing epidemiology of cystic fibrosis. *J Pediatr* 1993;122:1–9.
47. Cystic Fibrosis Foundation Patient Registry, 2004 *Annual Data Report*
48. Liou TG, Adler FR, Cahill BC, et al. Survival effect of lung transplantation among patients with cystic fibrosis. *JAMA* 2001;286:2683–2689.
49. Kerem B, Rommens JM, Buchanan JA, et al. Identification of the cystic fibrosis gene: genetic analysis. *Science* 1989;245:1073–1080.
50. Rowe SM, Miller S, Sorscher EJ. Mechanisms of Disease: Cystic Fibrosis. *N Engl J Med* 2005;352:1992–2001.
51. Goss CH, Rubenfeld GD, Otto K, et al. The Effect of Pregnancy on Survival in Women With Cystic Fibrosis. *Chest* 2003;124:1460–1468.
52. Ramsey BW. Drug Therapy: Management of Pulmonary Disease in Patients with Cystic Fibrosis. *N Engl J Med* 1996;335:179–188.
53. Hubbard RC, McElvaney NG, Birrer P, et al. A preliminary study of aerosolized recombinant human deoxyribonuclease I in the treatment of cystic fibrosis. *N Engl J Med* 1992;326:812–815.
54. Ramsey BW, Astley SJ, Aitken ML, et al. Efficacy and safety of short-term administration of aerosolized recombinant human deoxyribonuclease in patients with cystic fibrosis. *Am Rev Respir Dis* 1993;148:145–151.
55. Ramsey BW, Pepe MS, Quan JM, et al. Intermittent administration of inhaled tobramycin in patients with cystic fibrosis. *N Engl J Med* 1999;340:23–30.
56. Saiman L, Marshall BC, Mayer-Hamblett N, et al. Azithromycin in patients with cystic fibrosis chronically infected with Pseudomonas aeruginosa: a randomized controlled trial. *JAMA* 2003;290:1749–1756.
57. Kerem E, Reisman J, Corey M, et al. Prediction of mortality in patients with cystic fibrosis. *N Engl J Med* 1992;326:1187–1191.
58. FitzSimmons SC, Burkhart GA, Borowitz D, et al. High-dose pancreatic-enzyme supplements and fibrosing colonopathy in children with cystic fibrosis. *N Engl J Med* 1997;336:1283–1289.
59. Aris RM, Lester GE, Caminiti M, et al. Efficacy of Alendronate in Adults with Cystic Fibrosis with Low Bone Density. *Am J Respir Crit Care Med* 2004;169:77–82.
60. Wang EE, Prober CG, Manson B, et al. Association of respiratory viral infections with pulmonary deterioration in patients with cystic fibrosis. *N Engl J Med* 1984;311:1653–1658.
61. Anthonisen NR, Connett JE, Kiley JP, et al. Effects of smoking intervention and the use of an inhaled anticholinergic bronchodilator on the rate of decline of FEV1. The Lung Health Study. *JAMA* 1994;272:1497–1505.
62. Pauwels RA, Buist AS, Calverley PM, et al. Global strategy for the diagnosis, management, and prevention of chronic obstructive pulmonary disease. NHLBI/WHO Global Initiative for Chronic Obstructive Lung Disease (GOLD) Workshop summary. *Am J Respir Crit Care Med* 2001;163:1256–1276.

63. Gervais A, Begin P. Bronchodilatation with a metered-dose inhaler plus an extension, using tidal breathing vs jet nebulization. *Chest* 1987;92:822–824.

64. Ikeda A, Nishimura K, Izumi T. Bronchodilating effects of combined therapy with clinical dosages of ipratropium bromide and salbutamol for stable COPD. *Chest* 1996;109:294.

65. Calverley P, Pauwels R, Vestbo J, et al. Combined salmeterol and fluticasone in the treatment of chronic obstructive pulmonary disease: a randomised controlled trial. *Lancet* 2003;361:449–456.

66. Sin DD, Wu L, Anderson JA, et al. Inhaled corticosteroids and mortality in chronic obstructive pulmonary disease. *Thorax* 2005;60:992–997.

67. Cottrell JJ, Openbrier D, Lave JR, et al. Home oxygen therapy. A comparison of 2- vs 6-month patient reevaluation. *Chest* 1995;107:358–361.

68. Nici l, Donner C, Wouters E, et al. American thoracic society/european respiratory society statement on pulmonary rehabilitation. *Am J Respir Crit Care Med* 2006;173:1390–1413.

69. The Agency for Health Care Policy and Research Smoking Cessation Clinical Practice Guideline. *JAMA* 1996;275:1270–1280.

70. Hughes JR, Goldstein MG, Hurt RD, et al. Recent advances in the pharmacotherapy of smoking. *JAMA* 1999;281:72–76.

71. The tobacco use and dependence clinical practice guideline panel, staff, and consortium representatives. A clinical practice guideline for treating tobacco use and dependence. *JAMA* 2000;283:244–254.

72. Jorenby DE, Leischow SJ, Nides MA, et al. A Controlled Trial of Sustained-Release Bupropion, a Nicotine Patch, or Both for Smoking Cessation. *N Engl J Med* 1999; 340:685–691.

73. International Guidelines for the Selection of Lung Transplant Candidates. *Am J Respir Crit Care Med* 1998;158:335–339.

74. Yusen RD, Lefrak SS, Gierada DS, et al. A Prospective Evaluation of Lung Volume Reduction Surgery in 200 Consecutive Patients. *Chest* 2003;123:1026–1037.

75. A Randomized Trial Comparing Lung-Volume—Reduction Surgery with Medical Therapy for Severe Emphysema. National Emphysema Treatment Trial Research Group. *N Engl J Med* 2003;348:2059–2073.

76. ATS Statement. Standards for the diagnosis and care of patients with chronic obstructive pulmonary disease. *Am J Resp Crit Care Med* 1995;152:577–S120.

77. Gross NJ, Bankwala Z. Effects of an anticholinergic bronchodilator on arterial blood gases of hypoxemic patients with chronic obstructive pulmonary disease. Comparison with a beta-adrenergic agent. *Am Rev Respir Dis* 1987;136:1091–1094.

78. Saint S, Bent S, Vittinghoff E. Antibiotics in chronic obstructive pulmonary disease exacerbations. A meta-analysis. *JAMA* 1995;273:957–960.

79. Singh JM, Palda VA, Stanbrook MB et al. Corticosteroid therapy for patients with acute exacerbations of chronic obstructive pulmonary disease: a systematic review. *Arch Intern Med* 2002;162:2527–2536.

80. Aaron SD, Vandemheen KL, Hebert P, et al. Outpatient Oral Prednisone after Emergency Treatment of Chronic Obstructive Pulmonary Disease. *N Engl J Med* 2003; 348:2618–2625.

81. Brochard L, Mancebo J, Wysocki M, et al. Noninvasive ventilation for acute exacerbations of chronic obstructive pulmonary disease. *N Engl J Med* 1995;333:817–822.

82. Kramer, N, Meyer, TJ, Meharg, J, et al. Randomized, prospective trial of noninvasive positive pressure ventilation in acute respiratory failure. *Am J Respir Crit Care Med* 1995;151:1799–1806.

83. Schwartz DA, Helmers RA, Galvin JR, et al. Determinants of survival in idiopathic pulmonary fibrosis. *Am J Respir Crit Care Med* 1994;149:450–454.

84. American Thoracic Society. Idiopathic pulmonary fibrosis: diagnosis and treatment (international consensus statement). *Am J Respir Crit Care Med* 2000;161:646–664.

85. Sharma OP, Maheshwari A, Thaker K. Myocardial sarcoidosis. *Chest* 1993;103:253–258.

86. ATS/ERS/WASOG Statement on Sarcoidosis. *Am J Resp Crit Care Med* 1999;160:736–755.

87. Raghu G. Interstitial lung disease: a diagnostic approach. Are CT scan and lung biopsy indicated in every patient? *AmJ Respir Crit Care Med* 1995;151:909–914.
88. Katzenstein AL, Myers JL. Idiopathic pulmonary fibrosis: clinical relevance of pathologic classification. *Am J Respir Crit Care Med* 1998;157:1301–1315.
89. Ai-Ping C, Lee K, Lim T. In-Hospital and 5-Year Mortality of Patients Treated in the ICU for Acute Exacerbation of COPD: A Retrospective Study. *Chest* 2005;128:518–524.
90. Ziesche R, Hofbauer E, Wittmann K, et al. A Preliminary Study of Long-Term Treatment with Interferon Gamma-1b and Low-Dose Prednisolone in Patients with Idiopathic Pulmonary Fibrosis. *N Engl J Med* 1999;341:1264–1269.

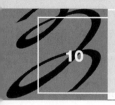

ALLERGY AND IMMUNOLOGY

Mitchell Grayson, Shirley Joo, Mario Castro,
Dorothy Cheung, and Ravi Aysola

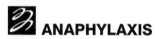 ANAPHYLAXIS

GENERAL PRINCIPLES

Definition

- **Anaphylaxis** is an immunoglobulin E (IgE)-mediated, rapidly developing, systemic allergic reaction.
- **Non-allergic anaphylaxis** (anaphylactoid) reactions mimic anaphylaxis but are not IgE mediated and are due to the degranulation of mast cells induced directly by the offending agent.

Classification

- The severity of anaphylaxis can be divided into the following three categories:
    - **Mild** (skin and subcutaneous tissues only): generalized erythema, urticaria, periorbital edema, or angioedema.
    - **Moderate** (features suggesting respiratory, cardiovascular, or gastrointestinal involvement): dyspnea, stridor, wheeze, nausea, vomiting, dizziness (presyncope), diaphoresis, chest or throat tightness, and abdominal pain.
    - **Severe** (hypoxia, hypotension, or neurologic compromise): cyanosis or PaO_2 $\leq 92\%$ at any stage, hypotension (systolic blood pressure [SBP] <90 mm Hg), confusion, loss of consciousness, or neurologic compromise.

Etiology

- Foods
- *Hymenoptera* (bees, wasps, and fire ants) stings
- Medications (including antibiotics, aspirin, and other nonsteroidal anti-inflammatory drugs)
- Latex rubber
- Blood products
- Seminal fluid
- Physical factors (such as cold temperature or exercise)
- Idiopathic

Pathophysiology

- Anaphylaxis is due to sensitization to an antigen and formation of specific IgE to that antigen. On re-exposure, the IgE on mast cells and basophils binds the antigen and cross-links the IgE receptor, which causes activation of the cells with subsequent release of pre-formed mediators, such as histamine.
- The release of these mediators ultimately causes capillary leakage, cellular edema, and smooth muscle contractions resulting in the constellation of physical symptoms described in the clinical presentation.

DIAGNOSIS

- Diagnosis is based primarily on history and physical examination, with confirmation in some cases provided by the laboratory finding of an elevated serum β-tryptase level. The absence of an elevated tryptase level does not exclude anaphylaxis.

Clinical Presentation

- The clinical manifestations of anaphylaxis and anaphylactoid reactions are the same. **Most serious reactions occur within minutes** after exposure to the antigen. However, the reaction may be delayed for hours. Some patients experience a biphasic reaction characterized by a recurrence of symptoms after 4–8 hours. A few patients have a protracted course that requires several hours of continuous treatment.
- Manifestations include pruritus, urticaria, angioedema, respiratory distress (due to laryngeal edema, laryngospasm, or bronchospasm), hypotension, abdominal cramping, and diarrhea.
- **The most common cause of death is airway obstruction,** followed by hypotension.
- The spectrum of reactions ranges from very severe and life-threatening to mild. However, left untreated, all reactions have the potential to become severe very rapidly. **A previous mild reaction does not predict the severity of future reactions with re-exposure to the offending agent.**

Differential Diagnosis

- **Anaphylaxis** due to pre-formed IgE and re-exposure: medications, *Hymenoptera* stings, and food are the most common causes of anaphylaxis.
- **Non-allergic anaphylaxis** (anaphylactoid), which are non–IgE-mediated anaphylaxis reactions:
  - **Radiocontrast sensitivity reactions** mimic anaphylaxis but are not IgE mediated. As a result of osmotic shifts, the contrast media is thought to lead to direct degranulation of mast cells in susceptible patients. Reactions can occur in 5%–10% of patients, with a fatal reaction occurring in 1 in 40,000 procedures. The following **risk factors** have been identified:
    - Age >50 years
    - Pre-existing cardiovascular or renal disease
    - History of allergy
    - History of a previous reaction to radiocontrast media
      - **Sensitivity to seafood or iodine does not predispose to radiocontrast media reactions.**
      - Although no predictive tests are available, if patients have a history of a reaction, the use of a low-ionic-strength contrast media and premedication is strongly suggested.
      - **Premedication regimen** includes prednisone (50 mg PO) given 13 hours, 7 hours, and 1 hour before the procedure and diphenhydramine (50 mg PO) given 1 hour before the procedure. An H2 blocker may also be given 1 hour before the procedure. It is important to remember that premedication is not 100% effective and that appropriate precautions for handling a reaction should be taken.
  - **Red man's syndrome** from vancomycin consists of pruritus and flushing of the face and neck. It can be prevented by slowing the rate of infusion and premedicating with diphenhydramine (50 mg PO) 30 minutes prior to the infusion.
  - Other drugs, including **opiates and flouroquinolones,** may cause anaphylactoid reactions. In all of these cases it is important to limit the number of anaphylactoid-inducing medications given to a patient. In addition, it is helpful to slow the rate of administration of these medications to avoid these unwanted responses.
- **Mastocytosis** should be considered in patients with recurrent unexplained anaphylaxis or flushing, especially with previous reactions to nonspecific mast cell degranulators such as opiates and radiocontrast media.

- **Ingestant-related** reactions mimic anaphylaxis, usually due to monosodium glutamate or sulfites or the presence of histamine-like substances in fish (scombroidosis).
- **Flushing syndromes** include flushing due to red man's syndrome, carcinoid, postmenopausal symptoms, alcohol use, and vasointestinal peptide (and other vasoactive intestinal peptide–secreting tumors).
- **Other forms of shock** such as hemorrhagic, hypoglycemic, cardiogenic, and septic.
- **Miscellaneous syndromes** such as C1 esterase (C1 INH) deficiency syndrome, pheochromocytoma, neurologic (seizure, stroke), and capillary leak syndrome.
- **Idiopathic anaphylaxis.**

Monitoring

- Observation for a minimum of 6 hours is indicated for patients with mild reactions limited to urticaria, angioedema, or mild bronchospasm.
- Patients with moderate to severe reactions should be admitted to the hospital for close observation of a possible biphasic reaction for at least 24 hours, and possibly as long as 72 hours.

TREATMENT

- **Immediate treatment of anaphylaxis and anaphylactoid reactions**
  - **Epinephrine** is the mainstay of therapy and should be administered immediately:
    - 0.3–0.5 mg (0.3–0.5 mL of a 1:1,000 solution) intramuscularly (IM) repeated at 10- to 15-minute intervals if necessary
    - 0.5 mL of 1:1,000 solution sublingually in cases of major airway compromise or hypotension
    - 3–5 mL of 1:10,000 solution via central line
    - 3–5 mL of 1:10,000 solution diluted with 10 mL of normal saline via endotracheal tube
    - For protracted symptoms that require multiple doses of epinephrine, an intravenous (IV) epinephrine drip may be useful; the infusion is titrated to blood pressure (BP).
- **Airway management** is a priority. Supplemental 100% oxygen therapy should be administered. Endotracheal intubation may be necessary. If laryngeal edema is not rapidly responsive to epinephrine, cricothyroidotomy or tracheotomy may be required.
- **Volume expansion** with IV fluids may be necessary. An initial bolus of 500–1,000 mL normal saline should be followed by an infusion that is titrated to BP and urine output.
- **β-Adrenergic antagonist** therapy increases the risk of anaphylaxis and anaphylactoid reactions and renders the reaction more difficult to treat.[1] Therefore, **glucagon**, given as a **1-mg (one-ampoule)** bolus and followed by a drip of up to 1 mg/hr, can be used to provide inotropic support for patients who are taking β-adrenergic antagonists.
- **α-Adrenergic or mixed-adrenergic agonist vasopressors must be avoided in this setting due to resultant unopposed α-mediated vasoconstriction.**
- **Inhaled β-adrenergic agonists** (albuterol 0.5 mL [2.5 mg] or metaproterenol 0.3 mL [15 mg] in 2.5 mL of normal saline) should be used to treat resistant bronchospasm.
- **Glucocorticoids** have no significant immediate effect. However, they may prevent relapse of severe reactions. Methylprednisolone, 125 mg IV, or hydrocortisone, 500 mg IV, can be administered.
- **Antihistamines** relieve skin symptoms but have no immediate effect on the reaction. They may shorten the duration of the reaction. The addition of an H2 antagonist may be useful.
- Self-administered epinephrine should be prescribed for all patients with a history of anaphylaxis to food or *Hymenoptera* sting. The patient should be instructed in its use.
- **Referrals** to an allergist for further evaluation should be offered to patients with a history of anaphylaxis. More importantly, patients with *Hymenoptera* sensitivity should be referred to an allergist for venom immunotherapy.

DRUG REACTIONS

- Adverse reactions to drugs are a very common problem. Only a subset of reactions is mediated immunologically; other drug reactions may be toxic or idiosyncratic. Many different mechanisms can account for immunologically mediated drug reactions (Table 10-1). These reactions can occur with relatively low doses of the drug, usually on re-exposure after an initial sensitization to the drug.
- **Beta-lactam sensitivity.** Penicillins and other beta-lactam antibiotics are commonly associated with immunologically mediated drug reactions.
    - **Penicillins** have a high incidence of immunologic reactivity as a result of their chemical structure.
        - The core structure consists of a reactive bicyclic β-lactam ring that serves as a hapten by covalently binding to tissue carrier proteins. Ninety-five percent of tissue-bound penicillin is found to be haptenated as the benzylpenicilloyl form and is called the **major determinant.**
        - Five percent of tissue-bound penicillin consists of three non–cross-reactive metabolites, termed the **minor determinants.**
        - Immediate allergic reactions are most often related to the major determinant.
        - In addition, some modified penicillins, such as ampicillin, can produce allergic reactions in which the antigenic determinant is the side chain.
        - Skin testing is available if there is a question of immediate hypersensitivity to penicillin. Ninety-seven percent of patients with a negative skin test to penicillin will not develop a significant immediate hypersensitivity reaction to penicillin.
        - A delayed, non–IgE-mediated reaction (e.g., a morbiliform rash or serum sickness) may still develop in these patients. **No case of penicillin-induced anaphylaxis has been reported in a patient who is skin test negative.** Seventy-five percent of patients who report a history of penicillin sensitivity are negative on skin testing and are not at risk for anaphylaxis. However, 4% of patients with unknown or negative histories of penicillin reactions have positive skin tests and are at risk of having an IgE-mediated event. Skin testing should only be performed by an allergist who has been appropriately trained to perform these tests.
    - **Cephalosporins** share cross-reactivity with penicillins because of their related structure.
        - Studies report a fourfold increased risk of hypersensitivity reactions to cephalosporins in penicillin-allergic patients as compared to the general population (8% vs. 2%).[2] The degree of cross-reactivity is related to the generation of the cephalosporin (first generation > second generation > third generation).
        - Although many of the reactions to second- and third-generation cephalosporins are directed at the side chains, skin testing to penicillin in these patients can be helpful because most severe anaphylactic reactions are directed against the reactive bicyclic core.

TABLE 10-1 Immunologically Mediated Drug Reactions

Type of reaction	Representative examples	Mechanism
Anaphylactic	Anaphylaxis Urticaria Angioedema	IgE-mediated degranulation of mast cell with resultant mediator release
Cytotoxic	Autoimmune hemolytic anemia Interstitial nephritis	IgG or IgM antibodies against cell antigens and complement activation
Immune complex	Serum sickness Vasculitis	Immune complex deposition and subsequent complement activation
Cell mediated	Contact dermatitis Photosensitivity dermatitis	Activated T cells against cell surface—bound antigens

- Patients with a history of a severe reaction to penicillin should be considered sensitive to cephalosporin unless they are skin test negative. Although patients with a history of a nonanaphylactic reaction to penicillin can often be given a second- or third-generation cephalosporin safely, it is advisable to precede the dose with an oral provocation challenge.
- **Other related antibiotics**
  - **Monobactams. Aztreonam** is the prototype antibiotic of this group with a mono-cyclic structure. No significant cross-reactivity is found between this group and the β-lactams.
  - **Carbapenems. Imipenem** is the prototype member of this group. A very high degree of cross-reactivity (50%) is found between imipenem determinants and penicillin determinants.
  - **Carbacephems** (e.g., loracarbef) are structurally related to cephalosporins. Few data exist in regard to cross-reactivity, but they are assumed to be related anti-genically and should be avoided in severely penicillin-sensitive patients.
- **Erythema multiforme (EM), Stevens-Johnson syndrome (SJS), and toxic epidermal necrolysis (TEN)** are all serious drug reactions involving primarily the skin.
  - EM is characterized most typically by target lesions.
  - SJS and TEN manifest with varying degrees of sloughing of the skin and mucous membranes (<10% of the epidermis in SJS and >10% in TEN).
  - Treatment focuses on the discontinuation of suspected drugs and treatment of any underlying infection. Other therapeutic maneuvers are directed at symptoms and may include hydration to maintain fluid balance, antihistamines to decrease pruritus, analgesics to relieve pain, and wet dressings to debride crusted erosions. Care in the burn unit or ICU may be required. Systemic corticosteroids are often used, but their efficacy is unproven. **Readministration or future skin testing with the offending drug is absolutely contraindicated.**

Management

- Use of the drug in question should always be avoided unless a definite medical indication exists.
- If use of the drug must be considered, a careful history of the reaction is helpful in defining the potential risk. The date of a reaction is useful, given that patients may lose their sensitivity to a drug over time. Timing of symptoms is important; symptoms occurring with the start of a drug course are more likely to be IgE mediated than are symptoms that develop several days after the completion of a course.
- On occasion, a history of an unrecognized, inadvertent re-exposure to a drug that had previously caused a reaction may be elicited. If this re-exposure was not associated with any reaction, it is due to lack of true IgE-mediated hypersensitivity or potentially a loss of sensitivity that may have developed.
- Finally, the type of symptoms must be detailed. Toxic reactions (e.g., nausea secondary to macrolide antibiotics or codeine) are not immunologic reactions and do not necessarily predict problems with other members in their respective class.

Treatment

- Discontinuation of the suspected drug or drugs is the most important initial approach in managing an allergic drug reaction.
- If the patient is taking the drug for a life-threatening illness (e.g., meningitis with penicillin allergy) and the reaction is a mild skin reaction, it may be reasonable to continue the medication and treat the reaction symptomatically. If the rash is progressive, however, the drug must be discontinued to avoid a desquamative process such as Stevens-Johnson syndrome.
- Similarly, anaphylactic reactions to a drug require evaluation of potential drug allergy before readministering the offending agent.

Referrals/Consultation

- A history of a true IgE-mediated reaction (anaphylaxis) does increase the likelihood of further IgE-mediated reactions.
- If no alternative drug is available and the patient has a history of an IgE-mediated reaction, the patient should be referred to an allergist for skin testing. Standard skin testing is available only for penicillin but may be useful for other β-lactam–related antibiotics and cephalosporins. If the patient has a positive skin test to penicillin, an allergist may perform desensitization.
- Results of testing to drugs other than penicillin must be interpreted within the clinical context of the case, and management may include a graded dose challenge under the direction of an allergist. A successful desensitization or graded challenge does not preclude the development of a non–IgE-mediated, delayed reaction (e.g., rash). Furthermore, if a dose of drug is missed following a desensitization procedure, the patient often will need to undergo a repeat desensitization.
- Patients who present to the emergency department with anaphylaxis for the first time should be given a prescription for self-injectable epinephrine and be referred to an allergist for further evaluation.

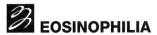 **EOSINOPHILIA**

GENERAL PRINCIPLES

- Peripheral blood **eosinophilia** is defined as an absolute eosinophil count of >450/microliter.
- Eosinophils are tissue-dwelling cells and are most abundant in mucosal tissues such as the respiratory and gastrointestinal tracts.

Epidemiology

- In industrialized nations, peripheral blood eosinophilia is most often due to atopic disease, whereas helminthic infections are the most common cause of eosinophilia in the rest of the world.

Etiology

- The **etiology** of eosinophilia may be classified by associated clinical context as shown in Table 10-2 or by the level of eosinophilia as shown in Table 10-3.

Classification

- **Eosinophilia associated with atopic disease.** Modest peripheral blood levels of eosinophils are often found in patients with allergic rhinitis, asthma, or atopic dermatitis.
- **Eosinophilia associated with pulmonary infiltrates.** This classification is inclusive of the pulmonary infiltrates with eosinophilia (PIE) syndromes and the eosinophilic pneumonias.
  - PIE syndromes refer to those diseases with pulmonary infiltrates and blood eosoinophilia. The **PIE syndromes** include allergic bronchopulmonary aspergillosis (ABPA), an IgE-dependent immunologic reaction to *Aspergillus fumigatus* consisting of pulmonary infiltrates, proximal bronchiectasis, and asthma- and drug-induced pneumonitis.
  - Eosinophilic pneumonias consist of pulmonary infiltrates with lung eosinophilia. It is important to note that eosinophilic pneumonias are only sometimes associated with blood eosinophilia. The **eosinophilic pneumonias** include acute and chronic eosinophilic pneumonias (idiopathic diseases that present with fever, cough, and dyspnea), Loffler syndrome (combination of blood eosinophilia and transient pulmonary infiltrates due to passage of helminthic larvae, usually *Ascaris lumbricoides*, through the lungs), and tropical pulmonary eosinophilia (a hypersensitivity response in the lung to lymphatic filariae).

TABLE 10-2 Causes of Eosinophilia

Eosinophilia associated with atopic disease
Allergic rhinitis
Asthma
Atopic dermatitis

Eosinophilia associated with pulmonary infiltrates
Passage of larvae through the lung (Loffler syndrome)
Chronic eosinophilic pneumonia
Acute eosinophilic pneumonia
Tropical pulmonary eosinophilia
Allergic bronchopulmonary aspergillosis (ABPA)
Coccidiomycosis

Eosinophilia associated with parasitic infection
Helminths (*Ascaris lumbricoides*, *Strongyloides stercoralis*, hookworm, *Toxocara canis or cati*, *Trichinella*)
Protozoa (only *Dientamoeba fragilis* and *Isospora belli*)

Eosinophilia associated with primary cutaneous disease
Atopic dermatitis
Eosinophilic fasciitis
Eosinophilic cellulitis
Eosinophilic folliculitis
Episodic angioedema with anaphylaxis

Eosinophilia associated with multiorgan involvement
Drug-induced eosinophilia
Churg-Strauss syndrome
Idiopathic hypereosinophilic syndrome
Eosinophilic leukemia

Miscellaneous causes
Eosinophilic gastroenteritis
Interstitial nephritis
HIV infection
Eosinophilia myalgia syndrome
Transplant rejection
Atheroembolic disease

- **Eosinophilia associated with parasitic infection.** Various multicellular parasites or helminths such as *Ascaris*, hookworm, or *Strongyloides* can induce blood eosinophilia, whereas single-celled protozoan parasites such as *Giardia lamblia* do not.
  - In cases of blood eosinophilia, **Strongyloides stercoralis** infection must be excluded because this helminth can set up a cycle of autoinfection leading to chronic infection with intermittent, sometimes marked, eosinophilia.
- **Eosinophilia associated with cutaneous disease**
  - **Atopic dermatitis** is classically associated with blood and skin eosinophilia.
  - **Eosinophilic fasciitis** is characterized by acute erythema, swelling, and induration of the extremities progressing to symmetric induration of the skin that spares the fingers, feet, and face.

 TABLE 10-3 Classification of Eosinophilia Based on the Peripheral Blood Eosinophil Count

Peripheral Blood Eosinophil Count (Cells/microliter)		
500–2,000	**2,000–5,000**	**>5,000**
Allergic rhinitis	Intrinsic asthma	Eosinophilia-myalgia syndrome
Allergic asthma	Allergic bronchopulmonary aspergillosis	Idiopathic hypereosinophilic syndrome
Food allergy	Helminthiasis	Episodic angioedema with eosinophilia
Urticaria	Churg-Strauss syndrome	Leukemia
Addison disease	Drug reactions	
Pulmonary infiltrates with eosinophilia syndromes	Vascular neoplasms	
Solid neoplasms	Eosinophilic fasciitis	
Nasal polyposis	HIV	

- Antibiotic therapy failure and recurrent swelling of an extremity without tactile warmth is characteristic of **eosinophilic cellulitis.**
- Patients with HIV are at risk for **eosinophilic pustular folliculitis.**
- A rare disease, **episodic angioedema with eosinophilia**, leads to recurrent attacks of fever, angioedema, and blood eosinophilia without other organ damage.

- **Eosinophilia associated with multiorgan involvement**
  - **Drug-induced eosinophilia.** Numerous drugs can cause blood and/or tissue eosinophilia. Drug-induced eosinophilia typically responds to cessation of the culprit medication. Asymptomatic drug-induced eosinophilia does not necessitate cessation of therapy. A list of medications most commonly associated with eosinophilia can be found elsewhere.[3]
  - **Churg-Strauss syndrome** (CSS) is a small-vessel vasculitis distinguished from other vasculitidies by tissue and blood eosinophilia, intravascular and extravascular eosinophilic granuloma formation, lung involvement with transient infiltrates on chest radiograph, and association with asthma. The onset of asthma and eosinophilia may precede the development of CSS by several years. Other manifestations include sinusitis, mono- or polyneuropathy, and rash.
    - Half of patients have anti-neutrophil cytoplasmic antibodies directed against myeloperoxidase (p-ANCA). Biopsy of affected tissue reveals a necrotizing vasculitis with extravascular granulomas and tissue eosinophilia.
    - Initial treatment involves high-dose glucocorticoids with the addition of cyclophosphamide if necessary. Leukotriene modifiers, like all systemic steroid-sparing agents (including inhaled steroids), have been associated with unmasking of CSS due to a decrease in systemic steroid therapy; however, no evidence exists that these drugs *cause* CSS.[4]
  - Idiopathic **hypereosinophilic syndrome** (HES) is a proliferative disorder of eosinophils characterized by specific organ damage due to infiltration of eosinophils, most notably in the heart.
    - HES occurs predominantly in men between the ages of 20 and 50 years and presents with insidious onset of fatigue, cough, and dyspnea and an associated eosinophil count of >1,500.
    - At presentation, patients typically are in the late thrombotic and fibrotic stages of eosinophil-mediated cardiac damage with signs of a restrictive cardiomyopathy and mitral regurgitation. An echocardiogram may detect intracardiac thombi, endomyocardial fibrosis, or thickening of the posterior mitral valve leaflet. Neurologic manifestations range from peripheral neuropathy to stroke or encephalopathy. Bone marrow examination reveals increased eosinophil precursors.
    - Initial treatment is with prednisone at 1 mg/kg/day; interferon-α has been shown to be effective as well.[5] More recently imatinib and anti-interleukin 5 treatment have shown great promise as the newest therapeutics for this disease (see later discussion).
  - **Acute eosinophilic leukemia** is a rare myeloproliferative disorder that is distinguished from HES by several factors: an increased number of immature eosinophils in the blood and/or marrow, >10% blast forms in the marrow, as well as symptoms and signs compatible with an acute leukemia. Treatment is similar to that for other leukemias (see Chapter 20: Medical Management of Malignant Disease).

Mechanism of Injury

- Activation of eosinophils leads to the release of stored granular components such as major basic proteins, eosinophil peroxidase, and eosinophil cationic protein, which are believed to be responsible for the tissue damage ascribed to these cells. In addition, these activated cells produce cytokines that can exacerbate the immunologic reaction.

DIAGNOSIS

- There are two approaches that are useful for evaluating eosinophilia, either by associated clinical context (Table 10-2) or by degree of eosinophilia (Table 10-3).

History

- The presence of cough, dyspnea, fever, or any symptoms of cancer should be determined, as should any history of rhinitis, wheezing, or rash.
- A complete medication list, including over-the-counter supplements, and a full travel history focused on countries where filariasis may be endemic (e.g., Southeast Asia, Africa, South America, or the Caribbean) should be obtained.
- Any pet exposure should be ascertained for possible exposure to toxocariasis.

Phyical Examination

- Physical examination should be guided by the history, with a special focus on the skin, upper and lower respiratory tracts, as well as cardiovascular and neurologic systems.

Laboratory Tests

- Mild **eosinophilia associated with symptoms of rhinitis or asthma** is indicative of underlying atopic disease, which can be comfirmed by skin testing.
- **Stool examination** for ova and parasites should be done on three separate occasions. Because only small numbers of helminths may pass in the stool and because tissue- or blood-dwelling helminths will not be found in the stool, **serologic tests** for antiparasite antibodies should also be sent. Such tests are available for strongyloidiasis, toxocariasis, and trichinellosis.
- Diagnosis at the time of presentation with Loffler syndrome can be made by detection of *Ascaris* larvae in respiratory secretions or gastric aspirates, but not stool.
- A history of asthma, significant peripheral blood eosinophilia (>10% of the leukocyte count), and pulmonary infiltrates suggests CSS. In this case, sinus computed tomography, nerve conduction studies, and testing for p-ANCA may aid in diagnosis.

Imaging

- **Chest x-ray** findings may also help to narrow the differential diagnosis. Peripheral infiltrates with central clearing are indicative of chronic eosinophilic pneumonia. Diffuse infiltrates in an interstitial, alveolar, or mixed pattern may be seen in acute eosinophilic pneumonia as well as drug-induced eosinophilia with pulmonary involvement. Transient infiltrates may be seen in Loffler syndrome, CSS, or ABPA. Central bronchiectasis is a major criterion in the diagnosis of ABPA. A diffuse miliary or nodular pattern, consolidation, or cavitation may be found in cases of tropical pulmonary eosinophilia.

Surgical Diagnostic Procedures and Pathologic Findings

- If no other cause of pulmonary infiltrates has been identified, a **bronchoscopy** may be necessary for analysis of bronchoalveolar lavage (BAL) fluid and lung tissue. The presence of eosinophils in BAL fluid or sputum with eosinophilic infiltration of the parenchyma is most typical of acute or chronic eosinophilic pneumonia.

Differential Diagnosis

- Various conditions can result in **eosinophilia associated with pulmonary infiltrates** (Table 10-2). The presence of asthma should lead to consideration of ABPA, CSS, or tropical pulmonary eosinophilia.
- The etiology of **eosinophilia associated with cutaneous lesions** (Table 10-2) is guided by the appearance of the lesions and results of the skin biopsy. The diagnosis of CSS cannot be made without a tissue biopsy showing infiltrating eosinophils and granulomas.
- When eosinophilia is marked and all other causes have been ruled out, the diagnosis of **idiopathic HES** should be considered. Diagnosis requires a blood eosinophilia of >1,500/microliter for >6 months with associated organ involvement. No specific test exists to identify these patients, and in general this is a diagnosis of exclusion.

TREATMENT

- When a drug reaction is suspected, discontinuation of the drug is both diagnostic and therapeutic. Other treatment options depend on the exact cause of eosinophilia because, with the exception of idiopathic HES, eosinophilia itself is a manifestation of an underlying disease.
- Recent trials have suggested efficacy of imatinib mesylate (Gleevec) and anti-interleukin 5 in the treatment of HES, especially in those patients with the FIP1L1 fusion protein.[6,7]
- Primary eosinophilia disorders should be followed by a specialist; any cases of unresolved or unexplained eosinophilia warrant evaluation by an allergist-immunologist.

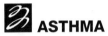 ASTHMA

GENERAL PRINCIPLES

Definition

- Asthma is a disease of the airways characterized by chronic airway inflammation and increased responsiveness (hyperreactivity) to a wide variety of stimuli (triggers).
- This hyperreactivity leads to obstruction of the airways, the severity of which may be widely variable in the same individual. As a consequence, patients have paroxysms of cough, dyspnea, chest tightness, and wheezing.
- Asthma is a chronic disease, with episodic acute exacerbations that are interspersed with symptom-free periods. Other conditions may present with wheezing and must be considered, especially in patients who are not responsive to therapy (Table 10-4).[8,9]

Anatomy

- The central and peripheral conducting airways of the lungs are primarily affected by asthma. Pathologic features of asthma include the following:
  - Inflammatory cell infiltration of the airways
  - Increased thickness of the bronchial smooth muscle
  - Partial or full loss of the respiratory epithelium
  - Subepithelial fibrosis
  - Hypertrophy and hyperplasia of the submucosal glands and goblet cells
  - Partial or full occlusion of the airway lumen by mucous plugs
  - Enlarged mucous glands and blood vessels[10]

Epidemiology

- The reported prevalence of asthma is quite variable and depends on the specific population being studied and criteria used to define asthma.

 TABLE 10-4   Conditions That Can Present as Refractory Asthma

Upper airway obstruction	Sinusitis
Tumor	Herpetic tracheobronchitis
Epiglottitis	Adverse drug reaction
Vocal cord dysfunction	Aspirin
Obstructive sleep apnea	β-Adrenergic antagonist
Tracheomalacia	Angiotensin-converting enzyme inhibitors
Endobronchial lesion	Inhaled pentamidine
Foreign body	Allergic bronchopulmonary aspergillosis
Congestive heart failure	Hyperventilation with panic attacks
Gastroesophageal reflux	

- The International Study of Asthma and Allergies in Childhood (ISAAC)[11] looked at the prevalence of symptoms, specifically wheezing, in 13- to 14-year-olds in 155 centers worldwide and found prevalence rates ranging from <5% to nearly 40%.
- In the United States:
  - At least one of every 20 individuals has asthma.
  - The prevalence of asthma has increased 61% over the last two decades.
  - Asthma is the leading chronic illness among children (10%–20%).
  - African-Americans are twice as likely as whites to be hospitalized due to asthma.
  - Asthma results in 10 million lost school days and 3 million lost work days.
  - Deaths from asthma have increased by 31% since 1980.
  - The death rate for African-Americans from asthma is three times higher than that for whites.[12,13]
- Risk factors for asthma can be broadly divided into host genetic and environmental factors.
  - There have been multiple genes and chromosomal regions associated with the development of asthma. Racial and ethnic differences have also been reported in asthma but are likely the result of socioeconomic and environmental factors rather than genuine racial predispositions.
  - There are multiple environmental factors that contribute to the development and persistence of asthma. Severe viral infection early in life, particularly respiratory syncytial virus (RSV), is associated with the development of asthma in childhood and may also play a role in its pathogenesis.
  - Childhood exposure and sensitization to a variety of allergens may contribute to the development of atopy and asthma; however, the exact nature of the relationship between allergen exposure and atopic sensitization is not clear.

Classification[8,9]

- **Mild intermittent asthma.**
  - This is characterized by mild asthma symptoms two or fewer times a week, nocturnal awakening fewer than two times a month, a peak expiratory flow (PEF) of >80% of personal best, and a forced expiratory volume over 1 second (FEV_1) of >80% predicted.
  - In this setting, a short-acting β_2-adrenergic agonist used on an as-needed basis (e.g., albuterol, 2–3 puffs) is appropriate.
- **Mild persistent asthma.**
  - These patients have asthma symptoms more than two times a week, nocturnal awakening more than two times a month but less than once per week, a PEF of >80% of personal best, and an FEV_1 of >80% predicted.
  - In addition to the short-acting β_2-adrenergic agonist, a long-term controller medication is required. A low dose of inhaled corticosteroid (Table 10-5) is the recommended long-term controller medication for this degree of severity. Alternative therapies, which are less effective, include a leukotriene antagonist, cromolyn, nedocromil, or theophylline.
- **Moderate persistent asthma.**
  - These patients have asthma symptoms daily, nocturnal awakening more than one time a week, a PEF of <60% to <80% of personal best, and an FEV_1 of >60% to >80% of predicted.
  - The use of a low to medium dose of inhaled corticosteroid together with a long-acting bronchodilator (salmeterol, 2 puffs twice daily) is the preferred therapy. Alternatives include increasing to a medium dose of inhaled corticosteroid (Table 10-5) or adding a leukotriene antagonist or theophylline to low to medium doses of inhaled corticosteroid.
- **Severe persistent asthma.**
  - These patients have asthma symptoms continuously, frequent nocturnal awakenings, PEF of <60% of personal best or FEV_1 of <60% predicted, or are limited in their physical activity.

TABLE 10-5 Comparative Daily Adult Dosages for Inhaled Corticosteroids[8,9]

Drug	Low dose	Medium dose	High dose
Triamcinolone (100 mcg/ puff)	4–10 puffs	10–20 puffs	>20 puffs
Beclomethasone dipropionate (42, 84 mcg/puff)	4–12 puffs: 42 mcg	12–20 puffs: 42 mcg	>20 puffs: 42 mcg
	2–6 puffs: 84 mcg	6–8 puffs: 84 mcg	>10 puffs: 84 mcg
Budesonide Turbuhaler (DPI: 200 mcg/dose)	1–2 inhalations	2–3 inhalations	>3 inhalations
Flunisolide (250 mcg/puff)	2–4 puffs	4–8 puffs	>8 puffs
Fluticasone	2–6 puffs: 44 mcg	2–6 puffs: 100 mcg	>6 puffs: 100 mcg
(MDI: 44, 110, 220 mcg/puff)	2 puffs: 110 mcg		>3 puffs: 220 mcg
(DPI: 50, 100, 250 mcg/ dose)	2–6 inhalations: 50 mcg	3–6 inhalations: 100 mcg	>6 inhalations: 100 mcg
			>2 inhalations: 250 mcg
Mometasone furoate (220 mcg/puff)	1 puff	2 puffs	3–4 puffs
Combination Agents			
Budesonide/Formeterol (DPI: 80/4.5 mcg/puff and 160/4.5 mcg/puff)	1–2 puff bid: 80/4.5 mcg/puff	2 puffs bid: 80/4.5 to 160/4.5 mcg/puff	2 puffs bid: 160/4.5 mcg/puff
Fluticasone/Salmeterol (DPI: 100/50, 250/50, 500/50 mcg/dose)	1 inhalation bid: 100/50 mcg	1 inhalation bid: 250/50 mcg	1 inhalation bid: 500/50 mcg

DPI = dry powder inhaler; MDI = metered-dose inhaler; bid = twice daily.

- A high dose of inhaled corticosteroid (Table 10-5) and a long-acting bronchodilator are the recommended therapies. These patients may require long-term oral corticosteroids (started at 2 mg/kg/d, not to exceed 60 mg/d), although repeated attempts should be made to reduce the dose while they are receiving high-dose inhaled corticosteroids.
- Patients who have severe persistent asthma in whom control is inadequate despite the use of oral or high-dose inhaled corticosteroids typically have chronic limitation of activity and require frequent bronchodilator use. These patients should be referred to an asthma specialist. The goal of therapy is to minimize symptoms and the need for oral corticosteroids.
- **Nocturnal symptoms.** These symptoms may necessitate the addition at night of either a long-acting inhaled β-adrenergic agonist (e.g., salmeterol, 2 puffs at bedtime) or sustained-release theophylline. Increased circadian variability in airflow obstruction (nighttime awakening) is a sign of heightened airway hyperreactivity; thus, an increase in the dose of anti-inflammatory medication also should be considered in these patients.

Pathophysiology

- Asthma results from multiple processes. The combination of these processes results in airway obstruction, hyperinflation and airflow limitation.[8,9]
  - Chronic airway inflammation characterized by infiltration of the airway wall, mucosa, and lumen by activated eosinophils, mast cells, macrophages, and T lymphocytes.
  - Bronchial smooth muscle contraction resulting from mediators released by a variety of cell types including inflammatory, local neural, and epithelial cells.
  - Epithelial damage manifested by denudation and desquamation of the epithelium leading to mucous plugs that obstruct the airway.
  - Airway remodeling characterized by the following findings:[10]
    - Subepithelial fibrosis, specifically thickening of the lamina reticularis from collagen deposition
    - Smooth muscle hypertrophy and hyperplasia
    - Goblet cell and submucosal gland hypertrophy and hyperplasia resulting in mucus hypersecretion
    - Possible airway wall thickening due to acute edema and cellular infiltration during asthma exacerbations

Etiology

- **Asthma attacks** are episodes of shortness of breath or wheezing that last minutes to hours. Patients may be completely symptom-free between attacks. Typically, attacks are triggered by acute exposure to irritants (e.g., smoke) or allergens.
- **Exacerbations** occur when airway reactivity is increased and lung function becomes unstable. During an exacerbation, attacks occur more easily and are more severe and persistent. Exacerbations are associated with factors that increase airway hyperreactivity, such as viral infections, allergens, and occupational exposures.
- A number of factors increase airway hyperresponsiveness and cause an acute and chronic increase in the severity of the disease.
  - **Allergens,** such as dust mites, cockroaches, and pet dander, cause an increase in airway inflammation and symptoms in allergic patients. Many occupational allergens and irritants cause asthma, even in small doses.
  - **Viral upper respiratory tract infections and sinusitis** are important causes of asthma exacerbations.
  - **Gastroesophageal reflux** can cause cough and wheezing in some patients. Some factors, such as tobacco and wood smoke, trigger acute bronchospasm and should be avoided by all patients.
  - **Cold air and exercise** can increase symptoms. Prophylactic use of cromolyn, nedocromil, or an inhaled β_2-adrenergic agonist (2–4 puffs 20 minutes before exposure) can minimize exercise-induced symptoms.

- **Aspirin and nonsteroidal anti-inflammatory drugs (NSAIDs)** can cause the sudden onset of severe airway obstruction. Patients with aspirin sensitivity and nasal polyps typically have the onset of asthma in the third or fourth decade of life.

DIAGNOSIS

History

- Recent emergency room visits and current oral corticosteroid use may indicate an exacerbation that has become refractory to outpatient management.
- Previous attacks that have required the use of oral corticosteroids, a previous episode of respiratory failure, use of more than two canisters per month of inhaled short-acting bronchodilator, and seizures with asthma attacks have been associated with severe and potentially fatal asthma. Most patients have a progressive worsening of symptoms over a period of days or weeks.[8,9]
- A precipitous onset of symptoms should raise the possibility of gastroesophageal reflux or a reaction to acute ingestion of aspirin or an NSAID.

Physical Examination

- A rapid assessment should be performed to identify those patients who require immediate intervention. The presence or intensity of wheezing is an unreliable indicator of the severity of an attack.
- A severe attack is suggested by respiratory distress at rest, difficulty in speaking in sentences, diaphoresis, or agitation. A respiratory rate of >28 breaths/minute, a pulse of >110 beats/minute, or a pulsus paradoxus of >25 mm Hg also indicates a severe episode.
- Patients with depressed mental status require intubation. Impending respiratory muscle fatigue may cause a depressed respiratory effort and paradoxical diaphragmatic movement.
- Subcutaneous emphysema should alert the examiner to the presence of a pneumothorax or pneumomediastinum.
- Pulmonary function tests (PFTs) are essential to the diagnosis of asthma. In patients with asthma, PFTs demonstrate an obstructive pattern, the hallmark of which is a decrease in expiratory flow rates.[8,9]
  - A reduction in FEV_1 and a proportionally smaller reduction in the forced vital capacity (FVC) occur. This produces a decreased FEV_1/FVC ratio (generally <0.75). With mild obstructive disease that involves only the small airways, the FEV_1/FVC ratio may be normal, with the only abnormality being a decrease in airflow at midlung volumes (forced expiratory flow 25%–75%).
  - The clinical diagnosis of asthma is supported by an obstructive pattern that improves after bronchodilator therapy. Improvement is defined as an increase in FEV_1 of >12% and 200 cc after 2–3 puffs of a short-acting bronchodilator.
  - In patients with chronic, severe asthma, the airflow obstruction may no longer be completely reversible. In these patients, the most effective way to establish the maximal degree of airway reversibility is to repeat PFTs after a course of oral corticosteroids (usually 40 mg/d for 10 days).
  - The lack of demonstrable airway obstruction or reactivity does not rule out a diagnosis of asthma. In cases in which spirometry is normal, the diagnosis can be made by showing heightened airway responsiveness to a methacholine or histamine challenge.

Laboratory Studies

- An objective measurement of airflow obstruction is essential to the evaluation of an asthma attack. The severity of the exacerbation should be classified as mild to moderate (PEF or FEV_1 >50% of predicted), severe (PEF or FEV_1 <50%), or impending or actual respiratory arrest. Hospitalization is recommended if the response to treatment is poor or incomplete. A low threshold for admission is appropriate for patients with recent hospitalization, a failure of aggressive outpatient management (with oral corticosteroids), or a previous life-threatening attack.[8,9]

- When spirometry is not available, peak flow rates can be obtained easily with a peak flowmeter. Generally, hospitalization is recommended if the PEF or FEV_1 is <50% of predicted, arterial carbon dioxide tension ($PaCO_2$) is >42 mm Hg, the symptoms are severe, or the patient is drowsy or confused. The response to initial treatment (60–90 minutes after three treatments with a short-acting bronchodilator) is a better predictor of the need for hospitalization than is the severity of an exacerbation.

- Arterial blood gas measurement should be considered in patients in severe distress or with an FEV_1 of <30% of predicted values after initial treatment. An arterial oxygen tension of <60 mm Hg is a sign of severe bronchoconstriction or of a complicating condition. Initially, the $PaCO_2$ is low, owing to an increase in respiratory rate. With a prolonged attack, the $PaCO_2$ may rise as a result of severe airway obstruction, increased dead-space ventilation, and respiratory muscle fatigue. A normal or increased $PaCO_2$ is a sign of impending respiratory failure and necessitates hospitalization. The patient requires aggressive bronchodilator therapy and should be monitored closely (often in an intensive care unit) to assess the need for mechanical ventilation.

Imaging

- Obtaining a chest radiograph is not routinely required and is performed only if a complicating pulmonary process, such as pneumonia or pneumothorax, is suspected, or to rule out other causes of dyspnea, cough, or wheezing in patients being evaluated for asthma.

Monitoring

- PEF monitoring provides an objective measurement of airflow obstruction and should be considered in patients with moderate to severe persistent asthma. Ideally, the PEF should be measured in the early morning and again after 12 hours, with additional measurements taken before and 20 minutes after bronchodilator therapy.

- The personal-best PEF (the highest PEF obtained when the disease is under control) is identified, and the PEF is checked when symptoms escalate or in the setting of an asthma trigger. This should be incorporated into an asthma action plan, setting 80%–100% of personal-best PEF as the "green" zone, 50%–80% as the "yellow" zone, and <50% as the "red" zone.[8,9]

- Patients should learn to anticipate situations that cause increased symptoms. For many individuals, monitoring symptoms instead of PEF is sufficient. In addition, it is useful for patients to monitor their PEF during times in which medications are changed.

TREATMENT

Medications

- Medical management involves chronic management and a plan for acute exacerbations. Most often it includes the daily use of an anti-inflammatory, disease-modifying medication (long-term-control medications) and as-needed use of a short-acting bronchodilator (quick-relief medications).

- **Supplemental oxygen** should be administered to the patient who is awaiting an assessment of arterial oxygen tension and should be continued to maintain an oxygen saturation of >90% (95% in patients with coexisting cardiac disease or pregnancy).

- **Bronchodilators** are first-line therapy in an asthma attack. Reversal of airflow obstruction is achieved most effectively by frequent administration of inhaled β_2-adrenergic agonists.
    - **Albuterol** is administered either via metered-dose inhaler (MDI) or nebulizer.

- For a mild to moderate exacerbation, initial treatment starts with 6–12 puffs of albuterol via MDI or 2.5 mg via nebulizer and is repeated q20min until improvement is obtained or toxicity is noted.
- For a severe exacerbation, albuterol, 2.5–5.0 mg q20min, and ipratropium bromide, 0.5 mg q3–4h, should be administered via nebulizer. Alternatively, albuterol, 10.0–15.0 mg, administered continuously over an hour, may be more effective in severely obstructed adults.
- The subsequent dosing schedule is adjusted according to the patient's symptoms and clinical presentation. Often, patients require a β_2-adrenergic agonist q2–4h during an acute attack. The use of an MDI with a spacer device under supervision of trained personnel is as effective as aerosolized solution by nebulizer. Cooperation may not be possible in the patient with severe airflow obstruction.
  - Parenteral administration of bronchodilators is unnecessary if inhaled medications can be administered quickly. In rare settings, aqueous epinephrine (0.3 mL of a 1:1,000 solution SC q20min) for up to three doses can be used. If epinephrine is administered, electrocardiograph monitoring is necessary.
- **Systemic corticosteroids** speed the resolution of exacerbations of asthma and should be administered to all patients with a moderate or severe exacerbation.
  - **Methylprednisolone** is the drug of choice for therapy. IV methylprednisolone, 125 mg, given on initial presentation decreases the rate of return to the emergency room of those patients who are discharged.[8,9]
  - The ideal dose of corticosteroid needed to speed recovery and limit symptoms is not well defined. Methylprednisolone, 40–60 mg IV q6h, is recommended. Oral corticosteroid administration may be as effective if given in equivalent doses (prednisone, 40–60 mg PO q12–24h).
  - For maximal therapeutic response, tapering of high-dose corticosteroids should not take place until objective evidence of clinical improvement is observed (usually 36–48 hour). Initially, patients are given a daily dose of oral prednisone, which is then reduced slowly. Dosing oral steroids twice a day may minimize symptoms.
  - A 7- to 14-day tapering dose of prednisone usually is successful in combination with an inhaled corticosteroid instituted at the beginning of the tapering schedule. In patients with severe disease or with a history of respiratory failure, a slower reduction in dose is appropriate.
  - Patients discharged from the emergency room should receive oral corticosteroids. A dose of prednisone, 40 mg/d for 5–7 days, can be substituted for a tapering schedule in selected patients. Either regimen should be accompanied by the initiation of an inhaled corticosteroid (or an increase in the previous dose of inhaled corticosteroid).
- **Methylxanthines** are generally not recommended for acute asthma attacks.
- **Antibiotics** have not been shown to have any benefit when administered routinely for acute asthma exacerbations. They can only be recommended as needed for treatment of comorbid conditions, such as pneumonia or bacterial sinusitis.[8,9]
- **Inhaled corticosteroids** are safe and effective for the treatment of chronic asthma (Table 10-5). They should be administered with a spacing device (if using MDI), and patients should be instructed to rinse their mouth with water after each administration to reduce the possibility of oral candidiasis and hoarseness.
  - The dose is increased as necessary according to symptoms and PEF. In patients with frequent β_2-adrenergic agonist use or other signs of poorly controlled disease, the dose should be increased by 50%–100% until symptoms are controlled.
  - If symptoms are severe, accompanied by nighttime awakening, or PEF is <65% of predicted values, a short course of oral corticosteroid (40–60 mg/d for 5–7 days) might be necessary to gain control of the disease quickly. Attempts should be made to decrease the dose of inhaled corticosteroid by 25% every 2–3 months to the lowest possible dose to maintain control.
  - Once-daily dosing of inhaled corticosteroids may be as effective as twice-daily dosing in the management of mild persistent asthma and may improve adherence.

- In patients who require regular use of oral corticosteroid, both **fluticasone,** 8 puffs/d (220 mcg/puff), and **mometasone,** 4 puffs/d (220 mcg/puff), are very effective in reducing symptoms and in minimizing the effects of oral corticosteroid use.
- Systemic corticosteroid absorption can occur in patients who use high doses of inhaled corticosteroids. Consequently, prolonged therapy with high-dose inhaled corticosteroids should be reserved for patients with severe disease or for those who otherwise require oral corticosteroids. Repeated efforts should be made at tapering the dose.
- **Cromolyn sodium** and **nedocromil sodium** are anti-inflammatory inhaled medications that are alternatives to inhaled corticosteroids in children with mild persistent asthma. The usual dosage is 8–12 puffs/d in three to four divided doses. Maximum improvement may be delayed for 4–6 weeks after initiation of therapy. Little additional benefit accrues from using these medications with an inhaled corticosteroid.
- **Leukotriene antagonists.** Montelukast (10 mg PO daily) and zafirlukast (20 mg PO bid) are oral leukotriene-receptor antagonists. These agents provide effective control of mild persistent asthma in the majority of patients. However, in comparison with inhaled corticosteroids, they are not as effective in improving asthma outcomes.
  - Leukotriene antagonists should be strongly considered for patients with aspirin-induced asthma or for individuals who cannot master the use of an inhaler.
  - Zileuton (600 mg qid) is a 5-lipoxygenase inhibitor that is available for the treatment of asthma (primarily reserved for severe asthma). Due to zileuton's potential to cause elevation of liver function enzymes, it is recommended that transaminases (ALT) be monitored at the initiation, once a month during the first 3 months, every 2–3 months for the first year, and then periodically.
- **Methylxanthines.** Theophylline provides mild bronchodilation in asthmatics. Sustained-release theophylline may be useful as adjuvant therapy to an anti-inflammatory agent in persistent asthma, especially for controlling nighttime symptoms.
  - It is essential that serum concentrations of theophylline be monitored on a regular basis, aiming for a level of 5–15 mcg/mL, because theophylline has a narrow therapeutic range with significant toxicities. Theophylline has many potential drug interactions, especially with antibiotics.
- **Long-acting β_2-adrenergic agonists,** such as salmeterol (1 puff bid) or formoterol (1 puff bid), added to low- or medium-dose inhaled corticosteroids have consistently been shown to improve lung function and symptoms.
  - Limited evidence shows that the addition of long acting β_2-adrenergic agonists can also reduce the required dose of inhaled corticosteroids in patients with moderate persistent asthma.[14]
  - The benefits of adding long-acting β_2-adrenergic agonists are more substantial than those achieved by leukotriene antagonists, theophylline, or increased doses of inhaled corticosteroid.[8]
  - A Food and Drug Administration advisory has been issued for all medications containing a long-acting β_2-agonist stating that they have been associated with an increased risk of severe asthma exacerbations and asthma-related death. The warning was issued in light of data from the Salmeterol Multi-center Asthma Research Trial (SMART), which showed a very low but significant increase in asthma-related deaths in patients receiving salmeterol (0.01%–0.04%). It is recommended that long-acting β_2-agonists should not be used as a substitute for inhaled corticosteroids in the management of asthma or to treat acute asthma symptoms.
  - **Anti-IgE therapy.** Omalizumab is a monoclonal antibody against IgE and has a role in the management of moderate and severe persistent asthma. Clinical trials have shown that the addition of omalizumab to a treatment regimen that included corticosteroids (inhaled or oral) and beta-agonists resulted in improvement in daily asthma symptom scores and asthma quality of life.[15] The use of omalizumab allowed reduction in the dose of oral and inhaled corticosteroids without a decline in daily asthma symptom scores and asthma-specific quality of life. Omalizumab should be considered as add-on therapy in those patients with moderate to severe allergic asthma who are inadequately controlled with appropriate combination therapy that includes

inhaled corticosteroids and long acting beta-agonists, have complications due to inhaled or oral corticosteroid use, or have significant disability due to their asthma symptoms. Omalizumab is administered subcutaneously and dosed based upon the patient's baseline IgE level (if between 30 and 700 International Units/mL) and weight.

■ **Alternative medications.** Immunosuppressive medications to reduce the need for oral corticosteroids, such as methotrexate, cyclosporine, tacrolimus, and mycophenolate mofetil, have been studied and may be useful in some patients. These individuals should be evaluated by an asthma specialist.

Referrals

■ Patients should be referred to a specialist in asthma care if they have life-threatening asthma; atypical signs or symptoms; comorbidities such as sinusitis, nasal polyps, aspergillosis, vocal cord dysfunction, gastroesophageal reflux, severe rhinitis; additional diagnostic testing is needed, such as rhinoscopy or bronchoscopy, bronchoprovocation testing, allergy skin testing; severe persistent asthma not responding to standard care, requirement of chronic oral corticosteroids; and a need for allergen immunotherapy.

Protocol

■ The goals of daily management are to control symptoms while maintaining normal activity and pulmonary function, to prevent exacerbations, and to minimize medication toxicity. Successful management requires patient education, objective measurement of airflow obstruction, and a medication plan for daily use and for exacerbations.

■ The severity of asthma varies over time in individual patients. Consequently, medication requirements vary over time. The National Heart, Lung, and Blood Institute consensus report classifies asthma into four different steps: mild intermittent, mild, moderate, and severe persistent.[9]

■ The goal of the stepwise approach is to gain control of symptoms as quickly as possible by assigning the patient to the most severe step in which any one feature occurs. Therapy is started at a level higher than the patient's severity to gain control and then decreased in follow-up once control has been achieved. Therapy should be reviewed every 1–6 months to check whether stepwise reduction is possible.[8,9]

Patient Education

■ Patient education should focus on the chronic and inflammatory nature of asthma, with identification of factors that contribute to increased inflammation.

   ■ The consequences of ongoing exposure to chronic irritants or allergens and the rationale for therapy should be explained. Patients should be instructed to avoid factors that aggravate their disease, how to manage their daily medications, and how to recognize and deal with acute exacerbations (known as an asthma action plan).

   ■ The use of a *written* daily management plan as part of the education strategy is recommended for all patients with persistent asthma.[8,9]

■ It is important for patients to recognize signs of poorly controlled disease.

   ■ These signs include an increased or daily need for bronchodilators, limitation of activity, waking at night because of asthma symptoms, and variability in the PEF.

   ■ Poorly controlled asthma is characterized by a greater need for bronchodilator therapy and by an increase in the circadian variation in PEF.

   ■ Specific instructions about handling these symptoms, including criteria for seeking emergency care, should be provided.

Follow-Up

- Close follow-up is required for patients discharged from the hospital or emergency room because increased airway hyperreactivity persists for 4–6 weeks after an asthma exacerbation. A return visit to the physician should be scheduled for 5–7 days after discharge. All patients with asthma should have follow-up care based on the control and severity of their disease: mild, 6 months; moderate, 3–5 months, severe, 1–2 months.[8,9]

URTICARIA AND ANGIOEDEMA

GENERAL PRINCIPLES

Definition

- **Urticaria** (hives) are raised, flat-topped, well-demarcated pruritic skin lesions with surrounding erythema. Central clearing can cause an annular lesion and is often seen after antihistamine use. An individual lesion usually lasts minutes to hours.
- **Angioedema** is a deeper lesion causing painful areas of skin-colored, localized swelling. It can be found anywhere on the body, but most often involves the tongue, lips, or eyelids. When angioedema occurs without urticaria, specific diagnoses must be entertained (see differential diagnosis).

Epidemiology

- Urticaria is a common condition that affects 15% to 24% of the U.S. population at some time in their life. Chronic idiopathic urticaria occurs in 0.1% of the U.S. population, and there does not appear to be an increased risk in persons with atopy.
- Angioedema generally lasts 12–48 hours and occurs in 40%–50% of patients with urticaria.

Classification

- **Acute urticaria (with or without angioedema)** is defined as an episode lasting <6 weeks. Usually, it is caused by an allergic reaction to a medication or food, but it may be related to underlying infection, recent insect sting, or exposure (contact or inhalation) to an allergen. A patient can develop a hypersensitivity to a food, medication, or self-care product that previously had been used without difficulty.
- **Chronic urticaria (with or without angioedema)** is defined as episodes that persist for >6 weeks. There are many possible causes of chronic urticaria and angioedema, including medications, autoimmunity, self-care products, and physical triggers. However, the etiology remains unidentified in >80% of cases.

Mechanism of Injury

- Mechanisms for initiation of urticaria and angioedema differ depending on the classification and are not fully understood, but the final common pathway is the degranulation of mast cells or basophils and the release of inflammatory mediators. Histamine is the primary mediator and elicits edema (wheal) and erythema (flare).

DIAGNOSIS

History

- A complete history and physical exam should elicit any identifiable triggers, including physical triggers such as pressure, cold, or heat.

■ The history should also attempt to rule out systemic causes. This includes determining whether any individual lesion lasts for >24 hours, in which case the diagnosis of urticarial vasculitis must be investigated by skin biopsy.

Physical Examination

■ The examiner should determine that the lesions in fact represent urticaria. A pen mark around the lesion may demonstrate the classic fading and appearance of new lesions. The presence of dermographism, an immediate wheal-and-flare response on stroking the skin, should be ascertained.
■ In addition, it is important to look for secondary causes of urticaria such as infection, vasculitis, connective tissue disease, lymphoproliferative disorders, and endocrine diseases.

Laboratory Evaluations

■ A complete blood count (CBC), erythrocyte sedimentation rate (ESR), urinalysis, and liver function tests should be obtained to screen for systemic etiologies of chronic urticaria, such as hematologic malignancies, autoimmune diseases, and occult infections, including hepatitis.

Pathologic Findings

■ A skin biopsy should be performed if individual lesions persist for >24 hours to rule out urticarial vasculitis.
■ Biopsy of acute urticarial lesions reveals dilation of small venules and capillaries located in the superficial dermis with widening of the dermal papillae, flattening of the rete pegs, and swelling of collagen fibers.
■ Chronic urticaria is characterized by a dense, nonnecrotizing, perivascular infiltrate consisting of T lymphocytes, mast cells, eosinophils, basophils, and neutrophils.
■ Angioedema shows similar pathologic alterations in the deep, rather than superficial, dermis and subcutaneous tissue.

Differential Diagnosis

■ **Mast cell releasability syndromes** such as systemic mastocytosis and cutaneous mastocytosis, including urticaria pigmentosa, should be considered.
■ **Urticarial vasculitis** presents with urticaria-like lesions that do not fade within 24 hours. It is a systemic vasculitis characterized by vascular damage with findings of fragmentation of neutrophils, red cell extavasation, and swelling of endothelial cells on biopsy.
■ **Angioedema without urticaria** should lead to consideration of specific entities.
  ■ Use of **angiotensin-converting-enzyme inhibitors** (ACEIs) or **angiotensin II-receptor blockers** (ARBs) can be associated with angioedema at any point in the course of therapy.
    • In this situation, both ACEIs and ARBs should be avoided and substitution with a different class of drugs should be made.
    • It is important to note that some patients continue to have episodic angioedema for years after discontinuation of these medications. The reason for this continued disease activity is unknown.
  ■ **Hereditary angioedema (HAE), or C1 esterase inhibitor (C1 INH) deficiency,** is inherited in an autosomal-dominant pattern.
    • Patients present with painful angioedema of any part of the body (including the abdominal tract) but never with urticaria.
    • All patients with angioedema without urticaria should be screened with a C4 level, which is reduced during and between attacks of HAE. If the C4 level is reduced, a quantitative and functional C1 INH assay should be performed. Measuring C1 INH levels alone is not sufficient because 15% of patients have normal levels

of a dysfunctional C1 INH protein; therefore, it is important to also obtain the functional assay.
- Treatment for attacks consists of supportive measures, including the use of fresh-frozen plasma and/or cryoprecipitate. Prophylactic treatment in consultation with an allergist may consist of recombinant human C1 INH or anabolic steroids.

■ **Acquired C1 INH deficiency** presents similarly to HAE but is typically associated with an underlying lymphoproliferative disorder or connective tissue disease. These patients have reduced C1q, C1 INH, and C4 levels. Other patients with the acquired form have an autoantibody to C1 INH with low C4 and C1 INH levels but a normal C1 level.

TREATMENT

■ Behavioral changes are an important mode of therapy.
  ■ **Elimination of all self-care products,** with the exception of those that contain no methylparaben, fragrance, or preservative, is useful when sensitivity to these products is a possibility.
  ■ Careful consideration should be given to the **elimination or substitution of each pre-scription or over-the-counter medication** or supplement. If a patient reacts to one medication in a class, the reaction likely will be triggered by all medications in that class. Exacerbating agents (such as NSAIDS, including aspirin, opiates, vancomycin, and alcohol) should be avoided because they may induce nonspecific mast cell de-granulation and exacerbate urticaria caused by other agents.
■ Medical therapy for acute uticaria
  ■ **In the presence of anaphylaxis, which consists of systemic symptoms** such as hy-potension, laryngeal edema, or bronchospasm, treatment with **epinephrine** (0.3–0.5 mL of a 1:1,000 solution intramuscularly) should be administered immediately. See Anaphylaxis section for additional information.
  ■ The ideal treatment of acute urticaria with or without angioedema is identification and avoidance of specific causes. **All potential causes should be eliminated.** Most cases resolve within 1 week. In some instances, it is possible to reintroduce an agent cautiously if it is believed not to be the etiologic agent. This trial should be done in the presence of a physician with epinephrine readily available.
    • Medications, especially antibiotics, are common offenders and should be dis-continued when possible. Agents such as aspirin, NSAIDS, opiates, vancomycin, contrast media, and alcohol should be avoided.
    • Foods that commonly cause urticaria with or without angioedema include peanuts, tree nuts, shellfish, non-shellfish fish, milk, eggs, wheat, soy, and fruits. However, any food may cause an allergic reaction and should be avoided if sus-pected.
    • In hospitalized patients, medications, intravenous contrast media, and latex should be considered as possible causes.
  ■ **A second-generation oral antihistamine** such as cetirizine, fexofenadine, desloratadine, or loratadine should be administered to patients until the hives have cleared. A first-generation antihistamine such as hydroxyzine may be added as an evening dose if needed in order to obtain control in refractory cases.
  ■ **Oral corticosteroids** should be reserved for patients with laryngeal edema or systemic symptoms of anaphylaxis after treatment with epinephrine. Corticosteroids will not have an immediate effect but may prevent relapse. They may also be helpful for patients with severe symptoms who have not responded to antihistamines.
  ■ If a patient presents with systemic symptoms, self-administered epinephrine should be prescribed for use in the case of accidental exposure to the same trigger in the future.
■ Medical therapy for chronic urticaria
  ■ **Antihistamines** for symptom control are the mainstay of treatment. Treatment should be continued for a period of 6 months, then lowered to the level needed to maintain symptom control.

- Second-generation H1 antihistamines, such as cetirizine, fexofenadine, loratadine, and desloratadine, are well tolerated and should be used as first-line agents. Cetirizine, the breakdown product of hydroxyzine, is often used for chronic urticaria treatment because it is thought to concentrate in the skin; however, it is minimally sedating. Loratidine is available over the counter.
- Classic H1 antihistamines, such as hydroxyzine, 25 mg PO q4–6h or prn, can be added for better control of lesions or for breakthrough lesions. The dose usually is limited by sedation.
- Doxepin, an antidepressant with H1- and H2-blocking effects, is a useful addition and often is less sedating than hydroxyzine.
- H2-blocking agents may be helpful in addition to H1 antihistamines to control breakthrough hives.
- Oral corticosteroids should be reserved for those patients in whom adequate control cannot be achieved with a combination of the aforementioned agents. Steroids should be used only for short periods of time.
- In regards to referrals, all patients with chronic urticaria or a history of anaphylaxis should be referred to an allergy specialist for evaluation of autoimmune triggers, including the presence of anti-thyroid antibodies or antibodies against the IgE receptor.

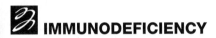

IMMUNODEFICIENCY

GENERAL MEASURES

Definition

- Immunodeficiency diseases are characterized by an increased susceptibility to infection. The type of infection and age of onset provide the first clues as to the type of immune defect.

Epidemiology

- The most common disease of immune deficiency is AIDS, which is not dealt with here (see Chapter 14, Human Immunodeficiency Virus Infection and Acquired Immunodeficiency Syndrome).
- In nonacquired immunodeficiencies, children and young adults present with abnormalities in T and B cells and are at risk for severe viral and bacterial infections.
- Adults usually present with defects in humoral immunity and are at increased risk of sinus or pulmonary infection from encapsulated bacteria.

Classifications

- Humoral immune deficiency
  - IgA deficiency
  - Common variable immunodeficiency (CVID)
  - Subclass deficiency
  - Hyper-IgE syndrome
- Cellular immune deficiency

Etiology

- There may be either hereditary or acquired defects in the production of immunoglobulins or abnormalities in B and T cell functions.
- The majority of immune defects of humoral immunity represent disorders in synthesis.
- However, increased degradation or catabolism of immunoglobulins can also be a mechanism of immunodeficiency in some disease states. Increased utilization of immunoglobulin may be seen in patients with severe underlying infection. Therefore, any formal

diagnosis and evaluation of humoral immunodeficiency should be postponed until infections are adequately treated.
- Protein-losing gastroenteropathy and renal glomeruli defects such as nephritic syndrome can result in the loss of large amounts of serum proteins, giving rise to hypogammaglobulinemia in addition to hypoalbuminemia.

Clinical Presentation

- **Immunoglobulin A (IgA) deficiency** is the most common immune deficiency, with a prevalence of 1 in 500 people.
  - Patients may be asymptomatic or present with recurrent sinus and pulmonary infections. Therapy is directed at early treatment with antibiotics because IgA replacement is not available.
  - In 15% of cases an associated immunoglobulin G (IgG) subclass deficiency is present.
  - Truly IgA-deficient patients (rather than those with very low levels) are at risk for developing a severe transfusion reaction because of the presence in some individuals of IgE anti-IgA antibodies; therefore these patients should be transfused with washed red blood cells or receive blood products only from IgA-deficient donors.
- **Common variable immunodeficiency (CVID)** includes a heterogeneous group of disorders in which patients present in the second to fourth decade of life with recurrent sinus and pulmonary infections and are discovered to have low or dysfunctional IgG, IgA, and IgM antibodies.
  - B cell numbers are usually normal, but there is decreased ability to produce immunoglobulin after immunization. Some patients may also exhibit T cell dysfunction and be anergic.
  - Patients may have associated gastrointestinal disease or autoimmune abnormalities (most commonly autoimmune hemolytic anemia, idiopathic thrombocytopenic purpura, pernicious anemia, and rheumatoid arthritis).
  - There is an increased incidence of malignancy, especially lymphoid and gastrointestinal malignancy.
  - Therapy consists of IV immunoglobulin (IVIG) replacement therapy as well as prompt treatment of infections with antibiotics.
- **Subclass deficiency.** Deficiencies of each of the IgG subclasses (IgG1, IgG2, IgG3, and IgG4) have been described.
  - These patients present with similar complaints as the CVID patients.
  - Total IgG levels may be normal. A strong association with IgA deficiency exists. There is disagreement as to whether this is a separate entity from CVID.
  - In most cases, there is no need to evaluate IgG subclass levels.
- **Hyper-IgE syndrome (Job syndrome)** is characterized by recurrent pyogenic infections of the skin and lower respiratory tract. This infection can result in severe abscess and empyema formation.
  - The most common organism involved is *Staphylococcus aureus*, but other bacteria and fungi have been reported.
  - Patients present with recurrent infections and have associated pruritic dermatitis, coarse (lion-like) facies, growth retardation, and hyperkeratotic nails. Laboratory data reveal the presence of normal levels of IgG, IgA, and IgM, but markedly elevated levels of IgE. A marked increase in tissue and blood eosinophils also may be observed.
  - The pathogenesis of the disorder is unknown, but it appears to be transmitted in an autosomal mode of inheritance with variable penetrance.
  - No specific therapy exists except for early treatment of infection with antibiotics.

DIAGNOSIS

- Workup begins with a CBC with differential, HIV test, quantitative immunoglobulin levels, and complement levels. Often the evaluation will need to include an assessment of B and T cell function.
- If immunoglobulin levels are normal and other possible precipitating factors such as allergy and anatomic abnormalities are ruled out, further evaluation should be pursued including an evaluation of B cell function. B cell response pre- and post-immunization

with both a protein antigen, such as tetanus, and polysaccharide antigen, such as pneumococcus (using the unconjugated 23-valent vaccine), should be tested because of the difference in how proteins and polysaccharides are handled by the immune system.

■ Titers of specific antibody are measured before and 4 weeks after immunization, with a good response defined as a fourfold increase in the antibody titer. Multiple serotypes of pneumococcus should be evaluated. A good response would be expected in greater than three of the serotypes.

■ A patient with normal or low IgG and a poor response to immunization is classified as having CVID.

TREATMENT OF HUMORAL IMMUNODEFICIENCY

■ IgA deficiency: no specific treatment is available. However, these patients should be promptly treated at the first sign of infection with an antibiotic that covers *Streptococcus pneumoniae* or *Haemophilus influenzae*.

■ CVID should be treated with IVIG. Numerous preparations of IVIG are available, all of which undergo viral inactivation steps.

  ▪ Replacement should be initiated with 400 mg/kg and infused slowly according to the manufacturer's suggestions (for most preparations, begin at 30 mL/hr and increase by 30 mL/hr every 15 minutes as tolerated to a maximum rate of 210 mL/hr).

  ▪ Possible side effects include myalgias, vomiting, chills, and lingering headache (due to immune complex–mediated aseptic meningitis).

  ▪ Patients, especially those with no detectable IgA, need to have vital signs monitored q15 minutes initially because anaphylaxis from IgE anti-IgA antibodies can develop in these patients. For these patients, it is best to use IVIG preparations that have very low IgA.

References

1. Lang DM, Alpern MB, Visintainer PF, Smith ST. Increased risk for anaphylactoid reaction from contrast media in patients on beta-adrenergic blockers or with asthma. *Ann Intern Med* 1991;115:270–276.
2. Petz LD. Immunologic cross-reactivity between penicillins and cephalosporins: a review. *J Infect Dis* 1978;137:S74–S79.
3. Chusid MJ. Eosinophilia in Childhood. *Immunol Allergy Clin North Am* 1999;19(2):327–346.
4. Wechsler ME, Flinn D, Gunawardena D, et al. Churg-Strauss syndrome in patients receiving montelukast as treatment for asthma. *Chest* 2000;117:708–713.
5. Malbrain ML, Vanden Bergh H, Zachee P. Further evidence for the clonal nature of the idiopathic hypereosinophilic syndrome: complete haematological & cytogenetic remission induced by interferon alpha in a case with a unique chromosomal abnormality. *Br J Haematol* 1996;92:176–183.
6. Cortes J, Auet P, Koller C, et al. Efficacy of imatinib mesylate in the treatment of idiopathic hypereosinophilic syndrome. *Blood* 2003;101(12):4714–4716.
7. Garrett JK, Jameson SC, Thomson B, et al. Anti-interleukin-5(mepolizumab) therapy for hyper eosinophilic syndromes. *J Allergy Clin Immunol* 2004;113(1):115–119.
8. Global Strategy for Asthma Management and Prevention. Global Initiative for Asthma (GINA). 2005.
9. Guidelines for the Diagnosis and Management of Asthma—expert panel report 2. National Asthma Education and Prevention Program, National Institutes of Health, National Heart, Lung and Blood Institute 2002.
10. Homer RJ, Elias JA. Airway remodeling in asthma: therapeutic implications of mechanisms. *Physiology* 2005;20:28–35.
11. Asher I, Weiland SK. The International Study of Asthma and Allergies in Childhood (ISAAC). ISAAC Steering Committee. *Clin Exp Allergy* 1998;28 Suppl 5:52–66.
12. Mannino DM, Homa DM, Akinbami LJ, et al. Surveillance for asthma—United States 1980–1999. *MMWR Morb Mortal Wkly Rep* 2002;51(SS-1):1–14.

13. Rabe KF, Adachi M, Lai CKW, et al. Worldwide severity and control of asthma in children and adults: the global Asthma Insights and Reality surveys. *J Allergy Clin Immunol* 2004;114:40–47.
14. Bateman ED, Boushey HA, Bousquet J, et al. Can guideline-defined asthma control be achieved? The Gaining Optimal Asthma Control Study. *Am J Respir Crit Care Med* 2004;170:836–844.
15. Busse WW. Anti-immunoglobulin E (omalizumab) therapy in allergic asthma. *Am J Respir Crit Care Med* 2001;164:S12–7.

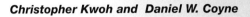

RENALDISEASES

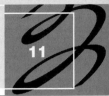

Christopher Kwoh and Daniel W. Coyne

EVALUATION OF THE PATIENT WITH RENAL DISEASE

DIAGNOSIS

Clinical Presentation

- Chronic kidney disease (CKD) frequently presents as abnormal routine laboratory data, such as an elevated serum creatinine (Cr) level (>1.0 mg/dL in women, or >1.3 mg/dL in men) or an abnormal urinalysis with proteinuria, hematuria, or pyuria.
- Acute renal failure (ARF) may manifest as abrupt onset of edema, malaise, oliguria, or hematuria, or may be detected as an asymptomatic laboratory finding. Initial evaluation should determine the need for emergent dialysis and then be directed at identifying reversible causes of renal dysfunction.

Laboratory Studies

- **Initial studies** in the evaluation of patients with suspected renal disease should include the following:
  - **Serum chemistries,** including electrolytes, Cr, blood urea nitrogen (BUN), calcium, magnesium, phosphate, uric acid, and albumin. If the serum Cr is stable, the glomerular filtration rate (GFR) can be estimated by using the **Cockcroft-Gault formula for Cr clearance (ClCr):**

$$\mathrm{Cl_{Cr}\ (mL/min)} = \frac{([140 - \mathrm{age}] \times [\mathrm{ideal\ body\ weight\ in\ kg}])}{72 \times \mathrm{Serum\ Cr\ (mg/dL)}} \times 0.85\ \mathrm{(for\ women)}$$

  - The **Modification of Diet in Renal Disease (MDRD) formula** is more accurate than the Cockroft-Gault formula in patients with significant renal disease, taking into account BUN, albumin, and race in addition to creatinine, age, and gender. It is unwieldy for hand calculation; however, an MDRD calculator can be found online at http://www.kidney.org/professionals/kdoqi/gfr_calculator.cfm. It is preferable to use the extended version and include serum albumin whenever available.
  - **Urine dipstick** for protein, occult blood, leukocytes, and pH, and microscopic examination of a freshly voided specimen for formed elements, such as crystals, red blood cells (RBCs), white blood cells (WBCs), and casts.
  - **Proteinuria** can be roughly quantitated by a **spot urine protein (mg/dL)–to–Cr (mg/dL) ratio** in a random urine specimen; the resulting ratio represents the amount of proteinuria in g/1.73 m^2 body surface area/d.
  - **Hematuria** may reflect a variety of conditions, including infection or inflammation of the prostate or bladder, malignancy (e.g., bladder or renal cell carcinoma), renal stones (see Nephrolithiasis), polycystic kidney disease, trauma with or without the presence of a bleeding diathesis, papillary necrosis, or glomerular disease (see Glomerulopathies).

■ **Urine sediment** should be examined. Epithelial cells and "muddy brown" granular casts are seen with ischemic damage of the tubules. Pyuria is seen with urinary tract infection or interstitial nephritis. WBC casts may be seen in pyelonephritis and interstitial nephritis. RBC casts are indicative of glomerulonephritis (GN). The presence of crystals may indicate stone disease or certain alcohol poisonings (see Chapter 25, Medical Emergencies).

■ **Supplementary studies** can be useful to assess renal function further and may aid in identifying specific disorders.

  ■ **Twenty-four-hour urine studies** include measurement of urine volume, Cr, and protein. The GFR can be estimated by calculation of the Cl_{Cr}:

$$Cl_{Cr} \text{ (mL/min)} = \frac{(\text{Urine Cr [mg/dL]} \times \text{Volume [mL]})}{(\text{Serum Cr [mg/dL]} \times \text{Time [min]})}$$

  • This value is useful in
    ◦ adjusting drug dosage
    ◦ predicting remaining renal function
    ◦ timing the placement of dialysis access

  ■ In adults under the age of 50 years, if the 24-hour Cr for women is <15–20 mg/kg lean body weight and for men is <20–25 mg/kg lean body weight, the collection may be incomplete, leading to an underestimation of the GFR. In severe renal failure, the measured Cl_{Cr} may overestimate the true GFR. In this setting, the mean of the Cl_{Cr} and urea clearance is a more accurate reflection of GFR.

  ■ Twenty-four-hour protein quantitation is necessary for confirmation of the nephrotic syndrome and is useful for following the response to treatment of certain glomerular diseases.

  ■ Measurements of 24-hour urinary volume, Cr, sodium, citrate, calcium, phosphate, oxalate, and uric acid are indicated in the evaluation of some patients with **nephrolithiasis**; this evaluation is best performed in the outpatient setting when the patient is on his or her usual diet.

  ■ **Blood tests**—including the erythrocyte sedimentation rate; antinuclear, antiglomerular basement membrane (anti-GBM), and antineutrophil cytoplasmic antibodies; complement levels; cryoglobulin studies; HIV and hepatitis B and C serologies; and antistreptococcal antibody titers—may be useful in evaluating glomerular disease.

    • Serum and urine protein **electrophoresis** should be performed in selected patients with proteinuria to exclude multiple myeloma and amyloid disease. Of note, a routine dipstick urinalysis is less sensitive to proteins other than albumin.

  ■ Urine **eosinophils** are seen in allergic interstitial nephritis, rapidly progressive glomerulonephritis (RPGN), acute prostatitis, and renal atheroemboli.

  ■ Urine **osmolality** and spot urine sodium and potassium may be useful in the evaluation and management of hyponatremia.

Imaging

■ **Renal ultrasonography** can assess kidney size, determine the presence of hydronephrosis, and identify renal cysts.

  ■ Small kidneys (<10 cm) generally reflect chronic renal disease, although kidney size may not be diminished in some common chronic processes, such as diabetes, HIV, amyloidosis, polycystic kidney disease, and multiple myeloma.

  ■ A discrepancy in kidney size of >2 cm may suggest unilateral renal artery stenosis, with atrophy of the kidney on the stenotic side.

  ■ The presence of hydronephrosis suggests obstructive nephropathy that may be chronic or acute in nature.

  ■ Multiple bilateral cortical cysts are suggestive of autosomal-dominant polycystic kidney disease.

■ **IV urography** is useful in the evaluation of nonglomerular hematuria, stone disease, and voiding disorders, but should be reserved for patients with normal or near-normal renal function.

- **Radionuclide scanning** uses technetium isotopes to assess the relative contribution of each kidney to overall renal function and provides important information if unilateral nephrectomy is being considered. Renal scanning is useful when disruption of renal blood flow is suspected; the absence of perfusion to either kidney should prompt further investigation of the renal vasculature. In addition, radionuclide studies can be used to follow renal function, leaks, and rejection in transplanted kidneys.
- **Magnetic resonance imaging (MRI) and magnetic resonance angiography** can be helpful in evaluating renal masses, detecting main renal artery stenosis, and diagnosing renal vein thrombosis. Unlike **standard arteriography,** magnetic resonance angiography does not require the administration of nephrotoxic contrast agents and possesses high sensitivity and specificity for atherosclerotic disease involving the proximal renal arteries.

Surgical Diagnostic Procedures

- **Renal biopsy** can determine diagnosis, guide therapy, and provide prognostic information in many settings, particularly in the evaluation of the nephrotic syndrome or glomerular hematuria.
  - **Biopsy may be indicated** in adults with glomerular diseases that present with proteinuria >2 g/d, hematuria, or RBC casts. It can be helpful in diseases such as systemic lupus erythematosus (SLE), pulmonary–renal syndromes, and paraproteinemias with renal involvement. Biopsy should also be considered in patients with renal failure and kidneys of normal size when other studies are nondiagnostic.
  - **Preparative measures for biopsy** include ultrasound imaging to establish the presence of two kidneys, urinalysis and culture to exclude urinary tract infection before biopsy, adequate blood pressure (BP) control, and correction of coagulation parameters. If renal function is significantly impaired, uremic platelet dysfunction may result in abnormal bleeding time (>10 minutes), which may increase the risk of significant postprocedure hemorrhage. IV desmopressin acetate (ddAVP; 0.3 mcg/kg) can be infused over 30 minutes before biopsy to correct an abnormal bleeding time. Packed RBCs should be available for transfusion. The patient should not take medications that interfere with platelet function (e.g., aspirin) before or immediately after the biopsy. Patients on dialysis who require a biopsy should have their dialysis sessions scheduled so as to avoid heparin anticoagulation immediately after the biopsy.

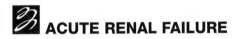 **ACUTE RENAL FAILURE**

GENERAL PRINCIPLES

Definition

- ARF is incited by many causes (Table 11-1), but all result in a sudden decline in the ability of the kidney to maintain fluid and electrolyte homeostasis.
- Renal failure may be **oliguric** (urine output <500 mL/d or <25 mL/hr × 4 hr) or **non-oliguric** (>500 mL/d).

Classification

- ARF may be classified as **prerenal, intrinsic,** or **postrenal** (obstructive).

Etiology

- **Prerenal azotemia** is the clinical result of renal hypoperfusion due to a decrease in effective arterial blood volume. Decreased effective circulating volume may result from volume depletion, peripheral vasodilation, or low cardiac output.
  - Table 11-2 includes laboratory tests that are helpful in differentiating oliguric prerenal azotemia from oliguric, intrinsic acute tubular necrosis (ATN).

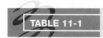

TABLE 11-1	Causes of Acute Renal Failure

Prerenal failure
Volume contraction
Hypotension
Heart failure (severe)
Liver failure (see Chapter 17, Liver Diseases)

Intrinsic renal failure
Acute tubular necrosis (prolonged ischemia; nephrotoxic agents, such as heavy metals, aminoglycosides, radiographic contrast media)
Arteriolar injury
Accelerated hypertension
Vasculitis
Microangiopathic disorder (thrombotic thrombocytopenic purpura, hemolytic–uremic syndrome)
Glomerulonephritis
Acute interstitial nephritis (drug induced)
Intrarenal deposition or sludging (uric acid, myeloma)
Cholesterol embolization (especially after an arterial procedure)

Postobstructive failure
Ureteral obstruction (clot, calculus, tumor, sloughed papillae, external compression)
Bladder outlet obstruction (neurogenic bladder, prostatic hypertrophy, carcinoma, calculus, clot, urethral stricture)

- Serum and urine samples should be obtained simultaneously before a fluid challenge or diuretic use is initiated. **Microscopic examination of a fresh urine sample is essential.**
- The prerenal state can be suggested by the presence of orthostasis or other signs of volume depletion on examination, by careful review of the patient's intake and urine output history, or by the presence of heart failure or liver failure, which may compromise effective circulating volume. Volume expansion, BP support, or treatment of heart failure may result in reversal of renal insufficiency.
- In prerenal states, the kidney avidly retains sodium, usually resulting in low urine sodium and a **fractional excretion of sodium (FE$_{Na}$)** of <1%. Other conditions in which an FE$_{Na}$ of <1% may be observed are radiocontrast-induced renal failure, acute GN, liver failure (see Chapter 17, Liver Diseases), pigment-induced nephrotoxicity, early obstructive nephropathy, vasculitis, and normal renal function. FE$_{Na}$ is particularly helpful in oliguric ARF. FE$_{Na}$ is calculated as follows:

$$FE_{Na} = ([U_{Na} \cdot P_{Cr}]/[P_{Na} \cdot U_{Cr}]) \cdot 100$$

where U = urine and P = plasma. Because loop diuretics force natriuresis, calculation of the FE$_{Na}$ is misleading in patients who are taking these agents. In patients with volume depletion and alkalosis from nasogastric suction or vomiting, bicarbonaturia

TABLE 11-2	Laboratory Examination in Oliguric Acute Renal Failure

Diagnosis	U/P$_{Cr}$	U$_{Na}$	FE$_{Na}$ (%)	U osmolality
Prerenal azotemia	>40	<20	<1	>500
Oliguric ATN	<20	>40	>1	<350

ATN, acute tubular necrosis; Cr, creatinine; FE$_{Na}$, fractional excretion of sodium; P, plasma; U, urine.

may also lead to concomitant sodium losses and an elevated FE_{Na}. The **fractional excretion of urea** (FE_{urea}) can be used to confirm the prerenal state in the presence of recent diuretic use, with an FE_{urea} of <35% suggestive of prerenal azotemia. FE_{urea} can be calculated using the FE_{Na} formula but replacing plasma sodium with BUN and urine sodium with urine urea.

■ **Postrenal failure or obstruction** of the upper or lower urinary tract may incite ARF. **Early diagnosis and relief of obstruction** are essential to prevent permanent renal damage.

■ **Lower urinary tract obstruction** is common in older men with enlarged prostates that cause bladder outlet obstruction. It can be assessed (and relieved) by temporary bladder catheterization and measurement of postvoid residual (>300 mL urine remaining in the bladder postvoid is highly suggestive of bladder outlet obstruction).

■ Renal ultrasonography usually identifies hydronephrosis in lower and **upper tract obstruction,** which may result from nephrolithiasis, tumor mass, retroperitoneal fibrosis, or other etiologies. Urine flow often increases dramatically with relief of bilateral obstruction. This postobstructive diuresis frequently is physiologic and reflects excretion of fluid, urea, and sodium accumulated during the period of obstruction. If the postobstructive diuresis appears excessive, fluid and electrolytes can be replaced with 0.45% saline. Potassium, calcium, and magnesium may also require replacement.

■ Unilateral obstruction with otherwise normal kidneys does not typically result in a significant elevation of the serum creatinine, since the remaining healthy kidney should be able to accommodate for the loss of the contralateral kidney.

■ **Micro-obstructive uropathy** with associated pyuria and eosinophiluria may be caused by **indinavir,** a protease inhibitor used in the treatment of HIV disease. Discontinuation of the drug can restore renal function.

■ **Intrinsic renal failure** results from a variety of injuries to the renal blood vessels, glomeruli, tubules, or interstitium (Table 11-1). These insults may be toxic, immunologic, or idiopathic. They may be iatrogenic or develop as part of a systemic disorder or as a primary renal disease.

■ **Ischemic ATN** may occur with decreased renal perfusion from any cause that results in ischemic damage and sloughing of the renal tubular epithelium. ATN is the most common cause of ARF in hospitalized patients and may frequently present postoperatively, after a hypotensive episode from sepsis or profound volume depletion, or may be induced by medications that cause renal arterial vasoconstriction or direct tubular toxicity.

• The classic findings in ATN may include evidence of a hypotensive episode, oliguria, rising serum Cr, "muddy brown" coarse granular casts on examination of the urine sediment, and FE_{Na} of >1%, reflecting tubular damage and inability to conserve sodium.

• **Management of ATN** is supportive, with volume repletion only until the patient is euvolemic, restriction of potassium-containing fluids, and close observation for the need to initiate dialytic support for electrolyte abnormalities, volume overload, acidosis, or uremia.

• If **volume overload** becomes evident, a **diuretic challenge** is reasonable, typically with 40–120 mg of furosemide IV. Because diuretics must be filtered and secreted to achieve efficacy, a high dose must be administered in the setting of decreased GFR. If urine output improves after administration of a bolus dose of loop diuretics, fluid management may be easier to achieve with a continuous infusion of loop diuretics (i.e., furosemide at 10–20 mg/hr) or with repeated bolus doses every 6–8 hours to convert the oliguric state to nonoliguric. Addition of a thiazide-type diuretic can further enhance diuresis in furosemide-responsive patients. However, this approach probably does not improve likelihood of renal recovery.

• In all cases of ATN, **supportive care** should focus on minimizing additional renal insults (avoidance of volume depletion, further hypotension, nonsteroidal anti-inflammatory drugs [NSAIDs], radiocontrast, aminoglycosides, and other nephrotoxins) and carefully assessing the need for dialytic intervention if volume overload, acidosis, uremia, or hyperkalemia cannot be managed otherwise.

• In most cases of ATN, recovery of renal function occurs over 1–6 weeks, although the patient may be left with some degree of CKD.

- **Radiocontrast nephropathy** occurs with increased frequency in patients with pre-existing renal insufficiency, particularly in the setting of diabetes mellitus. Volume depletion, multiple myeloma, use of NSAIDs, heart failure, and age >65 years may also be risk factors. Decreased GFR occurs immediately after contrast administration, and serum Cr is elevated by 24 hours. Patients often recover renal function over 7–14 days. To reduce the incidence of ARF, patients at risk should have measures taken to minimize contrast volume, use hypo- or iso-osmolar contrast if possible, and be hydrated with 1 mL/kg/hr of 0.45% saline beginning 12–24 hours before the contrast study and ending 12 hours after the study. **Sodium bicarbonate** may be a superior hydration agent given as 154 mEq/L, 3 mL/kg bolus 1 hour preprocedure and continuing for 6 hours postprocedure.[1] Furosemide should be reserved for patients in whom volume overload develops during hydration. **Acetylcysteine** (600 mg PO bid; four doses total, starting 1 day before the procedure) may reduce the incidence and severity of contrast nephropathy.[2]
- **Aminoglycoside nephrotoxicity** may cause ARF that is often nonoliguric and results from direct toxicity to the proximal tubules. Predisposing factors include prolonged exposure (usually >5 days) to these drugs, advanced age, volume depletion, liver disease, and pre-existing renal disease. The risk of aminoglycoside nephrotoxicity appears to be lower when the extended-interval dosing method is used (see Chapter 12, Antimicrobials), although this method should be avoided in patients with pre-existing renal insufficiency.
- **Pigment-induced renal injury** occurs during hemolysis or rhabdomyolysis. In **rhabdomyolysis,** aggressive IV fluid administration should be initiated to replace the fluid that is lost into necrotic muscle and to establish high urine flow. If sufficient urine flow can be established, alkalinization of the urine (urine pH >6.5) by IV infusion of 2–3 ampules of $NaHCO_3$ in 1 L 5% dextrose in water increases the solubility of heme pigments and may hasten recovery.
- **Acute uric acid nephropathy (tumor lysis syndrome)** may occur from cell lysis, with consequent hyperuricemia during cytotoxic therapy for hematologic malignancies. Uric acid production can be decreased by administration of **allopurinol,** 600 mg PO, before cytotoxic therapy, followed by 100–300 mg/d. The dosage should be adjusted for renal function. **Rasburicase,** 15 mg/kg IV, is highly effective and can be given prophylactically if the patient is at very high risk or after hyperuricemia develops despite prophylaxis. Forced alkaline diuresis to maintain a urine pH of 6.5–7.0 also helps to prevent uric acid precipitation; this can be accomplished with acetazolamide, 250 mg PO qid, or with IV infusion of 2–3 ampules of $NaHCO_3$ in 1 L 5% dextrose in water. If tumor lysis results in hyperphosphatemia, urine alkalinization greater than pH 7.0 increases the risk of calcium phosphate precipitation and thus should be avoided.
- **Acute interstitial nephritis** secondary to drugs may present with the classic signs of fever, rash, and renal dysfunction. When present, eosinophilia and eosinophiluria suggest the diagnosis. A high index of suspicion for interstitial nephritis must be maintained in patients who are taking drugs such as penicillins, sulfonamides, quinolones, and nonsteroidal anti-inflammatory drugs. In most cases, renal insufficiency resolves with discontinuation of the offending agent. A course of prednisone, initially at 60 mg PO daily, may hasten recovery. Streptococcal infections, leptospirosis, al infections, and sarcoidosis have also been implicated as causes of interstitial nephritis.
- **Hemolytic–uremic syndrome/thrombotic thrombocytopenic purpura** may be induced by bacterial toxins; medications such as mitomycin-C, clopidogrel, cyclosporine, tacrolimus (see Chapter 15, Solid Organ Transplant Medicine); OKT3; or radiation therapy; or may be associated with pregnancy or certain malignancies of the gastrointestinal (GI) tract. Diagnosis and therapy are discussed in Chapter 18, Disorders of Hemostasis.
- **Hepatorenal syndrome (HRS)** presents with renal failure in the setting of severe liver failure (see Chapter 17, Liver Disease).
- **Cholesterol emboli** are seen in patients with diffuse atherosclerotic disease who undergo aortic or other large arterial manipulation or who are receiving warfarin or

thrombolytic therapy. Physical findings may include retinal arteriolar plaques, lower extremity livedo reticularis, or necrotic areas of the distal digits. Laboratory findings that may aid in the diagnosis include eosinophilia, eosinophiluria, and hypocomplementemia, which usually resolve a week after the embolus. Renal cholesterol embolization frequently progresses to CKD and possible end-stage renal disease (ESRD). Anticoagulation can worsen embolic disease, and should be stopped if possible.

- **Abdominal compartment syndrome** can result in acute oliguric renal failure in the setting of increased intra-abdominal pressure (IAP), typically as a result of intra-abdominal fluid accumulation after fluid resuscitation following trauma or abdominal surgery, but may develop with massive ascites. IAP may be approximated by measuring bladder pressures by filling the bladder with 50 mL saline via an indwelling bladder catheter and applying a pressure transducer to a large-bore needle inserted into the aspiration port of the catheter. Compartment syndrome commonly develops with IAP >25 mm Hg; however, IAPs as low as 10 mm Hg have been implicated. Decompression of the abdominal compartment may be curative.
- **Acute GN** can result in ARF. **Rapidly progressive glomerulonephritis (RPGN)** presents with an acute deterioration in renal function, nephrotic or nonnephrotic proteinuria, and an active urinary sediment with hematuria and RBC casts (nephritic syndrome). Oliguria may be present. Many patients with idiopathic RPGN note a preceding viral-like illness. RPGN can be further characterized by the presence of immune complex deposition (e.g., systemic lupus erythematosus [SLE], poststreptococcal GN, immunoglobin [Ig] A nephropathy, endocarditis), the paucity of immune complex deposition (e.g., Wegener granulomatosis, microscopic polyangiitis, Churg-Strauss syndrome, idiopathic), or the presence of anti-GBM disease (see the section Glomerulopathies). Pathology is notable for crescent formation in >50% of glomeruli on renal biopsy. As many as 75% of patients with idiopathic RPGN may respond to high-dose, pulse glucocorticoid therapy—methylprednisolone, 7–15 mg/kg/d in divided doses for 3 days, followed by prednisone, 1 mg/kg/d for 1 month, gradually tapered over the next 6–12 months. In patients with extrarenal disease that is suggestive of vasculitis or a renal biopsy that demonstrates necrotizing GN, the addition of cyclophosphamide, 2 mg/kg/d PO adjusted for renal function, may be beneficial.

DIAGNOSIS

Monitoring

- Urine output should be continuously monitored. Electrolytes and serum Cr should be measured daily in most patients.
- **Hemodynamic monitoring** may be of value to ensure adequate volume expansion while avoiding overexpansion and to assess and manage poor cardiac function. Invasive monitoring with a central venous pressure or pulmonary artery catheter is indicated if an accurate assessment of intravascular volume cannot be determined by physical examination or an initial volume challenge.

TREATMENT

Medical Management

- **Drug dosages** of agents excreted by the kidney must be adjusted for the level of renal function.
- **Fluid management** is essential to avoid volume depletion, which may contribute to ARF by decreasing renal perfusion. When clinical assessment is unclear, invasive hemodynamic monitoring may be required. Once any volume deficit has been corrected, fluid and sodium balance must be carefully regulated to avoid volume overload.
  - **Fluid replacement** (usually 0.45% saline if IV) should be equal to insensible losses (approximately 500 mL/d in afebrile patients) plus urinary and other drainage losses.

Increased urine output and diuretic responsiveness in nonoliguric ARF allow more liberal administration of fluids (and nutrients). Because patients with nonoliguric ARF may lose significant amounts of fluid and electrolytes in the urine, careful attention to volume status and serum electrolyte levels is necessary to avoid electrolyte and water depletion. Hyponatremia in patients with ARF usually is secondary to volume expansion with hypotonic fluid, whereas hypernatremia is caused most often by overly aggressive diuresis in combination with inadequate intake of free water.

- **A fluid challenge** may be appropriate in oliguric patients who are not volume overloaded. The quantity of fluid to be given must be determined on an individual basis, but typically 500–1,000 mL normal saline is infused over 30–60 minutes. Frequent cardiopulmonary examination is necessary. Diuretic challenge may be appropriate if volume overload occurs in the setting of intrinsic renal failure.
- **Volume overload** may respond to **diuretics** as described for ischemic ATN. Volume overload that is unresponsive to diuretic therapy may require **dialysis or ultrafiltration**.
- **Dopamine** (<3 mcg/kg/min, a dosage that preferentially dilates the renal vasculature) occasionally initiates natriuresis and diuresis. However, clear evidence for a renal protective effect of dopamine is lacking and hence it is not routinely recommended in ARF.[3]

- **Dietary modification. Total enteral caloric intake** should be 35–50 kcal/kg/d to avoid catabolism. Patients who are highly catabolic (e.g., postsurgical and burn patients) or malnourished require higher protein intake and should be considered for early institution of dialysis. **Sodium intake** should be restricted to 2–4 g/d to facilitate volume management. **Potassium intake** should be restricted to 40 mEq/d, and **phosphorus intake** should be restricted to 800 mg/d. Ingestion of magnesium-containing compounds should be avoided.
- **Management of the recovery phase of ARF** usually requires careful monitoring of serum electrolytes, volume status, and urinary fluid and electrolyte losses. As with obstructive nephropathy, a diuretic phase may occur during recovery. Management is similar to that for postobstructive diuresis. Renal function may continue to improve over weeks to months

Dialysis

- **Indications for dialysis.** All patients with ARF should be evaluated daily to assess the need for dialysis. Technical aspects of dialysis are considered under the section Renal Replacement Therapies.
    - It is preferable to initiate dialytic support **before significant uremic signs or symptoms** are evident. Patients suffering from oliguric or anuric acute renal failure that is not anticipated to have a rapid recovery likely benefit from early initiation of dialytic therapy.
    - Severe **hyperkalemia, acidosis, or volume overload refractory to conservative therapy** mandates the initiation of dialysis.
    - Certain alcohol and drug intoxications should be treated with hemodialysis (see Chapter 25, Medical Emergencies).
    - **Additional absolute indications** for initiation of dialysis include uremic pericarditis, encephalopathy, neuropathy, and nutritional requirements (e.g., hyperalimentation) that may precipitate volume overload or uremia.
    - **Uremic signs and symptoms** become prominent as BUN rises. Neurologic manifestations, such as lethargy, seizures, myoclonus, asterixis, and peripheral polyneuropathies, may develop with uremia and are an indication for dialysis. **Uremic pericarditis** often manifests only as a pericardial friction rub and should be treated with intensive dialysis; heparin use during dialysis should be minimized in these patients.

Complications

- **Hyperkalemia** is common and, if mild (<6 mEq/L), can be treated with dietary restriction and potassium-binding resins (e.g., sodium polystyrene sulfonate). Marked hyperkalemia or hyperkalemia accompanied by electrocardiogram (ECG) abnormalities requires immediate medical therapy (e.g., calcium gluconate, insulin, glucose, and bicarbonate; see Chapter 3, Fluid and Electrolyte Management). **Severe hyperkalemia that is refractory to medical therapy is an indication for urgent dialysis.**
- **Phosphorus and calcium levels** are frequently abnormal in renal failure due to reduced renal excretion and excess release of cellular phosphate, despite dietary restriction. Serum calcium is often low but rarely requires specific treatment.
- Significant **metabolic acidosis** (serum bicarbonate level <18 mEq/L) may be treated with sodium bicarbonate, 650–1,300 mg PO tid. Severe acidosis (serum pH <7.2) requires prompt therapy with parenteral sodium bicarbonate (see Chapter 3, Fluid and Electrolyte Management) and a search for the underlying etiology. Sodium bicarbonate therapy should be used with care, as it may exacerbate volume overload and cause tetany by decreasing the ionized calcium concentration. **Acidosis that is unresponsive to medical therapy is an indication for dialysis.**
- **Hypertension** should be managed aggressively. Volume overload frequently contributes to hypertension. Antihypertensive medications that do not decrease renal blood flow (e.g., clonidine, prazosin, or calcium channel antagonists) are preferred. Hypertensive crisis can be managed with IV labetalol, fenoldopam, or sodium nitroprusside (see Chapter 4, Hypertension).
- **Anemia** is common in ARF and usually is caused by decreased RBC production and increased blood loss. GI bleeding is common in ARF, probably due to uremic platelet dysfunction and GI mucosal changes. Use of ddAVP, 0.3 mcg/kg IV over 30 minutes, may correct abnormal bleeding times. Transfusion is appropriate for patients with active bleeding or symptoms referable to anemia (see Chapter 19, Anemia and Transfusion Therapy). Erythropoietin is expensive and not effective as short-term therapy for anemia; data are lacking to support its use in ARF.
- **Infection** is the most common cause of death in patients with ARF. Antimicrobial therapy is dictated by the infectious process, and potentially nephrotoxic agents should not be withheld if their use is otherwise indicated. Most antimicrobial dosages need to be adjusted for the degree of renal failure.

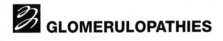 **GLOMERULOPATHIES**

DIAGNOSIS

Clinical Presentation

- Glomerulopathies may present with isolated hematuria or proteinuria, nephritic syndrome, or nephrotic syndrome. These syndromes may appear as a manifestation of primary glomerular disease or may be associated with systemic diseases, such as diabetes mellitus, amyloidosis, multiple myeloma, SLE, or others.
- The **nephritic syndrome** is characterized by hematuria, RBC casts, proteinuria, hypertension, edema, and deteriorating renal function.
- The **nephrotic syndrome** is characterized by proteinuria (>3.5 g/d), hypoalbuminemia, hyperlipidemia, and edema.

Surgical Diagnostic Procedures

- **Renal biopsy** often provides useful diagnostic, therapeutic, and prognostic information.

TREATMENT

General Principles

- **Edema and volume overload** can usually be managed with diuretics, as appropriate, and dietary sodium restriction.
- **Aggressive treatment of hypertension** with a goal BP of <125/75 in most cases has been associated with decreased proteinuria and slower progression of disease.
- **Proteinuria** should be monitored regularly via use of urinary protein-to-creatinine ratio or urinary microalbumin. A combination of angiotensin-converting enzyme (ACE) inhibitors and angiotensin-receptor blockers (ARBs) is more effective than either agent alone in reducing proteinuria, partially by reducing intraglomerular pressure. Use caution with these agents in patients with accelerating renal failure or a tendency toward hyperkalemia. Serum chemistries, including potassium and Cr, should be monitored within 1–2 weeks of initiation of therapy or an increase in dose.
- **Hyperlipidemia** in patients with long-standing nephrotic syndrome may increase the risk for atherosclerotic disease. Dietary restriction of cholesterol and saturated fat should be prescribed. HMG-CoA reductase inhibitors (see Chapter 5, Ischemic Heart Disease) are effective in improving the lipoprotein profile, may reduce cardiovascular risk, and may slow progression of renal disease.
- **Thromboembolic complications.** The nephrotic syndrome produces a hypercoagulable state, and the clinician should maintain a high index of suspicion for thromboemboli. Deep venous thrombosis of the upper and lower extremities, as well as renal vein thrombosis, may occur and should be treated with heparin anticoagulation, followed by long-term warfarin therapy (see Chapter 18, Disorders of Hemostasis and Thrombosis).
- **Dietary modifications** include modest dietary protein restriction (controversial) and dietary sodium restriction.

Disease-Specific Therapy

- The therapy is most often guided by results of renal biopsy and supplemental laboratory evaluation but frequently involves corticosteroid-based therapy for primarily nephrotic disorders and cytotoxic agents plus corticosteroids for primarily proliferative or nephritic disorders. The use of these agents is rapidly evolving and new immunomodulatory therapeutics are earning indications for glomerular diseases. These agents should be administered only in consultation with a nephrologist or other experienced physician with a current knowledge of the literature regarding indications and regimens.
- Initial dosages of cytotoxic drugs are suggested but may require adjustment to keep the WBC count above 3,000–3,500 cells/microliter. WBC counts should initially be checked at least weekly during the administration of cytotoxic agents.

PRIMARY GLOMERULOPATHIES

Minimal-Change Disease (MCD)

Diagnosis

Clinical Presentation

- MCD presents with nephrotic syndrome, quite often with normal serum creatinine levels.
- Certain neoplastic disorders, such as Hodgkin's disease and non-Hodgkin's lymphoma, have been associated with the development of MCD and should be considered in the appropriate setting. The combination of MCD and acute interstitial nephritis (AIN) induced by NSAIDs is well described. Progression to CKD is rare.

Pathologic Findings

- The kidney biopsy reveals normal light microscopy, negative immunofluorescence, and foot process fusion on electron microscopy.

Treatment

- Approximately 80% of adults with MCD respond to **prednisone**, 1 mg/kg/d PO, with a decrease in proteinuria to <3 g/d or a remission of the nephrotic syndrome. NSAID-induced MCD/AIN usually responds well to discontinuation of NSAIDs.
- In adult patients who respond, steroids should be tapered over 3 months and then discontinued.
- Failure to respond may reflect an error in diagnosis; MCD is most commonly confused with early focal segmental glomerulosclerosis.
- Urinary protein excretion should be carefully monitored during steroid taper. If relapse is documented, reinstitution of prednisone often is effective.
- Treatment with **cytotoxic agents** may be indicated in patients who are deemed steroid dependent, steroid resistant, or frequent relapsers.
  - Cyclophosphamide, 2 mg/kg/d PO for 8 weeks; chlorambucil, 0.2 mg/kg/d PO for 8–12 weeks; or cyclosporine, 5 mg/kg/d PO for 6–12 months, are typical regimens.

Focal Segmental Glomerulosclerosis

Diagnosis

Clinical Presentation

- Focal segmental glomerulosclerosis (FSGS) is usually characterized by hypertension, hematuria, renal insufficiency, and nephrotic syndrome.
- Although commonly idiopathic, there are well-described associated mutations in familial cases. FSGS may also be a secondary glomerular disease resulting from decreased nephron mass, obesity, or various other injuries.
- The disease frequently progresses to CKD and ESRD within 5–10 years of diagnosis.

Pathologic Findings

- Pathologic findings include focal and segmental sclerosis of glomeruli on light microscopy with focal or diffuse foot process effacement under electron microscopy.

Treatment

- It is generally not proven to be effective in the treatment of this disorder, but a trial of **prednisone**, 60 mg PO daily for at least 3 months, may be appropriate in an effort to reduce proteinuria and slow progression to ESRD in idiopathic FSGS.
- Resistant cases may respond to a combination of **glucocorticoids** and **cytotoxic agents** such as cyclosporine, 5 mg/kg/d PO, cyclophosphamide, 2 mg/kg/d PO, or mycophenolate mofetil 1,000–3,000 mg/d. These agents may also reduce the need for steroids in steroid-dependent cases.

Membranous Nephropathy

Diagnosis

Clinical Presentation

- Membranous nephropathy usually presents with the nephrotic syndrome, often with normal or near-normal GFR.
- Membranous nephropathy may be a primary renal disease or associated with a systemic disease (e.g., malignancy, SLE, or infections such as hepatitis B, syphilis, hepatitis C, or schistosomiasis) or drug ingestions (e.g., penicillamine, gold).
- Approximately one-third of patients with membranous nephropathy progress to ESRD; the remainder enter remission or have stable or very slowly declining renal function.

Pathologic Findings

- Pathologic findings include thickening of the GBM, often with GBM "spikes" on light microscopy with subepithelial deposits of IgG and C3 on immunofluorescence and electron microscopy.

Treatment

- Because of the generally good outcome, treatment usually is reserved for patients with poor prognostic factors (age >50, male gender, hypertension, reduced GFR, proteinuria >10 g/d, or marked interstitial fibrosis on renal biopsy) or severe symptomatic nephrotic syndrome.
- Treatment options include high-dose alternate-day **glucocorticoids** in conjunction with a **cytotoxic agent** (e.g., chlorambucil, 0.2 mg/kg/d, or cyclophosphamide, 1.5–2.5 mg/kg/d) for 6–12 months and, in nonresponders, cyclosporine, 3.5 mg/kg/d, for 12 months. Alternative agents include mycophenolate mofetil, rituximab, and possibly pentoxifylline.

IgA Nephropathy

Diagnosis

Clinical Presentation

- IgA nephropathy is most often an idiopathic disorder that is characterized by asymptomatic microscopic hematuria with mild proteinuria or recurrent episodes of gross hematuria that may be concomitant with an upper respiratory infection. It is the most common glomerular cause of hematuria.
- IgA nephropathy may be associated with hepatic cirrhosis, gluten enteropathy, or dermatitis herpetiformis.
- **Henoch-Schönlein purpura** is a systemic vasculitis that presents with the tetrad of palpable purpura (usually in the lower trunk or extremities), abdominal pain, joint inflammation, and renal failure due to IgA nephropathy. Fewer than 25% of cases progress to ESRD by 20 years.

Pathologic Findings

- Light microscopy is notable for increased mesangial cellularity and matrix. In severe cases crescents may form. Immunofluorescence and electron microscopy reveal mesangial deposition of IgA and C3.

Treatment

- **Glucocorticoids** may be helpful in patients who have progressive disease.
- The use of **omega-3 fatty acids,** found in fish oil (6 g PO bid including 1.8 g of eicosapentaenoic acid and 1.2 g of docosahexanoic acid), may be beneficial in preventing the deterioration of renal function. **Cyclophosphamide** has been used in severe crescentic disease.

Membranoproliferative Glomerulonephropathy

Diagnosis

Clinical Presentation

- Membranoproliferative glomerulonephropathy (MPGN) exhibits a variety of clinical presentations, including acute GN, nephrotic syndrome, and asymptomatic hematuria and proteinuria. The diagnosis should be suspected if these clinical findings are associated with low complement levels.
- **Hepatitis C (HCV)** accounts for most cases of MPGN and is often associated with cryoglobulinemia (see Chapter 23, Arthritis and Rheumatologic Diseases). SLE can cause the pathologic finding of MPGN. Idiopathic MPGN is a rare disorder.
- Fifty to sixty percent of patients with idiopathic MPGN progress to ESRD by 10–15 years.

Pathologic Findings

- Pathology includes mesangial proliferation with collapse of the capillary loop and alterations of the GBM with subendothelial (type I) or intramembranous (type II) electron-dense deposits. Mesangial interposition with the GBM may result in the appearance of "tram tracking."

Treatment

- For adult idiopathic MPGN, treatment has not been shown to improve disease-free survival, although the use of corticosteroids in children likely stabilizes disease. HCV-associated MPGN may improve with successful **antiviral therapy** including pegylated interferon alfa and ribavirin, unless the GFR is <50 mL/min, in which case only non-pegylated interferon alfa is currently approved (see Secondary Glomerulopathies).

SECONDARY GLOMERULOPATHIES

Diabetic Nephropathy

General Principles

- Diabetic nephropathy is the most common cause of ESRD in the United States (see Chapter 21, Diabetes Mellitus and Related Disorders).

Diagnosis: Pathologic Findings

- Although kidney biopsy is not usually indicated, findings include glomerular sclerosis and mesangial expansion with a nodular appearance (Kimmelstiel-Wilson nodules) on light microscopy, with GBM thickening on electron microscopy.

Treatment

- Treatment involves **aggressive glucose control** and **aggressive BP control** with ACE inhibitors or ARBs or both.

Systemic Lupus Erythematosus (SLE)

Diagnosis

Clinical Presentation

- SLE may involve the kidney and can present as slowly progressive azotemia with urinary abnormalities, as nephrotic syndrome, or as rapidly progressive renal insufficiency. Hypocomplementemia is often present during flares of nephritis.
- **Renal biopsy** is useful in SLE for evaluating disease activity and assessing irreversible changes such as glomerular sclerosis, tubular atrophy, and interstitial fibrosis. The clinical presentation is a poor predictor of the class of lupus nephritis involved.

Pathologic Findings

- A wide variety of **pathologic changes** may be seen on renal biopsy, including mesangial, membranous, focal or diffuse proliferative, and crescentic GN. Immunofluorescence is commonly positive for IgA, IgG, IgM, C3, and C4. A predominance of irreversible changes with little acute inflammation portends a poor response to therapy and should modify the aggressiveness of immunosuppressive treatment.

Treatment

- For patients with severe renal disease treatment is with **methylprednisolone**, 500 mg IV q12h for 3 days, followed by oral prednisone, 0.5–1.0 mg/kg PO daily. Prednisone should then be tapered over 6–8 weeks to the lowest dosage that controls disease activity, preferably using an alternate-day regimen.
- In moderate to severe lupus nephritis, induction with **mycophenolate mofetil**, 1,000 mg PO tid,[4] or **cyclophosphamide**, 0.5–1.0 g/m^2 IV monthly for 6 months, improves the likelihood of remission and appears to reduce the likelihood of progressive renal failure. Maintenance therapy minimizes relapse and should continue for 2 years with mycophenolate mofetil[5] or quarterly IV cyclophosphamide. Mycophenolate may have a more favorable side-effect profile compared to cyclophosphamide.

Dysproteinemias

General Principles
- Dysproteinemias include amyloidosis, light-chain and heavy-chain deposition diseases, and fibrillary/immunotactoid glomerulopathies.
- Dysproteinemias may be associated with multiple myeloma, Waldenström's macroglobulinemia, and other B-cell malignancies.

Diagnosis
- The diagnosis is often suggested by an abnormal serum protein electrophoresis or urine protein electrophoresis.
- Patients with dysproteinemias often have cardiac, hepatic, and neuropathic involvement in addition to kidney disease.
- **Amyloidosis** is characterized by the extracellular deposition of 10-nm fibrils composed of the variable region of monoclonal Ig light chains (typically λ) in a β-pleated configuration.
  - Pathologic diagnosis of amyloidosis can be made by Congo red–positive staining of the β-pleated fibrils. Fibrils can be seen under electron microscopy with 9- to 12-nm fibrils. Larger fibrils are seen in fibrillary and immunotactoid glomerulopathies.
- **Light-chain deposition disease** is characterized by the extracellular deposition of the constant region of monoclonal Ig (κ >80% of the time) light chains, whereas heavy and light chains are seen in **heavy-chain deposition disease**.
  - In **light-chain deposition disease,** a granular pattern of deposition that is negative for Congo red staining is seen. Immunofluorescence staining for λ and κ light chains and heavy chains aids in making the appropriate diagnosis.

Treatment
- **Melphalan** and **prednisone** have proved to be beneficial for amyloidosis and light-chain deposition disease.
- For dysproteinemias associated with multiple myeloma, high-dose chemotherapy may be effective in some patients.

Infection-Related GN

- Infection-related GN may occur in association with a variety of infectious processes, including **bacterial endocarditis, visceral abscesses, and infected shunts.** Treatment of the infection usually leads to the resolution of the active immune complex–mediated GN.
- **Poststreptococcal GN** is characterized by onset of edema, hypertension, and gross hematuria 7–28 days after a streptococcal pharyngeal or skin infection. It is associated with low complement levels and is usually self-limited with spontaneous resolution.
- **Hepatitis C** may cause MPGN, generally in association with **cryoglobulinemia.** Treatment with antivirals can be attempted (see Chapter 17, Liver Diseases), but its effectiveness in resolving the renal manifestations is variable.

Pulmonary–Renal Syndromes

The most common cause of pulmonary–renal syndrome is **pneumonia with ATN.**

Anti-GBM Antibody Disease

General Principles
- Anti-GBM antibody disease may present with pulmonary and renal involvement (**Goodpasture's syndrome**) or with renal disease alone. Anti-GBM disease often is rapidly progressive.

Diagnosis
- The diagnosis is based either on the presence of anti-GBM antibodies in the serum or on linear deposition of IgG antibody along the GBM on renal biopsy.

- Of these patients, 10%–30% may have a positive antineutrophil autoplasmic antibody (ANCA).

Treatment
- The goal is to clear anti-GBM antibodies from the serum while also suppressing formation of new antibodies.
- Treatment is with daily total volume **plasmapheresis** for approximately 2 weeks, in combination with:
  - **Cyclophosphamide,** 2 mg/kg PO daily for at least 8 weeks
  - **Methylprednisolone,** 7–15 mg/kg/d IV for 3 days, followed by **prednisone,** 60 mg PO daily tapered over at least 8 weeks
- Frequent clinical evaluation and measurement of anti-GBM antibody titers monitor progress. Immunosuppression should be continued until the anti-GBM antibody is undetectable. Relapse is common and tends to occur within the first several months.
- Poor response to therapy is predicted by the presence of oliguria, creatinine level >5.7 mg/dL, or >30% crescents on biopsy. Patients who require dialysis at presentation have a dismal renal prognosis. Even when the likelihood of renal recovery is poor, if there is evidence of pulmonary involvement, aggressive therapy is warranted.

Wegener's Granulomatosis and Microscopic Polyangiitis
(See also Chapter 23, Arthritis and Rheumatologic Diseases.)

Diagnosis
- Wegener's granulomatosis and microscopic polyangiitis often presents with nephritic renal failure with associated pulmonary disease and vasculitic skin lesions. Wegener's granulomatosis may also affect the sinuses.
- **Churg-Strauss syndrome** may be distinguished by the presence of asthma and eosinophilia (see also Chapter 10, Allergy and Immunology).
- **Wegener's** patients have a positive **cytoplasmic ANCA** directed against **proteinase-3** (anti-PR3) in 90% of cases. **Microscopic polyangiitis** patients typically have positive **perinuclear ANCA** directed against **myeloperoxidase** (anti-MPO).

Pathologic Findings
- Tissue biopsy (lung, kidney, or sinus) of Wegener's may reveal noncaseating granulomas.
- Light microscopy of the kidney in either diagnosis may reveal vasculitis and focal necrotizing or crescentic GN. Immunofluorescence on kidney biopsy shows a paucity of immune deposits.

Treatment
- Combined **cyclophosphamide,** 2 mg/kg/d PO, and **prednisone,** initially at 1 mg/kg/d and tapered, should be used for at least 3 months to induce remission. Treatment to prevent relapse should continue for at least 12 months of therapy using an oral steroid and either oral cyclophosphamide or azathioprine.
- **Trimethoprim-sulfamethoxazole,** 160 mg/800 mg (double strength) bid, has been shown to reduce extrarenal relapses in patients with Wegener's granulomatosis.

Sickle Cell Nephropathy

- Sickle cell nephropathy may present with microscopic or gross hematuria (which may be due to papillary necrosis), proteinuria, tubular dysfunction, and sclerosing glomerulopathy.

Treatment
- Treatment may include maintenance of high urine output, alkalinization of urine, and correction of fluid and electrolyte derangements as needed.
- **ACE inhibitor therapy** is beneficial in reducing proteinuria and possibly progression of sclerotic glomerular lesions.

HIV-Associated Nephropathy

- HIV-associated nephropathy is characterized by proteinuria, edema, and hematuria with or without azotemia.
- The histologic appearance on biopsy is similar to that of collapsing focal segmental glomerulosclerosis with proliferative podocytes. HIV infection has also been associated with other renal diseases, including membranous, membranoproliferative, proliferative, and crescentic GN; hemolytic–uremic syndrome/thrombotic thrombocytopenic purpura; and tubulointerstitial nephritis. Renal biopsy may be required to differentiate among these entities.

Treatment
- **Antiretroviral therapy** may stabilize renal function and reduce proteinuria.
- **Prednisone**, 60 mg/d for 3 months, may also improve renal function
- **ACE inhibitors** are beneficial in reducing proteinuria.

Autosomal-Dominant Polycystic Kidney Disease

General Principles
- Autosomal-dominant polycystic kidney disease (ADPKD) is a hereditary disorder resulting in cystic enlargement of the kidneys, with a prevalence of about 1/1,000. Mutations with PKD1 are most common (85% of cases) with most of the remainder attributed to PKD2, which is associated with a later onset of disease.

Diagnosis

Clinical Presentation
- Onset of renal failure is highly variable with about half of patients reaching ESRD by the age of 65. It is the fourth leading cause of ESRD in the United States.
- **Associated features** include hypertension, kidney stones (in 20%), cerebral aneurysms, hepatic cysts, mitral valve prolapse, aortic insufficiency, colonic diverticula, and abdominal hernias. Patients may present with episodes of gross hematuria due to cyst rupture into the collecting system, or flank pain sometimes with fever due to cyst infections or bleeding into a cyst.

Imaging
- Diagnosis is often made based on the finding of multiple bilateral renal cysts on ultrasound or computed tomography (CT) in the setting of a family history of PKD.
- Patients with PKD and a family history of **cerebral aneurysms** or symptoms attributable to cerebral aneurysms should undergo screening with a **brain magnetic resonance angiography** or contrast CT. The frequency of repeat examinations is not well established.

Treatment
- There are no proven therapies to reduce cyst formation; however, many physicians counsel against the use of caffeine.
- Episodes of **gross hematuria** may be treated with rest and hydration.
- **Cyst infections** should be treated with antibiotics that penetrate cysts such as trimethoprim/sulfamethoxazole, ciprofloxacin, or chloramphenicol. If pain from cysts is refractory to medical management, then percutaneous or surgical cyst reduction may be considered.

 # CHRONIC KIDNEY DISEASE

GENERAL PRINCIPLES

- CKD may result from many different etiologies and is often asymptomatic until severe renal insufficiency develops.

- The decline in GFR may be followed by plotting the reciprocal of serum Cr versus time. The resulting plot usually is linear, unless there is a superimposed renal insult, and is useful in end-stage planning and in predicting the time when dialysis is needed (typically, when GFR is <10 mL/min in individuals without diabetes and <15 mL/min in patients with diabetes).
- **Stages of CKD** are defined by the estimated GFR. A normal GFR is stage 1, 60–90 mL/min is stage 2, 30–60 mL/min is stage 3, 15–30 mL/min is stage 4, and <15 mL/min is stage 5. **Treatment goals are frequently guided by CKD stage.**
- Avoidance of factors that are known to cause an acute decline in renal function and early referral to a nephrologist for implementation of conservative medical treatment of CKD may preserve renal function and postpone the need for dialysis.

SPECIAL CONSIDERATIONS

Acute deterioration in CKD (i.e., a sudden decline in GFR that is more rapid than expected) should prompt a search for a superimposed, reversible process.

- **Decreased renal perfusion** may be due to volume depletion or decreased cardiac output. Afterload reduction may be useful in volume-replete patients with cardiac dysfunction, but caution should be taken to avoid decreased renal perfusion pressure. Hypotension induced by antihypertensive agents can exacerbate CKD, as can poorly controlled hypertension. Thus, all significant fluctuations in BP control should be investigated, especially if they are associated with a reduction in renal function.
- **Drugs** may cause direct toxicity to renal structures (e.g., aminoglycosides), decreased renal perfusion (e.g., nonsteroidal anti-inflammatory drugs, IV contrast), or allergic interstitial nephritis (e.g., allopurinol, antibiotics). Careful attention to drug dosing in patients with decreased GFR and avoidance of unnecessary use of nephrotoxic agents are appropriate.
- **Urinary tract obstruction and infections** should be considered in any patient with an unexplained sudden decline in renal function.
- **Progression of renal artery stenosis** may worsen pre-existing renal failure.
- **Cholesterol embolization** may worsen CKD and is seen most often in patients after procedures that require arterial catheterization (see Acute Renal Failure).
- **Renal vein thrombosis** may occur in nephrotic patients and exacerbate CKD and proteinuria.

TREATMENT

Conservative management of CKD includes measures to correct and prevent metabolic derangements of renal failure and preserve remaining renal function.

Special Therapy

Dietary Modification
- **Potassium** should be restricted to 40 mEq/d in individuals with hyperkalemia.
- **Hyperphosphatemia** may also play a role in the progression of renal failure. The goal is to maintain serum phosphorus levels between 2.7 and 4.6 mg/dL in stage 3–4 CKD and a phosphorous level between 3.5 and 5.5 mg/dL in stage 5 CKD. Dietary phosphorus should be restricted to 800–1,000 mg/d when GFR is <50 mL/min. As GFR falls further, phosphate restriction becomes less effective, and the addition of phosphate binders that prevent GI phosphate absorption is indicated.
- **Calcium carbonate** ($CaCO_3$), 500–1,000 mg (200 mg elemental Ca/500 mg $CaCO_3$), or calcium acetate, 667 mg (169 mg elemental Ca), PO with each meal, is effective in most patients. Serum calcium should be checked regularly, and administration of >1,500 mg of elemental calcium per day should be avoided. The non–calcium-containing binders, **sevelamer HCl** and **lanthanum carbonate**, can be used in dialysis-dependent patients. Sevelamer HCl in CKD patients not yet on dialysis may worsen metabolic acidosis.

- Lack of dietary phosphate restriction is the most common reason that phosphate binders fail to control hyperphosphatemia. $CaCO_3$ should be stopped if the calcium phosphate product is consistently >55, to avoid the possibility of metastatic calcification. If **hypocalcemia** (corrected for serum albumin) persists after phosphate has been controlled, nighttime supplementation of up to 500 mg of elemental calcium and supplementation with an active form of vitamin D may be indicated (see Chapter 3, Fluid and Electrolyte Management).
- **Sodium and fluid restriction** must be determined on an individual basis. For most patients, a no-added-salt diet (3 g sodium/d) is palatable and adequate. If necessary, 24-hour urinary sodium excretion can be determined to aid in sodium intake planning.
  - Once a patient has reached an acceptable volume status, fluid intake should equal daily urine output plus an additional 500 mL for insensible losses. Additional fluid restriction is appropriate only in patients with dilutional hyponatremia.
  - The presence of heart failure or refractory hypertension also may require greater restriction of salt and water. In nephrotic patients with edema, sodium restriction (2 g/d) and judicious use of diuretics should be implemented.
- **Magnesium** is excreted by the kidney and accumulates in CKD. Extra intake of magnesium (e.g., some antacids and cathartics) should be avoided.

Hypertension
- Hypertension accelerates the rate of decline of renal function in patients with CKD and should be **treated aggressively** (see Chapter 4, Hypertension).
- Target BP in most forms of CKD should be **130/80** or less.
  - **ACE inhibitors and ARBs** appear to have renoprotective properties beyond their antihypertensive effect.
  - **Diuretics** are beneficial for hypertension control in most CKD patients. Loop diuretics (e.g., furosemide) remain effective when the GFR is less than 25 mL/min, although dose increases may be required to maintain adequate diuretic response.

Metabolic Acidosis
- Metabolic acidosis is treated with oral **sodium bicarbonate** ($NaHCO_3$) 650–1,300 mg PO tid, to maintain serum bicarbonate at 22 mEq/L or greater. The additional sodium load from such therapy may require further dietary sodium restriction or administration of a diuretic (650 mg $NaHCO_3$ = 6.7 mEq or 170 mg sodium).
- Although **citrate** is converted by the liver to bicarbonate, it should not be used in CKD because it dramatically enhances GI absorption of aluminum and can lead to acute **aluminum neurotoxicity**.

RENAL OSTEODYSTROPHY AND SECONDARY HYPERPARATHYROIDISM

- Renal osteodystrophy refers to a number of skeletal disorders seen in chronic kidney disease and ESRD. Classifications include:
  - Osteitis fibrosa, associated with secondary hyperparathyroidism and an elevated parathyroid hormone (PTH), often with bone pain, fractures, and skeletal deformity.
    - Radiographic studies may show subperiosteal resorption and patchy osteosclerosis.
  - Low turnover or **adynamic bone** disease, which is associated with PTH levels often below target, is less common than osteitis fibrosa. It is more common among diabetics. It may result from low PTH levels, whether spontaneous or iatrogenic.
  - Osteomalacia may also develop from severe vitamin D deficiency or aluminum toxicity.
- **PTH levels**, calcium, and phosphorus should be measured periodically in all patients with a **GFR <60 mL/min**.

■ **Bone biopsy** may be necessary in certain cases to identify the type of bone disease and guide management.

Treatment

■ For **secondary hyperparathyroidism** treatment involves control of phosphorous, calcium, and PTH.
   ■ Correction of **hyperphosphatemia** and **hypocalcemia** will help reduce PTH levels.
   ■ Treatment involves **suppression of intact PTH** to normal (35–70 pg/mL) in stage 3 CKD, 70–110 pg/mL in stage 4 CKD, and 150–300 pg/mL in stage 5 CKD per Dialysis Outcomes Quality Initiative (DOQI) guidelines. The DOQI guidelines are based on data using the intact PTH; however, many laboratories are now using the **bio-intact PTH**, which is 50%–60% of the value of the intact PTH.
      • **Active vitamin D** preparations such as **calcitriol** (0.25–1.0 mcg PO daily) can be used to suppress PTH and correct hypocalcemia.
      • **19- nor-1,25-dihydroxyvitamin D$_2$ (paricalcitol),** 1–5 mcg PO daily in predialysis patients or 2–10 mcg IV with each dialysis, is a synthetic vitamin D analog with a lower incidence of hypercalcemia and may suppress hyperparathyroidism more effectively than calcitriol. **Doxercalciferol,** 1–5 mcg PO daily in predialysis patients, or 5–20 mcg PO three times per week with dialysis, is another synthetic vitamin D analog that may be used.
      • **Cinacalcet,** administered at 30–120 mg PO daily, is a calcimimetic that increases the sensitivity of the calcium-sensing receptor in the parathyroid. Use in dialysis patients results in reductions of PTH, serum calcium, and phosphorus. Its main side effects are nausea and vomiting. Approximately 5% of dialysis patients develop significant hypocalcemia (<7.5 mg/dL).
      • Patients with stage 3 or 4 CKD and PTH levels above target should have their **25-OH vitamin D levels** measured and, if these levels are low (<30 ng/mL), receive at least 6 months of supplementation with **ergocalciferol,** 50,000 International Units PO every week (for 12 weeks if 25-OH vitamin D level <5 ng/mL or 4 weeks for a level 5–15 ng/mL), then monthly.
      • When using any vitamin D preparation, **serum calcium and phosphorous** levels should be measured regularly and the dose adjusted accordingly at 1- to 2-month intervals to avoid hypercalcemia (calcium >10.2 mg/dL). If hyperphosphatemia cannot be controlled with diet and phosphate binders, then the vitamin D dose should be decreased or discontinued or the vitamin D supplement should be switched to a less hypercalcemic formulation (paricalcitol or doxercalciferol).
   ■ **Parathyroidectomy** may be required to control severe hyperparathyroidism. Indications include:
      • Certain cases of **calciphylaxis** (ischemic necrosis of skin or soft tissue associated with metastatic calcification) or extraskeletal calcification associated with significant hyperparathyroidism
      • Persistent severe hypercalcemia (after other causes of hypercalcemia are excluded)
      • Severe hyperparathyroidism (PTH >1,000) despite maximal medical therapy
■ Patients with **adynamic bone disease** should have their active vitamin D preparations discontinued and any calcium-based phosphate binders changed to non–calcium-based phosphate binders.

ANEMIA

■ Anemia is responsible for many symptoms of CKD. Maintenance of hemoglobin between 11 and 12 g/dL minimizes fatigue and improves quality of life.
■ **Epoetin** and **darbepoetin** can effectively treat anemia after ensuring that iron stores are adequate. Treatment should be initiated in most patients when hemoglobin is <11 g/dL. The initial dose of epoetin is 50–100 units/kg SC three times per week in dialysis patients and weekly in CKD patients. Extended intervals at up to every fourth week are effective in many CKD patients (see Chapter 19, Anemia and Transfusion Therapy). Darbepoetin

is dosed at 0.45 mcg/kg SC once a week or every other week, and dosing can be extended to every fourth week by doubling the dose when hemoglobin is in the target range.

■ **Iron stores** should be assessed before initiation of epoetin and periodically, with evaluation of transferrin saturation and ferritin. If transferrin saturation is <20% or ferritin is <200 mg/dL, consideration should be given to iron repletion with IV preparations of iron dextran (1,000 mg IV as a single dose, with an initial test dose of 25 mg), or ferric gluconate (125 mg IV · eight doses), or iron sucrose (100 mg IV · ten doses). Oral iron therapy is frequently effective in CKD patients not on dialysis. Iron replacement improves responsiveness to and requirements for epoetin.

PREPARATION FOR DIALYSIS

■ Patients should be counseled at an early stage to determine preferences for renal replacement therapies, including hemodialysis, peritoneal dialysis, and eligibility for renal transplantation.

■ Preparation for creation of a permanent vascular access for hemodialysis should be initiated by protecting the veins of the nondominant forearm from peripheral IVs and blood draws. This increases the likelihood of successful future arteriovenous (AV) fistula or graft placement. Timely referral to an access surgeon can facilitate creation of a primary AV fistula, the preferred vascular access for hemodialysis, which takes months to properly mature.

RENAL REPLACEMENT THERAPY

Renal replacement therapy is indicated when metabolic abnormalities can no longer be controlled with conservative management or when signs and symptoms of uremia develop; this generally occurs when Cl_{Cr} falls below 10 mL/min in nondiabetics and below 15 mL/min in diabetic patients. A variety of therapeutic options are available to the patient with ESRD.

HEMODIALYSIS

■ **Hemodialysis (HD)** works by diffusion of small molecular weight solutes across a semipermeable membrane. Fluid removal occurs via ultrafiltration.

■ Dialysis usually is performed three times a week. Efficiency of dialysis is best measured through changes in serum urea; serum creatinine is a poor measure of dialysis efficacy. Because urea distributes through total body water, larger patients require longer treatment times; hence, the duration of each treatment is adjusted to achieve a urea reduction ratio (URR) of at least 65%, with most treatments lasting 3–4 hours. URR is calculated as follows:

$$URR = \frac{(\text{pre-HD BUN} - \text{post-HD BUN})}{\text{pre-HD BUN}} \times 100$$

■ When HD is instituted, dietary protein intake should be increased to 1.0–1.2 g/kg/d, and fluid intake should be adjusted to permit a weight gain of approximately 2 kg between dialysis sessions. Antihypertensive medication may have to be reduced, and short-acting antihypertensives may need to be withheld on dialysis days. Diuretics and oral sodium bicarbonate can usually be discontinued.

■ **Vascular access** for blood outflow and return is necessary. Permanent vascular access requires creation of a primary AV anastomosis or placement of a synthetic AV graft.

  ■ **Primary AV fistulas** are considered the optimal form of permanent access; they have the lowest incidence of infection and thrombosis. Fistulas should be placed 3–6 months before anticipated dialysis because they take time to mature. In contrast, because **synthetic AV grafts** must merely heal and become incorporated, they usually are placed 1–3 months before anticipated dialysis. **Tunneled Silastic catheters** placed in the internal jugular vein are being increasingly used for long-term access; they have lower rates of infection than nontunneled catheters and fewer venous complications (stenosis, compromise of future arm grafts) than those placed in sub-clavian veins. Temporary access is usually via an internal jugular or femoral venous catheter.

■ **Infections** of vascular access sites are common and may produce local or systemic signs. Careful examination and ultrasonography of the access site may reveal a lo-cal abscess, which should be cultured and drained. Fevers, especially during HD treatment, should be promptly evaluated. Blood cultures should be obtained, and empiric antibiotic coverage should be considered even in patients who lack an obvi-ous source of infection. Initial therapy must include coverage for staphylococci and Gram-negative organisms. If blood cultures are positive, replacement of the catheter is almost always indicated. The catheter can be exchanged over a guidewire if there is no evidence of inflammation or infection at the exit site or along the tunnel. Doc-umented bacteremia should be treated with antibiotics for at least 3 weeks.

■ **Thrombosis** of a vascular access site can be recanalized by balloon catheter embolec-tomy, thrombolysis, or thrombectomy. The access site usually can be used immedi-ately after declotting.

Hypotension During Hemodialysis

■ Hypotension during hemodialysis is most commonly due to intravascular volume de-pletion and, less commonly, to the use of antihypertensives or nitrates before dialysis, allergic reactions to the dialyzer, left ventricular dysfunction, or autonomic insufficiency.

■ Acute **treatment** includes infusion of normal saline and reduction of the ultrafiltration rate. Other causes of hypotension, such as myocardial infarction, cardiac tamponade, sepsis, and bleeding, should be considered.

Active Bleeding and Coagulopathies

■ Active bleeding and coagulopathies may be exacerbated by the systemic anticoagulation used in HD.

■ The heparin dosage used for HD can usually be minimized or even withheld in patients with such disorders.

■ The platelet dysfunction seen in many uremic patients causes prolongation of the bleeding time and can be improved by the use of IV ddAVP (0.3 mcg/kg in 50 mL saline q4–8h), IV conjugated estrogen (0.6 mg/kg/d for 5 days), or intranasal ddAVP (see Chapter 18, Disorders of Hemostasis).

Dialysis Disequilibrium

■ Dialysis disequilibrium is a syndrome that may occur during the first few treatments of profoundly uremic patients and is attributed to central nervous system (CNS) edema from rapid osmolar shifts.

■ **Symptoms** include nausea, emesis, and headache, with occasional progression to con-fusion and seizures. This complication can be prevented or ameliorated by using lower blood flows and shorter treatment duration during initial dialysis sessions.

PERITONEAL DIALYSIS

Modalities

■ Peritoneal dialysis (PD) can be used in ARF and ESRD. It uses the peritoneum as a dialysis membrane, with solutes removed by diffusion into the dialysate. A typical dialysis exchange is performed by infusion of 2 L fluid into the peritoneal cavity, followed by an equilibration period and dialysate drainage. In ARF, PD exchanges can be performed as often as every hour.

■ PD should be avoided in patients with recent abdominal surgery or a history of multiple surgeries with adhesions. Strict sterile technique is mandatory when exchanges are being performed. Compared with HD, PD is less efficient and less useful in highly catabolic patients. PD may be better tolerated by patients with dilated cardiomyopathies because it causes fewer abrupt changes in BP and electrolytes, and fluid removal is continuous. PD also offers greater independence to patients on chronic dialysis than does HD.

- Fluid removal is controlled by adjusting the dextrose concentration in the dialysate (1.5%, 2.5%, or 4.25% glucose) to create an osmotic gradient for water. Higher dextrose concentrations increase the rate of fluid removal. **Icodextrin** is a glucose polymer that is minimally absorbed and maintains effective ultrafiltration gradients when used for 8- to 12-hour dwell times; some patients may have rashes and chemical peritonitis with icodextrin.
- **Continuous ambulatory PD** (CAPD) involves 2- to 3-L manual exchanges performed four to five times a day by the patient. There is also the option of including a single automated exchange during sleep.
- **Continuous cycling PD** (CCPD) uses an automatic cycler to perform several exchanges during sleep. It can be supplemented by daytime manual exchanges.
- The choice between CAPD and CCPD is often guided by characteristics of a patient's peritoneal membrane transport in addition to issues regarding lifestyle.

Complications of PD

- **Infections** are the most significant problem in PD and include peritonitis, infection of the catheter tunnel, and infection of the catheter exit site. **Peritonitis** typically causes increasing abdominal pain and cloudy peritoneal fluid. It is usually secondary to a break in sterile technique. Patients are trained to save cloudy fluid for cell count and culture and then to initiate antibiotic therapy on an outpatient basis.
  - A **neutrophil count** >100 cells/microliter in the dialysate is diagnostic of PD-associated peritonitis; however, peritonitis may be present with lower cell counts.
  - Because of the concern for emerging **vancomycin resistance**, initial empiric therapy should consist of cefazolin plus ceftazidime (Table 11-3) added to the PD fluid, which then should dwell for 5–6 hours.[6] Further antibiotic therapy should be guided by Gram stain and cultures.
- Hospitalization is indicated in patients with sepsis, resistant or recurrent infections, or suspicion of organ perforation or abscess formation.
- **Tunnel or exit site infections** involve skin organisms, frequently are difficult to treat, and may require catheter removal and temporary HD until the infection resolves.

 TABLE 11-3 **Intraperitoneal Antibiotics in Peritoneal Dialysis**

Antibiotic	Continuous dose (add to every exchange)	Intermittent dose (add to one exchange each day)
Cefazolin and cephalothin	Loading dose: 500 mg/L; maintenance dose: 125 mg/L	500 mg/L (or 15 mg/kg); if UO >500 mL/d, increase by 0.6 mg/kg body weight
Ceftazidime	Loading dose: 250 mg/L; maintenance dose: 125 mg/L	1,000 mg/d in one exchange
Gentamicin, netilmicin, tobramycin	Loading dose: 8 mg/L; maintenance dose: 4 mg/L	If UO >500 mL/d, give 1.5 mg/kg loading dose, then 0.6 mg/kg/d[a]; if UO <500 mL/d, give 0.6 mg/kg/d without load
Imipenem	Loading dose: 500 mg/L; maintenance dose: 200 mg/L	1,000 mg intraperitoneally bid

UO, urine output.
[a]Adjust dose based on blood levels (see Chapter 12, Antimicrobials).

- **Hyperglycemia** may occur as a result of systemic absorption of glucose from PD fluid.
  - Although regular insulin can be added to the dialysate, intraperitoneal insulin administration frequently results in unreliable dosing and an additional potential source of infectious contamination. Recent trends have favored traditional subcutaneous insulin administration for hyperglycemia in diabetic patients on PD. Using an icodextrin daytime exchange can reduce glucose exposure and uptake.
- **Protein loss** in PD can be excessive, and therefore dietary protein intake should be increased to 1.2–1.4 g/kg/d.

ULTRAFILTRATION AND HEMOFILTRATION

- **Dry ultrafiltration** is performed in a manner similar to that of standard HD, except that no dialysate is used and the concentration of toxins is not reduced. This is used when only volume removal is required. Negative pressure applied across the dialyzer membrane causes an ultrafiltrate of plasma to form and be removed. Large volumes of fluid may be removed in a short period. The patient may experience hypotension, but fluid removal is usually better tolerated by isolated dry ultrafiltration than with concomitant HD.
- **Slow, continuous renal replacement therapies** include **continuous venovenous hemofiltration** alone or with HD. These modalities were developed to treat critically ill patients in an intensive care unit (ICU) setting.
  - Continuous treatment permits the slow removal of large amounts of volume and solutes while minimizing hemodynamic compromise.
  - Continuous venovenous hemofiltration and continuous venovenous hemofiltration with HD use a blood pump that circulates blood though a double-lumen venous catheter, avoiding the need for an arterial line.
  - Both modalities usually require systemic anticoagulation, and patients are bedbound during treatment.
  - Fluid balance, electrolytes, and glucose must be closely monitored. Drug clearance may be higher than with HD or PD, and therefore drug levels should be monitored whenever possible.

RENAL TRANSPLANTATION

- Renal transplantation offers patients a lifestyle that is closest to normal and may lead to improved survival over HD and PD. One-year graft survival rates are >80% for cadaveric allografts and >90% for living-related donor grafts.
- **Pretransplantation evaluation** of the recipient includes assessment of cardiovascular status and structural abnormalities of the urinary tract, correction of potential sources of infection, human lymphocyte antigen typing, and evaluation for preformed antibodies against potential donor antigens. The latter, along with blood group compatibility testing, should prevent hyperacute rejection in most cases. Contraindications to transplantation include most malignancies, active infections, and significant cardiac or pulmonary disease.
- Immunosuppression, infectious complications, and long-term management of renal transplant recipients are discussed in Chapter 15, Solid Organ Transplant Medicine.

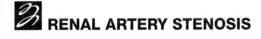 **RENAL ARTERY STENOSIS**

DEFINITION

- Renal artery stenosis (RAS) is the partial or complete occlusion of the renal artery resulting in ischemia to the kidney and renovascular hypertension.

DIAGNOSIS

Clinical Presentation

- RAS should be considered in the setting of poorly controlled hypertension despite four or more antihypertensive medications, hypertension with asymmetric kidney sizes, flash pulmonary edema, acute renal failure upon the initiation of ACE inhibitors or ARBs, or the presence of an abdominal bruit.

Imaging

- **Diagnosis** may be obtained via a Doppler ultrasound, magnetic resonance angiogram, or arteriogram of the renal artery. A stenosis >70% is considered potentially significant.

TREATMENT

- **Unilateral renal artery stenosis** alone rarely results in a significant decline in GFR, so the treatment goals are focused on resolution of hypertension and pulmonary edema.
  - For most patients, medical management of hypertension is sufficient. Treatment with **ACE inhibitors or ARBs**, sometimes with the addition of a diuretic, can often effectively control blood pressure in most patients.
  - If hypertension or pulmonary edema cannot be controlled medically, then angioplasty with stenting or surgical bypass may be considered.
- **Bilateral renal artery stenosis** may also result in ischemic renal failure. Angioplasty or bypass may also improve hypertension, but improvement in renal function is widely variable. Use of an ACE inhibitor or ARB may result in a decline in renal function.
  - Normal kidney sizes and textures on renal ultrasound and lack of proteinuria reflect normal underlying renal parenchyma and a higher likelihood of renal function improving with revascularization. Patients with high-grade stenoses and those with well-documented recent acute declines in GFR are also more likely to respond.

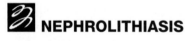 # NEPHROLITHIASIS

CLASSIFICATION

- Calcium-based kidney stones are most common (75%), usually **calcium oxalate**, less often **calcium phosphate**. Stones may also be composed of **uric acid**, **struvite** (magnesium ammonium phosphate associated with staghorn renal calculi and urea splitting bacterial infections involving *Proteus* or *Klebsiella*), and, rarely, **cystine** (with autosomal-recessive cystinuria).

DIAGNOSIS

Clinical Presentation

- Nephrolithiasis presents with hematuria, predisposition to urinary tract infection, and flank or costovertebral angle pain with passage of the stone.
- Renal stones may also be an incidental finding on radiographic studies. Oliguria and ARF may occur when both collecting systems are blocked by stones.

Imaging

- Diagnosis is made with plain abdominal radiogram. Calcium stones are radiopaque. Uric acid stones are radiolucent. Cystine and struvite stones have intermediate radiopacity.

■ **Noncontrast helical CT scanning** has largely supplanted IV pyelography for evaluation of renal colic and follow-up for patients with recurrent nephrolithiasis. Renal ultrasound may be useful to rule out obstruction of the collecting systems, particularly in the evaluation of pregnant patients with suspected nephrolithiasis.

Metabolic Evaluation

■ Urine should be cultured and examined for pH and crystals. Other initial studies include serum electrolytes, Cr, calcium, uric acid, and phosphorus levels. Urine should be strained and all passed stones should be saved for analysis.

■ The extent of the metabolic evaluation that should be undertaken for the patient with a single calcium stone has not been established, but recurrent calcium nephrolithiasis warrants complete investigation. Patients with noncalcium stones should undergo complete evaluation after the first episode.

■ **Additional studies** may include PTH levels (if hypercalcemia is present for calcium phosphate stones) and 24-hour urine studies for measurement of calcium, phosphate, urate, oxalate, citrate, Cr, sodium, urea nitrogen, and cystine. Yearly follow-up examination of the patient with nephrolithiasis includes abdominal radiographs or CT scanning to evaluate stone burden and repeat metabolic studies to assess the effects of specific therapies.

TREATMENT

■ Treatment is with analgesia, with ketoralac or narcotics such as meperidine, and hydration to increase urine output.

■ If the stone is obstructing outflow or is accompanied by infection, removal is indicated with **urgent urologic intervention**.

■ After passage of a stone, treatment is directed at prevention of recurrent stone formation. In most patients, the foundation of therapy is maintenance of high urine output (>2.5 L/d) through oral hydration. Evaluation and management depend on the type of stone and are best performed in the **outpatient setting**.

  ▪ Effective treatment of **calcium oxalate stones** includes a low-sodium diet (<2 g/d), low-protein and low-oxalate diet, normal calcium diet with no calcium supplements, and high urine output. Thiazide diuretics may reduce calciuria and potassium citrate may be given to correct hypocitraturia.

  ▪ Uric acid stones can be minimized by increased urine output, reduced uric acid production by low-protein diet and allopurinol if needed, and alkalinization of the urine with sodium bicarbonate or citrate supplementation.

  ▪ Struvite calculi frequently require surgical removal. Potassium citrate may be useful adjunctive therapy.

  ▪ Cystine stone reduction can be achieved by very high urine outputs (>3 L/d), urinary alkalinization, and low-sodium diet, and by breaking the disulfide bonds of cystine and increasing its solubility using tiopronin or captopril.

References
1. Merten GJ, Burgess WP, Gray LV, et al. Prevention of contrast-induced nephropathy with sodium bicarbonate: a randomized controlled trial. *J Amer Med Assoc* 2004;291:2328–2334.
2. Tepel M, van der Giet M, Schwarzfeld C, et al., Prevention of radiographic-contrast-agent-induced reductions in renal function by acetylcysteine. *N Engl J Med* 2000;343:180–184.
3. Denton MD, Chertow GM, Brady HR. "Renal-dose" dopamine for the treatment of acute renal failure: scientific rationale, experimental studies and clinical trials. *Kidney Int* 1996;50:4–14.

4. Ginzler EM, Dooley MA, Aranow C, et al. Mycophenolate mofetil or intravenous cyclophosphamide for lupus nephritis. *N Engl J Med* 2005;353:2219–2228.
5. Contreras G, Pardo V, Leclercq B, et al. Sequential therapies for proliferative lupus nephritis. *N Engl J Med* 2004;350:971–980.
6. Keane WF, Bailie GR, Boeschoten E, et al. Adult peritoneal dialysis-related peritonitis treatment recommendations: 2000 update. *Perit Dial Int* 2000;20:396–411.

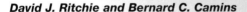

ANTIMICROBIALS
David J. Ritchie and Bernard C. Camins

12

GENERAL PRINCIPLES

Empiric antimicrobial therapy should be initiated based on expected pathogens for a given infection. As microbial resistance is increasing among many pathogens, a review of institution antibiograms as well as local, regional, national, and global susceptibility trends assists in the development of empiric therapy regimens. In addition, an accurate allergy history and pregnancy/lactation status should be elicited from the patient, as several agents are contraindicated in these settings. Antimicrobial therapy should be modified, if possible, based on results of culture and sensitivity testing to agent(s) that have the narrowest spectrum possible. Attention should be paid to the possibility of switching from parenteral to oral therapy where possible, as many oral agents have excellent oral bioavailability. Several antibiotics have major drug interactions or require alternate dosing in renal or hepatic insufficiency, or both. For antiretroviral and antiparasitic agents, see Chapter 14, Human Immunodeficiency Virus Infection and Acquired Immunodeficiency Syndrome, and Chapter 13, Treatment of Infectious Diseases, respectively.

 ANTIBACTERIAL AGENTS

PENICILLINS

- Penicillins (PCNs) irreversibly bind PCN-binding proteins in the bacterial cell wall, causing osmotic rupture and death. Once the mainstay of antimicrobial therapy, these agents have a somewhat diminished role today because of acquired resistance in many bacterial species through alterations in PCN-binding proteins or expression of hydrolytic enzymes.
- PCNs remain among the drugs of choice for syphilis, group A streptococci, *Listeria monocytogenes*, *Pasteurella multocida*, *Actinomyces*, susceptible enterococcus species, and some anaerobic infections.
- **Aqueous penicillin G** (2–4 million units IV q4h or 18–24 million units daily by continuous infusion) is the IV preparation of PCN. This formulation is the therapy of choice for neurosyphilis (see Chapter 13, Treatment of Infectious Diseases). Although the potassium salt is more commonly used, the sodium salt is available and can be given in the setting of hyperkalemia or azotemia.
- **Procaine penicillin G** is an IM repository form of penicillin G that can be used as an alternative treatment for neurosyphilis at a dose of 2.4 million units IM daily in combination with probenecid, 500 mg PO qid for 10–14 days.
- **Benzathine PCN** is a long-acting IM repository form of penicillin G that is commonly used for treating early latent syphilis (<1 year duration [1 dose, 2.4 million units IM]) and late latent syphilis (unknown duration or >1 year [2.4 million units IM every week for three doses]). It is occasionally given for group A streptococcal pharyngitis and prophylaxis after acute rheumatic fever or poststreptococcal glomerulonephritis.

- **Penicillin V** (250–500 mg PO qid) is an oral formulation of PCN that is typically used to treat group A streptococcal pharyngitis.
- **Ampicillin** (2–3 g IV q4–6h) is the drug of choice for treatment of infections caused by susceptible enterococcus species, group B streptococci, or *L. monocytogenes*. Oral ampicillin (250–500 mg PO qid) may be used for uncomplicated sinusitis, pharyngitis, otitis media, and urinary tract infections (UTIs), but amoxicillin is generally preferred.
- **Ampicillin/sulbactam** (1.5–3.0 g IV q6h) combines ampicillin with the β-lactamase inhibitor sulbactam, thereby extending its spectrum to include methicillin-sensitive *Staphylococcus aureus* (MSSA), anaerobes, and many Enterobacteriaceae. It is effective for infections of the upper and lower respiratory tract, genitourinary tract, and abdominal, pelvic, and polymicrobial soft tissue infections and is the IV antibiotic of choice for serious soft tissue infections due to human or animal bites.
- **Amoxicillin** (250–500 mg PO tid) is an oral antibiotic similar to ampicillin that is commonly used for uncomplicated sinusitis, pharyngitis, otitis media, and UTIs. **Amoxicillin/clavulanic acid** (875 mg PO bid, or 500 mg PO tid, or 90 mg/kg/d divided q12h [Augmentin ES-600 suspension], or 2,000 mg PO q12h [Augmentin XR]) is an oral antibiotic similar to ampicillin/sulbactam that combines amoxicillin with the β-lactamase inhibitor clavulanate. It is useful for treating complicated sinusitis, otitis media, and skin infections and is the oral antibiotic of choice for prophylaxis in human or animal bites after appropriate local treatment. It is often used as a step-down therapy from IV ampicillin/sulbactam.
- **Nafcillin and oxacillin** (2 g IV q4–6h) are penicillinase-resistant synthetic PCNs that are the drugs of choice for treating, MSSA, infections. These drugs have little activity against enterococci or Gram-negative bacteria. Dose reduction by one-half should be considered in decompensated liver disease.
- **Dicloxacillin and cloxacillin** (250–500 mg PO qid) are oral antibiotics with a spectrum of activity similar to that of nafcillin and oxacillin that are typically used to treat localized skin infections.
- **Piperacillin** (3 g IV q4h or 4 g IV q6h) is an extended-spectrum PCN derivative with enhanced Gram-negative activity as well as enterococcal activity. This agent has reasonable antipseudomonal activity but generally requires coadministration of an aminoglycoside for treatment of serious infections. Although piperacillin has significant enterococcal activity, ampicillin is still the treatment of choice for susceptible enterococcal infections.
- **Ticarcillin/clavulanic acid** (3.1 g IV q4–6h) combines ticarcillin with the β-lactamase inhibitor clavulanic acid. This combination extends the spectrum to include most Enterobacteriaceae, MSSA, and anaerobes, making it a useful antibiotic for intra-abdominal and complicated soft tissue infections. Ticarcillin/clavulanic acid also has a unique role in treatment of *Stenotrophomonas* infections. Alternative therapy with cefepime, a carbapenem, or a fluoroquinolone should be used when bacteria with *AmpC*-inducible β-lactamases (i.e., *Enterobacter*, *Citrobacter freundii*, *Serratia*, *Providencia*, and *Morganella* species) are identified as principal pathogens. Ticarcillin/clavulanic acid has a high sodium load and should be used cautiously in patients at risk for fluid overload.
- **Piperacillin/tazobactam** (3.375 g IV q6h or the higher dose of 4.5 g IV q6h for *Pseudomonas*) combines piperacillin with the β-lactamase inhibitor tazobactam. It has a similar spectrum and indications as ticarcillin/clavulanic acid but also has activity against ampicillin-sensitive enterococci. An aminoglycoside should generally be added to piperacillin/tazobactam for treatment of serious infections caused by *Pseudomonas aeruginosa* or for nosocomial pneumonia. Alternative therapy with cefepime, a carbapenem, or a fluoroquinolone should be used when bacteria with *AmpC*-inducible β-lactamases (i.e., *Enterobacter*, *Citrobacter freundii*, *Serratia*, *Providencia*, and *Morganella* species) are identified as principal pathogens.
- **Adverse effects.** All PCN derivatives have been associated with anaphylaxis, interstitial nephritis, anemia, and leukopenia. Oxacillin and nafcillin can cause hepatitis. Ticarcillin/clavulanic acid can aggravate bleeding by interfering with platelet adenosine diphosphate receptors. Prolonged high-dose therapy (>2 weeks) is typically monitored with weekly serum creatinine and blood counts (liver function tests (LFTs) are included with oxacillin/nafcillin). **All patients should be asked about PCN or cephalosporin**

allergy. These agents should not be used in patients with a reported serious PCN allergy without prior skin testing or desensitization, or both.

CEPHALOSPORINS

- Cephalosporins kill bacteria by interfering with cell wall synthesis by the same mechanism as PCNs.
- They are clinically useful because of their low toxicity and broad spectrum of activity. However, all currently available cephalosporins are devoid of activity against enterococci and methicillin-resistant *S. aureus* (MRSA).
- **First-generation cephalosporins** have activity against staphylococci, streptococci, and some *Escherichia coli*, *Klebsiella*, and *Proteus* species. They have limited activity against other enteric Gram-negative bacilli and anaerobes. These agents have similar spectrum of activity and indications and are commonly used for treating skin/soft tissue infections, UTIs, and OSSA infections. Cefazolin (1–2 g IV/IM q8h) is a parenteral formulation, and **cefadroxil** (500 mg–1 g PO bid), **cephalexin** (250–500 mg PO q6h), and **cephradine** (250–500 mg PO q6h) are oral preparations.
- **Second-generation cephalosporins** have expanded coverage against enteric Gram-negative rods and can be divided into above-the-diaphragm and below-the-diaphragm agents.
  - **Cefuroxime** (1.5 g IV/IM q8h) is a useful antibiotic for treatment of infections above the diaphragm. This agent has reasonable antistaphylococcal and antistreptococcal activity in addition to an extended spectrum against Gram-negative aerobes and can be used for skin/soft tissue infections, complicated UTIs, and community-acquired pneumonia. Cefuroxime does not reliably cover *Bacteroides fragilis*.
  - **Cefoxitin** (1–2 g IV q4–8h) is useful for treatment of infections below the diaphragm. This agent has less potent antistaphylococcal or antistreptococcal activity than first-generation cephalosporins but has reasonable activity against Gram-negative aerobes and anaerobes, including *B. fragilis*. Cefoxitin is typically used for intra-abdominal or gynecologic surgical prophylaxis and infections, including diverticulitis and pelvic inflammatory disease.
  - **Cefuroxime axetil** (250–500 mg PO bid), **cefprozil** (250–500 mg PO bid), and **cefaclor** (250–500 mg PO bid) are oral second-generation cephalosporins typically used for bronchitis, sinusitis, otitis media, UTIs, local soft tissue infections, and step-down therapy for pneumonia or cellulitis responsive to parenteral cephalosporins. **Loracarbef** (200–400 mg PO q12–24h) is chemically classified as a carbacephem rather than a cephalosporin but is generally used for the same indications as the oral second-generation cephalosporins.
- **Third-generation cephalosporins** have broad coverage against enteric, aerobic Gram-negative bacilli and retain significant activity against streptococci and MSSA. They have moderate anaerobic activity but generally not against *B. fragilis*. Ceftazidime is the only third-generation cephalosporin that is useful for treating serious *P. aeruginosa* infections. Several of these agents have substantial central nervous system (CNS) penetration and are useful in treating meningitis (see Chapter 13, Treatment of Infectious Diseases). Third-generation cephalosporins are not reliable for treatment of serious infections caused by organisms producing *AmpC* β-lactamases regardless of the results of susceptibility testing. These pathogens should be treated with cefepime, carbapenems, or quinolones.
  - **Ceftriaxone** (1–2 g IV/IM q12–24h), **cefotaxime** (1–2 g IV/IM q4–12h), and **ceftizoxime** (1–4 g IV/IM q8–12h) are very similar to one another in spectrum and efficacy. They can be used as empiric therapy for pyelonephritis, urosepsis, pneumonia (ceftriaxone or cefotaxime), intra-abdominal infections (combined with metronidazole), gonorrhea, and meningitis (ceftriaxone and cefotaxime). They can also be used for osteomyelitis, septic arthritis, endocarditis, and soft tissue infections once a susceptible organism has been identified.
  - **Cefpodoxime proxetil** (100–400 mg PO bid), **cefdinir** (300 mg PO bid), **ceftibuten** (400 mg PO daily), and **cefditoren pivoxil** (200–400 mg PO bid) are oral third-generation cephalosporins useful for the treatment of bronchitis and complicated

sinusitis, otitis media, and UTIs. These agents can also be used as step-down therapy for pneumonia that is responsive to parenteral third-generation cephalosporins. Cefpodoxime can be used as single-dose therapy for uncomplicated gonorrhea.

- **Ceftazidime** (1–2 g IV/IM q8h) may be used for treatment of infections caused by susceptible strains of *P. aeruginosa*.
- The fourth-generation cephalosporin has excellent aerobic Gram-negative bacillus coverage, including *P. aeruginosa* and other bacteria producing *AmpC* β-lactamases. Its Gram-positive activity is similar to that of the ceftriaxone and cefotaxime.
  - **Cefepime** (500 mg–2 g IV/IM q8–12h) is routinely used for empiric therapy in febrile neutropenic patients (see Chapter 20, Medical Management of Malignant Disease). It also has a prominent role in treating antibiotic-resistant Gram-negative bacteria and some infections involving Gram-negative and Gram-positive aerobes in most sites, although clinical experience for treatment of meningitis is more limited. Antianaerobic coverage should be added for treatment of infections where anaerobes are suspected.
- **Adverse effects.** All cephalosporins have been associated with anaphylaxis, interstitial nephritis, anemia, and leukopenia. **PCN-allergic patients have a 5%–10% incidence of a cross-hypersensitivity reaction to cephalosporins.** These agents should not be used in a patient with a reported allergy without prior skin testing or desensitization, or both. Prolonged therapy (>2 weeks) is typically monitored with a weekly serum creatinine and complete blood count (CBC). Ceftriaxone can cause biliary sludging and symptomatic gallbladder disease, requiring discontinuation of the medication.

MONOBACTAMS

- Aztreonam (1–2 g IV/IM q6–12h) is a monobactam that is active only against aerobic Gram-negative rods including *P. aeruginosa*.
  - It has minimal Gram-positive or anaerobic activity.
  - It is useful in patients with known PCN or cephalosporin allergies, as no apparent cross reactivity is present.

CARBAPENEMS

- Carbapenems exert their bactericidal effect by interfering with cell wall synthesis, similar to PCNs and cephalosporins. They are among the antibiotics of choice for infections caused by organisms producing *AmpC* β-lactamases. Carbapenems are also active against most Gram-positive and other Gram-negative bacteria, including anaerobes.
- Carbapenems are important agents for treatment of **antibiotic-resistant bacterial infections** at most body sites. These agents are commonly used for severe polymicrobial infections, including Fournier's gangrene, intra-abdominal catastrophes, and sepsis in compromised hosts.
- Notable bacteria that are **resistant** to carbapenems include ampicillin-resistant enterococci, MRSA, and *Stenotrophomonas* and *Burkholderia* species. In addition, ertapenem does not provide reliable coverage against *P. aeruginosa*, *Acinetobacter*, or enterococci; therefore, imipenem or meropenem would be preferred for empiric treatment of nosocomial infections when these pathogens are suspected.
- Meropenem is the preferred carbapenem for treatment of CNS infections.
- **Imipenem** (500 mg–1 g IV/IM q6–8h), **meropenem** (1 g IV q8h), and **ertapenem** (1 g IV q24h) are the currently available carbapenems.
- **Adverse effects.** Carbapenems can precipitate seizure activity, especially in older patients, individuals with renal insufficiency, and patients with pre-existing seizure disorders or CNS pathology. Carbapenems should be avoided in these patients unless no reasonable alternative therapy is available. Like cephalosporins, carbapenems have been associated with anaphylaxis, interstitial nephritis, anemia, and leukopenia.

- Patients who are allergic to PCNs/cephalosporins may have a cross-hypersensitivity reaction to carbapenems, and these agents should not be used in a patient with a reported severe PCN allergy without prior skin testing, desensitization, or both. Prolonged therapy (>2 weeks) is typically monitored with a weekly serum creatinine, LFTs, and CBC.

AMINOGLYCOSIDES

- Aminoglycosides exert their bactericidal effect by binding to the bacterial ribosome, causing misreading during translation of bacterial messenger RNA into proteins. These drugs are often used in combination with cell wall–active agents for treatment of severe infections caused by Gram-positive and Gram-negative aerobes. Prolonged low-dose therapy is indicated in combination therapy for endovascular infections caused by enterococcus species, PCN/cephalosporin-resistant streptococci, or Gram-negative endocarditis.
- Aminoglycosides tend to be synergistic with cell wall–active antibiotics such as PCNs, cephalosporins, and vancomycin. However, they do not have activity against anaerobes, and their activity is impaired in the low pH/low oxygen environment of abscesses. Resistance to one aminoglycoside is not routinely associated with resistance to all members of this class, and in cases of serious infections, susceptibility testing with each aminoglycoside is recommended. Use of these antibiotics is limited by significant nephrotoxicity and ototoxicity.

Dosing and Administration

- Traditional dosing of aminoglycosides involves standard divided daily dosing of aminoglycosides, 1–2 mg/kg IV q8h, with the upper end of the dose range reserved for life-threatening infections. Peak and trough concentrations should be obtained with the third or fourth dose and then every 3–4 days, along with regular serum creatinine monitoring. **Increasing serum creatinine or peak/troughs out of the acceptable range require immediate attention.** Traditional dosing, rather than extended-interval dosing, should be used for pregnant patients and for those with endocarditis, burns that cover more than 20% of the body, cystic fibrosis, anasarca, and creatinine clearance (Cr_{Cl}) of <20 mL/min.
- **Extended-interval dosing** of aminoglycosides is an alternative method of administration and is more convenient than traditional dosing for most indications. Extended-interval doses are provided in the following specific drug sections. A drug concentration is obtained 6–14 hours after the first dose, and a nomogram (Fig. 12–1) is consulted to determine the subsequent dosing interval. Monitoring includes obtaining a drug concentration 6–14 hours after the dosage at least every week and a serum creatinine three times a week. In patients who are not responding to therapy, a 12-hour concentration should be checked, and if that concentration is undetectable, extended-interval dosing should be abandoned in favor of traditional dosing. For obese patients (actual weight >20% above ideal body weight [IBW]), an obese dosing weight (obese dosing weight = IBW + 0.4 [actual body weight – IBW]) should be used for determining doses for both traditional and extended-interval methods.
- Specific agents
  - **Gentamicin** traditional dosing is an initial loading dose of 2 mg/kg IV (2–3 mg/kg in the critically ill) followed by 1.0–1.7 mg/kg IV q8h (peak, 4–10 mcg/mL; trough, <2 mcg/mL). Extended-interval dosing is an initial 5 mg/kg, with the subsequent dosing interval determined by a nomogram (Fig. 12–1).
  - **Tobramycin** traditional dosing is an initial loading dose of 2 mg/kg IV (2–3 mg/kg in the critically ill) followed by 1.0–1.7 mg/kg IV q8h (peak, 4–10 mcg/mL; trough, <2 mcg/mL). Extended-interval dosing is an initial 5 mg/kg, with the subsequent dosing interval determined by a nomogram (Fig. 12–1). Tobramycin is also available as an inhalational agent for adjunctive therapy for patients with cystic fibrosis or bronchiectasis complicated by *P. aeruginosa* infection (300 mg inhalation bid).

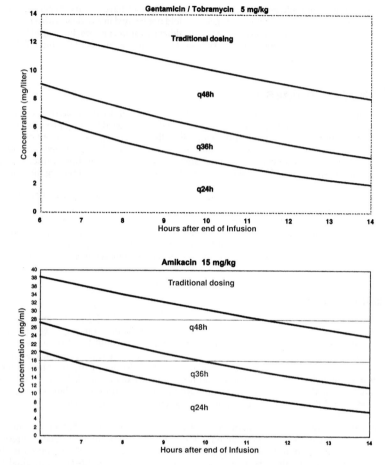

Figure 12-1. Nomograms for extended-interval aminoglycoside dosing. (Adapted from RM Reichley, JR Little, TC Bailey, Barnes-Jewish Hospital and Washington University School of Medicine.)

- **Amikacin** has an additional unique role for mycobacterial and *Nocardia* infections. Traditional dosing is an initial loading dose of 5.0–7.5 mg/kg IV (7.5–9.0 mg/kg in the critically ill) followed by 5 mg/kg IV q8h or 7.5 mg/kg IV q12h (peak, 20–35 mcg/mL; trough, <10 mcg/mL). Extended-interval dosing is 15 mg/kg, with the subsequent dosing interval determined by a nomogram (Fig. 12–1).
- **Streptomycin** is most commonly used for treating drug-resistant tuberculosis (TB; 15 mg/kg/d IM; the maximum dose per day is 1 g for daily dosing and 1.5 g for twice- or thrice-weekly dosing) and enterococcal endocarditis (7.5 mg/kg IM/IV q12h; maximum, 500 mg q12h). It generally has less Gram-negative activity than the other aminoglycosides and no activity against *P. aeruginosa*. Other indications for streptomycin (tularemia, brucellosis, plague) have largely been supplanted by gentamicin or other antibiotics.
- **Adverse effects. Nephrotoxicity** is the major adverse effect of aminoglycosides. If possible, prolonged therapy with aminoglycosides should be monitored by health care professionals who routinely administer home IV therapy and with systematic monitoring of laboratory studies. Nephrotoxicity is reversible when detected early

but can be permanent, especially in patients with tenuous renal function due to other medical conditions. Aminoglycosides should be used cautiously or avoided, if possible, in patients with decompensated kidney disease. **Ototoxicity** (vestibular or cochlear) is also possible and requires weekly hearing tests with extended therapy (>14 days). Streptomycin is unique in that it causes more ototoxicity with a lower risk of nephrotoxicity. Concomitant administration of aminoglycosides with other known nephrotoxic agents (i.e., amphotericin B, foscarnet, nonsteroidal anti-inflammatory drugs, pentamidine, polymyxins, cidofovir, and cisplatin) should be avoided if possible.

VANCOMYCIN

- Vancomycin (15 mg/kg IV q12h; up to 30 mg/kg IV q12h for meningitis) is a glycopeptide antibiotic that interferes with cell wall synthesis by binding to a D-alanyl-D-alanine precursor that is critical for peptidoglycan cross linking in most Gram-positive (not Gram-negative) bacterial cell walls. Vancomycin is bacteriostatic for enterococci. The **goal trough** concentration is at least 10–15 mcg/mL and perhaps up to 20 mcg/mL or more for other serious infections. Peak concentrations should generally only be measured in critically ill infected patients or in patients with endocarditis, osteomyelitis, meningitis, or other severe sequestered infections, with a goal of 30–45 mcg/mL. **Patients with end-stage renal disease** should receive a single 15-mg/kg dose and then be redosed when the concentration drops below 10–15 mcg/mL. Several factors, including the emergence of resistant nosocomial pathogens, low toxicity, and ease of administration, have led to an overuse of vancomycin and the evolution of vancomycin-resistant bacteria, most recently vancomycin-resistant *S. aureus* (VRSA).
- **Resistance.** Today, most hospitals have serious problems with vancomycin-resistant *Enterococcus faecium* (VRE), and there are now reports of clinical isolates of *S. aureus* that are intermediately resistant (VISA) and resistant to vancomycin (VRSA).
- **Indications for use** are detailed in Table 12–1.
- **Vancomycin should not be used routinely** in the following circumstances: (a) routine surgical prophylaxis, (b) empiric therapy for nonseptic neutropenic fever, (c) treatment of single blood culture isolates of coagulase-negative staphylococcus or treatment of coagulase-negative staphylococcus in cases in which the site of infection is inconsistent with the organism (e.g., community-acquired pneumonia or intra-abdominal infection), (d) routine treatment of *Clostridium difficile* colitis, (e) to complete a course of therapy in

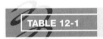

TABLE 12-1	Indications for Vancomycin Use

Treatment of serious infections caused by oxacillin-resistant *Staphylococcus aureus* (OSSA)

Treatment of serious infections caused by ampicillin-resistant enterococci

Treatment of serious infections caused by Gram-positive bacteria in patients who are allergic to all other appropriate therapies

Oral treatment of *Clostridium difficile* colitis that has not responded to two courses of metronidazole or is failing metronidazole with a potentially life-threatening colitis

Surgical prophylaxis for placement of prosthetic devices at institutions with known high rates of OSSA or in patients who are known to be colonized with OSSA

Empiric use in suspected Gram-positive meningitis until an organism has been identified and sensitivities confirmed

Life-threatening sepsis syndrome in a patient with known methicillin-resistant *S. aureus* colonization or extended hospitalization until pathogen(s) are identified

Documented coagulase-negative staphylococcal endocarditis or catheter related bloodstream infection

Empiric use for serious dialysis catheter–related bloodstream infections until the results of blood culture data are available

the absence of MRSA or ampicillin-resistant enterococci, (f) prophylaxis against catheter infections, and (g) use in topical application or irrigation. In dialysis patients, vancomycin use should be avoided in clinical situations in which MRSA is unlikely.

- **Adverse effects.** Vancomycin is typically administered by slow IV infusion over at least 1 hour. More rapid infusion rates can cause the **red man syndrome,** which is a histamine-mediated reaction that is typically manifested by flushing and redness of the upper body (see Chapter 10, Allergy and Immunology).

FLUOROQUINOLONES

- Fluoroquinolones exert their bactericidal effect by inhibiting bacterial DNA gyrase and topoisomerase, which are critical for DNA replication. In general, these antibiotics are well absorbed orally, with serum concentrations that approach those of parenteral administration. These agents typically have poor activity against enterococci, although they may have some efficacy for enterococcal UTIs when other agents are inactive or contraindicated. Newer fluoroquinolones have activity against MRSA but should be considered only when oxacillin, nafcillin, and first-generation cephalosporins are contraindicated or inactive. Concomitant administration with aluminum- or magnesium-containing antacids, sucralfate, bismuth, oral iron, oral calcium, and oral zinc preparations can markedly impair absorption of all orally administered fluoroquinolones.
- **Norfloxacin** (400 mg PO q12h) is useful for the treatment of UTIs caused by Gram-negative rods; however, other fluoroquinolones are preferred in this setting. This agent should not be used to treat systemic infections.
- **Ciprofloxacin** (250–750 mg PO q12h or 500 mg PO daily [Cipro XR] or 200–400 mg IV q8–12h), **levofloxacin** (250–750 mg IV/PO q24h), and **ofloxacin** (200–400 mg IV or PO q12h) are active against Gram-negative aerobes including many *AmpC* β-lactamase–producing pathogens. These agents are commonly used for UTIs, pyelonephritis, infectious diarrhea, prostatitis, and intra-abdominal infections (with metronidazole). Ciprofloxacin is the most active quinolone against *P. aeruginosa* and is the quinolone of choice for serious infections with that pathogen. However, ciprofloxacin has relatively poor activity against Gram-positive cocci and anaerobes and should not be used as empiric monotherapy for community-acquired pneumonia, skin and soft tissue infections, or intra-abdominal infections. Ciprofloxacin (500 mg), levofloxacin (250 mg), or ofloxacin (400 mg) can be used as single-dose therapy to treat gonorrhea. Oral and IV therapy with these agents give similar maximum serum levels; thus, oral therapy is appropriate unless contraindicated or concomitantly coadministered with polyvalent metallic cations.
- **Levofloxacin** (250–750 mg PO or IV q24h), **moxifloxacin** (400 mg PO/IV daily), and **gemifloxacin** (320 mg PO daily) are newer fluoroquinolones with improved coverage of aerobic Gram-positive bacteria (streptococci, staphylococci) and atypical respiratory pathogens (*Chlamydia pneumoniae, Mycoplasma, Legionella*) but less Gram-negative activity (especially against *P. aeruginosa*) than ciprofloxacin. Moxifloxacin and gemifloxacin also have reasonable anaerobic activity, possibly expanding their role in mixed aerobic/anaerobic infections. Moxifloxacin may be used as monotherapy of complicated intra-abdominal or skin and soft tissue infections. Each of these agents is useful for treatment of sinusitis, bronchitis, community-acquired pneumonia, and UTIs (except moxifloxacin, which is only minimally eliminated in the urine). They are reasonable therapy for uncomplicated soft tissue infections if PCNs or cephalosporins are inactive or contraindicated. Some of these agents have activity against mycobacteria and have a potential role in treating drug-resistant TB and atypical mycobacterial infections.
- **Adverse effects.** The principal adverse reactions with fluoroquinolones include nausea, CNS disturbances (drowsiness, headache, restlessness, and dizziness, especially in the elderly), rash, and phototoxicity. Moxifloxacin, levofloxacin, and gemifloxacin can cause prolongation of the QTc interval and should not be used in patients who are receiving class I or class III antiarrhythmics, in patients with known electrolyte or conduction abnormalities, or in those who are taking other medications that prolong the QTc interval or induce bradycardia. These agents should also be used cautiously in the elderly,

in whom asymptomatic conduction disturbances are more common. Fluoroquinolones should not be routinely used in patients younger than 18 years or in pregnant or lactating women due to the risk of arthropathy in pediatric patients. They may also cause an age-related arthropathy, particularly in elderly patients, and should be discontinued in individuals in whom joint pain or tendonitis (especially the Achilles tendon) develops. **This class of antibiotics has major drug interactions.**

MACROLIDE AND LINCOSAMIDE ANTIBIOTICS

- Macrolide and lincosamide antibiotics are bacteriostatic agents that block protein synthesis in bacteria by binding the 50S subunit of the bacterial ribosome. This class of antibiotics has activity against Gram-positive cocci, including streptococci and staphylococci, and some upper respiratory Gram-negative bacteria, but minimal activity against enteric Gram-negative rods. They are commonly used to treat pharyngitis, otitis media, sinusitis, and bronchitis, especially in PCN-allergic patients, and are among the drugs of choice for treating *Legionella*, *Chlamydia*, and *Mycoplasma* infections. The newer macrolides (azithromycin and clarithromycin) can be used as monotherapy for outpatient community-acquired pneumonia and have a unique role in the treatment and prophylaxis of *Mycobacterium avium* complex (MAC) infections in patients with HIV (see Chapter 14, Human Immunodeficiency Virus Infection and Acquired Immunodeficiency Syndrome). Many PCN-resistant strains of pneumococci are also resistant to macrolides.

- **Erythromycin** (250–500 mg PO qid or 0.5–1.0 g IV q6h) possesses activity against Gram-positive cocci (except enterococci) and can be used to treat bronchitis, pharyngitis, sinusitis, otitis media, and soft tissue infections in PCN-allergic patients. It is effective for treatment of atypical respiratory tract infections due to *Legionella pneumophila* (1 g IV q6h), *C. pneumoniae*, and *Mycoplasma pneumoniae*. However, there is significant resistance to erythromycin among *Haemophilus influenzae* species, and therefore, efficacy of this drug for upper and lower respiratory tract infections is limited. It can also be used for treatment of *Chlamydia trachomatis* infections (500 mg PO qid for 7 days) and as an alternate therapy for syphilis in PCN-allergic patients.

- **Clarithromycin** (250–500 mg PO bid or 1,000 mg XL PO daily) has a spectrum of activity similar to that of erythromycin but with enhanced activity against some respiratory pathogens (especially *Haemophilus*). It is commonly used to treat bronchitis, sinusitis, otitis media, pharyngitis, soft tissue infections, and community-acquired pneumonia. It has a prominent role in treating MAC infections in HIV patients and is an important component of regimens used to eradicate *Helicobacter pylori* (see Chapter 16, Gastrointestinal Diseases).

- **Azithromycin** (500 mg PO for 1 day, then 250 mg PO daily for 4 days; 250–500 mg PO daily; 500 mg PO daily for 3 days; 2,000 mg microspheres PO for one dose; 500 mg IV daily) has a similar spectrum of activity to clarithromycin and is commonly used to treat bronchitis, sinusitis, otitis media, pharyngitis, soft tissue infections, and community-acquired pneumonia. It has a prominent role in MAC prophylaxis (1,200 mg PO every week) and treatment (250–500 mg PO daily) in HIV patients. It is also commonly used to treat *C. trachomatis* infections (1 g PO single dose). A major advantage of azithromycin is that it does not have the numerous drug interactions seen with erythromycin and clarithromycin.

- **Clindamycin** (150–450 mg PO tid–qid or 600–900 mg IV q8h) is chemically classified as a lincosamide (related to macrolides), with a predominantly Gram-positive spectrum similar to that of erythromycin with additional inclusion of activity against most anaerobes, including *B. fragilis*. It has excellent oral bioavailability (90%) and penetrates well into bone and abscess cavities. It is also used for treatment of aspiration pneumonia and lung abscesses. Clindamycin is often active against community-acquired strains of methicillin-resistant *S. aureus* (CA-MSSA), and the agent has emerged as a treatment option for skin and soft tissue infections caused by this organism. Clindamycin may be used as a second agent in combination therapy for invasive streptococcal infections to decrease toxin production. The agent may also be used for treatment of suspected anaerobic infections (peritonsillar/retropharyngeal abscesses, necrotizing fasciitis), although metronidazole is used more commonly for intra-abdominal infections (clindamycin has less reliable activity against *B. fragilis*). Clindamycin has additional uses, including treatment of babesiosis (in combination with quinine), toxoplasmosis (in combination with pyrimethamine), and *Pneumocystis jiroveci* pneumonia (in combination with primaquine).

■ **Adverse effects.** Macrolides and clindamycin are associated with nausea, abdominal cramping, and LFT abnormalities (particularly erythromycin). Liver function profiles should be checked intermittently during extended therapy. Hypersensitivity reactions with prominent skin rash are more common with clindamycin, as is pseudomembranous colitis secondary to *C. difficile*. **Erythromycin and clarithromycin have major drug interactions** caused by inhibition of the cytochrome P-450 system.

SULFAMETHOXAZOLE, SULFADIAZINE, SULFISOXAZOLE, TRIMETREXATE, AND TRIMETHOPRIM

■ Sulfamethoxazole, sulfadiazine, sulfisoxazole, trimetrexate, and trimethoprim slowly kill bacteria by inhibiting folic acid metabolism. This class of antibiotics is most commonly used for uncomplicated UTIs, sinusitis, and otitis media. They also have unique roles in treatment of *P. jiroveci*, *Nocardia*, *Toxoplasma*, and *Stenotrophomonas* infections.

■ **Sulfamethoxazole** (2 g PO, then 1 g PO q12h), **sulfisoxazole** (1 g PO q6h), and **trimethoprim** (100 mg PO bid) are occasionally used as monotherapy for treatment of UTIs. These drugs are more often used in the combination preparations outlined in the following sections. Trimethoprim in combination with dapsone is an alternate therapy for mild *P. jiroveci* pneumonia (see Chapter 13, Treatment of Infectious Diseases).

■ **Trimethoprim/sulfamethoxazole** is a combination antibiotic (IV or PO) with a 1:5 ratio of trimethoprim to sulfamethoxazole. The IV preparation is dosed at 5 mg/kg IV q8h (based on the trimethoprim component) for serious infections. The oral preparations (160 mg trimethoprim/800 mg sulfamethoxazole per double-strength [DS] tablet) are extensively bioavailable, with similar drug concentrations obtained with IV and with PO formulations. Both components have excellent tissue penetration, including bone, prostate, and CNS. The combination has a broad spectrum of activity but typically does not inhibit *P. aeruginosa*, anaerobes, or group A streptococci. It is the therapy of choice for *P. jiroveci* pneumonia (see Chapter 14, Human Immunodeficiency Virus Infection and Acquired Immunodeficiency Syndrome), *Stenotrophomonas maltophilia*, *Tropheryma whippelii*, and *Nocardia* infections. It is commonly used for treating sinusitis, otitis media, bronchitis, prostatitis, and UTIs (1 DS PO bid). Trimethoprim/sulfamethoxazole is active against the majority of community-acquired strains of MSSA, and the agent has emerged as a viable treatment for uncomplicated cases of skin and soft tissue infections caused by this organism. It is used as *P. jiroveci* pneumonia prophylaxis (1 DS PO twice a week, three times a week, or single strength or DS daily) in HIV-infected patients, solid organ transplant patients, bone marrow transplant patients, and patients receiving fludarabine. Intravenous therapy is routinely converted to the PO equivalent for patients who require prolonged therapy. For serious infections, such as *Nocardia* brain abscesses, it may be useful to monitor sulfamethoxazole peaks (100–150 mcg/mL) and troughs (50–100 mcg/mL) occasionally during the course of therapy and to adjust dosing accordingly. In patients with renal insufficiency, doses can be adjusted by following trimethoprim peaks (5–10 mcg/mL). Prolonged therapy can cause bone marrow suppression, possibly requiring treatment with leucovorin (5–10 mg PO daily) until cell counts normalize.

■ **Sulfadiazine** (1.0–1.5 g PO q6h) in combination with pyrimethamine (200 mg PO followed by 50–75 mg PO daily) and leucovorin (10–20 mg PO daily) is the therapy of choice for toxoplasmosis. Sulfadiazine is also occasionally used to treat *Nocardia* infections.

■ **Trimetrexate** (45 mg/m^2 IV daily) combined with leucovorin (20 mg/m^2 PO or IV q6h continued for 3 days after the last dose of trimetrexate) is an alternate (salvage) therapy for *P. jiroveci* infections. Bone marrow suppression, renal insufficiency, and hepatotoxicity may occur.

■ **Adverse effects.** These drugs are associated with cholestatic jaundice, bone marrow suppression, interstitial nephritis, "false" elevations in serum creatinine, and severe hypersensitivity reactions (Stevens-Johnson syndrome/erythema multiforme). Nausea is common with higher doses. **All patients should be asked whether they are allergic to "sulfa drugs,"** and specific commercial names should be mentioned (i.e., Bactrim or Septra).

CHLORAMPHENICOL

■ Chloramphenicol (12.5–25.0 mg/kg IV q6h; maximum, 1 g IV q6h) is a bacteriostatic antibiotic that binds to the 50S ribosomal subunit, blocking protein synthesis in susceptible bacteria. It has broad-spectrum activity against aerobic and anaerobic Gram-positive and Gram-negative bacteria, including *S. aureus*, enterococci, and enteric Gram-negative rods. It also is active against spirochetes, *Rickettsia*, *Mycoplasma*, and *Chlamydia*. The drug may also be used for serious VRE infections. Because of its excellent CNS penetration, chloramphenicol also plays a role for treatment of meningitis caused by susceptible organisms in PCN-allergic patients and for meningitis caused by *Francisella tularensis* or *Yersinia pestis*.

■ **Adverse effects** include idiosyncratic aplastic anemia (~1/30,000) and dose-related bone marrow suppression. Peak drug levels (1 hour postinfusion) should be checked every 3–4 days (goal peak <25 mcg/mL) and doses adjusted accordingly. Dosage adjustment is necessary in the presence of significant liver disease. **This class of antibiotics has major drug interactions.**

METRONIDAZOLE

■ Metronidazole (250–750 mg PO/IV q6–12h) is only active against anaerobic bacteria and some protozoa. The drug exerts its bactericidal effect though accumulation of toxic metabolites that interfere with multiple biologic processes. It has excellent tissue penetration, including abscess cavities, bone, and CNS.

■ It has greater activity against Gram-negative than Gram-positive anaerobes but is active against *Clostridium perfringens* and *C. difficile*. It is the treatment of choice as monotherapy for *C. difficile* colitis and bacterial vaginosis, and it can be used in combination with other antibiotics to treat intra-abdominal infections and brain abscesses (see Chapter 13, Treatment of Infectious Diseases). Protozoal infections that are routinely treated with metronidazole include *Giardia*, *Entamoeba histolytica*, and *Trichomonas vaginalis*. A dose reduction may be warranted for patients with decompensated liver disease.

■ **Adverse effects** include nausea, dysgeusia, disulfiram-like reactions to alcohol, and mild CNS disturbances (headache, restlessness). Rarely, metronidazole causes seizures and peripheral neuropathy.

TETRACYCLINES

■ Tetracyclines are bacteriostatic antibiotics that bind to the 30S ribosomal subunit and block protein synthesis.

■ They have unique roles in the treatment of *Rickettsia*, *Ehrlichia*, *Chlamydia*, *Nocardia*, and *Mycoplasma* infections.

■ These agents are used as therapy for Lyme disease–related arthritis and as alternate therapy for syphilis and *P. multocida* infections in PCN-allergic patients. Their general use is limited because of widespread resistance among more common bacterial pathogens.

■ **Tetracycline** (250–500 mg PO q6h) is commonly used for severe acne and in some *H. pylori* eradication regimens (see Chapter 16, Gastrointestinal Diseases). It can also be used for treatment of acute Lyme borreliosis, Rocky Mountain spotted fever, ehrlichiosis, psittacosis, *Mycoplasma* pneumonia, *Chlamydia* pneumonia, and chlamydial infections of the eye or genitourinary tract, but these infections are generally treated with doxycycline or other antibiotics. Aluminum- and magnesium-containing antacids and preparations that contain oral calcium, oral iron, or other cations can significantly impair oral absorption of tetracycline and should be avoided within 2 hours of the dose.

- **Doxycycline** (100 mg PO/IV q12h) is the most commonly used tetracycline and is standard therapy for *C. trachomatis*, Rocky Mountain spotted fever, ehrlichiosis, and psittacosis. This agent also has a role for malaria prophylaxis and for treatment of community-acquired pneumonia.
- **Minocycline** (200 mg PO, then 100 mg PO q12h) is similar to doxycycline in its spectrum of activity and clinical indications. It is second-line therapy for pulmonary nocardiosis and cervicofacial actinomycosis. Minocycline also has activity against some multi–drug-resistant Gram-negative pathogens and may be used as an adjunctive agent in this setting as per results of susceptibility testing.
- **Adverse effects.** Nausea and photosensitivity are common side effects. Patients should be warned about sun exposure. Rarely, these medications are associated with pseudotumor cerebri. **They should not routinely be given to children or to pregnant or lactating women** because they can cause tooth enamel discoloration in young children. Minocycline is associated with vestibular disturbances.

GLYCYLCYCLINES

- Tigecycline (100 mg IV loading dose, then 50 mg IV q12h) is the only U.S. Food and Drug Administration (FDA)-approved antibiotic in this class. Its mechanism of action is similar to that of tetracyclines by inhibiting the translation of bacterial proteins by binding to the 30S ribosome. The addition of the glycyl side chain expands its activity against bacterial pathogens that are normally resistant to tetracycline and minocycline. It has a broad spectrum of bactericidal activity against Gram-positive, Gram-negative, and anaerobic bacteria except *P. aeruginosa* and *Proteus* species. It is currently only indicated for treatment of complicated skin and skin structure infections and complicated intra-abdominal infections. Tigecycline should be reserved for use in treatment of tissue infections due to resistant pathogens such as VRE, *Acinetobacter* spp., and *Enterobacter* spp. Until more data are available, it should not be used to treat primary bacteremias.
- **Adverse Effects.** Nausea and vomiting are the most common adverse events. Tigecycline has not been studied in patients younger than 18 years and is contraindicated in pregnant and lactating women. Since it has a similar structure to tetracyclines, photosensitivity, tooth discoloration, and rarely pseudotumor cerebri may occur.

STREPTOGRAMINS

Streptogramins are a class of antimicrobial agents that complex with bacterial ribosomes to inhibit protein synthesis.

- **Quinupristin/dalfopristin** (7.5 mg/kg IV q8h) is the first FDA-approved drug in this class.
- It has activity against antibiotic-resistant Gram-positive organisms, especially VRE, MRSA, VISA, VRSA, and antibiotic-resistant strains of *Streptococcus pneumoniae*. It has some activity against Gram-negative upper respiratory pathogens (*Haemophilus* and *Moraxella*) and anaerobes, but more appropriate antibiotics are available to treat these infections. Quinupristin/dalfopristin is bacteriostatic for enterococci and can be used for treatment of serious infections with VISA and VRE (however, it has little activity against *Enterococcus faecalis*). It can also be used for treatment of serious infections with MRSA and *S. pneumoniae* when vancomycin cannot be tolerated.
- **Adverse effects** include arthralgias and myalgias, which occur frequently and can necessitate discontinuation of therapy. IV site pain and thrombophlebitis are common when the drug is administered through a peripheral vein. It has also been associated with elevated LFTs and, as it is primarily cleared by hepatic metabolism, patients with significant

hepatic impairment require a dose adjustment. Quinupristin/dalfopristin is similar to erythromycin with regard to drug interactions.

OXAZOLIDINONES

- Oxazolidinones are a new class of antibiotics that block assembly of bacterial ribosomes and inhibit protein synthesis. **Linezolid** (600 mg IV/PO bid) is the first FDA-approved drug in this class, and IV and oral formulations produce equivalent serum concentrations. It has potent activity against Gram-positive bacteria, including drug-resistant enterococci, staphylococci, and streptococci. Its activity against MRSA is comparable to that of vancomycin. However, it has no meaningful activity against Enterobacteriaceae and borderline activity against *Moraxella* and *H. influenzae.*
- **Use of linezolid should be restricted** to serious infections with VRE, as an alternative to vancomycin for treatment of MRSA infections, for patients with an indication for vancomycin therapy who are intolerant of that medication, and as oral therapy of MRSA infections when IV access is unavailable. Supporting data for treatment of osteomyelitis, endocarditis, and meningitis are minimal, and routine use for these infections should be carefully undertaken. Resistance develops to this antibiotic, and it is imperative that abscesses be adequately drained to minimize this risk and that organism susceptibility is verified.
- **Adverse effects.** Side effects include diarrhea, nausea, and headache. Thrombocytopenia occurs frequently in patients who receive more than 2 weeks of therapy, and serial platelet count monitoring is indicated in this setting. A CBC, serum creatinine, and LFTs should be checked every 1–2 weeks during prolonged therapy with this new agent. Extremely prolonged therapy (typically longer than 6 months) has been associated with peripheral and optic neuropathy.
- **Linezolid has several important drug interactions.** It is a mild monoamine oxidase inhibitor, and patients should be advised not to take selective serotonin reuptake inhibitors (SSRIs) while on the drug to avoid the serotonin syndrome. Ideally, patients should be off the SSRI for at least a week before initiating linezolid. Over-the-counter cold remedies that contain pseudoephedrine or phenylpropanolamine should also be avoided, as coadministration with linezolid can elevate BP. Linezolid does not require dose adjustments for renal or hepatic dysfunction.

DAPTOMYCIN

- Daptomycin (4 mg/kg IV q24h for skin and skin structure infections; 6 mg/kg IV q24h for bloodstream infections) belongs to a new class of antibiotics called the cyclic lipopeptides. The drug exhibits rapid bactericidal activity against a wide variety of Gram-positive bacteria, including enterococci, staphylococci, and streptococci. Daptomycin also maintains activity against many of the bacteria that have become resistant to methicillin and vancomycin, and is currently FDA approved for treatment of complicated skin and skin structure infections as well as *Staphylococcus aureus* bacteremia and right-sided endocarditis. The drug should not be used to treat primary lung infections due to its decreased activity in the presence of pulmonary surfactant. Resistance develops to this antibiotic, and it is imperative that abscesses be adequately drained to minimize this risk and that organism susceptibility is verified.
- **Adverse effects** include GI disturbances, injection site reactions, elevated liver function tests, and elevated creatine phosphokinase. Serum creatine phosphokinase should be monitored weekly, as daptomycin has been associated with skeletal muscle effects. Patients should also be monitored for signs of muscle weakness and pain, and the drug should be discontinued if these symptoms develop in conjunction with marked creatine phosphokinase elevations. Consideration should also be given to avoiding concomitant use of daptomycin and HMG-CoA reductase inhibitors due to the potential increased risk of myopathy.

FOSFOMYCIN

- Fosfomycin (3-g sachet dissolved in cold water PO once) is a bactericidal oral antibiotic that kills bacteria by inhibiting an early step in cell wall synthesis. It has a spectrum of activity that includes most urinary tract pathogens, including *P. aeruginosa*, *Enterobacter* species, and enterococci (including VRE).
- It is most useful for treating uncomplicated UTIs in women with susceptible strains of *E. coli* and *E. faecalis*. It should not be used to treat pyelonephritis or systemic infections. It should only be administered once, as therapeutic drug levels are maintained in the urine for approximately 48 hours.
- **Adverse effects** include diarrhea. It should not be taken with metoclopramide, as that drug interferes with fosfomycin absorption.

NITROFURANTOIN

- Nitrofurantoin (50–100 mg PO macrocrystals qid or 100 mg PO dual-release formulation bid for 5–7 days) is a bactericidal oral antibiotic that is useful for uncomplicated UTIs except those caused by *Proteus*, *P. aeruginosa*, or *Serratia*. The drug is metabolized by bacteria into toxic intermediates that inhibit multiple bacterial processes. It has had a modest resurgence in use, as it is frequently effective against uncomplicated VRE UTIs.
- Although it was commonly used in the past for UTI prophylaxis, this practice should be avoided, as prolonged therapy is associated with chronic pulmonary syndromes that can be fatal. Nitrofurantoin should not be used for pyelonephritis or any other systemic infections.
- **Adverse effects.** Nausea is the most common adverse effect, and the drug should be taken with food to minimize this problem. Patients should be warned that their urine may become brown secondary to the medication. Furthermore, it should not be used in patients with an elevated serum creatinine, as the risk for development of treatment-associated adverse effects is increased. It should not be given with probenecid, as this combination decreases the concentration of nitrofurantoin in the urine.

METHENAMINE

- Methenamine hippurate or methenamine mandelate (one or two tablets [depending on the specific preparation] PO qid) is a urine/bladder antiseptic that is converted into formaldehyde in the urine when the pH is <6.0.
- Because the active drug is formaldehyde, most bacteria and fungi are potentially susceptible to therapy. The formaldehyde is generated while urine is retained in the bladder; therefore, methenamine is effective only in the lower urinary tract, and its efficacy is impaired in the setting of a draining Foley catheter. These drugs are rarely used because of the large number of alternative antibiotics that are available today. They do have a limited role in treating uncomplicated UTI caused by multiple drug–resistant bacteria or yeast.
- **Adverse effects** include bladder irritation, dysuria, and hematuria with prolonged use. Therapy should be limited to a maximum of 3 weeks at a time, and urine pH should be obtained once early during therapy to ensure an appropriately acidic pH. Vitamin C can be used to assist in urine acidification. It is **contraindicated** in the setting of glaucoma, significant renal insufficiency, and acidosis. It should not be given concomitantly with sulfonamides, as these drugs form an insoluble precipitate in the urine.

COLISTIN

- Colistimethate sodium; polymyxin E (IV therapy is 2.5–5.0 mg/kg/d divided into two to four doses; maximum dose, 5 mg/kg/d); and **polymyxin B** (12,000– 5,000 units/kg/d by continuous infusion [500,000 units in 500 mL 5% dextrose in water; adjust rate to achieve desired daily dosing]) are bactericidal polypeptide antibiotics that kill Gram-negative bacteria by disrupting the cell membrane. These drugs have roles in the treatment of multiple drug–resistant Gram-negative bacilli, predominantly *P. aeruginosa*, but are inactive against *Proteus* and *Serratia*.

■ **These medications should only be given under the guidance of an experienced clinician,** as parenteral therapy has significant CNS side effects and potential nephrotoxicity. Inhaled colistin (75 mg tid or 150 mg bid given by standard nebulizer) is better tolerated, with only mild upper airway irritation, and has some efficacy as adjunctive therapy for *P. aeruginosa* pulmonary infections. Inhaled colistin may also have a potential role as primary therapy for *Acinetobacter* pneumonias.

■ **Adverse effects** with parenteral therapy include paresthesias, slurred speech, peripheral numbness, tingling, and significant dose-dependent nephrotoxicity. The dosage should be carefully reduced in patients with renal insufficiency, as overdosage in this setting can result in neuromuscular blockade and apnea. If CNS side effects are significant with twice-daily dosing of colistin, four times daily dosing or continuous infusion (total daily dose in 500 mL 5% dextrose in water infused over 24 hours) should be arranged. Serum creatinine should be monitored daily early in therapy and then at a regular interval for the duration of therapy. **Concomitant use with aminoglycosides, other known nephrotoxins, or neuromuscular blockers should be avoided if possible.**

ANTIMYCOBACTERIAL AGENTS

Effective therapy of *Mycobacterium tuberculosis* (MTB) infections requires combination chemotherapy designed to prevent the emergence of resistant organisms and maximize efficacy. Increased resistance to conventional antituberculous agents has led to the use of more complex regimens and has made susceptibility testing an integral part of TB management (see Chapter 13, Treatment of Infectious Diseases).

ISONIAZID

■ Isoniazid (INH, 300 mg PO daily) exerts bacterialcidal effects on susceptible mycobacteria by interfering with the synthesis of the lipid components of the mycobacterial cell wall. It is well absorbed orally and has good penetration throughout the body including the CNS. INH is a component of nearly all treatment regimens and can be given twice a week in directly observed therapy (15 mg/kg/dose; 900 mg maximum). INH remains the drug of choice for treatment of latent tuberculosis infection (300 mg PO daily for 9 months).

■ **Adverse effects** include elevations in liver transaminases (20%). This effect can be idiosyncratic but is usually seen in the setting of advanced age, underlying liver disease, or concomitant consumption of alcohol and may be potentiated by rifampin. Transaminase elevations to greater than threefold the upper limit of the normal range necessitate holding therapy. Patients with known liver dysfunction should have weekly LFTs during the initial stage of therapy. INH also antagonizes vitamin B_6 metabolism and potentially can cause a peripheral neuropathy. This can be avoided or minimized by coadministration of pyridoxine, 25–50 mg PO daily, especially in the elderly, in pregnant women, and in patients with diabetes, renal failure, alcoholism, and seizure disorders.

RIFAMYCINS

Rifamycins exert bacterialcidal activity on susceptible mycobacteria by inhibiting DNA-dependent RNA polymerase, thereby halting transcription.

■ **Rifampin** (600 mg PO daily or twice a week) is active against many Gram-positive and Gram-negative bacteria in addition to MTB. It is also used as adjunctive therapy in staphylococcal prosthetic valve endocarditis (300 mg PO q8h), for prophylaxis of close contacts of patients with infection caused by *Neisseria meningitidis* (600 mg PO q12h), and as adjunctive treatment of bone and joint infections associated with prosthetic material or devices. The drug is well absorbed orally and is widely distributed throughout the body including the cerebrospinal fluid (CSF).

■ **Rifabutin** (300 mg PO daily) is principally used to treat TB and MAC infections in HIV-positive patients who are receiving highly active antiretroviral therapy, as it has less deleterious effects on protease inhibitor metabolism than does rifampin (see Chapter 14, Human Immunodeficiency Virus Infection and Acquired Immunodeficiency Syndrome).

■ **Rifapentine** (600 mg PO twice a week for 2 months, then every week to complete therapy) is a rifamycin that appears to be associated with more TB relapses than rifampin; therefore, it is typically not used as a first-line drug.

■ **Adverse effects.** Patients should be warned about reddish-orange discoloration of body fluids, and contact lenses should not be worn during treatment. Rash, GI disturbances, hematologic disturbances, hepatitis, and interstitial nephritis can occur. Uveitis has been associated with rifabutin and hyperuricemia with rifapentine. **This class of antibiotics has major drug interactions.**

PYRAZINAMIDE

■ Pyrazinamide (15–30 mg/kg PO daily; maximum, 2 g or 50–75 mg/kg PO twice a week; maximum, 4 g/dose) kills mycobacteria replicating in macrophages by an unknown mechanism.

■ It is well absorbed orally and widely distributed throughout the body including the CSF. Pyrazinamide is typically used for the first 2 months of therapy.

■ **Adverse effects** include hyperuricemia and hepatitis.

ETHAMBUTOL

■ Ethambutol (15–25 mg/kg PO daily or 50–75 mg/kg PO twice a week; maximum, 2.5 g/dose) is bacteriostatic with an unknown mechanism of action.

■ Doses should be reduced in the presence of renal dysfunction.

■ **Adverse effects.** These may include optic neuritis, which manifests as decreased red-green color perception, decreased visual acuity, or visual field deficits. Baseline and monthly visual examinations should be performed during therapy. Renal function should also be carefully monitored as drug accumulation in the setting of renal insufficiency can increase risk of ocular effects.

STREPTOMYCIN

■ Streptomycin is an aminoglycoside that can be used as a substitute for ethambutol and for drug-resistant MTB. It does not adequately penetrate the CNS and should not be used for TB meningitis (see Antibacterial Agents).

ANTIVIRAL AGENTS

Current antiviral agents only suppress viral replication. Viral containment or elimination requires an intact host immune response.

Anti-influenza drugs include not only **amantadine** and **rimantadine**, but also two newer drugs, zanamivir and oseltamivir, which block influenza A and B neuraminidases. This enzymatic activity is necessary for successful viral egress and release from infected cells. These drugs have shown modest activity in clinical trials, with a 1- to 2-day improvement in symptoms in patients who are treated within 48 hours of the onset of influenza symptoms. Although there are data showing that these agents are effective for prophylaxis of influenza, annual influenza vaccination remains the intervention of choice in all high-risk patients and health care workers (see Appendix C, Immunizations and Post-exposure Therapies).

■ **Amantadine and rimantadine** (100 mg PO bid for both; 100 mg PO daily in elderly patients, dialysis patients, or those with decompensated liver disease) prevent influenza A entry into cells by blocking endosomal acidification, which is necessary for fusion of the viral envelope with the host cell membrane. These agents have no activity against influenza B. They are effective when therapy is initiated within 48 hours of initial symptoms and continued for 7–10 days. Patients at high risk of complications (e.g., immunocompromised patients, the elderly, diabetics, dialysis patients, and patients with pulmonary or cardiac disease) should probably be treated even after 48 hours of symptoms in the absence of studies that specifically address the treatment of high-risk patients. These drugs can also be used for influenza prophylaxis in nonimmune individuals who have been exposed to the virus and in patients and staff members of nursing homes or hospitals during an epidemic.

   ■ **Adverse effects.** GI disturbances and CNS dysfunction, including dizziness, nervousness, confusion, slurring of speech, blurred vision, and sleep disturbances, may be experienced with use of these antivirals. Rimantadine has fewer side effects than amantadine.

■ **Zanamivir** (10 mg [two inhalations] q12h for 5 days, started within 48 hours of the onset of symptoms) is an inhaled neuraminidase inhibitor that is active against influenza A and B. Zanamivir is indicated for treatment of uncomplicated acute influenza infection in adults and children 7 years of age or older who have been symptomatic for <48 hours. When used within 30 hours of the onset of influenza symptoms, zanamivir reduces the duration of symptoms by an average of 1–2 days. Limited evidence of its successful use for influenza prophylaxis has been shown, although it is currently not FDA approved for this use.

   ■ **Adverse effects.** Headache, GI disturbances, dizziness, and upper respiratory symptoms are sometimes reported.

   ■ Bronchospasms or declines in lung function, or both, may occur in patients with underlying respiratory disorders and may require a rapid-acting bronchodilator for control.

■ **Oseltamivir** (75 mg PO bid for 5 days) is an orally administered neuraminidase inhibitor that is active against influenza A and B.

   ■ It is indicated for treatment of uncomplicated acute influenza in adults and children 1 year of age or older who have been symptomatic for <2 days and for prophylaxis of influenza after exposures. When used for treatment of influenza within 40 hours of the onset of influenza symptoms, oseltamivir was associated with a 1.3-day reduction in median time to clinical improvement. This agent is U.S. FDA approved for prophylaxis of influenza A and B in adults and children 1 year of age or older.

   ■ **Adverse effects.** Nausea, vomiting, and diarrhea have been reported. Dizziness and headache may also occur.

ANTIHERPETIC AGENTS

Antiherpetic agents are nucleotide analogs that inhibit viral DNA synthesis.

■ **Acyclovir** is active against herpes simplex virus (HSV) and varicella-zoster virus (VZV) (400 mg PO tid for HSV, 800 mg PO five times a day for localized VZV infections, 5 mg/kg IV q8h for severe HSV infections, and 10 mg/kg IV q8h for severe VZV infections and HSV encephalitis).

   ■ Acyclovir has no effect on herpes viruses that are latent.

   ■ It is indicated for treatment of primary and recurrent genital herpes, severe herpetic stomatitis, and herpes simplex encephalitis. It can be used as prophylaxis in patients who have frequent HSV recurrences (400 mg PO bid).

   ■ It is also used for herpes zoster ophthalmicus, disseminated primary VZV in adults (significant morbidity compared to the childhood illness), and severe disseminated primary VZV in children.

- **Adverse effects.** Reversible crystalline nephropathy may occur; pre-existing renal failure, dehydration, and IV bolus dosing increase the risk of this effect. Rare cases of CNS disturbances, including delirium, tremors, and seizures, may also occur, particularly with high doses, in patients with renal failure and in the elderly.
- **Valacyclovir** (1,000 mg PO q8h for herpes zoster, 1,000 mg PO q12h for initial episode of genital HSV infection, and 500 mg PO q12h or 1,000 mg daily for recurrent episodes of HSV) is an orally administered prodrug of acyclovir used for the treatment of acute herpes zoster infections and for treatment or suppression of genital HSV infection.
    - The most common **adverse effect** is nausea. Valacyclovir rarely can cause CNS disturbances, and high doses (8 g/d) have been associated with development of hemolytic–uremic syndrome/thrombotic thrombocytopenic purpura in immunocompromised patients, including those with HIV and bone marrow and solid organ transplants.
- **Famciclovir** (500 mg PO q8h for herpes zoster, 250 mg PO q8h for the initial episode of genital HSV infection, and 125 mg PO q12h for recurrent episodes of genital HSV infection) is an orally administered antiviral agent used for the treatment of acute herpes zoster reactivation and for treatment or suppression of genital HSV infections.
    - **Adverse effects** include headache, nausea, and diarrhea.
- **Ganciclovir** (5 mg/kg IV q12h for 14–21 days for induction therapy of cytomegalovirus [CMV] retinitis, followed by 6 mg/kg IV for 5 days every week or 5 mg/kg IV daily; the oral dose is 1,000 mg PO tid with food) is used to treat CMV.
    - It has activity against HSV and VZV, but safer drugs are available to treat those infections. The drug is widely distributed in the body, including the CSF.
    - It is indicated for treatment of CMV retinitis and other serious CMV infections in immunocompromised patients (e.g., transplant and AIDS patients). Chronic maintenance therapy generally is required to suppress CMV disease in patients with AIDS.
    - **Adverse effects.** Neutropenia, which may require the addition of granulocyte colony-stimulating factor for management (300 mg SC daily–qwk). Thrombocytopenia, rash, confusion, headache, nephrotoxicity, and GI disturbances may also occur. Blood counts and electrolytes should be monitored weekly while the patient is receiving therapy. Other agents with nephrotoxic or bone marrow suppressive effects may enhance the adverse effects of ganciclovir.
- **Valganciclovir** (900 mg PO daily–bid) is the oral prodrug of ganciclovir; it has excellent bioavailability and can be used for treatment of CMV retinitis and, thus, has supplanted the use of oral ganciclovir, which has poor oral bioavailability. Adverse effects are the same as those for ganciclovir.
- **Foscarnet** (60 mg/kg IV q8h or 90 mg/kg IV q12h for 14–21 days as induction therapy, followed by 90–120 mg/kg IV daily as maintenance therapy for CMV; 40 mg/kg IV q8h for acyclovir-resistant HSV and VZV) is used to treat CMV retinitis in patients with AIDS. It is typically considered for use in patients who are not tolerating or responding to ganciclovir.
    - It is occasionally used for CMV disease in bone marrow transplant patients to avoid the bone marrow–suppressive effects of ganciclovir. It also has a role in treatment of acyclovir-resistant HSV/VZV infections or ganciclovir-resistant CMV infections.
    - **Adverse effects.** Risk for nephrotoxicity is a major concern. Creatinine clearance should be determined at baseline and electrolytes (PO_4, Ca^{2+}, Mg^{2+}, K^+) and serum creatinine checked twice a week. Normal saline (500–1000 mL) should be given before and during infusions to minimize nephrotoxicity. It should be avoided in patients with a serum creatinine of >2.8 mg/dL or baseline Cr_{Cl} of <50 mL/min. Concomitant use of other nephrotoxins (e.g., amphotericin, aminoglycosides, pentamidine, nonsteroidal anti-inflammatory drugs, cisplatin, or cidofovir) also should be avoided. Foscarnet chelates divalent cations and can cause tetany even with normal serum calcium levels. Use of foscarnet with pentamidine can cause severe hypocalcemia. Other side effects include seizures, phlebitis, rash, and genital ulcers. **Prolonged therapy with foscarnet should be monitored by physicians who are experienced with administration of home IV therapy and can systematically monitor patients' laboratory results.**
- **Cidofovir** (5 mg/kg IV qwk for 2 weeks as induction therapy, followed by 5 mg/kg IV q14d chronically as maintenance therapy) is used to treat CMV retinitis in patients with

AIDS. Efficacy of the drug is not established for CMV in other organ systems or in patients without AIDS. It can be administered through a peripheral IV line.

- **Adverse effects.** The most common is nephrotoxicity. It should be avoided in patients with a Cr_{Cl} of <55 mL/min, a serum creatinine >1.5 mg/dL, significant proteinuria, or a recent history of receipt of other nephrotoxic medications.
- **Each cidofovir dose should be administered with probenecid** (2 g PO 3 hours before the infusion and then 1 g at 2 and 8 hours after the infusion) along with 1 L normal saline IV 1–2 hours before the infusion to minimize nephrotoxicity. Patients should have a serum creatinine and urine protein check before each dose of cidofovir is given. These patients should be followed by a physician regularly, as administration of this drug requires systematic monitoring of laboratory studies.

ANTIFUNGAL AGENTS

AMPHOTERICIN B

Amphotericin B is fungicidal by interacting with ergosterol to disrupt the fungal plasma membrane. Reformulation of this agent in various lipid complexes has decreased some of its adverse side effects.

- **Amphotericin B deoxycholate** (standard; 0.3–1.5 mg/kg/d as a single infusion over 2–6 hours) is the mainstay of antifungal therapy for severely ill patients with fungal disease.
- It is not effective for *Pseudallescheria boydii* or *Candida lositaniae* infections.
- **Lipid complexed preparations** of amphotericin B, including amphotericin B lipid complex (5 mg/kg IV daily), liposomal amphotericin B (3–5 mg/kg IV daily), and amphotericin B colloidal dispersion (3–4 mg/kg IV daily), have decreased nephrotoxicity and are generally associated with fewer infusion-related reactions than amphotericin B deoxycholate. Despite these advantages, lipid complexed preparations have not yet been directly compared to standard amphotericin B therapy for most fungal infections. Based on currently available clinical data, no clear evidence exists for increased efficacy with the use of lipid complexed preparations, and minimal data are available that compare the lipid complexed preparations to each other. However, studies have shown lipid preparations to be at least equivalent and possibly slightly superior to standard amphotericin B for empiric therapy in neutropenic fevers.
- **Adverse effects**
  - The major adverse effect of all amphotericin B formulations, including the lipid formulations, is **nephrotoxicity**. Patients should receive 500–1,000 mL normal saline before each infusion to minimize nephrotoxicity. Irreversible renal failure appears to be related to cumulative dosing. Therefore, concomitant administration of other known nephrotoxins should be avoided if possible.
  - Common **infusion-related effects** include fever/chills, nausea, headache, and myalgias. Premedication with 500–1,000 mg of acetaminophen and 50 mg of diphenhydramine may control many of these symptoms. More severe reactions may be prevented by premedication with hydrocortisone, 25–50 mg IV. Intolerable infusion-related chills can be managed with meperidine, 25–50 mg IV. Some advocate administration of a 1- to 5-mg test dose, but this is not routinely necessary.
  - Amphotericin B therapy is associated with **potassium and magnesium wasting** that generally requires supplementation. Serum creatinine and electrolytes (including Mg^{2+} and K^+) should be monitored at least two to three times a week.

FLUCYTOSINE

- Flucytosine (25.0–37.5 mg/kg PO q6h) kills susceptible *Candida* and *Cryptococcus* species by interfering with DNA synthesis.

- **Main clinical uses** are for the treatment of cryptococcal meningitis and severe *Candida* infections in combination with amphotericin B.
- **Adverse effects**
  - Adverse effects include dose-related bone marrow suppression and bloody diarrhea due to intestinal flora conversion of flucytosine to 5-fluorouracil.
  - Peak drug concentrations should be monitored to keep peak concentrations between 50 and 100 mcg/mL. Close monitoring of serum concentrations and dose adjustments are critical in the setting of renal insufficiency. LFTs should be obtained at least once a week.

AZOLES

Azoles are fungistatic agents **that inhibit ergosterol synthesis.**

- **Itraconazole** (200–400 mg PO daily or 200 mg IV q12h for four doses, then 200 mg IV daily) is a triazole with broad-spectrum antifungal activity.
  - It is commonly used to treat histoplasmosis, blastomycosis, and sporotrichosis.
  - It is considered to be an alternative therapy for *Aspergillus* and is often used to consolidate a course of conventional amphotericin B. It can also be used to treat infections caused by dermatophytes, including onychomycosis of the toenails (200 mg PO daily for 12 weeks) and fingernails (200 mg PO bid for 1 week, with a 3-week interruption, and then a second course of 200 mg PO bid for 1 week).
  - The capsules require adequate gastric acidity for absorption and, therefore, should be taken with food, whereas the liquid is not significantly affected by gastric acidity and is better absorbed on an empty stomach.
- **Fluconazole** (100–800 mg PO/IV daily) is the **drug of choice for many localized candidal infections,** such as UTIs, thrush, esophagitis, peritonitis, and hepatosplenic infection. It is also a viable agent for severe disseminated candidal infections (e.g., candidemia) and is a second-line agent for primary treatment of cryptococcal meningitis (400–800 mg PO daily for 10–12 weeks, then 200 mg PO daily).
  - It is commonly used to suppress cryptococcal meningitis in immunocompromised patients (200 mg PO daily) after initial therapy with amphotericin B and flucytosine. Single-dose therapy is effective for vaginal yeast infections (150 mg PO once). Fluconazole does not, however, have activity against *Aspergillus* species and therefore should not be used for treatment of those infections. Its absorption is not dependent on gastric acid.
- **Ketoconazole** (200–600 mg PO daily) is useful for treating histoplasmosis, blastomycosis, and chromomycosis infections outside of the CNS, but its use has been largely supplanted by the newer azole agents.
  - It is not effective for *Aspergillus* species.
  - Absorption is dependent on gastric acidity.
  - **Adverse side effects.** Ketoconazole antagonizes testosterone metabolism and antiandrogen side effects can occur with prolonged therapy.
- **Voriconazole** (loading dose of 6 mg/kg IV [2 doses 12 hours apart] followed by a maintenance dose of 4 mg/kg IV q12h or 200 mg PO bid [100 mg PO bid if <40 kg]) is a new triazole antifungal with a spectrum of activity against a wide range of pathogenic fungi. It has enhanced in vitro activity against all clinically important species of *Aspergillus*, as well as *Candida* (including non-*albicans*), *Scedosporium apiospermum*, and *Fusarium* species.
  - It is indicated for the treatment of invasive aspergillosis, for which it demonstrates typical response rates of 40–50% and superiority over conventional amphotericin B, candidemia, esophageal candidiasis, and *Scedosporium* and *Fusarium* infections.
  - An advantage of voriconazole is the easy transition from IV to PO therapy because of excellent bioavailability. For refractory diseases, a dose increase of 50% may be useful. The maintenance dose is cut in half for patients with moderate hepatic failure.
  - Because of its metabolism through the **cytochrome P-450** system (enzymes 2C19, 2C9, and 3A4), there are several **clinically significant drug interactions** that must

be considered. Rifampin, rifabutin, carbamazepine (markedly reduced voriconazole levels), sirolimus (increased drug concentrations), and astemizole (prolonged QTc) are contraindicated while the patient is receiving voriconazole. Concomitantly administered cyclosporine, tacrolimus, and warfarin require more careful monitoring.

■ Posaconazole (200 mg PO q8h) is a new oral azole antifungal agent that is U.S. FDA-approved for prophylaxis of invasive aspergillosis and candidiasis in hematopoetic stem cell transplant patients with graft versus host disease or in patients with hematologic malignancies experiencing prolonged neutropenia from chemotherapy. This oral drug is uniquely active against mucor spp. and may prove to be a useful agent for treatment of mucormycosis.

  • Each dose should be administered with a full meal or liquid supplement.
  • Rifabutin, phenytoin, and cimetidine significantly reduce the bioavailability of posaconazole and should not routinely be used concomitantly.
  • Posaconazole significantly increases bioavailability of cyclosporine, tacrolimas, and midazolam necessitating dosage reductions of these agents when used with posaconazole. Dosage reduction of vinca alkaloids, statins, and calcium channel blockers should also be considered.
  • Terfinadine, astemizole, pimozide, cisapride, quinidine, and ergot alkaloids are contraindicated with posaconazole.

■ **Adverse effects.** Nausea, diarrhea, and rash are mild side effects. Hepatitis is a rare but serious complication. Therapy must be monitored closely in the setting of compromised liver function (weekly LFTs) and should be monitored regularly with chronic use. Itraconazole levels should be checked after 1 week of therapy to confirm absorption. IV itraconazole should be avoided in patients with severe heart failure and in those with a Cr_{Cl} of <30 mL/min to avoid excessive accumulation of the hydroxyl-β-cyclodextrin vehicle. Similarly, the IV formulation of voriconazole should not be used in patients with a Cr_{Cl} of <50 mL/min because of the potential for toxicity from the vehicle. Transient visual disturbance is a common adverse effect (30%) of voriconazole. **This class of antibiotics has major drug interactions.**

ECHINOCANDINS

This class of antifungals inhibit the enzyme $(1,3)$-β-D-glucan synthase that is essential in fungal cell wall synthesis.

Caspofungin Acetate

■ Caspofungin acetate (70 mg IV loading dose, followed by 50 mg IV q24h) is the first available drug of the echinocandin class of antifungal agents, which act by inhibiting the synthesis of cell wall glucan.

■ It has fungicidal activity against most *Aspergillus* and *Candida* species, including azole-resistant *Candida* strains. However, *Candida guilliermondi* and *Candida parapsilosis* may be relatively resistant.

■ It does not have appreciable activity against *Cryptococcus*, *Histoplasma*, or *Mucor* species.

■ It is only available in an intravenous preparation, as it is not absorbed from the GI tract. Metabolism is mostly hepatic, although the cytochrome P-450 system is not significantly involved.

■ It is U.S. FDA approved for invasive aspergillosis and candidemia. Clinical studies have shown it to be at least as effective as, and better tolerated than, amphotericin B for the treatment of esophageal candidiasis, candidemia, and invasive candidiasis.

■ In vitro and limited clinical studies suggest a synergistic effect when caspofungin is given in conjunction with itraconazole, voriconazole, or amphotericin B for *Aspergillus* infections.

■ **Adverse effects.** Fever, rash, nausea, and phlebitis at the injection site are infrequent. An increased maintenance dosage is necessary with the use of drugs that induce hepatic metabolism (e.g., efavirenz, nelfinavir, phenytoin, rifampin, dexamethasone). The maintenance dose should be reduced to 35 mg for patients with moderate hepatic impairment; however, no dose adjustment is necessary for renal failure.

Micafungin Sodium

- Micafungin sodium (50–150 mg IV q24h) was recently approved by the FDA for treatment of esophageal candidiasis (150 mg IV q24h) and as fungal prophylaxis for patients undergoing hematopoietic stem cell transplantation (50 mg IV q24h). Data on its efficacy and safety are still limited. Although it increases serum concentrations of sirolimus and nifedipine, these increases may not be clinically significant. Micafungin does not interact with any other immunosuppressant or other drugs. No change in dosing is necessary in renal or hepatic dysfunction, but caution should be taken when administering to patients with severe hepatic dysfunction.
- **Adverse effects** include rash and delirium. Some patients were observed to have elevated LFTs while on therapy.

Anidulafungin

- Anidulafungin (100–200 mg IV loading dose, followed by 50–100 mg IV q24h) was recently approved by the FDA for treatment of candidemia and other systemic *Candida* infections (intra-abdominal abscess and peritonitis) as well as esophageal candidiasis. Data on its efficacy and safety are still limited. Anidulafungin is not a substrate, inhibitor, or inducer of cytochrome P-450 isoenzymes and is not expected to have clinically relevant drug interactions. No dosage change is necessary in any stage of renal or hepatic insufficiency.
- **Adverse effects,** Possible histamine-mediated reactions, elevations in liver function tests, and rarely hypokalemia may occur.

TERBINAFINE

- Terbinafine (250 mg PO daily for 6–12 weeks) is an allylamine antifungal agent that kills fungi by inhibiting ergosterol synthesis. It is approved for the treatment of onychomycosis of the fingernail (6 weeks of treatment) or toenail (12 weeks of treatment). It is not generally used for systemic infections.
- **Adverse effects.** Headache, GI disturbances, rash, LFT abnormalities, and taste disturbances may occur. This drug should not be used in patients with hepatic cirrhosis or a Cr_{Cl} of <50 mL/min because of inadequate data. It has only moderate affinity for cytochrome P-450 hepatic enzymes and does not significantly inhibit the metabolism of cyclosporine (15% decrease) or warfarin.

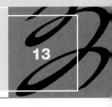
 PRINCIPLES OF THERAPY

GENERAL PRINCIPLES

- The decision to initiate, continue, and stop antimicrobial chemotherapy should be prudently made. Indiscriminate use of such therapy has been associated with adverse effects, the development of drug resistance, and excess costs.
- When antimicrobial therapy is indicated, a number of factors, reviewed in this chapter, must be considered. When antimicrobial agents are not readily available due to industry-related shortages, consultation with an infectious disease expert for alternative therapeutic options is prudent.

Choice of Initial Antimicrobial Therapy

- The infecting organism is often unknown when therapy is initiated. In these cases, empiric therapy should be directed against the most likely pathogens, using a regimen that possesses the narrowest spectrum that adequately covers the predicted organisms.
- Therapy should then be altered in accordance with the patient's course and laboratory results.

Procedures

- **During the initial evaluation,** a Gram stain of potentially infected material often permits a rapid presumptive diagnosis and may be essential for interpretation of subsequent culture results.
- **Local susceptibility patterns** must be considered in selecting empiric therapy because patterns vary widely among communities and individual hospitals.
- **Cultures** are usually necessary for precise diagnosis and are required for susceptibility testing. Whenever organisms with special growth requirements are suspected, the microbiology laboratory should be consulted to ensure appropriate transport and processing of cultures.
- **Antimicrobial susceptibility testing** facilitates a rational selection of antimicrobial agents and should be performed on most positive bacterial cultures.
- **Rapid diagnostic testing,** such as use of polymerase chain reaction (PCR) and antigen detection, may also provide early confirmation of an infectious etiologic agent.

STATUS OF THE HOST

- The clinical status of the patient contributes to the speed with which therapy must be instituted, the route of administration, and the type of therapy.
- Patients should be evaluated promptly for hemodynamic stability, rapidly progressive or life-threatening infections, and immune defects.

363

- **Timing of the initiation of antimicrobial therapy.** In acute clinical scenarios, empiric therapy is usually begun immediately after appropriate cultures have been obtained. However, if the patient's condition is stable, delaying the empiric use of antimicrobials might permit specific therapy based on the results of initial diagnostic testing and avoid adverse effects from the use of unnecessary drugs. Urgent therapy is indicated in febrile patients who are neutropenic or asplenic. In other immunosuppressed patients, fever alone seldom warrants urgent therapy; instead, the overall clinical assessment determines the need for empiric antimicrobials. Sepsis, meningitis, and rapidly progressive anaerobic or necrotizing infections should also be treated promptly with antimicrobials.
- **Route of administration.** Patients with serious infections should be given antimicrobial agents intravenously (IV). In less urgent circumstances, intramuscular (IM) or oral (PO) therapy often is sufficient. Oral therapy is acceptable when it is tolerated and able to achieve adequate drug concentrations at the site of infection.
- **Type of therapy.** Bactericidal therapy is preferred over bacteriostatic regimens for patients with immunologic compromise or life-threatening infection. It is preferred also for infections characterized by impaired regional host defenses, such as endocarditis, meningitis, and osteomyelitis. Examples of bactericidal antibiotics include beta-lactams and fluoroquinolones.
- **Pregnancy and the postpartum.** Although no antimicrobial agent is known to be completely safe in pregnancy, the penicillins and cephalosporins are used most often. **Tetracyclines and fluoroquinolones are among the agents specifically contraindicated,** and the sulfonamides and aminoglycosides should not be used if alternative agents are available (see Appendix B, Pregnancy and Medical Therapeutics). Most antibiotics that are administered in therapeutic doses appear in breast milk and, therefore, should be used with caution in patients who are breast-feeding.

ANTIMICROBIAL COMBINATIONS

- The indiscriminate use of antimicrobial combinations should be avoided because of the potential for increased toxicity, pharmacologic antagonism, and the selection of resistant organisms.
- The empiric use of multiple antimicrobials to provide broader coverage is justified in seriously ill patients under the following circumstances:
  - The identity of an infecting organism is not apparent.
  - The suspected pathogen has a variable antimicrobial susceptibility.
  - Failure to initiate effective antimicrobial therapy will likely increase morbidity or mortality.
- In addition, antimicrobial combinations are specifically indicated to produce synergism (e.g., in enterococcal endocarditis), to treat polymicrobial infections (e.g., peritonitis after rupture of a viscus), and to prevent the emergence of antimicrobial resistance (e.g., tuberculosis [TB]).

ASSESSMENT OF ANTIMICROBIAL THERAPY

- When therapy is initiated, continued, or discussed from the perspective of potential treatment failure, one should consider the following questions:
  - Is the isolated organism the etiologic agent?
  - Is adequate antimicrobial therapy being provided?
  - Is the concentration of antimicrobial agent adequate at the site of infection?
  - Have resistant pathogens emerged?
  - Is a persistent fever due to underlying disease, abscess formation, an iatrogenic complication, a drug reaction, or another process?

DURATION OF THERAPY

- The duration of therapy depends on the nature of infection and the severity of clinical presentation.
- Treatment of acute uncomplicated infections should be continued until the patient has been afebrile and clinically well, usually for a minimum of 72 hours.
- Infections at certain sites (e.g., endocarditis, septic arthritis, osteomyelitis) require prolonged therapy.

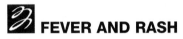 **FEVER AND RASH**

GENERAL PRINCIPLES

- Fever with rash is a common presentation of many infectious and noninfectious diseases that range from benign to life-threatening. This syndrome should be distinguished from infections of the skin or soft tissues, such as cellulitis.

Etiology

- The etiology of a febrile rash illness is often suggested by the type and distribution of the rash and historical data (travel; animal, insect, and drug exposures; immune status).

DIAGNOSIS

Physical Examination

- Gloves should be worn while examining the rash, and respiratory isolation precautions should be considered if a transmissible pathogen is suspected (e.g., varicella, meningococcemia, measles, and certain bioterrorism agents).

Diagnostic Procedures

- Blood cultures are useful to exclude bacteremia. Skin biopsy with Gram stain, culture, microscopy, or PCR may be helpful. Rashes may be atypical, more severe, and caused by unusual organisms (including fungi) in immunocompromised hosts.
- **Maculopapular** rashes may suggest drug hypersensitivity, secondary syphilis, typhoid (rose spots), Lyme disease, acute HIV infection, West Nile fever, dengue fever, or viral exanthems.
- **Vesicular** or **pustular** lesions can be seen with varicella, herpes simplex virus, disseminated gonococcal infection, endocarditis, monkeypox, and smallpox (see the Bioterrorism section).
- **Diffuse erythematous** rashes, often with desquamation, should raise suspicion of toxin-mediated diseases (see the Toxin-Mediated Infections section) or toxic epidermal necrolysis.
- **Petechial** and **purpuric** lesions often herald life-threatening infections (meningococcemia, pneumococcemia, Gram-negative bacterial sepsis, Rocky Mountain spotted fever [RMSF], malaria, viral hemorrhagic fevers) or autoimmune disorders.

TREATMENT

Empiric Therapy

- Empiric antimicrobial therapy should be initiated immediately for those with severe illness or a rash suggesting a potentially life-threatening infection such as meningococcemia or RMSF.

- Ceftriaxone, 2 g IV q12h, with **doxycycline**, 100 mg IV or PO q12h, is a reasonable empiric regimen. If a pathogen is isolated, therapy should be tailored according to susceptibilities.

SPECIFIC PATHOGENS

- *Neisseria meningitidis* septicemia (meningococcemia).
  - This can occur with or without meningitis and presents with maculopapular lesions and petechiae, which may rapidly progress to extensive ecchymotic lesions (purpura fulminans) and death.
  - **Diagnostic** tests include identification of Gram-negative diplococci in a Gram-stained specimen or growth in culture from blood, cerebrospinal fluid (CSF), or lesion scrapings.
  - **Treatment** of choice is a third-generation cephalosporin (e.g., ceftriaxone, 2 g IV q12h). Penicillin is an alternative if the isolate is sensitive. Chloramphenicol, 100 mg/kg/d IV (maximum, 4 g/d) divided q6h can be used in the severely beta-lactam-allergic patient.
  - Duration of therapy is generally 10–14 days.
- RMSF
  - Caused by *Rickettsia rickettsii* after a tick bite, which may go unrecognized.
  - Fever, headache, and myalgias are followed 1–5 days later with a petechial rash starting on the distal extremities that may be faint and difficult to detect.
  - **Death** can occur when treatment is delayed.
  - Antibiotic of choice is **doxycycline**, 100 mg q12h IV or PO for 7 days, or 2 days after becoming afebrile. **Chloramphenicol** is an alternative.

 SEPSIS

GENERAL PRINCIPLES

Definition

- **Sepsis,** a leading cause of death in the United States, involves a series of proinflammatory and procoagulant responses to invading pathogens.
- The mortality for patients with sepsis is 15%, and pathogens are bacteria more often than fungi and viruses.

DIAGNOSIS

- Sepsis is diagnosed when there is evidence of infection and criteria for the systemic inflammatory response syndrome are met.[1]

TREATMENT

- **Early use of appropriate antibiotics can reduce mortality from sepsis.** If a probable source of infection is evident, antimicrobials can be selected for the most likely pathogens and their anticipated antibiotic sensitivity pattern. If no obvious source is identified, empiric antimicrobial selection should be based on the clinical situation. Before therapy is initiated, specimens of potentially infected body fluids should be collected for Gram stain and culture. Two sets of blood cultures should be obtained from either separate venipuncture sites or one venipuncture and one central venous catheter (CVC) port. Empiric coverage usually includes a beta-lactam antimicrobial agent plus an aminoglycoside. Initial empiric coverage may also include vancomycin, particularly in a nosocomial setting or when a CVC is present.

■ **For community-acquired sepsis** with no obvious underlying disease, a third-generation cephalosporin plus vancomycin covers most potential pathogens.

■ **Asplenic patients** are at particular risk for fulminant sepsis with encapsulated organisms such as *Streptococcus pneumoniae, Haemophilus influenzae,* and *N. meningitidis.* A third-generation cephalosporin in high doses (e.g., ceftriaxone, 2 g IV q12h) should be administered promptly with or without vancomycin, 1 g IV q12h.

■ **Neutropenic hosts,** in whom *Pseudomonas aeruginosa* sepsis may be likely, should be initially treated with an antipseudomonal beta-lactam antimicrobial agent with or without an aminoglycoside.

SPECIAL CONSIDERATIONS

■ **Septic shock.** Beyond antimicrobial treatment, vasopressors, bolus IV fluids, physiologic doses of hydrocortisone, and activated protein C may play a role (see Chapter 8, Critical Care).

 # SKIN, SOFT-TISSUE, AND BONE INFECTIONS

GENERAL PRINCIPLES

■ Infections of intact skin are usually treated empirically; however, surgical sampling with culture is required for pathogen isolation in infections that are deep, severe, or will require prolonged antibiotics.

■ Because of the rising incidence of community-associated methicillin-resistant *Staphylococcus aureus* (CA-MRSA) and nosocomial MRSA, severe infections in which *S. aureus* is the likely primary pathogen should be treated empirically with vancomycin, 1 g IV q12h, until susceptibilities are available. Therapy should be switched to oxacillin or cefazolin if the strain proves susceptible.[2]

■ CA-MRSA has emerged in patients with no risk factors. It can cause necrotizing skin infections (associated with the Panton-Valentine leukocidin virulence factor), recurrent boils, or indurated skin lesions mistaken for spider bites. The organism is sensitive to vancomycin and usually to trimethoprim-sulfamethoxazole and clindamycin. Surgical drainage is necessary for most lesions.[3]

SKIN INFECTIONS

■ **Erysipelas** is a painful, superficial, erythematous, sharply demarcated lesion that is usually found on lower extremities and is caused by group A beta-hemolytic streptococci (GABHS) in the normal host.

■ Treatments of choice:
  ■ **Penicillin V,** 250–1000 mg PO qid or **penicillin G,** 1–2.0 million units IV q6h, depending on the severity of illness.
  ■ In **patients who are penicillin allergic,** erythromycin, 500 mg PO qid, or other macrolides are alternatives.

SOFT-TISSUE INFECTIONS

■ **Cellulitis** involves the skin and underlying soft tissue superficial to fascia, with less distinct margins than erysipelas.
  ■ GABHS and *S. aureus* are the usual pathogens and are clinically indistinguishable.
  ■ **Initial therapy** is oxacillin, 1–2 g IV q4h; cefazolin, 1–2 g IV q8h; or vancomycin, 1 g IV q12h. Alternatives for the severely penicillin-allergic patient include macrolides or

clindamycin. Mild disease can be treated with oral equivalents of the aforementioned. If present, coexisting **tinea pedis** should be treated with topical antifungals to prevent recurrence of lower extremity cellulitis.

■ **Diabetic patients** with cellulitis often require broader-spectrum coverage, including a beta-lactam/beta-lactamase inhibitor, third-generation cephalosporin, or a carbapenem, depending on severity.

■ **Water-borne pathogens.** Severe cellulitis is sometimes seen after exposure to fresh (*Aeromonas hydrophila*) or salt water (*Vibrio vulnificus*). In these settings, initial therapy should include ceftazidime, 2 g IV q8h; cefepime, 2 g IV q8h; or ciprofloxacin, 400 mg IV q8h or 750 mg PO bid. Doxycycline, 100 mg IV/PO q12h should be added for *Vibrio* infections, which have a strong predilection for patients with cirrhosis.

■ **Infected decubitus ulcers** and **limb-threatening diabetic foot ulcers** are usually polymicrobial; superficial swab cultures are unreliable. Osteomyelitis is a frequent complication and should be excluded.

■ **Treatment** consists of wound care and debridement.

■ Moderately severe decubitus ulcers and most diabetic foot infections require systemic antibiotics covering *S. aureus*, anaerobes, and enteric Gram-negative organisms.

■ Options include **clindamycin**, 450–900 mg IV q8h with either a third-generation **cephalosporin** or **ciprofloxacin**, 500–750 mg PO bid; a beta-lactam/beta-lactamase inhibitor combination, or imipenem-cilastatin, 500 mg IV q6h, depending on the severity of illness. Less severe diabetic foot infections are usually due to *S. aureus* with or without *Streptococcus* species and can often be managed with cephalexin, dicloxacillin, or clindamycin, unless MRSA is isolated, in which case vancomycin may be necessary.[4]

■ **Necrotizing fasciitis** is an infectious disease emergency with **high mortality** manifested by extensive soft-tissue infection and thrombosis of the microcirculation with resulting necrosis.

■ It may present initially like simple cellulitis, with rapid progression to necrosis with dusky, hypoesthetic skin and bulla formation. Infection spreads quickly along fascial planes and may be associated with sepsis or streptococcal toxic shock syndrome (TSS).

■ **Fournier gangrene** is necrotizing fasciitis of the perineum.

■ **Diagnosis** is mostly clinical. High suspicion should prompt **immediate surgical exploration** where lack of resistance to probing is diagnostic. Early in the disease process, computed tomography (CT) scans and plain films may demonstrate gas and fascial edema.

■ Bacterial etiology is either mixed anaerobic (*Bacteroides*, other anaerobes, aerobic Gram-negative organisms, and *Streptococcus* species) or GABHS with or without *S. aureus* and **CA-MRSA (as described above)**. Intraoperative Gram stain is used to differentiate among these.

■ **Treatment** includes volume support, IV antibiotics, and aggressive surgical debridement, which is imperative.

■ Initial empiric antibiotic therapy should include penicillin G (or ampicillin), clindamycin, and a third-generation cephalosporin (or aminoglycoside).

■ If the Gram stain or culture suggests mixed infection, imipenem or a beta-lactam/beta-lactamase inhibitor combination is an alternative. Penicillin and clindamycin should be continued if GABHS is the pathogen, but they should be replaced with vancomycin if MRSA is suspected by the Gram stain or culture.

■ Adjunctive hyperbaric oxygen may be useful.

■ **Anaerobic myonecrosis (gas gangrene)** usually is due to *Clostridium perfringens*, *Clostridium septicum*, *S. aureus*, GABHS, or other anaerobes. Distinguishing this condition from necrotizing fasciitis requires gross inspection of the involved muscle at the time of surgery.

■ **Treatment** requires prompt surgical debridement and combination antimicrobial therapy with intravenous penicillin and clindamycin.

■ A third-generation **cephalosporin, ciprofloxacin, or an aminoglycoside** should be added until the Gram stain excludes Gram-negative involvement.

OSTEOMYELITIS

■ This should be considered when skin or soft-tissue infections overlie bone and when localized bone pain accompanies fever or sepsis.[5]

Diagnosis

■ Diagnosis is made by detection of bone through a skin ulcer or by imaging with plain films, bone scintigraphy, or magnetic resonance imaging (MRI). Biopsy of the affected bone should be performed (before initiation of antimicrobials, if possible) to determine the microbial etiology.

■ If a causative organism is not identified, empiric therapy should be selected to cover *S. aureus* (oxacillin or vancomycin) and any other likely pathogens (see discussion below).

■ Cure typically requires at least 4–6 weeks of high-dose antimicrobial therapy. Parenteral therapy should be given initially; oral regimens may be considered after 2–3 weeks only if the pathogen is susceptible and adequate bactericidal levels can be achieved.

■ **Erythrocyte sedimentation rate and C-reactive protein** are usually markedly elevated and can be used to monitor the response to therapy.

    ▦ **Acute hematogenous osteomyelitis** is caused most frequently by *S. aureus*. In the absence of vascular insufficiency or a foreign body, it can be treated with antimicrobial therapy alone.

    ▦ **Vertebral osteomyelitis** may be due to *S. aureus*, Gram-negative bacilli, or *Mycobacterium tuberculosis*.

    ▦ **Osteomyelitis associated with a contiguous focus of infection** may be due to *S. aureus*, Gram-negative bacilli, coagulase-negative staphylococci (surgical-site infections), or anaerobes (infected sacral decubitus ulcers).

    ▦ **Osteomyelitis associated with vascular insufficiency** (e.g., in diabetic patients) seldom is cured by drug therapy alone; revascularization, debridement, or amputation often is required. Infections are generally polymicrobial, including anaerobes.

    ▦ **Osteomyelitis in the presence of orthopedic devices** is most often caused by *S. aureus* or coagulase-negative *Staphylococcus* species. It is rarely eradicated by antimicrobials alone. Cure typically requires the removal of the device. When removal is impossible, the addition of rifampin (RIF), 300 mg PO tid, is recommended.

    ▦ **Osteomyelitis associated with hemoglobinopathies** is caused most often by *S. aureus* or *Salmonella* species. *Salmonella* osteomyelitis may require surgical treatment and parenteral administration of a third-generation cephalosporin or ciprofloxacin.

    ▦ **Chronic osteomyelitis** usually is associated with a sequestrum of necrotic bone and frequently involves Gram-negative pathogens as well as *S. aureus*. Eradication requires a combination of medical and surgical treatment to remove the persistent nidus of infection. Long-term, suppressive antimicrobial therapy can be used if surgery is not feasible. Hyperbaric oxygen may be a useful adjunctive therapy.

 # TOXIN-MEDIATED INFECTIONS

CLOSTRIDIAL INFECTIONS

■ Botulism (see the **Bioterrorism section**).

■ **Tetanus** (intoxication with *Clostridium tetani* toxin) is a rare disease in the United States but should be diagnosed when the classic presentation of generalized rigidity, trismus, risus sardonicus, and painful convulsive spasms of skeletal muscles is followed by autonomic dysfunction. A prior injury or wound has usually occurred.

    ▦ **Treatment** consists of human tetanus immunoglobulin, 3,000–5,000 units IM. Benzodiazepines, and occasionally paralytics, can be used to control spasms.

    ▦ Ventilatory support is often necessary. Antimicrobial therapy remains controversial; however, metronidazole is often used. Tetanus is best prevented by immunization, and, for high-risk wounds, human tetanus immunoglobulin, 250 units IM, is used.

- *Clostridium difficile*–**associated diarrheal disease** is frequently seen after systemic antimicrobial therapy, usually in hospitalized patients. Diagnosis is made by detection of *C. difficile* toxins in stool or by colonoscopic visualization of **pseudomembranes**.
  - **Treatment** is primarily targeted toward elimination of *C. difficile* from the gut. **First-line therapy** for initial episodes is **metronidazole**, 500 mg PO tid for 10–14 days, and discontinuation of the offending antibiotic, if possible. Vancomycin, 125–500 mg PO (IV is not effective) qid, is used for severe or refractory disease.
  - Antimotility agents should be avoided in severe disease. IV **metronidazole** is a less effective alternative when enteral therapy is not possible.
  - Intracolonic **vancomycin** is sometimes used in severe cases in which gut motility is altered and surgical intervention is imminent.[6]
  - **Recurrence** is common, and well-established effective regimens are lacking. A first recurrence is usually treated with metronidazole as for initial episodes. Frequently recurrent disease is often treated with metronidazole or vancomycin in a regimen that is either of extended duration, tapered, or pulsed. Adjunctive therapy with oral RIF or bacitracin is sometimes used, and adjunctive use of probiotics, such as *Saccharomyces boulardii* and *Lactobacillus* GG, may be useful in selected patients but should be avoided in immunocompromised patients.

TOXIC SHOCK SYNDROME

- **Toxic shock syndrome (TSS)** is a life-threatening disease caused by exotoxins produced by *S. aureus* or GABHS.
- **Staphylococcal TSS** is most often associated with tampon use in young women, vaginitis, or colonization of surgical wounds.
  - **Diagnosis** is made by the presence of fever, hypotension, macular desquamating erythroderma usually involving the palms and soles, and multisystem involvement, such as vomiting, diarrhea, and renal failure. Blood cultures are often negative.
  - **Treatment is primarily supportive.** Tampons should be removed and avoided in the future. Oxacillin, cefazolin, or vancomycin is administered for 10–14 days to decrease the risk of relapse.
  - **Intravenous immunoglobulin (IVIG)**, 1 g/kg on day 1, followed by 0.5 g/kg on days 2 and 3, may be useful for severe cases.
- **Streptococcal TSS** is associated with invasive GABHS infections, particularly necrotizing fasciitis. It is defined by isolation of GABHS, hypotension, and multiorgan failure with or without desquamating rash.
  - **Treatment** is directed at the primary infection and should include penicillin G, 4 million units IV q4h, clindamycin, 900 mg IV q8h, and IVIG as described above.[7]

CENTRAL NERVOUS SYSTEM INFECTIONS

MENINGITIS

- **Acute bacterial meningitis** is a medical emergency. Meningitis should be considered in any patient with fever and stiff neck or neurologic symptoms, especially if another concurrent infection or head trauma is present. Therapy should not be delayed for diagnostic measures because prognosis depends on rapid initiation of antimicrobial treatment.

Diagnosis

- Diagnosis requires lumbar puncture with measurement of opening pressure and examination of CSF protein, glucose, cell count with differential, and Gram stain with culture.
- Blood cultures should always be obtained.

■ Depending on the clinical scenario, other potentially useful CSF studies include rapid plasma reagin (RPR), acid-fast stain, latex agglutination antigen detection, cryptococcal antigen, arbovirus antibodies, and PCR for herpes simplex virus (HSV) and enteroviruses.

■ The performance of a head CT scan before lumbar puncture is controversial but is generally not required for nonelderly, immunocompetent patients who present without focal neurologic abnormalities, seizures, or diminished level of consciousness.[8] Typical CSF findings include a neutrophilic pleocytosis, markedly elevated CSF protein, and decreased glucose level.

Treatment

■ Treatment consists of supportive measures and antimicrobial therapy. Whenever acute bacterial meningitis is suspected, high-dose parenteral antimicrobial therapy should be started as soon as possible.

■ Until the etiology of the meningitis is known, an empiric regimen should be based on the CSF Gram stain.

■ If no organisms are seen, high-dose third-generation cephalosporins (ceftriaxone, 2 g IV q12h, or cefotaxime, 2 g IV q4h) and vancomycin, 1 g IV q8–12h, are recommended while culture results are pending. Ampicillin, 2 g IV q4h, should be added for immunocompromised and older (>50 years of age) patients. In the postneurosurgical setting, or after head or spinal trauma, broad-spectrum coverage with high-dose vancomycin and ceftazidime, 2 g IV q8h, is indicated. Empiric regimens should be altered once culture and sensitivity data are known.

■ Dexamethasone, 10 mg IV q6h, started just before or during initial antibiotics and given for 4 days, reduces the risk of a poor neurologic outcome in patients with meningitis caused by S. pneumoniae. Steroids have not proven to be of benefit for bacterial meningitis caused by other organisms, and thus should be discontinued if a different pathogen is isolated.[9]

Therapy for Specific Infections

■ For *S. pneumoniae*, IV penicillin G, 4 million units q4h, for 10–14 days, is appropriate when the isolate is fully susceptible to penicillin. High-dose ceftriaxone or cefotaxime (as described above) is used for intermediate penicillin-resistant isolates, and vancomycin is added if there is ceftriaxone resistance or high-level penicillin resistance. Options for severely penicillin-allergic patients are vancomycin plus RIF, 300 mg PO tid; or chloramphenicol, 1.0 g IV q6h. Vancomycin should not be used alone.

■ For *N. meningitidis*, high-dose ceftriaxone or cefotaxime is continued for at least 5 days after the patient has become afebrile, usually a 7-day total course. Chloramphenicol is an option for the penicillin-allergic patient. Patients should be placed in a private room on respiratory isolation for at least the first 24 hours of treatment. Close contacts (e.g., persons living in the same household and health care workers having close contact with secretions, e.g., intubation) should receive prophylaxis with RIF, 600 mg PO bid for 2 days, or single-dose therapy with either ciprofloxacin, 500 mg PO, or ceftriaxone, 250 mg IM. Terminal component complement deficiency (C5–C9) should be ruled out in patients with recurrent meningococcal infections.

■ *Listeria monocytogenes* meningitis is seen in immunosuppressed adults and the elderly. Treatment is with ampicillin, 2 g IV q4h, in combination with a systemically administered aminoglycoside for at least 3–4 weeks. Trimethoprim/sulfamethoxazole (TMP/SMX; TMP, 5 mg/kg IV q6h) is an alternative for the penicillin-allergic patient.

■ **Gram-negative bacillary meningitis** usually is a complication of head trauma and neurosurgical procedures. High-dose ceftazidime or cefepime, 2 g IV q8h, is used for most pathogens, including *P. aeruginosa*. High-dose ceftriaxone or cefotaxime may be used for susceptible pathogens. Alternatives include meropenem and ciprofloxacin.

■ *S. aureus* meningitis is usually a result of high-grade bacteremia, direct extension from a parameningeal focus, or neurosurgical procedures. Oxacillin and nafcillin, 2 g IV q4h, are the drugs of choice. First-generation cephalosporins do not reliably penetrate into the CSF. Vancomycin should be used for penicillin-allergic patients and when methicillin resistance is likely or confirmed. RIF may also be necessary.

- **Ventriculitis and ventriculoperitoneal shunt infections** are typically caused by coagulase-negative staphylococci, *S. aureus*, and *Propionibacter* species. They are treated with IV vancomycin with or without RIF or intraventricular vancomycin, 10 mg daily to every other day. Removal of an infected shunt is often necessary for cure.
- **Aseptic meningitis** is usually milder than bacterial meningitis and is characterized by fever, headache, meningismus, and photophobia, often preceded by upper respiratory symptoms or pharyngitis. Viruses are common causes, as is drug-induced inflammation (e.g., nonsteroidal anti-inflammatory drugs, TMP/SMX). A lymphocytic CSF pleocytosis is common (although neutrophils may predominate very early in the disease course), and CSF PCR can detect enteroviruses, HSV, and HIV. For enteroviral meningitis, the treatment is supportive care. Acyclovir, 10 mg/kg IV q8h, is used for moderate to severe HSV-2 meningitis.

ENCEPHALITIS

- **HSV–1** is the most common and most important cause of sporadic infectious encephalitis. HSV encephalitis should be considered in any patient who presents with acute fever and neurologic abnormalities, particularly with personality change or seizures, and without meningeal signs. **Diagnosis** is confirmed by detection of HSV-1 in the CSF by PCR; however, a negative PCR does not rule out HSV encephalitis. Temporal lobe enhancement is typically seen on brain MRI. **Treatment** is acyclovir, 10 mg/kg IV q8h infused over 1 hour with adequate hydration, which should be initiated at first suspicion and continued for 14–21 days. Delayed initiation of therapy greatly increases the risk of poor neurologic outcomes.
- **West Nile virus** (WNV) (see the Arthropod-Borne Diseases, Zoonoses, and Bite Wounds section).

BRAIN ABSCESS

- **Brain abscesses** in the immunocompetent host are usually bacterial in origin and are a result of spread from a contiguous focus or septic emboli from endocarditis. Infection is often mixed, with oral streptococci, *S. aureus*, and anaerobes being the most common pathogens.
  - **Diagnosis** is radiographic, with ring-enhancing lesions seen on MRI or contrast CT scans. A microbiologic etiology must be determined by biopsy or at the time of surgery.
  - **Therapy** is often surgical with the addition of systemic antimicrobials. Empiric therapy should be chosen to cover the most likely pathogens based on the primary infection site. When no preceding infection can be found, a third-generation cephalosporin combined with metronidazole and vancomycin is a reasonable regimen until culture data are available.

NEUROCYSTICERCOSIS

- **Neurocysticercosis** can present as new-onset seizures, hydrocephalus, or focal neurologic abnormalities. It is acquired from eating undercooked pork that contains the eggs of *Taenia solium*, which is endemic in Mexico and Central America.
  - **Diagnosis** should be suspected in hosts with new-onset seizures of unknown etiology and exposure to endemic areas. Serologic tests are available at the Centers for Disease Control and Prevention (CDC). Brain imaging reveals multiple unilocular cysts that may or may not enhance.
  - **Treatment** may require surgery or high-dose albendazole or praziquantel, depending on the location of cysts and severity. Anticonvulsants and steroids are often necessary to control symptoms.

CARDIOVASCULAR INFECTIONS

INFECTIVE ENDOCARDITIS

Etiology

- Infective endocarditis (IE) usually is caused by Gram-positive cocci.
- Injection drug use and intravascular devices increase the risk for staphylococcal endovascular infection.
- Gram–negative and fungal IE occur infrequently and usually are associated with injection drug use or prosthetic valves.
- Patients may present within 3–10 days with critical illness (**acute bacterial endocarditis**) or weeks to months (**subacute bacterial endocarditis**) with constitutional symptoms, immune complex disease (nephritis, arthralgias), and emboli (renal, splenic, and cerebral infarcts; petechiae; Osler nodes; Janeway lesions).
- A deformed or previously damaged valve is the usual focus of infection in subacute bacterial endocarditis.
- Dental procedures and bacteremia from distant foci of infection are frequent seeding events; instrumentation of the genitourinary or gastrointestinal (GI) tract is a less common cause.

Diagnosis

Laboratory Studies

- The most reliable diagnostic criterion is continuous bacteremia in a compatible clinical setting. **Blood cultures** are positive in at least 90% of patients. The yield is reduced if the patient has received antimicrobial therapy within 1–2 weeks.
- Three culture samples should be taken from separate sites over at least a 1-hour period before empiric therapy is begun if the clinical situation allows. The diagnosis of IE remains essentially clinical and microbiologic rather than echocardiographic.

Imaging

- Patients with IE and vegetations seen by transthoracic echocardiography are at higher risk of embolism, heart failure, and valvular disruption; however, a negative transthoracic echocardiogram does not exclude the diagnosis of IE.
- When clinical evidence of IE exists, **transesophageal echocardiography** improves the sensitivity of the Duke criteria to diagnose and define IE, especially in hosts with prosthetic valves.[11] The role of delayed echocardiography in IE is to define surgical disease.
- Presence of vegetations alone does not mandate surgical intervention. Vegetations seen on echocardiography may persist unchanged for at least 3 years after clinical cure.

Treatment[10]

Medications

- High doses of antimicrobials for extended periods are standard.
- Quantitative susceptibility testing of the responsible organism(s) to multiple antibiotics is more reliable than disk diffusion testing and is essential to ensure that optimal treatment is administered.
- **Baseline audiometry** is recommended for patients who will receive 7 or more days of aminoglycoside therapy, with follow-up audiometry contingent on the duration of treatment or development of symptoms.
- **Acute bacterial endocarditis** requires empiric antimicrobial treatment before culture results become available. *S. aureus* and Gram-negative bacilli are the most likely pathogens. Initial treatment for *S. aureus* should include **vancomycin**, 1 g IV q12h, plus **gentamicin** or **tobramycin**, 1.0–1.5 mg/kg IV q8h. For isolates found to be methicillin sensitive, **oxacillin**, 2 g IV q4h, is superior to vancomycin and should be substituted. Therapy should then be modified on the basis of culture and susceptibility data.

- **Subacute bacterial endocarditis** is caused most often by streptococci. **Penicillin** therapy typically results in cure rates of >90%. *Streptococcus bovis* bacteremia and endocarditis are associated with lower GI disease, including neoplasms. Groups B and G streptococcal endocarditis may also be associated with lower intestinal pathology.
- **Prosthetic valve endocarditis**
  - Prosthetic valve endocarditis (PVE) occurs in 1%–4% of patients with prosthetic valves.
  - Early infections (within 2 months of surgery) commonly are caused by *S. aureus*, *S. epidermidis*, Gram-negative bacilli, *Candida* species, and other opportunistic organisms.
  - PVE must be considered in any patient with sustained bacteremia after valve surgery.
  - **Treatment** for methicillin-sensitive *S. aureus* consists of combination therapy with **oxacillin**, 2 g IV q4h, plus RIF, 300 mg PO q8h, for at least 6 weeks. For MRSA, **vancomycin**, 1 g IV q12h, with RIF is used. Gentamicin, 1 mg/kg IV q8h, should be given for the initial 2 weeks of therapy in either case.
  - Therapy should also be guided by the results of MIC testing. Late PVE (i.e., ≥2 months after surgery) usually is caused by organisms similar to those seen on native valves.

Therapy for Specific Infections

- For **viridans streptococci**, penicillin G, 12–18 million units/d IV continuous infusion or divided into 4–6 daily doses, for 4 weeks, is effective for penicillin-susceptible strains (minimal inhibitory concentration [MIC] <0.12 mcg/mL). Therapy with parenteral penicillin and an aminoglycoside for 2 weeks is an alternative, but extended aminoglycoside treatment should be avoided in the elderly and in patients who cannot tolerate the potential nephrotoxicity or ototoxicity. If the penicillin MIC is ≥0.12 mcg/mL but is ≤0.5 mcg/mL, the addition of streptomycin or gentamicin may be appropriate for the first 2 weeks of therapy, followed by penicillin G alone for 2 more weeks. Patients with endocarditis caused by streptococci with penicillin MIC of >0.5 mcg/mL may require combination therapy similar to that given for enterococcal IE (see below). Ampicillin, 2 g IV q4h, or ceftriaxone, 2 g IV q24h, can be substituted if penicillin G is unavailable. In patients who are allergic to penicillin, skin testing and desensitization should be considered because beta-lactam therapy is preferred. Vancomycin is an alternative, with maintenance of trough levels near 15 mcg/L; peak levels generally do not need to be monitored regularly.
- **GABHS and *S. pneumoniae*** should be treated with penicillin G, 2–4 million units IV for 4–6 weeks. Penicillin-resistant pneumococci should be treated with ceftriaxone, 2 g IV q24h for 4–6 weeks.
- ***Enterococcus* species** cause 10%–20% of cases of subacute bacterial endocarditis. Isolates from patients with enterococcal endocarditis should be screened for beta-lactamase production and susceptibility to vancomycin, quinupristin/dalfopristin, linezolid, and gentamicin. Recommended treatment regimens for susceptible isolates are ampicillin, 2 g IV q4h, or penicillin G, 3–5 million units IV q4h, in combination with gentamicin (if the isolate does not exhibit high-level gentamicin resistance), 1.0–1.5 mg/kg IV q8h, for 4–6 weeks. In susceptible strains, vancomycin in combination with an aminoglycoside is effective and should be used for penicillin-allergic patients or individuals with beta-lactamase–producing strains. Aminoglycoside and vancomycin levels should be monitored (see Appendix A, Barnes–Jewish Hospital Laboratory Reference Values). Baseline and weekly audiometry is recommended for patients who receive aminoglycosides for >7 days. Vancomycin-resistant enterococci (VRE) IE is difficult to treat, and infectious disease consult is recommended. For VRE isolates that are resistant to ampicillin, treatment with linezolid, daptomycin, or quinupristin/dalfopristin with or without doxycycline is advised.
- ***S. aureus*** should be treated with oxacillin, 2 g IV q4h for 6 weeks. An aminoglycoside can be added during the first 3–5 days of therapy or in patients who do not respond to beta-lactam therapy alone. For young hosts with right-sided IE, treatment with oxacillin for 4 weeks may be sufficient. Older patients with aortic valve infection have a high

mortality and often require surgical intervention. For IE caused by MRSA, vancomycin is the drug of choice, although daptomycin and linezolid are alternatives.

- *Staphylococcus epidermidis* (coagulase-negative staphylococcus) IE primarily occurs in patients with valvular prostheses. These organisms often are resistant to beta-lactam agents; thus, the treatment of choice is vancomycin, 1 g IV q12h, in combination with RIF, 300 mg PO q8h, for at least 6–8 weeks, along with gentamicin, 1 mg/kg IV q8h for the first 2 weeks of therapy. Vancomycin and aminoglycoside levels should be monitored. Because detection of beta-lactam resistance in coagulase-negative staphylococci is potentially difficult, beta-lactam therapy for serious coagulase-negative staphylococcal infections is controversial.
- HACEK is an acronym for a group of fastidious, slow-growing Gram-negative bacteria (*Haemophilus*, *Actinobacillus*, *Cardiobacterium*, *Eikenella*, and *Kingella* species) that have a predilection for infecting heart valves. The treatment of choice is ceftriaxone, 2 g IV q24h for 4 weeks. Ampicillin-sulbactam or ciprofloxacin are alternatives.
- Blood culture–negative IE is usually encountered when antimicrobials are initiated before cultures are obtained or, rarely, with fastidious pathogens, such as nutritionally deficient streptococci, HACEK organisms, *Coxiella burnetii* (Q fever), *Bartonella*, *Tropheryma whippelii* (Whipple's disease), and fungi. Empiric therapy can be initiated despite negative cultures with ceftriaxone 2 g IV q24h, or ampicillin-sulbactam, 3 g IV q6h, plus an aminoglycoside for 4–6 weeks. Vancomycin plus ciprofloxacin can be substituted for the beta-lactam agents in penicillin-allergic patients.

Response to Antimicrobial Therapy
- Frequently, clinical improvement is seen within 3–10 days.
- Daily blood cultures should be obtained until sterility is documented.
- Persistent or recurrent fever usually represents extensive cardiac infection but also might be due to septic emboli, drug hypersensitivity, or subsequent nosocomial infection. Such fever seldom represents the development of antimicrobial resistance.

Surgery
- Indications include uncontrolled infection as manifested by sustained bacteremia while on therapy, refractory heart failure, an unstable prosthetic valve, or prosthetic valve obstruction.
- Surgical intervention might also be necessary when native valve endocarditis is complicated by recurrent systemic emboli, mycotic aneurysm, persistent conduction defects, chordae tendineae or papillary muscle rupture, or early closure of the mitral valve on echocardiography, or when PVE is complicated by a periprosthetic leak.
- Fungal endocarditis is refractory to medical therapy and requires surgery for cure.
- Endocarditis due to Gram-negative bacilli may be refractory to antimicrobials alone. Although a 10-day course of preoperative antimicrobials is desirable, surgery must not be delayed in patients whose condition is deteriorating.

Special Considerations
- The American Heart Association recommends that prophylaxis for IE be provided to patients at risk who undergo procedures associated with bacteremia (Table 13-1).

MYOCARDITIS

General Principles
- When the heart is involved in an inflammatory process, the cause is often an infectious agent. Myocarditis may occur during and after viral, rickettsial, bacterial, and parasitic infection.
- It is also a rare complication following vaccination with vaccinia virus (smallpox vaccine).

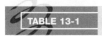

TABLE 13-1	Endocarditis Prophylaxis

Clinical scenario	Drug and dosage
I. Endocarditis prophylaxis is recommended for the following cardiac conditions: prosthetic valves, previous endocarditis, congenital heart disease, surgical shunts or conduits, valvular heart disease, hypertrophic cardiomyopathy, mitral valve prolapse with regurgitation.	
II. Regimens for dental, oral, or respiratory tract procedures (including dental extractions, periodontal or endodontal procedures, professional teeth cleaning, rigid bronchoscopy, surgery on respiratory mucosa, tonsillectomy.	
Standard prophylaxis	Amoxicillin, 2 g PO 1 hr before procedure
Unable to take PO	Ampicillin, 2 g IM or IV within 30 min before procedure
Penicillin-allergic patient	Clindamycin, 600 mg PO, or cephalexin or cefadroxil, 2 g PO,[a] or clarithromycin or azithromycin, 500 mg PO 1 hr before procedure
Penicillin-allergic and unable to take PO	Clindamycin, 600 mg IV, or cefazolin, 1 g IV within 30 min before procedure
III. Regimens for gastrointestinal and genitourinary procedures (esophageal, sclerotherapy or dilation, endoscopic retrograde cholangiopancreatography with biliary obstruction, biliary or intestinal surgery; cystoscopy, uretheral dilation, prostrate surgery.	
High-risk patient	Ampicillin, 2 g IM or IV, plus gentamicin, 1.5 mg/kg (maximum, 120 mg) within 30 min before procedure; 6 hr later, ampicillin, 1 g IM or IV, or amoxicillin, 1 g PO
High-risk, penicillin—allergic patient	Vancomycin, 1 g IV, plus gentamicin, 1.5 mg/kg (maximum, 120 mg), timed to be completed within 30 min before procedure
Moderate-risk patient	Amoxicillin, 2 g PO 1 hr before procedure, or ampicillin, 2 g IM or IV within 30 min before procedure
Moderate-risk, penicillin-allergic patient	Vancomycin, 1 g IV timed to finish within 30 min before procedure

Note: IM, intramuscularly; IV, intravenously; PO, orally.
[a]Cephalosporins should not be used in patients with anaphylactic or urticarial reactions to penicillin.
Adapted from AS Dajani, KA Taubert, W Wilson, et al. Prevention of bacterial endocarditis: recommendations by the American Heart Association. *JAMA* 277:1794, 1997.

Diagnosis

Clinical Presentation
■ Presentation varies greatly. Patients may be asymptomatic or may present with dysrhythmias, chest pain, or fulminant, fatal congestive heart failure.

Laboratory Studies
■ Nasopharyngeal swab testing, serology, and PCR studies may be performed for viruses.
■ Tissue diagnoses via endomyocardial biopsies may be helpful.

Treatment
■ Therapeutic regimens should be targeted to the identified agent. The role of IV immunoglobulin and antiviral agents in viral-mediated myocarditis remains anecdotal.

PERICARDITIS

- Acute pericarditis is a syndrome caused by inflammation of the pericardium and characterized by chest pain, a pericardial friction rub, and diffuse ST-segment elevations on ECG (see Chapter 5, Ischemic Heart Disease, and Chapter 6, Heart Failure, Cardiomyopathy, and Valvular Heart Disease).
- In most cases, viruses are implicated as the infectious etiologies of pericarditis. The role of antiviral therapies in viral pericarditis remains to be characterized. TB is another occasional cause (see the Tuberculosis section).

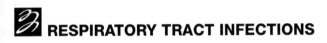 **RESPIRATORY TRACT INFECTIONS**

UPPER RESPIRATORY TRACT INFECTIONS

Pharyngitis

General Principles

- Most cases are caused by upper respiratory viruses, although distinction from streptococcal (GABHS) and gonococcal pharyngitis is difficult on clinical grounds.

Diagnosis

- Laboratory studies are reserved for symptomatic patients exposed to streptococcal pharyngitis, individuals with signs of significant infection (i.e., fever, pharyngeal exudate, and cervical adenopathy), patients whose pharyngeal infection fails to clear despite symptomatic therapy, and patients with a history of rheumatic fever.
- **Rapid antigen detection testing** (RADT) is useful for identifying GABHS, which requires therapy to prevent acute pyogenic complications and rheumatic fever. A negative test does not reliably exclude GABHS, making a culture necessary when RADT is negative.
- Serology for Epstein–Barr virus (e.g., heterophile agglutinin or monospot) and examination of a peripheral blood smear for atypical lymphocytes should be performed when infectious mononucleosis is suspected.
- Acute HIV infection should be considered in the differential diagnosis of pharyngitis with atypical lymphocytosis and negative streptococcus and Epstein–Barr virus testing.

Treatment

- Most cases of pharyngitis are self-limited and do not require antimicrobial therapy.
- Treatment for GABHS should be initiated in the setting of a positive culture or RADT, if the patient is at high risk for development of rheumatic fever, or if the diagnosis is strongly suspected, pending the results of culture.
- Treatment schedules include **penicillin V**, 250 mg PO qid or 500 mg PO bid for 10 days, **erythromycin**, 250 mg PO qid for 10 days, or **benzathine penicillin G**, 1.2 million units IM as a one-time dose.
- **Surgical** intervention and **parenteral therapy** may be necessary for severe cases involving airway compromise or inability to take oral medications.[12] For treatment of gonococcal pharyngitis, see the Sexually Transmitted Diseases section.

Epiglottitis

General Principles

- Epiglottitis should be considered in the febrile patient who complains of severe sore throat, odynophagia, new-onset drooling, and dysphagia but in whom minimal findings are noted on inspection of the pharynx.

Diagnosis
- Throat and blood cultures
- Lateral soft-tissue radiograph of the neck should be obtained to assess airway occlusion.

Treatment
- **Hospitalization and prompt otolaryngologic consultation for airway management are suggested in all suspected cases.**
- Antimicrobial therapy should include an agent that is active against *H. influenzae*, such as **ceftriaxone**, 1–2 g IV q24h, or **cefotaxime**, 1–2 g IV q6–8h.

Sinusitis

General Principles
- Sinusitis is caused by obstruction of the osteomeatal complex.
- The goals of medical therapy for acute and chronic sinusitis are to control infection, reduce tissue edema, facilitate drainage, maintain patency of the sinus ostia, and break the pathologic cycle that leads to chronic sinusitis.
- **Acute rhinosinisitis** is a clinical diagnosis that presents with cough, purulent nasal discharge, and sinus tenderness with or without fever.
  - It is most often caused by upper respiratory viruses. Bacterial pathogens, such as *S. pneumoniae, H. influenzae, Moraxella catarrhalis*, and anaerobes, should be considered if symptoms are severe or if they persist for more than a week.[13]
  - **Symptomatic treatment** is the mainstay of therapy, including systemic decongestants and analgesics with or without a short course of topical decongestant.
  - Empiric antibiotic therapy is indicated for severe symptoms or failure of symptomatic therapy. First-line antibiotics include a 10-day regimen of amoxicillin, 500 mg PO tid, or TMP/SMX, one double-strength (DS) tablet PO bid. Second-generation cephalosporins, amoxicillin/clavulanate, and macrolides are good second-line agents in case of primary treatment failure.
- With **chronic sinusitis**, patients experience nasal congestion or obstruction. Secondary complaints include pain, pressure, postnasal discharge, and fatigue.
  - Posttreatment coronal sinus CT with bone windows is the radiographic modality of choice; plain films are not recommended.
  - Nasal endoscopy may complement CT scan by permitting direct inspection of the surface mucosa of the ethmoid air cells.
  - The etiologic agents include those for acute sinusitis, as well as *S. aureus, Corynebacterium diphtheriae, Prevotella* species, and *Veillonella* species.
  - Therapy may include a nasal steroid spray; the role of antimicrobial agents is unclear.
  - Some chronic cases require endoscopic surgery.

Influenza Virus Infection

General Principles
- Influenza viruses cause an acute, self-limited febrile illness with myalgias, cough, and malaise. The virus is readily transmissible and associated with outbreaks of varying severity during the winter months.
- **Clinical sequelae** of influenza virus infection include viral pneumonia and secondary bacterial pneumonia.
- **H5N1 avian influenza** is transmitted to humans via close contact with infected birds and can cause severe pneumonia and acute respiratory distress syndrome with a case-fatality ratio >50%.

Diagnosis
- This condition is most commonly diagnosed clinically, with confirmation by nasopharyngeal swab for rapid antigen testing or direct fluorescent antibody test and culture.

Treatment

Medications
- Treatment must be initiated within 48 hours of the onset of symptoms to be effective in immunocompetent patients. Available antiviral treatment regimens are as follows:
  - The **neuraminidase inhibitors** are used in treatment and prophylaxis of influenza A and B.
  - Oseltamivir, 75 mg PO bid for 5 days, is well tolerated in capsule and elixir formulations.
  - Zanamivir, 10 mg inhaled twice a day for 5 days, is an inhalational agent that may occasionally cause bronchospasm in patients with asthma.
  - Amantadine and rimantadine, each 100 mg PO bid, are effective for the treatment and prophylaxis of some influenza A strains; however high levels of resistance emerged in H3N2 isolates in 2005, and thus these agents are **NOT recommended** for seasonal influenza.[14]

Vaccination
- Annual influenza vaccination is recommended for all adults >50 years old and persons with comorbidities. Vaccination has been shown to reduce all-cause mortality in elderly populations.[15] Vaccination of high-risk inpatients should be considered during influenza season if there is no underlying febrile illness.

LOWER RESPIRATORY TRACT INFECTIONS

Acute Bronchitis

Diagnosis

Clinical Presentation
- Acute bronchitis involves inflammation of the bronchi that causes the acute onset of cough, sputum production, and symptoms of upper respiratory tract infection.
- The usual causes are viral agents, such as coronavirus, rhinovirus, influenza, or parainfluenza. Uncommon causes include *Mycoplasma pneumoniae*, *Chlamydophilia pneumoniae*, and *Bordetella pertussis*.

Imaging
- Pneumonia should be routinely ruled out either clinically or radiographically, and diagnostic tests for influenza should be performed if it is suspected.

Laboratory Studies
- Cough that lasts for >2 weeks in an adult should be evaluated for pertussis with a nasopharyngeal swab for culture or PCR, or both.

Treatment
- Treatment is symptomatic and is directed most often at controlling cough (dextromethorphan, 15 mg PO q6h). Routine antimicrobial use is not recommended[16] unless influenza or pertussis is confirmed.
- **Erythromycin,** 500–1000 mg PO q6h for 14 days, or **azithromycin,** 500 mg PO single dose followed by 250 mg PO daily, is used for therapy.
- Pertussis cases should be reported to the local health department for contact tracing and administration of postexposure prophylaxis with erythromycin or azithromycin.

Acute Exacerbations of Chronic Bronchitis

Diagnosis
- Acute exacerbation of chronic bronchitis (AECB) is characterized by an increase in volume or purulence of sputum with increased cough or dyspnea.

- *H. influenzae* is the major pathogen, followed by *S. pneumoniae* and *M. catarrhalis*. Many episodes of AECB are incited by tobacco exposure, air pollution, occupational exposure, subclinical asthma, viral infection, or allergies.

Treatment
- Uniformly active oral antibiotics include amoxicillin/clavulanate, third-generation cephalosporins, macrolides (azithromycin and clarithromycin), and doxycycline.
- For hosts with severe underlying disease and compromised respiratory status, broader treatment with a third-generation cephalosporin or respiratory fluoroquinolone is indicated. See Chapter 9, Pulmonary Disease, for further details.

Pneumonia

General Principles
- Traditionally, pneumonia is categorized as community-acquired pneumonia (CAP), hospital-acquired pneumonia, or ventilator-associated pneumonia (VAP) (see the Nosocomial Infections section).

Diagnosis

Physical Examination
- Fever and respiratory symptoms, including cough with sputum production, dyspnea, and pleurisy, are common presenting features in immunocompetent patients. Signs include tachypnea, rales, or consolidation on auscultation.

Imaging
- Chest radiograph reveals a new pulmonary infiltrate.
- Fiberoptic bronchoscopy is used for detection of associated anatomic lesions, biopsy for histopathologic workup, or quantitative cultures of conventional bacteria.

Laboratory Studies
- Assessment of etiologic agents in all hospitalized patients should include **pretreatment expectorated sputum for Gram stain and culture and blood cultures.**
- Most patients can be treated as outpatients, although all should be evaluated for severity of illness, comorbid factors, and oxygenation.
- For patients with CAP, the predominant etiologic agent is *S. pneumoniae*, in which multidrug resistance is rapidly increasing.
- Pneumonia caused by atypical agents, such as *Legionella pneumophila*, *Chlamydophilia pneumoniae*, or *Mycoplasma pneumoniae*, cannot be reliably determined clinically. If an atypical agent is suspected, urinary *Legionella* antigen should be sent. PCR assays for detecting other atypical pathogens may be available in some areas.
- Acute and convalescent serologic testing can retrospectively identify several atypical pathogens including *C. pneumoniae, C. burnetii* (Q fever), and hantavirus.

Treatment

Medications
- Low-risk CAP patients may be effectively treated at home with oral antibiotics.[17]
- Guidelines giving detailed empiric treatment regimens have been published, with an emphasis on targeting the most likely pathogens within specific risk groups.[18]
  - **Treatment of immunocompetent outpatients** with no recent antibiotic exposure and no comorbidities should consist of **doxycycline** or a **macrolide.**
  - **Treatment of patients** with recent antibiotic exposure or comorbidities should include respiratory fluoroquinolone (e.g., moxifloxacin) monotherapy or advanced macrolide (azithromycin or clarithromycin) with or without high-dose amoxicillin.
  - Hospitalized patients should be treated with ceftriaxone, 1 g IV daily, or cefotaxime, 1 g IV q8h, plus azithromycin or clarithromycin, or monotherapy with a respiratory fluoroquinolone.

- For all critically ill patients, the addition of azithromycin or clarithromycin or a respiratory fluoroquinolone to a beta-lactam regimen is necessary to provide coverage for *L. pneumophila.*
- Antibiotic therapy should be narrowed if a specific microbiological etiology is obtained.
- Intravenously administered penicillin G, which reaches high concentrations in lung tissue, remains an effective treatment for sensitive *S. pneumoniae* isolates.[19]

Surgery
- Thoracentesis of pleural effusions should be performed, with analysis of pH, cell count, Gram stain and bacterial culture, protein, and lactate dehydrogenase (see Chapter 9, Pulmonary Disease). Empyemas should be drained.

Lung Abscess

General Principles
- Lung abscess typically results from macroaspiration of oral flora.
- Risk factors include periodontal disease and conditions that predispose patients to aspiration of oropharyngeal contents.
- Bacterial causes of lung abscess include oral anaerobes (*Prevotella* spp., *Actinomyces* spp., and anaerobic and microaerophilic streptococci), enteric Gram-negative bacilli, *S. aureus*, and *S. pneumoniae* serotype III.
- Polymicrobial infection is common.

Diagnosis

Clinical Presentation
- Typically lung abscess is indolent and reminiscent of pulmonary tuberculosis, with dyspnea, fever, chills, night sweats, weight loss, and cough productive of putrid or blood-streaked sputum.

Imaging
- Chest radiography is very sensitive and typically reveals infiltrates with cavitation and air-fluid levels in dependent areas of the lung.

Treatment
- Postural drainage of the involved lung segment and antibiotic treatment with an antipneumococcal fluoroquinolone plus clindamycin or a beta-lactam/beta-lactamase inhibitor.

Tuberculosis

General Principles

Etiology
- TB is a systemic disease caused by *M. tuberculosis.*
- Most cases are the result of reactivation of prior infection, and persons at highest risk include those with HIV infection, silicosis, diabetes mellitus, chronic renal insufficiency, malignancy, malnutrition, and other forms of immunosuppression, especially therapy with tumor necrosis factor (TNF) antagonists like infliximab and etanercept.[20]

Epidemiology
- The prevalence of TB, particularly multidrug-resistant forms (MDR-TB), is increased among immigrants from Southeast Asia, Sub-Saharan Africa, the Indian subcontinent, and Central America. Extreme multidrug resistant TB (XDR-TB) is becoming increasingly prevalent in Sub-Saharan Africa.

Diagnosis

Clinical Presentation
- The most frequent clinical presentation is pulmonary disease.

- Extrapulmonary disease may present as cervical lymphadenitis, genitourinary disease, osteomyelitis, miliary dissemination, meningitis, peritonitis, or pericarditis.

Laboratory Studies
- Positive fluorochrome or acid-fast bacteria (AFB) smears of sputum are presumptive evidence of active TB, although nontuberculous mycobacteria and some *Nocardia* species may give positive results with these techniques.
- Use of radiometric culture systems and species-specific DNA probes can provide results faster than traditional methods.
- Drug susceptibility testing should be performed on all initial isolates as well as on follow-up isolates from patients who do not respond to standard therapy.

Treatment[21]
- Treatment does not have to take place in a hospital setting, but hospitalization to initiate therapy provides an opportunity for intensive patient education.
- If a patient is hospitalized, proper isolation in a **negative-pressure room** is essential.
- **The local health department** should be notified of all cases of TB so that contacts can be identified and adherence to the regimen can be ensured by directly observed therapy.[22]

Medications
- Chemotherapy: At least two drugs to which the organism is susceptible must be used because of the high frequency with which primary drug resistance to a single drug develops. Extended therapy is necessary because of the prolonged generation time of mycobacteria.
- Because adherence to multidrug regimens for prolonged periods is difficult, directly observed therapy should be used for all patients.
- Initial therapy of uncomplicated pulmonary TB should include **four** drugs unless the likelihood of drug resistance is very low (i.e., the rate of isoniazid [INH] resistance in the community is <4% or the patient has not received prior therapy for TB, has not been exposed to any contacts with drug-resistant TB, and is not from an area where drug-resistant TB is prevalent)[23]:
    - **INH** (5 mg/kg; maximum, 300 mg PO daily),
    - **RIF** (10 mg/kg; maximum, 600 mg PO daily),
    - **pyrazinamide** (PZA, 15–30 mg/kg, maximum 2 g PO daily), and
    - either **ethambutol** (EMB, 15–25 mg/kg PO daily) or **streptomycin** (15 mg/kg; maximum, 1.5 g IM daily) should be administered initially.
    - If the isolate proves to be fully susceptible to INH and RIF, EMB (or streptomycin) can be dropped and INH, RIF, and PZA continued to finish 8 weeks, followed by 16 weeks of INH and RIF. Patients at high risk for relapse (cavitary pulmonary disease or positive TB cultures after 2 months of therapy) should be treated for 9 months.
    - After at least 2 weeks of daily therapy, the drugs can be administered two or three times per week at adjusted doses. **Pyridoxine** (vitamin B_6), 25–50 mg PO daily, should be considered for all patients who take INH to prevent neuropathy.
- **Organisms that are resistant** only to INH can be effectively treated with a 6-month regimen if a standard four-drug regimen consisting of INH, RIF, PZA, and EMB or streptomycin was started initially.
- When INH resistance is documented, the INH should be discontinued, and the remaining three drugs should be continued for the duration of therapy.
- Therapy for multidrug-resistant TB has been less well studied, and consultation with an expert in the treatment of TB should be considered.
- **Extrapulmonary disease** in adults can be treated in the same manner as pulmonary disease, with 6- to 9-month regimens. TB meningitis should be treated for 9–12 months.

- **Glucocorticoid administration.** In TB, the administration of glucocorticoids is controversial. Prednisone, 1 mg/kg PO daily initially, has been used in combination with antituberculous drugs for life-threatening complications such as meningitis and pericarditis.

Risk Management

- **Monitoring response to therapy.** Patients with pulmonary TB whose sputum AFB smears are positive before treatment should submit sputum for AFB smear and culture every 1–2 weeks until AFB smears become negative. Sputum should then be obtained monthly until two consecutive negative cultures are documented. Conversion of cultures from positive to negative is the most reliable indicator of a response to treatment. Continued symptoms or persistently positive AFB smears or cultures after 3 months of treatment should raise the suspicion of drug resistance or nonadherence and prompt referral to an expert in the treatment of TB.
- **Monitoring for adverse reactions.** Most patients should have a baseline laboratory evaluation at the start of therapy that includes hepatic enzymes, bilirubin, CBC, and serum creatinine. Routine laboratory monitoring for patients with normal baseline values is probably unnecessary except in patients with HIV, cases of alcohol consumption, in chronic liver disease, and in pregnant women. Monthly clinical evaluations with specific inquiries about symptoms of drug toxicity are essential. Patients who are taking EMB should be tested monthly for visual acuity and red–green color perception.

Special Considerations

- **Pregnant patients** should not receive PZA or streptomycin, and thus a 9-month course of therapy is recommended. Pregnancy-related TB should be treated with INH, RIF, EMB, and pyridoxine for 2 months, after which the EMB can be stopped if the isolate proves to be drug sensitive.

Latent Tuberculosis Infection[24]

General Principles

- Untreated, approximately 5% of persons with latent tuberculosis infection (LTBI) develop active TB disease within 2 years of infection.
- TB disease develops in an additional 5% of persons over the life span. Adequate prophylactic treatment can substantially reduce the risk of disease.
- LTBI is diagnosed by a positive tuberculin skin test (TST; 5TU [tuberculin units] of purified protein [PPD]).

Criteria for a Positive TST

- Maximum diameter of **induration** (not erythema) is used to grade the TST reference.
- A 5-mm induration is considered positive in patients with HIV infection or another defect in cell-mediated immunity, close contacts of a known case of TB, patients with chest radiographs that are typical for healed TB, and individuals with organ transplantation or other immunosuppression.
- A 10-mm induration is considered positive in immigrants from high-prevalence areas (Asia, Africa, Latin America, Eastern Europe), prisoners, the homeless, parenteral drug abusers, nursing home residents, low-income populations, patients with chronic medical illnesses or health and economic disparities, and those people who have frequent contact with these groups (e.g., health care workers, prison guards).
- For otherwise healthy individuals who are not in a high-prevalence group, 15-mm induration is a positive TST.

Chemoprophylaxis for LTBI

- This should be administered only after active disease has been ruled out by a proper evaluation (chest radiography, sputum collection, or both). **INH**, 300 mg PO daily for

9 months, should be administered, regardless of age, to persons with LTBI who have risk factors for progression to active TB disease.

- Groups that are considered highest priority for treatment are as follows:
  - Persons in whom a TST conversion develops within 2 years of a previously negative TST regardless of age.
  - Persons with a history of untreated TB or chest radiographic evidence of previous disease.
  - Persons with HIV infection, diabetes mellitus, end-stage renal disease, hematologic or lymphoreticular malignancy, conditions associated with rapid weight loss, chronic malnutrition, silicosis, or patients who are receiving immunosuppressive therapy.
  - Household members and other close contacts of patients with active disease who have a reactive TST.
- Persons with HIV infection who have had known contact with a patient with active TB should be treated for LTBI regardless of tuberculin status. Contacts with a nonreactive TST should undergo a repeat TST 3 months after the last exposure to the infectious person.
- A 9-month course of INH is adequate for all patients with LTBI even among those with HIV infection. Alternative regimens of shorter duration but higher toxicity can be considered in consultation with a TB expert. Referral to the health department for chemoprophylaxis is recommended to ensure adherence and to monitor for medication-related complications.

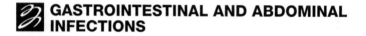 # GASTROINTESTINAL AND ABDOMINAL INFECTIONS

PERITONITIS

General Principles

Etiology

- **Primary or spontaneous bacterial peritonitis** is a common complication of cirrhosis with ascites, which is discussed in Chapter 16, Gastrointestinal Diseases. *Escherichia coli*, other aerobic enteric Gram-negatives, and *Streptococcus* species are the primary pathogens seen with primary or spontaneous bacterial peritonitis. *M. tuberculosis* and *Neisseria gonorrhoeae* (FitzHugh–Curtis syndrome in women) also occasionally cause peritonitis.
- **Secondary peritonitis** is caused by spillage of bacteria from a perforated viscus in the GI or genitourinary tract, usually resulting in an acute surgical abdomen. Infections are virtually always mixed, with *E. coli*, *Bacteroides fragilis*, and other facultative and anaerobic Gram-negatives predominating.

Treatment

- A third-generation cephalosporin, such as ceftriaxone, 2 g IV q24h, or cefotaxime, 2 g IV q8h, is generally the treatment of choice for **primary or spontaneous bacterial peritonitis**. Alternatives include beta-lactam/beta-lactamase inhibitor combinations or carbapenems.
- Surgery and supportive care (particularly volume support) are the primary interventions for **secondary peritonitis,** and **empiric antimicrobial therapy** must be broad in spectrum and should cover the likely pathogens from the presumed source. Optional regimens include monotherapy with a beta-lactam/beta-lactamase inhibitor combination or a carbapenem, depending on severity. Combination therapy options are metronidazole with ampicillin and an aminoglycoside or with a fluoroquinolone. Intra-abdominal abscess formation is a complication with secondary peritonitis that usually requires drainage.

HEPATOBILIARY INFECTIONS

General Principles

Etiology and Clinical Presentation

- **Acute cholecystitis** is typically preceded by biliary colic associated with cholelithiasis and characteristically presents with fever, right upper quadrant tenderness with Murphy's sign, and vomiting. Acalculous cholecystitis occurs in 5%–10% of acute cholecystitis patients.
- **Ascending cholangitis** is a sometimes fulminant infectious complication of an obstructed common bile duct. The classic presentation is the Charcot triad of fever, right upper quadrant pain, and jaundice. Bacteremia and shock are common.

Diagnosis

Imaging

- Ultrasonography is the diagnostic imaging modality of choice for diagnosing infections of the biliary tract.
- Technetium-99m-hydroxy iminodiacetic acid scanning and CT scanning may also be useful.

Treatment

- Management of **acute cholecystitis** includes parenteral fluids, restricted PO intake, analgesia (meperidine causes less spasm of the sphincter of Oddi than morphine), and surgery.
- The **role of antimicrobials** for uncomplicated cholecystitis is unclear; however, perioperative antibiotics such as a beta-lactam/beta-lactamase inhibitor combination may reduce the risk of postsurgical infections. Advanced age, severe disease, or the presence of complications such as gallbladder ischemia or perforation, peritonitis, or bacteremia requires broad-spectrum antibiotics. Initial regimens include a beta-lactam/beta-lactamase inhibitor such as ampicillin/sulbactam, 3 g IV q6h, or piperacillin/tazobactam, 3.375 g IV q6h; or metronidazole, 500 mg IV q8h, with a third-generation cephalosporin or ciprofloxacin, 400 mg IV q12h. Imipenem, 500 mg IV q6h, may be preferred for life-threatening disease or if the risk of *P. aeruginosa* is high. Immediate surgery is usually necessary for severe disease.
- The timing of cholecystectomy is controversial in uncomplicated cholecystitis and in many cases is delayed.
- The mainstay of therapy for **ascending cholangitis** is aggressive supportive care and surgical or endoscopic decompression and drainage in all but the mildest cases. Broad-spectrum antibiotics as recommended for cholecystitis are mandatory.

OTHER INFECTIONS

- **Diverticulitis** presents with left lower quadrant abdominal pain and fever and is diagnosed by abdominal/pelvic CT scan. Enteric Gram-negative bacilli and gut anaerobes are the causative organisms. The standard regimen for mild diverticulitis is TMP/SMX, 160 mg/800 mg (DS) PO bid, or ciprofloxacin, 500 mg PO bid, and metronidazole, 500 mg PO bid, for 7–10 days. Broader antimicrobial coverage (as for secondary peritonitis) and surgical intervention are warranted for more severe cases.
- **Appendicitis** requires surgical intervention, usually with adjuvant antimicrobial therapy as for secondary peritonitis.
- **Infectious diarrhea** (see Chapter 16, Gastrointestinal Diseases).
- Peritonitis related to **peritoneal dialysis** (see Chapter 11, Renal Diseases).
- **Hepatitis** (see Chapter 17, Liver Diseases).

GENITOURINARY INFECTIONS

- The diagnostic and therapeutic approaches to adult genitourinary infections are determined by gender-specific anatomic differences, prior antimicrobial exposures, and the presence of medical devices.

LOWER URINARY TRACT INFECTIONS

- Lower urinary tract infections (UTIs) are characterized by pyuria, often with dysuria, urgency, or frequency.
- A rapid presumptive diagnosis can be made by microscopic examination of a fresh, unspun, clean-voided urine specimen.
- A urine Gram stain can be helpful in guiding initial antimicrobial choices. Bacteriuria (>1 organism per oil-immersion field) or pyuria (>8 leukocytes per high-power field) correlates well with the presence of infection.
- Quantitative culture often yields $>10^5$ bacteria/mL, but colony counts as low as 10^2–10^4 bacteria/mL may indicate infection in women with acute dysuria.
- Acute uncomplicated cystitis in women[25]
  - Acute uncomplicated cystitis in women is caused primarily by *E. coli* (80%) and *Staphylococcus saprophyticus* (5%–15%).
  - If pyuria is present microscopically or by leukocyte esterase testing, empiric treatment with **TMP/SMX**, 160 mg/800 mg PO bid for 3 days, is recommended.
  - In patients who are **intolerant of sulfa, TMP**, 100 mg PO bid, or nitrofurantoin sustained release, 100 mg PO bid for 7 days, can be used. Nitrofurantoin is also effective for enterococcal UTIs, including those caused by VRE.
  - Second-generation fluoroquinolones (e.g., ciprofloxacin, 250 mg PO bid for 3 days) are more costly but should be considered in areas where *E. coli* resistance to TMP/SMX is >20%.[26]
  - A pretreatment urine culture is recommended for diabetics, patients who are symptomatic for >7 days, individuals with recurrent UTI, women who use a contraceptive diaphragm, and individuals older than 65 years. Therapy should be extended to 7 days in this subset of patients.
- Recurrent cystitis in women
  - Recurrent infections are due to host-dependent risk factors, which vary for young women, healthy postmenopausal women, and older women who are institutionalized.[27]
  - Relapses with the original infecting organism that occur within 2 weeks of cessation of therapy should be treated for 2 weeks and may indicate a urologic abnormality.
  - An alternative method of contraception might decrease the frequency of reinfection in women who use a diaphragm and spermicide.
  - **Prophylactic therapy** can be beneficial for patients who experience frequent reinfection. Sterilization of the urine with a standard treatment regimen is necessary before prophylaxis is initiated. For women with relapses that correlate with sexual intercourse, **TMP/SMX**, 80 mg/400 mg (one single-strength tablet), or **ciprofloxacin**, 250 mg, after coitus may provide adequate prophylaxis. TMP/SMX, 40 mg/200 mg or qod, usually is sufficient to decrease recurrences that are unrelated to coitus.
- UTIs in men
  - Cystitis is rare but does not necessarily indicate a urologic abnormality, but should prompt consideration of sexually transmitted infections.
  - Risk factors include anal intercourse, lack of circumcision, and intercourse with a sex partner who has vaginal colonization with uropathogens.
  - A pretreatment urine culture should be obtained routinely.
  - If no complicating factors are present, a 7-day course of **TMP/SMX, TMP** alone, or a second-generation **fluoroquinolone** can be prescribed. If the response to therapy is prompt, a urologic evaluation is unlikely to be useful.

- Urologic studies are appropriate when no underlying risk factor is identified, treatment fails, in the event of recurrent infections, or when pyelonephritis occurs.
- **Catheter-associated bacteriuria**
  - Catheter-associated bacteriuria is a common source of Gram-negative bacteremia in hospitalized patients.
  - **Prevention measures** include aseptic technique for urinary catheter insertion, use of a closed drainage system, and removal of the catheter as soon as possible.
  - When **candiduria** is present, it is crucial to distinguish infection from colonization, which usually does not require treatment other than optimization of host status (glucose control in diabetics, removal or change of Foley catheter). Symptomatic candiduria with pyuria and asymptomatic candiduria in patients at high risk for development of candidemia (e.g., severely immunosuppressed) should receive fluconazole, 100–200 mg PO daily, for 5 days. Amphotericin continuous bladder irrigations have not been proven to be efficacious.
  - In patients with **chronic indwelling catheters**, the development of bacteriuria is inevitable, and long-term antimicrobial suppression simply selects for multidrug-resistant bacteria. Such patients should be treated with systemic antimicrobials only when symptomatic infection with pyuria is evident.
- **Acute urethral syndrome**
  - This condition occurs in women who have lower UTI symptoms and pyuria with $<10^5$ bacteria/mL urine. These patients may have bacterial cystitis or urethritis caused by *Chlamydia trachomatis*, *Ureaplasma urealyticum*, or, less frequently, *N. gonorrhoeae*.
  - Specific cultures of the endocervix for sexually transmitted diseases should be performed (see the Sexually Transmitted Diseases section). If no specific etiology is found, **doxycycline**, 100 mg PO bid for 7 days, is recommended. **Azithromycin**, 1 g PO in a single dose, is an alternative.
- **Prostatitis**
  - **Acute prostatitis** is characterized by fever, chills, dysuria, and a boggy, tender prostate on examination.
  - Patients with **chronic prostatitis** are usually asymptomatic, but some experience low back pain, perineal or testicular discomfort, mild dysuria, and recurrent bacteriuria. Quantitative urine cultures before and after prostatic massage may be necessary for diagnosis. Prostatitis often is associated with $<10^3$ bacteria/mL of seminal fluid.
  - Infections usually are caused by enteric Gram-negative bacilli.
  - **TMP/SMX**, 160 mg/800 mg (DS) PO bid for 14 days, is an effective, economical treatment for acute infections. **Second-generation fluoroquinolones** are useful alternatives.
  - Patients with chronic bacterial prostatitis should receive prolonged therapy (for at least 1 month with the fluoroquinolones or 3 months with TMP/SMX).
- **Epididymitis**
  - This condition usually is caused by *N. gonorrhoeae* or *C. trachomatis* in sexually active young men and by Gram-negative enteric organisms in older men.
  - **Diagnosis** and **therapy** should be directed accordingly, with **ceftriaxone** and **doxycycline** in young men and **TMP/SMX** or **ciprofloxacin** in men older than 35 years.

PYELONEPHRITIS

Diagnosis

- Patients present with fever, flank pain, and lower UTI symptoms. Urine specimens characteristically demonstrate significant bacteriuria, pyuria, and occasional leukocyte casts.
- Urine cultures should be obtained in all patients. Blood cultures should be obtained in those who are hospitalized because bacteremia will be detected in 15%–20%. The causative agent usually is *E. coli*.[28]

Treatment

- Patients with **mild to moderate illness** who are able to take oral medication can be safely treated as outpatients with 7 days of a second-generation fluoroquinolone or, if the organism is susceptible, with TMP/SMX for 10–14 days.
- Patients with more **severe illness**, those who are nauseated and vomiting, and pregnant patients should be treated initially with parenteral therapy. Appropriate empiric parenteral regimens include third-generation cephalosporins, second-generation fluoroquinolones, or ampicillin plus gentamicin. The last-named regimen is preferred if **enterococcal infection** is suspected on the basis of a urine Gram stain.

Special Considerations

- **Evaluation for anatomic abnormalities** should be done for patients who do not respond to initial empiric treatment within 48 hours. Presence of an anatomic abnormality such as intrarenal abscess or renal calculi should be evaluated by ultrasonography, CT scan, or intravenous pyelogram (IVP).

 # SEXUALLY TRANSMITTED DISEASES

ULCERATIVE DISEASES

Genital Herpes

- Genital herpes is caused by **herpes simplex virus (HSV)**, usually type 2, and is characterized by painful grouped vesicles in the genital and perianal regions that rapidly ulcerate and form shallow tender lesions.
- The initial episode may be associated with inguinal adenopathy, fever, headache, myalgias, and aseptic (Mollaret) meningitis; recurrences usually are less severe.

Diagnosis

- The confirmation of HSV infection requires culture or PCR; however, clinical presentation is usually adequate for diagnosis.

Treatment

- **Acyclovir**, 400 mg PO tid (or 200 mg PO five times a day) for 7–10 days, is recommended for all primary genital HSV infections if begun within 1 week of symptoms. Alternative regimens include valacyclovir, 1,000 mg PO bid for 10 days, or famciclovir, 250 mg PO tid for 7–10 days.
- Treatment is indicated for severe recurrences, and options include acyclovir, 400 mg PO tid (or 200 mg PO five times a day) for 5 days, or 800 mg PO tid for 2 days; valacyclovir, 500 mg PO bid for 3 days; or famciclovir, 125 mg PO bid for 5 days. Suppressive therapy with acyclovir, 400 mg PO bid; valacyclovir, 500–1,000 mg PO daily; or famciclovir, 250 mg PO bid; may be useful in patients having >6 recurrences per year.[29] Topical acyclovir has no proven benefit in the treatment or prophylaxis of HSV infection.

Syphilis

General Principles

- Syphilis is caused by the *Treponema pallidum* spirochete.
- Primary syphilis may develop within several weeks of exposure and involves one or more painless, indurated, superficial ulcerations (chancre).
- Secondary syphilis develops after the chancre resolves and involves a rash, mucocutaneous lesions, adenopathy, and constitutional symptoms.
- Tertiary syphilis includes cardiovascular, gummatous, and neurologic disease (general paresis, tabes dorsalis, or meningovascular syphilis).

- There is a high degree of HIV coinfection in patients with syphilis, and HIV infection should be excluded with appropriate testing.[30]

Diagnosis
- In **primary syphilis,** dark-field microscopy of the lesion exudate, or a nontreponemal serologic test (e.g., RPR or Venereal Disease Research Laboratory [VDRL]), in combination with a treponemal serologic test (e.g., fluorescent treponemal antibody absorption test, microhemagglutinin antigen–*T. pallidum*) are confirmatory.
- Diagnosis of **secondary syphilis** is made on the basis of positive serologic studies and the presence of compatible clinical illness.
- In the absence of symptoms, **latent syphilis** is a serologic diagnosis–early latent syphilis is defined as serologically positive for <1 year, and late latent syphilis is defined as serologically positive for >1 year.
- Diagnosis of **tertiary disease** requires clinical correlation with cardiovascular, neurologic, or systemic symptoms. To exclude **neurosyphilis**, a lumbar puncture should be performed in the presence of neurologic or ophthalmic signs or symptoms, evidence of tertiary disease, treatment failure, or serum RPR or VDRL of 1:32 or greater (unless the duration of infection is <1 year). Patients with HIV and syphilis of >1 year's duration also should undergo a lumbar puncture.

Treatment
- To treat primary, secondary, and early latent disease, benzathine **penicillin G,** 2.4 million units IM in a single dose, is used. The alternative is **doxycycline,** 100 mg PO bid for 14 days.
- Treatment of late latent and tertiary disease should include benzathine penicillin G, 2.4 million units IM, one dose per week for 3 weeks. An alternative is doxycycline, 100 mg PO bid for 4 weeks.
- Neurosyphilis treatment should include aqueous penicillin G, 18–24 million units IV daily in divided doses or continuous infusion for 10–14 days; an alternative is procaine penicillin, 2.4 million units IM daily, plus probenecid, 500 mg PO qid for 10–14 days. Some practitioners follow this standard neurosyphilis regimen with an additional IM injection of benzathine penicillin G. Neurosyphilis patients with a penicillin allergy should be desensitized to allow for penicillin therapy. A less efficacious alternative if penicillin is not available is ceftriaxone, 2 g IV or IM daily for 14 days.

VAGINITIS AND VAGINOSIS

- **Trichomoniasis** is a parasitic infection caused by *Trichomonas vaginalis.*
  - Clinical symptoms include malodorous purulent vaginal discharge, dysuria, and genital inflammation.
  - Physical examination reveals profuse frothy discharge and cervical petechiae.
  - The pH of vaginal fluid usually is ≥4.5.
  - Diagnosis requires visualization of motile trichomonads on a saline wet mount of discharge.
  - **Treatment** is with metronidazole, 2 g PO in a single dose; intravaginal metronidazole gel is not effective. In the event of single-dose treatment failure, patients should receive metronidazole, 500 mg PO bid for 7 days. Metronidazole-resistant infection should be treated with tinidazole, 2 g PO in a single dose.
  - Because trichomoniasis is associated with adverse outcomes in **pregnancy**, it is recommended that pregnant women with symptoms of trichomoniasis be treated with single dose metronidazole, 2 g PO.[31]
- **Vulvovaginal candidiasis** (VVC) is generally not a sexually transmitted disease but commonly develops in relation to oral contraceptive use or antibiotic therapy.
  - If recurrent, it may be a presenting manifestation of unrecognized HIV infection.
  - It presents with thick, cottage cheese–like vaginal discharge in conjunction with intense vulvar inflammation, pruritus, and external dysuria.

- Definitive diagnosis requires **visualization of fungal elements** on a potassium hydroxide preparation of vaginal discharge fluid, but therapy often is initiated on the basis of the clinical presentation.
- **Treatment** is fluconazole, 150 mg PO × 1, or any of the intravaginal imidazole regimens (e.g., clotrimazole vaginal cream or suppository, 100 mg at bedtime for 7 days or 200 mg at bedtime for 3 days). For problematic recurrent VVC, fluconazole, 150 mg PO every 72 hours for three doses, followed by 150 mg PO weekly for at least 6 months, is usually effective.[32]
- Fluconazole failure could indicate the presence of a **non-*albicans* *Candida*** species.

CERVICITIS/URETHRITIS

- This is a frequent presentation of infection with ***N. gonorrhoeae*** or ***C. trachomatis*** and occasionally *Mycoplasma hominis*, *U. urealyticum*, and *T. vaginalis*. These infections frequently coexist, and the clinical presentations may be identical.
- Women with urethritis or cervicitis, or both, complain of mucopurulent vaginal discharge, dyspareunia, and dysuria. Men with urethritis complain of dysuria and a purulent penile discharge.
- A positive endocervical or urethral culture, endocervical DNA probe test, or urinary PCR is required for diagnosis. For gonorrhea, a Gram stain of endocervical or urethral discharge with Gram-negative diplococci can also establish the diagnosis.
- Because of frequent coinfection, **simultaneous therapy for chlamydia** is recommended when gonorrhea is diagnosed. Single-dose antigonococcal therapies include ofloxacin, 400 mg PO, ciprofloxacin, 500 mg PO, ceftriaxone, 125 mg IM, or spectinomycin, 2 g IM. Effective antichlamydial therapy includes azithromycin, 1 g PO in a single dose; doxycycline, 100 mg PO bid for 7 days; or erythromycin stearate, 500 mg PO qid (or enteric-coated erythromycin base, 666 mg PO tid) for 7 days.[33]
- Because of increasing resistance rates, fluoroquinolones should not be used to treat gonorrhea in men who have sex with men and for infections acquired in areas with high rates of resistance, including Asia, the Pacific Islands, California, England, and Wales.[34]

PELVIC INFLAMMATORY DISEASE

- Pelvic inflammatory disease (PID) is an upper genital tract infection in women, usually preceded by cervicitis that ranges from mild illness with lower abdominal pain and dyspareunia to peritonitis and tubo-ovarian abscess.
- Long-term consequences of untreated PID include chronic pain, infertility, and ectopic pregnancy. Cervical motion tenderness and the presence of at least 10 white blood cells per low-power field on endocervical smear Gram stain are consistent with PID. Endocervical cultures or probes for chlamydia and gonorrhea should be obtained. Severely ill, pregnant, HIV-infected, and severely nauseated patients should be hospitalized.
- **Treatment** for hospitalized patients should include either cefoxitin, 2 g IV q6h, or cefotetan, 2 g IV q12h, plus doxycycline, 100 mg IV or PO q12h. Clindamycin, 900 mg IV q8h, plus gentamicin is an alternative. Parenteral antibiotics are usually continued for at least 48 hours after the patient shows signs of improvement. Doxycycline, 100 mg PO bid for 14 days, should be used to complete the course of therapy.
- For outpatient therapy, several regimens are effective: (1) cefoxitin, 2 g IM single dose, with probenecid, 1 g PO, plus doxycycline, 100 mg PO bid for 14 days, with or without metronidazole, 500 mg PO bid for 14 days; (2) ceftriaxone, 250 mg IM single dose, plus doxycycline, 100 mg PO bid for 14 days, plus metronidazole, 500 mg PO bid for 7 days; or (3) ofloxacin, 400 mg PO bid, or levofloxacin 500 mg PO daily, for 14 days, plus metronidazole, 500 mg PO bid for 14 days. Intrauterine devices should be removed. Patients should abstain from sexual intercourse during therapy. All patients should receive follow-up within 72 hours to ensure adequate response to therapy.

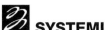 # SYSTEMIC MYCOSES

- These can often be identified by taking into account the clinical findings, site of infection, inflammatory response, and fungal appearance. Yeast-like fungi are typically round or oval and reproduce by budding, whereas molds are composed of tubular hyphae that grow by branching and longitudinal extension.
- Clinical presentations are protean and not pathogen specific.

CANDIDIASIS

General Principles

- Candidiasis is often associated with concurrent antibiotic use, contraceptive use, immunosuppressant and cytotoxic therapy, and indwelling foreign bodies. Mucocutaneous disease may resolve after elimination of the causative condition (e.g., antibiotic therapy) or may persist and progress in the setting of immunosuppressive conditions. Serious complications, such as skin lesions, ocular disease, and osteomyelitis, can occur.
- Systemic antifungal therapy is recommended for all forms of invasive candidiasis.

Diagnosis

- Candidiasis may present as mucocutaneous or invasive disease (e.g., candidemia with or without tissue dissemination).
- Mucocutaneous candidiasis is usually a clinical diagnosis, although a potassium hydroxide preparation of exudate provides confirmation. Cultures can be obtained in refractory cases to exclude the presence of non-*albicans Candida* species. Invasive candidiasis is diagnosed by positive cultures of blood or tissue.

Treatment[35]

- **Oral candidiasis,** or thrush, usually responds to topical therapy with clotrimazole troches, 10 mg dissolved in the mouth five times a day for 14 days. Fluconazole, 100–200 mg PO daily, is very effective and preferred over topical therapy if the patient has esophageal involvement. Amphotericin B, 10–20 mg IV daily for 7–14 days; voriconazole, 200 mg PO bid; and caspofungin, 50 mg IV daily, are effective alternatives for disease that is severe or failing fluconazole. The duration of therapy depends on clinical response and the reversibility of the underlying condition.
- **Isolated catheter-related candidemia** (see the Nosocomial Infections section).
- **Disseminated candidiasis** should be treated with more prolonged courses of either amphotericin B, 0.5 mg/kg/d IV for a total of 0.5–2.0 g, or a lipid formulation of amphotericin B. Fluconazole, 400 mg IV or PO daily, is an alternative for invasive disease caused by *C. albicans* and some non-*albicans* species including *Candida parapsilosis* and *Candida tropicalis* which are generally sensitive to fluconazole.[36] Echinocandins and newer generation azoles are alternatives if fluconazole fails and in patients who are intolerant of amphotericin B.

ASPERGILLOSIS

General Principles

Etiology
- This condition is caused by *Aspergillus* species, which are ubiquitous environmental fungi.
- **Allergic bronchopulmonary aspergillosis** has a natural history that includes remissions and exacerbations with eventual pulmonary bronchiectasis and fibrosis.
    - **Diagnosis** generally requires the presence of asthma, eosinophilia, immunologic evidence of *Aspergillus* colonization, and radiographic abnormalities.

- **Treatment** consists of allergen avoidance and the intermittent use of corticosteroids. Itraconazole, 200 mg PO daily, for 16 weeks, decreases exacerbations and improves lung function.[37]
- **Pulmonary aspergilloma** has a variable natural history, ranging from spontaneous resolution to locally invasive disease.
  - **Diagnosis** is made in the setting of a characteristic radiographic presentation ("fungus ball") and serum *Aspergillus* precipitins.
  - **Treatment** is controversial because antifungal therapy has not been proven beneficial; however, surgical resection or bronchial artery embolization may be necessary for massive hemoptysis.
- **Invasive aspergillosis** (IA) is a serious condition associated with vascular invasion, thrombosis, and ischemic infarction of involved tissues and progressive disease after hematogenous dissemination. IA is usually seen in severely immunocompromised patients.
  - **Diagnosis** requires characteristic histologic evidence of involved tissue and a positive culture.
  - The serum galactomannan assay can be used for prospective monitoring in high-risk patients.[38]
  - Infectious disease consultation should usually be obtained to assist with **treatment** of serious IA. Therapy traditionally required amphotericin B (1.0–1.5 mg/kg/d for 2.0–2.5 g total) or a better-tolerated but much more expensive lipid formulation of amphotericin B; however, newer agents are now available that exhibit similar or improved efficacy and less toxicity. Voriconazole, 6 mg/kg IV two doses 12 hours apart followed by a maintenance dose of 4 mg/kg IV q12h or 200 mg PO; and caspofungin, 70 mg IV loading dose followed by 50 mg IV q24h are two alternatives. Combination therapy, particularly with voriconazole and caspofungin, may improve outcomes, and is becoming standard of care for IA at some centers.[38] The newer azole agents and echinocandins may be useful alternatives in certain complicated infections, for which Infectious Disease consultation is recommended.

CRYPTOCOCCOSIS

- This mycosis occurs worldwide and is caused by *Cryptococcus neoformans*, a yeast associated with soil and pigeon excrement.
- Definitive **diagnosis** requires detection of encapsulated yeast in tissue or body fluids with culture confirmation. The latex agglutination test for cryptococcal antigen in serum or CSF provides a supportive diagnosis. Lumbar puncture is necessary in persons with systemic disease to exclude coexistent CNS involvement.
- **Treatment** depends on the patient's immune function and the site of infection.[39] In general, treatment is necessary for immunocompromised hosts, CNS or disseminated disease, and patients with symptomatic infection at any site. For patients without HIV infection, the treatment of choice for CNS disease is amphotericin B, 0.7–1.0 mg/kg IV daily, with flucytosine, 25 mg/kg PO q6h, for 2 weeks, followed by at least 10 weeks of fluconazole, 400 mg PO daily. Flucytosine dosage should be adjusted to achieve appropriate serum levels (peak, 70–80 mg/L, trough 30–40 mg/L) and to avoid serious adverse events.
- For non–CNS disseminated disease, including cutaneous involvement or cryptococcemia, fluconazole, 200–400 mg PO daily for 6–12 months, is recommended. Isolated asymptomatic pulmonary cryptococcosis in an immunocompetent host can usually be followed without specific therapy.

HISTOPLASMOSIS

- Major endemic mycosis associated with bird and bat excrement primarily in the Ohio and Mississippi River Valleys is caused by *Histoplasma capsulatum*.

- **Diagnosis** requires visualization of small yeasts in tissue or body fluids or a positive culture associated with positive complement fixation and immunodiffusion serology. Detection of *Histoplasma* antigen in urine, serum, or CSF is reliable in the diagnosis of disseminated infection of immunosuppressed hosts.[40] Disease ranges from asymptomatic to mild pulmonary involvement to severe disseminated disease.
- **Standard therapy** for most symptomatic infections is itraconazole, 200 mg PO tid loading dose for 3 days, followed by 200 mg PO bid for 6–12 months; the elixir formulation should be used given its more reliable absorption, and documentation of therapeutic levels is essential. More severe disease requires an initial course of amphotericin B, whereas mild pulmonary disease can be observed without specific therapy.

BLASTOMYCOSIS

- This endemic mycosis in North America is caused by *Blastomyces dermatitidis*.
- **Diagnosis** requires demonstration of large yeasts with broad-based buds or a positive culture from tissues or body fluids. Serologic studies are unreliable for diagnosis. Disease ranges from asymptomatic to chronic pulmonary involvement to severe disseminated disease.
- **Treatment** is usually itraconazole elixir, 200–400 mg PO daily following a loading dose of 200 PO tid, for a minimum of 6 months. Amphotericin B, 0.7–1.0 mg/kg/d for a total dose of 1.5–2.5 g, should be used for life-threatening or CNS disease, often followed by a course of itraconazole.[41]

COCCIDIOIDOMYCOSIS

- This major endemic mycosis of the southwestern United States and Central America is caused by *Coccidioides immitis*.
- **Diagnosis** requires visualization of an endosporulating spherule in tissue or body fluids, positive culture, or positive complement fixation serology. Lumbar puncture should be performed to rule out CNS involvement in persons with severe, rapidly progressive, or disseminated disease.
- **Treatment** is fluconazole, 400–600 mg PO daily, or itraconazole elixir, 200 mg PO, for at least 6 months for mild or moderate nonmeningeal disease. High-dose fluconazole, 800 mg PO, with or without intrathecal amphotericin, is preferred for meningitis. Patients with disease that is severe, progressive, or disseminated may benefit from amphotericin B, 1.0–1.5 mg/kg IV for a total of 1–3 g, depending on the clinical response. Some patients may require chronic maintenance therapy with itraconazole.[42]

SPOROTRICHOSIS

- This condition is caused by *Sporothrix schenckii* following traumatic inoculation, generally of the extremities, after contact with soil or plant material. Lymphocutaneous disease is the usual manifestation. Untreated disease can persist and slowly progress over time; hematogenous dissemination occurs rarely in immunocompromised hosts, and pneumonia, arthritis, or meningitis can develop.
- **Diagnosis** requires demonstration of yeast in tissue or body fluids, a positive culture, or positive serologic studies.
- **Treatment**[43] for lymphocutaneous disease is itraconazole elixir, 100–200 mg PO daily for 3–6 months, with documentation of therapeutic levels. A saturated solution of potassium iodide, 5 drops PO tid, increased to 40 drops tid as tolerated, for 3–6 months is an alternative. Severe and meningeal disease should be treated with amphotericin B, 0.5 mg/kg IV daily for 1–2 g total.

ARTHROPOD-BORNE INFECTIONS, ZOONOSES, AND BITE WOUNDS

TICK-BORNE INFECTIONS

- Tick-borne illnesses (TBIs) are common during the summer months in many areas of the United States; prevalences for specific diseases depend on the local population of vector ticks and animal reservoirs.
- **Coinfection** with multiple TBIs is common and should be considered when patients present with overlapping syndromes.
- Risk should be assessed by outdoor activity in endemic regions rather than known tick bite or attachment, which often go unnoticed.

Lyme Borreliosis (Lyme Disease)

General Principles
- This is the most common vector-borne disease in the United States and is a systemic illness of **variable severity** caused by the spirochete *Borrelia burgdorferi*.
- It is seen in endemic regions, including northeastern coastal states, the upper Midwest, and northern California.
- It has three distinct stages, which start after an incubation period of 7–10 days:
  - Stage 1 (**early local disease**) is characterized by erythema migrans, a slowly expanding macular rash >5 cm in diameter, often with central clearing, and by mild constitutional symptoms.
  - Stage 2 (**early disseminated disease**) occurs within several weeks to months and includes multiple erythema migrans lesions, neurologic symptoms (e.g., seventh cranial nerve palsy, meningoencephalitis), cardiac symptoms (atrioventricular block, myopericarditis), and asymmetric oligoarticular arthritis.
  - Stage 3 (**late disease**) occurs after months to years and includes chronic dermatitis, neurologic disease, and asymmetric monoarticular or oligoarticular arthritis. Chronic fatigue is not seen more frequently in patients with Lyme borreliosis than in control subjects.

Diagnosis
- **Diagnosis** rests on clinical suspicion in the appropriate setting but can be supported by two-tiered serologic testing (screening enzyme-linked immunosorbent assay [ELISA] followed by Western blot).
- A substantial degree of coinfection occurs with babesiosis and ehrlichiosis.

Treatment
- Treatment depends on stage and severity of disease.[44]
  - Oral therapy (doxycycline, 100 mg PO bid; amoxicillin, 500 mg PO tid; or cefuroxime axetil, 500 mg PO bid for 10–21 days) is used for early localized or disseminated disease without neurologic or cardiac involvement. The same agents, given for 28 days, are recommended for late Lyme disease.
  - Doxycycline has the added benefit of covering potential coinfection with ehrlichiosis.
  - Parenteral therapy (ceftriaxone, 2 g IV daily; cefotaxime, 2 g IV q8h; penicillin G, 3–4 million units IV q4h) for 14–28 days should be used for severe neurologic or cardiac disease, regardless of stage.
  - Prophylactic doxycycline, 200 mg PO single dose, may reduce the risk of Lyme disease in endemic areas following a bite by a nymph-stage deer tick.[45]

RMSF (see the Fever and Rash Section)

Ehrlichiosis and Anaplasmosis

- These are systemic TBIs caused by intracellular pathogens of the closely related *Ehrlichia* and *Anaplasma* genera. Two similar syndromes are recognized:
  - **Human monocytic ehrlichiosis (HME)**, caused by *Ehrlichia chafeensis*, is endemic in the south and south-central United States.
  - **Human granulocytic anaplasmosis (HGA, formerly HGE)**, caused by *Anaplasma phagocytophilum*, is found in the same regions as Lyme borreliosis due to a shared tick vector.
- Onset of illness usually occurs 1 week after exposure, with fever, headache, and myalgias.
- Rash is only occasionally seen.
- Severe disease can result in respiratory failure, renal insufficiency, and neurologic decompensation.
- Leukopenia, thrombocytopenia, and elevated liver transaminases are the hallmarks of moderately severe disease.
- **Identification of morulae** in circulating monocytes (HME) or granulocytes (HGA) is uncommon but diagnostic in the appropriate clinical setting. Confirmation is by acute and convalescent serology or PCR of blood or other fluids.
- Prompt initiation of **antimicrobial therapy** is likely to improve prognosis in severe disease. The drugs of choice are doxycycline, 100 mg PO or IV q12h, or tetracycline, 25 mg/kg/d PO divided qid, for 7–14 days.

Tularemia

- This condition is endemic to the south-central United States.
- It is caused by the Gram-negative *Francisella tularensis*.
- Disease onset with fever and malaise occurs 2–5 days after tick bite, exposure to infected animals (particularly rabbits), or to infectious aerosol. Presentation is one of several forms based on inoculation site and route of exposure. Painful regional lymphadenitis with (ulceroglandular form) or without (glandular) a skin ulcer is the **most common** finding. Systemic (typhoidal) and pneumonic disease are more likely to be severe, with high mortality if not treated promptly.
- **Diagnosis** can be confirmed by culture of blood, sputum, or pleural fluid but it is insensitive. **The microbiology laboratory must be alerted promptly of culture specimens from patients with suspected tularemia to allow for use of advanced biohazard precautions.** Acute and convalescent serologic studies provide a retrospective diagnosis.
- Streptomycin, 1 g IM q12h for 10 days, has been the **treatment of choice;** however, gentamicin, 5 mg/kg IV divided q8h, is nearly as effective and easier to administer. Doxycycline, 100 mg PO for 14–21 days, is an oral alternative but is more likely to result in relapse. Ciprofloxacin, 500–750 mg PO bid for 14–21 days, may also be effective.

Babesiosis

- This malaria-like illness is caused by the intraerythrocytic parasite *Babesia microti* after a tick bite. It is endemic in the same regions as Lyme borreliosis, with which patients may be coinfected.
- Disease ranges from subclinical to severe, with fever, chills, myalgias, headache, and dark urine due to hemolysis. Hemolytic anemia may also be present.
- **Diagnosis** is made by visualization of the parasite in erythrocytes on thick or thin blood smears. A serologic test is also available at the CDC.
- **Treatment** may be necessary for moderate or severe disease, especially in asplenic patients. Atovaquone, 750 mg PO bid, plus azithromycin, 600 mg PO daily, for

7–10 days is the first choice. Clindamycin, 600 mg PO/IV q8h, plus quinine, 650 mg PO tid, for 7–10 days should be considered for life-threatening disease.

MOSQUITO-BORNE INFECTIONS

Arboviral Meningoencephalitis

- This condition is caused by multiple viral agents (**West Nile virus [WNV]**, Eastern and Western equine encephalitis, La Crosse encephalitis, St. Louis encephalitis).
- Infections usually occur in the summer months, and **most are subclinical.**
- Symptomatic cases of WNV infection range from a mild febrile illness to aseptic meningitis, fulminant encephalitis, or a poliomyelitis-like presentation with flaccid paralysis. Long-term neurologic sequelae are common with severe disease.
  - In addition to mosquitoes, transmission can occur from blood transfusion, organ transplant, and breast-feeding.
  - **Diagnosis** is usually clinical or by acute and convalescent serologic studies. Specific IgM antibody detection in CSF is diagnostic for acute WNV.
- **Treatment** for all arboviral meningoencephalitides is supportive.

Malaria

- **Malaria** is a systemic parasitic disease that is endemic to most of the tropical and subtropical world.

General Principles

- *Plasmodium falciparum* malaria, the most severe form of the disease, is a potential medical emergency. The onset of illness occurs within weeks or up to 6–12 months after infection with fever, headache, myalgias, and fatigue. Malaria is sometimes characterized by triphasic, periodic (every 48 hours for *Plasmodium ovale* and *Plasmodium vivax*) paroxysms of rigors followed by high fever with headache, cough, and nausea, then culminating in profuse sweating. Complicated, or severe, falciparum malaria is diagnosed in the setting of: hyperparasitemia (>5%), cerebral malaria, hypoglycemia, lactic acidosis, renal failure, acute respiratory distress syndrome, or coagulopathy.

Diagnosis

- **Diagnosis** is by visualization of parasites on examination of Giemsa-stained thick blood smears. **Malaria should be suspected and excluded in all persons with fever who have been in an endemic area within the previous year.**

Treatment

- **Treatment** is dependent on the type of malaria, severity, and risk of chloroquine resistance where the infection occurred. Malaria remains chloroquine sensitive in Central America north of the Panama Canal, most of the Caribbean, and some of the Middle East. Updated information on geographic locations of chloroquine resistance can be found on the CDC Web site, http://www.cdc.gov/travel/. **Usual treatment regimens** are as follows:
  - Uncomplicated *P. falciparum* from chloroquine-sensitive areas and *P. malariae*: chloroquine, 600-mg base (1,000 mg chloroquine phosphate) PO single dose, followed by 300-mg base PO 6, 24, and 48 hours later.
  - **P. ovale** and most **P. vivax**: same as preceding, plus primaquine phosphate, 15.3-mg base (26.5 mg salt) PO daily, for 14 days to prevent relapse. Glucose 6-phosphate dehydrogenase deficiency must be ruled out before primaquine is initiated.
  - Uncomplicated *P. falciparum* from chloroquine-resistant areas and *P. vivax* from **Australia, Indonesia, or South America:** quinine sulfate, 650 mg PO tid, plus

doxycycline, 100 mg PO bid for 7 days. Alternatives are atovaquone, 1 g PO daily, plus proguanil, 400 mg PO daily, both for 3 days; mefloquine; or halofantrine.

- ■ **Complicated or severe** *P. falciparum*: quinidine gluconate, 10 mg salt/kg (maximum, 600 mg) IV over 1–2 hours, followed by 0.02 mg/kg/min as a continuous infusion for 72 hours or until parasitemia is <1%, at which time the 72-hour course can be completed with oral quinine sulfate as previously described. Exchange transfusion can be considered when *P. falciparum* parasitemia exceeds 15%, although the benefit has not been proven.
- ■ **Prophylaxis.** Pretravel advice and appropriate chemoprophylaxis regimens are available at the CDC Web site, http://www.cdc.gov/travel/.

Dengue Fever

- ■ Acute febrile illness; appears 4–7 days after transmission of dengue virus from a mosquito bite.
- ■ Fever, chills, severe musculoskeletal pain, and prominent frontal headache lead to prostration and malaise.
- ■ Hepatic involvement is common, and a hemorrhagic fever syndrome may occur.
- ■ **Diagnosis** is serologic, and **treatment** is supportive.

ZOONOSES

Cat-Scratch Disease (Bartonellosis)

- ■ This lymphadenitis syndrome is caused by the bacterium *Bartonella henselae*. A single or a few papulopustular lesions appear 3–10 days after a cat bite or scratch, followed by regional lymphadenitis (usually cervical or axillary) and mild constitutional symptoms.
- ■ **Atypical presentations** include oculoglandular disease, encephalopathy, arthritis, and severe systemic disease.
- ■ **Diagnosis** is made by exclusion of other causes of lymphadenitis and by detection of antibodies to *B. henselae* or PCR of infected tissue, skin, or pus.
- ■ **The role of routine antimicrobial therapy is not well established** because there is little evidence that therapy alters the natural course of disease, which usually resolves spontaneously over 2–4 months. If antimicrobial therapy is prescribed, azithromycin, 500 mg PO single dose followed by 250 mg PO for 4 more days, is recommended. Needle aspiration of suppurative lymph nodes may provide symptomatic relief.

Leptospirosis

- ■ This acute febrile illness with varying presentations is caused by *Leptospira interrogans*, a ubiquitous pathogen of wild and domestic mammals, reptiles, and amphibians.
- ■ **Onset** is 5–14 days after contact with infected animals or water contaminated with their urine.
- ■ **Anicteric leptospirosis,** which accounts for most cases, is a biphasic illness that starts with **influenza-like symptoms** and proceeds to conjunctival suffusion and aseptic meningitis after a brief defervescent period.
- ■ A minority of cases progress directly to **Weil's disease (icteric leptospirosis),** with multiorgan failure manifested by severe jaundice, uremia, and hemorrhagic pneumonitis.
- ■ **Diagnosis** is confirmed by specific cultures of urine or blood, PCR, or paired serologic studies.
- ■ **Therapy** for anicteric disease, which can shorten the duration of illness, is doxycycline, 100 mg PO bid, or amoxicillin, 500 mg PO q6h, for 7 days. Penicillin G, 1.5 million U IV q4–6h, or a third-generation cephalosporin, is used for treatment of severe disease, during which a Jarisch–Herxheimer reaction is possible.

Brucellosis

- This is a protean systemic infection caused by members of the *Brucella* genus of Gram-negative coccobacilli.
- It is usually preceded by direct contact with body fluids of livestock animals or by eating unpasteurized dairy foods.
- Symptoms are initially nonspecific, but complications within every organ system can occur (diarrhea, arthritis, meningitis, endocarditis, pneumonia). Growth on blood or tissue culture confirms the diagnosis.
- **Antimicrobial therapy** with doxycycline, 100 mg PO bid, for 6 weeks with or without gentamicin for 2–3 weeks, or RIF for 6 weeks, reduces duration and complications of the disease. Audiometry should be performed weekly while gentamicin therapy is administered.

H5N1 Avian Influenza

- Although primarily a pathogen of birds, H5N1 influenza virus can cause severe disease in humans after close contact with infected birds.
- Clinical manifestations include fever, cough, and dyspnea and often progresses with high mortality to severe pneumonia and acute respiratory distress syndrome.
- Antiviral therapy with oseltamivir or zanamivir may improve outcomes.

Anthrax (see the Bioterrorism Section)

Plague (see the Bioterrorism Section)

BITE WOUNDS

General Principles

- The wound should be assessed for the following:
  - Location and extent of injury
  - Functional disability
  - Evidence of infection
  - Need for rabies prophylaxis

Treatment

- Management includes obtaining cultures from visibly infected wounds, copious irrigation, and radiographic studies to exclude fracture, foreign body, or joint space involvement.
- Most wounds should not be sutured unless they are on the face and have been copiously irrigated. Wound **elevation** should be encouraged.
- **Antimicrobial** therapy is given to treat overt infection and as prophylaxis for high-risk bite wounds based on severity (moderate to severe), location (on hands, genitalia, or near joints), bite source (cats), immune status, and type of injury (puncture or crush). Tetanus booster should be given if none has been administered to the patient in the last 5 years.
- The need for **rabies vaccination** and immunoglobulin prophylaxis (see Appendix C, Immunizations and Postexposure Therapies) should be determined after any animal bite. Rabies causes an invariably fatal neurologic disease manifested by hydrophobia, pharyngeal spasm, seizures, and coma. A single case of survival after symptom onset by an aggressive coma-inducing regimen has been reported.[46] Risk of rabies depends on the animal species and the geographic location. **Regardless of species, if the animal is rabid or suspected to be rabid, the human diploid vaccine and rabies immunoglobulin should be administered immediately.** Endemic rabies is present in some wild animals, particularly bats, mandating immediate prophylaxis following bites from these animals. Bites by domestic animals rarely require prophylaxis unless the animal's condition is

unknown. Public health authorities should be consulted to determine whether prophylaxis is recommended for most other animals.

Human Bites

- Human bites are prone to infection and other complications, particularly clenched-fist injuries.
- The normal oral flora of humans includes viridans streptococci, staphylococci, *Bacteroides* species, *Fusobacterium* species, peptostreptococci, and *Eikenella corrodens*.
- Treatment
  - Prophylaxis with amoxicillin/clavulanate, 875 mg/125 mg PO bid for 5 days for uninfected wounds.
  - Infected wounds require parenteral therapy, such as ampicillin/sulbactam, 1.5 g IV q6h; cefoxitin, 2 g IV q8h; or ticarcillin/clavulanate, 3.1 g IV q6h, for 1–2 weeks.
  - Therapy should be extended to 4–6 weeks if osteomyelitis is present.

Dog Bites

- The normal oral flora includes *Pasteurella multocida*, streptococci, staphylococci, and *Capnocytophaga canimorsus*.
- Dog bites comprise 80% of animal bites, but only 5% of such bites become infected.
- **Prophylactic antibiotic therapy** with amoxicillin/clavulanate, 875 mg/125 mg PO bid, for 3–5 days should usually be administered, unless the bite is trivial.
- For infected dog-bite wounds, amoxicillin/clavulanate, or clindamycin plus ciprofloxacin, is effective.

Cat Bites

- Normal oral flora includes *P. multocida* and *S. aureus*.
- Because more than 80% of cat bites become infected, **prophylaxis** with amoxicillin/clavulanate should routinely be provided. Cephalosporins should not be used.
- For infected wounds, effective therapy includes amoxicillin/clavulanate, doxycycline, or cefuroxime axetil. Duration of therapy is 1–2 weeks for cellulitis and 4–6 weeks for osteomyelitis.
- Bartonellosis can also occur after bites.

Wild Animal Bites

- Need for **rabies vaccination** should be determined (see above).
- For most animals, amoxicillin/clavulanate is a good choice for prophylaxis and empiric treatment.
- **Monkey bites** should be treated with acyclovir because of the risk of *Herpesvirus simiae*.

NOSOCOMIAL INFECTIONS

GENERAL PRINCIPLES

- Nosocomial infections substantially contribute to morbidity, mortality, and excess health care costs.
- Efforts to control and prevent the spread of nosocomial infections require an institutional assessment of resources, priorities, and commitment to infection control practices (see Appendix G, Infection Control and Isolation Recommendations).

CATHETER-RELATED BLOODSTREAM INFECTIONS

Diagnosis

- Clinical findings that increase the suspicion of catheter-related bloodstream infections (CR–BSIs) are local inflammation or phlebitis at the central venous catheter (CVC) insertion site, sepsis, endophthalmitis, lack of another source of bacteremia, and resolution of fever after catheter removal.
- Paired blood cultures should initially be drawn through the IV catheter and percutaneously. Differential time to positivity between peripheral and CVC-drawn blood cultures of >120 minutes suggests CR-BSI.[47]
- Semiquantitative or quantitative catheter tip cultures may be helpful to confirm the diagnosis.
- After a positive culture and therapy is initiated, blood cultures should be repeated to document clearance of bacteremia.

Treatment

- *S. aureus, S. epidermidis (coagulase-negative staphylococci)*, aerobic Gram-negative species, and *Candida* species are most commonly associated with CR–BSIs.[48]
  - Initial empiric antimicrobial therapy.
    - Host factors, such as comorbidities, severity of illness, multidrug-resistant colonization, prior infections, and current antimicrobial agents, are important considerations when selecting the initial antimicrobial regimen.
    - **Vancomycin**, 1 g IV q12h, is usually appropriate for empiric therapy because the majority of CR-BSIs are caused by staphylococci.
    - Gram-negative bacilli should be treated broadly, e.g., cefepime 1 g IV q12h, to cover nosocomial pathogens until species identification and susceptibilities are known.
    - **Duration** of treatment depends on whether the infection is complicated or uncomplicated. Duration of treatment should be longer if the CVC remains in situ.
  - Pathogen-specific therapy.
    - Once the pathogen has been identified, antimicrobial therapy should be narrowed to the most effective regimen.
    - Methicillin-sensitive *S. aureus* CR-BSI should be treated with oxacillin, 2 g IV q4h, or alternatively with cefazolin, 1–2 g IV q8h. First-line therapy for MRSA is vancomycin, 1 g IV q12h. Linezolid, 600 mg PO or IV q12h, or daptomycin, 6 mg IV daily, are alternatives. Transesophageal echocardiography (TEE) should be considered to exclude endocarditis. Duration of therapy is 2 weeks if TEE is negative and 4–6 weeks if endocarditis is present.[48]
    - *S. epidermidis* (coagulase-negative staphylococci) CR-BSI is treated similarly to MRSA, with vancomycin being the drug of choice in most cases. Duration of therapy is 5–7 days after CVC removal or 10–14 days if the CVC is retained.
    - **Catheter-related candidemia** in hosts who are hemodynamically unstable or have had prolonged fluconazole therapy should be treated with amphotericin B, 0.5 mg/kg IV q24h, or caspofungin, 70 mg IV single dose followed by 50 mg IV daily. Patients who are hemodynamically stable, have had low fluconazole exposure, and have a *Candida* species that is usually sensitive to fluconazole can be treated with fluconazole, 400 mg IV or PO daily. Duration of antifungal treatment for candidemia should be for 14 days after the last positive blood culture result and when signs and symptoms of infection have resolved.
  - **CVC removal** may involve complex decision making with consideration of host status, need for and type of vascular access, and the identified pathogen.
    - CVCs **must be** removed in the setting of an insertion-site or tunnel-site infection (i.e., pus or significant inflammation at the site).
    - CVCs should be removed for *Candida* and most Gram-negative CR-BSIs.
    - Immunosuppressed patients with CVCs who have fever, neutropenia, and hemodynamic instability should also have CVCs removed.

- The majority of septic patients with short-term CVCs should have CVCs removed at the first signs of sepsis. Decisions for removal of long-term catheters are tailored to the clinical scenario.
- Nontunneled CVCs should generally be removed for CR-BSI caused by organisms other than coagulase-negative staphylococci.
- Antibiotic lock therapy is an option that may be used to help salvage CVCs.

Prevention

- Prevention of CR-BSI.
  - Aseptic insertion techniques are imperative with CVC placement.
  - Tincture of iodine skin preparation can reduce the risk of pseudobacteremia from coagulase-negative staphylococci. Subclavian vein CVCs are associated with lower CR-BSI rates than internal jugular CVCs, whereas femoral CVCs have the highest rates of CR-BSIs and should be removed within 72 hours of placement. Subcutaneous tunneling and use of antiseptic-impregnated CVCs may further reduce the incidence of CR-BSIs. Strategies for decreasing the incidence of CR-BSIs include the use of transparent dressings, strict adherence to aseptic technique and hand washing, antiseptic-impregnated catheter cuffs, topical antiseptic solutions, and routine catheter changes by experienced health care workers.
  - Topical antimicrobial ointment, inline membrane filters, and frequent dressing changes are interventions that have NOT been associated with reduced CR-BSIs. Routine exchange of CVCs over guidewires is not recommended.

HOSPITAL AND VENTILATOR-ASSOCIATED PNEUMONIA

General Principles

- Hospital- (HAP) and ventilator-associated (VAP) pneumonias occur in 0.3%–0.7% of hospitalized patients.
- On clinical presentation there is a new pulmonary infiltrate or increasing oxygen requirement in patients with fever, with or without cough, that occurs >48 hours after admission.

Diagnosis

- Optimal specimens are uncontaminated sterile body fluids (pleural or blood), bronchoscopy aspirates (cultured quantitatively), or aspirates from endotracheal tubes.
- The most frequent pathogens are Gram-negative bacilli and *S. aureus*.
- Fiberoptic bronchoscopy may be diagnostic (quantitative cultures) and therapeutic (re-expansion of lung segment) in these patients.

Treatment

- Initial empiric antimicrobial therapy should target treatment of nosocomially acquired pathogens, particularly *P. aeruginosa* and MRSA.
- Targeted therapy should be based on culture results and in vitro sensitivity testing.
- Empyemas require drainage.

MRSA INFECTIONS

- These should be distinguished from MRSA colonization.
- **First-line therapy** for most MRSA infections is vancomycin (dosed to therapeutic trough levels).
- Linezolid, 600 mg IV or PO q12h, is an alternative.
- Eradication of MRSA nasal carriage can be achieved with a 5-day course of twice-daily intranasal mupirocin.

VRE INFECTIONS

- A distinction exists between VRE colonization and infection. The majority of patients with VRE bloodstream infections are treated with linezolid, daptomycin, or quinapristin/dalfopristin.
- Most VRE-related lower UTIs can be treated with nitrofurantoin, ampicillin, ciprofloxacin, or other agents that achieve high urinary concentrations.
- Eradication of enteric VRE colonization has been attempted without success.

MULTIDRUG-RESISTANT GRAM NEGATIVE INFECTIONS

- Highly resistant gram negative organisms (e.g., *Acinetobacter, Klebsiella*, and *Pseudomonas* species) are becoming increasingly common causes of nosocomial infections.
- Antimicrobial choices are often limited. In addition to broad spectrum agents such as beta-lactam/beta-lactamase inhibitor combinations and carbapenems, tigecycline, and colistin may occasionally be useful.
- Infectious diseases consultation is recommended for such complicated multidrug resistant infections.

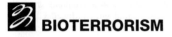 BIOTERRORISM

GENERAL PRINCIPLES

- Several highly fatal and easily produced microorganisms have the potential to be used as agents of bioterrorism. Six diseases have been designated as the most likely to be used for such a purpose. All can produce substantial illness in large populations via an aerosol route of exposure.
- Most of the likely diseases are rare, so a high index of suspicion is necessary to identify the first few cases.
- A bioterrorism-related outbreak should be considered if an unusually large number of patients present simultaneously with a respiratory, GI, or febrile rash syndrome; if several otherwise healthy patients present with unusually severe disease; or if an unusual pathogen for the region is isolated.
- Suspected or confirmed cases of anthrax or smallpox should be treated as an **epidemiologic emergency** and reported immediately to the local health department.

ANTHRAX

General Principles

- Caused by contact with spores from the Gram-positive *Bacillus anthracis*.
- Spores germinate at the site of entry into the body, primarily the lung (**inhalational anthrax**), the skin (**cutaneous anthrax**), or the intestinal mucosa (**gastrointestinal anthrax**).
- The inhalational (45% case-fatality rate) and cutaneous forms are the most likely to be encountered in an intentional release.

Diagnosis

- Inhalational anthrax presents with an early prodrome of an influenza-like illness (fevers, malaise, myalgias but without nasal symptoms), GI symptoms, or both, followed by fulminant respiratory distress, multiorgan failure, and death.
- Diagnosis is suggested by a **widened mediastinum** without infiltrates on chest radiography and confirmed by blood culture.
- Cutaneous anthrax is characterized by a painless black eschar with surrounding edema.

Treatment

- **Immediate antibiotic initiation** on first suspicion of inhalational anthrax reduces mortality. **Empiric therapy**[49] should be ciprofloxacin, 400 mg IV q12h, *or* doxycycline, 100 mg IV q12h, *and* one or two other antibiotics that are active against *B. anthracis* (RIF, clindamycin, penicillin, amoxicillin, vancomycin, imipenem, chloramphenicol).
- On improvement, therapy can be switched to oral ciprofloxacin, 500 mg PO bid, *or* doxycycline, 100 mg PO bid, *and* one other active agent. The total course of therapy should be 60 days to reduce the risk of delayed spore germination.
- Uncomplicated cutaneous anthrax can be treated with oral ciprofloxacin, 500 mg bid, *or* doxycycline, 100 mg bid, for the same duration.
- **Postexposure prophylaxis** consists of oral ciprofloxacin, 500 mg bid for 60 days after exposure. Doxycycline or amoxicillin is an alternative if the strain proves susceptible.

SMALLPOX

General Principles

- Smallpox is caused by variola virus.
- It was declared eradicated as a naturally occurring disease in 1979; however, remaining viral stocks pose a potential bioterrorism threat to an unimmunized population.
- **It is transmitted person to person** through respiratory droplets and carries a case-fatality ratio of 25%–30%.

Diagnosis

- High fever, myalgias, low back pain, and headache appear 7–17 days after exposure, followed by the distinctive rash 3–5 days later.
- The rash starts on the face and distal extremities, including palms and soles, with relative sparing of the trunk, and all lesions in one area are in the same stage of development. These features help to distinguish smallpox from chickenpox (varicella).
- Lesions progress through stages of macules, deep vesicles, pustules, scabs, and permanent pitting scars. Diagnosis is primarily clinical but can be confirmed by electron microscopy, PCR, and culture at reference laboratories.

Treatment

- Treatment consists of supportive care because **no specific antiviral treatment is available.**
- All suspected cases must be placed in contact and respiratory isolation until all scabs have separated to prevent secondary transmission.
- **Postexposure prophylaxis** with live vaccinia virus vaccine within 3 days of exposure offers near-complete protection for responders but is associated with uncommon severe adverse reactions. Progressive vaccinia, eczema vaccinatum, and severe cases of generalized vaccinia can be treated with vaccinia immunoglobulin.

PLAGUE

General Principles

- Plague is caused by the Gram-negative bacillus *Yersinia pestis* and takes one of three forms:
  - **Bubonic,** with a local lymphadenitis (bubo) and 14% case-fatality ratio.
  - **Septicemic,** with 30%–50% case-fatality ratio.
  - **Pneumonic,** with 57% case-fatality ratio, nearing 100% when treatment is delayed. Pneumonic disease can be transmitted from person to person and would be expected after inhalation of aerosolized *Y. pestis*.
- Naturally acquired plague occurs rarely in the southwestern United States after exposure to infected animals.

Diagnosis

- An initial **influenza-like illness** precedes dyspnea, cough, and hemoptysis that rapidly progresses to **fulminant pneumonia** and Gram-negative sepsis.
- Diagnosis is confirmed by isolation of *Y. pestis* from blood, sputum, or CSF.

Treatment

- Start at first suspicion of plague because rapid initiation of **antibiotics** improves survival.
  - Agents of choice are **streptomycin**, 1 g IM q12h; **gentamicin**, 5 mg/kg IV/IM q24h *or* a 2 mg/kg loading dose, then 1.7 mg/kg IV/IM q8h, with appropriate monitoring of drug levels; or **doxycycline**, 100 mg PO/IV bid. Alternatives include **ciprofloxacin** and **chloramphenicol**.[50]
  - The switch to oral therapy can be made after clinical improvement, for a total course of 10–14 days.
  - Respiratory droplet isolation precautions should be instituted on first suspicion.
- **Postexposure prophylaxis** is doxycycline, 100 mg PO bid, or ciprofloxacin, 500 mg PO bid, for 7 days after exposure.

TULAREMIA

See the Arthropod-Borne Diseases, Zoonoses, and Bite Wounds section.

BOTULISM

General Principles

- Botulism is the result of intoxication with botulinum toxin, produced by the anaerobic Gram-positive bacillus *Clostridium botulinum*.
- Rare sporadic outbreaks in the United States are due to ingestion of toxin from improperly canned foods (**food-borne botulism**). The toxin can also be inhaled directly from an aerosol source. Mortality is low when it is recognized early but may be very high in the setting of mass exposure if supportive care equipment supplies (i.e., ventilators) are exhausted.

Diagnosis

- The classic symptom triad is as follows:
  - Lack of fever.
  - Clear sensorium.
  - **Symmetric descending flaccid paralysis,** beginning with ptosis, diplopia, and dysarthria and progressing to loss of gag reflex and diaphragmatic function followed by diffuse skeletal muscle paralysis. Sensation remains intact. Paralysis lasts for weeks to months.
- Diagnosis is **confirmed** by detection of toxin in serum.

Treatment

- Primarily supportive, particularly **ventilatory support**.
- Although the degree of paralysis that is evident at the time of presentation is not reversible, further progression can be halted by administration of **botulinum antitoxin**, which is available from the local health department (one vial administered intravenously, with or without additional intramuscular administration, per package insert).
- **Postexposure prophylaxis** with antitoxin is not recommended because of the high incidence (10%) of hypersensitivity reactions and limited supply.

VIRAL HEMORRHAGIC FEVER

General Principles

- This syndrome is caused by many different RNA viruses, including filoviruses (**Ebola** and **Marburg**), flaviviruses (**dengue**), bunyaviruses (**hanta viruses, Congo-Crimean hemorrhagic fever** [CCHF]), and arenaviruses (**South American hemorrhagic fevers**). All cause sporadic disease in endemic areas, and most can be transmitted as an aerosol or contact with infected body fluids.
- Lassa, CCHF, and Ebola may be transmissible through **respiratory spread**.
- **Case-fatality ratios** are variable but can be as high as 90% for severe Ebola cases.

Diagnosis

- Early symptoms are fevers, myalgias, and malaise.
- Severity ranges from mild to fulminant, and symptomatology varies depending on the specific virus.
- All can severely disrupt vascular permeability and cause disseminated intravascular coagulation, manifested by edema, mucous membrane hemorrhage, petechiae, and shock. Thrombocytopenia, leukopenia, and hepatitis are common. Serologic tests can differentiate most agents of viral hemorrhagic fever from malaria, rickettsial diseases, meningococcemia, and other causes of disseminated intravascular coagulation.

Treatment

- Primarily supportive, particularly management of fluid and blood product status.
- IV **ribavirin** is an experimental treatment that has been used for CCHF, Lassa, and Rift Valley fevers.
- **All patients suspected of having viral hemorrhagic fever should be placed in respiratory and contact isolation** to prevent secondary transmission.
- **Postexposure prophylaxis** with oral ribavirin has been studied for CCHF and Lassa fever.

References

1. Hotchkiss RS, Karl IE. The Pathophysiology and Treatment of Sepsis. *N Engl J Med* 2003;348:138–150.
2. Stevens DL, Bisno AL, Chambers HF, et al. Practice Guidelines for the Diagnosis and Management of Skin and Soft-Tissue Infections. *Clin Infect Dis* 2005;41:1373–1406.
3. Fridkin SK, Hagemann JC, Morrison M, et al. Methicillin-resistant Staphylococcus aureus disease in three countries. *N Engl J Med* 2005;352:14:1436–1444.
4. Lipsky BA, Berendi R, Deery HG. Diagnosis and Treatment of Diabetic Foot Infections. *Clin Infect Dis* 2004;39:885–910.
5. Lew DP, Waldvogel FA. Osteomyelitis. *Lancet* 2004;364:369–379.
6. Apisarnthanarak A, Razavi B, Mundy LM. Adjunctive Intracolonic Vancomycin for Severe *Clostridium difficile* Colitis: Case Series and Review of the Literature. *Clin Infect Dis* 2003;690–696.
7. Darenberg J, Ihendyane N, Sjölin J, et al. Intravenous Immoglobulin G Therapy in Streptococcal Toxic Shock Syndrome: A European Randomized, Double-Blind, Placebo-Controlled Trial. *Clin Infect Dis* 2003;37:333–340.
8. Hasbun R, Abrahams J, Jekel J, et al. Computed Tomography of the Head before Lumbar Puncture in Adults with Suspected Meningitis. *N Engl J Med* 2001;345:1727–1733.
9. de Gans J, van de Beek D. Dexamethasone in Adults with Bacterial Meningitis. *N Engl J Med* 2002;347:1549–1556.
10. Baddour LM, Wilson WR, Bayer AS. Infective Endocarditis: Diagnosis, Antimicrobial Therapy, and Management of Complications: A Statement for Healthcare Professionals From the Committee on Rheumatic Fever, Endocarditis, and Kawasaki Disease, Council on Cardiovascular Disease in the Young, and the Councils on Clinical Cardiology,

Stroke, and Cardiovascular Surgery and Anesthesia, American Heart Association. *Circulation* 2005;111:e394–e433.

11. Li JS, Sexton DJ, Mick N, et al. Proposed Modifications on the Duke Criteria for the Diagnosis of Infective Endocarditis. *Clin Infect Dis* 2000;30:633–638.

12. Bisno AL, Gerber MA, Gwaltney Jr, JM, et al. Practice Guidelines for the Diagnosis and Management of Group A Streptococcal Pharyngitis. *Clin Infect Dis* 2002;35:113–125.

13. Gonzales R, Bartlett JG, Besser RE, et al. Principles of Appropriate Antibiotic Use for Treatment of Acute Respiratory Tract Infections in Adults: Background, Specific Aims, and Methods. *Ann Intern Med* 2001;134:479–486.

14. Centers for Disease Control and Prevention. High Levels of Adamantane Resistance Among Influenza A (H3N2) Viruses and Interim Guidelines for Use of Antiviral Agents—United States, 2005–06 Influenza Season. *MMWR* 2006;55:44–46.

15. Voordouw ACG, Sturkenboom CJM, Dieleman JP, et al. Annual Revaccination Against Influenza and Mortality Risk in Community-Dwelling Elderly Persons. *JAMA* 2004;2089–2095.

16. Gonzales R, Bartlett JG, Besser RE, et al. Principles of Appropriate Antibiotic Use for Treatment of Uncomplicated Acute Bronchitis: Background. *Ann Intern Med* 2001;134:521–529.

17. Carratala J, Fernandez-Sabe N, Ortega L, et al. Outpatient Care Compared with Hospitalization for Community-Acquired Pneumonia. *Ann Intern Med* 2005;142:165–172.

18. Mandell LA, Bartlett JG, Dowell SF, et al. Update of Practice Guidelines for the Management of Community-Acquired Pneumonia in Immunocompetent Adults. *Clin Infect Dis* 2003;37:1405–1433.

19. Yu VL, Chiou CCC, Feldman C, et al. Correlation with In Vitro Resistance, Antibiotics Administered, and Clinical Outcome. *Clin Infect Dis* 2003;37:230–237.

20. Keane J. Editorial Commentary: Tumor Necrosis Factor Blockers and Reactivation of Latent Tuberculosis. *Clin Infect Dis* 2004;39:300–302.

21. Blumberg HM, Leonard Jr MK, Jasmer RM. Update on the Treatment of Tuberculosis and Latent Tuberculosis Infection. *JAMA* 2005;293:22:2776–2784.

22. Horsbrough CR, Feldman S, Ridzon R. Practice Guidelines for the Treatment of Tuberculosis. *Clin Infect Dis* 2000;31:3:633–639.

23. American Thoracic Society, Centers for Disease Control and Prevention, Infectious Diseases Society of America. Treatment of Tuberculosis. *MMWR* 2003;52 (RR-11).

24. Horsburgh Jr. CR. Priorities for the Treatment of Latent Tuberculosis Infection in the United States. *N Engl J Med* 2004;350:2060–2067.

25. Fihn SD. Acute Uncomplicated Urinary Tract Infection in Women. *N Engl J Med* 2003;349:259–266.

26. Raz R, Cazan B, Kennes R, et al. Empiric Use of Trimethoprim-Sulfamethoxazole (TMP-SMX) in the Treatment of Women with Uncomplicated Urinary Tract Infections, in a Geographical Area with a High Prevalence of TMP-SMX Resistant Uropathogens. *Clin Infect Dis* 2002;34:1165–1169.

27. Raz R, Gennesin Y, Wasser J, et al. Recurrent Urinary Tract Infections in Postmenopausal Women. *Clin Infect Dis* 2000;30:152–156.

28. Scholes D, Hooton TM, Roberts PL, et al. Risk Factors Associated with Acute Pyelonephritis in Healthy Women. *Ann Intern Med* 2005;142:20–27.

29. Workowski KA, Levine WC. Sexually Transmitted Diseases Treatment Guidelines-2002. *MMWR* 2002;Vol. 51 (RR-6).

30. Golden MR, Marra CM, Holmes KK. Update on Syphilis: Resurgence of an Old Problem. *JAMA* 2003;290:11:1510–1514.

31. Workowski KA, Levine WC. Sexually Transmitted Diseases Treatment Guidelines—2002. *MMWR* 2002;Vol. 51 (RR-6).

32. Sobel JD, Wiesenfeld HC, Martens M, et al. Maintenance Fluconazole Therapy for Recurrent Vulvovaginal Candidiasis. *N Engl J Med* 2004;351:876–883.

33. Peipert JF. Genital Chlamydial Infections. *N Engl J Med* 2003;349:2424–2430.

34. Centers for Disease Control and Prevention. Increases in Fluoroquinolone-Resistant Neisseria gonorrhoeae Among Men Who Have Sex with Men-United States, 2003, and Revised Recommendations for Gonorrhea Treatment, 2004. *MMWR* 2004;53:335–338.

35. Spellberg BJ, Filler SG, Edwards Jr. JE. Current Treatment Strategies for Disseminated Candidiasis. *Clin Infect Dis* 2006;42:244–251.
36. Rex JH, Walsh TJ, Sobel JD, et al. Practice Guidelines for the Treatment of Candidiasis. *Clin Infect Dis* 2000;30:662–678.
37. Stevens DA, Schwartz HJ, Lee JY, et al. Randomized Trial of Itraconazole in Allergic Bronchopulmonary Aspergillosis. *N Engl J Med* 2000;342:756–762.
38. Marr KA, Boeckh M, Carter RA. Combination Antifungal Therapy for Invasive Aspergillosis. *Clin Infect Dis* 2004;39:797.
39. Saag MS, Graybill RJ, Larsen RA, et al. Practice Guidelines for the Management of Cryptococcal Disease. *Clin Infect Dis* 2000;30:710–718.
40. Wheat J, Sarosi G, McKinsey D, et al. Practice Guidelines for the Management of Patients with Histoplasmosis. *Clin Infect Dis* 2000;30:688–695.
41. Chapman SW, Bradsher Jr. RW, Campbell Jr. GD, et al. Practice Guidelines for the Management of Patients with Blastomycosis. *Clin Infect Dis* 2000;30:679–683.
42. Galgiani JN, Ampel NM, Blair JE, et al. Coccidioidomycosis. *Clin Infect Dis* 2005;41:1217–1223.
43. Lyon GM, Zurita S, Casquero J, et al. Population-Based Surveillance and a Case-Control Study of Risk Factors for Endemic Lymphocutaneous Sporotrichosis in Peru. *Clin Infect Dis* 2003;36:34–39.
44. Wormser GP, Dattwyler RJ, Shapiro ED, et al. The Clinical Assessment, Treatment, and Prevention of Lyme Disease, Human Granulocytic Anaplasmosis, and Babesiosis: Clinical Practice Guidelines by the Infectious Diseases Society of America. *Clin Infect Dis* 2006;43:1089–1134.
45. Nadelman RB, Nowakowski J, Fish D, et al. Prophylaxis with Single-Dose Doxycycline for the Prevention of Lyme Disease after an Ixodes scapularis Tick Bite. *N Engl J Med* 2001;345:79–84.
46. Willoughby Jr. RE, Tieves KS, Hoffman GM, et al. Survival after Treatment of Rabies with Induction of Coma. *N Engl J Med* 2005;352:2508–2514.
47. Raad I, Hanna HA, Alakech B, et al. Differential Time to Positivity: A Useful Method for Diagnosing Catheter-Related Bloodstream Infections. *Ann Intern Med* 2004;140:18–25.
48. Mermel LA, Farr BM, Sherertz RJ, et al. Guidelines for the Management of Intravascular Catheter-Related Bloodstream Infections. *Clin Infect Dis* 2001;32:1249–1272.
49. Inglesby TV, O'Toole T, Henderson DA, et al. Anthrax as a Biological Weapon, 2002: Updated Recommendations for Management. *JAMA* 2002;287:2236–2252.
50. Mwengee W, Butler T, Mgema S, et al. Treatment of Plague with Gentamicin or Doxycycline in a Randomized Clinical Trial in Tanzania. *Clin Infect Dis* 2006;42:614–621.

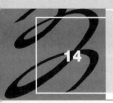

HUMAN IMMUNODEFICIENCY VIRUS INFECTION AND ACQUIRED IMMUNODEFICIENCY SYNDROME
Diana Nurutdinova and E. Turner Overton

GENERAL PRINCIPLES

Definition

- HIV type 1 is a human retrovirus that infects predominantly lymphocytes that bear the CD4 surface protein, as well as coreceptors belonging to the chemokine receptor family. Other cell populations may serve as an important reservoir of the virus. Infection usually leads to lymphopenia, CD4 T-cell depletion, and impaired cell-mediated immunity.
- Over time, this immune dysfunction gives rise to AIDS, which is characterized by development of opportunistic infections (OIs), malignancies, and wasting. The time from onset of HIV infection to development of AIDS varies from months to years (depending on host and viral factors), with a median incubation period of 10 years.
- The virus is transmitted sexually or parenterally, and perinatally.
- HIV type 2 is endemic to regions in West Africa. It is characterized by much slower progression to AIDS and resistance to nonnucleoside reverse transcriptase inhibitors (NNRTIs).

DIAGNOSIS

History

- **Initial evaluation** of persons with a confirmed HIV infection should include the following measures:
  - **Complete history,** with emphasis on previous OIs, viral coinfections, and other complications
  - **Psychological and psychiatric history.** Depression and substance use are common and should be identified and treated as necessary.
  - Family and social support assessment

Laboratory Studies

- **Before checking an individual's HIV serology,** informed consent should be obtained. Informed consent is required in most states and countries.
  - Serology. HIV serology should be checked in the following persons:
    - **Persons in high-risk categories,** including IV drug users, homosexual and bisexual men, hemophiliacs, sexual partners of the aforementioned patients, sexual partners of a known HIV patient, persons involved in sex trading and their sexual partners, persons with sexually transmitted diseases, persons who received blood products between 1977 and 1985, persons who have multiple sexual partners or who engage in unprotected intercourse, persons who consider themselves at risk, and patients with findings that are suggestive of HIV infection
    - **Pregnant women**
    - **Patients with active tuberculosis (TB)**

- **Hospitalized patients** between the ages of 15 and 54 years if the community seroprevalence rate exceeds 1% or AIDS cases number more than 1 per 1,000 discharges
- **Donors of blood, semen, and organs**
- **Health care workers** who perform invasive procedures (depending on the policy of the institution in which they work)
- **Persons with occupational exposures** (e.g., needlesticks) and source patients of the exposures

- Screening is performed with an **enzyme-linked immunosorbent assay (ELISA)**. The current HIV test used in the United States is a combination HIV-1/HIV-2 enzyme immunoassay test kit that is also sensitive to antibodies to HIV-2. The Centers for Disease Control and Prevention offer special tests for HIV-2 and HIV-1 non-B subtypes.
- A positive screening test is confirmed by a repeat positive ELISA and a positive **Western blot** (presence of at least two of the following bands: p24, gp41, gp120/160).
- **An isolated positive ELISA result should not be reported to the patient until this result is confirmed by a Western blot.** An indeterminate test is one for which the ELISA is positive but the criteria for a positive Western blot are not fulfilled. A rapid HIV-1 antibody test has been approved by the U.S. Food and Drug Administration and can be considered for use outside of traditional laboratory and clinical settings.

- **Complete blood count (CBC), routine chemistry**
- **CD4 cell count** (normal range, 600–1500 cells/microliter) and CD4 percentage
- **Virologic markers.** Several quantitative HIV type 1 RNA viral load assays are currently in use, including a branched DNA assay and a nucleic acid sequence amplification assay. The reverse transcriptase polymerase chain reaction (PCR) assay is the most widely used. Regular PCR has a lower limit of detection of 400 viral copies/mL, whereas the ultrasensitive assay has a lower limit of detection of 40 copies/mL.
- **Tuberculin skin test**
- **Rapid plasma reagin (RPR) test**
- **Toxoplasma and cytomegalovirus (CMV) immunoglobin (Ig) G and hepatitis A, B (HBsAg, HBsAb, HBcAb), and C serologies**
- **Chlamydia/gonococcal urine/cervical probe**
- **Cervical Papanicolaou smear** (most commonly using the thin prep method)
- **HIV resistance testing** at baseline, with treatment failure, and particularly for pregnant women

Monitoring

- Plasma HIV RNA load is used for monitoring of therapy. The goal is to reduce the viral load levels below the detection limits. CD4 cell counts should be checked periodically to assess the immune status of the patient and to define the start of prophylactic therapy. After starting or changing antiretroviral therapy (ART), the viral load should be checked at 4–6 weeks, and the regimen should be reassessed. When the ultrasensitive HIV RNA becomes undetectable and the patient is on a stable regimen, monitoring can be done every 3 months.
- **HIV resistance testing** is done using two different types of assays: genotypic, in which the reverse transcriptase and the polymerase genes are sequenced using different techniques, and phenotypic, in which the HIV replication in vitro in the presence of antiretroviral drugs is examined. Results of resistance testing can be used to guide ART.

TREATMENT

Medications

- Immunizations
  - **Pneumococcal vaccine.** Efficacy has not been clearly established in this population. Antibody responses are better when CD4 cell counts are >200 cells/microliter. Revaccination after 5 years should be considered.

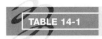

TABLE 14-1	General Principles for Treatment of Human Immunodeficiency Virus Infection

Ongoing HIV replication leads to immune system damage and progression to AIDS.

Plasma HIV RNA levels indicate the magnitude of HIV replication and its associated rate of CD4 cell destruction; CD4 counts indicate the extent of HIV-induced immune damage that has already been experienced.

Treatment decisions should be individualized by level of risk indicated by plasma HIV RNA levels and CD4 counts.

Complete suppression of HIV replications (measured by the ultrasensitive assay) should be the goal of therapy once it is initiated.

The most effective means of suppressing HIV replication is the simultaneous initiation of potent combination antiretroviral therapy.

Each drug should be used according to optimum schedules and dosages.

Any change in antiretroviral therapy increases future therapeutic constraints and potential drug resistance.

Women, especially if pregnant, should receive optimal antiretroviral therapy to reduce the risk of vertical transmission.

The same principles of antiretroviral therapy apply to HIV-infected children and adults.

Persons with acute primary HIV infections should be treated with potent antiretroviral therapy.

All HIV-infected persons, even those with viral loads below detectable limits, should be considered infectious.

Source: 2005 Guidelines for the use of antiretroviral agents in HIV-infected adults and adolescents. Available at: http://aidsinfo.nih.gov/guidelines/.

- ▪ **Hepatitis A and B virus (HAV and HBV).** Vaccination for HAV is recommended for HIV-seropositive subjects who are negative for HAV antibodies, as hepatitis A superinfection can cause fulminant hepatitis in hepatitis C virus (HCV)–coinfected subjects who are not vaccinated or did not respond to immunization. HIV-positive patients are at higher risk of becoming chronic carriers of HBV after having an acute HBV infection. Therefore, if antibodies against hepatitis B core and hepatitis B surface antigens are negative, HBV vaccination is indicated. Coinfection with HCV is very prevalent in this population (especially among IV drug abusers); no vaccine for HCV currently exists. Antibody response is improved with undetectable HIV viral load and higher CD4 count.[1]
- ▪ **Influenza.** Influenza vaccination has been recommended in patients infected with HIV; however, vaccination may promote HIV replication and produce a transient increase in the viral load for up to 3 months after vaccination.
- ■ Antiretroviral Therapy
  - ▪ **General principles** for the treatment of HIV infection are outlined in Table 14–1.
  - ▪ **ART** should be individualized and closely monitored by measuring plasma HIV viral load. Reductions in plasma viremia correlate with increased CD4 cell counts and AIDS-free survival.
  - ▪ **Indications** for the initiation of ART include the following:
    - • **Therapy should be initiated in patients with a CD4 count of <200 cells/microliter or in the symptomatic patient** (with AIDS, thrush, or unexplained fever) regardless of the CD4 count or viral load.
    - • **In the asymptomatic patient, if the CD4 count is between 200 and 350 cells/microliter,** initiation of ART is recommended, although some controversy still exists. Initiation of ART depends on the patient's readiness, comorbidities, and drug toxicities.
    - • **In the asymptomatic patient, if the HIV RNA is >100,000 copies/mL,** initiation of highly active ART is recommended although some controversy exists. Initiation of ART depends on the patient's readiness, comorbidities, and drug toxicities.

- In the asymptomatic patient, if the CD4 count is >350 cells/microliter, there is no strong evidence of clinical benefit of early initiation of ART, and many experts would delay the initiation of treatment. Patients with viral loads >55,000 copies/mL should be monitored closely.

■ **Antiretroviral drugs.** Specific drug information is summarized in Tables 14–2, 14–3, and 14–4. Approved antiretroviral drugs are grouped into four categories.

▧ **Nucleoside analog reverse transcriptase inhibitors (NRTIs)** constrain HIV replication by incorporating into the elongating strand of DNA, causing chain termination. All nucleoside analogs have been associated with **lactic acidosis,** presumably related to mitochondrial toxicity.

▧ **NNRTIs** inhibit HIV by binding noncompetitively to the reverse transcriptase. A single dosage of nevirapine at the time of labor has been shown to decrease perinatal transmission of the virus. Side effects of NNRTIs include rash, increased aspartate transaminase (AST) and alanine transaminase (ALT), and Stevens-Johnson syndrome (more likely with nevirapine). Central nervous system (CNS) side effects are commonly experienced with the use of efavirenz.

▧ **Protease inhibitors (PIs)** are a very potent group of drugs that block the action of the viral protease required for protein processing late in the viral cycle. They are used in combination regimens. Gastrointestinal (GI) intolerance is one of the most commonly encountered adverse effects. All PIs can produce increased bleeding in hemophiliacs; these agents have also been associated with metabolic abnormalities such as glucose intolerance, increased cholesterol and triglycerides, and body fat redistribution. Due to their metabolism via cytochrome P-450, **PIs have important drug interactions,** and concomitant medications should be reviewed carefully (see Table 14–5). Boosting with ritonavir is a common practice in order to achieve better therapeutic concentrations.

▧ **HIV entry inhibitors** belong to a new class of antiretroviral agents that target different stages of the HIV entry process. T-20 **(enfuvirtide)** is a fusion inhibitor only available for use as a subcutaneous injection, 90 mg bid. The most frequent side effect is a local reaction at the injection site.

▧ **Initial therapy.** ART is usually started in the outpatient setting by a physician with expertise in the management of patients with HIV infection. Adherence is the key factor for success of ART. Treatment should be individualized and adapted to the patient's lifestyle. Any treatment decision influences future therapeutic options because of the possibility of drug cross resistance. Potent ART generally consists of a combination of two NRTIs plus one or two PIs or a nonnucleoside reverse transcriptase receptor.

▧ **Treatment failure** is defined as (a) less than a log (10-fold) reduction of the viral load 4–6 weeks after starting a new antiretroviral regimen; (b) failure to reach an undetectable viral load after 4–6 months of treatment; (c) detection of the virus after initial complete suppression of viral load, which suggests development of resistance; or (d) persistent decline of CD4 cells or clinical deterioration. Confirmed treatment failure should prompt changes in ART, based on results of genotype testing. In this situation, at least two of the drugs should be substituted with other drugs that have no expected cross resistance.

▧ **HIV resistance testing** at this stage may help determine a salvage regimen in the patients with prior antiretroviral therapy. The importance of adherence should be stressed. Referral to an HIV specialist is highly recommended in this situation.

▧ **Drug interactions.** Antiretroviral medications, especially PIs, have multiple drug interactions. **PIs and delavirdine both inhibit and induce the P-450 system,** and thus interactions are frequent with other inhibitors of the P-450 system, including macrolides (erythromycin, clarithromycin) and antifungals (ketoconazole, itraconazole), as well as other inducers, such as rifamycins (rifampin, rifabutin) and anticonvulsants (phenobarbital, phenytoin, carbamazepine). **Drugs with narrow therapeutic indexes that should be avoided or used with extreme caution** include antihistamines (although loratadine is safe), antiarrhythmics (flecainide, encainide, quinidine), long-acting opiates (fentanyl, meperidine), long-acting benzodiazepines (midazolam, triazolam),

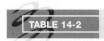

NRTIs	Dosage[a]	Food restrictions	Common side effects
Abacavir (ABC)	300 mg PO bid or combination tablets: ABC 300 mg + 3TC 150 mg + AZT 300 mg (Trizivir) one tablet bid or ABC 600 mg + 3TC 300 mg (Epzicom) 1 tablet daily	No	Hypersensitivity reaction; if hypersensitivity reaction occurs, rechallenge can be fatal[b]
Didanosine (ddI)	Preferred as an enteric-coated formula (Videx EC); >60 kg: 400 mg PO daily, <60 kg: 250 mg PO daily	On empty stomach	Pancreatitis, peripheral neuropathy, diarrhea
Emtricitabine (FTC)[c]	Closely related to 3TC (cross resistance possible); 200 mg PO daily	No	No common severe side effects; may have gastrointestinal (GI) intolerance
Lamivudine (3TC)	150 mg PO bid 300 mg PO daily	No	Rare
Stavudine (d4T)	>60 kg: 40 mg PO bid, <60 kg: 30 mg PO bid; extended-release form: >60 kg: 100 mg PO daily, <60 kg: 75 mg PO daily	No	Peripheral neuropathy, pancreatitis, lipoatrophy
Zidovudine (ZDV, AZT)	300 mg PO bid or combination tablet AZT + 3TC (Combivir) one tablet bid or AZT + 3TC + ABC (Trizivir) one tablet bid	No	Bone marrow suppression, GI intolerance
Tenofovir (TDF)[d]	300 mg PO daily or combination tablet TDF 300 mg + FTC 200 mg one tablet daily or combination tablet TDF 300 mg + FTC 200 mg + Efavirenz 600 mg one tablet daily	No	Rare cases of renal toxicity

[a]Dose adjustment required in patients with renal failure for most NRTIs.
[b]ABC-related hypersensitivity reaction: flulike symptoms, fever, rash, upper respiratory symptoms, GI intolerance.
[c]Zalcitabine (ddC) belongs to this class of NRTIs; however, it is rarely used in clinical practice.
[d]Tenofovir (TDF) is a nucleotide that is available as tenofovir disoproxil fumarate.

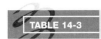

| TABLE 14-3 | Nonnucleoside Reverse Transcriptase Inhibitors (NNRTIs) | | |

NNRTI[a]	Dosage	Food restrictions	Side effects
Efavirenz (EFV)	600 mg PO daily	On empty stomach; avoid taking after high-fat meals because of increased peak concentration	Central nervous system symptoms (dizziness, somnolence, insomnia, abnormal dreams), teratogenicity; false-positive urine cannabinoid test[b]
Nevirapine (NVP)[c]	200 mg PO daily for 2 wk, then 200 mg PO bid or 400 mg daily	No	Skin rash; hepatitis; severe life-threatening hepatotoxicity observed when used with initial CD4 count >250 cells/mm³ in women and >400 cells/mm³ in men

[a]See Table 14-5 for interactions with other antiretrovirals.
[b]Use of gas chromatography or mass spectroscopy is recommended if screening for cannabis is desired.
[c]Delavirdine is rarely used in clinical practice in the United States.

warfarin, 3-hydroxy-3-methylglutaryl coenzyme A (HMG-CoA) reductase inhibitors (pravastatin is the safest), and oral contraceptives. Sildenafil concentrations are increased, and methadone and theophylline concentrations are decreased with concomitant administration of certain PIs and NNRTIs. Grapefruit juice can increase levels of saquinavir and decrease levels of indinavir. See Tables 14–5 and 14–6 for interactions between antiretroviral drugs and other medications.

Protocol

Treatment of HIV infection and AIDS includes ART, prophylaxis for and treatment of opportunistic infections, and treatment and prophylaxis of neoplasias.

Patient Education

■ **Contraception, safer sex practices,** educational issues, and substance abuse treatment when necessary
■ **Social worker referral** and open discussions about aggressiveness of care when the disease advances

Complications

■ **Complications of ART.** The long-term use of antiretrovirals has been associated with toxicity, the pathogenesis of which is only partially understood at this time.
  ■ **Lipodystrophy syndrome** is an alteration in body fat distribution and can be stigmatizing to individuals. Changes consist of the accumulation of visceral fat in the abdomen, neck (buffalo hump), and pelvic areas, and/or the depletion of subcutaneous fat, causing facial or peripheral wasting. Lipodystrophy has been associated in particular with PIs and NRTIs, but other factors also may be important. Changes in the patient's ART regimen and lifestyle modifications such as exercise may

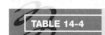

TABLE 14-4 Protease Inhibitors (PIs)

PI	Dosage[a]	Food restrictions	Side effects
Fosamprenavir (fAPV)[b]	1,400 mg PO bid; combined with RTV(r): fAPV/r, 700/100 mg bid or fAPV/r, 1,400/200 mg daily	No	Rash, diarrhea, nausea
Atazanavir (ATV)	400 mg PO daily; combined with RTV(r): ATZ/r, 300/100 mg daily if prior experience with PIs or taken with tenofovir (TDF)	Take with food	Increased indirect bilirubin, fewer metabolic effects
Indinavir (IDV)	800 mg PO tid usually with RTV(r): IDV/r, 800/100 mg bid; IDV/r, 800/200 mg bid	No food if taken alone, can be taken with or without food if combined with RTV(r)	Nephrolithiasis, increased indirect bilirubin, headache
Lopinavir (LPV)	Only available in fixed combination with RTV(r): LPV/r, 400/100 mg PO bid (Kaletra) or 533/133 mg (if used with EFV or NVP) New formulation 200/50 mg tablet, two tablets bid daily regimens may be used in treatment-naïve patients only	Take with food; new formulation can be taken with or without food	Diarrhea, hyperlipidemia, hyperglycemia
Nelfinavir (NFV)	750 mg PO tid or 1,250 mg PO bid	Take with food	Diarrhea, nausea
Ritonavir (RTV)[c]	Usually added to achieve booster effect in combination with other PIs; in full dose, 600 mg PO bid (rarely used)	Take with food	Nausea and vomiting, paresthesias, hepatitis, taste perversion, asthenia
Saquinavir (SQV)	1,200 mg PO tid (soft gel, Fortovase) usually with RTV(r): SQV/r, 1,000/100 mg PO bid or SQV/r, 400/400 mg bid	Take with food	Headache, diarrhea
Tipranavir (TPV)	Used only with RTV boosting: TPV/r, 500/200 mg bid	Take with food	Hepatitis, skin rash, hyperlipidemia, hyperglycemia

[a]See Tables 14-5 and 14-6 for interactions with antiretrovirals and other medications.
[b]fAPV is the prodrug of amprenavir; amprenavir is being phased out, and fAPV should be used instead.
[c]RTV is usually added using a lower dose to achieve a booster effect, especially with LPV, SQV, fAPV, and IDV.

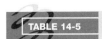

TABLE 14-5	Selected Interactions between Antiretrovirals (ARVs)

ARV	Interactions
Protease Inhibitors	
Lopinavir/ritonavir (LPV/r)	Do not coadminister with fAMP, TPV
Atazanavir (ATV)	Do not use with IDV due to additive risk of ↑ bilirubin in previously PI-experienced patients use RTV boosting
	If given with ddI EC should be given at different times
Nelfinavir (NFV)	If coadministered with LPV/r, decrease NFV to 100 mg bid
Ritonavir (RTV)	Used as a boosting agent for most of the PIs
Tipranavir (TPV)	Doses for coadministration with all PIs except RTV are not established
	Doses for coadministration with ABC and AZT are not established
Nonnucleoside Reverse Transcriptase Inhibitors	
Efavirenz (EFV)	Requires RTV boosting when used with SQV, ATV, fAMP, IDV
Nevirapine (NVP)	Do not coadminister with ATV
	Requires boosting with RTV when used with IDV, SQV
Nucleoside Reverse Transcriptase Inhibitors	
Tenofovir (TDF)	ATV should be boosted with RTV when coadministered with TDF
	Caution when used in combination with ddI and NNRTIs in treatment-naïve patients (potential virologic failure)
Didanosine (ddI)	Separate administration from other agents by 2 hours
	When coadministered with TDF increased ddI levels can cause CD4 lymphocyte suppression: decrease ddI dose to 250 mg
	Increased incidence of lactic acidosis with d4T
Zidovudine (AZT)	Do not coadminister with d4T due to antagonistic effect
Lamivudine (3TC)	Do not coadminister with FTC

Source: U.S. Food and Drug Administration. Available at: http://www.fda.gov/cder/drug/default.htm and National Institutes of Health. Available at: http://www.aidsinfo.nih.gov/.
Complete updated HIV clinical guidelines available at: http://www.aidsinfo.nih.gov/Guidelines/Default.aspx?Menuitem=Guidelines.

improve morphologic changes. Other supplemental therapies such as rosiglitazone and cosmetic surgery are currently under investigation.

■ **Hyperlipidemia**, especially hypertriglyceridemia, is associated mainly with PIs (especially ritonavir). Improvement has been seen after treatment with atorvastatin, pravastatin, and/or gemfibrozil.

■ **Peripheral insulin resistance, impaired glucose tolerance, and hyperglycemia** have been associated with the use of PI-based regimens, mainly indinavir. Lifestyle changes or changing ART can be considered in these cases.

■ **Lactic acidosis** with liver steatosis is a rare but sometimes fatal complication associated with NRTIs. The mechanism appears to be part of mitochondrial toxicity. Higher rates of lactic acidosis have been reported with the use of stavudine and

TABLE 14-6 Selected Interactions between Antiretrovirals and Other Medications

ARV	Interactions
Protease Inhibitors	
	Do not coadminister with simvastatin, lovastatin: levels increased; can cause myopathy and rhabdomyolysis. Atorvastatin can be administered with PIs with close monitoring
	Rifampin and rifapentine cannot be coadministered with PIs due to decreased plasma concentrations
	St. John's Wort should not be used with any PIs: reduces PI plasma concentration
	Decrease in methadone levels observed with most of the PIs
	Caution when coadministered with sildenafil: increased concentration with all PIs
Lopinavir/ritonavir (LPV/r)	Inhibitor of P-450 system
	Fluticasone use can result in suppressed adrenal function
	Decrease rifabutin to 150 mg every other day or three times per week
Atazanavir (ATV)	Decreases clarithromycin dose by 50%
	PPIs significantly decrease ATV concentration: should not be coadministered
	When coadministered with H_2 blockers, should be given 12 hours apart
	Caution due to increased levels of antiarrhythmics
	Decrease rifabutin to 150 mg every other day or three times per week
	Monitor anticonvulsant levels
Nelfinavir (NFV)	Monitor anticonvulsant levels
	Decrease rifabutin to 150 mg every other day or three times per week
Ritonavir (RTV)	Fluticasone use can result in suppressed adrenal function
	Do not coadminister with amiodarone and voriconazole
Tipranavir (TPV)	Inhibitor of P-450 system
	Fluticasone use can result in suppressed adrenal function
	Do not coadminister with amiodarone, quinidine, flecainide
	Do not coadminister with oral contraceptives
	Decrease rifabutin to 150 mg every other day or three times per week
Nonnucleoside Reverse Transcriptase Inhibitors	
	St. John's Wort should not be coadministered due to suboptimal levels of NNRTIs
	Decreased levels of oral contraceptives when coadministered
Efavirenz (EFV)	Inducer/inhibitor of the P-450 system
	Do not coadminister with voriconazole: decreases voriconazole levels
	Decreases methadone levels; can cause opiate withdrawal
Nevirapine (NVP)	Inducer of the P-450 system
	Rifabutin lowers NVP levels; do not coadminister with rifampin
	Decreases methadone levels; can cause opiate withdrawal
Nucleoside Reverse Transcriptase Inhibitors	
Tenofovir (TDF)	Coadministration with cidofovir, acyclovir, valacyclovir, ganciclovir, and valganciclovir may increase serum concentrations of either tenofovir or the coadministered drug
Didanosine (ddI)	Do not coadminister with allopurinol (decreased didanosine concentrations), ribavirin (hepatic failure)
	Monitor for didanosine toxicity when coadministered with ganciclovir or valganciclovir
Zidovudine (AZT)	Avoid concomitant ribavirin and interferon use
	Increased hematologic toxicity with ganciclovir, valganciclovir, cidofovir

Source: U.S. Food and Drug Administration. Available at: http://www.fda.gov/cder/drug/default.htm and National Institutes of Health. Available at: http://www.aidsinfo.nih.gov/.
Complete updated HIV clinical guidelines available at: http://www.aidsinfo.nih.gov/Guidelines/Default.aspx? Menuitem=Guidelines.

didanosine in pregnant women. The clinical picture can range from asymptomatic hyperlactatemia to severe lactic acidosis with hepatomegaly and steatosis. Suspected drugs should be discontinued and supportive care given as needed.

■ **Osteopenia and osteoporosis** are described in HIV-infected individuals. The pathogenic mechanism of this problem is likely related to the inflammatory milieu of HIV itself. The role of ART is being further studied.

■ **Osteonecrosis, particularly of the hip,** has been increasingly associated with HIV disease.

 # OPPORTUNISTIC INFECTIONS

GENERAL PRINCIPLES

Definition

■ Potent ART has decreased the incidence, changed the manifestations, and improved the outcome of OIs.

■ A new clinical syndrome associated with the immune enhancement induced by potent ART, **immune reconstitution syndrome,** has been described and generally presents as local inflammatory reactions. Examples include paradoxical reactions with TB reactivation, localized *Mycobacterium avium* complex adenitis, and CMV vitreitis immediately after the initiation of potent ART. Hepatitis virus infections can be aggravated with the immune reconstitution associated with ART.

Monitoring

■ Careful monitoring is important after starting ART.

■ In the case of immune reconstitution syndrome, ART is usually continued, and the addition of low-dose steroids might decrease the degree of inflammation.

Medications

■ **Prophylaxis for OIs** can be divided into primary and secondary prophylaxis.

■ **Primary prophylaxis** is established before an episode of OI occurs. Institution of primary prophylaxis depends on the level of immunosuppression as judged by the patient's CD4 cell count and percentage. The following interventions are considered standards of care and should be applied in every patient.[2]

■ *Pneumocystis jiroveci* pneumonia **(PCP) prophylaxis** should be initiated when the CD4 count is <200 cells/microliter, if the CD4% has decreased to 15% or less, or if the patient has unexplained fever for more than 2 weeks or experiences an episode of oral candidiasis. Trimethoprim/sulfamethoxazole (TMP/SMX), 160 mg/800 mg (one double-strength [DS] tablet) PO once a day or three times a week, is the preferred regimen. If TMP/SMX is contraindicated, dapsone, 100 mg PO daily (after ruling out glucose 6-phosphate dehydrogenase deficiency); atovaquone, 1,500 mg PO daily; or inhaled pentamidine, 300 mg once a month, are alternatives.

■ **TB prophylaxis** should be given to patients with a positive purified protein derivative (PPD) test (>5 mm of induration), a history of a previous untreated PPD test, or recent contact with an individual with active TB. Isoniazid (INH), 300 mg PO daily, plus pyridoxine, 50 mg PO daily, for 9 months is the regimen of choice. Rifampin, 600 mg PO daily, with pyrazinamide, 20 mg/kg daily, for 2 months is an alternative. In INH-resistant TB, rifampin for 4 months is indicated. Monitoring of liver toxicity is mandatory, especially in patients who are coinfected with hepatitis viruses.

■ *Toxoplasma gondii* **prophylaxis** is indicated for seropositive patients with CD4 cell counts of <100 cells/microliter. TMP/SMX DS, one tablet daily, is the preferred regimen. A combination of dapsone, 50 mg PO daily, plus pyrimethamine, 50 mg PO weekly, and leucovorin, 25 mg PO weekly, is an alternative.

■ *Mycobacterium avium* **complex prophylaxis** is indicated if CD4 cell counts are <50 cells/microliter and consists of azithromycin, 1,200 mg PO weekly, or clarithromycin, 500 mg PO bid. Rifabutin, 300 mg PO daily, is an alternative, but its use may be limited by potential drug interactions.

■ **Varicella-zoster virus (VZV) prophylaxis** is indicated if a significant exposure to chickenpox or shingles occurs, the patient does not have a history of chickenpox, and the patient is VZV seronegative. VZV immunoglobulin (five vials of 1.25 mL each) should be given IM within 96 hours of exposure.

■ **Primary prophylaxis is not routinely recommended** for the following OIs: recurrent bacterial pneumonia, mucosal candidiasis, CMV retinitis, cryptococcosis, and endemic fungal infections such as histoplasmosis and coccidioidomycosis.

■ **Secondary prophylaxis** is instituted after an episode of infection has been adequately treated. Most OIs in AIDS are incurable, and the patient usually requires lifelong therapy.

■ **Withdrawal of prophylaxis.** Recommendations suggest withdrawing primary and secondary prophylaxis for most opportunistic infections if sustained immunologic recovery has occurred (CD4 cell counts consistently above 150–200 cells/microliter).

VIRAL INFECTIONS

Cytomegalovirus Infection

General Principles

■ CMV retinitis occurs very frequently and accounts for 85% of CMV disease in patients with AIDS.

Treatment

■ **Treatment of CMV retinitis** can be local or systemic and is administered in two phases, induction and maintenance.

■ **Valganciclovir,** a ganciclovir prodrug, has been approved for use in CMV retinitis. Drug levels are equivalent to those of IV ganciclovir. For induction, 900 mg PO bid for 21 days is given, followed by 900 mg once a day. **Treatment is indefinite unless immunologic recovery occurs.** Adverse effects are similar to those of ganciclovir.

■ **Ganciclovir** is given at an induction dosage of 5 mg/kg IV bid for 14–21 days and a maintenance dosage of 5 mg/kg IV daily indefinitely (unless immune reconstitution occurs). The most common side effect of ganciclovir is myelotoxicity resulting in neutropenia. The neutropenia may respond to granulocyte colony-stimulating factor therapy. An intraocular ganciclovir implant is effective but does not provide systemic CMV therapy.

■ **Foscarnet** is given at an induction dosage of 60 mg/kg IV q8h or 90 mg/kg IV bid for 14–21 days, followed by a maintenance dosage of 90–120 mg/kg IV daily indefinitely, unless immune reconstitution occurs. Nephrotoxicity is the major side effect; therefore, adequate hydration and electrolyte monitoring (including calcium) are required.

■ **Cidofovir** is effective at an induction dosage of 5 mg/kg IV weekly for 2 weeks, followed by a maintenance dosage of 5 mg/kg IV every 2 weeks. Probenecid (2 g PO 3 hours before and 1 g PO 2 and 8 hours after cidofovir is given) and generous saline hydration must be used to reduce the renal toxicity of cidofovir. Urinalysis and electrolytes should be monitored closely.

■ **Fomivirsen** is an antisense oligonucleotide given intraocularly, 330 mcg, on days 1 and 15 and then monthly. It does not provide systemic therapy.

■ **Combination regimens** (ganciclovir and foscarnet) may be more effective than either drug alone, but together they are poorly tolerated.

- For other invasive CMV disease, the optimal therapy is with IV ganciclovir, PO valganciclovir, IV foscarnet, or a combination of two drugs (in persons with prior anti-CMV therapy), for at least 3–6 weeks. Foscarnet has the best cerebrospinal fluid (CSF) penetration and is the drug of choice for CMV encephalitis and myelopathy. Maintenance therapy is indicated.

Herpes Virus Infection

Diagnosis
- Herpes simplex virus infections can be associated with large genital and perirectal lesions, esophagitis, proctitis, and pulmonary disease.
- HIV-infected individuals are more likely to have severe diseases and treatment failures due to the development of resistance.

Treatment
- Administration of acyclovir (400 mg PO tid), famciclovir (250 mg PO tid), or valacyclovir (500 mg PO tid) for 1 week is usually effective. For more severe disease, IV acyclovir, 5 mg/kg q8h, is recommended.
- Relapses are frequent, and acyclovir, 400 mg PO bid, may prevent their recurrence.
- Herpes simplex virus can become resistant to acyclovir, in which case foscarnet, 40 mg/kg IV q8h for 10–14 days, or one dose of cidofovir, 5 mg/kg IV, should be used.

Varicella-zoster Virus

Diagnosis
- VZV may cause typical dermatomal lesions or disseminated infection. It may also cause encephalitis, which is more common with ophthalmic distribution of facial nerve.

Treatment
- Acyclovir, 10 mg/kg IV q8h for 7–14 days, is the recommended therapy. For milder cases, administration of acyclovir (800 mg PO five times a day), famciclovir (500 mg PO tid), or valacyclovir (1 g PO tid) for 1 week is usually effective.

Epstein-Barr Virus Infection

Diagnosis
- Epstein-Barr virus (EBV) causes oral hairy leukoplakia, for which no treatment is required.
- It is also associated with primary CNS lymphoma in patients with advanced AIDS.

JC Virus

General Principles
- JC virus is a papovavirus associated with progressive multifocal leukoencephalopathy.

Diagnosis
- Symptoms include mental status changes, weakness, and disorders of gait.
- Characteristic periventricular and subcortical white matter lesions are seen on magnetic resonance imaging (MRI).

Treatment
- Potent ART has improved the survival of patients with progressive multifocal leukoencephalopathy.

Parvovirus B19

General Principles
- Chronic parvovirus infections can cause pure red blood cell (RBC) aplasia.

Treatment

- Treatment is with IV **immunoglobulin**, 0.4 g/kg IV daily for 10 days.
- Relapses are frequent.

Chronic Hepatitis C

General Principles

- **Chronic hepatitis C** has a significant impact on morbidity and mortality in HIV-infected patients.

Treatment

- Treatment using a combination of pegylated interferon-α and ribavirin is effective in HIV-positive patients, but sustained virologic response rates are much lower, specifically in genotype 1.
- New antiviral drugs against the hepatitis C virus are in development.

BACTERIAL INFECTIONS

These are common in HIV-infected patients and often recur or follow atypical or aggressive courses. Intensive therapy generally is necessary, followed by chronic suppression.

Bacillary Angiomatosis

General Principles

- **Bacillary angiomatosis** is caused by *Bartonella henselae*.

Diagnosis

- Infection is characterized by multiple nodular, purplish lesions in the skin and other organs.

Treatment

- Erythromycin, 500 mg PO q6h, is the drug of choice.
- Doxycycline, 100 mg PO bid, is also effective.
- Other macrolides and ciprofloxacin, 500 mg PO bid, are alternatives.

Campylobacter jejuni

General Principles

- *C. jejuni* can produce GI or disseminated infections in HIV-infected patients.

Treatment

- Either **erythromycin**, 500 mg PO qid, or **ciprofloxacin**, 500 mg PO bid, can be used for treatment.

Rhodococcus equi

General Principles

- *R. equi* can cause necrotizing cavitary pneumonia.

Treatment

- Treatment consists of **vancomycin**, 1 g IV q12h, followed by chronic suppression with **erythromycin**, 500 mg PO qid, plus **rifampin**, 600 mg PO daily, or with ciprofloxacin, 500 mg PO bid.

Salmonella Species

General Principles

- *Salmonella* can result in recurrent bacteremia in AIDS patients. It occurs more commonly in men who have sex with men due to risk factors.

Treatment
- Antibacterial therapy should be **based on susceptibility.**
- Ceftriaxone, 1 g IV daily; ampicillin, 1 g IV q6h; TMP/SMX, 1 DS tablet PO bid; and ciprofloxacin, 500 mg PO bid, are options, depending on the sensitivities of the organism.

Bacterial Pneumonias

General Principles
- Bacterial pneumonias occur frequently in HIV-infected patients, and the risk for bacterial pneumonia is several times higher in HIV-infected individuals than in HIV-seronegative patients.
- If more than one episode occurs in 12 months, it is considered AIDS defining.

Etiology
- Usually, they are due to *Streptococcus pneumoniae* or *Haemophilus influenzae.*
- Gram-negative rods (especially *Pseudomonas aeruginosa*) may also produce pneumonia in advanced HIV disease.

Syphilis

General Principles
- **Syphilis** can have an atypical course in HIV-infected patients, and treatment failures are more frequent in this population.

Diagnosis
- A spinal tap is recommended in HIV-infected patients with latent syphilis to rule out neurosyphilis.

Treatment
- **Benzathine penicillin,** 2.4 million units IM one time for primary syphilis or weekly for 3 weeks for secondary or latent syphilis (of >1 year in duration), is the regimen of choice.
- **Doxycycline,** 100 mg PO bid for 14 days, is an alternative.
- If neurosyphilis is present, penicillin G, 12–24 million units IV daily for 14 days, is the treatment of choice. Patients who are allergic to penicillin should be desensitized. Data regarding the use of ceftriaxone, 1–2 g IV daily for 14 days, are limited.

Follow-up
- Close monitoring and follow-up using the nontreponemal test at 3, 6, and 12 months are necessary in all cases.
- Persons with a sustained positive nontreponemal titer should receive retreatment and be considered for CSF evaluation to rule out neurosyphilis.[3]

Special Considerations
- **Other sexually transmitted diseases** are treated as they would be in non–HIV-infected patients (see Chapter 13, Treatment of Infectious Diseases).

MYCOBACTERIAL INFECTIONS

Mycobacterium tuberculosis

General Principles
- *M. tuberculosis*[2,4,5] is especially frequent among HIV-infected patients, particularly IV drug abusers. Primary as well as reactivated disease occurs.

Diagnosis

- Clinical manifestations depend on the level of immunosuppression. Patients with higher CD4 cell counts tend to exhibit classic presentations with **apical cavitary disease**.
- More immunosuppressed patients may demonstrate atypical presentations that can resemble disseminated primary infection, with diffuse or localized pulmonary infiltrates and hilar lymphadenopathy.
- Extrapulmonary dissemination is common.

Treatment

- For treatment recommendations, see Chapter 13, Treatment of Infectious Diseases.
- Current recommendations suggest the **substitution of rifabutin for rifampin** in patients who are receiving concomitant ART, especially PIs.
- The dosage for rifabutin should be reduced to 150 mg daily if the patient is receiving ritonavir, indinavir, nelfinavir, or fosamprenavir, whereas it should be increased to 450 mg daily when combined with nevirapine or efavirenz.
- In subjects who are ART naïve, ART can be delayed for a few weeks after TB-specific therapy is started.

M. avium Complex (MAC) Infection

General Principles

- *M. avium* complex (MAC) infection is the most commonly occurring mycobacterial infection in AIDS patients and is responsible for significant morbidity in patients with advanced disease (CD4 cell count <100 cells/microliter).

Diagnosis

- Disseminated infection with fever, weight loss, and night sweats is the most frequent presentation.
- MAC infection can result in bacteremia in AIDS patients.

Laboratory Studies

- Anemia and an elevated alkaline phosphatase level are the usual laboratory abnormalities.

Treatment

- Initial therapy should include a macrolide (clarithromycin, 500 mg PO bid) and ethambutol, 15 mg/kg PO daily.
- Rifabutin, 300 mg PO daily, or ciprofloxacin, 500 mg PO bid, can be added in severe cases.
- Secondary prophylaxis for disseminated MAC can be discontinued if the CD count had a sustained increase >100 cells/microliter for 6 months or longer in response to ART, and if 12 months of therapy for MAC is completed and there are no symptoms or signs attributable to MAC.[5]

Mycobacterium kansasii Infection

General Principles

- *M. kansasii* frequently occurs in HIV patients and should always be considered significant.

Diagnosis

- Clinically, the infection appears similar to TB.

Treatment
- A combination of **rifampin**, 600 mg PO daily, **ethambutol**, 15 mg/kg/day PO, and **INH**, 300 mg PO daily, is the recommended therapy
- Consultation with an infectious disease specialist is recommended.

Mycobacterium haemophilum Infection
Diagnosis
- *M. haemophilum* can produce ulcerative skin lesions in AIDS patients.

Treatment
- It requires treatment with a macrolide, rifampin, and two other drugs active against the organism.

FUNGAL INFECTIONS

P. jiroveci Pneumonia
General Principles
- *P. jiroveci* pneumonia (PCP) is the most common infection in patients with AIDS and is the leading cause of death in this population.

Treatment
- TMP/SMX is the treatment of choice. The dosage is 5 mg/kg of the TMP component IV q6–8h for severe cases, with a switch to oral therapy when the patient's condition improves. Total duration of therapy is 21 days. Prednisone should be added if the patient has an arterial oxygen tension (PaO_2) of <70 mm Hg or an alveolar-arterial oxygen gradient ($P[A-a]O_2$) in excess of 35 mm Hg. The most frequently prescribed prednisone regimen is 40 mg PO bid on days 1–5 and 20 mg bid on days 6–10, followed by 20 mg daily on days 11–21. For patients who cannot receive TMP/SMX, the following alternatives are available:
  - For mild to moderately severe disease (PaO_2 >70 mm Hg or $P[A-a]O_2$ <35 mm Hg)
    - Trimethoprim, 20 mg/kg/d PO, and dapsone, 100 mg PO daily. Glucose 6-phosphate dehydrogenase deficiency should be ruled out before dapsone is used.
    - Clindamycin, 600 mg IV or PO tid, plus primaquine, 15 mg PO daily. Glucose-6-phosphate-dehydrogenase deficiency should be ruled out before primaquine is used.
    - Atovaquone, 750 mg PO tid. This drug should be administered with meals to increase absorption.
  - For severe disease (PaO_2 <70 mm Hg or $P[A-a]O_2$ >35 mm Hg)
    - Pentamidine, 4 mg/kg IV daily, should be infused over 2 hours. Hypoglycemia or hyperglycemia is common, and monitoring of glucose and serum electrolytes (including calcium) is essential. Nephrotoxicity, hematologic toxicity, and hypotension also are frequent.
    - Trimetrexate, 45 mg/m^2 IV daily over 90 minutes, and leucovorin, 20 mg/m^2 IV or PO q6h, can be given.
    - Prednisone taper should be added.
- Prophylaxis is indicated as described in the OI section. Secondary PCP prophylaxis can be discontinued if the CD4 count is >200 cells/microliter for more than 3 months as a result of ART treatment.

Candidiasis
General Principles
- The severity of infection depends on the degree of the patient's immunosuppression.
- Candidiasis is common in the HIV-infected host.

Diagnosis
- Location of infection can be oral, esophageal, or vaginal.

Treatment
- Oral and vaginal candidiasis usually responds to local therapy with troches or creams (**nystatin** or **clotrimazole**).
- For patients who do not respond or who have esophageal candidiasis, **fluconazole**, 100–200 mg PO daily, is the treatment of choice.

Special Considerations
- **Fluconazole-resistant candidiasis** is becoming increasingly frequent, especially in patients with advanced disease who have been receiving antifungal agents for prolonged periods.
- **Itraconazole** oral suspension (200 mg bid) is occasionally effective. Many patients require amphotericin B, either as an oral suspension (100 mg/mL swish and swallow qid) or parenterally.
- **Caspofungin**, an echinocandin, can be considered for refractory cases using an induction dose of 70 mg IV the first day and then 50 mg IV daily for maintenance.
- **Voriconazole** may also be useful.

Cryptococcus Neoformans

General Principles
- The severity of infection depends on the degree of the patient's immunosuppression.
- Cryptococcal meningitis is the most frequent CNS fungal infection in AIDS patients

Diagnosis
- Patients with CNS infection usually present with headaches, fever, and possibly mental status changes, but presentation can be more subtle.
- Cryptococcal infection can present as pulmonary or cutaneous disease.

Laboratory Studies
- Diagnosis is based on **lumbar puncture** results and on the determination of latex cryptococcal antigen, which is usually positive in the serum and in the CSF.
- CSF opening pressure should always be measured to assess the possibility of elevated intracranial pressure.

Treatment
- Initial treatment is with **amphotericin B**, 0.7 mg/kg/d IV, and **5-flucytosine**, 25 mg/kg PO q6h for 2–3 weeks, followed by **fluconazole**, 400 mg PO daily for 8–10 weeks and then 200 mg PO daily indefinitely.
- The 5-flucytosine level should be monitored during therapy to avoid toxicity. A lipid preparation of **amphotericin** can be used in patients with renal insufficiency.

Special Therapy
- Repeat lumbar punctures (removing up to 30 mL CSF until the pressure is below 20–25 cm H_2O) may be required to relieve elevated intracranial pressure.
- In persons who have persistent elevation of intracranial pressure, a temporary lumbar drain is indicated.

Histoplasma capsulatum Infections

General Principles
- The severity of infection depends on the degree of the patient's immunosuppression.
- Histoplasmosis often occurs in AIDS patients who live in endemic areas such as the Mississippi and Ohio River Valleys.
- Such infections are usually disseminated at the time of diagnosis.

Diagnosis
- Suspect histoplasmosis in patients with fever, hepatosplenomegaly, and weight loss.
- Pancytopenia develops due to bone marrow involvement.

Laboratory Studies
- Diagnosis is made by a positive culture, but the urine *Histoplasma* antigen can also be used for diagnosis and to monitor treatment.

Treatment
- Treatment is with **amphotericin B**, 0.5 mg/kg IV daily for a total dose of 0.5–1.0 g, followed by **itraconazole**, 300 mg PO bid for 3 days for induction therapy, followed by 200 mg PO bid indefinitely.
- **Itraconazole absorption** should be documented by a serum drug level.
- Discontinuation of itraconazole is possible if sustained increase in CD4 count is observed >100–200 cells/microliter for more than 6 months.[2]

Coccidioides immitis Infections
General Principles
- *Coccidioides* infection is frequent in AIDS patients in endemic areas of the southwestern United States.
- Extensive disease with extrapulmonary spread is common.

Diagnosis
- Diagnosis is made by a positive culture, serum detection of IgM and IgG by immunodiffusion, and complement fixation.
- Urine *Histoplasma* antigen can also be used for diagnosis and to monitor treatment.

Treatment
- **Amphotericin B** therapy is indicated initially, followed by lifelong suppression with **fluconazole**, 400 mg PO daily, or **itraconazole**, 200 mg PO bid.
- Coccidioidal meningitis requires intracisternal or intraventricular therapy with amphotericin B. Fluconazole may also be effective.

Aspergillosis
General Principles
- This infection can involve the lungs, CNS, heart, kidneys, and sinuses.
- Aspergillosis is increasing among HIV-infected patients, especially those who are neutropenic and those with advanced disease (<50 CD4 cells/microliter).

Diagnosis
- Diagnosis requires a biopsy of the tissue involved.

Treatment
- **Voriconazole** is the treatment of choice.
- Alternatives include **amphotericin B** and **itraconazole**.
- **Caspofungin** can be used for refractory disease using an induction dose of 70 mg IV the first day and subsequently 50 mg IV daily for maintenance.
- Combination therapy is under study. Prognosis is poor for patients with invasive aspergillosis.

PROTOZOAL INFECTIONS

Toxoplasma gondii

Diagnosis
- Toxoplasmosis typically causes multiple CNS lesions and presents with encephalopathy and focal neurologic findings.

Laboratory Studies
- Disease represents reactivation of a previous infection, and the serologic workup usually is positive.

Imaging
- MRI of the brain is the best radiographic technique for diagnosis.
- Often, the diagnosis relies on response to empiric treatment, as seen by a reduction in the size of the mass lesions.

Treatment
- Sulfadiazine, 25 mg/kg PO q6h, plus pyrimethamine, 100 mg PO on day 1 followed by 75 mg PO daily, is the therapy of choice.
- Leucovorin, 5–10 mg PO daily, should be added to prevent hematologic toxicity. For patients who are allergic to sulfonamides, clindamycin (600 mg IV or PO q8h) can be used instead of sulfadiazine.
- Doses are reduced after 3–6 weeks of therapy.
- Secondary prophylaxis can be discontinued among patients with a sustained increase in CD4 count >200 cells/microliter for more than 6 months as a result of response to ART, and if the initial therapy is complete and there are no symptoms or signs attributable to *Pneumocystis*.

Cryptosporidium

Diagnosis
- *Cryptosporidium* causes chronic watery diarrhea with malabsorption in HIV-infected patients.

Laboratory Studies
- Diagnosis is based on the visualization of the parasite in an acid-fast stain of stool.

Treatment
- No effective specific therapy has been developed.
- **Nitazoxanide**, 500 mg PO bid, may be effective.
- Potent **ART** also has been reported to be effective.

Cyclospora

Diagnosis
- *Cyclospora* causes chronic diarrhea.

Treatment
- TMP/SMX, one DS tablet PO bid for 7–10 days, is usually effective.

Isospora belli

Diagnosis
- *Isospora* causes chronic diarrhea.

Treatment
- Treatment with TMP/SMX, one DS tablet PO qid for 10 days, followed by chronic suppression with TMP/SMX, one DS tablet PO daily, is effective.

Microsporidia

Diagnosis
- *Microsporidia* can produce diarrhea and biliary tree disease in patients with advanced infection.

Laboratory Studies
- Diagnosis is difficult and requires special staining of the stool. *Enterocytozoon bieneusi* and *Encephalitozoon intestinalis* are the microsporidia most commonly found. *E. intestinalis* can cause disseminated disease.

Treatment
- Conventional therapy is with albendazole, 400 mg PO bid, but this regimen has only modest success for *E. bieneusi* infections. Relapses are common when therapy is stopped.

Strongyloides

General Principles
- *Strongyloides* presents as disseminated infection in AIDS patients from endemic areas (southeastern United States, immigrants from tropical and subtropical countries).

Treatment
- **Thiabendazole**, 22 mg/kg (maximum, 1.5 g) PO daily for 7–14 days, is the drug of choice for disseminated strongyloidiasis.

ASSOCIATED NEOPLASMS

Kaposi's Sarcoma

General Principles
- Kaposi's sarcoma usually presents as a cutaneous lesion; the GI tract and lungs are the usual visceral organs involved.
- Kaposi's sarcoma is associated with human herpesvirus 8 infection.

Diagnosis
- In AIDS patients, it commonly presents as skin lesions but can be disseminated, even visceral.

Treatment
- Local therapy with liquid **nitrogen** or intralesional injection with alitretinoin or vinblastine has been used. Cryotherapy or radiation may be useful as well.
- Systemic therapy involves chemotherapy (e.g., liposomal doxorubicin, paclitaxel, liposomal daunorubicin, thalidomide, retinoids), radiation, and interferon-α.

Lymphoma

General Principles
- Lymphomas commonly associated with AIDS are non-Hodgkin's lymphoma, CNS and systemic lymphoma, and lymphomas of B-cell origin.
- EBV appears to be the associated pathogen.

Diagnosis
- Primary CNS lymphomas are common and can be multicentric.
- Diagnosis is based on clinical symptoms, the presence of enhancing brain lesions, brain biopsy, and a positive EBV-PCR of the CSF.
- Other OIs need to be ruled out.

■ Other potential extranodal sites of involvement including bone marrow, GI tract, and liver require tissue biopsy to confirm the diagnosis.

Treatment
■ Treatment involves **chemotherapy** and **radiation**.

Cervical and Perianal Neoplasias

General Principles
■ Both HIV-infected men and women are at high risk for human papilloma virus–related disease.
■ Certain human papilloma virus subtypes such as 16 and 18 are oncogenic.
■ Cancer can also arise from perianal condyloma acuminata.

Diagnosis
■ Screening for vaginal dysplasia with a Papanicolaou smear is indicated every 6 months during the first year and, if results are normal, annually afterwards.
■ Screening for anal intraepithelial neoplasms is currently under evaluation.

References
1. Overton ET, Sungkanuparph S, Powderly WG, et al. Undetectable plasma HIV RNA load predicts success after hepatitis B vaccination in HIV-infected persons. *Clin Infect Dis* 2005;41:1045–1048.
2. Kaplan JE, Masur H, Holmes KK. Guidelines for Preventing Opportunistic Infections Among HIV-Infected Persons—2002. Recommendations of the U.S. Public Health Service and the Infectious Diseases Society of America. *MMWR Morb Mortal Wkly Rep* 2002; 51(RR08):1–46.
3. Workowski KA, Levine WC. Sexually Transmitted Diseases Treatment Guidelines—2002. *MMWR Morb Mortal Wkly Rep* 2002; 51(RR06):1–80.
4. Notice to Readers: Updated Guidelines for the Use of Rifabutin or Rifampin for the Treatment and Prevention of Tuberculosis Among HIV-Infected Patients Taking Protease Inhibitors or Nonnucleoside Reverse Transcriptase Inhibitors. *MMWR Morb Mortal Wkly Rep* 2000;49(09):185–189.
5. Prevention and Treatment of Tuberculosis Among Patients Infected with Human Immunodeficiency Virus: Principles of Therapy and Revised Recommendations. *MMWR Morb Mortal Wkly* 1998;47(RR20):1–51.

SOLID ORGAN TRANSPLANT MEDICINE
Brent W. Miller

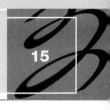

$\mathcal{T}$he objective of this chapter is to provide an overview of topics relevant to the delivery of general medical care to the solid organ transplant recipient.

GENERAL PRINCIPLES

Indications/Contraindications

- Solid organ transplantation is a **treatment, not a cure,** for end-stage organ failure of the kidney, liver, pancreas, heart, and lung. However, the benefits of organ replacement coexist with the risks of chronic immunosuppression. Thus, not all patients with organ failure are transplant candidates.
- All organs remain in short supply with increasing waiting times for potential recipients. **Living-donor transplants** are increasingly common in kidney transplantation and are being evaluated in liver and lung transplantation as a partial solution to this shortage. Xenotransplantation is **not** a viable option in the near future.
- For indications and contraindications of heart, lung, kidney, and liver transplantations, see Chapter 6, Heart Failure, Cardiomyopathy, and Valvular Disease; Chapter 9, Pulmonary Disease; Chapter 11, Renal Diseases; and Chapter 17, Liver Diseases, respectively.
- **Immunologic considerations** prior to the transplant must be fully evaluated including ABO compatibility with the donor, human leukocyte antigen (HLA) typing, and some degree of immune response testing. Newer protocols using plasmapheresis and aggressive immunosuppression have had some success in overcoming immunologic barriers.[1]

Patient Preparation

Immunosuppressive medications are used to promote acceptance of a graft (induction therapy), to reverse episodes of acute rejection (rejection therapy), and to prevent rejection (maintenance therapy). These agents are associated with immunosuppressive effects, immunodeficiency toxicity (e.g., infection and malignancy), and nonimmune toxicity (e.g., nephrotoxicity, diabetes mellitus, or neurotoxicity).[2,3]

Immunosuppressive medications should only be prescribed and administered by physicians and nurses who have appropriate knowledge and expertise. Many variables factor into the choice and dose of drug, and the guidelines for each specific organ are different.

- **Glucocorticoids** are immunosuppressive and anti-inflammatory. Their mechanisms of action include inhibition of cytokine transcription, induction of lymphocyte apoptosis, down-regulation of adhesion molecule and major histocompatibility complex expression, and modification of leukocyte trafficking.[4]
- The **side effects** of chronic glucocorticoid therapy are well known (see Chapter 23, Arthritis and Rheumatologic Diseases). As a result of the associated morbidity, steroids are tapered rapidly in the immediate posttransplant period to achieve maintenance doses of 0.1 mg/kg or less. Four further strategies are developing to minimize side effects: steroid-free immunosuppression, steroid avoidance, rapid steroid tapering, and steroid

withdrawal. Although most long-term transplant recipients have abnormalities in the adrenal axis, increases in glucocorticoid therapy are not indicated for routine surgery or illness.[5]

■ **Antiproliferative agents**

■ **Azathioprine** is a purine analog that is metabolized by the liver to 6-mercaptopurine (active drug), which, in turn, is catabolized by xanthine oxidase. Azathioprine inhibits the synthesis of DNA and thereby suppresses the proliferation of activated lymphocytes. The major dose-limiting toxicity of this agent is myelosuppression, which is usually reversible after dose reduction or discontinuation of the drug. The usual maintenance dose is 1.5–2.5 mg/kg/d in a single dose. Drug levels are generally not obtained.

■ **Mycophenolate** is converted to an active metabolite, mycophenolic acid (MPA). MPA inhibits the rate-limiting step in de novo purine synthesis. Because lymphocytes are relatively dependent on the de novo pathway for purine synthesis, lymphocyte proliferation is selectively inhibited by MPA.

  • The **major adverse effects** of MPA are gastrointestinal (GI) disturbances, including nausea, diarrhea, and abdominal pain, and hematologic disturbances, namely, leukopenia and thrombocytopenia. Antacids that contain magnesium and aluminum interfere with the absorption of MPA and should not be given concurrently. The usual dose is 1–2 g daily in divided doses, although lesser doses may be used with concomitant tacrolimus than cyclosporine because of drug interactions affecting MPA levels. Additionally, the dosage of MPA should be reduced in the presence of renal impairment. Drug levels can be obtained to verify absorption or compliance, but the clinical utility of MPA levels has not been determined.

■ **Sirolimus** is a macrocyclic antibiotic produced by *Streptomyces hygroscopics*. Sirolimus forms a complex with the same receptor-binding protein as tacrolimus; this complex inhibits the activation of a regulatory kinase, mammalian target of rapamycin (mTOR), and thus prohibits T-cell progression from the G1 to the S phase of the cell cycle. Unlike the calcineurin inhibitors, sirolimus does not affect cytokine transcription but inhibits cytokine and growth factor–induced cell proliferation. A second mTOR inhibitor, everolimus, is in development.

  • The **major adverse effects** of this drug include hyperlipidemia, anemia, proteinuria, difficulty with wound healing, cytopenias, peripheral edema, oral ulcers, and gastrointestinal symptoms, although other less common side effects are present. Sirolimus is not nephrotoxic, although it may compound the vasoconstriction of calcineurin inhibitors and potentiate their nephrotoxicity. Thus, sirolimus is best utilized alone, or with steroids and/or other antiproliferative agents. Further, it interacts with cyclosporine metabolism, making monitoring of both drugs difficult. The typical dose is 2–5 mg daily in a single dose. Therapeutic drug monitoring is being perfected, with current trough levels between 5 and 15 ng/mL most commonly being used. Sirolimus should be avoided in advanced chronic kidney disease and immediately postoperatively.

■ **Calcineurin inhibitors** bind to immunophilins (intracellular binding proteins). The calcineurin inhibitor–immunophilin complex inhibits a key phosphatase that is involved in transducing the signal from the T-cell receptor to the nucleus. The net effect is blockade of interleukin-2 and other cytokine transcription, leading to inhibition of T-lymphocyte activation and proliferation. Current strategies are being developed for calcineurin withdrawal and avoidance in solid organ transplantation. Intravenous calcineurin inhibitors should be avoided because of their extreme toxicity and must never be given as a bolus under any circumstances.

■ **Cyclosporine (CsA)** is a cyclic 11–amino acid peptide derived from a fungus. Its major nonimmune side effect is nephrotoxicity due to glomerular afferent arteriolar vasoconstriction. This action leads to an immediate decline in glomerular filtration rate of up to 30% and a long-term vaso-occlusive fibrotic renal disease that often results in chronic kidney disease in recipients of all organ transplants. Angiotensin-converting enzyme inhibitors, sirolimus, volume depletion, and other nephrotoxins may potentiate this toxicity. Acute nephrotoxicity is reversible with dose reduction; chronic nephrotoxicity is generally irreversible and nearly universally present in all patients after 8–10 years of therapy.

■ Other **adverse effects** include gingival hyperplasia, hirsutism, tremor, hypertension, glucose intolerance, hyperlipidemia, hyperkalemia, and, rarely, thrombotic microangiopathy. CsA has a narrow therapeutic window, and doses are adjusted based on blood levels (recommended maintenance trough levels of 100–300 ng/mL: and 2-hour levels <800–1,200 ng/mL). Usual doses are 6–8 mg/kg/d in divided doses, with careful attention to levels and toxicities.

■ **Tacrolimus** is a macrolide antibiotic and, like CsA, is nephrotoxic. Tacrolimus is more neurotoxic and diabetogenic than CsA, but it is associated with less hirsutism, hypertension, and gingival hyperplasia. Tacrolimus dosing is based on trough blood levels (recommended maintenance levels of 5–10 ng/mL). Usual starting dose is 0.15 mg/kg/d in divided doses.

■ Biologic agents
  ■ Polyclonal antibodies
    • **Antithymocyte globulin** is produced by injecting human thymocytes into animals and collecting sera. This generates antibodies against a wide variety of human immune system antigens. When subsequently infused into human patients, T lymphocytes are depleted as a result of complement-mediated lysis and clearance of antibody-coated cells by the reticuloendothelial system. Lymphocyte function is also disrupted by blocking and modulating the expression of cell surface molecules by the antibodies. Infusion is through a central vein over 4–6 hours. The most common side effects are fever, chills, and arthralgias. Other important adverse effects include myelosuppression, serum sickness, and, rarely, anaphylaxis. Two preparations are available: horse antithymocyte globulin (ATGAM) and rabbit antithymocyte globulin (Thymoglobulin). Current literature suggests that rabbit antithymocyte globulin is more efficacious. These drugs can be utilized at the time of transplantation to promote engraftment ("induction") or as a subsequent treatment for acute rejection. The long-term risk of increased malignancy, particularly lymphoma, remains a concern with these agents.
  ■ Monoclonal antibodies
    • **Anti–interleukin-2 receptor monoclonal antibodies.** Daclizumab (humanized) and basiliximab (chimeric) are monoclonal antibodies that competitively inhibit the alpha subunit of the interleukin-2 receptor (CD25) and thereby inhibit activation of T cells. Humanization and chimerization reduce the murine sequences of these genetically engineered antibodies, respectively. This results in antibodies with an extended half-life and minimizes the chances of developing human antimurine antibodies. These drugs are administered by a peripheral vein perioperatively at the time of transplantation and are associated with few side effects.
    • **OKT3** is a murine monoclonal antibody directed against the CD3 E chain associated with the T-cell receptor. It is administered as a bolus injection via a peripheral vein. OKT3 depletes $CD3^+$ T cells and modulates CD3 expression. The most common side effect is cytokine release syndrome, characterized by fever, chills, nausea, vomiting, diarrhea, myalgia, and, occasionally, hypotension and noncardiogenic pulmonary edema. Other side effects include encephalopathy, seizures, and aseptic meningitis. OKT3 is rarely used because of the efficacy and safety of newer agents.
    • **Alemtuzumab** is a monoclonal antibody against CD52, a molecule present on B and T cells. Subsequent antibody-mediated cell lysis occurs, causing lymphocyte depletion. Alemtuzumab has been utilized extensively in B-cell chronic lymphocytic leukemia and has been utilized off-label in transplantation as induction therapy. Its precise role is being investigated.

PROPHYLAXIS

■ **Immunization.** Pneumococcal and hepatitis B vaccination should be given at the time of pretransplant evaluation. Influenza A vaccination should be administered yearly. Live vaccines should be avoided after transplantation.[6]

- **Trimethoprim/sulfamethoxazole** prevents urinary tract infections, *Pneumocystis jiroveci* pneumonia, and *Nocardia* infections. The optimal dose and duration of prophylaxis have not been determined. In sulfa allergic patients, dapsone and aerosolized pentamidine are alternatives.
- **Acyclovir** prevents reactivation of herpes simplex virus (HSV) but is ineffective in cytomegalovirus (CMV) prophylaxis. HSV can be a serious infection in immunosuppressed individuals and some form of prophylaxis should be utilized during the first year. Patients with recurrent HSV infections (oral or genital) should be considered candidates for long-term prophylaxis. Lifetime acyclovir should also be used in Epstein-Barr virus (EBV)–seronegative patients who receive an EBV-positive organ.
- **Ganciclovir** or **valganciclovir** prevents CMV infection when administered to patients who were previously CMV seropositive or received a CMV-positive organ, or both. Typically, they are administered from 3 months to 12 months following transplantation. CMV hyperimmune globulin or IV ganciclovir can also be used for this purpose.
- **Fluconazole** or **ketoconazole** can be given to patients with a high risk of systemic fungal infections or recurrent localized fungal infections. Both medications increase cyclosporine and tacrolimus levels (see Immunosuppressive Medications). **Nystatin suspension, clotrimazole** troches, or weekly fluconazole are used to prevent oropharyngeal candidiasis (thrush).

PEARLS AND PITFALLS

Important drug interactions are always a concern given the polypharmacy associated with transplant patients. Before prescribing a new medication to a transplant recipient, always investigate drug interactions.

- The combination of allopurinol and azathioprine should be avoided or used cautiously due to the risk of profound myelosuppression.
- CsA is metabolized by cytochrome P-450 (3A4). Therefore, CsA levels are decreased by drugs that induce cytochrome P-450 activity, such as rifampin, isoniazid, barbiturates, phenytoin, and carbamazepine. Conversely, CsA levels are increased by drugs that compete for cytochrome P-450, such as verapamil, diltiazem, nicardipine, azole antifungals, erythromycin, and clarithromycin. Similar effects are seen with tacrolimus and sirolimus.
- Tacrolimus and CsA should not be taken together because of the increased risk of severe nephrotoxicity.
- Lower doses of MPA should be used when either tacrolimus or sirolimus is taken concurrently.
- Concomitant administration of CsA and sirolimus may result in a twofold increase in sirolimus levels; to avoid this drug interaction, CsA and sirolimus should be dosed 4 hours apart.

COMPLICATIONS

- Acute rejection
  - **Kidney** allograft rejection currently occurs in only 10% of patients and is defined as an immunologically mediated, acute deterioration in renal function associated with specific pathologic changes on renal biopsy including lymphocytic interstitial infiltrates, tubulitis, and arteritis. Patients who do not receive induction therapy have a 20%–30% incidence of acute rejection.
    - Most episodes of acute rejection occur in the first 6 months after transplantation. The low incidence of acute rejection today usually entails a careful search for inadequate drug levels, noncompliance, or unusual forms of rejection (antibody-mediated rejection). Late acute rejection (>1 year after transplantation) usually results from inadequate immunosuppression or patient noncompliance.

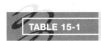

TABLE 15-1	Differential Diagnosis of Renal Allograft Dysfunction

<1 wk posttransplant	< 3 mo posttransplant	> 3 mo posttransplant
Acute tubular necrosis	Acute rejection	Prerenal azotemia
Hyperacute rejection	Calcineurin inhibitor toxicity	Calcineurin inhibitor toxicity
Accelerated rejection	Prerenal azotemia	Acute rejection (noncompliance, low levels)
Obstruction	Obstruction	Obstruction
Urine leak (ureteral necrosis)	Infection	Recurrent renal disease
Arterial or venous thrombosis	Interstitial nephritis	De novo renal disease
Atheroemboli	Recurrent renal disease	Renal artery stenosis (anastomotic or atherosclerotic)

- **Manifestations** include an elevated serum creatinine, decreased urine output, increased edema, or worsening hypertension. Initial symptoms are often absent except for the rise in creatinine. Constitutional symptoms (fever, malaise, arthralgia, painful or swollen allograft) are uncommon in current practice.
- **Differential diagnosis** varies with duration after transplantation (Table 15-1). Diagnosis of acute renal allograft rejection is made by percutaneous renal biopsy after excluding prerenal azotemia via hydration and repeating laboratory tests, calcineurin inhibitor nephrotoxicity (trough and/or peak levels and associated signs), infection (urinalysis and culture), and obstruction (renal ultrasound).
■ **Lung** transplant rejection occurs frequently and most commonly in the first few months after transplantation. The majority of patients have at least one episode of acute rejection. Multiple episodes of acute rejection predispose to the development of chronic rejection (bronchiolitis obliterans syndrome).
  - **Manifestations** are nonspecific and include fever, dyspnea, and a nonproductive cough. The chest radiograph is usually unchanged, and, if it is abnormal in the early phase of rejection, the findings are generally nondiagnostic (perihilar infiltrates, interstitial edema, pleural effusions). Abnormal pulmonary function testing is not specific for rejection, but a 10% or greater decline in forced vital capacity or forced expiratory volume in 1 second, or both, is usually clinically significant.
  - **Differential diagnosis.** It is important to attempt to distinguish rejection from infection, because the treatments are markedly different.
  - **Diagnosis** is generally made by fiberoptic bronchoscopy with bronchoalveolar lavage and transbronchial biopsies.
■ **Heart** transplant recipients typically have two to three episodes of acute rejection in the first year after transplantation with a 50%–80% chance of having at least one rejection episode, most commonly in the first 6 months.
  - **Manifestations** may include symptoms and signs of left ventricular dysfunction, such as dyspnea, paroxysmal nocturnal dyspnea, orthopnea, syncope, palpitations, new gallops, and elevated jugular venous pressure, but many patients are asymptomatic. Acute rejection may also be associated with a variety of tachyarrhythmias, atrial more often than ventricular.
  - **Diagnosis** is established by endomyocardial biopsy performed during routine surveillance or as prompted by symptoms. None of the noninvasive techniques has demonstrated sufficient sensitivity and specificity to replace the endomyocardial biopsy.
■ **Liver** transplant recipients commonly experience acute allograft rejection, with at least 60% having one episode. Acute rejection typically occurs within the first

3 months after transplant and often in the first 2 weeks after the operation. Acute rejection in the liver is generally reversible and does not portend a potentially serious adverse outcome as in other organs. Recurrent viral hepatitis is a much more frequent and morbid problem.

- **Manifestations** may be absent with only a slight elevation in transaminases, or the patients may have signs and symptoms of liver failure, including fever, malaise, anorexia, abdominal pain, ascites, decreased bile output, elevated bilirubin, and/or transaminases.
- **Differential diagnosis** of early liver allograft dysfunction includes primary graft nonfunction, preservation injury, vascular thrombosis, biliary anastomotic leak, or stenosis. These should be excluded clinically or by Doppler ultrasonography. Late allograft dysfunction may be due to rejection; recurrent hepatitis B or C, CMV, or EBV infection; cholestasis; or drug toxicity.
- **Diagnosis** is made by liver biopsy after technical complications are excluded.

■ **Treatment of acute allograft rejection** depends on the histologic severity (grade). Mild rejection of heart and lung transplants is often left untreated.

- First-line therapy for acute rejection usually consists of either pulse methylprednisolone or high-dose prednisone, with a 60%–80% response rate.
- Rejection that is more severe, recurrent, or refractory to glucocorticoid therapy is generally treated with antilymphocyte antibody preparations.
- Maintenance immunosuppressive agents are often added or substituted after an episode of acute rejection.

■ **Chronic allograft dysfunction** (formerly chronic rejection) is a slowly progressive, insidious decline in function of the allograft characterized by gradual vascular and ductal obliteration, parenchymal atrophy, and interstitial fibrosis. Diagnosis is often difficult and generally requires a biopsy. The process is mediated by immune and nonimmune factors. Chronic allograft dysfunction accounts for the vast majority of late graft losses and is the major obstacle to long-term graft survival. The manifestations of chronic rejection are unique to each organ system. To date, no effective therapy is available for established immune-mediated chronic allograft dysfunction. Current investigational strategies are aimed at prevention.

■ **Infections (Table 15-2)**[7]

  ■ **CMV infection** from reactivation of CMV in a seropositive recipient or new infection from a CMV-positive organ can lead to a wide range of presentations from a mild viral syndrome to allograft dysfunction, invasive disease in multiple organ systems, and even death. CMV-seronegative patients who receive a CMV-seropositive organ are at substantial risk, particularly in the first year. Because of the potential progression and severity of untreated disease, treatment is usually indicated in the transplant patient without tissue diagnosis of invasive disease. Shell-vial culture of the buffy coat is accurate only when plated within 24 hours of sample collection. Seroconversion with a positive immunoglobulin (Ig) M titer or a fourfold increase in IgM or IgG titer suggests acute infection; however, many centers now use polymerase chain reaction–based diagnostic techniques from blood samples, and treatment usually is administered in the patient with evidence of viral replication.[8]

- Treatment is with oral valganciclovir, 450–900 mg PO bid (adjusted for renal function) or IV ganciclovir, 2.5–5.0 mg/kg bid (adjusted for renal function), for 3–4 weeks. Hyperimmune globulin is often used in combination with ganciclovir for patients with organ involvement.
- Foscarnet and cidofovir are more toxic alternatives and should be reserved for ganciclovir-resistant cases.
- Prophylaxis during the highest incidence of severe CMV infection episodes (e.g., 3–12 months after transplantation in patients who are either seropositive or receive a seropositive organ) with oral ganciclovir (1,000 mg PO tid) or valganciclovir (450 mg daily) has markedly reduced the incidence of life-threatening CMV infections.
- Routine monitoring of CMV viremia in the blood followed by prompt preemptive treatment with valganciclovir has also been shown to be successful at preventing life-threatening CMV infections.

TABLE 15-2 Timing and Etiology of Posttransplant Infections

Time period	Infectious complication	Etiology
<1 mo posttransplant	Nosocomial pneumonia, wound infection, urinary tract infection, catheter-related sepsis	Bacterial or fungal infections
1–6 mo posttransplant	Opportunistic infections	Cytomegalovirus _Pneumocystis jiroveci_ _Aspergillus_ spp. _Toxoplasma gondii_ _Listeria monocytogenes_ West Nile virus Varicella-zoster virus
	Reactivation of pre-existing infections	_Mycobacteria_ spp. Endemic mycoses
>6 mo posttransplant	Community-acquired infections	Bacterial
	Chronic progressive infection	Hepatitis B Hepatitis C Cytomegalovirus Epstein-Barr virus Papillomavirus Polyoma virus (BK)
	Opportunistic infections	_P. jiroveci_ _L. monocytogenes_ _Nocardia asteroides_ _Cryptococcus neoformans_ _Aspergillus_ spp. West Nile virus

- **Hepatitis B and C.** Patients with active hepatitis or cirrhosis are not considered for nonhepatic transplantation. Immunosuppression increases viral replication in organ transplant recipients with either hepatitis B or C.
  - **Hepatitis B** can recur as fulminant hepatic failure even in patients with no evidence of viral DNA replication before transplantation. In liver transplantation, the risk of recurrent hepatitis B virus infection can be reduced by the administration of hepatitis B immunoglobulin during and after transplantation. Experience with lamivudine therapy initiated before transplantation to lower viral load has shown decreased likelihood of recurrent hepatitis B virus.
  - **Hepatitis C** typically progresses slowly in nonhepatic transplants, and the effect of immunosuppression remains to be determined on mortality due to liver disease. Treatment protocols for hepatitis C in the nonhepatic transplant population are not yet established. Hepatitis C nearly always recurs in liver transplant recipients whose original disease was due to hepatitis C. Therapy for recurrent hepatitis C virus with a combination of ribavirin and interferon results in histopathologic improvement of disease, although dosage and duration of therapy remain controversial.
- **EBV** plays a role in the development of posttransplant lymphoproliferative disease. This life-threatening lymphoma is treated by withdrawal or reduction in immunosuppression and often aggressive chemotherapy (see Long-Term Complications of Transplantation).

■ The role of newly discovered **viral agents** such as HHV-6, HHV-7, HHV-8, and polyoma (BK and JC) virus after transplantation remains to be established, although BK virus is known to cause interstitial nephritis resulting in renal allograft loss.

■ **Fungal and parasitic infections,** such as *Cryptococcus*, *Mucor*, aspergillosis, and *Candida* species, result in increased mortality after transplantation and should be aggressively diagnosed and treated. The role of prophylaxis with oral fluconazole has not been established.

Long-Term Complications of Transplantation

■ Cardiovascular complications
- **Hypertension** occurs in up to 80% of renal transplant patients and to a lesser degree in other solid organ transplant recipients. Blood pressure (BP) should be monitored and maintained below 130/80. Certain calcium channel blockers significantly increase CsA and tacrolimus levels and drug levels should be carefully monitored. Angiotensin-converting enzyme inhibitors should usually be avoided in the early posttransplant period because of the potential for increased nephrotoxicity when patients are receiving high doses of cyclosporine or tacrolimus. However, these agents may be renoprotective in the long term. When suspected, anastomotic or atherosclerotic renal artery stenosis should be excluded.
- **Coronary heart disease.** Graft atherosclerosis in cardiac allografts is partially immunologic in nature. Cardiac disease is the leading cause of death in renal transplant recipients and should be screened aggressively before transplantation, with aggressive modification of risk factors after transplantation.

■ Endocrine and metabolic complications
- **Obesity** is a common problem in the late posttransplant period, with average weight gains in excess of 40 lb by 1 year. The approach should be multidisciplinary and include dietary and exercise counseling. Most medications that promote weight loss, however, impair BP control. Most studies show that withdrawal of steroids has little impact on weight reduction, thus emphasizing lifestyle as a key component to controlling obesity after transplant.
- **Hyperlipidemia** occurs in as many as 60% of solid organ transplant recipients. Elevated lipid levels may be related to medications (glucocorticoids, CsA, thiazides), comorbidity, and genetic factors. Hyperlipidemia is associated with cardiovascular disease and may also have a role in chronic allograft vasculopathy. Dietary intervention alone is often insufficient to achieve a therapeutic target, and treatment should follow the National Cholesterol Education Program guidelines.
- **Diabetes mellitus.** Glucocorticoids, calcineurin inhibitors, and obesity all contribute to diabetes after transplantation. Tacrolimus may have a higher incidence of diabetes versus cyclosporine (approximately 20% vs. 5%, respectively). Patients should be screened with fasting plasma glucose levels as recommended by the American Diabetes Association.
- **Bone disease.** Avascular necrosis and steroid-induced osteoporosis can be disabling, leading to multiple fractures and often requiring joint replacement. Bone densitometry at regular intervals monitors osteopenia, although cortical bone loss can occur rapidly within the first months of high-dose glucocorticoid therapy. Transplant recipients should be in positive calcium balance with calcium supplementation (calcium carbonate, 1,000–1,500 mg/d between meals or at bedtime). Vitamin D insufficiency should be treated (25 hydroxy vitamin D levels <30 pg/mL). Vitamin D supplements, calcitonin, and bisphosphonates have been used in transplant recipients. Secondary hyperparathyroidism must be excluded in all patients with renal impairment or previous renal failure.

■ **Renal disease.** Chronic allograft dysfunction is the leading cause of allograft loss in renal transplant recipients. Calcineurin inhibitor (CsA or tacrolimus) nephrotoxicity or recurrent native disease may also develop in these patients. Chronic calcineurin inhibitor nephrotoxicity may also lead to chronic renal insufficiency and end-stage renal disease (ESRD), requiring dialysis or transplantation in recipients of lung, heart, liver, or pancreas transplants. The incidence of ESRD secondary to calcineurin inhibitor toxicity in recipients of solid organ transplants is at least 10%, and the incidence of significant chronic kidney disease approaches 50%.[9]

- **Malignancy** occurs in transplant patients with an overall incidence that is threefold to fourfold higher than that seen in the general population (age matched). Some cancers occur at the same rate, whereas other neoplasms have a much higher frequency than normal. The spontaneous malignancies that occur most frequently in transplant recipients include cancers of the skin and lips, lymphoproliferative disease, bronchogenic carcinoma, Kaposi sarcoma, uterine/cervical carcinoma, renal cell carcinoma, and anogenital neoplasms.[10]
    - **Skin and lip cancers** are the most common malignancies (40%–50%) seen in transplant recipients, with an incidence 10–250 times that of the general population. Risk factors include immunosuppression, ultraviolet radiation, and human papillomavirus infection. These cancers develop at a younger age, and they are more aggressive in transplant patients than in the general population. Using protective clothing and sunscreens and avoiding sun exposure are recommended. Examination of the skin is the principal screening test, and early diagnosis offers the best prognosis.
    - **Posttransplant lymphoproliferative disease** accounts for one-fifth of all malignancies after transplantation, with an incidence of approximately 1%. This is 30- to 50-fold higher than in the general population, and the risk increases with the use of antilymphocyte therapy for induction or rejection. The majority of these neoplasms are large-cell non-Hodgkin lymphomas of the B-cell type. Posttransplant lymphoproliferative disease results from EBV-induced B-cell proliferation in the setting of chronic immunosuppression. The presentation is often atypical and should always be considered in the patient with new symptoms. Diagnosis requires a high index of suspicion followed by a tissue biopsy. Treatment includes reduction or withdrawal of immunosuppression and chemotherapy.

SPECIAL CONSIDERATIONS

Evaluation of the Transplant Patient with Medical Problems

- The evaluation of the transplant recipient with general medical or surgical problems should always encompass the details of the patient's organ transplant and treatment. Thus, the following should always be reviewed when taking a history from an organ transplant recipient:
    - Cause of organ failure
    - Treatment for organ failure prior to transplantation
    - Type and date of transplant
    - CMV status of donor and recipient
    - Initial immunosuppression, particularly use of antibody-based induction therapy
    - Initial function of transplant (e.g., nadir creatinine, FEV_1, ejection fraction, synthetic function and transaminases, etc.)
    - Current function of allograft
    - Complications of transplantation (surgical problems, acute rejection, infections, chronic organ dysfunction, etc.)
    - Current immunosuppression regimen and recent drug levels

References

1. Primer on Transplantation, 2nd ed. Norman DA and Turka LA, (Eds). Blackwell Publishing, Malden, MA, 2001.
2. Halloran PF. Immunosuppressive durgs for kidney transplantation. *N Engl J Med* 2004;351:2715–2729.
3. Miller BW, Brennan DC. Maintenance immunosuppressive therapy in renal transplantation in adults. In: UpToDate, Rose BD (Ed), UptoDate, Waltham, MA 2006.
4. Rhen T, Cidlowski JA. Antiinflammatory action of glucocorticoids-new mechanisms for old drugs. *N Engl J Med* 2005;353:1711–1723.

5. Miller BW, Brennan DC. Withdrawal or avoidance of corticosteroids after renal transplantation. In: UptoDate, Rose BD (Ed), UptoDate, Waltham, MA 2006.
6. Guidelines for vaccination of solid organ transplant candidates and recipients. *Am J Transplant* 2004;4(sup10):160–163.
7. Fishman JA, Rubin RH. Infection in organ-transplant receipients. *N Engl J Med* 1998;338:1741–1751.
8. Brennan DC. Cytomegalovirus in renal transplantation. *J Am Soc Nephrol* 2001;12:848–855.
9. Ojo AO, Held PJ, Port FK, et al. Chronic renal failure after transplantation of a non-renal organ. *N Engl J Med* 2003;349:931–940.
10. Penn I. Cancers complicating organ transplantation. *N Engl J Med* 1990;323:1767–1769.

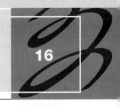
 GASTROINTESTINAL BLEEDING

GENERAL PRINCIPLES

Definitions

- Gastrointestinal (GI) bleeding may manifest as passage of bright or altered blood with emesis or bowel movements. Acute GI bleeding typically presents with overt blood loss that can be readily recognized by the patient or treating physician.
- **Overt GI bleeding** is the passage of fresh or altered blood in emesis or in the stool.
- **Occult bleeding** refers to a positive fecal occult blood test (stool guaiac) or iron-deficiency anemia without visible blood in the stool.
- **Obscure bleeding** consists of GI blood loss of unknown origin that persists or recurs after negative initial endoscopic evaluation; obscure bleeding can be either overt or occult.

    The following segments refer primarily to overt bleeding.

DIAGNOSIS

Clinical Presentation

- **Hematemesis,** coffee-ground emesis, and aspiration of blood or coffee grounds from a nasogastric (NG) tube suggest an upper GI source of blood loss.
- **Melena,** black sticky stool with a characteristic odor, indicates an upper GI source of blood loss, although small-bowel and sometimes right colonic bleeds can result in melena.
- Various shades of red blood are seen in the stool with distal small-bowel or colonic bleeding, depending on the rate of blood loss and colonic transit.
- **Bleeding from the anorectal area** typically results in bright blood coating the exterior of formed stool, sometimes associated with distal colonic symptoms (e.g., rectal urgency, straining or pain with defecation).
- Although patients with **upper GI bleeding** can also present with red blood in their stool, this is almost invariably associated with hemodynamic compromise and circulatory shock.
- **Other symptoms** may include fatigue, weakness, abdominal pain, pallor, or dyspnea.
- Estimation of **amount of blood lost** can be attempted, but is often inaccurate. If the baseline hematocrit is known, the drop in hematocrit provides a rough estimate of blood loss. In general, patients with lower GI bleeding have less hemodynamic compromise compared to those with upper GI bleeding.
- **Emesis** preceding upper GI bleeding may suggest a Mallory-Weiss tear.
- **Hypotension** and hypovolemic shock preceding the bleeding episode may suggest ischemic colitis.
- **Radiation therapy** to the prostate or pelvis suggests radiation proctopathy, and prior aortic graft surgery raises suspicion of an aortoenteric or aortocolonic fistula.

439

- **Chronic constipation** may suggest bleeding from stercoral (stool-induced) ulceration of the rectum.
- Recent **polypectomy** may indicate postpolypectomy bleeding.
- Chronic renal disease may be associated with GI angiodysplasia, while patients with hereditary hemorrhagic telangiectasia can have GI telangiectasia as a source for blood loss.
- **Coagulation abnormalities** can propagate bleeding from a pre-existing lesion in the GI tract. Disorders of coagulation, such as liver disease, von Willebrand disease, vitamin K deficiency, and disseminated intravascular coagulation can influence the course of GI bleeding (see Chapter 18, Disorders of Hemostasis).
- **Medications** known to affect the coagulation process include warfarin, heparin, aspirin, nonsteroidal anti-inflammatory drugs (NSAIDs), clopidogrel (Plavix), and thrombolytic agents. Newer antithrombotic agents can also propagate bleeding and include glycoprotein IIb/IIIa receptor antagonists (abciximab [ReoPro], eptifibatide [Integrilin], tirofiban [Aggrastat]) (see Chapter 5, Ischemic Heart Disease) and direct thrombin inhibitors (argatroban, bivalirudin). NSAIDs and aspirin can result in mucosal damage anywhere in the GI tract.

Physical Examination

- **Color of stool.** Direct examination of spontaneously passed stool or stool obtained during a digital rectal examination can provide important clues as to the level of bleeding. In addition to assessing the color of stool, a **digital rectal** examination may identify a potential source of bleeding in the anorectum. Anal fissures, typically seen in the posterior midline, can result in extreme pain during a rectal examination.
- **NG aspiration.** An NG aspirate is useful in the diagnosis of upper GI bleeding. Hemoccult testing of a normal-appearing NG aspirate is of no clinical utility; the aspirate should be considered positive only if blood or dark particulate matter ("coffee grounds") is seen. Gastric lavage with water or saline may be useful in assessing the activity and severity of upper GI bleeding and in clearing the stomach of blood and clots before endoscopic examination. After a diagnosis of upper GI bleeding is made, the NG tube is not required further in a stable patient, especially if endoscopy is to follow. In a small fraction of patients, a bleeding source in the duodenum can result in a negative NG aspirate.
- **Intravascular volume and hemodynamic status.** Constant monitoring or frequent assessment of vital signs is necessary early in the evaluation, as a sudden increase in pulse rate or decrease in blood pressure (BP) may be an early indicator of recurrent or ongoing blood loss.
- If the baseline BP and pulse are within normal limits, sitting the patient up or having the patient stand may result in **orthostatic hemodynamic changes** (drop in systolic BP of >10 mm Hg, rise in pulse rate of >15 bpm). Orthostatic changes in pulse and BP are seen with loss of 10%–20% of the circulatory volume; supine hypotension suggests a >20% loss. Hypotension with a systolic blood pressure of <100 mm Hg or baseline tachycardia suggests significant hemodynamic compromise that requires urgent volume resuscitation.

Laboratory Studies

- Complete blood count
- **Coagulation parameters** (prothrombin time, partial thromboplastin time, platelet count)
- **Blood group, cross matching** of 2–4 units of blood
- Comprehensive chemical profile (including liver function tests, serum creatinine)

MANAGEMENT

- **Restoration of intravascular volume.** Two large-bore IV lines with 14- to 18-gauge catheters or a central venous line should be urgently placed. Isotonic saline, lactated Ringer solution, or 5% hetastarch can be initiated; patients in shock may require volume administration using pressure infusion devices or hand infused using large syringes and stopcocks. **Packed red blood cell (RBC) transfusion** should be used for volume replacement whenever possible; O-negative blood or simultaneous multiple-unit transfusions may be indicated if bleeding is massive. Transfusion should be continued until hemodynamic stability is achieved and the hematocrit reaches ≥25%; patients with cardiac or pulmonary disease may require transfusion to a hematocrit of ≥30%. The rate of volume infusion should be guided by the patient's condition and the rate and degree of volume loss. Vasopressors are generally not indicated, although transient IV pressor therapy is sometimes beneficial until enough volume is infused.

■ **Correction of coagulopathy.** Discontinuation of anticoagulant, if possible, followed by infusion of fresh frozen plasma (FFP) can be used to correct prolonged coagulation parameters from warfarin. An initial infusion of 2–4 units of FFP can be supplemented with further infusion based on reassessment of the coagulation parameters. Parenteral vitamin K (10 mg SC or IM) may be indicated for prolonged prothrombin time from warfarin therapy or hepatobiliary disease but takes several hours to days for adequate reversal; it should be repeated daily for a total of three doses in hepatobiliary disease. Protamine infusion (1 mg antagonizes ∼100 units of heparin) can be used for immediate reversal of anticoagulation from heparin infusion. Platelet infusion may be indicated when the platelet count is <50,000/mm^3.

■ **Airway protection.** Endotracheal intubation to prevent aspiration should be considered when altered mental status (shock, hepatic encephalopathy), massive hematemesis, or active variceal hemorrhage is present.

Specific Tests for Localizing and Treating the Bleeding Source

■ Endoscopy
  ■ **Esophagogastroduodenoscopy (EGD)** is the preferred method of investigation and therapy of upper GI bleeding and is associated with high diagnostic accuracy, therapeutic capability, and low morbidity. Volume resuscitation or blood transfusion should precede endoscopy in hemodynamically unstable patients. Patients with ongoing bleeding benefit most from urgent EGD, while stable patients with minimal bleeding (e.g. "coffee ground" emesis with stable hematocrit) can have the procedure performed electively during the hospitalization.
  ■ Early **colonoscopy** can be performed after a rapid bowel purge in patients whose condition has clinically stabilized and who can tolerate an adequate bowel purge. The yield of finding a potential bleeding source in the colon is greatest if colonoscopy is performed within the initial 24 hours of presentation.
    • Patients unable to drink adequate amounts of the balanced electrolyte solution can have an NG tube placed for infusion of the bowel purge. All patients with acute lower GI bleeding from an unknown source should eventually undergo endoscopic evaluation of the colon during the initial hospitalization, regardless of the initial mode of investigation. Although early diagnostic endoscopy does not reduce mortality, therapeutic endoscopy reduces transfusion requirements, need for surgery, and length of hospital stay.
  ■ **Anoscopy** may be useful in the detection of internal hemorrhoids and anal fissures. In an outpatient or emergency room setting, **anoscopy** and **sigmoidoscopy** may be useful in rapid diagnosis of the level of bleeding before patient triage, but is usually followed by colonoscopy after bowel preparation.
  ■ **Push enteroscopy** allows evaluation of the proximal small bowel if a bleeding source is not seen within reach of a standard upper endoscope, especially if the colon has been excluded as a bleeding source by careful colonoscopy.

■ **Tagged red blood cell (TRBC) scanning.** RBCs labeled with technetium-99m remain in circulation for as long as 48 hours and extravasate into the bowel lumen with active bleeding. This extravasation can be detected as pooling of the radioactive tracer on gamma camera scanning. The pattern of peristaltic movement of the pooled tracer can help identify the potential site of bleeding.
  ■ A positive TRBC scan identifies patients likely to require invasive intervention and with high in-hospital morbidity, while a negative test may imply a better short-term prognosis. However, the scan is only positive 45% of the time. When positive, it

is accurate in identification of the location of the bleeding source in 80% of cases. The false localization rate of approximately 20% precludes use of this test alone in directing surgical resection of the bleeding bowel segment. Therefore, the clinical utility of this test is for assessing location and intensity of bleeding before more invasive tests are performed, especially in patients who demonstrate evidence of ongoing active bleeding.

- **Arteriography** allows rapid localization and potential therapy of GI bleeding by demonstrating extravasation of the dye into the intestine when bleeding rates exceed 0.5 mL/min.
  - Arteriography may also identify the bleeding lesion, especially bleeding diverticula or angiodysplasia. A tumor blush or a late draining vein of angiodysplasia may be seen even in the absence of active bleeding.
  - When an actively bleeding lesion is found during angiography, intra-arterial infusion of vasopressin can cause vasoconstriction and stop bleeding. Superselective cannulation and embolization of the bleeding artery is sometimes performed.
  - In upper GI bleeding, arteriography is reserved for situations where brisk bleeding makes endoscopy difficult.
  - In small-bowel or lower GI bleeding, arteriography is utilized for both diagnosis and therapy of the bleeding lesion, typically after initial localization with TRBC scanning. Immediate or early extravasation on TRBC scanning carries the greatest likelihood of a positive arteriogram.
  - In stable patients with recurrent, difficult-to-localize GI bleeding, infusion of anticoagulants (e.g., heparin), thrombolytic agents (e.g., streptokinase), or intra-arterial vasodilators in a controlled fashion may increase the diagnostic yield of angiography. These provocative measures can be associated with excessive bleeding and should only be used in specialized centers in stable patients without comorbid illnesses.
- **Capsule endoscopy.** A tiny camera, a light source, and a transmitter sealed in a biocompatible capsule resistant to digestive juices collect 50,000 images over 8 hours, mostly from the small bowel. This technique is most useful after the upper gut and the colon have been thoroughly examined, and the bleeding source is expected in the small bowel. Disadvantages are that the images cannot be viewed in real time, exact localization within the small bowel cannot be pinpointed, and therapy cannot be administered.
- **Intraoperative enteroscopy.** When an actively bleeding source is identified within the small bowel, endoscopic therapy or surgical intervention can be facilitated by performing intraoperative enteroscopy. The surgeon, through an abdominal incision, advances the endoscope (inserted either through the mouth, the anus, or an enterotomy) by pleating bowel over the instrument.
- **Double balloon enteroscopy.** This is a new technique that allows visualization of most of the small bowel, using a special endoscope with an overtube. Balloons at the endoscope tip and the overtube can be consecutively inflated and deflated while inserting and pulling out the endoscope to allow bowel to pleat over the overtube, thus allowing deep endoscope insertion into the small bowel, either through the mouth or the anus. This procedure is only available in advanced centers.

Medications

- **Nonvariceal upper GI bleeding**
  - Intravenous proton pump inhibitors (PPIs) or high-dose PPIs administered orally (e.g., omeprazole, 40 mg PO bid) reduce the rate of recurrent bleeding and the need for surgery in patients with upper GI bleeding awaiting endoscopic treatment or if endoscopy is contraindicated or postponed; mortality is reduced in peptic ulcer bleeding, but not other causes of upper GI bleeding. Conventional oral doses of PPIs may suffice after endoscopic therapy has been administered. PPI therapy, oral or IV, is better than IV histamine-2 receptor antagonist (H_2RA) therapy in bleeding peptic ulcers.
- **Variceal bleeding**
  - When variceal bleeding is suspected, **octreotide** infusion should be initiated immediately (50- to 100-mcg bolus, followed by infusion at 25–50 mcg/hr). Octreotide infusion acutely reduces portal pressures and controls variceal bleeding with very few

side effects, improving the diagnostic yield and therapeutic success of subsequent endoscopy.

- **Vasopressin (0.3 units/min IV, titrated by increments of 0.1 units/min q30min until hemostasis is achieved, side effects develop, or the maximum dose of 0.9 units/min is reached)** is an alternative agent, rarely used because of significant cardiovascular complications including cardiac arrest and myocardial infarction. Concomitant infusion of **nitroglycerin** may reduce undesirable cardiovascular side effects and provide more effective control of bleeding. Nitroglycerin is administered only if the systolic BP is >100 mm Hg, at a dose of 10 mcg/min IV, increased by 10 mcg/min q10–15min until the systolic BP falls to 100 mm Hg or a maximum dose of 400 mcg/min is reached.

Endoscopic Therapy

- **Therapeutic endoscopy** offers the advantage of immediate treatment and should be implemented in all patients early in the hospital course (within 24 hours). Fluid resuscitation and hemodynamic stability are essential before endoscopy. Administration of promotility agents such as metoclopramide (10 mg IV) or erythromycin (150–250 mg IV) may accelerate gastric emptying, and thereby help clear the stomach of blood or clots prior to endoscopy in patients with significant or ongoing bleeding.
- **Variceal ligation** or **banding** is the endoscopic therapy of choice for esophageal varices. **Intensive care unit (ICU) admission** and **endotracheal intubation** for airway protection should be considered when active bleeding from varices is suspected. It is effective in controlling active hemorrhage and achieves variceal eradication rapidly, with lower rates of rebleeding and fewer complications compared to sclerotherapy. Complications of banding include superficial ulceration, dysphagia, transient chest discomfort, and, rarely, esophageal strictures.
- **Sclerotherapy** is also effective but is used less frequently because of complications (ulcerations, strictures, perforation, pleural effusions, adult respiratory distress syndrome, sepsis). Recurrent bleeding may be seen in up to 50% of patients but usually responds to repeat sclerotherapy. Fever may be seen in 40% of patients within the first 2 days of therapy; fever that lasts longer than 2 days should prompt investigation for bacteremia.

Other Therapy

- **Transjugular intrahepatic portosystemic shunt (TIPS)** is a radiologic procedure wherein an expandable metal stent is deployed between the hepatic veins and the portal vein to decompress the portal system and reduce portal venous pressure. Indications include refractory variceal bleeding unresponsive to variceal ligation or sclerotherapy, and bleeding from gastric varices in the setting of portal hypertension. Encephalopathy may occur in up to 25% of patients but is usually controlled with medical therapy (see Complications of Hepatic Insufficiency, Chapter 17, Liver Diseases). Shunt stenosis is another significant complication that may respond to balloon dilation. Screening for shunt stenosis with duplex Doppler ultrasound is recommended if the patient redevelops variceal bleeding or has recurrence of esophageal or gastric varices on endoscopy.

Surgery

- **Emergent total colectomy** may rarely be required as a lifesaving maneuver for massive, unlocalized, colonic bleeding; this should be preceded by emergent EGD to rule out a rapidly bleeding upper source whenever possible. Certain lesions (e.g., neoplasia, Meckel's diverticulum) require surgical resection for a cure.
- **Splenectomy** is curative in bleeding gastric varices from splenic vein thrombosis. Ongoing bleeding with transfusion requirements exceeding 4–6 units over 24 hours or 10 units overall, or more than two to three recurrent bleeding episodes from the same source have been considered indications for surgery.
- **Shunt surgery** (portacaval or distal splenorenal shunt) should be considered in patients with good hepatic reserve if the patient (a) fails endoscopic or pharmacologic therapy, (b) is unable to return for follow-up visits, (c) is at high risk of death from recurrent

bleeding because of cardiac disease or difficulty in obtaining blood products, or (d) lives far from medical care. Although bleeding may be controlled in 95% of cases, hospital death rates are high, and there is a significant incidence of postoperative encephalopathy, especially among patients with higher grades of Child's classification (see Chapter 17, Table 17-5).

 ESOPHAGEAL DISORDERS

GASTROESOPHAGEAL REFLUX DISEASE

General Principles

Definition

- Gastroesophageal reflux disease (GERD) is defined as symptoms or tissue damage resulting from reflux of gastric acid into the esophagus and more proximal structures.

Diagnosis

Clinical Presentation

- The predominant symptoms of GERD are heartburn and regurgitation.
- **Atypical symptoms** include cough, asthma, hoarseness, chest pain, hiccups, and dental erosions.
- Symptom response to a therapeutic trial of PPIs can be diagnostic.

Endoscopy

- Endoscopic evaluation is recommended for patients with **warning symptoms** of dysphagia, odynophagia, early satiety, weight loss, or bleeding, and **atypical symptoms** (cough, asthma, hoarseness, chest pain, aphthous ulcers, hiccups, dental erosions).
- Patients with symptoms refractory to empiric acid suppression or requiring continuous medication for prolonged periods should also undergo endoscopy.
- Ambulatory pH monitoring is used to establish elevated esophageal acid exposure and symptom-reflux correlation in patients with ongoing symptoms despite acid suppression (especially if endoscopy is negative) or those with atypical symptoms. It is also used to determine adequacy of acid suppression in patients with established GERD and ongoing symptoms.

Management

Lifestyle Modification

- The basics of **lifestyle modification** include eating small meals; refraining from eating for 2–3 hours before lying down; elevating the head of the bed 4–6 in.; decreasing intake of fatty foods, chocolate, coffee, cola, and alcohol; and smoking cessation.
- Lifestyle modification also includes **avoiding medications** such as calcium channel blockers, theophylline, sedatives/tranquilizers, and anticholinergics, as they may potentiate reflux.
- Lifestyle modifications alone are unlikely to resolve symptoms in the majority of GERD patients, but should be recommended in conjunction with medications.

Medications

- In patients with mild or intermittent symptoms, over-the-counter **antacids** and **H_2RAs** can be used intermittently or prophylactically if necessary.
- PPIs have been demonstrated to be more effective than placebo or standard-dose H_2RA in symptomatic relief as well as endoscopic healing of GERD. Higher doses (omeprazole, 20–40 mg PO bid or equivalent) may be required in severe esophagitis or persistent symptoms. Continuous long-term PPI therapy is safe and effective in maintaining remission of GERD symptoms, and is recommended for patients with erosive esophagitis, Barrett's esophagus, and severe symptoms.

■ Standard doses of **H₂RAs** (Table 16-1) can result in symptomatic benefit in up to 60% of patients and endoscopic healing in 50%. Higher doses of H₂RAs (equivalent to ranitidine, 600 mg daily) improve the healing rate to 75% at a higher cost. Dosage adjustments are required in renal insufficiency.

Surgery
■ Indications for **fundoplication** include the need for continuous or increasing doses of medication in patients who are good surgical candidates. Patients who require aggressive long-term medical therapy should be offered the surgical option. Other indications include patient preference for surgery and noncompliance with medical therapy.
  ■ The success rate of laparoscopic fundoplication in controlling GERD symptoms exceeds 90%, with fewer complications compared to the open technique. Elevated esophageal acid exposure and correlation of symptoms to reflux events on ambulatory pH monitoring predict a higher likelihood of a successful outcome.
  ■ Patients with medical treatment failures need careful evaluation to determine whether symptoms are indeed related to acid reflux before surgical options are considered; these patients often have other diagnoses including visceral hypersensitivity and functional heartburn.

Complications
■ Esophageal ulceration and stricture formation can occur in patients with GERD. Iron-deficiency anemia is less common.
■ GERD can contribute to laryngitis, laryngeal ulcers, asthma, and dental caries.
■ Barrett's esophagus is a change in the esophageal mucosa from normal squamous epithelium to specialized intestinal metaplastic epithelium due to longstanding acid related injury. It carries a small risk of progression to esophageal adenocarcinoma. Endoscopic surveillance for Barrett's esophagus should be considered in patients with a symptom history that exceeds 5 years.

Differential Diagnosis
Other disorders that can result in esophagitis include:

| **TABLE 16-1** | **Dosage of Acid-Suppressive Agents** |

Medication therapy	Peptic ulcer disease	GERD	Parenteral
Cimetidine[a]	300 mg qid 400 mg bid 800 mg at bedtime	400 mg qid 800 mg bid	300 mg q6h
Ranitidine[a]	150 mg bid 300 mg at bedtime	150–300 mg bid–qid	50 mg q8h
Famotidine[a]	20 mg bid 40 mg at bedtime	20–40 mg bid	20 mg q12h
Nizatidine[a]	150 mg bid 300 mg at bedtime	150 mg bid	
Omeprazole	20 mg daily	20–40 mg daily–bid	
Esomeprazole	40 mg daily	20–40 mg daily–bid	20–40 mg q24h
Lansoprazole	15–30 mg daily	15–30 mg daily–bid	30 mg q12–24h
Pantoprazole	20 mg daily	20–40 mg daily–bid	40 mg q12–24h or 80 mg IV, then 8 mg/hr infusion

GERD, gastroesophageal reflux disease.
[a]Dosage adjustment required in renal insufficiency.

Eosinophilic Esophagitis

■ Eosinophilic esophagitis is an idiopathic disorder characterized by eosinophilic infiltration of the esophageal mucosa, resulting in mucosal changes (furrows, corrugations, whitish plaques) as well as luminal narrowing (narrow-caliber esophagus, strictures, solid food dysphagia). Food antigens are thought to play a role in the pathogenesis. The diagnosis should be suspected in young men with solid food dysphagia, episodes of food impaction, or reflux symptoms not responsive to maximal antisecretory therapy. Mucosal biopsies during endoscopy will demonstrate marked eosinophilic infiltration. Management includes topical and systemic corticosteroids, leukotriene receptor antagonists, elimination diets, and cautious dilation of tight strictures.

Infectious Esophagitis

■ Infectious esophagitis is seen most often in immunocompromised states (AIDS, organ transplant recipients), esophageal stasis (abnormal motility [e.g., achalasia, scleroderma]; mechanical obstruction [e.g., strictures]), malignancy, diabetes mellitus, and antibiotic use. However, herpes simplex virus (HSV) and varicella esophagitis can occur in the normal healthy host. The presence of typical oral lesions (thrush, herpetic vesicles) may suggest an etiologic agent. The usual presenting symptoms are dysphagia and odynophagia.

   ■ *Candida* **esophagitis** results from fungal overgrowth of the esophagus, impaired cell-mediated immunity, or both. Fungal overgrowth typically occurs in the setting of esophageal stasis, impaired cell-mediated immunity from immunosuppressive therapy (e.g., with steroids or cytotoxic agents), malignancies, or AIDS. Chronic mucocutaneous candidiasis is a congenital immunodeficiency state that is also associated with *Candida* esophagitis.

   ■ Symptomatic relief can be achieved with 2% viscous **lidocaine** swish and swallow (15 mL PO q3–4h PRN) or **sucralfate** slurry (1 g PO qid). Concomitant acid suppression should also be administered.

   ■ **Fluconazole** 100–200 mg/d or **itraconazole** 200 mg/d for 14–21 days is recommended as initial therapy for *Candida* esophagitis. For infections refractory to azoles, a short course of parenteral **amphotericin B** (0.3–0.5 mg/kg/d) should be considered.

   ■ **HSV** esophagitis can be treated with **acyclovir** 400–800 mg PO five times a day for 14–21 days or 5 mg/kg IV q8h for 7–14 days. **Famciclovir** and **valacyclovir** are alternate agents.

   ■ IV therapy with **ganciclovir**, **foscarnet**, or **cidofovir** are all effective for a variety of GI cytomegalovirus (CMV) infections in immunocompromised hosts (see Chapter 15, Solid Organ Transplant Medicine). **Ganciclovir** 5 mg/kg IV q12h or **foscarnet** 90 mg/kg IV q12h for 3–6 weeks can be used as initial therapy. Oral **valganciclovir** may also be effective.

Chemical Esophagitis

■ Ingestion of caustic agents (alkalis, acids) or medications such as oral potassium, doxycycline, quinidine, iron, NSAIDs, aspirin, and bisphosphonates can result in mucosal irritation and damage.

■ Cautious early endoscopy is recommended to evaluate the extent and degree of mucosal damage. With caustic ingestions, the optimal time to perform endoscopy is 24–72 hours from ingestion.

■ The offending medication should be discontinued if possible. Mucosal coating agents (sucralfate) and acid suppressive agents may help. A second caustic agent to neutralize the first is contraindicated.

Nonspecific Ulceration. Nonspecific ulceration can be seen with medications, malignancy, or AIDS (idiopathic ulcer).

■ Multiple biopsies, brushings, and culture specimens should be obtained at endoscopy.

■ Idiopathic ulcer of AIDS may respond to oral steroid or thalidomide therapy.

■ Concomitant acid suppression should always be administered.

ACHALASIA

General Principles

Definition
- **Achalasia** is the most easily recognized motor disorder of the esophagus, characterized by failure of the lower esophageal sphincter (LES) to relax completely with swallowing and aperistalsis of the esophageal body.

Diagnosis

Clinical Presentation
- Presenting symptoms can include dysphagia, regurgitation, chest pain, weight loss, and aspiration pneumonia.

Objective Testing
- **Esophageal manometry** is the gold standard for diagnosis. The characteristic findings include a nonrelaxing LES and aperistalsis of the esophageal body.
- **Barium radiographs** may demonstrate a typical appearance of a dilated intrathoracic esophagus with impaired emptying, an air–fluid level, absence of gastric air bubble, and tapering of the distal esophagus with the appearance of a bird's beak.
- **Endoscopy** may help exclude a stricture or neoplasia of the distal esophagus; the esophageal body may be dilated and contain food debris, whereas the LES, although pinpoint, typically allows passage of the endoscope into the stomach with minimal resistance.

Treatment

Medications
- **Smooth muscle relaxants** such as nitrates or calcium channel blockers administered immediately before meals may afford short-lived symptom relief. Overall, **medications are not very effective** and are only indicated as temporizing measures.
- **Botulinum toxin** injection into the LES at endoscopy can result in relief of achalasia symptoms that can last several weeks to months. This approach may be useful in elderly and frail patients who are poor surgical risks or as a bridge to more definitive therapy. Botulinum toxin injection may induce fibrosis in the region of the LES, making subsequent surgery more cumbersome.

Surgery
- Disruption of the circular muscle of the LES using **pneumatic dilation** can result in lasting reduction of LES pressure and symptomatic relief. Gastroesophageal reflux can result, treated with lifelong acid suppression. Esophageal perforation occurs in 3%–5%, requiring prompt surgical repair.
- A **surgical (Heller) myotomy** offers good efficacy and lasting symptom relief. It can be performed laparoscopically with minimal complications. Laparoscopic myotomy is typically combined with an antireflux procedure to prevent symptoms from acid reflux.

Complications
- Complications include aspiration pneumonia and weight loss.
- Achalasia is associated with a 0.15% risk of squamous cell cancer of the distal esophagus, a 33-fold higher risk relative to the nonachalasic population.

DIFFUSE ESOPHAGEAL SPASM

General Principles

Definition
- Diffuse esophageal spasm is a spastic disorder characterized by simultaneous, nonperistaltic contractions in the esophageal body.
- Concomitant incomplete LES relaxation may be present. The major symptoms are dysphagia and chest pain.

Diagnosis

- **Esophageal manometry** is essential for diagnosis.
- **Barium studies** may show a beaded or "corkscrew" esophagus, sometimes with epiphrenic diverticula.

Treatment

Medications
- **Smooth muscle relaxants** such as nitrates and calcium channel blockers are commonly used.
- Low-dose **tricyclic antidepressants (TCAs)** can be effective for symptom relief not only in diffuse esophageal spasm, but also in other nonspecific spastic motor disorders of the esophagus.
- **Botulinum toxin injection** may be required for resistant cases.

Surgery
- Resistant cases may require **empiric esophageal dilation.**
- **Surgical myotomy** is rarely indicated for patients with severe symptoms.

ESOPHAGEAL HYPOMOTILITY DISORDERS

General Principles

Definition
- Esophageal hypomotility disorders are characterized by feeble or absent esophageal peristalsis, with LES hypomotility, leading to severe GERD.

Etiology
- While typically idiopathic, hypomotility disorders can be associated with connective tissue diseases, Barrett's esophagus, and diabetes mellitus.
- Scleroderma can cause fibrosis that results in aperistalsis and atony of the distal esophagus and LES; the esophagus is involved in 75%–85% of cases.

Diagnosis

- **Dysphagia** and **heartburn** are the predominant symptoms.
- **Esophageal manometry** may demonstrate weak or absent peristaltic sequences and LES hypomotility.
- **Barium swallow** may reveal a dilated esophageal body, an open LES, and free reflux of gastric contents into the esophagus.
- **Endoscopy** may show a dilated esophagus with gaping gastroesophageal junction and evidence of GERD.

Treatment

- No specific therapy exists for esophageal hypomotility from connective tissue diseases.
- Acid suppression with a **proton pump inhibitor** is recommended for acid reflux. Fundoplication is relatively contraindicated.
- Periodic dilation may be necessary for strictures.

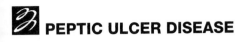 **PEPTIC ULCER DISEASE**

GENERAL PRINCIPLES

Definition

- Peptic ulcer disease (PUD) is characterized by breaks in the lining of the stomach and duodenum when corrosive effects of acid and pepsin overwhelm mucosal defense mechanisms. Peptic ulcers can also occur in the esophagus, in the small bowel adjacent to gastroenteric anastomoses, and within a Meckel's diverticulum.

Etiology

- *Helicobacter pylori*, a spiral, Gram-negative urease-producing bacillus, is thought to be responsible for 80% of ulcers that are not due to NSAIDs.
- NSAIDs and aspirin can result in mucosal damage anywhere in the GI tract and are responsible for most peptic ulcers not due to *H. pylori*. Past history of PUD, age >60 years, concomitant corticosteroid or anticoagulant therapy, high-dose or multiple NSAID therapy, and presence of serious comorbid medical illnesses all increase risk for PUD.
- A gastrin-secreting tumor or gastrinoma can result in uncontrolled acid secretion, and accounts for <1% of all peptic ulcers.
- When none of the above etiologies is evident, the ulcer is designated idiopathic.
- Cigarette smoking doubles the risk for peptic ulcers.

DIAGNOSIS

Clinical Presentation

- Epigastric pain or dyspepsia may be presenting symptoms; however, symptoms are not always predictive of the presence of ulcers.
- Epigastric tenderness may be elicited on abdominal palpation.
- Ten percent may present with a complication. The important complications are gastrointestinal bleeding, perforation, penetration, and gastric outlet obstruction.
- In the presence of alarm symptoms (weight loss, early satiety, bleeding, anemia, and lack of appropriate response to acid suppression), endoscopy is indicated to evaluate for a complication or an alternate diagnosis.

Investigation

- **Endoscopy** is the gold standard for diagnosis of peptic ulcers.
- **Barium studies** also have good sensitivity for diagnosis of ulcers, but smaller ulcers and erosions may be missed; further, biopsies cannot be taken.
- **Serum *H. pylori* antibody testing** is the cheapest noninvasive test for diagnosing *H. pylori* infection; the antibody remains detectable as long as 18 months after successful eradication, and therefore this test cannot be used to document successful eradication of the organism.
- **Stool *H. pylori* antigen testing** also has high sensitivity and specificity for the diagnosis of *H. pylori* infection. This test can be used to confirm eradication of *H. pylori* after triple therapy.
- **Rapid urease assay** (*Campylobacter*-like organism [CLO] test) and histopathologic examination of endoscopic biopsy specimens are commonly used for diagnosis in patients undergoing endoscopy; these tests may be falsely negative in patients on PPI therapy.
- **Carbon-labeled urea breath testing** is the most accurate noninvasive test for diagnosis. This test is often used to document successful eradication after therapy in patients with ongoing dyspeptic symptoms or complicated ulcer disease.

TREATMENT

Medications

- Regardless of etiology, **acid suppression** forms the mainstay of therapy of PUD. Gastric ulcers are typically treated for 12 weeks, and duodenal ulcers for 8 weeks.
  - Oral PPI or H_2RA therapy will suffice in most instances; parenteral administration of PPIs may be necessary, especially in the presence of GI bleeding or when oral administration is not tolerated or not possible (see Table 16-1). Dosage intervals should be prolonged for H_2RAs in the presence of renal insufficiency. Side effects are uncommon, but headache and mental status abnormalities (lethargy, confusion, depression, hallucinations) can result from H_2RA therapy; abdominal pain and diarrhea are common side effects of PPI therapy. Rare hepatotoxicity, thrombocytopenia, and leukopenia have been observed with H_2RA use. Cimetidine can impair metabolism of many drugs, including warfarin anticoagulants, theophylline, and phenytoin (see Appendix C).
- **Sucralfate** acts by coating the mucosal surface without blocking acid secretion and can be as effective as H_2RAs or high-dose antacids in healing duodenal ulcers. Side effects include constipation and reduction of bioavailability of certain drugs (e.g., cimetidine, digoxin, fluoroquinolones, phenytoin, and tetracycline) when administered concomitantly.
- **Antacids** are rarely used as primary therapy for PUD but can be useful as supplemental therapy for pain relief. The choice of antacid is determined by buffering capacity, formulation, and side effects. A typical dose is 30 mL of a high-potency liquid antacid, administered four to six times a day. Magnesium-containing antacids should be avoided in renal failure.
- **Antimicrobial therapy** in addition to antisecretory medication for eradication of *H. pylori* promotes healing and markedly reduces recurrence of gastric and duodenal ulcers. Several antimicrobial and antisecretory agent regimens are available (Table 16-2), and eradication is recommended in all *H. pylori*–infected patients with PUD. Metronidazole resistance (predominantly in females and patients of Asian descent) and poor compliance with therapy may affect eradication rates.
- **Nonpharmacologic measures.** Dietary modification should only include the avoidance of foods that are reproducibly associated with dyspeptic symptoms. Cigarette smoking doubles the risk of peptic ulcer development, delays healing, and promotes recurrence; therefore, cessation of cigarette smoking should be encouraged in all instances. Alcohol in high concentrations can damage the gastric mucosal barrier, but no evidence exists to link alcohol with ulcer recurrence.
- NSAIDs and aspirin should be avoided if possible.

Surgery

- Surgery is still occasionally required for intractable symptoms, GI bleeding, Zollinger-Ellison syndrome, and other complications of PUD. Surgical options vary depending on the location of the ulcer and the presence of associated complications.
- Significant morbidity can occur after surgical therapy of PUD, and adequate therapy requires a thorough understanding of the postsurgical complications.

Follow-Up

- EGD or upper GI series should be performed 8–12 weeks after initial diagnosis of all gastric ulcers to document healing; repeat endoscopic biopsy should be considered for nonhealing ulcers to exclude the possibility of a malignant ulcer.
- Duodenal ulcers are almost never malignant, and therefore documentation of healing is unnecessary in the absence of symptoms.

Complications

- **GI bleeding** (see Gastrointestinal Bleeding)

TABLE 16-2	Examples of Regimens Used for Eradication of *Helicobacter pylori*	

Medications	Dose	Comments
Clarithromycin	500 mg bid	First line
Amoxicillin	1 g bid	
PPI[a]	bid	
Pepto-Bismol	524 mg qid	First line in penicillin-allergic patients
Metronidazole	250 mg qid	Salvage regimen if three-drug regimen
Tetracycline	500 mg qid	fails
PPI[a] or H$_2$RA[b]	bid	
Clarithromycin	500 mg bid	Alternate regimen if four-drug therapy
Metronidazole	500 mg bid	is not tolerated
PPI[a]	bid	
Levofloxacin	250 mg bid	Alternate salvage regimen
Amoxicillin	1 g bid	
PPI[a]	bid	
Rifabutin	300 mg daily	Alternate salvage regimen
Amoxicillin	1 g bid	
PPI[a]	bid	

PPI, proton pump inhibitor.
Duration of therapy: 10–14 days. When using salvage regimens after initial treatment failure, choose drugs that have not been used before.
[a]Standard doses for PPI: omeprazole 20 mg, lansoprazole 30 mg, pantoprazole 40 mg, rabeprazole 20 mg, all twice a day. Esomeprazole is used as a single 40-mg dose once a day.
[b]Standard doses for H$_2$RA: ranitidine 150 mg, famotidine 20 mg, nizatidine 150 mg, cimetidine 400 mg, all twice a day.

- **Gastric outlet obstruction** is more likely to occur with ulcers that are close to the pyloric channel. Nausea and vomiting, sometimes several hours after meals, may occur. Plain abdominal radiographs often show a dilated stomach with an air–fluid level. NG suction should be maintained for 2–3 days to decompress the stomach while repleting fluids and electrolytes intravenously.
  - Although medical management may be temporarily effective, recurrence is common, and endoscopic balloon dilation or surgery is often necessary for definitive correction.
- **Perforation** occurs in a small number of PUD patients and usually necessitates emergency surgery. Perforation may occur in the absence of previous symptoms of PUD, and may be asymptomatic in patients who are receiving glucocorticoids. A plain upright radiograph of the abdomen may demonstrate free air under the diaphragm.
- **Pancreatitis** can result from penetration into the pancreas, most commonly seen with ulcers in the posterior wall of the duodenal bulb. The pain becomes severe and continuous, radiates to the back, and is no longer relieved by antisecretory therapy. Serum amylase may be elevated. Computed tomography (CT) scanning may be diagnostic. These patients frequently require surgery.

Postsurgical Complications

- **Abdominal symptoms.** Postoperative abdominal discomfort or vomiting after meals can be secondary to recurrent ulcer, afferent loop obstruction, bile reflux gastritis, gastric outlet obstruction, or stump carcinoma (a late complication). **Dumping syndrome** is caused by rapid gastric emptying of a large osmotic load into the small intestine and occurs after gastroenteric anastomosis with or without subtotal gastrectomy, vagotomy, and pyloroplasty.

- **Early dumping syndrome** occurs 15–30 minutes after eating and is due to osmotic fluid shifts into the gut lumen. Symptoms can be abdominal (nausea, vomiting, abdominal pain) or vasomotor (palpitations, sweating, dizziness).
- **Late dumping syndrome** consists of similar symptoms 2–4 hours after meals, due to excessive serum insulin response to rapid delivery and absorption of sugars from the small intestine.
- Dietary modification to multiple small meals high in protein and low in refined carbohydrates can be beneficial; liquids with meals should be avoided. Anticholinergics, fiber supplements, and ephedrine may relieve the vasomotor symptoms. In refractory situations, SC administration of octreotide may be necessary.
- **Malabsorption.** Mild steatorrhea can occur as a result of decreased intestinal transit time and inadequate mixing of food with bile and pancreatic secretions. Bacterial overgrowth due to afferent loop stasis can also lead to steatorrhea (see Other Gastrointestinal Disorders).
- **Anemia.** Deficiencies of folate, vitamin B_{12}, and iron can lead to anemia. Postoperative iron-deficiency anemia is usually a result of dietary iron malabsorption, but blood loss from gastritis or recurrent ulcers may contribute.

SPECIAL CONSIDERATIONS

- **Zollinger-Ellison syndrome** is caused by a gastrin-secreting, non-β islet cell tumor of the pancreas or duodenum. Multiple endocrine neoplasia type I can be associated with this syndrome in 25% of patients. The resultant hypersecretion of gastric acid can cause multiple peptic ulcers in unusual locations, ulcers that fail to respond to standard medical therapy, or recurrent ulceration after surgical therapy. Diarrhea and gastroesophageal reflux symptoms are common.
- Gastric acid output is typically >15 mEq/L, and gastric pH <1.0. A fasting serum gastrin level while off acid suppression for at least 5 days serves as a screening test; a value >1,000 pg/mL is seen in 90% of patients. When serum gastrin is elevated but <1,000 pg/mL, a secretin stimulation test may demonstrate a paradoxical 200-pg increment in serum gastrin level after IV secretin in patients with gastrinomas. PPIs are generally required in higher doses than those used for PUD. Specialized nuclear medicine scans (octreotide scans) can be useful in localizing the neoplastic lesion for curative resection.

INFLAMMATORY BOWEL DISEASE

GENERAL PRINCIPLES

Definition

- **Ulcerative colitis** (UC) is an idiopathic chronic inflammatory disease of the colon and rectum, characterized by mucosal inflammation and typically presenting with bloody diarrhea. Rectal involvement is almost universal.
- **Crohn's disease** is characterized by transmural inflammation of the gut wall and can affect any part of the tubular GI tract.

DIAGNOSIS

Clinical Presentation

- Both disorders can present with diarrhea, weight loss, and abdominal pain. Ulcerative colitis typically presents with bloody diarrhea. Crohn's disease can also present with fistula formation, strictures, abscesses, or bowel obstruction.
- Endoscopy and imaging studies are useful diagnostic modalities.

TREATMENT

Medications

- 5-Aminosalicylic acid (ASA) compounds
  - **Sulfasalazine** reaches the colon intact, where it is metabolized to 5-ASA and a sulfapyridine moiety. It is therefore used for colonic disease (UC and Crohn's disease limited to the colon), either as initial therapy (0.5 g PO bid, increased as tolerated to 0.5–1.5 g PO qid) or to maintain remission (1 g PO bid–qid).
  - Adverse effects are mainly caused by the sulfapyridine moiety and include headache, nausea, vomiting, and abdominal pain; a reduction in dose may be beneficial.
  - Hypersensitivity reactions are less common and include skin rash, fever, agranulocytosis, hepatotoxicity, and aplastic anemia. Reversible reduction in sperm counts can be seen in males. Paradoxic exacerbation of colitis is a rare adverse effect.
  - Folic acid supplementation is recommended, as sulfasalazine impairs folate absorption.
- **Newer 5-ASA preparations** lack the sulfa moiety of sulfasalazine and are associated with fewer side effects.
  - **Mesalamine** (5-ASA) is available in several formulations. An oral preparation released at pH >7 (Asacol, 800–1,600 mg PO tid) is useful in UC as well as ileocecal/colonic Crohn's disease. A second preparation, balsalazide (Colazal, 2.25 g PO tid for active disease, 1.5 g PO bid for maintenance), is cleaved by colonic bacteria to mesalamine and an inert carrier molecule and is useful for colonic inflammation. A third preparation with time- and pH-dependent release of the active ingredient throughout the GI tract (Pentasa, 0.5–1.0 g PO qid) is useful in diffuse Crohn's disease that also affects the small bowel; it can be used in UC as well. Rare hypersensitivity reactions occur and include pneumonitis, pancreatitis, hepatitis, and nephritis. Mesalamine preparations can be used for initiation and maintenance therapy.
  - **Olsalazine** is a 5-ASA dimer that is cleaved by bacteria in the colon and can be used in UC and Crohn's colitis. Diarrhea is a major side effect and can limit its use.
- **Glucocorticoids** are beneficial in inducing remission of active UC and Crohn's disease. They are not recommended for mild disease; they can be used concurrently with other anti-inflammatory agents in moderate to severe disease, especially with flare-ups of disease activity. Extracolonic manifestations of inflammatory bowel disease (ocular lesions, skin disease, and peripheral arthritis) also respond to glucocorticoids.
  - A typical starting oral dose of **prednisone** is 40–60 mg given once a day in the morning. Depending on response, the dose can be reduced by 10 mg every 5–10 days and tapered off in 3–6 weeks. In severe disease or in patients who cannot tolerate oral medication, IV administration (methylprednisolone, 20–40 mg daily to bid, up to 1 mg/kg/d) may be necessary for brief periods; higher doses are used in refractory disease. Glucocorticoids are not recommended for maintenance therapy, and alternatives should be sought for the patient who appears dependent on these medications.
  - **Oral or parenteral glucocorticoids should not be prescribed before ruling out an infectious process and should not be initiated for the first time over the telephone.**
  - **Budesonide** (Entocort, 9 mg/d) may have less systemic side effects compared to glucocorticoids when used for mild to moderate ileocolonic Crohn's disease.
- Immunosuppressive agents
  - **6-Mercaptopurine,** a purine analog, and **azathioprine,** its S-imidazole precursor, cause preferential suppression of T-cell activation and antigen recognition. They are used orally in doses of 1.0–1.5 mg/kg body weight daily. Both agents have more favorable side effect profiles than do glucocorticoids and are used as steroid-sparing agents in severe or refractory inflammatory bowel disease (IBD). Response may be delayed for up to 1–2 months. Side effects include reversible bone marrow suppression, pancreatitis, and allergic reactions.
  - **Methotrexate** (15–25 mg IM or PO weekly) has also been used as a steroid-sparing agent in Crohn's disease. Side effects include hepatic fibrosis, bone marrow suppression, alopecia, pneumonitis, allergic reactions, and teratogenicity.

- IV **cyclosporine** has been used in refractory cases of UC; however, the benefit is temporary. Side effects include nephrotoxicity, hepatotoxicity, hypertrichosis, seizures, and lymphoproliferative disorders.
- **Antibiotics**
  - **Metronidazole** (250–500 mg PO tid) can be used as an alternate first-line agent or adjunctive therapy in mild to moderate Crohn's disease. Peripheral neuropathy is a concern with long-term use.
  - **Ciprofloxacin** (500 mg PO bid) has also been used in Crohn's disease. The two agents can be used concurrently in perianal Crohn's disease for prolonged periods with good results.
  - An alternative agent that is sometimes used is **sulfamethoxazole-trimethoprim.**
- **Infliximab** (Remicade) is a monoclonal antibody against tumor necrosis factor-α that induces inflammatory cell lysis by binding to tumor necrosis factor receptors on the cell surface. Infliximab (IV infusions of 5 mg/kg) is used for therapy of fistulous Crohn's disease, refractory inflammatory-type Crohn's disease unresponsive to conventional therapy, and more recently, severe ulcerative colitis.
  - Induction regimens typically consist of doses at 0, 2, and 6 weeks, with maintenance doses every 8 weeks. Congestive heart failure may worsen after therapy.
  - Sepsis and reactivation of latent tuberculosis or histoplasmosis may occur; a tuberculin test may be indicated to evaluate for latent tuberculosis.
  - Serious infusion reactions may occur, and constant monitoring is essential during infusion.
- **Sargramostim** (granulocyte macrophage colony stimulation factor [GM-CSF], 6 mcg/kg/day SC for continuous periods of up to 2 months) may benefit patients with refractory Crohn's disease by stimulating the innate immune system in the gastrointestinal tract. Side effects can include injection site reactions and bone pain.
- **Local therapy.** UC that is limited to the rectum or distal left colon can be treated effectively with 5-ASA and/or glucocorticoid enemas or suppositories administered once to twice a day; concurrent systemic therapy may be required in severe cases. Symptomatic benefit may be achieved in perianal Crohn's disease with sitz baths, analgesic, and hydrocortisone creams and local heat, in addition to systemic anti-inflammatory agents and antibiotics.
- **Antidiarrheal agents** may be useful as an adjunctive therapy in selected patients with mild exacerbations or postresection diarrhea. They are contraindicated in severe exacerbations and toxic megacolon.
- **Other measures.** A low-roughage diet often provides symptomatic relief in patients with mild to moderate disease or in patients with strictures. Elemental diets have been used in acute phases of the diseases, especially Crohn's disease, but are unpalatable and disliked by patients.
  - **Total parenteral nutrition** and bowel rest may be required in severe disease, for nutritional maintenance and symptom relief while waiting for the effects of medical treatment, or as a bridge to surgery.
  - Patients with Crohn's ileitis or ileocolonic resection may need **vitamin B$_{12}$** supplementation. Specific oral replacement of **calcium, magnesium, folate, iron, vitamins A and D, and other micronutrients** may be necessary in patients with small-bowel Crohn's disease.

Surgery

- Surgery is generally reserved for patients with fistulas, obstruction, abscess, perforation, or bleeding, and rarely for medically refractory disease and neoplastic transformation.
- Recurrence close to the resected margins is common after bowel resection. Efforts should be made to avoid multiple resections in Crohn's disease because of the risk of short-bowel syndrome. Immunosuppressive agents should be discontinued before surgery and reinstituted if necessary during the postoperative period.

SPECIAL CONSIDERATIONS

■ **Colon cancer surveillance.** In patients with colitis lasting longer than 8–10 years (both UC and Crohn's colitis), annual colonoscopic surveillance for neoplasia with four-quadrant mucosal biopsies every 5–10 cm is recommended. Histopathologic evidence of any grade of dysplasia is an indication for total colectomy.

■ **Intestinal obstruction.** Stricture formation can result in intestinal obstruction in Crohn's disease. Presentation may resemble a flare, and a careful history, physical examination, and imaging studies are essential for diagnosis. NG tube decompression, parenteral hydration, and bowel rest may resolve minor episodes, but surgery may be necessary. Strictureplasty is an accepted procedure for focal tight strictures; biopsies should be obtained to rule out cancer at stricture sites. Patients with intermittent obstructive symptoms should avoid highly indigestible foods such as nuts, pits, hulls, skins, seeds, and pulps that may precipitate obstruction.

■ **Fulminant colitis** and **toxic megacolon.** Acute fulminant colitis presents as severe diarrhea with abdominal pain, bleeding, fever, sepsis, electrolyte disturbances, and dehydration. Toxic megacolon occurs in 1%–2% of patients with UC; the colon becomes atonic and modestly dilates, but systemic toxicity is the dominant feature.

- Patients should be kept NPO, with NG suction if there is evidence of small-bowel ileus.
- Dehydration and electrolyte disturbances should be treated vigorously.
- Anticholinergic and opioid medication should be discontinued.
- Intensive medical therapy with IV corticosteroids (hydrocortisone, 100 mg IV q6h or equivalent) and broad-spectrum antimicrobials should be initiated.
- Clinical deterioration/lack of improvement despite 7–10 days of intensive medical management, evidence of bowel perforation, or peritoneal signs are indications for urgent total colectomy.

FUNCTIONAL GASTROINTESTINAL DISORDERS

GENERAL PRINCIPLES

Definition

■ Functional GI disorders are characterized by the presence of abdominal symptoms in the absence of a demonstrable organic disease process. Symptoms can arise from any part of the luminal gut.

■ **Irritable bowel syndrome (IBS),** primarily characterized by abdominal pain linked to altered bowel habits, is the best-recognized functional bowel disease and the most commonly diagnosed GI illness.

DIAGNOSIS

Clinical evaluation and investigation should be directed toward prudently excluding organic processes in the involved area of the gut while initiating therapeutic trials when functional symptoms are suspected.

■ Older patients with new-onset bowel symptoms, patients with longstanding symptoms or symptoms not responsive to empiric therapy, and patients with alarm symptoms (gastrointestinal bleeding, anemia, weight loss, early satiety) need further workup with **endoscopy** and **imaging studies.**

■ In young individuals with short-lived symptoms and no other explanation for dyspepsia, **noninvasive testing for** *H. pylori* (serology or urea breath test) can be considered.

TREATMENT

Nonspecific Measures

Patient education, reassurance, and help with diet and lifestyle modification are key to an effective physician–patient relationship. The psychosocial contribution to symptom exacerbation should be determined, and its management may be sufficient for many patients.

Medications

- Neuromodulators
  - Low-dose TCAs (e.g., amitriptyline, nortriptyline, imipramine, doxepin: 25–100 mg at bedtime) have neuromodulatory and analgesic properties that are independent of their psychotropic effects and can be beneficial, especially in pain-predominant functional GI disorders.
  - Selective serotonin reuptake inhibitors (e.g., fluoxetine, 20 mg; paroxetine, 20 mg; sertraline, 50 mg, duloxetine 20–60 mg) are less effective but have better side effect profiles.
- Symptomatic management
  - Antiemetic agents are useful in functional nausea and vomiting syndromes, in addition to neuromodulators.
  - When pain and bloating are the predominant symptoms, antispasmodic or anticholinergic medications (hyoscyamine, 0.125–0.25 mg PO/sublingual up to qid; dicyclomine, 10–20 mg PO qid) may be beneficial.
  - Constipation-predominant IBS may benefit from increased dietary fiber (25 g/d) supplemented with laxatives PRN.
  - Loperamide (2–4 mg, up to qid/PRN) can reduce stool frequency, urgency, and fecal incontinence.
  - Newer $5-HT_4$ receptor agonists such as tegaserod (Zelnorm, 6 mg bid) may be useful in women with constipation-predominant IBS, but studies in men are inconclusive.
  - Alosetron (Lotronex, 1 mg daily to bid), a $5-HT_3$ antagonist, is useful in women with diarrhea-predominant IBS; its use is restricted to women with symptoms refractory to other measures because of the potential for ischemic colitis in a small proportion of patients.
- Patients with cyclic vomiting syndrome (stereotypic episodes of vigorous vomiting with asymptomatic intervals between episodes) benefit from treatment with low-dose TCAs or antiepileptic medications (Zonegran, Keppra) as maintenance options. Anecdotal evidence suggests that these patients may also benefit from sumatriptan (25–50 mg PO, 5–10 mg transnasally, or 6 mg SC at the beginning of an episode), especially if it is administered during a prodrome or early in the episode.

ACUTE INTESTINAL PSEUDO-OBSTRUCTION (ILEUS)

GENERAL PRINCIPLES

Definition

- Acute intestinal pseudo-obstruction or ileus consists of obstructive symptoms (nausea, vomiting, abdominal distension, lack of bowel movements) and intestinal dilation on imaging studies without a mechanical explanation.
- Ogilvie syndrome or acute colonic pseudo-obstruction describes colonic dilation without a mechanical obstruction in the presence of a competent ileocecal valve, which may be complicated by cecal rupture when dilation is rapid or massive.

Etiology

■ Predisposing causes include virtually any medical insult, particularly life-threatening systemic diseases, infection, vascular insufficiency, surgery, and electrolyte abnormalities.

DIAGNOSIS

■ A careful history and physical exam are essential in the initial evaluation of these patients.
■ Conventional laboratory studies (blood count, complete metabolic profile, amylase, lipase) help in assessing for a primary intra-abdominal inflammatory process.
■ **Obstructive series** (supine and upright abdominal radiograph with a chest radiograph) determines the distribution of intestinal gas and assesses for the presence of free intraperitoneal air.
■ **Additional imaging studies** may be required to assess for mechanical obstruction and inflammatory processes and include **CT scanning, contrast enema**, and **small-bowel series.**

TREATMENT

Nonspecific Measures

■ Basic supportive measures consist of nothing by mouth (NPO), fluid replacement, and correction of electrolyte imbalances. Prompt antimicrobial therapy is indicated if an infectious process is suspected. Medications that slow GI motility (adrenergic agonists, TCAs, sedatives, narcotic analgesics) should be withdrawn or doses reduced. The ambulatory patient is encouraged to remain active and to undertake short walks.
■ **Intermittent NG suction** prevents swallowed air from passing distally. In protracted cases, gastric decompression, either using an NG tube or a percutaneous endoscopic gastrotomy tube, eliminates upper GI secretions and decreases vomiting and gastric distension.
■ **Rectal tubes** help decompress the distal colon; more proximal colonic distension may necessitate **colonoscopic decompression**, especially when the cecal diameter approaches 9–10 cm. A flexible decompression tube can be left in the proximal colon during colonoscopy. Turning the patient from side to side may potentiate the benefit of colonoscopic decompression.
■ Temporary total parenteral nutrition may be required in protracted cases.

Medications

■ **Neostigmine** (2 mg IV administered slowly over 3–5 minutes) is beneficial in selected patients with acute colonic distension. The drug can induce rapid re-establishment of colonic tone and is contraindicated if mechanical obstruction remains in the differential diagnosis. Side effects include abdominal pain, excessive salivation, symptomatic bradycardia, and syncope. A trial of neostigmine may be warranted before colonoscopic decompression in patients without contraindications.
■ **Erythromycin** (200 mg IV) acts as a motilin agonist and stimulates upper gut motility; it has been used with some success in refractory postoperative ileus.
■ **Guanethidine, bethanechol,** and **metoclopramide** have all been used with mixed results.

Surgery

■ **Surgical consultation** is required when the clinical picture is suggestive of mechanical obstruction or if peritoneal signs are present.
■ **Cecostomy** is rarely required when colonoscopic decompression fails in acute colonic distension.
■ Surgical exploration is reserved for **acute cases** with peritoneal signs, ischemic bowel changes, or other evidence for perforation.

PANCREATICOBILIARY DISORDERS

ACUTE PANCREATITIS

General Principles

Definition
- Acute pancreatitis is inflammation of the pancreas and peripancreatic tissue from activation of potent pancreatic enzymes within the pancreas, particularly trypsin.

Etiology
- The most common causes are alcohol and gallstone disease. Less common causes include abdominal trauma, hypercalcemia, hypertriglyceridemia, and a variety of drugs. Postendoscopic retrograde cholangiopancreatography (ERCP) pancreatitis occurs in 5%–10% of patients undergoing ERCP.

Diagnosis

Imaging
- **Dual-phase (pancreatic protocol) CT scanning** is useful in the initial evaluation of severe acute pancreatitis. The Ranson criteria (Table 16-3) may provide prognostic information.

Treatment

General Measures
- Aggressive volume repletion with IV fluids must be undertaken, with careful monitoring of fluid balance and awareness of the potential for significant fluid sequestration within the abdomen. Serum electrolytes, calcium, and glucose levels should be monitored and supplemented as necessary. Patients with severe pancreatitis and hemodynamic instability often require admission to the ICU.

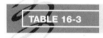 **Ranson Criteria for Severity Assessment in Acute Pancreatitis[a]**

	Alcoholic pancreatitis	Nonalcoholic pancreatitis
On admission		
Age	>55 yr	>70 yr
WBC count	>16,000/mcL	>18,000/mcL
Blood glucose	>200 mg/dL	>220 mg/dL
LDH	>350 International Units/L	>400 International Units/L
AST	>250 units/L	>440 units/L
During the first 48 hr of admission		
Fall in hematocrit	>10%	>10%
Serum calcium	<8 mg/dL	<8 mg/dL
Base deficit	>4.0 mEq/L	>5.0 mEq/L
Increase in blood urea	>5 mg/dL	>2 mg/dL
Fluid sequestration	>6 L	>6 L
Arterial PO$_2$	<60 mm Hg	<60 mm Hg

AST, aspartate aminotransferase; LDH, lactic dehydrogenase; PO$_2$ = oxygen tension; WBC, white blood cell.
[a]The presence of three or more criteria indicates severe pancreatitis.

- Urine output, hemodynamics, and laboratory parameters help assess adequacy of volume repletion.
- Patients should receive **nothing by mouth** until they are free of pain and nausea. NG suction is reserved for patients with ileus or protracted emesis. Total parenteral nutrition (TPN) may be necessary when inflammation is slow to resolve. Enteral nutrition through a tube placed distal to the ligament of Treitz is usually tolerated, and may be safer than TPN.
- **Acid suppression** may be necessary in severely ill patients with risk factors for stress ulcer bleeding (see Gastrointestinal Bleeding).

Medications
- **Narcotic analgesics** are usually necessary for pain relief.
  - **Meperidine** is the most commonly used agent. Though **morphine** is frequently avoided, there is no conclusive evidence that morphine has deleterious effects on sphincter of Oddi pressure. Patient-controlled analgesia is frequently necessary for adequate relief of pain.

Endoscopic Therapy
- Urgent **ERCP and biliary sphincterotomy** within 72 hours of presentation can improve the outcome of severe gallstone pancreatitis in the presence of elevated liver numbers and/or a dilated common bile duct. This is thought to result from reduced biliary sepsis rather than true improvement of pancreatic inflammation.

Complications
- **Necrotizing pancreatitis** represents a severe form of acute pancreatitis, usually identified on dynamic dual-phase CT scanning with IV contrast. The presence of radiologically identified pancreatic necrosis increases the morbidity and mortality of acute pancreatitis. Increasing abdominal pain, fever, marked leukocytosis, and bacteremia suggest infected pancreatic necrosis that requires broad-spectrum antibiotics and often surgical debridement. CT-guided percutaneous aspiration for Gram stain and culture can confirm the diagnosis of infected necrosis.
- The presence of **pseudocysts** is suggested by persistent pain or hyperamylasemia. Complications include infection, hemorrhage, rupture (pancreatic ascites), and obstruction of adjacent structures. Generally, asymptomatic nonenlarging pseudocysts can be followed clinically with serial imaging studies. Decompression of symptomatic, rapidly enlarging, or complicated pseudocysts can be performed by percutaneous, endoscopic, or surgical techniques.
- **Infection.** Potential sources of fever include pancreatic necrosis, abscess, infected pseudocyst, cholangitis, and aspiration pneumonia. Cultures should be obtained, and broad-spectrum antimicrobials that are appropriate for bowel flora should be administered. In the absence of fever or other clinical evidence for infection, prophylactic antimicrobial therapy has no clear role in acute pancreatitis.
- **Pulmonary complications.** Atelectasis, pleural effusion, pneumonia, and acute respiratory distress syndrome can develop in severely ill patients (see Chapter 9, Pulmonary Disease).
- **Renal failure.** Severe intravascular volume depletion or acute tubular necrosis can cause renal failure.
- **Other complications.** Metabolic complications include hypocalcemia, hypomagnesemia, and hyperglycemia. Gastrointestinal bleeding can result from stress gastritis, pseudoaneurysm rupture, or gastric varices from splenic vein thrombosis.

GALLSTONE DISEASE

General Principles

Definition
- **Asymptomatic cholelithiasis** is a common incidental finding for which no specific therapy is generally necessary.

- **Symptomatic cholelithiasis,** when upper abdominal symptoms are thought to be related to the presence of gallstones, is typically treated surgically with cholecystectomy.
- **Acute cholecystitis** is caused most often by obstruction of the cystic duct by gallstones, but acalculous cholecystitis can occur in severely ill or hospitalized patients.

Diagnosis

Clinical Presentation

- Cholelithiasis may present as **biliary colic,** a constant pain lasting for hours, located in the right upper quadrant, radiating to the back or right shoulder, and sometimes associated with nausea or vomiting.
- Other presentations of gallstone disease include acute cholecystitis, acute pancreatitis, and cholangitis. Gallstone disease may rarely be associated with gallbladder cancer.
- Patients with **acute ascending cholangitis** present with right upper quadrant pain, fever with chills, and jaundice (Charcot's triad), usually in the setting of biliary obstruction (choledocholithiasis, neoplasia, sclerosing cholangitis, biliary stent occlusion). Elderly patients may lack abdominal symptoms.

Imaging

- **Ultrasound scans** have a high degree of accuracy in diagnosis.
- Hydroxyiminodiacetic acid (HIDA) scan can demonstrate nonfilling of the gallbladder in patients with acute cholecystitis.

Treatment

Surgery

- **Cholecystectomy** is the therapy of choice for symptomatic gallstone disease and acute cholecystitis. Laparoscopic cholecystectomy compares favorably with the open procedure, with lower morbidity, shorter hospital stay, and better cosmetic results.

Nonoperative

- **Supportive measures** include IV fluid resuscitation and broad-spectrum antimicrobial agents, especially in the event of complications such as acute cholecystitis with sepsis, perforation, peritonitis, abscess, or empyema formation.
- Percutaneous cholecystotomy and decompression of the gallbladder can be performed under fluoroscopy in severely ill patients with acute cholecystitis who are not surgical candidates.
- **Ursodeoxycholic acid** (8–10 mg/kg/d PO in two to three divided doses for prolonged periods) might be prudent in a small select group of patients with small cholesterol stones in normally functioning gallbladders who are at high risk for complications from surgical therapy. Side effects include diarrhea and reversible elevation in serum transaminase levels.
- Another option is percutaneous instillation of contact solvents such as methyl-tertiary-butyl ether into the gallbladder and extracorporeal shock-wave lithotripsy combined with oral bile acid dissolution therapy. Experience with these therapies is limited, and neither is definitive as the gallbladder remains in place.

Complications

- **Acute pancreatitis.** See section on acute pancreatitis above.
- **Choledocholithiasis.** In patients who have undergone cholecystectomy, retained common bile duct stones can complicate the postoperative course. Common bile duct obstruction, jaundice, biliary colic, cholangitis, or pancreatitis can result. The diagnosis can be made on ultrasonography, CT scanning, or magnetic resonance cholangiography. ERCP with sphincterotomy and stone extraction is curative.
- **Acute ascending cholangitis** can present with right upper quadrant pain, fever with chills, and jaundice (Charcot's triad), usually in the setting of biliary obstruction (choledocholithiasis, neoplasia, sclerosing cholangitis, biliary stent occlusion). Cholangitis represents a medical emergency with high morbidity and mortality if biliary decompression

is not performed urgently. The condition should be stabilized with IV fluids and broad-spectrum antibiotics. Drainage of the biliary tree can be performed through the endoscopic (ERCP with sphincterotomy) or percutaneous approach under fluoroscopic guidance.

CHRONIC PANCREATITIS

General Principles

Definition
- Chronic pancreatitis represents changes resulting from recurrent acute or chronic inflammation of the pancreas. This is commonly seen with chronic alcohol abuse.
- **Endocrine insufficiency** may result from destruction of islet cells.

Diagnosis

Clinical Presentation
- Pain, **exocrine insufficiency** (manifesting as weight loss and steatorrhea), and **endocrine insufficiency** (manifesting as brittle diabetes) are the main clinical manifestations.

Laboratory Studies
- In the presence of steatorrhea, a serum trypsinogen level of <10 ng/mL is diagnostic of chronic pancreatitis.

Treatment

Medications
- **Narcotic analgesics** are frequently required for control of pain, and narcotic dependence is common. In patients with mild to moderate exocrine insufficiency, the addition of oral **pancreatic enzyme** supplements may be beneficial for pain control.
- **Pancreatic enzyme supplements** are the mainstay of management of pancreatic exocrine insufficiency, in conjunction with a low-fat diet (<50 g fat/d). Enteric-coated preparations (Pancrease or Creon, one to two capsules with meals) are stable at acid pH and should not be given with concomitant acid suppression.
- Fat-soluble vitamin supplementation may be necessary.
- **Insulin** therapy is generally required for endocrine insufficiency, as the resultant diabetes mellitus is characteristically brittle.

Surgery
- Patients with pancreatic duct obstruction from stones, strictures, or papillary stenosis may benefit from ERCP and sphincterotomy.
- Intractable pain may necessitate celiac ganglion block or even surgery.

 # DYSPHAGIA AND ODYNOPHAGIA

GENERAL PRINCIPLES

Definition

- **Oropharyngeal dysphagia:** Difficulty in transferring food from the mouth to the esophagus, often associated with symptoms of nasopharyngeal regurgitation and pulmonary aspiration.
- **Esophageal dysphagia:** The sensation of difficulty in passage of food down the esophagus.
- **Odynophagia:** Pain on swallowing food and fluids; may indicate the presence of esophagitis, particularly infectious esophagitis and pill esophagitis.

Etiology

- **Oropharyngeal dysphagia** is typically caused by neuromuscular or structural disorders involving the oropharynx and proximal esophagus.
- **Esophageal dysphagia** can occur from an obstructive process in the esophagus. Progressive dysphagia may be seen with neoplasia, while intermittent symptoms can result from webs or rings. Acute onset of dysphagia in temporal relationship to a meal may suggest food impaction. In the absence of a structural obstructive process, esophageal manometry may be necessary to exclude a motility disorder (achalasia, diffuse esophageal spasm).

DIAGNOSIS

Oropharyngeal Dysphagia

- Assessment is initiated with a detailed neurologic exam.
- Barium videofluoroscopy (modified barium swallow) evaluates the oropharyngeal swallow mechanism, and may identify laryngeal penetration.
- Ear, nose, and throat exam including flexible nasal endoscopy may identify structural etiologies.
- Imaging studies (CT scans) may demonstrate a structural process.
- Laboratory tests for polymyositis, myasthenia gravis, and other neuromuscular disorders can be considered.

Esophageal Dysphagia

- Endoscopy is typically used for initial investigation of esophageal dysphagia. Endoscopy provides information on mucosal abnormalities, allows tissue sampling, and offers the option of dilation if a narrowing is seen.
- Barium swallow is also a suitable initial test for esophageal dysphagia, although biopsies and esophageal dilation require endoscopy. Subtle rings and webs may not be visualized unless a barium swallow is performed using a solid bolus or a barium pill.
- Esophageal manometry can characterize esophageal motor disorders when other studies are normal or suggest a motility disorder.
- Acute esophageal obstruction is best investigated with endoscopy.

TREATMENT

General Measures

- Modification of diet and swallowing maneuvers may benefit patients with dysphagia, especially oropharyngeal dysphagia.
- Enteral feeding through a gastrostomy tube may be indicated in patients with frank tracheal aspiration on attempted swallowing.
- Endoscopic retrieval of an obstructing food bolus can result in dramatic resolution of acute dysphagia from food impaction.
- Nutrition needs to be addressed in patients with prolonged dysphagia causing weight loss; patients with dysphagia are typically advised to chew their food well and eat foods of soft consistencies.

Medications

- Mucosal inflammation from reflux disease can be treated with acid suppression, typically with a PPI.
- Odynophagia generally responds to specific therapy of the condition causing esophagitis (e.g., PPIs for reflux disease, antimicrobial agents for infectious esophagitis). Viscous lidocaine swish-and-swallow solutions may afford symptomatic relief.
- Patients with oropharyngeal dysphagia and drooling of saliva can be treated with **anticholinergic** medication (e.g., transdermal scopolamine).

- Glucagon (2- to 4-mg IV bolus) can be attempted in patients with acute dysphagia from food impaction, but is frequently unsuccessful. Sublingual **nitroglycerin** can also be given, but meat tenderizer should not be administered.

Endoscopic Therapy

- Esophageal dilation is performed for anatomic narrowings visualized during endoscopy. Empiric dilation is sometimes performed even when a defined narrowing is not identified, and may result in symptomatic benefit.
- Aggressive pneumatic dilation of the LES is sometimes performed for achalasia, but laparoscopic myotomy is gaining popularity over pneumatic dilation. Botulinum toxin injections to the LES may result in temporary symptom relief in achalasia.
- Esophageal stent placement can alleviate dysphagia in inoperable neoplasia.

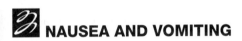 **NAUSEA AND VOMITING**

GENERAL PRINCIPLES

Etiology

- Nausea and vomiting may result from side effects of medications, systemic illnesses, central nervous system (CNS) disorders, and primary GI disorders.
- Vomiting that occurs during or immediately after a meal can result from a pyloric channel ulcer or from functional disorders.
- Vomiting within 30–60 minutes after a meal may suggest gastric or duodenal pathology.
- Delayed vomiting after a meal with undigested food from a previous meal can suggest gastric outlet obstruction or gastroparesis.

History

- Bowel obstruction and pregnancy should be ruled out.
- The patient's medication list should be scrutinized.

TREATMENT

General Measures

- Correction of fluid and electrolyte imbalances is an important supportive measure.
- Oral intake should be withheld or limited to clear liquids. Many patients with self-limited illnesses require no further therapy.
- NG decompression may be required for patients with bowel obstruction or protracted nausea and vomiting of any etiology.
- Patients with protracted nausea and vomiting may sometimes require enteral feeding through jejunal tubes, or rarely even total parenteral nutrition.

Medications

Empiric pharmacotherapy is often initiated while investigation is in progress, or when the etiology is thought to be self-limited.

- **Phenothiazines and related agents.** Prochlorperazine (Compazine), 5–10 mg PO tid–qid, 10 mg IM or IV q6h, or 25 mg PR bid; promethazine (Phenergan), 12.5–25.0 mg PO, IM, or PR q4–6h; and trimethobenzamide (Tigan), 250 mg PO tid–qid, 200 mg IM tid–qid, or 200 mg PR tid–qid are effective. Drowsiness is a common side effect, and acute dystonic reactions or other extrapyramidal effects may occur.
- **Dopamine antagonists** include metoclopramide (10 mg PO 30 minutes before meals and at bedtime), a prokinetic agent that also has central antiemetic effects. IV metoclopramide

can be used in nausea and vomiting associated with chemotherapy (see Chapter 20, Medical Management of Malignant Disease). Metoclopramide can also be tried in chronic cases where dysmotility of the upper GI tract is thought to play a significant role in symptoms. Drowsiness and extrapyramidal reactions may occur; tachyphylaxis may limit long term efficacy. Domperidone is an alternate agent that does not cross the blood-brain barrier and therefore has no CNS side effects; however, it is not uniformly available.

■ **Antihistaminic agents** are most useful for nausea and vomiting related to motion sickness, but may also be useful for other causes. Agents used include diphenhydramine (Benadryl, 25–50 mg PO q6–8h, or 10–50 mg IV q2–4h), dimenhydrinate (Dramamine, 50–100 mg PO or IV q4–6h), and meclizine (Antivert, 12.5–25 mg 1 hour before travel).

■ **Serotonin 5-HT$_3$ receptor antagonists.** Ondansetron (Zofran, 0.15 mg/kg IV q4h for three doses or 32 mg IV infused over 15 minutes beginning 30 minutes before chemotherapy) is effective in chemotherapy-associated emesis. It can also be used in emesis that is refractory to other medications (4–8 mg PO or IV up to q8h). Constipation may occur (see Chapter 20, Medical Management of Malignant Disease). **Granisetron**(Kytril, 10 mcg/kg IV for one to three doses 10 minutes apart, or 1 mg PO bid) is also effective.

■ **Neurokinin-1 (NK-1) receptor antagonist. Aprepitant** (Emend, 125 mg PO day 1, 80 mg PO days 2 and 3) is an alternative agent currently indicated **only for chemotherapy-induced nausea and vomiting.**

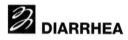 **DIARRHEA**

GENERAL PRINCIPLES

Definition

■ **Acute diarrhea** consists of increased frequency and/or fluidity of bowel movements of abrupt onset. Infectious agents, toxins, and drugs are the major causes of acute diarrhea. In hospitalized patients, pseudomembranous colitis, antibiotic- or drug-associated diarrhea, and fecal impaction should be considered.

■ **Chronic diarrhea** consists of passage of loose stools with or without increased stool frequency for more than 3–4 weeks.

Clinical Presentation and Etiology

Acute Diarrhea

■ **Bacterial and viral infections.** Viral enteritis and bacterial infections with *Escherichia coli*, *Shigella*, *Salmonella*, *Campylobacter*, and *Yersinia* species constitute the most common causes of acute diarrhea.

　■ **Pseudomembranous colitis** is usually seen in the setting of antimicrobial therapy and is caused by toxins produced by *Clostridium difficile*.

■ Parasitic infections

　■ **Amebiasis** may cause acute diarrhea, especially in travelers to areas with poor sanitation and in homosexual men. Demonstration of trophozoites or cysts of *Entamoeba histolytica* in the stool, or a serum antibody test, confirms the diagnosis.

　■ **Giardiasis** is confirmed by identification of *Giardia lamblia* trophozoites in the stool, in duodenal aspirate, or in small-bowel biopsy specimens. A stool immunofluorescence assay is also available for rapid diagnosis.

■ **Diarrhea related to medication use.** Common offending agents include laxatives, antacids, cardiac medications (e.g., digitalis, quinidine), colchicine, and antimicrobial agents. Symptoms usually respond to discontinuation of the offending agent.

■ **Graft versus host disease** needs to be considered in patients who develop diarrhea after organ transplantation, especially bone marrow transplantation.

Chronic Diarrhea

- After a careful history, thorough physical examination, and routine laboratory tests, chronic diarrhea can typically be classified into one of the following categories: watery diarrhea (secretory or osmotic), inflammatory diarrhea, or fatty diarrhea (steatorrhea).

Investigation

- Stool cultures, *C. difficile* toxin assay, ova and parasite examinations, and flexible sigmoidoscopy may be warranted in patients with severe, prolonged, or atypical symptoms.
- The fecal osmotic gap can be calculated in patients with chronic diarrhea and voluminous watery stools as follows: $290 - 2(\text{stool } [Na^+] + \text{stool } [K^+])$.
    - **Secretory diarrhea:** Stool osmotic gap is <50 mOsm/kg.
    - **Osmotic diarrhea:** Stool osmotic gap is >125 mOsm/kg.
- A positive fecal occult blood test or fecal leukocyte test suggests inflammatory diarrhea.
- Steatorrhea is traditionally diagnosed by demonstration of fat excretion in stool of >7 g/d in a 72-hour stool collection while the patient is on a 100-g/d fat diet. Sudan staining of a stool specimen is an alternate test; >100 fat globules per high-power field is suggestive of steatorrhea.
- Laxative screening should be considered in any patient with chronic diarrhea that remains undiagnosed.

TREATMENT

General Measures

- Adequate hydration is an essential part of the therapy of diarrheal disease. IV hydration is required in severe cases.
- Long-term IV fluids or parenteral nutrition is sometimes necessary in refractory diarrhea.
- Symptomatic therapy is recommended in simple self-limiting GI infections where diarrhea is frequent or troublesome, while diagnostic workup is in progress, when specific management fails to improve symptoms, or when a specific etiology is not identified.
    - **Loperamide,** 2–4 mg up to four times a day, **opiates** (tincture of opium; belladonna; and opium capsules), and **anticholinergic agents** (diphenoxylate and atropine [Lomotil], 15–20 mg/d of diphenoxylate in divided doses) are the most effective nonspecific antidiarrheal agents.
    - **Pectin** and **kaolin** preparations (bind toxins) and **bismuth subsalicylate** (antibacterial properties) are also useful in symptomatic therapy of acute diarrhea.
    - **Bile acid–binding resins** (e.g., cholestyramine, 1 g up to qid) are beneficial in bile acid–induced diarrhea.
    - **Octreotide** (100–200 μg bid–qid PRN) is useful in hormone-mediated secretory diarrhea, but can be of benefit in refractory diarrhea.

Medications

- **Empiric antibiotic therapy** is only recommended in patients with moderate to severe disease and associated systemic symptoms, while awaiting stool cultures.
    - **Fluoroquinolones** (ciprofloxacin, 500 mg PO bid for 3 days, or norfloxacin, 400 mg PO bid for 3 days)
    - **Trimethoprim-sulfamethoxazole** (160 mg/800 mg PO bid for 5 days)
- Oral **metronidazole** is the treatment of choice for pseudomembranous colitis. Oral **vancomycin** is reserved for resistant cases or intolerance to metronidazole (see Chapter 13, Treatment of Infectious Diseases, for further details).
- Treatment of symptomatic amebiasis is with **metronidazole,** 750 mg PO tid or 500 mg IV q8h for 5–10 days. This should be followed by **paromomycin,** 500 mg PO tid for 7 days, or **iodoquinol,** 650 mg PO tid for 20 days, to eliminate cysts.

- Therapy for giardiasis consists of metronidazole, 250 mg PO tid for 5–7 days, or tinidazole, 2-g single dose. Quinacrine, 100 mg PO tid for 7 days, is an alternative agent. More prolonged therapy may be necessary in the immunocompromised patient.

SPECIAL CONSIDERATIONS

- **Diarrhea in HIV disease**
  - Opportunistic agents, including *Cryptosporidium*, *Microsporidium*, CMV, *Mycobacterium avium* complex, and *Mycobacterium tuberculosis*, may cause diarrhea in patients with advanced HIV and should be looked for specifically.
  - Venereal infections (syphilis, gonorrhea, chlamydiosis, HSV infection) as well as other nonvenereal infections (amebiasis, giardiasis, salmonellosis, shigellosis) may also cause diarrhea.
  - Other causes of diarrhea in this population include intestinal lymphoma and Kaposi's sarcoma. Stool studies (ova and parasites, culture), endoscopic biopsies, and serologic testing may assist diagnosis.
  - The most likely cause of undiagnosed diarrhea is **missed pathogens;** however, drugs, antibiotics, HIV acting as a pathogen, autonomic disturbance, and abnormal intestinal motility may also contribute to diarrhea. Management consists of specific therapy if pathogens are identified; symptomatic measures may be of benefit in idiopathic cases.

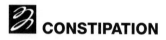 **CONSTIPATION**

GENERAL PRINCIPLES

Definition

- Constipation consists of infrequent (and frequently incomplete) bowel movements.

Etiology

- A recent change in bowel habits may indicate an organic cause, whereas constipation of several years' duration is more likely due to a functional disorder.
- Medication (e.g., calcium blockers, opiates, anticholinergics, iron supplements, barium sulfate) and systemic disease (e.g., diabetes mellitus, hypothyroidism, systemic sclerosis, myotonic dystrophy) may contribute.
- Other predisposing factors include lack of exercise, disorders that cause pain on defecation (e.g., anal fissures, thrombosed external hemorrhoids), and prolonged immobilization.

Investigation

- Colonoscopy and barium studies help rule out structural disease and may be particularly important in older individuals.
- Colonic transit studies, anorectal manometry, and defecography are reserved for resistant cases without an organic explanation.

TREATMENT

- Regular exercise and adequate fluid intake are nonspecific measures that may be of benefit.
- **Fiber supplementation.** An increase in dietary fiber intake to 20–30 g/d may be beneficial in many adults with constipation. Fecal impactions should be resolved before fiber supplementation is initiated. A fiber supplement such as wheat bran or psyllium with

water two to four times a day can be initiated; fluid intake should be increased with these preparations. Transient bloating often occurs.

Medications

- Laxatives
  - **Emollient laxatives** consist of docusate salts and mineral oil. Docusate sodium, 50–200 mg PO daily, and docusate calcium, 240 mg PO daily, allow water and fat to penetrate the fecal mass. Mineral oil (15–45 mL PO q6–8h) can be given orally or by enema. Tracheobronchial aspiration of mineral oil can result in lipoid pneumonia.
  - **Stimulant cathartics** such as castor oil, 15 mL PO, stimulate intestinal secretion and increase intestinal motility. Anthraquinones (cascara, 5 mL PO daily; senna, one tablet PO daily to qid) stimulate the colon by increasing fluid and water accumulation in the proximal colon. Chronic use can result in benign staining of the colonic mucosa (melanosis coli) and colonic atony from smooth muscle atrophy and damage to the myenteric plexus. Bisacodyl (10–15 mg PO at bedtime, 10-mg rectal suppositories) is structurally similar to phenolphthalein and stimulates colonic peristalsis. Lubiprostone (24 mcg PO bid) is a selective intestinal chloride channel activator, causing movement of fluid into the bowel lumen and stimulating peristalsis.
  - **Osmotic cathartics** include nonabsorbable salts or carbohydrates that cause water retention in the lumen of the colon. Magnesium salts include milk of magnesia (15–30 mL q8–12h) and magnesium citrate (200 mL PO); they should be avoided in renal failure. Lactulose (15–30 mL PO bid–qid) can cause bloating as a side effect.
- **Enemas.** Sodium biphosphate (Fleet) enemas (one to two rectally PRN) can be used for mild to moderate constipation and for bowel cleansing before sigmoidoscopy. However, these should be avoided in patients with renal failure because of the risk of developing hyperphosphatemia and subsequent hypocalcemia. Tap water enemas (1 L) are also useful for bowel cleansing. Oil-based enemas (cottonseed Colace, Hypaque) are reserved for refractory constipation.
- **Other agents.** Polyethylene glycol in powder form (MiraLax, 17 g PO daily to bid) can be used regularly or intermittently for the treatment of constipation. Serotonin 5-HT$_4$ receptor agonists (tegaserod, 6 mg bid) may be of benefit for some women with constipation-predominant irritable bowel syndrome. Lubiprostone (Amitiza, 24 mcg bid) is a newly available bicyclic fatty acid that increases frequency of bowel movements.
- **Bowel-cleansing agents.** Patients should be placed on a clear liquid diet the previous day and kept NPO for 6–8 hours or overnight prior to the bowel examination (colonoscopy or barium enema).
  - An iso-osmotic **polyethylene glycol solution** (GoLYTELY or NuLYTELY, 1 gallon, administered at a rate of 8 oz every 10 minutes) is commonly used as a bowel-cleansing agent before colonoscopy. This agent has a mildly salty taste, and can be more palatable if chilled; it can also be administered through an NG tube if necessary. Flavored preparations are also available.
  - **Nonabsorbable phosphate** (Fleet phosphosoda, 20–45 mL with 10–24 oz liquid, taken the day before and morning of the procedure) produces bowel movements in 0.5–6 hours. The dose can be taken with 4 oz of liquid and followed with at least 8 oz more of liquid, or 15 mL each can be mixed with three 8-oz glasses of liquid and taken within 30 minutes. Phosphosoda can result in severe dehydration, hyperphosphatemia, hypocalcemia, hypokalemia, hypernatremia, and acidosis. It should be avoided in the elderly and patients with electrolyte imbalances, congestive heart failure, and ascites; it is contraindicated in renal failure and hepatic dysfunction.
  - **Two-day bowel preparation** is sometimes indicated in elderly or debilitated individuals when the above agents are contraindicated. This consists of magnesium citrate (120–300 mL PO) administered on 2 consecutive days while the patient remains on a clear liquid diet; bisacodyl (30 mg PO or 10-mg suppository) can also be administered on both days. Oral bowel-cleansing agents should be avoided in patients with suspected bowel obstruction, ileus, bowel perforation, toxic colitis, or toxic megacolon. **Tap water enemas** (1-L volume, repeated one to two times) can cleanse the distal colon when colonoscopy is indicated in patients with proximal bowel obstruction.

OTHER GASTROINTESTINAL DISORDERS

GASTROPARESIS

General Principles

Definition
- Gastroparesis consists of abnormally delayed emptying of stomach contents into the small bowel, usually as a result of damage to the nerves or smooth muscle involved in gastric emptying.

Etiology
- Gastroparesis can result from chronic disorders (diabetes mellitus, scleroderma, intestinal pseudo-obstruction, previous gastric surgery) or, less frequently, from acute metabolic derangements (hypokalemia, hypercalcemia, hypocalcemia, hyperglycemia) or medications (narcotic analgesics, anticholinergic agents, chemotherapy agents).
- Mechanical obstruction should always be excluded.

Diagnosis

Clinical Presentation
- Symptoms include nausea, bloating, and vomiting, usually hours after a meal.

Investigation
- A gastric-emptying study consisting of gamma camera scanning after a radiolabeled meal can help with the diagnosis.
- Endoscopic evidence of retained food debris in the stomach after an overnight fast may be an indirect indicator of delayed gastric emptying.

Treatment

- Underlying metabolic derangements should be corrected.
- Patients should avoid high-fat, high-fiber meals.
- High-calorie liquid iso-osmotic meals may be beneficial in refractory situations.

Medications
- **Prokinetic agents** have been used with varying degrees of success.
  - **Metoclopramide** (10 mg PO qid half an hour before meals) has variable efficacy, and side effects (drowsiness, tardive dyskinesia, parkinsonism) may be limiting.
  - **Erythromycin** (250 mg PO tid or 200 mg IV) also stimulates gastric motility.
  - **Tegaserod**, a 5-HT$_4$ agonist with prokinetic properties, is being studied for use in gastroparesis.

CELIAC SPRUE

General Principles

Definition
- Celiac sprue is a sensitivity to gluten, the protein found in wheat, barley, and rye. The resulting inflammation in the small-bowel mucosa causes malabsorption of dietary nutrients.

Diagnosis

Investigation
- Noninvasive tests include antiendomysial and antitissue transglutaminase antibodies.

- Endoscopic biopsy revealing severe blunting or complete absence of villi is highly suggestive.

Treatment

- A gluten-free diet results in prompt improvement in symptoms.
- If symptoms persist despite strict gluten-free diet, radiologic and endoscopic evaluation of the small bowel should be performed to rule out complications including collagenous colitis and **small-bowel lymphoma.**

Medications
- Patients may require iron, folate, calcium, and vitamin supplements.
- **Corticosteroids** (prednisone, 10–20 mg/d) may be required in refractory cases, although the most common cause of refractory disease is dietary indiscretion.

LACTOSE INTOLERANCE

General Principles

Definition
- Selective deficiency of lactase in the intestinal brush border results in prompt symptoms upon ingestion of dairy products.
- Temporary lactase deficiency may result from bacterial or viral enteritis.

Diagnosis

Clinical Presentation
- Undigested lactose in the intestinal lumen causes osmotic diarrhea, abdominal cramps, and flatulence.
- Symptom resolution on avoidance of dairy products is usually sufficient for diagnosis.

Investigation
- Lactose tolerance and hydrogen breath tests can be used for diagnosis in difficult cases.

Treatment

- Patients are advised to avoid dairy products.

Medications
- Lactase supplements (two to four tablets or capsules with each lactose meal)

SMALL INTESTINAL BACTERIAL OVERGROWTH

General Principles

Etiology
- Bacterial overgrowth of the small intestine can result from any condition that causes intestinal stasis (small-bowel diverticulitis, afferent loop obstruction, scleroderma, intestinal pseudo-obstruction, strictures, adhesions). Hypochlorhydria and immunodeficiency are other predisposing conditions.
- Deconjugation of bile salts by the bacteria causes fat malabsorption. The bacteria also may compete for dietary vitamin B_{12}, causing anemia.

Diagnosis

- The diagnosis is suspected from patient presentation.
- Imaging of the abdomen may demonstrate intestinal stasis.
- Lactulose-hydrogen breath testing may confirm the diagnosis.
- Culture of small-bowel aspirate obtained at endoscopy is rarely required.

Treatment

Medications

- **Broad-spectrum antimicrobials** (tetracycline, 250 mg PO qid; amoxicillin/clavulanate, 250–500 mg PO tid; ciprofloxacin, 250 mg PO bid) can be used in 2-week courses intermittently.
- Vitamin supplementation may be necessary.

Surgery

- Surgical correction of the predisposing disorder may be indicated.

DIVERTICULOSIS

General Principles

Definition

- **Diverticula** consist of outpouchings in the bowel, most commonly in the colon, but also rarely seen elsewhere in the gut.
- **Diverticular bleeding** can rarely occur from an artery at the mouth of the diverticulum.
- **Diverticulitis** results from microperforation of a diverticulum and resultant extracolonic or intramural inflammation.

Diagnosis

Clinical Presentation

- Diverticulosis is most frequently asymptomatic. Though diverticulosis may be found in patients being investigated for symptoms of abdominal pain and altered bowel habits, a causal link is difficult to establish.
- Diverticular bleeding can be profuse, and presentation can consist of bright red blood per rectum associated with hemodynamic compromise.
- Typical symptoms of diverticulitis include left lower quadrant abdominal pain, fevers and chills, and alteration of bowel habits.

Investigation

- Diverticula are frequently seen on screening colonoscopy.
- Presentation with GI bleeding may require investigation as outlined at the beginning of this chapter.
- Diverticulitis may be associated with an elevated white blood cell (WBC) count with a left shift.
- Imaging studies, most commonly CT scans, are useful in the diagnosis of diverticulitis. A sodium diatrizoate (Hypaque) enema may demonstrate extracolonic leakage of contrast in difficult cases.
- Colonoscopy is contraindicated for 4–6 weeks after acute diverticulitis.

Treatment

General Measures

- Increased dietary fiber is generally recommended in patients with diverticulosis, although no hard data exist to support its benefit.
- Management of diverticular bleeding may require invasive measures, including angiography, intra-arterial vasopressin infusion, or surgery for control (see Gastrointestinal Bleeding).
- A low-residue diet is recommended for mild diverticulitis.

Medications

- Oral **antibiotics** (e.g., ciprofloxacin, 500 mg PO bid, and metronidazole, 500 mg PO tid for 10–14 days) may suffice for mild diverticulitis.

- Hospital admission, bowel rest, IV fluids, and broad-spectrum IV antimicrobial agents are typically required in moderate to severe cases.

Surgery
- Surgical resection of the bleeding segment may be necessary if diverticular bleeding cannot be controlled conservatively.
- Surgical consultation should be obtained early in moderate to severe diverticulitis, as operative intervention may be necessary should complications arise.

ISCHEMIC INTESTINAL INJURY

General Principles

Definition
- Acute mesenteric ischemia results from arterial (or rarely venous) compromise to the superior mesenteric circulation.
- Emboli and thrombus formation are the most common causes of acute mesenteric ischemia, although **nonocclusive mesenteric ischemia** from vasoconstriction can also give rise to the disorder.
- Ischemic colitis results from mucosal ischemia in the inferior mesenteric circulation during a low-flow state (hypotension, arrhythmias, sepsis, aortic vascular surgery) in patients with atherosclerotic disease.
- Vasculitis, sickle cell disease, vasospasm, and marathon running can also predispose to ischemic colitis.

Diagnosis

Clinical Presentation
- Patients with acute mesenteric ischemia may present with abdominal pain, but physical examination and imaging studies can be unremarkable until infarction has occurred. As a result, diagnosis is late and mortality is high.
- Ischemic colitis may manifest as transient bleeding or diarrhea; severe insults can lead to stricture formation, gangrene, and perforation.

Investigation
- Urgent angiography is indicated if the suspicion for acute mesenteric ischemia is high.
- In patients with ischemic colitis, characteristic "thumbprinting" of the involved colon may be seen on plain radiographs of the abdomen.
- Colonoscopy may reveal mucosal erythema, edema, and ulceration, sometimes in a linear configuration; evidence of gangrene or necrosis is an indication for surgical intervention.

Treatment
- Treatment of acute mesenteric ischemia is essentially surgical.
- In patients with ischemic colitis, in the absence of peritoneal signs or evidence of gangrene or perforation, expectant management with fluid and electrolyte repletion, broad-spectrum antimicrobials, and maintenance of an adequate BP usually suffices.
- Evidence of gangrene or necrosis in the setting of ischemic colitis is an indication for surgery.

ANORECTAL DISORDERS

- **Thrombosed external hemorrhoids** present as acutely painful, tense, bluish lumps covered with skin in the anal area. The thrombosed hemorrhoid can be surgically excised under local anesthesia for relief of severe pain. In less severe cases, oral analgesics, sitz baths (sitting in a tub of warm water), stool softeners, and topical ointments may provide symptomatic relief.

■ **Internal hemorrhoids** commonly present with either bleeding or a prolapsing mass with straining. Bulk-forming agents such as fiber supplements are useful in preventing straining at defecation. Sitz baths and Tucks pads (cotton soaked in witch hazel) may provide symptomatic relief. Ointments and suppositories that contain topical analgesics, emollients, astringents, and hydrocortisone (e.g., Anusol-HC Suppositories, one per rectum bid for 7–10 days) can also be used to decrease edema. Hemorrhoidectomy or band ligation can be curative, and is indicated in patients with recurrent or constant bleeding.

■ **Anal fissures** present with acute onset of pain during defecation and are often caused by passage of hard stool. Anoscopy reveals an elliptical tear in the skin of the anus, usually in the posterior midline. Acute fissures generally heal in 2–3 weeks with the use of stool softeners, oral or topical analgesics, and sitz baths. Topical nitroglycerin ointment, 0.2%, applied three times a day may be beneficial. Chronic fissures often require surgical therapy.

■ **Perirectal abscess** commonly presents as a painful induration in the perianal area. Patients with IBD and immunocompromised states are particularly susceptible. Prompt drainage is essential to avoid the serious morbidity associated with delayed treatment. Antimicrobials directed against bowel flora (metronidazole, 500 mg PO tid, and ciprofloxacin, 500 mg PO bid) should be administered in patients with significant inflammation, systemic toxicity, or immunocompromised states.

Suggested Readings

Gibril F, Reynolds JC, Doppman JL, et al. Somatostatin receptor scintigraphy: its sensitivity compared with that of other imaging methods in detecting primary and metastatic gastrinomas. A prospective study. *Ann Intern Med* 1997;126(9):741–742.

Khuroo MS, Farahat KL, Kagevi IE. Treatment with proton pump inhibitors in acute non-variceal upper gastrointestinal bleeding: a meta-analysis. *J Gastroenterol Hepatol* 2005;20:11–25.

Barkun A, Mardou M, Marshall JK. Consensus recommendations for managing patients with nonvariceal upper gastrointestinal bleeding. *Ann Intern Med* 2003;139:843–857.

Leontiadis GI, McIntyre L, Sharma VK, et al. Proton pump inhibitor treatment for acute peptic ulcer bleeding. *Cochrane Database Syst Rev* 2004;(3):CD002094.

Saad R, Chey WD. A clinician's guide to managing Helicobacter pylori infection. *Cleve Clin J Med* 2005;72:109–118.

Hoedema RE, Luchtefeld MA. The management of lower gastrointestinal hemorrhage. *Dis Colon Rectum* 2005;48:2010–2024.

Green BT, Rockey DC, Portwood G, et al. Urgent colonoscopy for evaluation and management of acute lower gastrointestinal hemorrhage: a randomized controlled trial. *Am J Gastroenterol* 2005;100:2395–2402.

DeVault KR, Castell DO. Updated guidelines for the diagnosis and treatment of gastroesophageal reflux disease. *Am J Gastroenterol* 2005;100:190–200.

Clouse RE. Spastic disorders of the esophagus. *Gastroenterologist* 1997;5:112–127.

Korzenik JR, Dieckgraefe BK, Valentine JF, et al. Sargramostim for active Crohn's disease. *N Engl J Med* 2005;352:2193–2201.

Schiller LR. Chronic diarrhea. *Gastroenterology* 2004;127:287–293.

Brandt LJ, Prather CM, Quigley EM, et al. Systematic review on the management of chronic constipation in North America. *Am J Gastroenterol* 2005;100(Suppl 1):S5–21.

Brandt LJ, Bjorkman D, Fennerty MB, et al. Systematic review on the management of irritable bowel syndrome in North America. *Am J Gastroenterol* 2002;97(Suppl 11): S7–26.

Ponec RJ, Saunders MD, Kimmey MB. Neostigmine for the treatment of acute colonic pseudoobstruction. *N Engl J Med* 1999;341:137.

LIVER DISEASES
Shelby Sullivan and Mauricio Lisker-Melman

17

 EVALUATION OF LIVER FUNCTION

GENERAL PRINCIPLES

Classification

- Liver disease is classified according to the duration of abnormalities as either **acute** (<6 months) or **chronic** (>6 months).

DIAGNOSIS

Laboratory Studies

- **Serum enzymes.** Hepatic disorders associated predominantly with elevation in **aminotransferases** are referred to as **hepatocellular;** hepatic disorders with predominant elevation in **alkaline phosphatase (AP)** are referred to as **cholestatic.**
  - Elevation of **serum aspartate and alanine aminotransferases (AST and ALT, respectively)** indicates hepatocellular injury and necrosis. Markedly elevated levels (>1,000 U/L) typically occur with acute hepatocellular injury (e.g., viral, drug induced, or ischemic), whereas mild to moderate elevations may be seen in a variety of conditions (e.g., acute or chronic hepatocellular injury, infiltrative diseases, biliary obstruction). The ratio of serum AST to ALT is typically >2 in alcoholic liver disease. In viral hepatitis, this ratio is characteristically <1.
  - **AP** is an enzyme that is present in a variety of tissues (bone, intestine, kidney, leukocytes, liver, and placenta). The concomitant elevation of other hepatic enzymes (e.g., **γ-glutamyl transpeptidase (GGT) or 5′-nucleotidase**) assists in establishing the hepatic origin of AP. Serum AP level is often elevated in biliary obstruction, space-occupying lesions or infiltrative disorders of the liver, and conditions that cause intrahepatic cholestasis (primary biliary cirrhosis, primary sclerosing cholangitis, drug-induced cholestasis). The degree of elevation of AP does not differentiate the site or cause of cholestasis.
  - **GGT** is an enzyme that is present in a variety of tissues. Increases in GGT and AP tend to occur in similar hepatic diseases. GGT may be elevated in individuals who ingest barbiturates, phenytoin, or alcohol even when other liver enzyme and bilirubin levels are normal.
  - **5′-nucleotidase** is comparable to AP in sensitivity in detecting biliary obstruction, cholestasis, and infiltrative hepatobiliary diseases.
- **Synthetic products**
  - **Serum albumin** concentration is frequently decreased in chronic liver disease. However, chronic inflammation, expanded plasma volume, and gastrointestinal or renal losses may also lead to hypoalbuminemia. Because the half-life of albumin is relatively long (20 days), serum levels may be normal in acute liver disease.

■ Several important proteins involved in **hemostasis** and **fibrinolysis** (coagulation factors [except factor VIII, which is produced by the liver and endothelium] α_2-antiplasmin, antithrombin, heparin cofactor II, high molecular weight kininogen, prekallikrein, protein C, and protein S) are synthesized by the liver. The synthesis of factors II, VII, IX, and X and proteins C and S depends on the presence of vitamin K. The adequacy of hepatic synthetic function can be estimated by the **prothrombin time (PT)** and the **international normalized ratio (INR)** (see Chapter 18, Disorders of Hemostasis). PT/INR prolongation may result from impaired coagulation factor synthesis or vitamin K deficiency. Normalization of PT/INR after administration of vitamin K indicates vitamin K deficiency.

■ **Cholesterol** is synthesized in the liver. Patients with advanced liver disease may have very low cholesterol levels. However, in primary biliary cirrhosis, levels of serum cholesterol may be markedly elevated.

■ Other synthetic products whose levels can be measured in specific liver diseases are α_1-antitrypsin and ceruloplasmin.

■ Excretory products
  ■ **Bilirubin** is a degradation product of hemoglobin and nonerythroid hemoproteins (e.g., cytochrome, catalase). Total serum bilirubin is composed of **conjugated (direct)** and **unconjugated (indirect)** fractions. Unconjugated hyperbilirubinemia occurs as a result of **excessive bilirubin production** (neonatal or physiologic jaundice, hemolysis and hemolytic anemias, ineffective erythropoiesis, and resorption of hematomas), **reduced hepatic bilirubin uptake** (Gilbert's syndrome and drugs such as rifampin and probenecid), or **impaired bilirubin conjugation** (Gilbert's or Crigler-Najjar's syndrome). Elevation of conjugated and unconjugated fractions occurs in Dubin-Johnson's and Rotor's syndromes and in conditions associated with **intrahepatic** (from hepatocellular, canalicular, or ductular damage) and **extrahepatic** (from mechanical obstruction) **cholestasis**.

  ■ **Bile acids** are produced in the liver and are secreted into the intestine, where they are required for lipid digestion and absorption. Elevated levels of serum bile acids are specific but not sensitive markers of hepatobiliary disease. Levels of individual bile acids are not useful in the differential diagnosis of liver disorders.

  ■ **α-Fetoprotein** is normally produced by fetal liver cells. Its production falls to normal adult levels of <10 ng/mL within 1 year of life. An α-fetoprotein level of >400 ng/mL or a rapid doubling time is very suggestive of hepatocellular carcinoma (HCC); however, mild to moderate elevations can also be seen in states of acute and chronic liver inflammation.

Imaging

■ **Ultrasonography** is used to screen for dilation of the biliary tree and to detect gallstones and cholecystitis in patients with right-sided abdominal pain associated with abnormal liver blood tests. It can reveal and characterize liver masses, abscesses, and cysts. Color-flow doppler ultrasonography can assess patency and direction of blood flow in the portal and hepatic veins. Ultrasonography is a frequently used modality for screening of hepatocellular carcinoma.

■ **Helical computed tomography (CT)** scan with IV contrast is useful in the evaluation of parenchymal liver disease. It has the added feature of contrast enhancement to define space-occupying lesions (e.g., abscess and tumor) and allows calculation of liver volume. Triple-phase CT (noncontrast, arterial phase, and venous phase) is indicated for liver mass evaluation. A delayed phase is useful when cholangiocarcinoma is suspected.

■ **Magnetic resonance imaging (MRI)** offers information similar to that provided by CT scan and the additional advantage of better characterization of liver lesions, fatty infiltration, and iron deposition. It is the modality of choice in patients with an allergy to iodinated contrast and renal failure.

■ **Magnetic resonance cholangiopancreatography (MRCP)** is a specialized version of MRI that provides an alternative noninvasive diagnostic modality for visualizing the intra- and extrahepatic bile ducts.

- Percutaneous transhepatic cholangiography (PTC) and endoscopic retrograde cholangiopancreatography (ERCP) involve the instillation of contrast into the biliary tree. They are most useful after the preliminary determination of biliary tree abnormalities detected by ultrasonography, CT, or MRI/MRCP.
- Technetium-99m red blood cell (RBC) scan is helpful in confirming the diagnosis of hepatic hemangioma. Other imaging techniques have diminished its usefulness.
- Positron emission tomography (PET) is an emerging modality that uses differences in metabolism among normal, inflammatory, and malignant tissues. PET scans are helpful in assessing the presence of hepatic metastasis in colorectal cancer. PET scans may also be helpful in diagnosing cholangiocarcinoma.

Liver Biopsy

- Percutaneous liver biopsy can be performed with or without radiographic (ultrasound or CT) guidance. In the presence of coagulopathy, thrombocytopenia, and/or ascites, a biopsy can be obtained by the transjugular route. Suspicious liver lesions are usually biopsied with ultrasonographic or CT guidance. Laparoscopy is an alternative method for obtaining liver tissue. Percutaneous liver biopsy is generally safe and usually is performed as an outpatient procedure. Bleeding, pain, infection, injury to neighboring organs, and (rarely) death are potential complications.

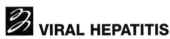 # VIRAL HEPATITIS

GENERAL PRINCIPLES

- The hepatotropic viruses include hepatitis A (HAV), hepatitis B (HBV), hepatitis C (HCV), hepatitis D (HDV), and hepatitis E (HEV) (Tables 17-1 and 17-2). Nonhepatotropic viruses (viruses that indirectly affect the liver) include Epstein-Barr virus, cytomegalovirus, herpes virus, measles, Ebola, and others.

Definitions

- Acute viral hepatitis is defined by the sudden onset of significant aminotransferase elevation as a consequence of diffuse necroinflammatory liver injury. Symptoms may be variable. This condition may resolve or progress to fulminant failure or chronic hepatitis.
- Chronic viral hepatitis is defined as the presence of persistent (at least 6 months) necroinflammatory injury that can lead to cirrhosis. Histopathologic classification of chronic viral hepatitis is based on etiology, grade, and stage. Grading and staging are measures of the severity of the necroinflammatory process and fibrosis, respectively.

HEPATITS A VIRUS

General Principles

Epidemiology

- HAV is the most common cause of viral hepatitis worldwide.
- Approximately 30% of acute viral hepatitis in the United States is caused by HAV.
- High-risk groups include people living in or traveling to underdeveloped countries, men having sex with men, and staff and attendees at daycare centers.
- HAV is an RNA virus that belongs to the picornavirus family.

Mode of Transmission

- HAV infection is usually transmitted via the fecal–oral route.
- Large-scale outbreaks due to contamination of food and drinking water can occur.
- The period of greatest infectivity is 2 weeks before the onset of clinical illness; fecal shedding continues for 2–3 weeks after the onset of symptoms.

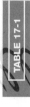

TABLE 17-1 Clinical and Epidemiologic Features of Hepatotropic Viruses

Organism	Hepatitis A	Hepatitis B	Hepatitis C	Hepatitis D	Hepatitis E
Incubation	15–45 d	30–180 d	15–150 d	30–150 d	30–60 d
Transmission	Fecal–oral	Blood Sexual Perinatal	Blood Sexual (rare) Perinatal (rare)	Blood Sexual (rare)	Fecal–oral
Risk groups	Residents of and travelers to endemic regions Children and caregivers in daycare centers	Injection drug users Multiple sexual partners Men having sex with men Infants born to infected mothers Health care workers Transfusion recipients	Injection drug users Transfusion recipients	Any person with hepatitis B virus Injection drug users	Residents of and travelers to endemic regions
Fatality rate	1.0%	1.0%	<0.1%	2%–10%	1%
Carrier state	No	Yes	Yes	Yes	No
Chronic hepatitis	None	2%–10% in adults; 90% in children <5 yr	70%–85%	Variable	None
Cirrhosis	No	Yes	Yes	Yes	No

| **TABLE 17-2** | **Viral Hepatitis Serologies** |

Hepatitis	Acute	Chronic	Recovered/latent	Vaccinated
HAV	IgM anti-HAV+	NA	IgG anti-HAV+	IgG anti-HAV+
HBV	IgM anti-HBc+ HBeAg+ HBsAg+ HBV DNA+	IgG anti-HBc+ HBeAg± Anti-HBe±[a] HBsAg+ HBV DNA±[a]	IgG anti-HBc+ HBeAg− Anti-HBe ±[a] HBsAg− Anti-HBs Ab+ HBV DNA−	Anti-HBs+ only
HCV	All tests possibly negative HCV RNA+ Anti-HCV Ab+ in 8–10 wk	Anti-HCV Ab+ HCV RNA+	Anti-HCV Ab+ HCV RNA−[b]	NA
HDV	IgM anti-HDV+[c] HDV Ag+[c]	IgG anti-HDV+[c]	IgG anti-HDV+[c]	NA+[d]
HEV	Available from CDC and research specialty laboratories	NA	Available from CDC and research specialty laboratories	NA

Ab, antibody; CDC, Centers for Disease Control and Prevention; HAV, hepatitis A virus; HBc, hepatitis B core antigen; HBeAg, hepatitis B e antigen; HBsAg, hepatitis B surface antigen; HBV, hepatitis B virus; HCV, hepatitis C virus; HDV, hepatitis D virus; HEV, hepatitis E virus; NA, not applicable.
[a]HBeAg is present during periods of high replication along with HBV DNA. Anti-HBe is present during periods of low replication when HBeAg and HBV DNA may be undetectable.
[b]Negative HCV RNA results should be interpreted with caution. Differences are found in thresholds for detection among assays and among laboratories.
[c]Markers of HBV infection are also present, because HDV cannot replicate in the absence of HBV.
[d]Although no vaccine is available for HDV, immunity to HBV protects against HDV infection.

- Although the period of viremia is brief, sexual transmission and parenteral transmission may occur.

Clinical Features
- HAV can be silent (subclinical), especially in children and young adults. Symptoms vary from mild illness to fulminant hepatic failure (FHF). Malaise, fatigue, pruritus, headache, abdominal pain, myalgias, arthralgias, nausea, vomiting, anorexia, and fever are common but nonspecific symptoms.
- **Physical examination** may reveal jaundice, hepatomegaly, and in rare cases lymphadenopathy, splenomegaly, or a vascular rash.

Diagnosis
- The diagnosis of acute HAV is made by the detection of **IgM anti-HAV antibody.**
- The **recovery phase** and **immunity phase** are characterized by **IgG anti-HAV antibody.**
- Liver biopsy is rarely needed.

Clinical Course
- Almost all cases of acute HAV hepatitis will resolve in 4–6 weeks.
- Prolonged cholestatic disease, characterized by persistent jaundice, is more frequently seen in adults.

- **Acute liver failure** is relatively rare, but risk increases with age: 0.1% in patients younger than 15 years old to >1% in patients older than 40 years old.
- HAV does not induce chronic hepatitis or cirrhosis.

Treatment

- No specific treatment is available.
- Supportive treatment is recommended.
- Liver transplantation may be an option for FHF.

Prophylaxis

- **Preexposure prophylaxis** (Appendix C, Immunizations and Postexposure Therapies)
  - **HAV vaccine** should be given to travelers to endemic areas, men who have sex with men, illegal drug users, persons with high occupational risk for infection (research personnel working with HAV or HAV-infected primates), persons who have clotting factor disorders, and persons with chronic liver disease. In the United States, children residing in areas where the incidence of hepatitis A is twice the national average and people living in communities with local outbreaks of HAV should be vaccinated. Vaccinations should be administered at 0 and 6 months.
  - **Vaccination** should be initiated at least 4 weeks before travel to an endemic area. For individuals who require immediate protection, the first dose of HAV vaccine can be administered concomitantly with immunoglobulin (Ig) 0.02 mL/kg IM **injection,** at different anatomic injection sites.
  - Travelers who are allergic to a vaccine component or who elect not to undergo vaccination should receive a single dose of Ig (0.02 mL/kg IM if the desired duration of protection is up to 3 months or 0.06 mL/kg if the desired duration is 2–5 months). The dose should be repeated if the travel period exceeds 5 months.
- **Postexposure prophylaxis.** (Appendix C, Immunizations and Postexposure Therapies.)
  - Ig (0.02 mL/kg IM) should be given within 2 weeks of the last exposure to unvaccinated individuals.
  - Household and sexual contacts and persons who have shared illegal drugs with a person who has serologically confirmed acute HAV should receive Ig and the first dose of vaccine at different anatomic sites.
  - **Ig** should be administered to all previously unvaccinated staff and attendees of day-care centers if one or more cases of HAV are recognized in children or employees or if cases are recognized in two or more households of center attendees. HAV vaccine can be administered at the same time as Ig at different anatomic sites.
  - If a food handler is diagnosed with HAV, Ig should be administered to other food handlers at the same establishment and to patrons who can be identified and treated within 2 weeks of exposure.

HEPATITIS B VIRUS

General Principles

Epidemiology

- Two billion people worldwide have been infected and more than 350 million people are chronic carriers.
- In endemic areas such as Asia and sub-Saharan Africa, infection is usually acquired in childhood, while in Western countries where HBV is relatively rare, the infection is acquired in adulthood.
- HBV causes 60%–80% of **hepatocellular carcinoma** worldwide.
- **High-risk groups** include individuals with a history of multiple blood transfusions, patients on hemodialysis, health care workers, injection drug users, household and heterosexual contacts of hepatitis B carriers, men having sex with men, residents and employees of residential care facilities, travelers (>6 months) to hyperendemic regions, and natives of Alaska, Asia, and the Pacific Islands.

Mode of Transmission

- **Parenteral routes** (e.g., needlestick injury, injection drug use, and transfusion)
- **Sexual contact**
- **Vertical or perinatal transmission** (from mother to infant)

Clinical Features

- **Acute hepatitis B** can be silent (subclinical), especially in children and young adults. Symptoms vary from mild illness to FHF. Malaise, fatigue, pruritus, headache, abdominal pain, myalgias, arthralgias, nausea, vomiting, anorexia, and fever are common but nonspecific symptoms.
- **Chronic hepatitis B** runs an indolent course, sometimes for decades. Fatigue is a common symptom. The disease may only become clinically apparent late in the natural course, when symptoms typically seen in end-stage liver disease (ESLD) appear.
- **Extrahepatic manifestations** include polyarteritis nodosa, glomerulonephritis, cryoglobulinemia, serum sickness–like illness, papular acrodermatitis (predominantly in children), and aplastic anemia.

Diagnosis

- **HBV is a DNA virus** that belongs to the **hepadnavirus family.** It contains a number of antigens that elicit a corresponding antibody response.
  - **Hepatitis B surface antigen (HBsAg)** is detectable in serum in acute and chronic HBV infection and disappears after clearance of the virus.
  - **Hepatitis B core antigen (HBcAg)** is not found in serum but can be detected within liver cells by immunoperoxidase staining during active viral replication.
  - **Hepatitis B e antigen (HBeAg)** appears shortly after HBsAg in the serum and its persistence is indicative of active viral replication and a high degree of infectivity.
  - **Antibody against HBsAg (anti-HBs)** appears after the disappearance of HBsAg and after vaccination. Anti-HBs confers immunity (except in rare cases of chronic HBV infection with very low titers of heterotypic anti-HBs).
  - **IgM antibody against HBcAg (IgM anti-HBc)** usually is present in acute infection and occasionally can be detected during periods of high viral replication in chronic disease.
  - **IgG anti-HBc** is detectable in chronic infection and, in association with anti-HBs, after recovery. Rarely, patients with isolated IgG anti-HBc can reactivate HBV in the setting of immunosuppression (e.g., transplantation).
  - **Antibody against HBeAg (anti-HBe)** usually indicates low-level replication and a lower degree of infectivity. Some patients harbor HBV mutants (e.g., precore, core promoter), in which case the conventional serologic markers may vary.
  - **HBV viral DNA (HBV DNA)** is the most accurate marker of viral replication. It is detected by polymerase chain reaction (PCR) and reported as copies per milliliter or International Units per milliliter.
- For use of HBV markers in clinical practice, see Table 17-3.
- Genotype determination is not part of the daily practice of most clinicians; however, their clinical significance is growing.
- **Liver biopsy** is useful to score the degree of inflammation (grade) and fibrosis (stage) in patients with chronic hepatitis. Special staining techniques are helpful to identify HBsAg and HBcAg.

Clinical Course

- Incubation period after HBV infection ranges from 30–160 days.
- Depending on the age of the person at infection, people may have spontaneous resolution or progression to chronicity.
  - Children younger than 5 years old: 90% will develop chronic HBV infection.
  - Adults: 5%–10% will develop chronic HBV.
- Chronic hepatitis B
  - Spontaneous clearance of HBsAg occurs in 1% of patients annually.
  - Thirty percent progress to **cirrhosis.**

TABLE 17-3 Use of HBV Markers in Clinical Practice

Test	Acute hepatitis B	Resolved acute hepatitis B	High-replication chronic HBV	Low-replication chronic HBV	HBV precore mutant	Vaccination
HBsAg	+	−	+	+	+	−
HBeAg	+	−	+	−	−	−
Anti-HBs	−	+	−	−	−	+
Anti-HBe	−	+	−	+	+	−
IgM anti-HBc	+	−	−	−	−	−
IgG anti-HBc	−	+	+	+	+	−
HBV DNA	$>10^5$ copies/mL	Negative	$>10^5$ copies/mL	10^2–10^4 copies/mL	$>10^4$ copies/mL	Negative
ALT/AST	+++	Normal	+++	Normal	+/++	Normal

ALT, alanine transaminase; AST, aspartate transaminase; HBc, hepatitis B core antigen; HBeAg, hepatitis B e antigen; HBsAg, hepatitis B surface antigen; HBV, hepatitis B virus.

- Five to ten percent progress to **HCC** with or without preceding cirrhosis. The risk of HCC is dependant on the degree of viral replication.

Treatment

- Goals of treatment
  - **Clearance** of HBV DNA
  - **HBeAg and HBsAg seroconversion** (i.e., antigen disappearance and appearance of antibodies)
  - **Normalization** of **liver enzymes**
  - **Normalization** of **histology**
- Current treatment options
  - The interferons (IFN) are glycoproteins with antiviral, immunomodulatory, and antiproliferative actions. The addition of polyethylene glycol (PEG) to the standard IFN (α2a and 2b) molecules (pegylation) results in prolonged half-life with improved bioavailability. **IFN-α2a and 2b is administered subcutaneously thrice weekly for 4–6 months, or peginterferon alfa for 48 weeks.** HBeAg seroconversion is achieved in 30% of treated patients, and HBsAg seroconversion in 5%–10%. They do not induce resistant mutations. Their use is contraindicated in patients with decompensated liver disease. Common adverse events from IFN therapy include flu-like syndrome (headache, fatigue, myalgias, arthralgias, fever, and chills), neuropsychiatric disorders (depression, irritability, and concentration impairment), reversible bone marrow suppression (neutropenia, thrombocytopenia, and anemia), and other effects (alopecia, thyroiditis, injection site reactions).
  - **Lamivudine** is a nucleoside analog with antiviral activity. It is administered orally at 100 mg daily. Treatment success is proportional to treatment duration. Its use has been diminished by a high rate of induction of resistant mutants (15%–20% per year of treatment).
  - **Adefovir** is a nucleotide analog with antiviral activity. It is administered orally at 10 mg daily. Treatment success is proportional to treatment duration. Adefovir can be used as a treatment option for patients with lamivudine resistance. It is safely used in patients with advanced or decompensated liver disease. In patients with renal impairment, dose adjustment is needed. Fifteen to twenty-nine percent of nucleotide naïve patients will develop resistance to adefovir after 4–5 years of treatment.
  - **Entecavir** is a nucleoside analog with antiviral activity. It is admistered orally at 0.5 mg daily in naïve nucleoside patients and 1 mg daily in patients with known lamivudine resistance mutations. In patients with renal impairment, dosage adjustment is needed. Resistant mutants are very rare in nucleoside-naïve treated patients after 3 years of therapy. In lamivudine resistant patients, resistance mutations to entecavir are more frequent (15% after 3 years of treatment).
  - **Telbivudine** is a nucleoside analog. It was recently approved for treatment of HBV in the United States. Preliminary reports show robust antiviral activity with a mild to moderate rate of induction of resistant mutants at 2 years of therapy.
  - New agents, regimens, and combination therapies are currently under investigation.
  - **Liver transplantation** is indicated for patients with advanced liver disease due to infection with HBV. Immunoprophylaxis with hepatitis B immunoglobulin (HBIg) combined with a nucleoside or nucleotide analog is obligatory to diminish hepatitis B recurrence.

Prophylaxis

- Preexposure prophylaxis (See Appendix C, Immunizations and Postexposure Therapies)
  - **HBV vaccine** should be considered for everyone, particularly in individuals with a history of multiple blood transfusions, patients on hemodialysis, health care workers, injection drug users, household and heterosexual contacts of hepatitis B carriers, men having sex with men, residents and employees of residential care facilities, travelers (>6 months) to hyperendemic regions, and natives of Alaska, Asia, and the Pacific Islands.

- Many countries have included HBV vaccination (0, 1, and 6 months) in their infant or adult immunization programs. The Centers for Disease Control and Prevention has recommended a universal vaccination program for infants and sexually active adolescents in the United States.
- Prevaccination screening for previous exposure or infection is recommended in high-risk groups to avoid vaccinating recovered individuals or those with chronic infection.
- For patients who require rapid immunity, the dosage schedule can be escalated to 0, 1, and 2 months, but a follow-up booster at 6 months is required for long-lasting immunity.
- Additional doses, higher doses, or revaccination can be considered in nonresponders and hyporesponders (anti-HBs <10 International Units/mL) to elicit protective levels of immunity. Booster doses may be needed in immunosuppressed individuals in whom anti-HBs levels fall below 10 International Units/mL on annual testing.
- Postexposure prophylaxis (see Appendix C)
  - Infants born to HBsAg-positive mothers should receive HBV vaccine and HBIg, 0.5 mL, within 12 hours of birth. Immunized infants should be tested at approximately 12 months of age for HBsAg, anti-HBs, and anti-HBc. The presence of HBsAg indicates that the infant is actively infected. The presence of both anti-HBs and anti-HBc suggests that infection occurred but was probably modified by immunoprophylaxis and that immunity is likely to be prolonged. The presence of anti-HBs alone is indicative of vaccine-induced immunity.
  - Susceptible sexual partners of individuals with HBV and victims of needlestick injury (with HBV contamination) should receive HBIg (0.04–0.07 mL/kg) and the first dose of HBV vaccine at different sites on the body as soon as possible (preferably within 48 hours but no more than 7 days after exposure). A second dose of HBIg can be administered 30 days after exposure, and the vaccination schedule should be completed.
  - Postexposure prophylaxis with HBIg and lamivudine or adefovir should be used after liver transplantation for ESLD that results from HBV (see Chapter 15, Solid Organ Transplant Medicine).

HEPATITIS C VIRUS

General Principles

Epidemiology

- HCV is a global health problem with approximately **200 million carriers worldwide.**
- HCV is an RNA virus that belongs to the Flaviviridae family.
- The incidence of HCV in the U.S. has decreased from 240,000 cases per year in 1985 to 18,000 cases in 2003.
- In the United States, 4 million people have been infected with this virus, and 8,000–10,000 people die of HCV-related chronic liver disease per year.
- HCV is a frequent cause of **HCC.**
- **Risk factors for HCV infection** include a history of multiple blood transfusions, hemodialysis, injection drug use, multiple sexual partners, and occupational exposure with blood and blood-derived products. Other risk factors may include tattooing, body piercing, sharing "straws" for intranasal cocaine use, sharing razors, and history of military service.

Modes of Transmission

- **Parenterally** (e.g., transfusion, injection drug use, needlestick injury)
- **Sexually** and **from mother to offspring,** although at a much lower frequency than HBV

Clinical Features

- **Acute hepatitis** can be silent (subclinical), especially in children and young adults. Symptoms vary from mild illness to FHF. Malaise, fatigue, pruritus, headache, abdominal pain, myalgias, arthralgias, nausea, vomiting, anorexia, and fever are common but nonspecific symptoms.

- Chronic hepatitis runs an indolent course, sometimes for decades. **Fatigue is a common symptom.** The disease may only become clinically apparent late in the natural course, when symptoms typically seen in ESLD appear.
- **Extrahepatic manifestations** include mixed cryoglobulinemia (10%–25% of patients with HCV), glomerulonephritis, porphyria cutanea tarda, cutaneous necrotizing vasculitis, lichen planus, lymphoma, and other autoimmune disorders.

Diagnosis

- **Antibodies against HCV (anti-HCV)** may be undetectable for the first 8 weeks after infection. Positive tests are usually diagnostic in patients with elevated liver enzymes and with risk factors for the infection. **The antibody does not confer immunity.** The test has a sensitivity of 95%–99% and a lower specificity. A false-positive test in the setting of autoimmune hepatitis or hypergammaglobulinemia may be detected. A false-negative test may be seen in immunosuppressed individuals and in patients on hemodialysis.
- **HCV RNA** can be detected by **PCR** in serum as early as **1–2 weeks after infection.** It determines the presence of actual virus and ongoing infection. Different HCV RNA tests are available and vary in detection sensitivity. Viral concentrations are expressed in international units per milliliter (International Units/mL). This test is useful both for diagnosis and treatment follow-up/response.
- Tests to detect **HCV genotypes, subtypes, or serotypes** are commercially available. HCV genotype influences the duration, dosage, and response to treatment. Genotype 1 accounts for 75% and genotypes 2 and 3 account for 20% of HCV infection in the United States.
- The **recombinant immunoblot assay (RIBA)** is a supplementary test that has been replaced by PCR.
- **Liver biopsy** is useful to score the degree of inflammation (grade) and fibrosis (stage) in the liver of chronically infected patients.

Clinical Course

- The incubation period is 15–150 days.
- **Acute hepatitis** is frequently **clinically silent.**
- **Fifteen percent** of people infected with HCV will have **spontaneous resolution.**
- **Chronic HCV** will occur in 85% of infected people.
- **Progression to cirrhosis** is slow (two to three decades) and is seen in a quarter of patients with chronic HCV.
- HCC develops in approximately **1%–2% of patients per year,** and rarely occurs in the absence of cirrhosis.

Treatment

- Acute infection
  - **IFN-α (standard or pegylated)** for 6 months has been associated with a high rate of sustained HCV RNA clearance.
  - The role of **ribavirin** in addition is under investigation.
- Chronic infection
  - A combination of SC **pegylated-interferon (PEG-IFN)** and **oral ribavirin 400–600 mg twice daily** is administered for 6–12 months. **Peginterferon alfa-2a 180 mcg/wk** and **peginterferon alfa-2b 1.5 mcg/kg/wk** are both efficacious. Sustained virologic response (SVR), defined as clearance of HCV RNA from serum 6 months after completion of treatment, occurs in approximately 55% of all patients. **HCV genotype, viral load, and fibrosis score** determination are important in patient management. **Genotype 1** HCV infection is less susceptible to treatment and requires 12 months of therapy with a 35%–45% SVR. **Genotypes 2 and 3** are more susceptible to treatment and require 6 months of therapy with an 80%–85% SVR. Side effects of ribavirin include teratogenicity, hemolytic anemia, and pulmonary symptoms (dyspnea, cough, and pneumonitis). Contraindications to treatment with ribavirin include pregnancy

or unwillingness to practice birth control, chronic renal insufficiency, and the inability to tolerate anemia (15%–30%).
- Liver transplantation may be indicated in advanced viral disease, but disease recurrence is frequent (see Chapter 15, Solid Organ Transplant).

Prophylaxis

- No preexposure prophylaxis or vaccine exists.

HEPATITIS D VIRUS

- HDV is a small **RNA virus** with an envelope consisting of HBsAg.
- It is found throughout the world, and is endemic to the Mediterranean basin, the Middle East, and portions of South America. Outside these areas, infections occur primarily in individuals who have received transfusions or in injection drug users. **HDV requires the presence of HBV for infection and replication.**
- **High-risk groups** are similar to HBV (see HBV Epidemiology).
- HDV infection clinically presents as **a coinfection** (acute hepatitis B and D), as a **superinfection** (chronic hepatitis B with acute hepatitis D), or as a **latent infection** (e.g., in the liver transplant setting).
- Diagnosis is made by finding HDV RNA or HDV antigen in serum or liver and by detecting antibody to the HDV antigen.
- In patients with coinfection, the course is transient and self-limited. The rate of progression to chronicity is similar to the one reported for acute HBV. In superinfection, the HBV carriers may present with a severe acute hepatitis exacerbation with frequent progression to chronic HDV infection.
- **IFN-α** is the **treatment of choice** for chronic hepatitis D.
- Although there is no vaccine to prevent HDV in carriers of HBV, both infections can be prevented by timely administration of the HBV vaccine.

HEPATITIS E VIRUS

- HEV is an **RNA virus** that belongs to the **Caliciviridae family.**
- It has been implicated in epidemics in India, Southeast Asia, Africa, and Mexico. Reported cases in the United States have been in travelers to endemic areas.
- Transmission closely resembles that of HAV (i.e., **fecal–oral route**).
- Acute hepatitis E is clinically indistinguishable from other acute viral hepatitis. HEV infection is associated with a high fatality rate in pregnant women in the second and third trimesters.
- There is no chronic infection associated with HEV.
- Treatment is supportive.
- There is not pre- or postexposure prophylaxis.

DRUG-INDUCED LIVER TOXICITY

GENERAL PRINCIPLES

- Drug-induced liver toxicity (DILT) is the most common circumstance for a drug to be removed from the market.
- DILT causes approximately 50% of the cases of acute liver failure in the United States, with acetaminophen being the most common causative agent.
- Less commonly DILT can cause chronic liver disease, cirrhosis, and hepatocellular carcinoma.

Pathophysiology

- **Intrinsic hepatotoxicity** results from the **direct hepatotoxic effects** of the drug or its metabolite. This mechanism is predictable and dose dependent. Examples include carbon tetrachloride, elemental phosphorus, and acetaminophen in supratherapeutic doses.
- **Idiosyncratic hepatotoxicity** can be divided into **hypersensitivity (allergic)** responses and **metabolic hepatotoxicity mechanisms (nonallergic)**. These reactions depend on multiple variables and are not predictable.
  - **Hypersensitivity responses** occur as a result of stimulation of the immune system by a metabolite of a drug alone or after haptenization (covalently binding) to a liver protein. (e.g., allopurinol, diclofenac). The latency of the reaction is variable. Repeated challenge with the same agent leads to prompt recurrence of the reaction.
  - **Metabolic hepatotoxicity** occurs in susceptible patients as a result of altered drug clearance or accelerated production of hepatotoxic metabolites (e.g., isoniazid, ketoconazole). The latency of the reaction is variable.

Mechanisms of Injury

- There are three major classifications of DILT that occur as a result of both intrinsic and idiosyncratic hepatotoxicity:
  - **Hepatocellular injury** refers to injury to the **liver cell.**
  - **Cholestatic injury** refers to injury to the **biliary system.**
  - **Mixed hepatocellular** and cholestatic refers to injury to both the liver cell and the biliary system.
- Other less common types of DILT include formation of chronic hepatitis, chronic cholestasis, granulomatous formation, fibrosis or cirrhosis, and carcinogenesis.

Clinical Presentation

- The acute presentation can be clinically silent. When symptoms are present they are nonspecific and include nausea/vomiting, general malaise, fatigue, and abdominal pain.
- In the acute setting, the majority of patients will recover after cessation of the offending drug.
- Fever and rash may also be seen in association with hypersensitivity reactions.

DIAGNOSIS

- Clinical suspicion
- **Temporal relation** of the injury to drug initiation
- **Biochemical abnormalities**
  - Hepatocellular injury: **AST and ALT elevation** more than two times the upper limit of normal
  - Cholestatic injury: **alkaline phosphatase** and **conjugated bilirubin elevation** more than two times the upper limit of normal
  - Mixed injury includes increases in all of the above biochemical abnormalities to more than two times the upper limit of normal.
- Resolution of injury after the offending drug has been stopped
- Liver biopsy is sometimes needed

TREATMENT

- Treatment includes cessation of exposure to the offending drug and institution of supportive measures.
- An attempt to remove the agent from the gastrointestinal (GI) tract should be made in most cases of acute toxic ingestion using lavage or cathartics (see Chapter 25, Medical Emergencies, Overdoses).
- Liver transplantation may be an option for patients with FHF.
- Management of acetaminophen overdose is a medical emergency (see Chapter 25, Medical Emergencies, Overdoses).

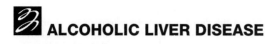 ALCOHOLIC LIVER DISEASE

GENERAL PRINCIPLES

- **Alcohol** is a **toxic substance** to the liver.
- The **spectrum** of alcoholic liver disease is broad, and a single patient may be affected by more than one of the following conditions: **fatty liver, alcoholic hepatitis,** or **alcoholic cirrhosis.**

Epidemiology

- A significant medical and socioeconomic problem. Although ethyl alcohol exerts a direct toxic effect on the liver, significant liver damage develops in only 10%–20% of chronic alcoholics. Average alcohol consumption can be measured by units per week. **One unit** is equal to 7 g of alcohol, one glass of wine, or one 240-mL can of 3.5%–4% beer. Approximately 30–40 units of alcohol per week can induce cirrhosis in 3%–8% of individuals over 12 years.
- **Fatty liver** is the most commonly observed abnormality, and occurs in up to 90% of alcoholics.
- **Alcoholic cirrhosis** is a common cause of ESLD, cirrhosis, and hepatocellular carcinoma.
- Additional factors (e.g., genetic, nutritional, environmental) may be important in the pathogenesis of alcoholic liver disease.

DIAGNOSIS

Clinical Presentation

- Fatty liver
  - Patients are usually asymptomatic.
  - Clinical findings include hepatomegaly and mild liver enzyme abnormalities.
  - Fatty liver may be reversible with abstinence.
- Alcoholic hepatitis
  - Alcoholic hepatitis may be clinically silent or severe enough to lead to rapid development of hepatic failure and death.
  - Clinical features include fever, upper abdominal pain, anorexia, nausea, vomiting, weight loss, and jaundice.
  - In severe cases, patients may have hepatic encephalopathy, ascites, and gastrointestinal bleeding.
  - Patients frequently give a history of drinking up until the onset of symptoms.
  - Prognosis depends on the severity of presentation and alcohol abstinence. The **in-hospital mortality** for severe cases is up to **50%.**
- Alcoholic cirrhosis
  - The presentation is variable, from **clinically silent disease** to decompensated cirrhosis with complications of **portal hypertension** (see Portal Hypertension).
  - Patients have a history of current or past long-term alcohol use.
  - **Prognosis is variable** and depends on the degree of decompensation and alcohol abstinence.

Laboratory Studies

- In alcoholic fatty liver laboratory tests may be normal or may demonstrate mild elevation in serum aminotransferases (**AST higher than ALT**) and **AP.**
- In alcoholic hepatitis, liver laboratory test typically demonstrates elevation in serum aminotransferases (**AST higher than ALT**) and **AP. Hyperbilirubinemia** and **prolongation of PT** may also be seen.

- Laboratory abnormalities associated with a **poor prognosis** include renal failure, leukocytosis, a markedly elevated total bilirubin, and prolongation of the PT that does not normalize with vitamin K.
- A discriminant function $(DF) = 4.6 \times (PT_{patient} - PT_{control}) + serum\ bilirubin,$ can be determined to assess in-hospital mortality.

■ In alcoholic cirrhosis, liver abnormalities may vary depending on disease severity.

Liver Biopsy

■ The typical histopathologic findings in alcoholic liver disease include Mallory hyaline bodies, neutrophilic infiltrate, necrosis of hepatocytes, collagen deposition, and fatty change.

■ The indication of liver biopsy depends on the clinical assessment of the patient. It may be helpful for differential diagnosis.

TREATMENT

Behavioral

■ **Abstinence from alcohol**

■ **Rehabilitation** (i.e., Alcoholics Anonymous, private counseling, etc.)

Medications

■ **Treatment** of acute alcoholic hepatitis with **corticosteroids is controversial.** However, there is evidence that patients with a DF >32 and **hepatic encephalopathy** may benefit from steroid therapy.

■ Oral prednisone can be started at 40–60 mg/d and subsequently tapered as clinically indicated.

■ **Pentoxifylline (400 mg PO tid)** is a nonselective phosphodiesterase inhibitor with anti-inflammatory properties and an excellent safety profile that has shown improved survival in severe (DF >32) alcoholic hepatitis.

■ *S*-Adenosylmethionine, antioxidants, tumor necrosis factor inhibitors, and glutathione prodrugs are under investigation in alcoholic liver disease.

Surgical

■ Patients with cirrhosis and ESLD may be evaluated for liver transplant, but are required to abstain from alcohol for 6 months.

Complications

■ Potentially dangerous interactions may occur between alcohol and a variety of medications, including sedative-hypnotics, anticoagulants, and acetaminophen, even in the absence of alcoholic liver disease, because of shared metabolic pathways.

 # IMMUNE-MEDIATED LIVER DISEASE

AUTOIMMUNE HEPATITIS

General Principles

Definition
■ Autoimmune hepatitis (AIH) is **a chronic inflammation** of the liver of unknown cause, associated with circulating auto-antibodies and hypergammaglobulinemia.

Epidemiology
■ AIH occurs worldwide.

- It occurs most often in women (10–30 years and late middle age).
- In North America, cirrhosis is present at initial presentation more often in black patients than in Caucasian patients.

Diagnosis

Clinical Presentation
- In approximately 30% of cases, the presentation is **acute** and similar to viral hepatitis. Patients may present in **FHF** or with **asymptomatic elevation** of serum **ALT**. It **presents** with **cirrhosis** in at least **25%** of patients.
- The most common symptoms at presentation include fatigue, jaundice, myalgias, anorexia, diarrhea, acne, and right upper quadrant abdominal discomfort.
- Extrahepatic manifestations may be found in 30%–50% and include celiac sprue, Coombs' positive hemolytic anemia, autoimmune thyroiditis, Graves' disease, rheumatoid arthritis, ulcerative colitis, and other less common presentations.
- Autoimmune hepatitis is not associated with any specific physical examination findings.
- Patients with AIH may **overlap** with findings consistent with other liver diseases (e.g., primary biliary cirrhosis, primary sclerosing cholangitis, and autoimmune cholangitis).

Laboratory Studies
- Elevated levels of **serum aminotransferases, circulating autoantibodies** (antinuclear antibody, smooth muscle antibody, and liver–kidney microsomal antibody), and **hypergammaglobulinemia.**

Liver Biopsy
- **Liver biopsy** is **essential** for the diagnosis.
- "Piecemeal necrosis" or interface hepatitis with lobular or panacinar inflammation (lymphocytic and plasmacytic infiltration) are the histologic hallmarks of the disease.

Treatment

Medications
- **Therapy** is initiated with either **prednisone** alone (40–60 mg/d) or a **combination of prednisone** (40–60 mg/d) and **azathioprine** (1–2 mg/kg/d).
- Prednisone is tapered with biochemical and clinical improvement to an eventual discontinuation of treatment. Some patients require lifelong low-dose therapy.
- **Remission** (normalization of serum bilirubin, immunoglobulin levels, AST, ALT; disappearance of symptoms; resolution of histologic changes) is achieved in **65%** and **80%** of patients within **1.5** and **3 years,** of treatment, respectively.
- **Relapses** occur in at least **20%–50%** of patients after cessation of therapy. Relapses require retreatment.
- **Refractory disease** (i.e., remission not achieved with standard-dose prednisone or azathioprine) may require "salvage" therapy with cyclosporine, tacrolimus, or mycophenolate mofetil.

Surgery
- **Liver transplantation** should be considered in patients with ESLD.
- After transplantation, **recurrent AIH** is seen in **17% of patients. De novo AIH,** defined as AIH in patients transplanted for nonautoimmune diseases has been described in **3%–5% of transplant recipients.**

PRIMARY BILIARY CIRRHOSIS

General Principles

Definition
- Primary biliary cirrhosis (PBC) is a **cholestatic** hepatic disorder of unknown etiology with autoimmune features.

Epidemiology
- It most often affects **middle-aged women** (90%–95%).
- Although PBC is seen worldwide, it is more commonly described in North America and Northern Europe.

Diagnosis

Clinical Presentation
- The **course** is highly **variable.**
- **Fatigue, jaundice,** and **pruritus** are often the most troublesome symptoms.
- **Extrahepatic manifestations** include keratoconjunctivitis sicca, renal tubular acidosis, gallstones, thyroid disease, scleroderma, Raynaud's phenomenon, CREST syndrome.
- PBC progresses along a path of increasingly severe histologic damage (florid bile duct lesion, ductular proliferation, fibrosis, and cirrhosis). Ultimately, patients progress to **cirrhosis with liver failure in 10–15** years from diagnosis.

Laboratory Studies
- **Antimitochondrial antibodies** are present in >90% of patients.
- Typical features include elevated levels of **AP, hyperbilirubinemia, cholesterol, IgM,** and **bile acids.**

Liver Biopsy
- **Liver biopsy** may be helpful for both diagnosis and staging.

Treatment

Medications
- **Ursodeoxycholic acid** (13–15 mg/kg/d PO) improves liver function test abnormalities and appears to delay progression of disease when given long term (>4 years).
- Symptom-specific therapy for pruritus, steatorrhea, and malabsorption are outlined below.
- No curative therapy is available.

Surgery
- **Liver transplantation** may be necessary in advanced disease.
- Recurrent PBC after transplantation has been documented.

PRIMARY SCLEROSING CHOLANGITIS

General Principles

Definition
- **Primary sclerosing cholangitis (PSC)** is a **cholestatic** liver disorder characterized by inflammation, fibrosis, and eventual obliteration of the extrahepatic and intrahepatic bile ducts.

Epidemiology
- Most patients are **middle-aged men.**
- **PSC is frequently associated with inflammatory bowel disease (70% with ulcerative colitis).**

Diagnosis

Clinical Presentation
- **Clinical manifestations** include intermittent episodes of jaundice, hepatomegaly, pruritus, weight loss, and fatigue.
- **Cholangitis** is a frequent complication in patients with severe strictures of the biliary ducts.

- Patients may progress to **cirrhosis** and **ESLD.**
- **Cholangiocarcinoma** is the most frequent neoplasm associated with PSC and occurs in 6%–20% of patients.

Laboratory Studies
- **PSC** should be considered in individuals with **inflammatory bowel disease** who have increased levels of **AP** even in the absence of symptoms of hepatobiliary disease.

Imaging
- PSC is confirmed by demonstration of **strictures or irregularities** of the **intrahepatic** and **extrahepatic bile ducts** by **ERCP or MRCP.**

Liver Biopsy
- Liver biopsy is helpful in the diagnosis of small-duct PSC, in the exclusion of other diseases, and in staging.

Treatment
Medical
- High-dose **ursodeoxycholic acid** (20 mg/kg) may be beneficial in improving ductal damage and liver fibrosis.
- Episodes of cholangitis should be managed with IV antibiotics and endoscopic therapy as outlined below.

Endoscopic Therapy
- ERCP can be performed to **dilate** and **stent dominant strictures.**

Surgery
- Colectomy for ulcerative colitis does not affect the course of PSC.
- Patients with advanced disease or recurrent cholangitis should be referred for liver transplantation.
- Cholangiocarcinoma is in general a contraindication to liver transplantation.
- Recurrent PSC after liver transplantation has been documented.

COMPLICATIONS OF CHOLESTASIS

GENERAL PRINCIPLES
- Any condition that blocks bile excretion (in the liver cells or biliary ducts) is defined as cholestasis. Laboratory manifestations of cholestasis include elevated levels of AP and bilirubin.
- Cholestasis can lead to **nutritional deficiencies, osteoporosis,** and **pruritus.**

NUTRITIONAL DEFICIENCIES
Etiology
- **Nutritional deficiencies** result from fat malabsorption (see Chapter 2, Nutritional Support).
- **Fat-soluble vitamin deficiency** (vitamins A, D, E, K) is often present in advanced disease and is particularly common in patients with steatorrhea.

Diagnosis
- Patients may give a history of **oily** or **foul-smelling diarrhea.**
- Stool can be tested for **fecal fat.** Both spot tests and 24-hour collections can be done.

■ **25-hydroxy vitamin D serum concentrations** reflect the **total body stores** of **vitamin D.** Vitamin D deficiency in the setting of malabsorption and steatorrhea is a good clinical marker for total body concentrations of other fat-soluble vitamins.

Treatment

■ In patients with steatorrhea, a **low-fat diet** (40–60 g/d) helps to decrease symptoms but may compromise total energy intake.
■ Fat-soluble vitamin replacement can be accomplished by water-soluble preparations of **vitamin A,** 10,000–50,000 International units PO daily; **vitamin K,** 5–10 mg PO daily; and **vitamin E,** 30–100 International Units PO daily.
■ Vitamin D deficiency can be corrected by **25-hydroxyvitamin D3 (25-cholecalciferol),** 50,000 Units PO 3× weekly.
■ Serum levels of **25-hydroxy vitamin D** should be **monitored** to assess the adequacy of replacement therapy and avoid toxicity.
■ **Zinc deficiency** may occur in some patients and is corrected with **zinc sulfate,** 220 mg PO daily (50 mg elemental zinc) for 4 weeks.

OSTEOPOROSIS

Definition

■ **Osteoporosis** is defined as a decrease in the amount of bone (mainly trabecular bone), leading to a decrease in the integrity of the bone and an increase in the risk of fractures.

Etiology

■ Osteoporosis is more commonly seen in clinical cholestasis due to **PBC.**
■ It may result from **increased bone resorption, decreased bone formation, or both.**

Diagnosis

■ Bone mineral density through **dual energy x-ray absorptiometry (DEXA)** should be measured in all patients at the time of diagnosis and during follow-up.

Treatment

■ Treatment of bone disease includes exercise, oral calcium supplementation (1.0–1.5 g/d), bisphosphonate therapy, and vitamin D supplementation.

PRURITUS

Pathophysiology

■ The pathophysiology is debated and may be due to the accumulation of bile acid compounds or endogenous opioid agonists.

Diagnosis

■ Patients with cholestasis may present with itching in the setting of a normal or elevated bilirubin level.

Treatment

Medications

■ **Pruritus** is best treated with **cholestyramine,** a basic anion exchange resin. It binds bile acids and other anionic compounds in the intestine and inhibits their absorption. The dose is 4 g mixed with water before and after the morning meal, with additional doses before lunch and dinner to control symptoms. The maximum recommended dose is 16 g/d.

- Cholestyramine should not be given concurrently with vitamins or other medications, as it may impair absorption.
- **Colestipol,** another similar resin, is also available.
- **Antihistamines** (diphenhydramine or doxepin, 25 mg PO at bedtime) and petrolatum may provide symptomatic relief.
- **Rifampin** (300–600 mg/d) and **naltrexone** (25–50 mg/d) are reserved for intractable pruritus.

Other
- Plasmapheresis, charcoal hemoperfusion, and partial external biliary diversion are invasive therapeutic procedures that can also be administered when medical therapy has failed.
- Liver transplantation is a last resort option for intractable pruritus

 # METABOLIC LIVER DISEASE

GENERAL PRINCIPLES

- A number of treatable metabolic disorders present with hepatocellular dysfunction, including **Wilson's disease** and **hereditary hemochromatosis.**
- Other infrequent disorders include **glycogen storage disease, phospholipidosis,** and α_1-antitrypsin deficiency.

WILSON'S DISEASE

General Principles

- **Wilson's disease (WD)** is an **autonomic-recessive disorder** (ATP7B gene on chromosome 13) that results in progressive **copper overload** in the liver, brain, kidney, and cornea.
- Incidence is 1 in 30,000.
- WD is a rare cause of **FHF, chronic hepatitis,** and **cirrhosis** in the United States.

Diagnosis

Clinical Presentation
- The diagnosis of WD should be considered in patients with unexplained liver disease with or without neuropsychiatric symptoms, first-degree relatives with WD, or individuals with FHF (with or without hemolysis).
- The average **age at presentation** of liver dysfunction is **6–20 years,** but it can manifest later in life.
- **Neuropsychiatric disorders** usually occur later, most of the time in association with cirrhosis. The manifestations include **asymmetric tremor, dysarthria, ataxia, and psychiatric features.**
- Other **extrahepatic manifestations** include Kayser-Fleischer rings on slit-lamp examination (gold to brown rings due to copper deposition in the Descemet membrane in the periphery of the cornea), hemolytic anemia, renal tubular acidosis, arthritis, and osteopenia.

Laboratory Data
- Data include low serum ceruloplasmin level (<20 mg/dL), elevated serum free copper level (>25 mcg/dL), and elevated 24-hour urinary copper level (>100 mg).

Radiology Studies
- Brain imaging (basal ganglia changes) findings are nonspecific.

Liver Biopsy

■ The **liver histology** (massive necrosis, steatosis, glycogenated nuclei, chronic hepatitis, fibrosis, cirrhosis) findings are **nonspecific** and depend on the presentation and stage of the disease.

■ Elevated hepatic copper levels of >250 mcg/g dry weight (normal <40 mcg/g) on biopsy are highly suggestive of WD.

Treatment

Medical

■ Treatment is with copper-chelating agents.

  ▪ **Zinc salts** 50 mg tid are indicated in patients with chronic hepatitis and cirrhosis in the absence of hepatic failure. Zinc may be associated with the use of penicillamine and trientine. Other than gastric irritation, zinc has an excellent safety profile.

  ▪ **Penicillamine** 1–2 g/d (in divided doses bid or qid) **plus pyridoxine** 25 mg/d to avoid its deficiency during treatment. It is indicated in patients with hepatic failure. Use may be limited by side effects (hypersensitivity, bone marrow suppression, proteinuria, systemic lupus erythematosus, Goodpasture syndrome). **Penicillamine should never be given as initial treatment to patients with neurologic symptoms.**

  ▪ **Trientine** 1–2 g/d (in divided doses bid or qid). This has similar side effects as penicillamine, but at a lower frequency. The risk of neurologic worsening with trientine is less than with penicillamine.

  ▪ **Tetrathiomolybdate (TM)** 120 mg/d (20 mg tid with meals and 60 mg at bedtime away from food) with **zinc therapy.** This is the treatment of choice for patients presenting with neurologic symptoms. TM has a good safety profile. Anemia, leukopenia, and mild elevations of aminotransferases may be seen during treatment.

Liver Transplantation

■ Liver transplantation is the only therapeutic option in FHF or in progressive dysfunction despite chelation therapy.

■ In the absence of neurologic symptoms, liver transplantation has a good prognosis and requires no further medical treatment.

HEREDITARY HEMOCHROMATOSIS

General Prinicples

■ **Hereditary hemochromatosis (HH)** is an autosomal-recessive disorder of iron overload. The gene responsible (**HFE gene**) is on chromosome 6. This systemic disorder is related to abnormal iron absorption in the duodenum that leads to excessive and damaging iron deposition in the liver, heart, pancreas, skin, and endocrine system.

■ This is the most common inherited form of iron overload affecting Caucasian populations.

■ One in 200–400 Caucasian individuals are homozygous for the HFE gene mutations.

■ It is usually not diagnosed until middle age (40–60 years).

Diagnosis

Clinical Presentation

■ Presentation varies from **asymptomatic disease** to **cirrhosis.**

■ Associated findings include slate-colored skin, diabetes, cardiomyopathy, arthritis, hypogonadism, or hepatic dysfunction.

■ Patients with cirrhosis are at increased risk for the development of **hepatocellular carcinoma** despite therapy.

Laboratory Data

- The diagnosis is suggested by **high fasting transferrin saturation (>45%).**
- The diagnosis is subsequently confirmed by the presence of specific mutations in the **HFE.** The most common mutation associated with HH is **C282Y.** Less frequent mutations include the **H63D** and **S65C** and the compound heterozygous **C282Y/H63D.**
- Iron overload in the presence of genotypes not associated with HH requires further assessment with ancillary tests.

Imaging

- **MRI** is the modality of choice for noninvasive quantification of iron storage in the liver. It allows for repeated measures and minimizes sampling error.

Liver Biopsy

- Biochemical tests, HFE genotype determination, and imaging have replaced the role of liver biopsy in establishing the diagnosis.
- Liver biopsy is most helpful in staging the disease, especially in individuals who are at increased risk of having advanced fibrosis or cirrhosis.
- In patients with iron overload without typical HFE gene mutations, liver biopsy is still a valuable diagnostic tool.

Treatment

- Therapy consists of **phlebotomy** (500 mL blood/wk) until iron depletion is confirmed by a ferritin level <50 ng/mL and a transferring saturation of <40%. Thereafter, maintenance phlebotomy of 1–2 units of blood three to four times a year is continued for life.
- Deferoxamine is an iron-chelating agent used in the setting of HH if the patient's hemodynamics cannot tolerate phlebotomy. It binds free iron and facilitates urinary excretion.

Liver Transplantation

- Liver transplantation may be considered in cases of HH with cirrhosis.

Screening

- Once a diagnosis has been made, the **patient's family members** should **undergo screening** for HH by measuring fasting transferrin saturation and ferritin levels.
- Genetic testing may also be performed.

Prognosis

- The survival rate in appropriately treated noncirrhotic patients is identical to that of the general population.
- Patients who undergo liver transplantation for hemochromatosis tend to have poorer 1- and 5-year survival rates when compared to other liver transplant recipients.

α_1-ANTITRYPSIN DEFICIENCY

General Principles

- α_1-Antitrypsin deficiency (α1AT) is an autosomal-recessive disease associated with accumulation of misfolded α_1-antitrypsin in the endoplasmic reticulum of hepatocytes. The gene associated with the disease is located on chromosome 14. α1AT can also be associated with emphysema in early adulthood, as well as other extrahepatic manifestations including panniculitis, pancreatic fibrosis, and membranoproliferative glomerulonephritis.
- Incidence is 1 in 1,600.
- The most common allele is **protease inhibitor M (PiM—normal variant), followed by** PiS and PiZ (deficient variants). Blacks have lower frequency of these alleles.
- The disease may present as **neonatal cholestasis** or later in life as **chronic hepatitis, cirrhosis,** or **hepatocellular carcinoma.**

Diagnosis

Clinical Presentation

- Patients may present with cholestasis, mild abnormalities in aminotransferases, and cirrhosis.
- The presence of significant pulmonary and hepatic disease in the same patient is very rare (1%–2%).
- Chronic hepatitis, cirrhosis, or hepatocellular carcinoma may develop in 10%–15% of patients with the PiZZ phenotype during the first 20 years of life. Controversy exists as to whether liver disease develops in heterozygotes (PiMZ, PiSZ, PiFZ, etc.).

Laboratory Data

- Low serum α_1-antitrypsin level (10%–15% of normal)
- Decreased α-1 globulin level on serum electrophoresis
- The patient should also be tested for α1AT phenotype.

Liver Biopsy

- The liver biopsy is essential for the diagnosis and shows characteristic periodic acid-Schiff–positive, diastase-resistant globules in the periportal hepatocytes.

Treatment

- Currently, there is no specific medical treatment.
- Gene therapy for α1AT deficiency is a potential future alternative.
- Transplantation is curative, with survival rates of 90% at 1 year and 80% at 5 years.

 # MISCELLANEOUS DISORDERS

ISCHEMIC HEPATITIS

General Principles

- **Ischemic hepatitis** results from liver hypoperfusion. Synonyms include shock liver and hypoxic hepatitis.
- Clinical circumstances include severe blood loss, severe burns, cardiac failure, heat stroke, sepsis, and sickle cell crisis.

Diagnosis

Clinical Presentation

- Ischemic hepatitis presents as acute and transient rise of liver enzymes in the thousands during or following a hypotensive episode.

Laboratory Studies

- Laboratory studies show a rapid rise and fall in levels of serum AST, ALT (>1,000 mg/dL), and lactic dehydrogenase within 1–3 days of the insult with subsequent slow decline in aminotransferases if the underlying cause is corrected.
- Total bilirubin, alkaline phosphatase, and INR may initially be normal but subsequently rise as a result of reperfusion injury.

Liver Biopsy

- Liver biopsy is not usually needed for diagnosis.
- Centrilobular necrosis and sinusoidal distortion with inflammatory infiltrates in zone 3 (central areas) are the classic histologic features.

Treatment

- Correct the underlying condition that caused the circulatory collapse.

Prognosis

- Prognosis is determined by the rapid and effective treatment of the underlying cause.

VASCULAR DISEASES

General Principles

- Vascular diseases of the liver can be due to impaired arterial or venous blood flow. The portal vein and the hepatic artery provide two-thirds and one-third of hepatic blood flow, respectively.

Hepatic Vein Thrombosis

Definition

- Hepatic vein thrombosis (HVT; previously known as Budd-Chiari's syndrome) causes a hepatic venous outflow obstruction with multiple etiologies and a variety of clinical consequences.

Etiology

- Thrombosis is the main factor leading to obstruction of the hepatic venous system, frequently in association with myeloproliferative disorders, antiphospholipid antibody syndrome, paroxysmal nocturnal hemoglobinuria, factor V Leiden, protein C and S deficiency, and contraceptive use.
- Another cause is membranous obstruction of the inferior vena cava (IVC).
- HVT can occur during pregnancy and in the postpartum period.
- Less than 20% of cases are idiopathic.

Diagnosis

Clinical Presentation

- Patients may present with an acute, subacute, or chronic illness characterized by **ascites, hepatomegaly,** and **right upper quadrant abdominal pain.**
- Other symptoms may include jaundice, encephalopathy, gastrointestinal bleeding, and lower extremity edema.

Laboratory Studies

- Serum-to-ascites albumin gradient is >1.1 g/dL. Serum albumin, bilirubin, AST, ALT, and PT are mildly abnormal.
- Laboratory evaluation of prothrombotic conditions should be performed (see Chapter 18, Disorders of Hemostasis).

Imaging

- Doppler ultrasound can be used as a screening test.
- Definitive diagnosis is made with magnetic resonance venography or hepatic venography.

Treatment

Nonsurgical

- Nonsurgical treatment includes anticoagulants, thrombolytics, diuretics, angioplasty, stents, and transjugular intrahepatic portosystemic shunt (TIPS).

Surgical

- Decompression procedures and liver transplantation are therapeutic options.

Sinusoidal Obstruction Syndrome

Definition
- Sinusoidal obstruction syndrome (SOS; previously known as veno-occlusive disease) refers to alterations in the liver microcirculation that may occur in the absence of vascular occlusion.

Etiology
- It is seen in bone marrow transplant recipients after conditioning therapy with total body irradiation and high-dose cytoreductive chemotherapy, in renal transplant recipients who are immunosuppressed with azathioprine, and in association with ingestion of pyrrolizidine alkaloids (Jamaican bush teas).

Diagnosis

Clinical Presentation
- Diagnosis is based on the triad of **hepatomegaly, weight gain** (2%–5% of baseline body weight), **and hyperbilirubinemia** (>2 mg/dL), generally occurring within 3 weeks after bone marrow transplantation.
- The severity of SOS varies from mild to moderate to severe disease.
- The clinical presentation depends on the severity of the disease.

Laboratory Studies
- The laboratory findings correlate with the clinical disease, from mild to significant elevations in aminotransferases and bilirubin.

Procedures
- A useful approach to the diagnosis is the transjugular measurement of the hepatic venous pressure. A concomitant liver biopsy can be performed during the same procedure.
- The typical histology shows centrilobular congestion with hepatocellular necrosis and accumulation of hemosiderin-laden macrophages. The terminal hepatic venules exhibit minimal edema without obvious fibrin deposition or thrombosis.

Treatment
- Treatment is largely supportive.
- Defibrotide, a single-stranded polydeoxyribonucleotide drug, has shown promise in uncontrolled clinical trials.

Prophylaxis
- Altering the myeloablative therapy and reducing the dose of radiation may decrease the incidence of SOS.
- Other preventative measures like anticoagulation, pretreatment with ursodeoxycholic acid, pentoxifylline, and prostaglandin E have not been proven to be consistently effective.

Prognosis
- Prognosis depends on the severity of disease.

Portal Vein Thrombosis

Etiology
- **Portal vein thrombosis (PVT)** is a disease of both children and adults. In adults it is seen in a variety of clinical settings, including abdominal trauma, cirrhosis, malignancy, hypercoagulable states, and intra-abdominal infections, pancreatitis, and after portocaval shunt surgery or splenectomy.

Diagnosis

Clinical Presentation
- PVT can present as an acute or a chronic condition.

- The acute phase may go unrecognized. Symptoms include abdominal pain/distension, nausea, anorexia, weight loss, diarrhea, or features of the underlying disorder.
- Chronic PVT may present with variceal hemorrhage or other manifestations of portal hypertension.

Imaging
- **Ultrasonographic Doppler** examination is sensitive and specific for establishing the diagnosis.
- Angiography, CT, or magnetic resonance angiography can also be used.

Laboratory Data
- In patients with no obvious etiology, a prothrombotic workup should be performed.

Treatment

Medical
- Anticoagulation should be considered in the setting of acute PVT.

Other
- In the chronic setting treatment should focus on the complications of portal hypertension including nonselective beta-blockers, endoscopic banding for varices, and diuretics for ascites.
- Transjugular intrahepatic portosystemic shunt (TIPS) should be considered in selected cases.
- Portosystemic surgery carries a high morbidity and mortality, especially in patients with PVT in association with cirrhosis.

HEPATIC ABSCESS
- Hepatic abscess may be classified as either **pyogenic** or **amebic**.

Pyogenic Abscess

Etiology
- **Pyogenic abscess** can result from hematogenous infection, spread from intra-abdominal infection, or ascending infection from the biliary tract.
- Approximately 20% of cases are cryptogenic in origin.

Diagnosis

Clinical Presentation
- Clinical features include fever, chills, weight loss, jaundice, and abdominal pain from tender hepatomegaly.

Laboratory Studies
- Laboratory studies may demonstrate leukocytosis and elevated AP.
- More than half the patients have positive blood cultures at the time of presentation.

Imaging
- Diagnosis is confirmed by CT, MRI, or ultrasonography.

Treatment

Medications
- Treatment includes a prolonged course of antibiotic therapy.

Drainage
- In select cases, treatment is by imaging-guided percutaneous or surgical drainage.

Follow-Up
- Repeated imaging is recommended to document resolution.

Amebic Abscess

- Amebic abscess should be considered in patients from endemic areas.

Diagnosis

Clinical Presentation
- Diagnosis requires a high index of clinical suspicion.
- Clinical features include fever, chills, and tender hepatomegaly.

Laboratory Studies
- Specific serologic tests for *Entamoeba histolytica* such as the indirect hemagglutination determination are helpful in establishing the diagnosis in low-prevalence areas.

Treatment

Medication
- Amebic abscesses are treated with metronidazole.

Drainage
- Imaging-guided drainage is reserved for amebic abscesses at risk for rupture or when pyogenic coinfection is suspected.

GRANULOMATOUS HEPATITIS

Definition
- Granulomatous hepatitis is the consequence of a nonspecific reaction to a wide spectrum of diverse etiologic stimuli.

Etiology
- Etiologies include infections (e.g., brucellosis, syphilis, mycobacterial, fungal, and rickettsial diseases), sarcoidosis, drug-induced injury, lymphoma, and idiopathic causes.

Diagnosis

Clinical Presentation
- Patients may present with fever, hepatosplenomegaly, and signs of portal hypertension on physical examination.

Laboratory Studies
- Laboratory studies show elevated liver enzyme levels (particularly AP).

Liver Biopsy
- Liver biopsy is the most accurate and specific way to diagnose granulomatous hepatitis.

Treatment

Medical
- Specific therapy is directed at the underlying cause.
- If the clinical suspicion for tuberculosis is high, an empiric trial of antituberculous therapy may be warranted despite negative mycobacterial cultures.

NONALCOHOLIC FATTY LIVER DISEASE

GENERAL PRINCIPLES

- Nonalcoholic fatty liver disease (NALFD) is a clinicopathologic syndrome that encompasses several clinical entities that range from simple steatosis to steatohepatitis, fibrosis, and end-stage liver disease in the absence of significant alcohol consumption.
- Nonalcoholic steatohepatitis (NASH) is part of the spectrum of NAFLD and is defined as steatosis with hepatocellular ballooning plus lobular inflammation. Pathologic findings in NASH also include pericellular or perisinusoidal fibrosis.
- The exact mechanisms leading to excess hepatic fat and hepatic cellular damage are incompletely understood.

Epidemiology

- NAFLD is a worldwide phenomenon.
- It is the most common liver disease in the United States, affecting 20%–35% of the adult population.
- NAFLD is associated with an increasing prevalence of type II diabetes, metabolic syndrome, and obesity in the U.S. population.
- It affects both children and adults, and the incidence increases with age.
- Approximately 25% of patients with NASH progress to cirrhosis over a 10- to 15-year period.
- Up to 70% of cases of **cryptogenic cirrhosis** have NASH as the underlying etiology.
- Cirrhosis due to NALFD may also by complicated by HCC (13% of all cases of HCC).

Etiology

- It is usually associated with insulin resistance to glucose metabolism and features of the metabolic syndrome (see Chapter 21, Diabetes Mellitus and Related Disorders).
    - Secondary causes include hepatotoxic drugs (amiodarone, nifedipine, estrogens), surgical procedures (jejunoileal bypass, extensive small-bowel resection, biliary and pancreatic diversions), and miscellaneous conditions (total parenteral nutrition, hypobetalipoproteinemia, environmental toxins).

DIAGNOSIS

Clinical Presentation

- The disease may vary from asymptomatic to advanced ESLD and HCC.

Laboratory Data

- Liver enzyme elevations are mild. Up to 80% of patients will have normal liver enzymes.
- Biochemical abnormalities may reflect the stage of the disease (e.g., cholestasis, hypoalbuminemia, increased INR).

Imaging

- Imaging studies such as ultrasonography, CT scan, and MRI may detect moderate to severe steatosis.
- Magnetic resonance spectroscopy offers a quantitative measurement of liver fat content, but is not commonly available.

Liver Biopsy

- Liver biopsy remains the gold standard by which the diagnosis is made. However, the decision to perform a liver biopsy should take into account the specific clinical questions that are relevant to each case.

TREATMENT

Medical

- No established specific treatment is available for NAFLD.
- Therapies to correct or control associated conditions are warranted (weight loss through diet and exercise, tight control of diabetes and insulin resistance, appropriate treatment of hyperlipidemia, and discontinuation of possible offending agents).

Liver Transplantation

- Liver transplantation should be considered in patients with ESLD, although recurrence can develop.

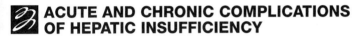 **ACUTE AND CHRONIC COMPLICATIONS OF HEPATIC INSUFFICIENCY**

ACUTE HEPATIC INSUFFICIENCY

Fulminant Hepatic Failure

General Principles
- FHF is defined as the acute onset of altered mental status and coagulopathy within 8–24 weeks of initial symptoms of liver disease in an otherwise healthy individual.

Epidemiology
- Acetaminophen hepatotoxicity and viral hepatitis are the most common causes of FHF.
- Other causes include AIH, drug and toxin exposure, ischemia, acute fatty liver of pregnancy, WD, and Reye's syndrome.
- In 20% of cases, no clear cause is identified.

Diagnosis

Clinical Presentation
- Patients may present with mild to severe mental status changes in the setting of moderate to severe acute hepatitis and coagulopathy.
- Jaundice may or may not be initially present.
- A history of acetaminophen overdose, toxin ingestion, or risk factors for viral hepatitis may be obtained.
- Patients can develop cardiovascular collapse, acute renal failure, cerebral edema, and sepsis.

Laboratory Data
- Aminotransferases are typically elevated, and in many cases are >1,000 International Units/L.
- INR is ≥1.5.
- Initial workup to determine the etiology of FHF should include:
  - Acute viral hepatitis panel
  - Serum drug screen, which includes acetaminophen
  - Ceruloplasmin
  - AIH serologies
  - Pregnancy test

Treatment
- Supportive therapy in the intensive care unit (ICU) setting of a tertiary center with liver transplant capabilities is essential.
- Precipitating factors should be identified and treated if possible.
- Blood glucose, electrolytes, acid-base, coagulation parameters, and fluid status should be monitored serially.

- Vitamin K, fresh frozen plasma, and the use of recombinant activated factor VIIa should be considered in the setting of active bleeding or when invasive procedures are required.
- Cerebral edema and intracranial hypertension are related to severity of encephalopathy. In patients that reach grade III or IV encephalopathy, intracranial pressure monitoring should be considered (intracranial pressure should be maintained below 20–25 mm Hg, cerebral perfusion pressure should be maintained above 50 mm Hg). Therapies to decrease cerebral edema include mannitol (0.5–1 g/kg IV), hyperventilation (reduce $PaCO_2$ to 25–30 mm Hg), hypothermia (32–34°C), and barbiturates.
- Transplantation should be urgently considered in cases of FHF.

Prognosis
- Prior to transplantation survival was <15%; in the posttransplant era survival is >65%.
- Death often results from progressive liver failure, GI bleeding, cerebral edema, sepsis, or arrhythmia.
- Poor prognostic indicators in acetaminophen-induced FHF include arterial pH <7.3, INR >6.5, creatinine >2.3 mg/dL, and encephalopathy grade III–IV.

CHRONIC HEPATIC INSUFFICIENCY

- Cirrhosis is a chronic diffuse condition characterized by replacement of liver cells by fibrotic tissue, which creates a nodular-appearing distortion of the normal liver architecture. This fibrosis represents the end result of a variety of etiologies of liver injury.

Hepatic Encephalopathy

- **Hepatic encephalopathy** is the syndrome of disordered consciousness and altered neuromuscular activity that is seen in patients with acute or chronic hepatocellular failure or portosystemic shunting.

Mechanisms of Injury
- The pathogenesis of hepatic encephalopathy is controversial, and numerous mediators have been implicated.
- **Precipitating factors** include azotemia; acute liver failure; use of a tranquilizer, opioid, or sedative-hypnotic medication; GI hemorrhage; hypokalemia and alkalosis (diuretics and diarrhea); constipation; infection; high-protein diet; progressive hepatocellular dysfunction; and portosystemic shunts (surgical or TIPS).

Diagnosis
- Presentation varies from subtle mental status changes to coma.
- Asterixis (flapping tremor) is present in stages I–II of encephalopathy. This motor disturbance is not specific to hepatic encephalopathy.
- The electroencephalogram shows slow, high-amplitude, and triphasic waves.
- Determination of blood ammonia level is not a sensitive or specific test for hepatic encephalopathy.

Treatment
Diet
- The rationale and benefit of dietary protein restriction is controversial. Once the patient is able to eat, a diet containing 30–40 g of protein per day is initiated. Special diets (vegetable protein or branched-chain amino acid enriched) may be beneficial in patients with encephalopathy that is refractory to the usual measures.

Medications
- Medications include **nonabsorbable disaccharides** (lactulose, lactitol, and lactose in lactase-deficient patients) and **antibiotics** (neomycin, metronidazole, and rifaximin).
- The initial dose of lactulose is 15–45 mL PO bid–qid. Maintenance dose should be adjusted to produce three to five soft stools per day. Oral lactulose should not be given to patients with an ileus or possible bowel obstruction.

- **Lactulose enemas** (prepared by the addition of 300 mL lactulose to 700 mL distilled water) can also be administered.
- **Neomycin** can be given by mouth (500–1,000 mg q6h) or as a retention enema (1% solution in 100–200 mL isotonic saline). Approximately 1%–3% of the administered dose of neomycin is absorbed, with the attendant risk of ototoxicity and nephrotoxicity. The risk of toxicity is increased in patients with renal insufficiency. Because lactulose is as effective as neomycin, it is preferred for initial and maintenance therapy.
- **Metronidazole** (250 mg PO q8h) is useful for short-term therapy when neomycin is unavailable or poorly tolerated. Long-term metronidazole is not recommended due to its associated toxicities.
- **Rifaximin** 400 mg PO tid is a new antibiotic with a very good safety profile that is used as an alternative to neomycin and metronidazole.
- Combination therapy with lactulose and any of the antibiotics mentioned above should be considered in cases that are refractory to either agent alone.

Portal Hypertension

- Portal hypertension is the main complication of cirrhosis, and is characterized by increased resistance to portal flow and increased portal venous inflow. Portal hypertension is established by determining the pressure difference between the hepatic vein and the portal vein (pressure gradient >10 mm Hg).
- Direct and indirect clinical consequences of portal hypertension include esophageal and gastric varices, portal hypertensive gastropathy, ascites, hepatorenal syndrome, and spontaneous bacterial peritonitis.

Etiology

- Causes of portal hypertension in patients without cirrhosis include idiopathic portal hypertension, schistosomiasis, congenital hepatic fibrosis, sarcoidosis, cystic fibrosis, arteriovenous fistulas, splenic and portal vein thrombosis, myeloproliferative diseases, nodular regenerative hyperplasia, and focal nodular hyperplasia.

Diagnosis

Clinical Presentation

- **Portal hypertension** frequently complicates cirrhosis and presents with ascites, GI bleeding from esophageal or gastric varices or portal hypertensive gastropathy, and splenomegaly.

Imaging

- Ultrasonography, CT, and MRI showing cirrhosis, splenomegaly, collateral venous circulation, and ascites are suggestive of portal hypertension.

Diagnostic Procedures

- Upper endoscopy showing varices (esophageal or gastric) or portal hypertensive gastropathy
- Transjugular portal pressure measurements

Treatment

- Treatment of gastrointestinal bleeding due to portal hypertension is covered in Chapter 16, Gastrointestinal Diseases.

Ascites

- **Ascites** is the abnormal (>25 mL) accumulation of fluid within the peritoneal cavity. Causes of ascites besides cirrhosis include cancer (peritoneal carcinomatosis), heart failure, tuberculosis, pancreatic disease, nephrotic syndrome, surgery or trauma to the lymphatic system or ureters, and serositis.

Diagnosis

Clinical Presentation

- Presentation ranges from ascites detected only by imaging methods to a distended, bulging abdomen on physical examination. Percussion of the abdomen reveals shifting dullness.

Imaging

- Ultrasonography, CT, and MRI are sensitive methods to detect ascites.

Laboratory Studies

- A serum to ascites albumin gradient (SAAG) that is >1.1 g/dL indicates portal hypertension–related ascites (97% specificity).
- An SAAG of <1.1 g/dL is found in nephrotic syndrome, peritoneal carcinomatosis, serositis, tuberculosis, and biliary or pancreatic ascites.

Diagnostic Procedures

- **Paracentesis** should be performed for diagnosis (e.g., new-onset ascites, suspicion of malignant ascites, or spontaneous bacterial peritonitis [SBP]) or as a therapeutic maneuver when tense ascites causes significant discomfort or respiratory compromise.
  - Routine diagnostic testing should include fluid cell and differential counts, albumin, total protein, and culture.
  - Amylase and triglyceride measurement, cytology, and mycobacterial smear/culture can be performed to confirm specific diagnoses.
  - **Bleeding** and **intestinal perforation** are possible complications.
  - Rapid large-volume paracentesis (>5 L) may lead to circulatory collapse, encephalopathy, and renal failure. Concomitant administration of IV albumin (5–8 g/L ascites removed) can be used to minimize these complications, especially in the setting of renal insufficiency or the absence of peripheral edema.

Treatment

Dietary

- **Dietary salt restriction** (2 g salt or 88 mmol Na^+/d) should be initiated and continued thereafter unless the renal ability to excrete sodium spontaneously improves.
  - In selected cases, it may be necessary to restrict sodium intake further.
  - The use of potassium-containing salt substitutes can lead to serious hyperkalemia.
  - Routine water restriction is not necessary. If dilutional hyponatremia (serum Na^+ <120 mmol/L) occurs, fluid restriction to 1,000–1,500 mL/d usually suffices.

Medications

- **Diuretic therapy** can be initiated along with salt restriction. The goal of diuretic therapy should be a daily weight loss of no more than 1.0 kg in patients with edema and approximately 0.5 kg in those without edema until ascites is adequately controlled. Diuretics should not be administered to individuals with an increasing serum creatinine level.
- **Spironolactone** (100 mg PO in a single daily dose with food) is the diuretic of choice. The daily dose can be increased by 50–100 mg every 7–10 days until satisfactory weight loss, a maximum dose of 400 mg, or side effects occur. Hyperkalemia and gynecomastia are common side effects. Amiloride or triamterene (potassium-sparing diuretics) are substitutes that can be used in patients in whom painful gynecomastia develops.
- **Loop diuretics,** such as furosemide (20–40 mg, increasing to a maximum dose of 160 mg PO daily) or bumetanide (0.5–2.0 mg PO daily), can be added to spironolactone.
- Patients should be observed closely for signs of dehydration, electrolyte disturbances, encephalopathy, muscle cramps, and renal insufficiency. Nonsteroidal anti-inflammatory agents may blunt the effect of diuretics and increase the risk of renal dysfunction.

Nonoperative
- **TIPS** has been proven effective in the management of refractory ascites (fluid overload that is nonresponsive to a sodium-restricted diet and high-dose diuretic therapy).
  - Complications include shunt occlusion, bleeding, infection, cardiopulmonary compromise, and hepatic encephalopathy.

Spontaneous Bacterial Peritonitis

- **SBP** is an infectious complication of portal hypertension–related ascites. Risk factors for SBP include ascitic fluid protein concentration <1 mg/dL, variceal hemorrhage, and a prior episode of SBP.

Diagnosis
Clinical Manifestations
- Clinical manifestations include abdominal pain and distention, fever, decreased bowel sounds, and worsening of hepatic encephalopathy. However, the disease may be present in the absence of specific clinical signs. Cirrhotic patients with ascites and evidence of any clinical deterioration should undergo diagnostic paracentesis to exclude SBP.

Laboratory
- The diagnosis is likely when the ascitic fluid contains >250 neutrophils/microliter Gram stain reveals the organism in only 10%–20% of samples. A positive culture confirms the diagnosis.
  - Cultures are more likely to be positive when 10 mL ascitic fluid is inoculated into two blood culture bottles at the bedside.
  - The most common organisms are *Escherichia coli, Klebsiella,* and *Streptococcus pneumoniae.* Blood cultures are positive in approximately one-half of cases with SBP. Polymicrobial infection is uncommon and should lead to the suspicion of secondary bacterial peritonitis.

Treatment
- In suspected cases (fever, abdominal pain, or tenderness) without more than 250 neutrophils/microliter, empiric **antibiotic therapy** with a third-generation cephalosporin (e.g., ceftriaxone, 1 g IV daily, or cefotaxime, 1–2 g IV q6–8h, depending on renal function; see Appendix E) or a quinolone (ciprofloxacin, 400 mg IV q12h) is appropriate for 5 days. Paracentesis should be repeated if no clinical improvement occurs in 48–72 hours, especially if the initial ascitic fluid culture was negative.
- Concomitant use of albumin 1.5 g/kg body weight at diagnosis and 1 g/kg body weight on day 3 improves survival and prevents renal failure in SBP.
- **Norfloxacin** (400 mg PO daily) can be used as secondary prophylaxis by reducing the frequency of recurrent episodes of SBP. However, the use of antibiotic prophylaxis has not been clearly shown to improve survival and does select resistant gut flora.

Hepatorenal Syndrome

- Hepatorenal syndrome (HRS) is a unique form of functional renal impairment in the setting of acute or, more commonly, chronic liver disease. Common precipitating factors include systemic bacterial infections, SBP, and large-volume paracentesis without volume expansion.

Diagnosis
- Major and minor diagnostic criteria are summarized in Table 17-4.
  - **Type I** HRS is characterized by the acute onset of rapidly progressive (<2 weeks), oliguric renal failure unresponsive to volume expansion. There is a doubling of the initial serum creatinine to a level >2.5 mg/dL or a 50% reduction in the creatinine clearance to a level <20 mL/min.
  - **Type II** HRS progresses more slowly but relentlessly and often clinically manifests as diuretic-resistant ascites.

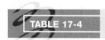

TABLE 17-4	Diagnostic Criteria of Hepatorenal Syndrome

Major criteria

Low glomerular filtration rate, as indicated by serum creatinine >1.5 mg/dL or 24-hr creatinine clearance <40 mL/min

Absence of shock, ongoing bacterial infection, fluid losses, and current treatment with nephrotoxic drugs

No sustained improvement in renal function (decrease in serum creatinine to 1.5 mg/dL or increase in creatinine clearance to 40 mL/min) after diuretic withdrawal and expansion of plasma volume with 1.5 L of a plasma expander

Proteinuria <500 mg/dL and no ultrasonographic evidence of obstructive uropathy or parenchymal renal disease

Additional criteria

Urine volume <500 mL/d

Urine sodium <10 mEq/L

Urine osmolality greater than plasma osmolality

Urine red blood cells <50/high-power field

Serum sodium concentration <130 mEq/L

Note: All major criteria must be present for the diagnosis of hepatorenal syndrome. Additional criteria are not necessary for the diagnosis but provide supportive evidence.
Adapted from Arroyo V, Gines P, Gerbes AL, et al. Definition and diagnostic criteria of refractory ascites and hepatorenal syndrome in cirrhosis. International Ascites Club. *Hepatology* 1996;23:164.

Treatment

Medical
- No clear or established treatments are available for HRS. Systemic vasoconstrictors including vasopressin analogs (terlipressin), somatostatin analogs (octreotide), and α-adrenergic agonists (midodrine and norepinephrine) with plasma expansion have shown a beneficial role in uncontrolled studies.

Nonmedical
- TIPS is a potential treatment alternative; however, data are limited.
- Hemodialysis may be indicated in patients listed for liver transplantations.

Liver Transplantation
- In suitable candidates, liver transplantation may be curative.

Prognosis
- Without treatment, patients with type I HRS have a short-term fatal prognosis, with death occurring within 2–3 months of onset. Patients with type II HRS have a median survival of approximately 6 months.

Hepatocellular Carcinoma (HCC)

Epidemiology
- HCC frequently occurs in patients with cirrhosis, especially when associated with viral hepatitis (HBV or HCV), alcoholic cirrhosis, α1AT deficiency, and hemochromatosis.
- HCC is the fifth most common cancer in men and the ninth most common cancer in women worldwide.
- It constitutes 84% of primary liver cancer in the United States (mean age at diagnosis is 65).

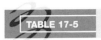

| TABLE 17-5 | Child-Turcotte-Pugh Scoring System to Assess Severity of Liver Disease | | |

Clinical and biochemical measurements	Points scored for increasing abnormality		
	1	2	3
Albumin	>3.5	2.8–3.5	<2.8
Bilirubin (mg/dL)	<2	2–3	>3
For cholestatic diseases: bilirubin (mg/dL)	<4	4–10	>10
PT (seconds prolonged)[a] or	<4	4–6	>6
INR[a]	<1.7	1.7–2.3	>2.3
Ascites	Absent	Mild	Moderate
Encephalopathy (grade)	0	1 and 2	3 and 4
Class	**Total points**		
A	5–6		
B	7–9		
C	10–15		

[a]Either the prothrombin time (PT) or international normalized ratio (INR) can be used for scoring.

Diagnosis

Clinical Presentation
- Clinical presentation is directly proportional to the stage of disease. Early disease is asymptomatic, while patients with late-stage disease may present with right upper quadrant abdominal pain, weight loss, and hepatomegaly.
- Suspect HCC in a well-controlled cirrhotic patient who develops manifestations of liver decompensation.

Laboratories
- α-Fetoprotein is the most widely used screening test. The sensitivity and specificity of the test are dependant on the cutoff value. A cutoff of 400 ng/mL or a rapid doubling time (weeks to months) is highly specific.

Imaging
- Liver ultrasound, triple-phase CT, and MRI are adequate and frequently used for detection of HCC.

Liver Biopsy
- Liver biopsy should be considered for those cases where the combination of imaging and α-fetoprotein values are not diagnostic.

Treatment
- Hepatic resection is the treatment of choice in noncirrhotic patients and may also be considered in well-compensated cirrhotic patients (Child-Pugh class A; see Table 17-5).
- Liver transplantation is the treatment of choice for cirrhotic patients (single HCC <5 cm or up to three nodules <3 cm).
- Alternative therapy for unresectable tumors includes percutaneous alcohol or acetic acid injection, arterial chemoembolization, microwave coagulation therapy, or radiofrequency ablation.

Prognosis
- Early diagnosis is essential, as surgical resection and liver transplantation can improve long-term survival. However, survival remains very poor: 1-year and 3-year survival rates are 36% and 17%, respectively.

LIVER TRANSPLANTATION

General Principles

- Liver transplantation is an effective therapeutic option for both irreversible acute and chronic liver diseases for which available therapies have failed.
- Whole cadaveric livers and partial livers (split-liver, reduced-size, and living-related) are used in the United States as sources for liver transplantation.

Epidemiology

- In the United States, over 17,000 patients are awaiting liver transplants, approximately 5,000 transplants are performed in the United States each year, and approximately 2,000 patients per year die while on the waiting list.
- The disparity between supply and demand of suitable livers for transplantation continues to increase.

Indications

- Patients that fulfill criteria for FHF are potential candidates for liver transplantation.
- Patients with chronic liver disease should be considered for transplant evaluation when they have a decline in hepatic synthetic or excretory functions, ascites, hepatic encephalopathy, or complications such as HRS, hepatocellular carcinoma, recurrent SBP, or variceal bleeding.
- The prioritization for liver transplantation in chronic liver disease is determined by the **Model for End-Stage Liver Disease (MELD)** score. The MELD score is determined by the use of an equation that takes into account serum bilirubin, serum creatinine, and INR.

Contraindications

- Severe and uncontrolled extrahepatic infection
- Advanced cardiac or pulmonary disease
- Extrahepatic malignancy
- Multiorgan failure
- Unresolved psychosocial issues
- Medical noncompliance issues
- Ongoing substance abuse (e.g., alcohol and illegal drugs)

Protocol

- Candidates for liver transplantation are evaluated by a multidisciplinary team that includes hepatologists, transplant surgeons, transplant nurse coordinators, social workers, psychologists, and financial coordinators.
- Immunosuppressive, infectious, and long-term complications are discussed in Chapter 15, Solid Organ Transplant Medicine.

Suggested Readings

Adams LA, Angulo P. Recent concepts in non-alcoholic fatty liver disease. *Diabet Med* 2005;22:1129–1133.

Brewer GJ, Askari FK. Wilson's disease: clinical management and therapy. *J Hepatol* 2005;42(Suppl):S13–21.

Cardenas A. Hepatorenal syndrome: a dreaded complication of end-stage liver disease. *Am J Gastroenterol* 2005;100:460–467.

Czaja AJ, Bianchi FB, Carpenter HA, et al. Treatment challenges and investigational opportunities in autoimmune hepatitis. *Hepatology* 2005;41:207–215.

Garcia-Tsao G. Portal hypertension. *Curr Opin Gastroenterol* 2005;21:313–322.

Harrison SA, Bacon BR. Relation of hemochromatosis with hepatocellular carcinoma: epidemiology, natural history, pathophysiology, screening, treatment, and prevention. *Med Clin North Am* 2005;89:391–409.

Jalan R. Acute liver failure: current management and future prospects. *J Hepatol* 2005;42(Suppl):S115–123.

Maddrey WC. Drug-induced hepatotoxicity: 2005. *J Clin Gastroenterol* 2005;39:S83–89.

Marrero JA. Screening tests for hepatocellular carcinoma. *Clin Liver Dis* 2005;9:235–251.

Polson J, Lee WM. AASLD position paper: the management of acute liver failure. *Hepatology* 2005;41:1179–1197.

Runyon BA. Management of adult patients with ascites due to cirrhosis. *Hepatology* 2004;39:841–856.

Schilsky ML, Oikonomou I. Inherited metabolic liver disease. *Curr Opin Gastroenterol* 2005;21:275–282.

Sobhonslidsuk A, Reddy KR. Portal vein thrombosis: a concise review. *Am J Gastroenterol* 2002;97:535–541.

Willner IR, Reuben A. Alcohol and the liver. *Curr Opin Gastroenterol* 2005;21:323–330.

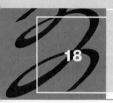

18

DISORDERS OF HEMOSTASIS AND THROMBOSIS

Roger Yusen, Charles Eby, and Richard Walgren

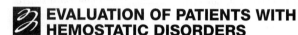

EVALUATION OF PATIENTS WITH HEMOSTATIC DISORDERS

GENERAL PRINCIPLES

Definition

- **Normal hemostasis** involves a complex sequence of interrelated reactions, leading to platelet aggregation (primary hemostasis) and activation of the coagulation cascade (secondary hemostasis) to produce a durable vascular seal.
  - **Primary hemostasis** is an immediate but temporary response to vessel injury. Platelets and von Willebrand factor (vWF) interact to form a primary plug, after which platelet activation occurs and blood vessels constrict, limiting flow.
  - **Secondary hemostasis (coagulation)** is a slower process that results in the formation of a fibrin clot (Fig. 18-1). Coagulation is initiated when vascular damage exposes extravascular tissue factor initiating activation of factor VII, factor X, and prothrombin with subsequent activation of factors V, VIII, IX, XI, and XIII, leading to accelerated and sustained generation of thrombin, conversion of fibrinogen to fibrin, and formation of a durable clot.[1]

DIAGNOSIS

History

- A detailed history is crucial for determining whether a bleeding disorder is present and whether it is likely to be congenital or acquired, mild or severe, and involving primary or secondary hemostasis.
  - Prolonged bleeding after challenges such as dental extractions, circumcision, menstruation, labor and delivery, trauma, or surgery may suggest an underlying bleeding disorder, especially if blood transfusion or hospital admission for control of hemostasis is required.
  - Self-reporting of easy bruising and prolonged bleeding with minor cuts is often noninformative unless accompanied by more serious bleeding events.
  - A detailed family history may reveal evidence to support an inherited bleeding disorder.
  - Acquired bleeding disorders may be suggested by recent onset and comorbid conditions (liver disease, alcohol consumption, autoimmune disease) or commonly implicated medications.

Physical Examination

- Primary hemostasis defects are suggested by mucosal bleeding and bruising.
  - Bruising manifests as areas (<2 mm) of subcutaneous bleeding that do not blanch with pressure, called **petechiae;** larger patches (<1 cm), designated **purpura;** or

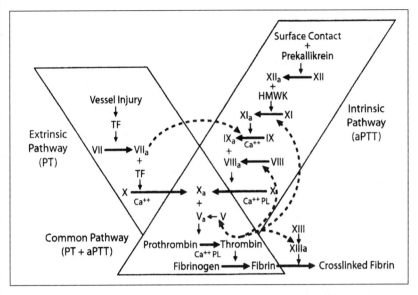

Figure 18-1. Coagulation cascade. *Solid arrows* indicate activation, and *dashed lines* indicate additional substrates activated by factor VIIa or thrombin. aPTT, activated partial thromboplastin time; HMWK, high molecular weight kininogen; PL, phospholipid; PT, prothrombin time; TF, tissue factor.

extensive areas of bruising (>1 cm), called **ecchymoses.** Petechiae typically present in areas that are subjected to increased hydrostatic force typically involving the lower legs or the periorbital area after coughing or vomiting.

■ Disorders of secondary hemostasis usually produce deep ecchymoses, hematomas, hemarthroses, or delayed bleeding after trauma or surgery.

Laboratory Studies

■ Selection of laboratory tests in patients with suspected hemostatic disorders is guided by the history and physical examination. Initial studies should include a platelet count, prothrombin time (PT), activated partial thromboplastin time (aPTT), and peripheral blood smear review.

Primary Hemostasis

■ The **platelet count** should be determined in all patients suspected of a hemostatic disorder. A low platelet count on a complete blood count (CBC) report requires a manual slide review to rule out a platelet clumping artifact due to the anticoagulant ethylene diamine tetra-acetic acid (EDTA), platelet glycoprotein IIb/IIIa receptor inhibitor drugs, or unusually large platelets that are misclassified as red cells or lymphocytes by the automated hematology instrument.

■ The **bleeding time (BT)** may detect qualitative or quantitative disorders of platelets or vWF, or abnormalities of capillary integrity. It is generally not prolonged by disorders of secondary hemostasis.

　■ The BT is not useful for predicting the risk of bleeding complications before invasive procedures in unselected patients.[2]

　■ BT may be prolonged after ingestion of medications that interfere with platelet function, such as aspirin. Other variables that can prolong the BT include differences in technician performance, subcutaneous edema, thinning of the skin, and anemia.

Therefore, when platelet dysfunction is suspected and the BT is prolonged, additional platelet function assays may be appropriate.

- The **PFA-100** (Dade Behring, Deerfield, IL) instrument simulates primary hemostasis at sites of small vessel injury by assessing vWF-dependent platelet activation in citrated whole blood. In addition to qualitative platelet disorders, abnormal results may be due to thrombocytopenia, anemia, and qualitative and quantitative vWF defects.
  - PFA-100 may be used to detect moderate to severe congenital and acquired platelet dysfunction and as part of a panel of tests to screen for von Willebrand disease.
  - However, this test currently cannot be used to predict bleeding risk or monitor antiplatelet agents since adequate clinical investigations have not been performed.[3]
- In vitro platelet aggregation studies measure platelet secretion and aggregation in response to purified platelet agonists. They are used to evaluate patients who are suspected of having an inherited qualitative platelet disorder. Performance requires considerable technical expertise, and nonspecific abnormal results are typical when platelet aggregation tests are performed on acutely ill patients receiving multiple medications.
- **von Willebrand factor antigen (vWF:Ag)** is a measure of circulating vWF protein by immunoassay.
- **von Willebrand factor activity, ristocetin cofactor (vWF:RCo)** is a functional assay of vWF-mediated agglutination of control platelets in the presence of the antibiotic ristocetin.
- **von Willebrand factor multimer analysis** by agarose gel electrophoresis separates vWF multimers by size.

Secondary Hemostasis

- The **prothrombin time (PT)** measures the time to form a fibrin clot after the addition of thromboplastin (tissue factor and phospholipid) and calcium to citrated plasma.
  - This test is sensitive to deficiencies of **"extrinsic pathway"** factor VII and common pathway (factors X, V, prothrombin) coagulation factors and fibrinogen.
  - Reporting PT ratios as an international normalized ratio (INR) reduces interlaboratory variation. Using plasma samples from patients taking warfarin, manufacturers compare the sensitivity of each lot of thromboplastin to a World Health Organization reference thromboplastin and assign an international sensitivity index (ISI). Laboratories convert PT ratios to INR using the equation $INR = (\text{patient PT/mean normal PT})^{ISI}$.[4] Several point-of-care instruments accurately measure PT/INR from a drop of whole blood for use in coagulation clinics or home monitoring.
- The **activated partial thromboplastin times (aPTT)** is also used to screen for secondary hemostasis disorders. aPTT measures the time to form a fibrin clot after activation of citrated plasma by calcium, phospholipid, and negatively charged particles.
  - aPTT is prolonged by deficiencies of coagulation factors of the **"intrinsic pathway"** (high molecular weight kininogen, prekallikrein, factor XII, factor XI, factor IX, and factor VIII) and **"common pathway"** (factor V, factor X, prothrombin), and fibrinogen.
- The **thrombin time (TT)** measures time to clot formation after the addition of thrombin to citrated plasma. It is sensitive to quantitative and qualitative deficiencies of fibrinogen, fibrin degradation products, some monoclonal antibodies, heparin, and direct thrombin inhibitor drugs. The presence of heparin is confirmed if a prolonged TT corrects after adding a reagent to absorb, neutralize, or degrade heparin.
- **Fibrinogen (Clauss method)** concentration is determined by a clotting assay and is inversely proportional to the prolongation of the TT performed on diluted plasma.
- **Clot urea stability** is a qualitative functional test used to screen for severe congenital or acquired deficiency of factor XIII (<5%) in patients who have a clinical bleeding disorder but no evidence of a primary hemostasis defect and normal PT, aPTT, and TT. After activation by thrombin, FXIIIa forms covalent cross links between fibrin molecules to produce a durable clot.
- **Mixing studies** are performed to determine if a prolonged PT or aPTT is due to a factor deficiency or an inhibitor. When patient plasma is mixed 1:1 with normal pooled plasma

TABLE 18-1	Factor Deficiencies that Cause Prolonged Prothrombin Time (PT), Activated Partial Thromboplastin Time (aPPT), or Both
Abnormal assay	**Suspected factor deficiencies**
aPTT	XII, XI, IX, or VIII
PT	VII
PT and aPTT	II, V, X, or fibrinogen

(all factor activities = 100%), deficient factors are restored to at least 50%, sufficient to **normalize or nearly normalize** the PT or aPTT. The next step is to perform selected factor activity assays (Table 18-1) to identify the deficiency. Most inhibitor antibodies are still detectable after a 1:1 mix, and the prolonged PT or aPTT does not completely correct.

- **Coagulation factor activities** are determined by performing a PT or aPTT on a mixture of patient plasma and plasma deficient in the factor of interest and comparing the result to clotting times of plasmas with known factor activities.

 # PLATELET DISORDERS

THROMBOCYTOPENIA

General Principles

Definition

- **Thrombocytopenia** is defined as a platelet count of <140,000/microliter at Barnes-Jewish Hospital. A helpful diagnostic strategy is to differentiate disorders of marrow production from conditions that result in increased platelet destruction or sequestration. A bone marrow examination, which can be performed safely at platelet counts >10,000/mL, may be helpful in making this distinction. Agents such as aspirin, nonsteroidal anti-inflammatory drugs (NSAIDs), and anticoagulants that further impair hemostasis are relatively contraindicated in patients with thrombocytopenia.

Differential Diagnosis

Disorders Resulting in Decreased Platelet Production

> Bone marrow failure syndromes
> Myelodysplastic syndrome
> Marrow infiltration
> Drug suppression or chemotherapy induced
> Irradiation induced
> Nutritional deficiency
> Chronic alcoholism
> Viral infection (Parvovirus, HIV)

Disorders Resulting in Increased Platelet Clearance

> Immune thrombocytopenic purpura (idiopathic, autoimmune, drug induced)
> Thrombotic thrombocytopenic purpura
> Heparin-induced thrombocytopenia
> Disseminated intravascular coagulation
> Posttransfusion purpura
> Mechanical destruction (aortic valve dysfunction, mechanical valves, extracorporeal bypass)

Acute hemorrhage with crystalloid volume replacement
Infection (HIV; ehrlichiosis; rickettsia; HHV-6)

Disorders Resulting from Increased Sequestration of Platelets

Hypersplenism

General Considerations

Thrombocytopenia can be the end result of a series of systemic illnesses affecting the bone marrow, including primary bone marrow failure, bone marrow infiltration, vitamin deficiencies, and infectious processes.

- **Bone marrow failure,** either congenital (Fanconi's anemia, dyskeratosis congenital, Schwachman-Diamond syndrome, etc.) or acquired (aplastic anemia, paroxysmal nocturnal hemoglobinuria), generally presents with bi- or trilineage cytopenias but can on occasion present with an isolated thrombocytopenia.
- **Marrow infiltration (myelophthisis)** by tumors, storage diseases, chronic myeloproliferative disorders, or granulomatous disease may interfere with normal platelet production.
  - The diagnosis is confirmed by examination of a bone marrow biopsy and aspirate. The presence of nucleated red blood cells (RBCs), teardrop red cells, and immature myeloid forms on a peripheral smear may indicate a myelophthisic process.
  - Treatment is directed toward the underlying cause of the marrow infiltration.
  - **Myelodysplastic syndrome (MDS)** is a clonal hematopoietic stem cell disorder that manifests as cytopenia and dysplasia of one or more cell lineages.
- **Prolonged vitamin B_{12} or folate deficiency** usually causes pancytopenia but may result in isolated thrombocytopenia, which resolves with appropriate supplementation.
- **Infections** can cause thrombocytopenia in a variety of ways. Some organisms, such as fungi and mycobacteria, infiltrate the bone marrow.
  - HIV is commonly associated with thrombocytopenia, either through direct infection of megakaryocytes or by accelerated peripheral destruction secondary to an immune thrombocytopenia.[4] HIV is known to be associated with thrombotic thrombocytopenic purpura (TTP), and thrombocytopenia may arise as a result of opportunistic infections or as a complication of antiretroviral therapy.
  - Human herpesvirus (HHV)-6 causes thrombocytopenia in immunosuppressed patients by suppressing production of megakaryocyte progenitor cells.[5]
- Usually, increased bleeding is not attributable to thrombocytopenia until the count drops below 50,000/microliter. The risk of spontaneous life-threatening (e.g., central nervous system [CNS], gastrointestinal [GI]) bleeding increases at counts below 20,000/mL and substantially at counts below 10,000/microliter.

Specific Causes of Thrombocytopenia

Immune Thrombocytopenic Purpura

- Immune thrombocytopenic purpura (ITP) is an acquired autoimmune disorder in which antiplatelet antibodies result in platelet destruction, leading to thrombocytopenia and an increased risk of serious bleeding.

Epidemiology

- The annual incidence of adult ITP is estimated to be 32 cases per 10^6 persons,[7] most commonly affecting women during the second and third decades. Estimates of the incidence of serious drug-induced thrombocytopenia, excluding cytotoxic drugs and heparin, are typically around 10 per 10^6 persons.

Etiology

- **Immune thrombocytopenia** is caused by the binding of autoantibodies (usually IgG) to platelet surface antigens, resulting in premature clearance by the reticuloendothelial system. Immune thrombocytopenia may arise as a result of other underlying diseases, such as systemic lupus erythematosus (SLE), antiphospholipid antibody (APA) syndrome,

HIV, hepatitis C virus, or lymphoproliferative disorders, and testing for these diseases is performed based on history, physical examination, and laboratory findings.[8]

- Drug-induced **thrombocytopenia** may be idiosyncratic or dose dependent. Of the several mechanisms of drug-induced thrombocytopenia, the most common are antibody mediated.[9] The most common medications that are reported to cause thrombocytopenia include quinidine, quinine, rifampin, trimethoprim/sulfamethoxazole, and methyldopa.[10] Some drugs, such as ethanol, directly inhibit thrombopoiesis.

Clinical Presentation
- In adults, **ITP** typically presents as mild mucocutaneous bleeding that develops over several weeks. However, patients may have an asymptomatic mild or moderately decreased platelet count that is discovered incidentally when a CBC is ordered for other indications.

Laboratory testing
- The diagnosis of idiopathic or primary **ITP** is suggested by isolated thrombocytopenia in the absence of a likely underlying causative disease or medication.
  - Serologic tests for antiplatelet antibodies generally are not helpful in diagnosing **ITP** because of poor sensitivity.[11]
  - Bone marrow biopsy and aspirate studies are not required in most patients suspected of ITP but can be useful in selected patients to exclude primary bone marrow disorders, especially in individuals older than 60 years and patients who do not respond to therapy.[12]
  - Platelet antibody tests may be modified to detect drug-dependent platelet antibodies but are insensitive due to weak binding of drug, unknown optimal concentration of drug, or antibodies recognizing a metabolite of the parent drug.

Treatment
- Not all patients with **immune thrombocytopenia** require treatment. Initial therapy, when indicated, consists of glucocorticoids (typically prednisone 1 mg/kg/d) with the addition of IVIg (1 g/kg × 2 days) in nonresponders or if the patient is bleeding. Most patients who are treated respond to therapy within 1–3 weeks. Of the patients who respond to glucocorticoid therapy, 30%–40% will relapse during a steroid taper, and these individuals are considered to have chronic ITP.
- **Drug-induced thrombocytopenia** is a diagnosis of exclusion and is confirmed only after normalization of platelet counts with discontinuation of the drug. Intravenous immunoglobulin (IVIg), steroids, and platelet transfusions can be administered if thrombocytopenia is life threatening.
- ITP patients who are **refractory to initial therapy or relapse** are treated either with splenectomy or immunosuppressive therapy. Splenectomy, ideally laparoscopic, is the treatment of choice, as two-thirds of patients with refractory ITP will obtain a durable complete response.
  - There is an approximately 15% relapse rate, which may be balanced by the rate of late postsplenectomy remissions.
  - Pneumococcal, meningococcal, and *Haemophilus influenzae* type B vaccines should be administered at least 2 weeks before splenectomy.
  - If a patient is a poor surgical candidate or unwilling to undergo splenectomy, medical salvage therapy may include prednisone, anti-D immunoglobulin (WinRho) in Rh-positive patients, androgen therapy with danazol, or immunosuppressive agents, such as vincristine, cyclophosphamide, rituximab, or azathioprine.[12,13]
  - The minority of patients who fail splenectomy are managed similarly to those with primary refractory ITP, with the exception of the use of WinRho, which is ineffective in the absence of a spleen.
  - Several small-molecule thrombopoietin receptor (TPO-R) agonists are currently in various stages of development and in clinical trials in patients with refractory ITP.[14]

Special Considerations

- ITP during pregnancy may be difficult to distinguish from gestational thrombocytopenia, pre-eclampsia, and HELLP (hemolysis, elevated liver enzymes, low platelets) syndrome and is a diagnosis of exclusion. Guidelines for treatment are similar to those for nonpregnant ITP patients and are reserved for platelet counts <30,000/microliter or bleeding complications.
  - IVIg is recommended for initial therapy, but glucocorticoids can also be used if an appropriate response to IVIg does not occur.
  - Patients who fail initial therapy with IVIg and glucocorticoids and who have a platelet count of <10,000 or are bleeding can be considered for splenectomy.
  - Pregnant patients with ITP can safely undergo vaginal delivery or cesarean section if the platelet count is >50,000/microliter.
  - Platelet transfusion before delivery is recommended in patients for whom a cesarean section is planned, if the platelet count is <10,000, or if the patient is bleeding.
  - Because most antiplatelet antibodies are IgG and are able to cross the placenta, approximately 5% of neonates who are born to affected mothers have severe thrombocytopenia and may be at risk for intracranial hemorrhage during delivery.
    - Centers with high-risk obstetric services can perform fetal blood sampling either by percutaneous umbilical vein sampling or fetal scalp vein sampling to determine the fetal platelet count before delivery. Some experts endorse cesarean section when the fetal platelet count is <20,000,[12] while others recommend a conservative approach to labor and delivery management and would not monitor fetal platelet counts.[15] Neonatal platelet counts may nadir several days postpartum.

Gestational Thrombocytopenia

General Principles

Definition

- Gestational thrombocytopenia is a benign, mild thrombocytopenia associated with pregnancy.

Epidemiology

- Gestational thrombocytopenia spontaneously occurs in approximately 5%–7% of otherwise uncomplicated pregnancies.

Etiology

- The mechanism of gestational thrombocytopenia is unknown.

Clinical Presentation and Treatment

- Gestational thrombocytopenia is a common (5%–10%) finding in the third trimester. Platelet counts are typically >70,000/microliter, and the mother is asymptomatic. Neonates are unaffected by gestational thrombocytopenia.
  - Other causes of thrombocytopenia during pregnancy include ITP, pre-eclampsia (in 15%–20% of cases), eclampsia (in 40%–50% of cases), HELLP syndrome, TTP, and disseminated intravascular coagulation (DIC), and a thorough evaluation for evidence of hemolysis, infection, hypertension, and liver dysfunction is required to distinguish between these syndromes.
  - Gestational thrombocytopenia, pre-eclampsia, and eclampsia usually resolve promptly after delivery; the management of gestational TTP is similar to that of TTP in the nonpregnant patient.[16]

Thrombotic Thrombocytopenic Purpura (TTP)

General Principles

Definition
- TTP is a type of microangiopathic hemolytic anemia produced by platelet vWF aggregates in the microcirculation. When TTP is suspected, the differential diagnosis of thrombotic microangiopathy includes DIC, malignant hypertension, vasculitis, and, during pregnancy, pre-eclampsia/eclampsia and HELLP syndrome.

Epidemiology
- The incidence of sporadic TTP is approximately 11.3 cases per 10^6 persons, and is higher in women and African Americans.[17]

Etiology
- Sporadic TTP is typically a result of autoantibody-mediated removal of plasma vWF-cleaving protease (ADAMTS13), leading to elevated levels of abnormal high molecular weight vWF multimers.[18] Unusually large vWF multimers spontaneously adhere to platelets and are necessary, but not sufficient, to produce occlusive vWF platelet aggregates in the microcirculation and subsequent microangiopathy. Second—hit events may involve endothelial dysfunction or injury.
- Secondary causes of TTP (drug induced; postorgan and stem cell transplantation) are not due to severe ADAMTS13 deficiency.

Clinical Presentation
- The complete clinical pentad of TTP, which is present in <30% of cases, includes consumptive thrombocytopenia, microangiopathic hemolytic anemia, fever, renal dysfunction, and fluctuating neurologic deficits.
  - Thrombocytopenia and microangiopathic hemolytic anemia are sufficient to raise suspicion for TTP in the absence of other identifiable causes.
  - TTP may occur during pregnancy and postpartum, has been associated with HIV, and can be drug induced (e.g., cyclosporine, ticlopidine, quinine). Rare autosomal-recessive inherited deficiencies of ADAMTS13 with chronic relapsing TTP also exist.
  - The **hemolytic–uremic syndrome** is usually immediately preceded by diarrhea and often hemorrhagic colitis due to shiga toxin-producing bacteria (*Shigella*, *Escherichia coli* O157:H7) and is associated with more pronounced renal dysfunction.

Laboratory Evaluation
- Laboratory evaluation of TTP shows evidence of intravascular hemolysis (anemia, low or undetectable haptoglobin, elevated lactate dehydrogenase), thrombocytopenia, normal coagulation studies, and renal insufficiency.
- The peripheral smear is significant for evidence of mechanical red cell damage (schistocytes) and thrombocytopenia.
- Assays for ADAMTS13 activity are offered by some reference laboratories; most patients with sporadic TTP will not have detectable plasma ADAMTS13 enzyme activity, and many will have detectable ADAMTS13 inhibitory antibodies. The utility of measuring ADAMTS13 activity/inhibition for diagnosis and management of TTP is currently under investigation.

Treatment
- **Rapid treatment of TTP is critical** to prevent serious morbidity or mortality from thrombotic complications. **Plasma exchange** of 1.0–1.5 plasma volumes daily is the mainstay of therapy. Remission rates are as high as 90% when plasma exchange is initiated without delay.
  - If plasma exchange is not available or will be delayed, fresh frozen plasma (FFP) should be infused immediately to replace ADAMTS13.

- The addition of **glucocorticoids** has become common practice, ranging from prednisone, 1 mg/kg PO daily, to methylprednisolone, 1 g IV daily.
- RBC transfusion can be given as needed.
- Platelet transfusion in the absence of significant bleeding is relatively contraindicated because of the potential risk of additional microvascular occlusion.
- The end point of therapy is not well defined, but plasma exchange is usually continued for at least 5 days or for 2 days after normalization of the platelet count and lactate dehydrogenase, resolution of neurologic signs, and improvement in microangiopathy.
- Schistocytes may persist for several weeks into a durable remission.
- Renal failure may be slower to improve, and persistent azotemia does not necessarily indicate treatment failure. Patients who do not respond initially to plasma exchange usually receive a trial of plasma exchange with cryosupernatant (depleted of vWF) in place of FFP.
- Relapse occurs most commonly within 1 month after discontinuing plasma exchange.
- **Immunosuppression** with cyclophosphamide, azathioprine, or vincristine may be beneficial for relapsed TTP.[19]
- **Rituximab**, an anti-CD20 monoclonal antibody, has proved effective in achieving durable remissions, according to several case reports[20] and clinical trials are under way to determine the optimal use of this drug.
- **Splenectomy** may salvage some patients with **TTP** who are initially refractory to plasma exchange or may reduce the frequency of relapses in patients who experience recurrent episodes.[21]

Heparin-Induced Thrombocytopenia

General Principles

Definition

- Heparin-induced thrombocytopenia (HIT) is an acquired hypercoagulable disorder caused by antibodies that target heparin and platelet factor 4 (PF4) complexes. HIT presents with a drop in platelet count of >50% during exposure to unfractionated heparin (UFH) or low molecular weight heparin (LMWH); it may produce clinical sequelae including arterial or venous thrombosis, skin necrosis at UFH/LMWH injection sites, or acute systemic reactions after IV bolus administration.

Epidemiology

- The incidence of **HIT** varies in different clinical settings, ranging from <1% to 2% in medical patients receiving prophylactic and therapeutic heparin, respectively, to 5% in patients receiving prophylactic heparin after total hip or knee replacement surgery. The incidence of HIT is considerably lower when patients are treated with low molecular weight heparins or the synthetic pentasaccharide fondaparinux.

Etiology

- HIT is a unique form of drug-induced thrombocytopenia. Immune-responsive patients produce autoantibodies to PF4, a protein contained in platelet *a* granules, when complexed with heparin. In a subset of patients who form antibodies, immune complexes bind to platelet IgG Fc receptors, leading to platelet activation, thrombocytopenia, and clot formation.[22]

Clinical Presentation

- The **diagnosis** of HIT is suggested by the development of thrombocytopenia during heparin therapy by any route (including heparin flushes) in the absence of other causes of thrombocytopenia, and a prompt recovery of platelet count after cessation of heparin.
  - The diagnosis is suspected when thrombocytopenia (<140,000) or a decrease in the platelet count of 50% or more from baseline develops in patients who are receiving heparin.
  - HIT usually develops between 5 and 14 days after heparin exposure. Exceptions include delayed onset of HIT after heparin is discontinued and HIT starting within

the first 24 hours in patients with recent exposure to heparin (within the past 30 days).[23]

■ Thrombocytopenia is rarely severe, bleeding is uncommon, and **venous or arterial thromboembolic complications occur in 30%–50% of patients.**

Laboratory Evaluation

■ When the clinical evidence for or against **HIT** is not compelling, laboratory testing for HIT antibodies is recommended. Two types of assays are available: **functional** (platelet aggregometry or serotonin release assay to detect activation of control platelets in the presence of patient serum and heparin) and **antigenic** (enzyme-linked immunosorbent assays [ELISAs] to detect antibodies against heparin–PF4 complexes).

　■ Functional assays are generally considered to be more specific and ELISA more sensitive. A positive ELISA is not sufficient to diagnose HIT since antibody-mediated platelet activation only occurs in a subset of PF4 antibody-positive patients.

　■ A positive antigenic test should be confirmed by a functional test.

　■ If clinical suspicion for HIT persists despite an initial negative PF4 ELISA, repeat testing is appropriate since some patients may convert to positive.

　■ Results for both types of HIT tests are rarely immediately available, and initial management decisions must be made based on clinical judgment.

Treatment

■ Treatment of **HIT** begins with elimination of all heparin exposure. Patients with thromboses, or at high risk of thrombotic complications, require alternative anticoagulation with a parenteral direct thrombin inhibitor, either hirudin (lepirudin) or argatroban (see Anticoagulants).

■ In **HIT** therapy, LMWH should be avoided due to high rates of cross reactivity with HIT antibodies.

■ Thrombocytopenia is generally not regarded as a contraindication to anticoagulation, unless the patient is bleeding.

■ In one series, 50% of patients with thrombocytopenia due to HIT were found to have subclinical lower extremity deep venous thromboses (DVTs). Therefore, screening lower extremity Doppler ultrasound in such patients is reasonable, as the finding of a DVT mandates anticoagulation for 3–6 months.[22] If clinically indicated, screening for pulmonary embolism (PE) may also be considered.

■ Oral anticoagulation therapy with warfarin should not be initiated until the platelet count normalizes and should overlap with ongoing anticoagulation with a direct thrombin inhibitor, because of the risk of limb gangrene.

■ Indications for, duration, and type of alternative anticoagulant for HIT patients without thrombotic complications following resolution of thrombocytopenia are uncertain at this time. Contrary to initial impressions, the synthetic pentasaccharide fondaparinux does induce heparin–PF4 antibodies in 1.5%–2.8% of treated patients.[24] While the clinical significance of these antibodies is uncertain, fondaparinux cannot be recommended as an alternative anticoagulant for HIT patients at this time.

Posttransfusion Purpura (PTP)

General Principles

Definition

■ PTP is a rare syndrome characterized by the formation of alloantibodies against platelet surface antigens, most commonly the antigen HPA-1a (PL^{A1}), resulting in severe thrombocytopenia.

Epidemiology

■ PTP occurs in HPA-1a—negative patients who receive blood or platelet transfusions from HPA-1a—positive donors.

Etiology
- **PTP** typically occurs in HPA-1a–negative multiparous women who are re-exposed to the antigen when transfused. Alloantibodies to the HPA-1a epitope appear to recognize the patient's HPA-1a–negative platelets causing thrombocytopenia. In some cases of PTP, the alloantibody is against a different platelet epitope.

Clinical presentation and laboratory evaluation
- In **PTP**, severe thrombocytopenia presenting with petechiae and bleeding occurs within approximately 7–10 days of transfusion.
- Confirmation of suspected **PTP** requires detection of platelet alloantibodies. Selected reference laboratories offer comprehensive serologic, flow cytometry, and molecular diagnostic testing to determine platelet alloantibody specificity, typically anti-HPA.

Treatment
- PTP treatment options include IVIg or plasmapheresis. HPA-1a–negative platelets are rarely available and posttransfusion platelet increments are likely to be poor regardless of HPA-1 phenotype; transfusion with platelets of unknown HPA-1 status should be reserved for severe bleeding.

Hypersplenism

General Principles

Definition
- **Hypersplenism** is a syndrome characterized by splenomegaly and sequestration of up to 90% of circulating platelets.
   - A variety of disorders, such as portal hypertension, infiltrative processes, and Felty's syndrome, may result in **hypersplenism,** but most produce only a modest decrease in the platelet count.
   - Treatment of **hypersplenism** is directed toward the underlying condition. Splenectomy is a consideration if the cause of splenomegaly is not remediable, if the splenomegaly is symptomatic, or as a diagnostic procedure in idiopathic splenomegaly.

Platelet Transfusion
- **Platelet transfusion guidelines.** Platelets can be separated from a unit of donated whole blood (random-donor platelets) or collected by apheresis (single-donor platelets). In patients with thrombocytopenia resulting from a platelet production defect, transfusion of either one single-donor apheresis unit or six random-donor units typically results in an immediate increment of approximately 30,000/microliter.
- **Reaction to platelets.** Removing white blood cells (WBCs) by filtration can reduce the risk of febrile reactions, alloimmunization, and refractoriness to platelet transfusion in patients who are likely to require chronic platelet support.
   - Single-donor apheresis platelet products are free of significant WBC contamination.
   - Platelets are infused over 30 minutes, and premedication with acetaminophen and diphenhydramine (Benadryl) is indicated if the patient has had a prior platelet transfusion reaction.
   - Many of the risks and complications of RBC transfusion (see Chapter 19, Anemia and Transfusion Therapy) apply to platelet transfusion as well.
- **Transfusion threshold.** Prophylactic platelet transfusion is appropriate for asymptomatic outpatients with platelet counts of <20,000/microliter and asymptomatic inpatients with platelet counts of <10,000/microliter. If a major invasive procedure is performed, a 50,000/microliter threshold is generally used. High-risk surgery (e.g., neurosurgery, ophthalmic surgery, cardiopulmonary bypass) may warrant prophylactic transfusion to keep the platelet count >100,000/microliter.
   - Platelet transfusion thresholds change if there is evidence of bleeding. For minor mucosal bleeding (minor epistaxis, occult GI bleeding, petechiae), the goal for platelet transfusion is a platelet count >20,000/microliter.
   - In the event of major bleeding (postoperative, CNS bleeding), the goal is a level of approximately 100,000/microliter.

- Unless the platelet half-life is shortened severely, there is no rationale for monitoring counts and transfusing more frequently than every 24 hours.
- Shortened platelet survival can be due to sepsis, fever, active bleeding, splenic sequestration, or alloantibody development in multiply transfused patients.
  - Antibody-mediated refractoriness is assessed by measuring the platelet count before and 60 minutes after transfusion of an apheresis unit or six random-donor platelets. An increment of <5000/microliter is consistent with antibody-mediated refractoriness rather than shortened survival due to another mechanism.
  - Using HLA-matched single-donor platelets, ABO-compatible platelets, or IVIg before transfusion may improve platelet increments.

THROMBOCYTOSIS

General Principles

Definition

- **Reactive thrombocytosis,** typically <1,000,000/microliter, may occur in response to resolving thrombocytopenia (after surgery or HIT), postsplenectomy, or conditions such as iron deficiency, chronic infectious or inflammatory states, and malignancies, either overt or occult. Patients with reactive thrombocytosis apparently do not have an increased risk of bleeding or thrombosis. No specific therapy is required except for correction of the underlying disorder.
- **Essential thrombocythemia (ET)** is a chronic myeloproliferative disorder characterized by persistent thrombocytosis and an increased susceptibility to thrombosis and hemorrhage. Like the other myeloproliferative disorders (e.g., chronic myelogenous leukemia, polycythemia vera, and myelofibrosis), ET is a clonal disorder of hematopoietic stem cells.[25]

Diagnosis

Clinical Presentation

- Thrombocytosis is often an incidental discovery in an asymptomatic patient. Thromboses may be arterial or venous, and involve both small and large vessels. The risk of thrombosis increases with age, prior thrombosis, duration of disease, and comorbidities.[26] Erythromelalgia, due to microvascular occlusive platelet thrombi, presents as intense burning or throbbing of the extremities, typically involving the feet, and is usually relieved with cold exposure. Hemorrhage is typically associated with platelet counts >1,000,000 and is secondary to an acquired deficiency of large vWF multimers.[27] Median age at diagnosis is 60 years, and 3%–5% of patients ultimately progress to acute myeloid leukemia.

Physical Examination

- Mild splenomegaly is present in almost 50% of ET patients. Typical signs of erythromelalgia include erythema and warmth of affected digits.

Laboratory Studies

- ET is typically a diagnosis of exclusion after dismissing reactive thrombocytosis or an alternative form of myeloproliferative disease.
  - Diagnostic criteria for ET include a platelet count of >600,000, a normal hematocrit, adequate iron stores, absence of Philadelphia chromosome on karyotype analysis, no evidence in the bone marrow of myelofibrosis or myelodysplastic syndrome, and no secondary cause.[28]
  - Megakaryocyte hyperplasia, often in clumps, is usually identified on bone marrow biopsy.
  - While ET patients typically have a normal karyotype, approximately 50% are positive for an acquired point mutation in the Janus kinase 2 (JAK2) gene. This mutation was only recently discovered.[29] As more is learned about its role in the pathogenesis

and prognosis of myeloproliferative disorders, including ET, determining JAK2 status is likely to become a definitive test when evaluating patients with unexplained thrombocytosis.

Treatment

- Management of **ET** must be individualized.
  - Younger asymptomatic patients without excess risk of thrombosis can be observed. Erythromelalgia usually responds to low-dose aspirin.
  - Older patients, particularly those with history of prior thrombosis, require treatment. The majority of thrombotic complications occur at modest elevations of platelets. Therefore, a reasonable treatment goal is platelet count of 400,000 or less. This can be accomplished with the use of platelet-lowering agents such as **hydroxyurea or anagrelide,** or with interferon-α in patients who are either pregnant or in their child-bearing years.[30]
    - The leukemogenic potential of long-term hydroxyurea therapy is unknown, but indirect evidence suggests that it is quite low.
    - Anagrelide specifically inhibits platelet production via incompletely understood mechanisms. Common side effects include palpitations, atrial fibrillation, fluid retention, and headache.
    - Results from a recent randomized study comparing hydroxyurea to anagrelide in ET patients showed equivalent platelet count control but more thrombotic and hemorrhagic complications and bone marrow transformation to myelofibrosis with anagrelide.[31]
    - Low-dose aspirin can be prescribed, but its additional benefit to cytoreduction is unclear. Acute arterial thrombosis is managed best with platelet pheresis in combination with aspirin. Platelet transfusion is appropriate for life-threatening hemorrhage.

QUALITATIVE PLATELET DISORDERS

General Principles

- **Qualitative platelet disorders** are suggested by mucocutaneous bleeding and excessive bruising in the setting of an adequate platelet count and normal screening tests for secondary hemostasis defects and von Willebrand's disease. Bleeding time and/or PFA-100 closure time may be prolonged, but neither test is adequately sensitive to rule out a mild to moderate platelet defect. If normal results are obtained with these tests and clinical suspicion remains high, in vitro platelet aggregation studies are appropriate. Acquired defects are more common than hereditary platelet qualitative disorders.

Classification

- **Inherited disorders** of platelet function are uncommon and are categorized as receptor defects, aberrant signal transduction, cyclooxygenase defects, secretory (e.g., storage pool disease), and adhesion or aggregation defects. In vitro platelet aggregation studies are useful for identifying patterns of agonist responses that are consistent with a particular category, although additional specialized testing may be required to confirm a specific diagnosis. Platelets from patients with Bernard-Soulier's syndrome and Glanzmann's thrombasthenia, two rare, autosomal-recessive, and clinically significant disorders, lack glycoprotein (GP) IbIX (vWF receptor) and GP IIb/IIIa (fibrinogen receptor), respectively.
- **Acquired** platelet function defects generally cause milder symptoms than do the inherited disorders. Patients with isolated platelet dysfunction may not bleed abnormally unless superimposed thrombocytopenia or coagulation defects are present.
  - Categories of acquired defects include clonal hematopoietic diseases (myeloproliferative disease, myelodysplasia, acute leukemia, and monoclonal gammopathy), metabolic disorders (uremia, liver failure), trauma (postcardiopulmonary bypass), and the most common, drug induced.

- Defects in every aspect of platelet function have been reported in **uremia,** but their individual and cumulative clinical significance is usually mild. The BT can be prolonged in uremic patients; however, the associated risk of bleeding is variable. The BT is also prolonged by anemia, which frequently accompanies renal insufficiency.
- Evidence for platelet dysfunction due to **liver disease** is not definitive. However, multiple hemostatic derangements (hyperfibrinolysis, DIC, coagulopathy, thrombocytopenia, anemia) accompany fulminant and end-stage liver disease, giving rise to abnormal bleeding and a prolonged bleeding time.
- **Drug-induced** platelet dysfunction is a side effect of a wide variety of drugs, including high-dose penicillin, bismuth subsalicylate (Pepto-Bismol), aspirin, other NSAIDs, and ethanol. Numerous other drugs, such as beta-lactam antibiotics, beta-blockers, calcium channel blockers, nitrates, antihistamines, psychotropic drugs, tricyclic antidepressants, and selective serotonin reuptake inhibitors, cause platelet dysfunction in vitro but rarely are associated with bleeding complications. Platelet dysfunction is the therapeutic mechanism of other drugs: aspirin, dipyridamole, thienopyridines, and GP IIb/IIIa antagonists.
- Certain **foods and herbal products** may affect platelet function[32] including omega-3-fatty acids, garlic and onion extracts, ginger, gingko, ginseng, and black tree fungus.

Treatment

Medications

- Patients with inherited bleeding disorders are managed conservatively, with platelet transfusions reserved for significant bleeding.
  - Patients with Bernard-Soulier Syndrome or Glanzmann thrombasthenia can become refractory to platelet transfusion due to alloantibodies that recognize the surface glycoprotein that they lack. There are anecdotal reports of successful control of bleeding in such patients following infusion of recombinant factor VIIa.
- Treatment of **uremic** patients is generally reserved for individuals with bleeding complications. Several interventions shorten prolonged BT and may improve hemostasis, although appropriate clinical trials have not been done: Hemodialysis and peritoneal dialysis improve uremia and shorten BT; increasing the hematocrit to at least 30%, either with the use of RBC transfusion or erythropoietin, shortens bleeding time.
  - Desmopressin (diamino-8-D-arginine vasopressin [DDAVP], **0.3 mcg/kg IV**), stimulates release of vWF from endothelial cells and shortens a prolonged BT, and is commonly administered before renal biopsy or during a bleeding episode.
  - Conjugated estrogens (0.6 mg/kg IV daily for 5 days) may improve platelet function for up to 2 weeks.
  - Transfused platelets acquire the uremic defect rapidly but can have transient utility in actively bleeding patients.

Special Considerations

Due to the possibility of hemostasis inhibition, all herbal medications and dietary supplements should be discontinued at least 2 weeks before major surgery.[33]

- **Antiplatelet agents** are useful for their antithrombotic effects.
- **Aspirin** is an irreversible cyclooxygenase-1 and -2 inhibitor. After aspirin is discontinued, its effects gradually diminish over approximately 7 days as new platelets are produced.
  - Patients receiving aspirin who are scheduled to undergo elective procedures are advised to stop the medication 5–7 days before surgery. However, the risk of significant bleeding in most patients on aspirin who require urgent surgery is probably too low to warrant a delay, excluding ophthalmologic and neurosurgery.[34]
  - All other **NSAIDs** reversibly inhibit cyclooxygenase-1 and -2 and their effect lasts only as long as they remain in plasma. **Cyclooxygenase-2 inhibitors** have antiplatelet activity in large doses but at therapeutic doses have a minimal effect on platelets, and one drug in this class, rofecoxib (Vioxx), was recently withdrawn from the market due to evidence of increased risk of arterial thromboembolic events.

- **Thienopyridines** (clopidogrel) inhibit platelet aggregation by blocking the platelet adenosine diphosphate receptor P2Y12. Because of its prolonged half-life, clopidogrel should be withheld beginning 10 days before elective invasive procedures.
- **Dipyridamole** inhibits platelet function by increasing intracellular cyclic adenosine monophosphate (cAMP), and is available either alone or in combination with aspirin (Aggrenox).
- The antiplatelet agents **abciximab, eptifibatide,** and **tirofiban** block platelet IIb/IIIa–dependent aggregation and are approved for use in acute coronary syndromes (see Chapter 5, Ischemic Heart Disease). Platelet transfusion compensates for drug-induced platelet dysfunction described above, except that caused by tirofiban and eptifibatide, and is thus effective therapy for patients with significant bleeding.

 # INHERITED BLEEDING DISORDERS

HEMOPHILIA A

General Principles

Definition
- **Hemophilia A** is an X-linked coagulation disorder that leads to impaired intrinsic pathway coagulation secondary to defects in the gene encoding factor VIII.

Classification
- **Hemophilia A** affects approximately 1 in 5,000 live male births. Approximately 40% of cases occur in families with no prior history of hemophilia, reflecting the high rate of spontaneous germ line mutations in the factor VIII gene.[35]
  - The clinical phenotype is determined by the factor VIII activity level: severe (<1% activity), moderate (1%–5% activity), and mild (>5% activity).
  - Patients with severe hemophilia (<1% activity) experience frequent spontaneous hemorrhages, including hemarthroses, hematomas, hematuria, and delayed posttraumatic and postoperative bleeding.
  - Repeated bleeding into a "target" joint can cause chronic synovitis and hemophilic arthropathy.
  - Moderate hemophiliacs have fewer spontaneous bleeding episodes, and mild hemophiliacs may only bleed excessively after trauma or surgery.

Treatment

Medications
- Primary therapy of **hemophilia A** is determined by the severity of the patient's disease and the type of hemorrhage. Usually patients with mild to moderate hemophilia A and a minor bleeding episode can be treated with **DDAVP**, which increases plasma factor VIII levels by three- to fivefold within 30 minutes, with a half-life of 8–12 hours. The usual DDAVP dose is 0.3 mcg/kg IV (in 50–100 mL normal saline infused over 30 minutes) or SC, or 300 mcg intranasally (Stimate, 1.5 mg/mL) dosed every 12 hours. Tachyphylaxis may occur after several doses.[36]
- Patients with mild to moderate hemophilia A with major bleeding episodes or those with severe hemophilia A with any prolonged source of hemorrhage require **FVIII replacement** for bleeding challenges.
  - This treatment may consist of either purified FVIII concentrate from pooled plasma or recombinant FVIII (rFVIII). The choice of replacement is determined by the availability of product, the patient's history of viral exposure, and patient preference.
  - Testing for viral pathogens combined with viral inactivation procedures has dramatically improved the safety of plasma-derived coagulation factor concentrates.
  - In general, previously untreated patients and those who are HIV and hepatitis B and C negative receive the more expensive rFVIII to minimize the risk of viral transmission.

- Typically, FVIII levels increase 2% for every 1 unit/kg factor VIII concentrate infused with a half-life of 8–12 hours. Thus, a 50-units/kg IV bolus would be expected to raise factor VIII levels to approximately 100% over baseline. This dosage can be followed by a 25-units/kg IV bolus q12h.
- To stop most mild hemorrhages, infusion of FVIII to achieve peak activities of 30%–50% of normal is necessary.
- Home therapy with factor replacement allows outpatient therapy of minor hemorrhages. One to three doses of factor usually suffice.
- Moderate to severe hemorrhages require infusions of FVIII to achieve peak activities of 50%–100% for adequate hemostasis. Inpatient treatment and dose adjustments guided by daily monitoring of peak and trough FVIII activity may be necessary to ensure adequate hemostasis and efficient use of expensive concentrates.[37]

HEMOPHILIA B

General Principles

Definition
- Hemophilia B is an X-linked coagulation disorder that leads to impaired intrinsic pathway coagulation secondary to defects in the gene encoding factor IX. The incidence of hemophilia B is approximately 1 in 30,000 male births.

Classification and Treatment
- Hemophilia B is clinically indistinguishable from hemophilia A, but the distinction is important, as the therapy consists of factor IX replacement with either FIX concentrate from pooled plasma or recombinant FIX (BeneFIX).
  - DDAVP does not increase FIX levels.
  - Postinfusion peak and trough targets, duration of replacement, and laboratory monitoring for treatment of hemophilia B–related bleeding episodes are similar to the guidelines provided for hemophilia A. Each unit of FIX replacement per kilogram of body weight typically generates a 1% increase in factor IX levels, with a half-life of 18–24 hours. For moderate to severe bleeding events, a loading dose of 100 units/kg is administered followed by 50 units/kg every 18–24 hours until hemostasis is achieved or 10–14 days postoperatively.

Complications of Therapy for Hemophilia

- **Inhibitors.** Alloantibodies to FVIII and FIX develop in approximately 20% and 12% of severe hemophilia A and B patients, respectively, in response to replacement therapy. These alloantibodies bind to and neutralize the activity of infused FVIII or FIX and prevent correction of the coagulopathy.
- Determining the titer of a FVIII inhibitor, using a laboratory assay that reports inhibitor strength in Bethesda units (BUs), is useful for predicting inhibitor behavior and for guiding therapy. Patients with high inhibitor titers (>5 BU) frequently have rapid anamnestic responses to repeat exposures and are defined as "high responders." Low responders (<5 BU) usually have minimal anamnesis on repeat exposure to FVIII or FIX. Several treatment options are available for hemophiliacs with FVIII or FIX inhibitors.
  - **Recombinant factor VIIa (rFVIIa, NovoSeven)** is currently approved for use in patients with hemophilia A and B in whom inhibitors to factor replacement have developed, and in patients with congenital factor VII deficiency. rFVIIa promotes hemostasis by activating the tissue factor/extrinsic pathway. It is available in 1.2-, 2.4-, or 4.8-mg vials and is dosed at 90 mcg/kg every 2 hours until hemostasis is achieved for hemophiliacs with inhibitors.[38]
  - An alternative replacement product is activated prothrombin complex concentrate (FEIBA VH), which contains partially activated vitamin K–dependent coagulation factors XI, X, and VII, and thrombin. However, dose and duration of treatment should be limited due to potential for thrombotic complications.

▧ Large doses of FVIII or FIX concentrates may be effective in hemophiliacs with weak inhibitors (BU <5–10).

von WILLEBRAND'S DISEASE

General Principles

Definition

- **von Willebrand's disease (vWD)**, results from an inherited qualitative or quantitative defect of vWF. The inheritance of most forms of **vWD** is autosomal dominant, although autosomal-recessive forms (types 2N and 3) exist. The spectrum of bleeding is broad and is related to the inherited form. vWF has two important functions: to facilitate adherence of platelets to injured vessel walls and to stabilize factor VIII in plasma.

Classification

- vWD is the most common inherited bleeding disorder, affecting an estimated 0.1% of the population.
- The characteristic clinical findings are mucocutaneous bleeding (epistaxis, menorrhagia, GI bleeding) and easy bruising.
  - ▧ Trauma, surgery, or dental extractions may result in life-threatening bleeding in severely affected individuals.
  - ▧ Patients with mild disease may remain undiagnosed into adulthood.[39]
  - ▧ Classification follows a revised nomenclature for vWD that recognizes three main types:
    - **Type 1 vWD, partial quantitative deficiency**
      - Type 1 accounts for 70%–80% of cases, and vWF:Ag and activity are proportionately low.
    - **Type 2 vWD, qualitative deficiency**
      - In most subtypes of type 2 vWD, FVIII activity is normal, vWF:Ag is mildly low, and vWF:RCo is decreased out of proportion to vWF:Ag levels.
    - **Type 3 vWD, severe quantitative deficiency**
      - In type 3 vWD, levels of vWF:Ag and vWF:RCo are extremely low or undetectable and FVIII is <5%.[39]

Diagnosis

Laboratory Studies

- vWF:Ag tests measure circulating vWF protein by immunoassay. A deficiency of vWF:Ag is sensitive for type 1 and 3 **vWD** and may be low normal for type 2 forms.
- vWF:RCo is a functional test of **patients'** vWF-mediated agglutination of **control** platelets in the presence of the antibiotic ristocetin. Decreased agglutination is due either to a deficiency of vWF (type 1 and 3) or vWF mutations that cause a selective loss of large multimers (type 2A and 2B), or defective platelet binding despite a normal multimer pattern (type 2M).
- Factor VIII activity may be low due to a quantitative deficiency of vWF (type 1 and 3) or due to a vWF mutation that reduces FVIII binding to vWF (type 2N).
- If a qualitative defect in vWF is suspected due to a vWF:Ag greater than vWF:RCo, obtain vWF multimer analysis by gel electrophoresis to determine if large vWF multimers are absent (type 2A and 2B) and a ristocetin-induced platelet aggregation test (**patient's plasma and platelets plus ristocetin**) to distinguish types 2A and 2M (attenuated) from type 2B (exaggerated) platelet aggregation responses.

Therapy and Monitoring

- Management of **vWD** consists of raising vWF:RCo and factor VIII to levels that ensure adequate hemostasis. **Minor bleeding** in **type 1 vWD** usually responds to **DDAVP**. A test dose should be administered, and clinically acceptable vWF:RCo and FVIII increases confirmed, to determine each patient's responsiveness. vWF:RCo levels of >50% are sufficient to correct most hemorrhages.

- DDAVP is not effective in some type 2A, 2M, and 2N vWD patients, is contraindicated in type 2B due to the risk of postinfusion thrombocytopenia, and is not useful in type 3 vWD.
- Oral contraceptives increase vWF levels and may be useful for management of menorrhagia.
- **Severe bleeding** and **major surgery** in vWD patients require vWF replacement provided by infusion of vWF as intermediate purity FVIII concentrates (Alphanate or Humate-P) or cryoprecipitate q12–24h to raise vWF:RCo levels to 100% initially and maintain them between 50% and 100% until healing is complete (typically 5–10 days).
  - Factor VIII activity is usually used as a surrogate marker because stat measurement of vWF:RCo is rarely available.
  - In general, 50 International Units vWF:RCo/kg raises the plasma vWF:RCo activity level to 100%.
  - Cryoprecipitate contains significant amounts of vWF and FVIII and is an alternative replacement product; however, it does not undergo viral inactivation.
  - High-purity (monoclonal) plasma-derived and recombinant FVIII concentrates do not contain vWF and should not be used for vWD.
  - Type 1 vWD patients who are undergoing minor invasive procedures can receive DDAVP 1 hour before surgery and q12–24h for 2–3 days postoperatively, with or without the oral antifibrinolytic drug aminocaproic acid (Amicar), but for more extensive surgery vWF should be administered.
  - In type 3 vWD, platelet transfusions may complement infusions of vWF to control bleeding by releasing vWF stored in α granules at the site of vascular injury.[39]

 # ACQUIRED COAGULATION DISORDERS

VITAMIN K DEFICIENCY

- **Vitamin K deficiency** is usually caused by malabsorption states or poor dietary intake combined with antibiotic-associated loss of intestinal bacterial colonization. Hepatocytes require vitamin K to complete the synthesis (γ-carboxylation) of clotting factors (X, IX, VII, prothrombin) and the natural anticoagulant proteins C and S.
  - Vitamin K deficiency is suspected when an at-risk patient has a prolonged PT that corrects after a 1:1 mix with normal pooled plasma.
  - **Vitamin K replacement** can be given orally, subcutaneously, or intravenously. Vitamin K absorption is variable when administered subcutaneously, especially in edematous patients, and intravenous vitamin K is effective but carries the risk of anaphylaxis. Oral administration is superior to subcutaneous vitamin K for reversing the effects of warfarin in outpatients.[40] With adequate replacement therapy, the PT should begin to normalize within 12 hours and should normalize completely in 24–48 hours.
  - **FFP** rapidly but only temporarily corrects acquired coagulopathies secondary to vitamin K deficiency and is indicated in patients who are actively bleeding or who require immediate invasive procedures.
    - The usual starting dose is 2–3 units (400–600 mL), with measurement of the PT and aPTT after the infusion to determine the need for additional therapy. Up to 10–15 mL/kg may be needed for severe bleeding with significant PT prolongation.
    - Because factor VII has a half-life of only 6 hours, the PT may again become prolonged and require additional FFP.
    - Vitamin K replacement should be initiated concomitantly with FFP.

LIVER DISEASE

- **Liver disease** can seriously impair hemostasis because coagulation factors, with the exception of vWF, are produced in the liver. Hemostatic abnormalities associated with liver disease are usually stable unless liver synthetic function is rapidly worsening, as in fulminant hepatic failure. Other complications of end-stage liver disease that may lead to abnormal hemostasis include hyperfibrinolysis, thrombocytopenia due to splenic sequestration, DIC, spontaneous bacterial peritonitis, gastrointestinal hemorrhage, and cholestasis, which impairs vitamin K absorption (see Chapter 17, Liver Diseases).

- **Vitamin K** replacement may be helpful in correcting mild prolongation of the PT in liver dysfunction; however, this is not effective if hepatic hyposynthesis is the underlying etiology.
- **FFP** is indicated for patients who are bleeding or require an invasive procedure and have abnormal coagulation parameters (PT or aPTT >1.5 times control).
- **Cryoprecipitate**, a concentrated source of fibrinogen, can be given at a dose of 1.5 units/10 kg body weight to correct severe hypofibrinogenemia (<100 mg/dL) if there is bleeding or the need for invasive procedures. This should be followed by periodic measurement of the fibrinogen level.
- **Platelet transfusion** is indicated for bleeding in the setting of thrombocytopenia.

DISSEMINATED INTRAVASCULAR COAGULATION

- **Disseminated intravascular coagulation** (DIC) is seen in a variety of systemic illnesses, including sepsis, trauma, burns, shock, obstetric complications, and malignancies (notably, acute promyelocytic leukemia).
  - The underlying cause is exposure of tissue factor to the circulation, which leads to uncontrolled generation of thrombin and its consequences: consumption of coagulation factors and regulators (protein C, protein S, antithrombin), platelet activation, fibrin generation, generalized microthrombi, and reactive fibrinolysis.
  - Consequences of **DIC** include diffuse bleeding, global organ dysfunction secondary to microvascular thrombi and ischemia, and, less often, large arterial and venous thrombosis.[41]
  - Although no one test confirms a diagnosis of **DIC**, affected patients commonly have prolonged PT and aPTT, thrombocytopenia, low fibrinogen levels, elevated fibrin degradation products, and a positive D-dimer.
  - DIC treatment consists of supportive care, correction of the underlying disorder if possible, and administration of FFP, cryoprecipitate, and platelets as needed. The use of heparin to prevent thrombosis in DIC is controversial, but adjusted-dose **heparin** (see Anticoagulants) is appropriate therapy for large-vessel thrombosis in DIC. Recombinant activated protein C (drotrecogin) reduces mortality in patients with severe sepsis due to its anticoagulant and anti-inflammatory activity (see Chapter 8, Critical Care).

ACQUIRED INHIBITORS OF COAGULATION FACTORS

- **Acquired inhibitors of coagulation factors** may arise de novo or may develop in hemophiliacs who have been exposed to factor replacement. The most common acquired specific inhibitor is directed against factor VIII. Patients present with an abrupt onset of bleeding, prolonged aPTT that does not correct after 1:1 mixing, markedly decreased FVIII activity, and a normal PT.
  - Bleeding complications in patients with factor VIII inhibitors (autoantibodies) are managed in the same manner as for hemophiliacs with alloantibodies to factor VIII (see Inherited Bleeding Disorders). Long-term therapy consists of immunosuppression with cyclophosphamide, prednisone, rituximab, or vincristine to reduce production of the autoantibody.[42]

DISORDERS OF FIBRINOGEN

- **Disorders of fibrinogen** may be acquired or inherited. Fibrinogen is an acute-phase reactant whose synthesis in liver is increased by inflammatory states or malignancy.
- Hypofibrinogenemia, secondary to decreased liver synthesis or consumption, and dysfibrinogenemia, secondary to synthesis of fibrinogen molecules with excess carbohydrate,[43] can cause impaired coagulation.

- Inherited dysfibrinogenemias are rare, and most are asymptomatic. However, approximately 40% are associated with hemorrhagic (20%) and thrombotic (20%) complications.
- Characteristic laboratory findings for **dysfibrinogenemia** consist of prolonged PT, aPTT, and thrombin time.
- When clinically indicated, hypofibrinogenemia and dysfibrinogenemia are corrected with cryoprecipitate infusions.

SPECIAL CONSIDERATIONS

- **Use of anticoagulants.** Hospitalized patients may have blood drawn through heparinized lines. Heparin contamination is confirmed by observing correction of a prolonged aPTT or TT after adding protamine to neutralize the heparin or by adding Hepzyme to degrade the heparin. Most PT reagents contain heparin-neutralizing substances.
- Use of direct thrombin inhibitors in patients suspected of HIT will prolong PT, PTT, and TT.
- Coagulation studies consistent with the predicted effects of warfarin and an otherwise negative evaluation may indicate accidental or surreptitious ingestion of warfarin. Detection of warfarin metabolites in serum is a confirmatory test.
- Ingestion of anticoagulant rodenticides containing "superwarfarin" (brodifacoum) causes prolonged elevation of the PT lasting up to 1 year. FFP and vitamin K are indicated for patients with associated bleeding. Standard doses of vitamin K are usually not sufficient to correct this coagulopathy, and high doses (100–150 mg/d orally) are required until the PT normalizes.[44]

 # VENOUS THROMBOEMBOLIC DISORDERS

GENERAL PRINCIPLES

Definition

- **Venous thromboembolism (VTE)** refers to the presence of **deep vein thrombosis (DVT)** or **pulmonary embolism (PE)**.
- **Superficial thrombophlebitis** may occur in any superficial veins.
- **APA syndrome** is defined by clinical and laboratory criteria, with at least one of each required to confirm the diagnosis.[45]
  - **Clinical criteria** consist of (a) the occurrence of arterial or venous thrombosis in any tissue or organ, and (b) pregnancy morbidities (unexplained late fetal death; premature birth complicated by eclampsia, pre-eclampsia, or placental insufficiency; at least three unexplained consecutive spontaneous abortions).
  - **Laboratory criteria** consist of persistent (at least 12 weeks apart) detection of autoantibodies (lupus anticoagulant [LA], anticardiolipin antibody, and β_2 glycoprotein-1 antibodies) that react with negatively charged phospholipids.
  - The APA syndrome may include other features, such as thrombocytopenia, valvular heart disease, livedo reticularis, neurologic manifestations, and nephropathy, though they are not part of the diagnostic criteria.

Anatomy

- The anatomic location of DVT and PE may affect prognosis and treatment recommendations.
  - Thromboses can be classified as **deep** or **superficial** and as **proximal** or **distal.**
    - The **superficial femoral vein** is actually a deep vein, and its preferred term is **femoral vein.**

- A lower extremity DVT found in or superior to the popliteal vein (or the confluence of tibial and peroneal veins) is considered **proximal,** whereas a DVT that is found inferior to the popliteal vein (or the confluence of tibial and peroneal veins) is considered **distal.**
  - PEs are often characterized as central (main pulmonary artery, lobar, or segmental) or distal (subsegmental or smaller) based on location in the pulmonary arterial system.

Epidemiology

- Symptomatic DVTs most commonly develop in the lower limbs.
- Calf vein DVTs uncommonly cause significant emboli, unless they propagate proximally.
- Without treatment, calf DVTs may extend to become proximal DVTs.
- Without treatment, approximately 50% of patients with proximal lower extremity DVT develop PE.
- DVTs in the proximal lower extremities and pelvis produce most PEs.
- DVTs that occur in upper extremities, often secondary to an indwelling catheter, may also cause PEs.
- Superficial thrombophlebitis may have concomitant DVT.

Etiology

- Venous thromboemboli arise under conditions of **stasis, hypercoagulability,** and venous **endothelial injury.**
  - Conditions leading to prolonged **immobilization** (trauma, surgery, and other major medical illnesses) predispose to development of VTE.
  - Hypercoagulable states may be inherited or acquired.
    - **Acquired hypercoagulable states** may arise secondary to malignancy, nephrotic syndrome, estrogen use, and pregnancy.
    - Both **HIT** and the **APA syndrome** can cause arterial or venous thrombi.
- **Superficial thrombophlebitis** is associated with varicose veins, trauma, infection, and hypercoagulable disorders.
- Other causes of pulmonary arterial occlusion include in situ thrombi (e.g., sickle cell disease), marrow fat embolism, and amniotic fluid embolism.

DIAGNOSIS

Risk Factors

- **Inherited thrombophilic disorders** are suggested by a history of spontaneous VTE at a young age (<50 years), recurrent VTE, documented VTE in first-degree relatives, thrombosis in unusual anatomic locations, and recurrent fetal loss.
  - The established inherited risk factors for VTE include two gene polymorphisms that are common in whites (factor V Leiden and prothrombin gene G20210A) and deficiencies of the natural anticoagulants protein C, protein S, and antithrombin.
  - Hyperhomocysteinemia is an uncommon inborn error of metabolism associated with extremely high plasma homocysteine and arterial and venous thromboembolic events in childhood. More commonly, milder homocysteine elevations arise from an interaction between genetic mutations that affect enzymes involved in homocysteine metabolism and acquired factors such as inadequate folate consumption.[46]
  - Unusual spontaneous venous thromboses, such as cavernous sinus thrombosis, mesenteric vein thrombosis, or portal vein thrombosis, may be the initial presentation of paroxysmal nocturnal hemoglobinuria (**PNH**) or myeloproliferative disorders.

- **Spontaneous (idiopathic) thrombosis,** despite the absence of an inherited thrombophilia and detectable autoantibodies, predisposes patients to the development of future thromboses.[46]
- **Autoantibodies** associated with HIT and the APA syndrome can cause arterial or venous thrombi. (See Heparin-induced Thrombocytopenia)
  - At least 10% of patients with SLE have evidence of LAs; however, most patients with LAs do not have SLE.

Clinical Presentation

- Symptoms and signs of **DVT** are neither sensitive nor specific. However, pretest assessment of the probability of a DVT is still useful when combined with the results of compression ultrasound or a D-dimer test, or both, in determining whether to exclude or accept the diagnosis of DVT or perform additional imaging studies.[47]
  - DVT may produce pain and edema in the affected extremity.
  - **Superficial thrombophlebitis** presents as a tender, warm, erythematous, and often palpable thrombosed vein. Accompanying DVT may produce additional symptoms and signs.
- Symptoms and signs of **PE** are neither sensitive nor specific.
  - PE may produce shortness of breath, chest pain (pleuritic), hypoxemia, hemoptysis, pleural rub, new right-sided heart failure, and tachycardia.[48]
  - Validated **clinical risk factors** for a PE in outpatients who present to an emergency department include signs and symptoms of DVT, high suspicion of PE by the clinician, tachycardia, immobility in the past 4 weeks, history of VTE, active cancer, and hemoptysis.[48]
  - **Clinical suspicion of DVT or PE should lead to objective testing.**

Differential Diagnosis

- The differential diagnosis for **unilateral lower extremity** symptoms and signs of **DVT,** such as swelling and pain, includes Baker cyst, hematoma, venous insufficiency, postphlebitic syndrome, lymphedema, sarcoma, arterial aneurysm, myositis, cellulitis, rupture of the medial head of the gastrocnemius, and abscess.
- **Bilateral lower extremity edema** often suggests the presence of heart, renal, or liver failure.
- Additional diseases to consider in association with **lower extremity pain** include musculoskeletal and arteriovascular disorders.
- The **differential diagnosis** of symptoms and signs of PE includes dissecting aortic aneurysm, pneumonia, acute bronchitis, bronchocarcinoma, pericardial or pleural disease, heart failure, costochondritis, and myocardial ischemia.

Laboratory Studies

- D-**dimer** is a cross-linked fibrin degradation product that may be increased during acute illness or VTE.
  - Various assays are available, and each differs in accuracy.
  - D-dimer testing for DVT or PE has a low positive predictive value and specificity; **patients with a positive test require further evaluation.**
  - The negative predictive value of a sensitive quantitative D-dimer assay is high enough to exclude a DVT when the objectively defined clinical probability is low and/or a noninvasive test is negative.[49,50]
  - A negative D-dimer in combination with low pretest probability can exclude almost all PEs.[51]
  - In settings in which the pretest probability is moderate or high, such as in some patients with cancer, a negative D-dimer test is not useful because it does not have a sufficient negative predictive value for excluding the presence of **DVT or PE.**[52,53]
- Hypercoagulability testing. See Table 18-2.
  - Testing for **APA** is indicated when clinical findings of the APA syndrome are present.

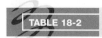

TABLE 18-2	Laboratory Evaluation of Thrombophilic States
Inherited thrombophilia	**Laboratory assessment**
Prothrombin gene mutation G20210A	G20210A mutation
Partial protein C deficiency	Protein C activity
Partial protein S deficiency	Free protein S antigen, Protein S activity
Partial antithrombin deficiency	Antithrombin heparin cofactor activity
Factor V Leiden	Activated protein C resistance, if positive confirm with factor V Leiden PCR
Hyperhomocysteinemia	Fasting plasma homocysteine level
Acquired thrombophilias	**Laboratory assessment**
Antiphospholipid antibody syndrome	Anticardiolipin antibody, Beta$_2$ glycoprotein 1, lupus anticoagulant
Paroxysmal nocturnal hemoglobinuria	RBC or WBC flow cytometry for loss of CD55, CD59
Myeloproliferative disorder	JAK-2 mutation

PCR, polymerase chain reaction; RBC, red blood cell; WBC, white blood cell.

- APAs are a heterogeneous group of autoantibodies that are detected with serologic tests (IgG and IgM β_2 glycoprotein-1 antibodies, and IgG and IgM cardiolipin antibodies) or clotting assays (LA), which are prolonged in their presence.
  - Performing both serologic and clotting assays improves sensitivity.
  - The aPTT or PT/INR may be elevated in LA patients, but these do not predispose to bleeding.
- To assess for **PNH** in the setting of unusual spontaneous venous thromboses, perform flow cytometry to detect missing antigens on red cells or leukocytes.

Imaging

DVT-Specific Testing
- The initial diagnostic test for symptomatic acute DVT should be a **noninvasive test,** typically **compression ultrasound** (called *duplex examination* when performed with Doppler testing).[54]
- In addition to assessing for DVT, compression ultrasound, MR venography, and CT venography may detect other pathology (see Differential Diagnosis).
  - Compression ultrasound is not sensitive at detecting **calf** DVT and may fail to visualize other veins, especially parts of the deep femoral vein, part of the upper extremity venous system, and the pelvic veins.
  - Noninvasive testing is also difficult to interpret in the setting of an **old DVT,** unless the original thrombus is known to have resolved.
  - **Lower extremity compression ultrasonography** is useful in a patient with a suspected PE who has a nondiagnostic ventilation/perfusion (V/Q) scan and in a patient with a nondiagnostic or negative chest CT scan with high suspicion of disease, because proximal DVT can serve as a surrogate for PE; ultrasonography also serves as a useful surrogate for PE, if positive, in patients who have contraindications to or difficulty completing imaging for PE (see Pulmonary Embolism Specific Testing).
  - Noninvasive testing has a low sensitivity in **asymptomatic** patients.
  - **Serial testing** can improve the diagnostic yield. If the initial noninvasive test is negative in a patient with a clinically suspected lower extremity DVT, anticoagulant therapy may typically be withheld, provided that testing is repeated at least once 3–14 days later.
  - **Simplified compression ultrasound** limited to only the common femoral vein in the groin and the popliteal vein (down to the trifurcation of the calf veins) is not as sensitive as a **complete** examination.

- Repeating simplified noninvasive tests within a few weeks improves sensitivity.
- When noninvasive testing or patient follow-up is unreliable, complete noninvasive testing or venography should be used.

■ **Venography** is the gold-standard technique for diagnosing DVT, although it requires placement of an IV catheter, administration of iodinated contrast, and exposure to radiation.
  ■ Noninvasive tests are preferred in symptomatic patients with suspected DVT.
  ■ Contraindications to venography include renal dysfunction and dye allergy.
■ **MRI** is noninvasive, and small studies have shown good sensitivity for acute, symptomatic proximal DVT.
  ■ Contraindications to MRI include gadolinium allergy, severe claustrophobia, certain implanted devices, and cerebral aneurysm.
■ **CT venography** is most commonly used to diagnose DVT in conjunction with a contrast-enhanced spiral CT for diagnosis of PE.[55,56]
  ■ Contraindications to spiral CT include renal dysfunction and dye allergy.
  ■ CT venography allows for visualization of the veins in the abdomen, pelvis, and proximal lower extremities.
  ■ Spiral CT used solely for DVT evaluation has been less accurate than CT used solely for PE diagnosis.[55,56]

PE-Specific Testing

■ **Nondefinitive tests** such as electrocardiography (e.g., right-sided strain pattern, with characteristic S wave in lead I, and Q wave in lead III, and T wave inversion in lead III), troponin levels, blood gases, and chest radiography may help determine the pretest probability, focus the differential diagnosis, and assess the cardiopulmonary reserve, but they do not rule in or rule out PE with acceptable certainty.
  ■ Unless there is an objectively low clinical probability of PE combined with a negative D-dimer test, the suspicion of PE requires an imaging evaluation.
■ **Contrast-enhanced spiral (helical) chest CT**
  ■ PE protocol chest CT requires IV administration of iodinated contrast and exposure to radiation.
  ■ Contraindications to spiral CT include renal dysfunction and dye allergy.
  ■ **Multidetector CT** is more sensitive than single-detector CT for detecting PE.
  ■ Used according to standardized protocols in conjunction with expert interpretation, spiral CT is relatively accurate for large (proximal) PEs, but the sensitivity is lower for small (distal) emboli.[55,56]
  ■ The sensitivity of CT for VTE improves by combining the CT pulmonary angiography results with (a) objective grading of clinical suspicion and (b) proximal lower extremity CT venography that assesses for DVT.
    - If CT venography is not performed, lower extremity compression ultrasonography would likely provide additional useful information.
  ■ **Clinical suspicion that is discordant with the objective test finding** (e.g., high suspicion with a negative CT scan, or low suspicion with a positive CT scan) **should lead to further testing.**
  ■ Advantages of CT scan over V/Q scan include more diagnostic results (positive or negative), with fewer indeterminate or inadequate studies, and the detection of alternative diagnoses, such as dissecting aortic aneurysm, pneumonia, and malignancy.
■ **V/Q scanning**
  ■ V/Q scanning requires administration of radioactive material (via both inhaled and IV routes).
  ■ V/Q scans may be classified as normal, nondiagnostic (i.e., very low probability, low probability, intermediate probability), or high probability for PE.
  ■ V/Q scanning is most useful in a patient with a normal chest radiograph, because nondiagnostic scans are extremely common in the setting of an abnormal chest radiograph.
  ■ Use of clinical suspicion improves the accuracy of V/Q scanning: In patients with normal or high-probability V/Q scans and matching pretest clinical suspicion, the positive predictive value is 96%.[57]

- When the V/Q findings and the clinical suspicion of PE are discordant, further testing should be performed.
- MR angiography (MRA)
  - MRI requires IV administration of a nonionic contrast agent (e.g., gadolinium).
  - MRI appears to be sensitive for diagnosing acute PE, though large studies have not been performed, and the PIOPED III study aims to better define the accuracy of MRI.
  - Similar to spiral CT, MRA may provide alternative diagnoses.
- Pulmonary angiography (PA)
  - Angiography requires placement of a pulmonary artery catheter, infusion of IV contrast, and exposure to radiation.
  - Similar to venography and PE-protocol CT scanning, contraindications to angiography include renal dysfunction and dye allergy.
  - Though PA is the gold standard for diagnosing PE, it can be inadequate or inaccurate in some situations, and less invasive tests are preferred for the initial evaluation.

PREVENTION

- The ideal strategy for management of VTE (DVT or PE) is prevention by identifying patients at high risk of thromboembolism and instituting prophylactic measures (see Chapter 1, Patient Care in Internal Medicine).

TREATMENT

- The goals of VTE therapy are to prevent recurrent VTE, consequences of VTE (i.e., post-phlebitic syndrome [i.e., pain, edema, and ulceration], pulmonary arterial hypertension, and death) and complications of therapy (e.g., bleeding and HIT).
- Standard laboratory tests (i.e., CBC and PT/aPTT) should be performed before starting UFH/LMWH/pentasaccharide to detect pre-existing cytopenias, coagulopathies, or evidence of LA. The laboratory values also serve as baselines during monitoring of UFH infusions and during assessment for HIT or bleeding.
- Unless contraindications exist, **initial treatment of VTE should consist of parenteral anticoagulation,** either with IV or SC UFH, SC LMWH, or SC pentasaccharide (fondaparinux).

Anticoagulants

- **Warfarin** is an oral anticoagulant that inhibits reduction of vitamin K to its active form and leads to depletion of the vitamin K–dependent clotting factors II, VII, IX, and X and proteins C and S.
  - Though warfarin has good oral absorption, it requires 4–5 days to achieve the full anticoagulant effect.
    - The initial INR rise primarily reflects warfarin-related depletion of factor VII, though the depletion of factor II takes several days due to its relatively long half-life.
    - Due to the rapid depletion of the anticoagulant protein C and slower onset of anticoagulant effect, patients might develop increased hypercoagulability during the first few days of warfarin therapy if warfarin is not combined with a parenteral anticoagulant.[58]
  - The typical recommended **starting dose** of warfarin is 5 mg PO daily, but depends upon age and habitus (e.g., ~3 mg in older, petite patients, ~7 mg in younger, robust patients). Patients with polymorphisms in genes for cytochrome P-450 2C9 or vitamin K epoxide reductase may benefit from cautious warfarin initiation (see www.NewWarfarin.com). The INR is used to adjust dosing (Table 18-3).
  - **Treatment solely with warfarin without a parenteral anticoagulant is inadequate for acute DVT/PE;** parenteral anticoagulant (UFH, LMWH, or pentasaccharide) should

TABLE 18-3	Warfarin Nomogram	

Day	INR	Dosage (mg)
2	<1.5	5
	1.5–1.9	2.5
	2.0–2.5	1.0–2.5
	>2.5	0
3	<1.5	5–10
	1.5–1.9	2.5–5.0
	2–3	0–2.5
	>3	0
4	<1.5	10
	1.5–1.9	5
	2–3	0–3
	>3	0
5	<1.5	10
	1.5–1.9	7.5–10.0
	2–3	0–5
	>3	0

INR, international normalized ratio.
Starting dose 5 mg PO daily on day 1.
Source: Adapted from *Ann Intern Med* 1997;127:333.

be continued for at least 4.5 days and until INRs of at least 2 are achieved on 2 consecutive days with warfarin therapy.
- For most indications, the **target INR** is 2.5 and the **therapeutic range** is 2–3.
- Patients with **mechanical heart valves** require a higher level of anticoagulation (INR target range, 2.5–3.5) (Table 18-4).

■ **Warfarin nomogram dosing** is likely more successful than non-standardized dosing (Table 18-3).
- **INRs** should be monitored frequently during the first month because multiple warfarin dose adjustments are usually necessary to determine a stable dose that will achieve a therapeutic INR.
  - Once a stable warfarin dose is achieved, INR monitoring should be performed at least every 4 weeks, though more frequent monitoring (e.g., weekly) is recommended in those with labile INRs.
  - Frequent INR monitoring is required when medications are added or discontinued, especially antibiotics, due to potential interactions with warfarin metabolism.

TABLE 18-4	Anticoagulation with Artificial Heart Valves	

Material	Type/location	INR
Tissue	Any	2.5 for 3 mo, then ASA 325 mg lifelong
Mechanical	St. Jude aortic	2–3[a]
	St. Jude mitral	3
	Caged-ball/caged disc	3, add ASA 81 mg

ASA, acetylsalicylic acid.
[a]May add ASA for coronary artery disease, h/o embolism, or mitral valve repair (MVR).

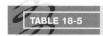

TABLE 18-5	Weight-Based Heparin Dosing[a]
Initial therapy[a]	
Bolus[b]	80 units/kg
Infusion[b]	18 units/kg/hr
Adjustments[c]	
aPTT <40	80 units/kg bolus; increase infusion by 3 units/kg/hr
aPTT 40–50	40 units/kg bolus; increase infusion by 2 units/kg/hr
aPTT 51–59	Increase infusion by 1 units/kg/hr
aPTT 60–94	No change
aPTT 95–104	Decrease infusion by 1 units/kg/hr
aPTT 105–114	Hold for 0.5 hr; decrease infusion by 2 units/kg/hr
aPTT >115	Hold for 1 hr; decrease infusion by 3 units/kg/hr

Note: Target activated partial thromboplastin time (aPTT) can vary among hospitals depending on reagents and instruments used.
[a]For patients with ST-segment elevation myocardial infarction, typical bolus dose is 60 units/kg (max. 5,000 units), and typical initial infusion dose is 12 units/kg/hr (max. 1,000 units/hr)
[b]Round all doses to nearest 100 units.
[c]Draw aPTT 6 hours after any bolus or change in infusion rate.
Source: Barnes-Jewish Hospital Pharmacy, St. Louis, MO.

- **Long-term anticoagulation with SC LMWH or fondaparinux** is an option for patients who are compliant with warfarin but have unacceptable INR lability, or those with LA and difficulty monitoring due to an elevated baseline INR.
- UFH is derived from porcine intestinal mucosa or bovine lung tissue.
  - UFH catalyzes the inactivation of thrombin and factor Xa by antithrombin.
  - At usual doses, UFH prolongs the TT and aPTT, and it has a minimal effect on the PT/INR.
  - Because the anticoagulant effects of UFH normalize within hours of discontinuation and UFH is **reversible with protamine sulfate,** it is the anticoagulant of choice for patients with increased risk of bleeding.
  - Dosing is not typically affected by renal function.
  - For **DVT prophylaxis,** the typical dosage is 5,000 units SC q8–12h, and aPTT monitoring is not necessary.
  - For **therapeutic anticoagulation,** UFH is usually administered IV with a bolus followed by continuous infusion.
    - Nomogram-driven weight-based dosing provides the most rapid and reliable prolongation of the aPTT into the therapeutic range (Table 18-5).[59]
    - Bleeding risks lead to use of different-intensity nomograms for different types of patients; patients with VTE often receive larger boluses and higher initial drip rates than patients with unstable angina who are also receiving acetylsalicylic acid (ASA) and other medications that increase the bleeding risk.
    - Dose-adjusted UFH may be administered SC q8h (e.g., 12,000 units UFH) or q12h (e.g., 16, 000 units UFH), and the aPTT should be drawn 6 or more hours after the injection.
- LMWHs are produced by chemical or enzymatic cleavage of UFH.
  - Since LMWH inactivates factor Xa to a greater extent than it does thrombin (IIa), LWMH minimally prolongs the aPTT.
  - Extensive clinical trials have confirmed the efficacy and safety of weight-based SC LMWH for the treatment of VTE.
  - Given a linear dose response, factor Xa monitoring is not normally recommended.
    - In patients experiencing renal dysfunction, obesity, or pregnancy, factor Xa level monitoring may be prudent.

- For therapeutic anticoagulation, factor Xa levels, measured 4 hours after an SC dose, should be 0.6–1.0 International Units/mL for q12h dosing and 1–2 International Units/mL for q24h dosing.[60]
■ Different LMWH preparations have different dosing recommendations (Table 18-6).
■ Given the renal clearance of LMWHs, they are generally contraindicated in patients with CrCl <10 mL/min and dose adjustments are required in patients with a CrCl <30 mL/min. Dose adjustments may also be required in patients with cachexia or obesity, or in women who are pregnant.
■ Though initial SC LMWH overlap therapy with PO warfarin is typically converted to sole PO warfarin long-term therapy, patients with cancer may have reduced recurrent VTE when treated long term solely with LMWH[61] at a slightly reduced dose.
■ LMWHs are only partially reversible with protamine.
■ **Because of the SC dosing route, LMWH** may be used for outpatient VTE therapy.
  - Patients selected for outpatient DVT therapy should have no other indications for hospitalization (i.e., complications of VTE or concomitant disease), be low risk for VTE recurrence and bleeding, have adequate cardiopulmonary reserve, have received instruction in the warning signs of bleeding and VTE recurrence, have access to a telephone and transportation, be able to inject the drug or have a responsible caretaker, and have adequate outpatient follow-up with a health care provider who can manage frequent lab testing, complications, etc.[62] Selection criteria for outpatient PE therapy have not been well validated.
■ **Long-term anticoagulation with SC LMWH** is the first choice in **pregnant** women (without artificial heart valves) with thrombosis, and it is an alternative for patients with cancer[61] and patients who have clearly **failed oral anticoagulation** (objectively confirmed new DVT/PE despite consistently therapeutic INRs).
■ **Fondaparinux** is a synthetic pentasaccharide that is structurally similar to the region of the heparin molecule that binds antithrombin and functions as a selective inhibitor of factor Xa.
  ■ Since fondaparinux inhibits factor Xa and does not inhibit thrombin, the aPTT is not significantly prolonged.
  ■ Large clinical trials have confirmed the efficacy and safety of weight-based subcutaneously dosed fondaparinux for the treatment of VTE.
  ■ Similar to the LMWHs, factor Xa monitoring is not normally recommended, but may be necessary for patients with renal dysfunction.
  ■ Fondaparinux may be used for outpatient VTE therapy.
  ■ The recommended dose for VTE therapy[63,64] is 7.5 mg SC daily, but dose adjustments are made for weight <50 and >100 kg (Table 18-6).
  ■ Fondaparinux is not reversible with protamine.

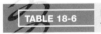

TABLE 18-6	**Low Molecular Weight Heparin and Pentasaccharide Dosages for Treatment of Venous Thromboembolism**

Drug	Dosage
Enoxaparin	Outpatient: 1 mg/kg SC q12h
	Inpatient: 1 mg/kg SC q12h *or* 1.5 mg/kg SC q24h
Tinzaparin	175 International Units/kg SC daily[a]
Dalteparin	200 International Units/kg SC daily[b]
Fondaparinux	5 mg SC daily for weight <50 kg, 7.5 mg SC daily for weight 50–100 kg, and 10 mg SC daily for weight >100 kg

IU, anti-Xa units; for enoxaparin, 1 mg = 100 anti-Xa units.
[a]U.S. Food and Drug Administration (FDA) approved for treatment of PE without DVT.
[b]Not an FDA-approved indication. 200 International Units/kg SC daily for month 1, followed by 150 International Units/kg SC daily during months 2–6 for patients with cancer undergoing prolonged LMWH therapy.
Caution with use of fondaparinux, tinzaparin, dalteparin or enoxaparin if Cr Cl <30 mL/min; anti-Xa level monitoring is recommended in this setting.

TABLE 18-7	Initial Lepirudin Infusion Rates in Renal Impairment[a]	
Creatinine clearance (mL/min)	Serum creatinine (mg/dL)	Adjusted infusion rate (mg/kg/hr)
45–60	1.6–2.0	0.075
30–44	2.1–3.0	0.045
15–29	3.1–6.0	0.0225
<15	>6	Avoid or stop infusion

[a]Dose adjustment is required for patients on hemodialysis or continuous venovenous hemodialysis.

- **Lepirudin** (**Refludan, recombinant hirudin**) is a direct thrombin inhibitor that is used for the treatment of **HIT.**
  - Lepirudin has a half-life of 1.5 hours, and a reversal agent is not available.
  - Lepirudin is cleared by kidneys, and **requires cautious use and dose adjustments in patients with renal insufficiency** (Table 18-7).
  - The treatment for HIT is a bolus of 0.4 mg/kg (up to 110 kg body weight, maximum dose 44 mg) followed by 0.15 mg/kg/hr (up to 110 kg body weight, maximum dose 16.5 mg) as a continuous IV infusion (see Fig. 18-2 for a dose adjustment algorithm); some experts advise against using the bolus to reduce drug accumulation in patients with renal dysfunction and to reduce the risk of anaphylaxis.

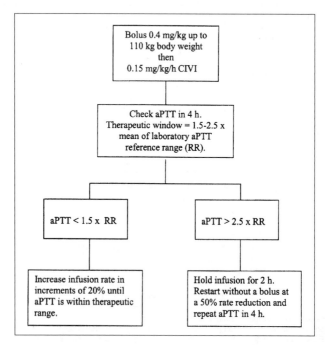

Figure 18-2. Lepirudin dosing algorithm. aPTT, activated partial thromboplastin time; CIVI, continuous intravenous infusion. (Adapted from Alving BM. How I treat heparin-induced thrombocytopenia and thrombosis. *Blood* 2003;101:31–37.)

- The aPTT is monitored 4 hours after a dose change and the dose is adjusted to obtain a target range 1.5–2.5 times the patient's baseline or the mean of the laboratory normal range.
  - Doses are adjusted in a manner similar to that of UFH therapy.
  - A lower target aPTT range (1.5–2.0 times baseline) may have similar efficacy and less bleeding risk.
- The increased PT/INR caused by lepirudin must be taken into account when interpreting INRs of patients receiving warfarin.[65]
- **Argatroban** is a synthetic direct thrombin inhibitor that is used for **HIT** therapy.
  - Argatroban has a half-life of <1 hour, and a reversal agent is not available.
  - The treatment for HIT is an intravenous infusion (without a bolus) of 2 mcg/kg/min, not to exceed 10 mcg/kg/min.
  - An aPTT is obtained 2 hours after beginning the infusion, and the infusion rate is adjusted to achieve a steady-state therapeutic aPTT (1.5–3.0 times the patient's normal baseline aPTT, not to exceed 100 seconds).
  - Argatroban is cleared by the liver, and it **requires dose adjustment in patients with hepatic dysfunction.**
    - Critically ill patients with possibly impaired hepatic function should possibly be given a starting dose of 0.5–1.0 mcg/kg/min.
  - Argatroban increases the PT/INR, and special warfarin dosing is required during coadministration.
    - After warfarin is coadministered, argatroban should be discontinued when the INR is >4, and the INR should be measured again within 4–6 hours.
      - If the INR is subtherapeutic (<2), argatroban should be resumed and the warfarin dose should be adjusted daily until a therapeutic INR (2–3) is achieved when off argatroban for 4–6 hours.
    - If the argatroban dose is >2 mcg/kg/min during warfarin coadministration, the effect of warfarin on the INR is less predictable, and the argatroban infusion should be temporarily reduced to 2 mcg/kg/min when planning to check the INR 4–6 hours later.[65]
      - If the INR is subtherapeutic (<2), argatroban should be resumed at the higher dose, and the warfarin dose should be adjusted daily until a therapeutic INR (2–3) is achieved when off the lower (2 mcg/kg/min) dose argatroban for 4–6 hours.

Thrombolytic Therapy

- **Thrombolytic therapy** may be appropriate for a small proportion of patients with VTE, but the risk of significant bleeding should be outweighed by the potential benefits.
  - The main indication for thrombolytic therapy of **PE** is refractory-associated systemic hypotension, and some experts advocate lytic therapy for patients with PE associated with right ventricular dysfunction.
    - Though many experts believe that thrombolytic therapy for PE saves lives, clinical trials have failed to demonstrate a survival benefit.
  - Though thrombolytic therapy is uncommonly used for **DVT,** the main indication for DVT is venous congestion that compromises the arterial supply to the limb, which is most often seen with massive iliofemoral DVT.
    - Compared to heparin alone, thrombolytic therapy for DVT produces more rapid and complete vein patency rates, but it causes more bleeding complications.
    - Debate exists whether thrombolytic DVT therapy reduces the incidence and severity of the postphlebitic syndrome.

Other Treatments

- **Leg elevation** is useful for the treatment of edema associated with DVT, though it is not an adequate sole therapy.

- **Ambulation** is encouraged for patients with DVT, especially after pain and edema are minimized, though strenuous lower extremity activity should initially be avoided.
- **Fitted graduated compression stockings** help to reduce the incidence of postphlebitic syndrome in patients with lower extremity DVT.
- In patients with **congenital antithrombin III (ATIII) deficiency,** infusion of **ATIII** concentrate should be considered for use during an acute thrombosis.[66]
- Treatment of **superficial thrombophlebitis** consists of heat, NSAIDs, and compression stockings.
  - Most superficial venous thromboses resolve within a few weeks.
  - Recurrent superficial thrombophlebitis may be treated with anticoagulation or vein stripping.[67]

Duration of Anticoagulation

- **Duration of anticoagulation** must be individualized for each patient based on patient preferences and an assessment of the patient's risk of recurrent VTE off therapy versus the risk of bleeding complications with continued anticoagulation.[68]
  - Patients with a **first episode of DVT due to reversible risk factors** (surgery, major trauma) are at very low risk of recurrence, and anticoagulation is recommended for 3 months.
  - For patients with a **first episode of idiopathic VTE** associated with less compelling risk factors, such as prolonged travel, oral contraceptive pills/hormone replacement therapy, or minor injuries, at least 6–12 months of anticoagulation is recommended.
  - For patients with **cancer** and DVT, LMWH for the first 3–6 months of long-term therapy is recommended, and extension of long-term therapy should be considered, especially if the cancer remains present.
  - Patients with a **first VTE and one inherited hypercoagulable risk factor** should receive anticoagulation for at least 6–12 months.
  - Patients with a **first VTE and antiphospholipid antibodies or two inherited risk factors** should receive 12 months of anticoagulation and be considered for indefinite therapy.
  - **After completion of the standard course** of oral anticoagulant therapy (INR 2–3) for proximal DVT or PE, options include stopping anticoagulation, long-term anticoagulation at an INR of 2–3,[69] or long-term anticoagulation at a lower target INR (1.5–2.0).[70]
  - **Isolated calf vein DVT** is often treated with a short duration (e.g., 3 months) of anticoagulation, especially if it is symptomatic.
  - Patients with **recurrent idiopathic VTE** should receive anticoagulation indefinitely, unless a contraindication develops, the risks appear to outweigh the benefits, or patient preferences dictate otherwise.
    - **Additional secondary prophylaxis** should be considered *after* completion of treatment of VTE.
  - For patients with a history of VTE, especially those with ongoing risk factors, temporary prophylactic anticoagulation should be considered during **periods of increased VTE risk,** including surgery, trauma, immobilization, hospitalization for medical illnesses, and postpartum.
    - In patients with **congenital ATIII deficiency,** infusion of **ATIII concentrate** should be considered during a high-risk period (e.g., surgery, pregnancy).[66]

Special Therapy

- **IVC filters** are mainly indicated for acute DVT situations in which there are **absolute contraindications to anticoagulation** (e.g., active bleeding, severe thrombocytopenia, urgent surgery) or **recurrent thromboemboli despite therapeutic (i.e., INR at least 2) anticoagulation.**
  - Though prophylactic IVC filters in patients with acute DVT/PE reduce the risk of recurrent PE, a reduction in overall mortality has not been demonstrated, and they do increase DVT recurrence rates.[71]

- Relative indications for IVC filters that require individualized decision making include primary or metastatic CNS cancer or limited cardiopulmonary reserve.
  - In patients who had **IVC filters** placed due to **temporary contraindications to anticoagulation,** anticoagulation therapy should be initiated when it is safe to do so to reduce the risk of filter-related thromboses.
  - Several types of removable **IVC filters** are now available, providing the option of a temporary physical barrier against emboli from the lower extremities, though filter removal requires a second invasive procedure, and supporting data are limited.
- **Catheter embolectomy, possibly combined with local thrombolytic therapy,** has been proposed for specific types of PE and DVT, but large-scale trials showing superiority of this approach have not been conducted.
- **Surgical embolectomy** should be considered for patients with life-threatening massive PE that have contraindications to thrombolytic therapy. Mortality is high, and patient selection is very important.

Risk Management and Complications

- **Bleeding** is the major complication of anticoagulation.
  - Up to 2% of patients who receive short-term UFH, LMWH, or pentasaccharide for VTE therapy experience major bleeding.
  - For patients receiving chronic oral anticoagulant therapy, the annual incidence of major bleeding is approximately 1%–3%.
  - Concomitant use of **antiplatelet agents** increases the risk of bleeding, and it should be avoided if possible.
- **Clinically significant bleeding should lead to the discontinuation of anticoagulation and consideration of IVC filter placement.**
- Asymptomatic INR elevation on warfarin
  - Asymptomatic minor INR elevations <5 should be managed by holding or reducing warfarin dose until the INR returns to the appropriate range and then resuming warfarin at a lower dose (Table 18-8).
  - Moderate ($\geq$5, <9) and marked $\geq$9 elevation of the INR in asymptomatic patients should be treated by holding one or more warfarin doses, giving vitamin K_1 (1–5 mg PO for moderate INR elevation, and 5–10 mg PO for marked INR elevation), and monitoring INRs.
- Bleeding with warfarin.
  - See Table 18-9 for risk factor–dependent major bleeding rates in patients treated with warfarin.
  - Serious hemorrhages should be treated with vitamin K (10 mg) by slow IV infusion and FFP.
  - Though expensive and potentially thrombogenic, **recombinant factor VIIa** may stop life-threatening bleeding.[72]
- For patients receiving **parenteral anticoagulants:**
  - Discontinuation is usually sufficient to restore normal hemostasis.
  - With moderate to severe bleeding, give **FFP.**
  - For patients receiving **UFH** who develop major bleeding, heparin can be completely reversed by infusion of **protamine sulfate** in situations where the potential benefits outweigh the risks (e.g., intracranial bleed, epidural hematoma, retinal bleed).
    - Heparin serum concentrations decline rapidly due to a short half-life after IV administration, and the amount of protamine required decreases over time.
    - Approximately 1 mg protamine sulfate IV neutralizes 100 units of heparin, up to a maximum dose of 250 mg. The dose can be given as a loading dose of 25–50 mg by slow intravenous injection over 10 minutes, with the rest of the calculated dose over 8–16 hours by intravenous infusion.
    - If 30 minutes to 1 hour has elapsed since a heparin dose, the protamine dose should be reduced to approximately 0.5 mg/100 units heparin.
    - If more than 2 hours has elapsed since a heparin dose, 0.25 mg protamine/100 units heparin should be administered.
    - If heparin was administered subcutaneously, the same reductions in the protamine dose are adequate.

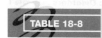

TABLE 18-8 **Treatment of Elevated INR >5**

Bleeding	INR	Action
None	>5	Hold warfarin
		Search for occult bleeding
		Evaluate for food and drug interactions or dosing errors
		Follow daily INR
	5–9	Vitamin K 1–2.5 mg PO if INR rising or at risk for bleeding
		Recheck INR in 24 and 48 hr
		Redose Vitamin K if INR remains high
	>9	Vitamin K 3–10 mg PO, IVPB
		INR q8h
		Repeat Vitamin K as needed
Minor	Any	Hold warfarin
		Vitamin K 1–5 mg PO or IVPB
		INR q8–24h; repeat Vitamin K as needed
		If bleeding not controlled in 24 hr, treat as major bleeding
Major	Any	Hold warfarin
		Vitamin K 10 mg IV over 20 min
		Give FFP or factor VII concentrate
		Follow INR q6–24h and continue vitamin K and FFP until INR <1.3 AND bleeding has stopped
		Surgical intervention for hemostasis

FFP, fresh frozen plasma; INR, international normalized ratio; IVPB, IV Piggyback.
Source: Barnes-Jewish Hospital Pharmacy, *Tool Book 2006.*

TABLE 18-9 **HEMORRHAGES Score**

Hepatic or renal disease	Albumin <3.6, CrCl <30 mL/min
EtOH abuse	
Malignancy	
Older age	>75 yr
Reduced platelets/platelet function	Plt <75 K, or on ASA
Rebleeding	2 points for prior major bleed, 1 point for prior minor bleed
Hypertension	SBP >160
Anemia	HCT <30
Genetic factors	
Excessive falls	
Stroke	

HEMORRHAGES Score

Score	Bleeding rate per 100 patient years warfarin (95% CI)
0	1.9 (0.6–4.4)
1	2.5 (1.3–4.3)
2	5.3 (3.4–8.1)
3	8.4 (4.9–13.6)
4	10.4 (5.1–18.9)
>5	12.3 (5.8–23.1)

CrCl, creatinine clearance; EtOH, ethyl alcohol; HCT; Plt, SBP, systolic blood pressure.
One point for each bleeding risk factor, except a prior major bleed (2 points).
CI, confidence interval.
Adapted from Gage BF, Yan Y, Milligan PE, et al. Clinical classification schemes for predicting hemorrhage. *Am Heart J* 2006;151:713–719.

- For major bleeding associated with **LWMH** protamine sulfate is less effective, neutralizing only approximately 60% of LMWH,[73] and it is not effective for reversing **pentasaccharide.**
  - For patients with very serious bleeding receiving fondaparinux, **concentrated factor VIIa** may be used.
- Anticoagulants should be used cautiously in patients undergoing **neuraxial procedures (lumbar puncture and epidural/spinal anesthesia, and epidural catheter removal)** because of the risk of development of **epidural hematomas and subsequent spinal cord compression and paralysis.**
  - Guidelines for the administration of each specific drug before and after such procedures should be followed.[74]
- **Occult GI or genitourinary bleeding** is a relative and not absolute contraindication to anticoagulation, though its presence prior to or during anticoagulation warrants an investigation for underlying disease.
- **Warfarin-induced skin necrosis** is a rare complication that can occur during initiation of warfarin therapy because of rapid depletion of protein C.
  - Necrosis occurs most often in areas with a high percentage of adipose tissue, such as breast tissue, and it can be life threatening.
  - Warfarin-induced skin necrosis can be prevented by first achieving therapeutic anticoagulation with an immediate-acting anticoagulant (UFH, LMWH, etc.) and avoiding "loading doses" of warfarin.
- **Warfarin is absolutely contraindicated in early** (i.e., first trimester) **pregnancy because of teratogenicity,** and it is often avoided during the entire pregnancy, though it is safe for infants of nursing mothers.[75]
- **Osteoporosis** is a potential complication of long-term heparin or warfarin use.[76]

Follow-Up

- If the clinical presentation is highly suspicious, **testing for intrinsic hypercoagulable risk factors** ideally should be delayed until some future time when the patient is in stable health and off anticoagulation therapy for at least 2 weeks **to avoid false-positive results** for some tests.
  - If there is a compelling reason to screen for hypercoagulable risk factors immediately, blood for **protein C, protein S, antithrombin, activated protein C resistance, and lupus anticoagulant** should be collected before initiating anticoagulation therapy.
  - Although normal protein C, protein S, and antithrombin tests rule out congenital deficiencies, abnormally low results require confirmation through repeat testing or screening first-degree relatives to rule out a temporary deficiency related to the acute thrombosis.
- For patients with suspected lower extremity DVT, an initial negative compression ultrasound, and no satisfactory alternative explanation, **serial testing** within 1–2 weeks can improve the diagnostic yield.
- If a **calf DVT** is detected and therapy is withheld due to patient preferences or risk of bleeding or contraindications, serial compression ultrasonography over 10–14 days is recommended to assess for proximal extension, which would mandate therapy.
- Though testing for PE in patients with DVT and testing for DVT in patients with PE will produce many positive findings, limited existing data do not strongly support such testing. However, baseline results may be useful for comparison in patients that return with symptoms of VTE and have positive findings on imaging studies.
- **Echocardiography** may be used to assess cardiopulmonary reserve and evidence of end-organ damage (right ventricular dysfunction) in patients with PE.

SPECIAL CONSIDERATIONS

Perioperative management of VTE requires close coordination with the surgical service (see Perioperative Medicine in Chapter 1, Patient Care in Internal Medicine). The benefit of treatment should be weighed against the risk of hemorrhage for each patient.

- **Invasive procedures** require discontinuation of warfarin.
  - If an invasive procedure is planned, warfarin therapy should be discontinued 4–5 days before the procedure, allowing the INR to drift below 1.5.[77]
  - If a temporary interruption of anticoagulation is unacceptable, parenteral anticoagulation can be initiated approximately 3 days after the last warfarin dose, to be stopped 6–24 hours prior to the procedure, depending on the half-life of the drug.
    - In some instances, intravenous UFH is the preferred choice of therapy (e.g., pregnant woman with a mechanical heart valve undergoing a procedure).
  - After the procedure, warfarin (at the previous dose) and/or parenteral anticoagulation are resumed as soon as adequate hemostasis and low bleeding risk has been achieved, typically within 24 hours.

References

1. Broze GJ Jr. Tissue factor pathway inhibitor and the revised theory of coagulation. *Annu Rev Med.* 1995;46:103–112.
2. Gewirtz AS, Miller ML, Keys TF. The clinical usefulness of the preoperative bleeding time. *Arch Pathol Lab Med.* 1996;120(4)353–356.
3. Hayward CP, Harrison P, Cattaneo M, et al. Platelet function analyzer (PFA)-100 closure time in the evaluation of platelet disorders and platelet function. *J Thromb Haemost.* 2006;4(2):312–319.
4. Kirkwood TB. Calibration of reference thromboplastins and standardisation of the prothrombin time ratio. *Thromb Haemost.* 1983;49(3):238–244.
5. Scaradavou A. HIV-related thrombocytopenia. *Blood. Rev.* 2002;16(1):73–76.
6. Isomura H, Yoshida M, Namba H, et al. Suppressive effects of human herpesvirus-6 on thrombopoietin-inducible megakaryocytic colony formation in vitro. *J Gen Virol.* 2000;81(Pt 3):663–673.
7. Frederiksen H, Schmidt K. The incidence of idiopathic thrombocytopenic purpura in adults increases with age. *Blood.* 1999;94(3):909–913.
8. Cines DB, Blanchette VS. Immune thrombocytopenic purpura. *N Engl J Med.* 2002; 346(13):995–1008.
9. Aster RH. Drug-induced immune thrombocytopenia: an overview of pathogenesis. *Semin Hematol.* 1999;36(1 Suppl 1):2–6.
10. George JN, Raskob GE, Shah SR, et al. Drug-induced thrombocytopenia: a systematic review of published case reports. *Ann Intern Med.* 1998;129(11):886–890.
11. Davoren A, Bussel J, Curtis BR, et al. Prospective evaluation of a new platelet glycoprotein (GP)-specific assay (PakAuto) in the diagnosis of autoimmune thrombocytopenia (AITP). *Am J Hematol.* 2005;78(3):193–197.
12. George, JN, Woolf, SH, Raskob, GE et al. Idiopathic Thrombocytopenic Purpura: A Practice Guideline Developed by Explicit Methods for the American Society of Hematology. *Blood.* 1996;88(1):3–40.
13. Stasi R, Pagano A, Stipa E, et al. Rituximab chimeric anti-CD20 monoclonal antibody treatment for adults with chronic idiopathic thrombocytopenic purpura. *Blood.* 2001;98(4):952–957.
14. Kojouri K, George JN. Recent advances in the treatment of chronic refractory immune thrombocytopenic purpura. *Int J Hematol.* 2005;81(2):119–125.
15. Cines DB, McMillan R. Management of adult idiopathic thrombocytopenic purpura. *Annu Rev Med.* 2005;56:425–442.
16. Kwaan HC, Soff GA. Management of thrombotic thrombocytopenic purpura and hemolytic uremic syndrome. *Semin Hematol.* 1997;34(2):159–166.
17. Terrell DR, Williams LA, Vesely SK, et al. The incidence of thrombotic thrombocytopenic purpura-hemolytic uremic syndrome: all patients, idiopathic patients, and patients with severe ADAMTS-13 deficiency. *J Thromb Haemost.* 2005;3(7):1432–1436.
18. Furlan, M, Robles R, Galbusera M, et al. von Willebrand Factor-Cleaving Protease in Thrombotic Thrombocytopenic Purpura and the Hemolytic-Uremic Syndrome. *New Engl J Med.* 1998;339:1578–1584.
19. Ferrara F, Annunziata M, Pollio F, et al. Vincristine as treatment for recurrent episodes

of thrombotic thrombocytopenic purpura. *Ann Hematol.* 2002;81(1):7–10. Epub 2001 Dec 8.

20. Zheng X, Pallera AM, Goodnough LT, et al. Remission of chronic thrombotic thrombocytopenic purpura after treatment with cyclophosphamide and rituximab. *Ann Intern Med.* 2003;138(2):105–108.

21. George JN. How I treat patients with thrombotic thrombocytopenic purpura-hemolytic uremic syndrome. *Blood.* 2000;96(4):1223–1229.

22. Alving BM. How I treat heparin-induced thrombocytopenia and thrombosis. *Blood.* 2003;101(1):31–37. Epub 2002 Aug 15.

23. Warkentin TE, Greinacher A. Heparin-induced thrombocytopenia: recognition, treatment, and prevention: the Seventh ACCP Conference on Antithrombotic and Thrombolytic Therapy. *Chest.* 2004;126(3 Suppl):311S–337S.

24. Warkentin TE, Cook RJ, Marder VJ, et al. Anti-platelet factor 4/heparin antibodies in orthopedic surgery patients receiving antithrombotic prophylaxis with fondaparinux or enoxaparin. *Blood.* 2005;106(12):3791–3796. Epub 2005 Aug 18.

25. Harrison CN. Essential thrombocythaemia: challenges and evidence-based management. *Br J Haematol.* 2005;130(2):153–165.

26. Harrison CN, Gale RE, Machin SJ, Linch DC. A large proportion of patients with a diagnosis of essential thrombocythemia do not have a clonal disorder and may be at lower risk of thrombotic complications. *Blood.* 1999;93(2):417–424.

27. Budde U, Scharf RE, Franke P, et al. Elevated platelet count as a cause of abnormal von Willebrand factor multimer distribution in plasma. *Blood.* 1993;82(6):1749–1757.

28. Murphy S, Peterson P, Iland H, Laszlo J. Experience of the Polycythemia Vera Study Group with essential thrombocythemia: a final report on diagnostic criteria, survival, and leukemic transition by treatment. *Semin Hematol.* 1997;34(1):29–39.

29. Baxter EJ, Scott LM, Campbell PJ, et al. Acquired mutation of the tyrosine kinase JAK2 in human myeloproliferative disorders. *Lancet.* 2005;365(9464):1054–1061.

30. Storen EC, Tefferi A. Long-term use of anagrelide in young patients with essential thrombocythemia. *Blood.* 2001;97(4):863–866.

31. Harrison CN, Campbell PJ, Buck G, et al. Hydroxyurea compared with anagrelide in high-risk essential thrombocythemia. *N Engl J Med.* 2005;353(1):33–45.

32. Basila D, Yuan CS. Effects of dietary supplements on coagulation and platelet function. *Thromb Res.* 2005;117(1–2):49–53.

33. Hodges PJ, Kam PC. The peri-operative implications of herbal medicines. *Anaesthesia.* 2002;57(9):889–899.

34. George JN, Shattil SJ. The clinical importance of acquired abnormalities of platelet function. *N Engl J Med.* 1991;324(1):27–39.

35. Mannucci PM, Tuddenham EG. Medical Progress: The hemophiliac—from royal genes to gene therapy. *New Engl J Med.* 2001;3441773–1779.

36. Mannucci PM. Desmopressin (DDAVP) in the treatment of bleeding disorders: the first 20 years. *Blood.* 1997;90(7):2515–2521.

37. DiMichele D, Neufeld EJ. Hemophilia. A new approach to an old disease. *Hematol Oncol Clin North Am.* 1998;12(6):1315–1344.

38. Hedner U. Recombinant factor VIIa (Novoseven) as a hemostatic agent. *Semin Hematol.* 2001;38(4 Suppl 12):43–47.

39. Mannucci PM. How I treat patients with von Willebrand disease. *Blood.* 2001;97(7): 1915–1919.

40. Crowther MA, Douketis JD, Schnurr T, et al. Oral vitamin K lowers the international normalized ratio more rapidly than subcutaneous vitamin K in the treatment of warfarin-associated coagulopathy. A randomized, controlled trial. *Ann Intern Med.* 2002;137(4):251–254.

41. Levi M, Ten Cate H. Disseminated intravascular coagulation. *N Engl J Med.* 1999; 341(8):586–592.

42. Wiestner A, Cho HJ, Asch AS, et al. Rituximab in the treatment of acquired factor VIII inhibitors. *Blood.* 2002;100(9):3426–3428.

43. Martinez J, MacDonald KA, Palascak JE. The role of sialic acid in the dysfibrinogenemia associated with liver disease: distribution of sialic acid on the constituent chains. *Blood.* 1983;61(6):1196–1202.

44. Chua JD, Friedenberg WR. Superwarfarin poisoning. *Arch Intern Med*. 1998;158(17): 1929–1932.

45. Miyakis S, Lockshin MD, Atsumi T, et al. International consensus statement on an update of the classification criteria for definite antiphospholipid syndrome (APS). *J Thromb Haemost*. 2006;4(2):295–306.

46. Seligsohn U, Lubetsky A. Genetic susceptibility to venous thrombosis. *N Engl J Med*. 2001;344(16):1222–1231.

47. Wells PS, Anderson DR, Bormanis J, et al. Value of assessment of pretest probability of deep-vein thrombosis in clinical management. *Lancet*. 1997;350(9094):1795–1798.

48. Wells PS, Ginsberg JS, Anderson DR, et al. Use of a clinical model for safe management of patients with suspected pulmonary embolism. *Ann Intern Med*. 1998;129(12):997–1005.

49. Stein PD, Hull RD, Patel KC et al. D-Dimer for the exclusion of acute venous thrombosis and pulmonary embolism; a systematic review. *Ann Intern Med* 2004; 140:589–602.

50. Wells PS, Owen C, Doucette S, et al. Does this patient have deep vein thrombosis? *JAMA*. 2006;295(2):199–207.

51. Ginsberg JS, Wells PS, Kearon C, et al. Sensitivity and specificity of a rapid whole-blood assay for D-dimer in the diagnosis of pulmonary embolism. *Ann Intern Med*. 1998;129(12):1006–1011.

52. Lee AY, Julian JA, Levine MN, et al. Clinical utility of a rapid whole-blood D-dimer assay in patients with cancer who present with suspected acute deep venous thrombosis. *Ann Intern Med*. 1999;131(6):417–423.

53. Goldstein NM, Kollef MH, Ward S, Gage BF. The impact of the introduction of a rapid D-dimer assay on the diagnostic evaluation of suspected pulmonary embolism. *Arch Intern Med*. 2001;161(4):567–571.

54. Tapson VF, Carroll BA, Davidson BL, et al. The diagnostic approach to acute venous thromboembolism. Clinical practice guideline. American Thoracic Society. *Am J Respir Crit Care Med*. 1999;160(3):1043–1066.

55. Stein PD, Fowler SE, Goodman LR, et al. Multidetector computed tomography for acute pulmonary embolism. *N Engl J Med*. 2006;354(22):2317–2327.

56. Rathbun SW, Raskob GE, Whitsett TL. Sensitivity and specificity of helical computed tomography in the diagnosis of pulmonary embolism: a systematic review. *Ann Intern Med*. 2000;132(3):227–232.

57. The PIOPED Investigators. Value of the ventilation/perfusion scan in acute pulmonary embolism. Results of the prospective investigation of pulmonary embolism diagnosis (PIOPED). *JAMA*. 1990;263(20):2753–2759.

58. Sallah S, Thomas DP, Roberts HR. Warfarin and heparin-induced skin necrosis and the purple toe syndrome: infrequent complications of anticoagulant treatment. *Thromb Haemost* 1997;78:785–790.

59. Raschke RA, Reilly BM, Guidry JR, et al. The weight-based heparin dosing nomogram compared with a "standard care" nomogram. A randomized controlled trial. *Ann Intern Med*. 1993;119(9):874–881.

60. Hirsh J, Lee AY. How we diagnose and treat deep vein thrombosis. *Blood*. 2002; 99(9):3102–3110.

61. Lee AY, Levine MN, Baker RI, et al. Low-molecular-weight heparin versus a coumarin for the prevention of recurrent venous thromboembolism in patients with cancer. *N Engl J Med*. 2003;349(2):146–153.

62. Yusen RD, Haraden BM, Gage BF, et al. Criteria for outpatient management of proximal lower extremity deep venous thrombosis. *Chest*. 1999;115(4):972–979.

63. Büller HR, Davidson BL, Decousus H, et al. Fondaparinux or enoxaparin for the initial treatment of symptomatic deep venous thrombosis: a randomized trial. *Ann Intern Med*. 2004;140(11):867–873.

64. Büller HR, Davidson BL, Decousus H, et al. Subcutaneous fondaparinux versus intravenous unfractionated heparin in the initial treatment of pulmonary embolism. *N Engl J Med*. 2003;349(18):1695–1702.

65. Büller HR, Agnelli G, Hull RD, et al. Antithrombotic therapy for venous thromboembolic disease: the Seventh ACCP Conference on Antithrombotic and Thrombolytic Therapy. *Chest*. 2004;126(3 Suppl):401S–428S.

66. Mannucci PM, Boyer C, Wolf M, et al. Treatment of congenital antithrombin III deficiency with concentrates. *Br J Haematol.* 1982;50(3):531–535.
67. Belcaro G, Nicolaides AN, Errichi BM, et al. Superficial thrombophlebitis of the legs: a randomized, controlled, follow-up study. *Angiology.* 1999;50(7):523–529.
68. Kearon C, Ginsberg JS, Kovacs MJ, et al. Comparison of low-intensity warfarin therapy with conventional-intensity warfarin therapy for long-term prevention of recurrent venous thromboembolism. *N Engl J Med.* 2003;349(7):631–639.
69. Ridker PM, Goldhaber SZ, Danielson E, et al. Long-term, low-intensity warfarin therapy for the prevention of recurrent venous thromboembolism. *N Engl J Med.* 2003;348(15):1425–1434. Epub 2003 Feb 24.
70. Decousus H, Leizorovica A, Parent F et al. A clinical trial of vena caval filters in the prevention of pulmonary embolism in patients with proximal deep-vein thrombosis. *NEJM* 1998;338:409–416.
71. Mayer SA. Recombinant activated factor VII for acute intracerebral hemorrhage. *N Engl J Med* 2005;352:777–785.
72. Crowther MA, Berry LR, Monagle PT, et al. Mechanisms responsible for the failure of protamine to inactivate low-molecular-weight heparin. *Br J Haematol.* 2002;116(1):178–186.
73. Horlocker TT, Wedel DJ, Benzon H, et al. Regional anesthesia in the anticoagulated patient: defining the risks (the second ASRA Consensus Conference on Neuraxial Anesthesia and Anticoagulation). *Reg Anesth Pain Med.* 2003;28(3):172–197.
74. Ansell J, Hirsh J, Poller L, et al. The pharmacology and management of the vitamin K antagonists: the Seventh ACCP Conference on Antithrombotic and Thrombolytic Therapy. *Chest* 2004;126:204S–233S.
75. Gage BF. Risk of osteoporotic fracture in elderly patients taking warfarin. *Arch Intern Med* 2006;166:241–246.
76. White RH, McKittrick T, Hutchinson R, et al. Temporary discontinuation of warfarin therapy: changes in the international normalized ratio. *Ann Intern Med.* 1995;122(1):40–42.

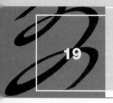

ANEMIA AND TRANSFUSION THERAPY
Morey Blinder and Joshua Field

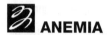 **ANEMIA**

GENERAL PRINCIPLES

Definition

- Anemia is defined as a decrease in the circulating red blood cell (RBC) mass (**<12 g/dL [hematocrit (Hct) <36%] in women** and **<14 g/dL [Hct <41%] in men**).

Etiology

- Defective RBC production
  - Substrate deficiency: iron, folate, B_{12} deficiency
  - Stem cell dysfunction: myelodysplastic syndrome, aplastic anemia
  - Dysregulation: decreased erythropoietin production
  - Bone marrow infiltration: infection, malignancy, fibrosis
- RBC loss or destruction
  - Bleeding
  - **Hemolysis:** autoimmune, microangiopathic, red cell membrane disorders (hereditary spherocytosis, elliptocytosis), enzyme deficiencies (G6PD deficiency), hemoglobinopathies (sickle cell disease)

DIAGNOSIS

Clinical Presentation

- **Clinical manifestations** of anemia vary depending on the etiology, severity, and rapidity of onset.
- Other underlying disorders such as cardiopulmonary disease may contribute to the severity of symptoms. Severe anemia may be well tolerated if it develops gradually, but patients with a hemoglobin (Hb) of <7 g/dL generally have symptoms of tissue hypoxia (fatigue, headache, dyspnea, lightheadedness, angina).
- Pallor, visual impairment, syncope, and tachycardia may signal **anemic hypovolemia**, which requires immediate attention.

Laboratory Studies

- Complete blood count (CBC):
  - Hb and Hct
  - The CBC estimates **RBC mass**, but its interpretation must take into consideration the volume status of the patient. Immediately after acute blood loss, the Hb and Hct are

unchanged because compensatory mechanisms have not had time to restore normal plasma volume.
- Reticulocyte count:
    - This indicates the **level of production of RBCs** and is an indicator of the bone marrow response to the anemia.
    - It usually is reported as reticulocytes/100 RBCs $\times$ 100 (% reticulocytes)
    - **Absolute reticulocyte count** = % reticulocytes RBC count (per mm^3)
    - Absolute reticulocyte count >100,000/mm^3 suggests a hyperproliferative bone marrow associated with loss or destruction of RBCs.
    - Anemia with a low absolute reticulocyte count suggests impaired RBC production.
- Mean cellular volume (MCV):
    - This is used in **classifying anemia** (microcytic, normocytic, and macrocytic for anemia with low, normal, and high MCV, respectively). Proper use of the MCV in establishing a diagnosis depends on examination of the peripheral smear for the following reasons:
        - Small and large cells may be present simultaneously, resulting in a normal MCV.
        - Reticulocytes are larger than mature RBCs and raise the MCV.
        - Abnormal cells may be present in numbers that are too small to affect the MCV.
        - RBC shape abnormalities and inclusions are not reflected in the MCV.
- **Peripheral blood smear**
    - RBC **morphology** is best evaluated in a portion of the smear where the RBCs are nearly touching one another. Heterogeneity in RBC size (anisocytosis) and shape (poikilocytosis) may be seen. Specific morphologic abnormalities should be sought, as well as any abnormalities in the white blood cells (WBCs) or platelets.
- **Additional testing** to establish an exact diagnosis should be guided by the initial findings, and, whenever possible, some tests should be performed before blood transfusions (peripheral smear, glucose-6-phosphate dehydrogenase [G6PD] level, Hb analysis, iron studies).
- Evaluation of anemia also requires consideration of the WBC and platelet count because bicytopenia or pancytopenia often suggests other causes.

ANEMIAS ASSOCIATED WITH DECREASED RED BLOOD CELL PRODUCTION

IRON-DEFICIENCY ANEMIA

General Principles

Etiology
- **Menstrual blood loss and increased iron requirements of pregnancy** are the most common causes in the developed world.
- **Gastrointestinal (GI) blood loss** is the presumed etiology in most other patients.
- **Decreased iron absorption** (celiac disease, postgastrectomy, *Helicobacter pylori*) or increased iron requirements (lactation) may also lead to iron deficiency.
- Chronic **intravascular hemolytic anemia** may lead to iron deficiency (e.g., long-distance running).
- Iron-deficiency anemia is the most common cause of anemia in the geriatric patient.
- A complete analysis of iron deficiency requires identification of the underlying cause.

Diagnosis

History
- Blood loss (melena, menorrhagia, frequent blood donation).
- **Pica** (consumption of substances such as ice, starch, or clay) may be present.

Physical Examination

- Splenomegaly, koilonychia ("spoon nail"), and the Plummer-Vinson's syndrome (glossitis, dysphagia, and esophageal webs) are rare findings. The presence of telangiactasias or heme-positive stool may help to identify the source of blood loss.

Laboratory Studies

- MCV is usually normal in early iron deficiency. As the **Hct** falls below 30%, anisocytosis increases and hypochromic microcytic cells appear, followed by a decrease in the MCV.
- Platelet count may be increased.
- **Peripheral smear** demonstrates **hypochromic, microcytic red cells** and occasional **pencil cells** and **target cells.**
- Iron testing
  - **Serum ferritin** level of <10 ng/mL in women or 20 ng/mL in men is indicative of **iron deficiency.**
    - Ferritin is an acute-phase reactant, so that normal levels may be seen in inflammatory states, liver disease, or malignancy despite low iron stores. A serum ferritin level of >200 ng/mL generally indicates adequate iron stores regardless of other underlying conditions.
  - **Serum iron** is usually low (<50 mcg/dL), and **total iron-binding capacity** is increased (>420 mcg/dL) in iron deficiency, but these values may fluctuate in a number of common clinical conditions and hence are less reliable indicators of iron stores than the serum ferritin.
  - **Bone marrow aspirate** is the definitive test for iron deficiency.
    - It is the earliest indicator of iron deficiency.
    - It is useful when diagnosis of iron deficiency is not clear.
  - **Therapeutic challenge** with supplemental iron can help to identify anemias that are iron responsive when diagnosis is uncertain.

Treatment

Medications

- Oral iron
  - **Ferrous sulfate, 325 mg (65 mg elemental iron) PO tid** taken between meals to maximize absorption, usually corrects the anemia and repletes iron stores (as determined by normalization of the serum ferritin) over approximately 6 months.
  - Concomitant use of acid-neutralizing medications is an underappreciated cause of an impaired response to oral iron.
  - **GI side effects,** such as constipation, cramping, diarrhea, or nausea, develop in approximately 25% of patients. These side effects can be decreased by initially administering the drug with meals or once a day and increasing the dose as tolerated.
  - Ferrous gluconate and fumarate at a similar dose may be better-tolerated alternative therapies.
  - Iron polysaccharide complex (Niferex) contains 150 mg of elemental iron and, given twice daily, is as effective as other preparations at a similar cost and seems to have fewer GI side effects.
  - Ferric forms of oral iron, sustained-release or enteric-coated preparations, dissolve poorly and generally should not be recommended.
  - Lower doses of ferrous sulfate are better tolerated and as effective in geriatric patients.
  - **Noncompliance** is the most common reason for a poor response to oral therapy.
- Parenteral iron
  - Indications for parenteral iron include poor enteral absorption, continued blood loss, or intolerance to oral iron.
  - Iron dextran (Infed)
    - **Test dose:** Allergic reactions or **anaphylaxis** to iron dextran occur in about 1 in 300 patients, thus a 25-mg test dose in 50 mL of normal saline over 5–10 minutes should be administered initially. If a reaction does not occur within 1 hour, proceed with administration of the total dose.

- **Total dose:** Dose in mL = (0.0442 × (desired hemoglobin − current hemoglobin) × ideal body weight) + (0.26 × ideal body weight)
- The total dose (generally between 1 and 2 g) should be diluted in 500 mL of normal saline and administered over 4–6 hours.
- For an online dose calculator, go to www.globalrph.com/irondextran.htm
- **Ferric gluconate (Ferrlecit)** is dosed at 125 mg and may be administered weekly or up to three times per week with hemodialysis. The risk of anaphylaxis is significantly less with ferric gluconate.
- With therapy, the reticulocyte count peaks in 5–10 days, and the Hb rises over 1–2 months.

THE THALASSEMIAS

General Principles

Definition
- The thalassemias comprise a group of inherited anemias caused by decreased production of alpha- or beta-globin chains of the hemoglobin tetramer (Table 19-1).

Epidemiology
- Thalassemia occurs in persons of Mediterranean, African, Middle Eastern, Indian, and Asian descent.

Classification
- **Alpha-thalassemia** is due to decreased synthesis of alpha-globin chains caused by deletions in one or more of the four alpha-globin genes.
- **Beta-thalassemia** is due to a reduced or absent production of one or two of the two beta-globin genes.

Etiology
- In beta-thalassemia, the excess alpha-globin chains form insoluble tetramers in the RBCs, resulting in membrane damage, ineffective erythropoiesis, and hemolytic anemia.
- A similar process in alpha-thalassemia occurs with an excess of beta-globin chains; however, tetramers of beta-globin are soluble, and thus the disease is less severe.

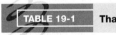

| TABLE 19-1 | Thalassemias |

	Number of affected genes	Hemoglobin (g/dL)	MCV (fL)	Transfusion dependent
Alpha-thalassemia				
Alpha-thal-2 trait	1	Normal	None	No
Alpha-thal-1 trait	2	>10	<80	No
Hemoglobin H	3	7–10	<70	+/−
Hydrops fetalis	4	Incompatible with life		
Beta-thalassemia				
Beta-thal minor (trait)	1	>10	<80	No
Beta-thal intermedia[a]	2	7–10	65–75	+/−
Beta-thal major	2	<7	<70	Yes

MCV, mean corpuscular volume.
[a]Beta-thalassemia intermedia has two mutated beta-globin genes with impaired but not absent synthesis.

Diagnosis

Physical Examination

- Splenomegaly and bone abnormalities caused by the expanded marrow are common in more severe forms of thalassemia.
- Hepatomegaly, signs of congestive heart failure, short stature, and hypogonadism are commonly due to transfusion-related iron overload.

Laboratory Studies

- Microcytic, hypochromic cells with poikilocytosis, target cells, and nucleated RBCs may be present on the peripheral smear.
- In thalassemia trait, iron studies are normal, as is the red cell distribution width (RDW), which help to differentiate the condition from the microcytosis of iron-deficiency anemia.
- Hemoglobin analysis (electrophoresis or high-performance liquid chromatography [HPLC]):
  - Beta-thalassemia: elevated hemoglobin A2 and/or hemoglobin F
  - Alpha-thalassemia: hemoglobin analysis normal. Diagnosis requires alpha-globin gene analysis.

Treatment

Transfusion Therapy

- **Packed RBCs (PRBCs):** A Hb of >9 g/dL improves exercise tolerance and prevents skeletal deformities and can usually be achieved with 1 unit of RBCs every 2–3 weeks or 2 units every month
- In severe forms of thalassemia, the transfusions result in tissue iron overload, which may cause congestive heart failure (CHF), hepatic dysfunction, glucose intolerance, and secondary hypogonadism. **Iron chelation therapy** delays or prevents these complications. Once clinical organ deterioration has begun, it may not be reversible.
- **Chelation therapy** is indicated for transfusion-associated iron overload from any cause. It is indicated in patients with iron infusion burden >20 units PRBCs and ferritin consistently >1,000 ng/mL. Deferoxamine, 40 mg/kg subcutaneously (SC) or intravenously (IV) over 8–12 hours continuous infusion.[1] Deferasirox, 20 mg/kg PO daily dissolved in water or juice. Side effects include nausea, vomiting, diarrhea, and abdominal pain. Efficacy is similar to that of deferoxamine.

Surgery

- **Splenectomy** removes the primary site of extravascular hemolysis and should be considered if RBC transfusion requirements increase and **exceed one and a half times the previous levels.**
  - To decrease the risk of **postsplenectomy sepsis**, immunization against *Pneumococcus*, *Haemophilus influenzae*, and *Neisseria meningitidis* should be administered at least 2 weeks before surgery if not previously vaccinated (see Appendix C, Immunizations and Postexposure Therapies).
  - **Not** recommended if the patient is younger than 5–6 years because of the risk of sepsis.

Stem Cell Transplant

- **Stem cell transplant (SCT)** should be considered in young patients with beta-thalassemia major who have an HLA-identical sibling.

MYELODYSPLASTIC SYNDROME

General Principles

Definition

- Myelodysplastic syndrome (MDS) **is a clonal stem cell disorder** characterized by ineffective hematopoiesis resulting in **peripheral cytopenias.** Some patients progress to develop **acute leukemia.**

World Health Organization Classification[2]

- **Refractory anemia:** Erythroid dysplasia <5% myeloblasts in bone marrow
    - With ring sideroblasts, >15% of nucleated marrow cells
    - Without ring sideroblasts
- **Refractory cytopenia with multilineage dysplasia:** Evidence of dysplasia in non-erythroid cell lines and <5% myeloblasts in bone marrow.
- **Refractory anemia with excess blasts:** 5%–20% myeloblasts in bone marrow.
- **5q-syndrome:** Favorable prognosis, may have thrombocytosis.
- Myelodysplastic syndrome, unclassifiable.

Prognosis

- Prognosis is based on WHO classification.
- See Table 19-2 for the international prognostic scoring system in MDS based on three laboratory features.[3]

Etiology

- **Idiopathic** (70% of patients).
- **Secondary** (30% of patients) to prior radiation, chemotherapy, or toxin exposure.

Diagnosis

Laboratory Studies

- Complete blood count:
    - **Cytopenias; anemia is most common** but any combination of low blood counts is possible.
    - Macrocytosis may be present.
- Peripheral smear:
    - **Dysplasia: hypogranular or hypolobulated neutrophils** (pseudo-Pelger-Hüet anomaly), basophilic stippling, and megaloblastic changes in red cells.
    - **Circulating blasts**

TABLE 19-2	**International Prognostic Scoring System**		
Score	**Bone marrow blasts (%)**	**Karyotype**[a]	**Cytopenias**
0	< 5	Good	0–1
0.5	5–10	Poor	2–3
1			
1.5	11–20		
2	21–30		

Risk group	**Total score**[b]	**Median survival (yr)**
Low	0	5.7
INT-1	0.5–1	3.5
INT-2	1.5–2	1.2
High	>2.5	0.4

INT, intermediate.
[a]Good: normal, -Y, 5q, 20q; poor: complex (>3 abnormalities), chromosome 7 abnormalities.
[b]Score—total score of bone marrow blasts, karyotype and cytopenia.

- **Bone marrow examination** with chromosomal analysis is necessary for diagnosis and classification.
  - Iron stain to evaluate for ring sideroblasts.
  - Vitamin B_{12} and folate levels to exclude megaloblastic anemia.

Special Considerations
- Bone marrow blast count >20% is diagnostic for acute leukemia.
- Supportive care including RBC transfusions as needed.
- Epo (40,000 units SC every week) or darbepoetin (200–300 mcg SC every 2–3 weeks) may provide some improvement in erythropoiesis.
- Pyridoxine 50–200 PO daily response rate 20% in patients with ring sideroblasts.

Treatment
Medications
- **5-Azacitidine (Vidaza)**, 75 mg/m^2 SC × 7 days of a 28 day cycle.[4]
  - Response rate 15.7% (complete remission + partial remission).
  - Slows progression to acute myeloid leukemia (AML) and improves survival versus best supportive care.[4]
  - Indicated for high-risk MDS (class INT-2 and high) and for patients who are transfusion dependent.
  - Most common side effects are neutropenia, anemia, and thrombocytopenia.
- **Immunosuppressive therapy** with antithymocyte globulin, cyclosporine, and glucocorticoids are most effective in patients with a hypocellular (referring to bone marrow cellularity) MDS.
- **Iron chelation therapy** should be considered in patients with a **low or Int-1 risk** after 50–100 units of RBCs have been transfused.
- **Lenolidamide** (10 mg PO daily for 21 days of a 28-day cycle) is effective in patients with MDS and 5q-syndrome.

Special Therapy
- **Stem cell transplant** should be considered in patients <50 years of age who have an HLA-identical sibling.

SIDEROBLASTIC ANEMIAS
General Principles
Definition
- **Sideroblastic anemias** are **hereditary** or **acquired** RBC disorders characterized by **abnormal iron metabolism** occasionally associated with the presence of ring sideroblasts in the bone marrow aspirate and normal cytogenetics.

Etiology
- Drugs (see Table 19-4, page 560)
- Lead toxicity
- Chronic ethanol use
- Copper deficiency

Diagnosis

- **CBC:** Anemia with low-normal MCV
- **A bone marrow examination including cytogenetics** may be necessary to evaluate for the presence of ring sideroblasts or other abnormal marrow forms.

Treatment

- **Remove any possible offending agent.**
  - **Pyridoxine 50–200 mg PO daily** to treat any underlying nutritional deficiency.

MEGALOBLASTIC ANEMIAS

General Principles

Definition
- **Megaloblastic anemias** are disorders characterized by altered morphology of hematopoietic cells and other rapidly dividing cells because of abnormalities in DNA synthesis.

Etiology
- **Folic acid deficiency** may develop within a few months.
  - Decreased intake often associated with **chronic alcohol use**
  - Malabsorption
  - Increased utilization (**hemolytic anemia, pregnancy**)
  - Drugs (**ethanol, trimethoprim, pyrimethamine, methotrexate, sulfasalazine, oral contraceptives,** and **anticonvulsants**) may lead to perturbed folate metabolism.
- **Vitamin B$_{12}$ deficiency** takes years to develop. Causes of vitamin B$_{12}$ deficiency include the following:
  - Dietary insufficiency
  - **Pernicious anemia**
  - Gastrectomy or partial gastrectomy
  - Disorders of proximal intestine
  - Bacterial overgrowth (blind loop)
  - Pancreatic insufficiency:
    - Chronic pancreatitis
  - Disorders of distal small intestine:
    - Ileitis or ileal resection
  - **Intestinal parasites:** Fish tapeworm (*Diphyllobothrium latum*)

Diagnosis

Clinical Presentation
- Symptoms are primarily attributable to anemia, although if secondary to B$_{12}$ or folate deficiency, glossitis, jaundice, and splenomegaly may be present.
- Vitamin B$_{12}$ deficiency may cause decreased vibratory and positional sense, ataxia, paresthesias, confusion, and dementia. Folate deficiency does not cause neurologic symptoms.

Laboratory Studies
- CBC: macrocytic anemia, leukopenia, and thrombocytopenia may also occur.
- **Peripheral smear:**
  - RBC macro-ovalocytes.
  - Hypersegmented neutrophils (containing ≥ 5 nuclear lobes).
- Elevated **lactate dehydrogenase (LDH)** and **indirect bilirubin** reflect ineffective erythropoiesis and premature destruction of RBCs.
- **Serum vitamin B$_{12}$ and RBC folate levels.** RBC folate is a more accurate indicator of body folate stores than serum folate, particularly if measured after folate therapy or improved nutrition has been initiated.
- **Serum methylmalonic acid (MMA) and homocysteine (HC)** are useful when the vitamin B$_{12}$ or folate level is indeterminate. **MMA and HC are elevated in vitamin B$_{12}$ deficiency; only HC is elevated in folic acid deficiency.**
- **The Schilling test** may be useful in the diagnosis of pernicious anemia due to vitamin B$_{12}$ deficiency but rarely affects the therapeutic approach.
- **Demonstrating antibodies to intrinsic factor** is specific for the diagnosis of pernicious anemia.
- **Bone marrow biopsy** may be necessary to rule out MDS and hematologic malignancy; these disorders may present with findings similar to those of megaloblastic anemia on peripheral smear.

- **Thyroid function studies** for patients with pernicious anemia.
  - Pernicious anemia is often associated with autoimmune thyroid disease.

Treatment

Medications
- **Folic acid** 1 mg PO daily until the deficiency is corrected. High doses of folic acid (5 mg PO daily) may be needed in patients with malabsorption syndromes.
- **Vitamin B_{12} deficiency** is corrected by administering vitamin B_{12}. A typical schedule is 1 mg IM daily for 7 days, then weekly for 1–2 months or until normalization of the Hb occurs. Long-term therapy is 1 mg IM monthly.
- Consider B_{12} at 1 mg PO daily for long-term management.
  - With therapy, reticulocytosis should begin within 1 week, followed by a rise in Hb over 6–8 weeks.

Special Considerations

- Neurologic complications may occur in the absence of anemia and may not resolve completely despite adequate treatment.
- Coexisting iron deficiency is present in one-third of patients with vitamin B_{12} deficiency and is a common cause for an incomplete response to therapy.

ANEMIA OF CHRONIC RENAL INSUFFICIENCY

General Principles

Etiology
- This condition is attributed primarily to **decreased endogenous erythropoietin production** and may occur as the creatinine clearance declines below approximately 50 mL/min (see Chapter 11, Renal Diseases).

Diagnosis

Laboratory Studies
- CBC: Normocytic anemia
- Peripheral smear: The RBCs are often hypochromic, with the occasional presence of echinocytes (burr cells).

Treatment

Medications
- **Erythroid growth factors** (Table 19-3), erythropoietin (Epo), darbepoetin
  - IV (hemodialysis patients) or SC (predialysis or peritoneal dialysis patients).
  - Most patients increase their Hct by 10 points or to a level >32% within 12 weeks of therapy.
  - **Adverse reactions** are uncommon. Hypertension may develop or worsen in some patients while the Hct is increasing. Seizures may occur, although the etiology is not well characterized.
  - **Suboptimal responses** may occur with coexisting iron deficiency or iron-restricted erythropoiesis; thus, many patients benefit from IV iron supplementation despite normal serum ferritin. Sodium ferric gluconate or iron sucrose, 100–125 mg one to three times per week IV, is typically used in this setting.

Special Considerations

- Treatment of anemia is indicated in predialysis and dialysis patients who are symptomatic.

	Agent and initial dose (SC or IV)	
Indication	**Erythropoietin**[a]	**Darbepoetin**[b]
Chemotherapy-induced anemia from nonmyeloid malignancy, multiple myeloma, lymphoma; anemia secondary to malignancy or MDS	40,000 units/wk or 150 units/kg three times a week	2.25 mcg/kg/wk or 100 mcg/wk or 200 mcg/2 wk or 500 mcg/3 wks
Anemia associated with renal failure	50–150 units/kg three times a week	0.45 mcg/kg/wk
Anemia associated with HIV infection	100–200 units/kg three times a week	Not approved
Anemia of chronic disease	150–300 units/kg three times a week	Not approved
Anemia in patients unwilling or unable to receive red blood cells; anemic patients undergoing major surgery	600 units/kg/wk × 3 300 units/kg/d × 1–2 wk	Not recommended

TABLE 19-3   Erythropoietin Dosing

MDS, myelodysplastic syndrome; tiw, thrice weekly.
[a]Dose increase after 48 wk up to 900 units/kg/wk or 60,000 units/wk; discontinue if hematocrit (Hct) is >40%; resume when Hct is <36% at 75% of previous dose.
[b]Dose increase after 6 wk up to 4.5 mg/kg/wk or 150 mg/wk or 300 mg/2 wk; hold dose if Hct is >36%; then resume when Hct is <36% at 75% of previous dose.

- Serum erythropoietin level is not indicated prior to initiation of therapy with Epo in chronic renal insufficiency and has no role in monitoring.

ANEMIA OF CHRONIC DISEASE

General Principles

Definition
- These anemias are associated with long-standing inflammatory diseases, malignancy, autoimmune disorders, and chronic infection.

Etiology
- Disorder of iron availability characterized by decreased absorption of iron in the duodenum and sequestration of stored iron in the reticuloendothelial cells.

Diagnosis

Laboratory Studies
- On CBC, **normochromic normocytic anemia** is typical.
- The peripheral smear is usually normal, although microcytes may be present.
- Ferritin is generally normal but may be elevated because it is an acute-phase reactant.
- **Serum transferrin receptor** may help to distinguish iron-deficiency anemia from anemia of chronic disease (elevated in iron deficiency, normal in anemia of chronic disease).

- Epo level is not useful for diagnosis, but levels <200 mU/mL suggests patient benefit from Epo
- Bone marrow exam may be needed to exclude other causes of anemia.

Treatment

- Treatment is directed at the underlying cause and at eliminating exacerbating factors such as nutritional deficiencies and marrow-suppressive drugs.

Medications
- Epo can be effective in patients with a pretreatment serum Epo level <200 mU/mL
  - Effective doses of Epo are higher than those reported in anemia from renal insufficiency.
  - If no response has been observed at 900 units/kg/wk, further dose escalation is unlikely to be effective.

ANEMIA ASSOCIATED WITH HIV INFECTION

General Principles

Epidemiology
- Anemia is the most common cytopenia in persons with HIV; the prevalence increases as the disease progresses and the CD4 count drops.[5]

Etiology
- Similar mechanism as anemia of chronic disease in which inflammatory mediators cause decreased erythropoiesis.

Diagnosis

Laboratory Studies
- CBC: **Normochromic, normocytic anemia,** although zidovudine and stavudine induce a macrocytic anemia.
- Decreased reticulocyte count
- Bone marrow exam rarely needed. (See Special Considerations)
- Dysplasia similar to MDS is common

Treatment

Medications
- Epo (Table 19-3) improves the Hct in patients with an endogenous Epo level of ≤500 mU/mL.

Special Considerations

- *Mycobacterium avium* **complex** infections are frequently associated with severe anemia. Diagnosis is established on bone marrow (BM) exam or culture. Treatment of *M. avium* complex is described in Chapter 14, Human Immunodeficiency Virus and Acquired Immunodeficiency Syndrome.
- **Parvovirus B19** should be considered in HIV-infected patients with transfusion-dependent anemia and a low reticulocyte count.
  - Laboratory studies: **parvovirus by polymerase chain reaction (PCR) from blood (serum) or BM.**
  - Treatment with IV immunoglobulin (0.4 g/kg IV daily for 5–10 days) results in erythropoietic recovery. Relapses have occurred between 2 and 6 months and can be successfully managed with intermittent IV immunoglobulin at an empiric maintenance dose of 0.4 g/kg IV for 1 day given every 4 weeks.[6]

PANCYTOPENIA

General Principles

- This condition may occur in a variety of situations, including megaloblastic anemia, MDS, acute leukemia, HIV infection, and infiltration of the marrow with tumor or granuloma.
- In immunocompromised patients, pancytopenia is frequently due to immunosuppressive agents or viral infection.
- A **bone marrow** examination is frequently required to establish the diagnosis.

APLASTIC ANEMIA

General Principles

Definition
- Aplastic anemia is an acquired abnormality of hematopoietic stem cells that usually presents with pancytopenia.

Etiology
- Most cases are idiopathic
- Approximately 20% of cases are associated with drug or chemical exposure (Table 19-4).
- Ten percent of cases are associated with viral illnesses (e.g., viral hepatitis, Epstein-Barr virus, cytomegalovirus [CMV]).

Diagnostic Criteria[7]
- Severe aplastic anemia
  - Bone marrow cellularity <30% with normal cytogenetics
  - Two of three peripheral blood criteria:
    - Absolute neutrophil count <500/mm^3
    - Platelet count <20,000/mm^3
    - Reticulocyte count <40,000/mm^3
  - No other hematologic disease
- Considered moderate aplastic anemia if patients have pancytopenia but do not fulfill criteria.

Diagnosis

Clinical Presentation
- Usually presents with **pancytopenia**.
- Presenting symptoms are usually due to anemia (fatigue, malaise, dyspnea) or thrombocytopenia (mucosal bleeding, bruising), although some patients present with **fever** and **leukopenia**.

Laboratory Studies
- Bone marrow biopsy is required for diagnosis.
  - Morphology of bone marrow biopsy may be difficult to distinguish from hypocellular MDS and paroxysmal nocturnal hemoglobinuria.

Treatment

- Suspected offending drugs should be discontinued and exacerbating factors corrected.
- Once the diagnosis is established, care should be provided in a center experienced with aplastic anemia.

TABLE 19-4 Drugs That Induce Red Blood Cell Disorders

| | | | Immune hemolytic anemia | | |
			Autoantibody	Hapten	Immune complex[b]
Sideroblastic anemia	Aplastic anemia[a]	Hemolytic episode in G6PD deficiency			
Chloramphenicol	Acetazolamide	Dapsone	α-Methyldopa	AK-Fluor 25%	Amphotericin B
Cycloserine	Antineoplastic agents	Furazolidone	Cephalosporins	Cephalosporins	Antazoline
Ethanol	Carbamazepine	Methylene blue	Diclofenac	Penicillins	Cephalosporins
Isoniazid	Chloramphenicol	Nalidixic acid	Ibuprofen	Tetracycline	Chlorpropamide
Pyrazinamide	Gold salts	Nitrofurantoin	Interferon-alpha	Tolbutamide	Diclofenac
	Hydantoins	Phenazopyridine	L-Dopa		Diethylstilbestrol
	Penicillamine	Primaquine	Mefenamic acid		Doxepin
	Phenylbutazone	Sulfacetamide	Procainamide		Hydrochlorothiazide
	Quinacrine	Sulfamethoxazole	Teniposide		Isoniazid
		Sulfanilamide	Thioridazine		p-Aminosalicylic acid
		Sulfapyridine	Tolmetin		Probenecid
					Quinidine
					Quinine
					Rifampin
					Sulfonamides
					Thiopental
					Tolmetin

G6PD, glucose-6-phosphate dehydrogenase.
[a]Drugs with >30 cases reported; many other drugs rarely are associated with aplastic anemia and are considered low risk.
[b]Some sources list the mechanism for many of these drugs as unknown.
Source: Data compiled from multiple sources. Agents listed are available in the United States.

Medications
- Immunosuppressive treatment with cyclosporine, glucocorticoids, and antithymocyte globulin should be considered in patients who do not undergo an SCT.[8]

Stem Cell Transplant
- Early referral to a center that is experienced in managing aplastic anemia is recommended. When feasible, SCT from an HLA-identical sibling is generally recommended and has achieved a long-term survival rate of 60%–70%.

Transfusions in Aplastic Anemia
- **Transfusions** with RBCs should be kept to a minimum in patients. Prophylactic platelet transfusions are generally recommended if the platelet count is below 10,000/mm³. Transfusion with blood products from family members should be avoided while SCT is being considered.

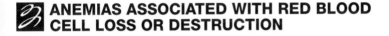

ANEMIAS ASSOCIATED WITH RED BLOOD CELL LOSS OR DESTRUCTION

GENERAL PRINCIPLES

Definition
- Anemias associated with increased erythropoiesis (i.e., an elevated reticulocyte count) are caused by bleeding or destruction of RBCs (hemolysis) and may exceed the capacity of normal bone marrow to correct the Hb. Bleeding is much more common than hemolysis.

Classification and Differential Diagnosis
- Blood loss
  - Sites of blood loss are usually readily clinically evident.
    - Suspect occult loss into GI tract, retroperitoneum, thorax, and deep compartments of thigh depending on history (recent instrumentation, trauma, hip fracture, coagulopathy).
- Hemolytic anemias are characterized by the predominant site of hemolysis.
  - **Intravascular hemolysis** may present with fever, chills, tachycardia, and backache.
    - ABO-incompatible RBC transfusion
    - Microangiopathic hemolytic anemia
      - Thrombotic thrombocytopenic purpura (TTP)
      - Disseminated intravascular coagulation (DIC)
      - Mechanical heart valve
      - Malignant hypertension
      - Vasculitis
    - Cold autoimmune hemolytic anemia (cold agglutinin disease)
    - RBC infection (malaria, babesiosis)
  - **Extravascular hemolysis** is characterized by RBC destruction in the reticuloendothelial system, primarily the spleen.
    - Warm autoimmune hemolytic anemia
    - Hereditary spherocytosis

DIAGNOSIS

Laboratory Studies
- CBC: Anemia **usually normocytic,** but MCV may be increased because of increased reticulocyte count.

- Reticulocyte count, bilirubin, and LDH may help to distinguish the bleeding patient (normal) from the patient with hemolysis (increased).
- All patients with suspected hemolysis should have a **direct antiglobulin test** (DAT, or direct Coombs' test). This test detects the presence of immunoglobulin G (IgG) and the third component of complement (C3) on the surface of RBCs and usually differentiates between immune and nonimmune causes of hemolysis.
- Peripheral smear may be diagnostic.
    - Microangiopathic hemolytic anemia: schistocytes, reticulocytes, and thrombocytopenia.
    - Autoimmune hemolytic anemia: spherocytes and reticulocytes.

Complications of Chronic Hemolysis

- **Aplastic crisis** is characterized by a sudden decrease in Hb and reticulocyte count.
    - This crisis is usually a complication of infection with **parvovirus B19**.
    - **Transfusion with RBCs is the mainstay of therapy,** and most patients recover in 10–14 days.
- **Cholelithiasis,** primarily with bilirubin stones, is present in most adult patients, and biliary pain is common.
    - Elective **laparoscopic cholecystectomy** is generally effective and should be considered in most patients. Acute cholecystitis should be treated medically, and cholecystectomy should be performed when the attack subsides (see Chapter 16, Gastrointestinal Diseases).
- Pulmonary hypertension

SICKLE CELL DISEASE

General Principles

Definition
- Sickle cell disease is molecularly characterized by a single amino acid substitution (Glu-Val) at position 6 in the beta-globin chain resulting in a structurally abnormal Hb molecule (HbS) that polymerizes under reduced oxygen conditions.

Classification
- **Sickle cell trait:** heterozygous for HbS.
    - Typically, carriers are asymptomatic.
    - The disease is associated with sudden death on extreme exertion (football, basketball, military basic training).
    - Renal complications: hyposthenuria, hematuria, urinary tract infection with or without pregnancy.
- **Sickle cell disease:** Homozygous for HbS or HbS beta-thalessemia
    - HbSC is milder.
    - HbS beta-thalassemia is mild

Diagnosis

Clinical Presentation
- Chronic hemolytic anemia; see prior discussion.
- **Vaso-occlusive pain crises** are the most common manifestation of sickle cell disease. Pain typically occurs in the back, ribs, and limbs and lasts for 5–7 days. The pattern of pain is usually consistent in any one patient from crisis to crisis.

Laboratory Studies
- CBC:
    - Normocytic anemia with Hb range from 5 to 10 g/dL in HbSS, and the MCV may be slightly elevated due to the increased reticulocyte count.

- Chronic neutrophilia (10,000–20,000/mm^3) is often present, and the platelet count may be increased.
- **Peripheral smear**
  - Classic distorted sickle-shaped erythrocytes
  - Target cells may be present, particularly in HbS beta-thalassemia and HbSC.
- **Hemoglobin analysis** by electrophoresis or HPLC distinguishes HbSS from sickle cell trait and other abnormal HbS.

Treatment

Medications

- **Antimicrobial prophylaxis** with penicillin VK, 125 mg PO bid up to age 3 years, then 250 mg PO bid until 5 years, is effective in reducing the risk of infection. Patients who are allergic to penicillin should receive erythromycin, 10 mg/kg PO bid. In most patients, antimicrobial prophylaxis should be discontinued after 5 years of age.[9]
- **Opioids** (see Chapter 1, Patient Care in Internal Medicine, Opioids) are typically used and are effectively administered by a **patient-controlled analgesia pump**, allowing for the patient to self-administer medication within a set limit of infusions (lockout interval) and basal rate.
  - Morphine (2 mg/hr basal rate with boluses of 2–10 mg every 6–10 minutes) is the drug of choice for moderate or severe pain. If patient-controlled analgesia is not used, morphine (0.1–0.2 mg/kg IV q2–3h) or hydromorphone (0.02–0.04 mg/kg IV q2–3h) is recommended.
- **Folic acid,** 1 mg PO daily, should be administered to patients with sickle cell disease because of chronic hemolysis.
- The full NIH guidelines for pain management are available at www.nhlbi.nih.gov/health/prof/blood/sickle/sc_mngt.pdf

Surgery

- For major surgery, RBC transfusions to increase the Hb concentration to 10 g/dL seem to be as effective as more aggressive transfusion regimens in most circumstances.[10]

Special Therapy

- Supplemental oxygen does not benefit acute pain crisis unless hypoxia is present.
- Patients who experience severe recurrent pain crisis that requires frequent medical intervention may benefit from chronic transfusion therapy or treatment with hydroxyurea.
  - **RBC transfusions** are indicated for patients with strokes, transient ischemic attacks, acute chest syndrome, aplastic crisis, priapism that is unresponsive to supportive care, and in preparation for general anesthesia (as discussed earlier).
  - **Hydroxyurea** (15–35 mg/kg PO daily) has been shown to increase levels of fetal Hb and decrease the incidence of vaso-occlusive pain episodes by approximately 50% and acute chest syndrome by approximately 70% in adults with sickle cell anemia.[16]
- **Iron chelation therapy** can be used as dictated by transfusion frequency (see Chelation Therapy section).

Health Maintenance

- **Dehydration and hypoxia** should be avoided because they may precipitate or exacerbate sickling (intense exercise, activities at high altitude, and flying in unpressurized aircraft should be strongly discouraged).
- **Regular yearly ophthalmologic examinations** are recommended in adults because of a high incidence of proliferative retinopathy leading to vitreous hemorrhage and retinal detachment. Laser photocoagulation is effective in preventing these complications.
- Immunizations in adults should include a polyvalent pneumococcal vaccine. Hepatitis B vaccine is recommended for hepatitis B surface antibody-negative patients. Yearly influenza vaccine is recommended (see Appendix C, Immunizations and Postexposure Therapies).

Complications

- Vaso-occlusive pain episode
  - This is the most common complication, accounting for >90% of hospitalizations in adults.
- **Acute chest syndrome** is associated with chest pain, pulmonary infiltrates, leukocytosis, and hypoxia and is indistinguishable from pneumonia.
  - *Chlamydia pneumoniae*, *Mycoplasma* species, respiratory syncytial virus, and *Staphylococcus aureus* are the most frequent organisms identified.
  - Initial management should include hospitalization, administration of supplemental oxygen to correct hypoxia, and adequate analgesia, and empiric coverage with **antimicrobials** such as a cephalosporin and a macrolide is recommended.
  - Transfusion of RBCs is recommended in most cases, and **exchange transfusion** to lower HbS concentration <30% should be considered in patients with multiple-lobe involvement, worsening disease, or hypoxemia (arterial oxygen tension <60 mm Hg).[11]
- **Splenic sequestration crisis** is associated with rapid onset of splenomegaly due to pooling of blood into the spleen causing severe anemia.
  - In adults, this complication generally occurs in patients with an **intact spleen**, such as those with **HbSC** or **HbS beta-thalassemia**.
  - **Hemodynamic support and RBC transfusions** are usually required.
  - **Splenic infarction**, causing severe left upper quadrant pain, may also result.
  - **Splenectomy should be considered** for recurrent events.
- **Priapism** refers to painful erection from vaso-occlusion, which may respond to hydration and analgesics. Transfusions and surgical drainage should be considered for acute events that last longer than 24 hours.
- **Osteonecrosis** of the femoral and humeral heads causes considerable morbidity in approximately one-third of patients.
  - Treatment consists of local heat, analgesics, and avoidance of weight bearing.
  - Hip and shoulder arthroplasty are often effective in decreasing symptoms and improving function and should be considered.
- **Stroke** occurs most commonly in children **younger than 10 years** and is usually caused by cerebral infarction.
  - Without treatment approximately **two-thirds of patients experience recurrent stroke**.
  - Long-term transfusions to maintain the HbS concentration at <50% for a minimum of 5 years reduce the incidence of recurrence. This is typically accomplished by chronic exchange transfusion.
- Leg ulcers
- **Renal tubular defects** caused by sickling lead to an inability to concentrate urine (hyposthenuria) and hematuria in sickle cell disease and sickle cell trait.
  - These conditions predispose patients to dehydration, which increases the risk of vaso-occlusive events.
  - Renal insufficiency occurs in 10%–20% of patients.

G6PD DEFICIENCY

General Principles

Definition

- This enzymatic deficiency of glucose-6-phosphate dehydrogenase results in RBCs that are more susceptible to oxidant stress than normal RBCs, leading to chronic or episodic hemolysis.

Epidemiology

- This is the most common of the hereditary RBC enzyme deficiencies.
- It is a sex-linked disorder that typically affects men.
- Over 500 different mutations have been identified with variable severity.

Classification
- A mild form of the deficiency occurs in approximately 10% of men of African heritage and is characterized by hemolytic episodes that are triggered by infections or drug exposure (Table 19-4).
- A more severe enzyme deficiency, such as the Mediterranean variety, results in hemolysis when susceptible individuals are exposed to fava beans.
- The most severe type causes a chronic, hereditary, nonspherocytic hemolytic anemia in the absence of an inciting cause.

Diagnosis

Laboratory Studies
- The peripheral smear shows "bite cells;" denatured Hb inclusions (**Heinz bodies**) are seen with special stains.
- Measurement of enzyme levels usually establishes the diagnosis but is inaccurate in the acute setting because senescent RBCs contain less G6PD and are more easily destroyed than are younger cells during a hemolytic episode.

Treatment
- Avoid offending medications
- Provide adequate hydration to protect renal function during hemolysis
- Conduct RBC transfusion for more severe forms

AUTOIMMUNE HEMOLYTIC ANEMIA

General Principles

Definition
- In autoimmune hemolytic anemia (AIHA) autoantibody is targeted to antigens on the patient's own red cells resulting in **extravascular hemolysis**.

Classification
- **Warm AIHA** antibodies interact best with RBCs at 37°C.
- **Cold AIHA** antibodies are most active at temperatures below 37°C.

Etiology
- **Warm antibody AIHA** is usually caused by an IgG autoantibody.
  - It may be idiopathic or associated with an **underlying malignancy** (lymphoma, chronic lymphocytic leukemia), collagen vascular disorder, or drug (Table 19-4).
- **Cold antibody AIHA** is typically IgM (in cold agglutinin disease).
  - **The acute form** often secondary to an **infection** (*Mycoplasma*, Epstein-Barr virus), which is usually transient.
  - **The chronic form** is due to a **paraprotein** (lymphoma, CLL, Waldenstom's macroglobulinemia) in approximately one-half of cases and is usually idiopathic in the others.

Diagnosis

Clinical Presentation
- Weakness, jaundice, and splenomegaly.
- Severe hemolysis may be associated with fever, chest pain, syncope, CHF, and hemoglobinuria.
- Episodic cold-induced intravascular hemolysis and vaso-occlusive events resulting in cyanosis of the ears, nose, fingers, and toes occur specifically in cold agglutinin disease.

Laboratory Studies
- Decrease in **haptoglobin**
- Increase in **LDH** and **bilirubin**, which may not be dramatic due to extravascular hemolysis

- Positive direct antiglobulin test DAT:
  - Warm AIHA: IgG+, C3+ or IgG+, C3−
  - Cold AIHA: IgG−, C3+
- Cold agglutinin titers
- Flow cytometry to rule out **paroxysmal nocturnal hemoglobinuria.**
- Peripheral smear shows **spherocytes,** polychromasia.
- Consider workup for underlying malignancy.

Treatment

- Both warm and cold AIHA therapy should be directed at identifying and treating any underlying cause.
- Warm AIHA
  - **Glucocorticoids,** such as prednisone 1 mg/kg. If patients are sensitive to glucocorticoids, response is typically seen in 7–10 days. When hemolysis has abated, glucocorticoids can be tapered over 2–3 months. Rapid steroid tapers can result in relapse.
  - **IVIG** is less effective than in ITP, with a response rate of about 40%.[12]
  - **Splenectomy** should be considered for steroid-resistant AIHA.
  - **Rituximab,** 375 mg/m^2 IV weekly for four doses, has shown efficacy in small case series.[13]
- Idiopathic cold AIHA
  - Glucocorticoids and splenectomy are not efficacious.
  - **Rituximab** has been demonstrated to be effective in a case reports.[14]
  - In severe cases, **plasma exchange** may be used to remove offending IgM antibody (which is 80% intravascular) to control the disease while other therapies are administered.
  - Warm RBC transfusions to 37°C; keep the patient and room warm to prevent exacerbation of hemolysis.

RBC Transfusion in AIHA

- **RBC transfusions** may not be as effective in increasing RBC mass due to hemolysis of transfused cells.
  - Transfuse RBCs only when patient is symptomatic/there is decreased oxygen-carrying capacity (e.g., Hb <6).
- Autoantibodies may confound plasma antibody screens and conventional cross-matches, and, therefore, alloantibodies may go undetected.

MICROANGIOPATHIC HEMOLYTIC ANEMIA

General Principles

Definition

- This is a syndrome of traumatic (microangiopathic) intravascular hemolysis.

Differential Diagnosis

- **Mechanical heart valves** can cause direct RBC shear stress, especially if the valve is dysfunctional; this may be difficult to diagnose.
- Disseminated intravascular coagulation (DIC), thrombotic thrombocytopenic purpura, hemolytic-uremic syndrome, severe hypertension, vasculitis, eclampsia, and some disseminated malignancies (see Chapter 20, Medical Management of Malignant Disease).

Diagnosis

Laboratory Studies

- CBC: normocytic anemia with thrombocytopenia
- Elevated LDH, reticulocyte count, bilirubin
- Decreased haptoglobin
- Peripheral smear shows schistocytes, polychromasia

Treatment

■ The treatment depends on the underlying etiology of microangiopathy. (For specific recommendations for thrombotic thrombocytopenic purpura/hemolytic uremic syndrome, see Chapter 18, Disorders of Hemostasis.)

 # TRANSFUSION THERAPY

GENERAL PRINCIPLES

■ The benefits and risks of transfusion therapy must be carefully weighed in each situation because blood products are a limited resource with potentially life-threatening side effects.

Indications/Contraindications

■ **RBC transfusion** is indicated to increase the oxygen-carrying capacity of blood in anemic patients. Transfusion threshold (in general):
  ■ **Hemoglobin 7–8 g/dL** with no cardiac risk.
  ■ **Hemoglobin 10 g/dL** with a history of **coronary artery disease** or risk of ischemia.
■ **One unit of RBCs increases the Hb by 1 g/dL in the average adult.**
■ If the cause of anemia is easily treatable (e.g., iron or folic acid deficiency) and no cerebrovascular or cardiopulmonary compromise is present, it is preferable to avoid transfusions.

Pretransfusion

■ The **type and screen procedure** tests the recipient's RBCs for the A, B, and D (Rh) antigens and also screens the recipient's serum for antibodies against other RBC antigens.
■ **Cross-matching** tests the patient's serum for antibodies against antigens on the donor's RBCs and is performed before a specific unit of blood is dispensed for a patient.

Manipulation of Blood Products

■ **Leukoreduced blood products** are recommended in the following circumstances:
  ■ If the patient has a history of one or more nonhemolytic febrile transfusion reactions that were not responsive to acetaminophen. Blood products are often leukoreduced at the time of collection or preparation. If they are not leukoreduced, bedside filters can leukoreduce the unit as it is being transfused; however this is not effective in the prevention of nonhemolytic febrile transfusion reactions, which are due to cytokines released from WBCs.
  ■ To prevent CMV infection in patients who require CMV-negative blood products that are not available.
  ■ To prevent the formation of platelet alloantibodies.
■ **Irradiation of blood products** eliminates immunologically competent lymphocytes and is recommended for immunocompromised bone marrow or organ transplant recipients or for any patient who is receiving directed donations from HLA-matched donors or first-degree relatives.
■ **Washed RBCs** are rarely indicated but should be considered in patients in whom plasma proteins may cause a serious reaction (e.g., IgA-deficient recipients or other anaphylactic reactions).
■ **CMV-negative blood products** are indicated in immunocompromised bone marrow or organ transplant recipients who are CMV antibody negative. If only CMV-positive products are available, the risk of CMV transmission can be minimized with prestorage leukoreduced units issued with a leukoreduction filter.

Procedures

- **Patient and blood product identification** procedures must be carefully followed to avoid mishandling errors.
- The IV catheter should be at least **18 gauge** to allow adequate flow.
- All blood products should be administered through a 170- to 260-mcm "standard" filter to prevent infusion of macroaggregates, fibrin, and debris.
- Patients should be observed for 5–10 minutes of each transfusion for adverse side effects and at regular intervals thereafter.
- Each unit of packed RBCs should be **completed within 4 hours of delivery to the bedside.**
- Infusion is typically administered over 2 hours.

COMPLICATIONS

Transfusion-Transmitted Infections

- **Transfusion-transmitted infections** include HIV-1/2, human T-lymphotropic virus type 1/2, hepatitis B virus, hepatitis C virus, syphilis, and West Nile virus.
- Risk of infectious transmission:
  - Risk of HIV- 1, HIV-2, human T-lymphotropic virus type 1, and hepatitis C is estimated to be 1 in 2,000,000–3,000,000.
  - Risk of hepatitis B virus transmission is approximately 1 in 50,000.
- Viral infections occur when donors are in the window period (undetectable to testing).
- CMV transmission from RBC and platelet transfusion is an important risk in immunocompromised patients.
- Bacterial transmission may occur from either a donor infection or a contaminant at the time of collection.
  - Platelet transfusions are more likely than RBCs to have bacterial contamination because they are stored at room temperature.
  - Most common organism identified in RBCs is *Yersinia enterocolitica* and in platelets is *Staphylococcus aureus*.

Noninfectious Hazards of Transfusion

- Hemolytic transfusion reactions
  - **Acute hemolytic reactions** are usually caused by **preformed antibodies** in the recipient and are characterized by intravascular hemolysis of the transfused RBCs soon after administration of ABO-incompatible blood.
    - **Fever, chills, back pain, chest pain, nausea, vomiting,** and symptoms related to hypotension may develop. **Acute renal failure** with hemoglobinuria may occur. In the unconscious patient, hypotension or hemoglobinuria may be the only manifestation.
    - If a hemolytic transfusion reaction is suspected, the **transfusion should be stopped immediately** and all **IV tubing should be replaced.** Clotted and EDTA-treated samples of the patient's blood should be delivered to the blood bank along with the remainder of the suspected unit for repeat of the cross-match. Direct and indirect Coombs' tests are performed, and the plasma and freshly voided urine should be examined for free Hb.
    - **Management** includes preservation of intravascular volume and protection of renal function. Urine output should be maintained at 100 mL/hr or greater with the use of IV fluids and diuretics or mannitol, if necessary. The excretion of free Hb can be aided by alkalinization of the urine. Sodium bicarbonate can be added to IV fluids to increase the urinary pH to ≥ 7.5 (see Chapter 11, Renal Diseases).
  - **Delayed hemolytic transfusion reactions** typically occur **3–10 days after transfusion** and are caused by either a primary or an amnestic antibody response to specific RBC antigens on donor RBCs.
    - Hb and Hct may fall.
    - DAT is positive, resulting in confusion with AIHA.

- Delayed hemolytic transfusion reaction may at times be severe; these cases should be treated similarly to acute hemolytic reactions.
- **Nonhemolytic febrile transfusion reactions** are characterized by fevers and chills.
  - Decreased incidence with leukoreduced products
  - White cells or cytokines released from white cells are thought to be the cause.
  - The symptoms may be treated with acetaminophen.
  - Prophylaxis with **acetaminophen** and **prestorage leukoreduced blood products** may prevent future febrile reactions.
- **Allergic reactions** are characterized by urticaria and in severe cases bronchospasm and hypotension.
  - The reactions are due to plasma proteins that elicit an **IgE-mediated response**. The reaction may be specific to the plasma proteins of a particular donor, and, therefore, the reaction may occur infrequently to blood products or never again.
  - If the symptoms are mild, pretreatment with **diphenhydramine** may prevent future reactions.
  - **Anaphylactic reactions** necessitate the addition of pretreatment **glucocorticoids** and **washed RBCs or volume-reduced platelets**.
  - If anaphylaxis occurs, check serum immunoglobulins because patients with **IgA deficiency** who receive IgA-containing blood products may experience anaphylaxis with small exposure to donor plasma.
- **Volume overload** with signs of CHF may be seen when patients with cardiovascular compromise are transfused with RBCs. Slowing the rate of transfusion and judicious use of diuretics help to prevent this complication.
- **Transfusion-related acute lung injury (TRALI)** is indistinguishable from acute respiratory distress syndrome and occurs within **4 hours** of a transfusion.
  - Symptoms include **dyspnea, hypotension, fever, chills, and hypoxemia**.
  - **Ventilatory assistance** may be required.
  - **Anti-human leukocyte antigen (HLA)** or **anti-granulocyte antibodies** in the donor's serum directed to the recipient's white blood cells cause the disorder.
  - Despite clinical or radiographic findings that suggest edema, data indicate that **diuretics have no role and may be detrimental**.[15]
  - **Hypoxemia resolves rapidly,** typically in about 24 hours.
  - On recognition, **transfusions must be stopped** and the blood bank notified so that **other products from the donor(s) in question may be quarantined**.
- **Transfusion-associated graft-versus-host disease** is usually seen in immunocompromised patients and is thought to result from the infusion of immunocompetent T lymphocytes.
  - Symptoms include **rash, elevated liver function tests, and severe pancytopenia**.
  - The **mortality is >80%**.
  - This has been reported in immunocompetent patients who share an HLA haplotype with HLA-homozygous blood donors (usually a relative or members of inbred populations).
  - **Irradiation of blood products** prevents this disease. Because the chances of shared HLA haplotypes with a random blood donor are extremely low, irradiation of nonrelated blood products is not indicated for the immunocompetent patient.
- **Posttransfusion purpura** is a rare syndrome of severe thrombocytopenia and purpura or bleeding that starts 7–10 days after exposure to blood products that contain platelets. The disorder is described in Chapter 18, Disorders of Hemostasis, the section Platelet Disorders.

Adverse Effects Due to Massive Transfusion

- Administration of blood products greater than the normal blood volume of the patient in a 24-hour period (**massive transfusion**) may be associated with several additional complications.
- **Hypothermia** caused by rapid infusion of chilled blood may cause cardiac dysrhythmias. A blood-warming device can prevent this problem.
- **Citrate intoxication** occurs in patients with hepatic dysfunction.

- This results in **hypocalcemia**, causing paresthesias, tetany, hypotension, and decreased cardiac output. On rare occasions the patient may require calcium gluconate, 10 mL of a 10% solution IV. Calcium should never be added directly to the transfusion product because it may cause the blood to clot.
- Hyperkalemia
  - Hyperkalemia is not usually significant **unless the patient was hyperkalemic before transfusion** (e.g., because of renal failure or muscle injury).
  - Twenty-four hours after massive transfusion, **hypokalemia may occur** as RBCs become more metabolically active and take up potassium from the plasma.
- **Bleeding complications** from dilution of platelets and plasma coagulation factors may be seen during massive transfusion. Correction of platelet and coagulation factor deficiencies should be based on clinical findings and laboratory monitoring rather than an empiric formula.

SPECIAL CONSIDERATIONS

- Long-term RBC transfusion therapy.
  - If the patient has received >20 units of RBCs, iron chelation therapy should be considered (see the section Anemias Associated with Decreased Red Blood Cell Production).
  - Consideration should also be given to performing an expanded RBC antigen panel to determine RBC phenotypic matches and decrease the risk of RBC alloimmunization and delayed hemolytic transfusion reactions.
- **Emergency RBC transfusions** should be used only in situations in which massive blood loss has resulted in cardiovascular compromise.
  - Volume expansion with normal saline should be attempted initially.
  - Blood typing can be performed in 10 minutes and cross-matching within 30 minutes in emergency situations.
  - If unmatched blood must be used, it should be group O/Rh-negative type that has been previously screened for reactive antibodies.
  - At the first sign of a transfusion reaction, the infusion should be stopped.
- **Approach to patients who are unwilling or unable to receive RBC transfusions** (e.g., Jehovah's Witness):
  - Management includes reducing blood loss by phlebotomy and obtaining necessary testing in pediatric tubes.
  - Epo is often of benefit (Table 19-3).
  - In most cases, concurrent use of oral or parenteral iron is also recommended (see Anemias Associated with Decreased Red Blood Cell Production). An increase in Hb of 1–2 g/dL over approximately a week is generally observed.

References

1. Olivieri NF, Berriman AM, Tyler BJ, et al. Reduction in tissue iron stores with a new regimen of continuous ambulatory intravenous deferoxamine. *Am J Hematol* 1992;41(1):61–63.
2. Harris NL, Jaffe ES, Diebold J, et al. World Health Organization of neoplastic diseases of the hematopoietic and lymphoid tissues: report of the clinical advisory committee meeting. Airlie House, Virginia, November 1997. *J Clin Oncol* 1999;17:3835–49.
3. Greenberg P, Cox C, LeBeau MM, et al. International Scoring System for Evaluating Prognosis in Myelodysplastic Syndromes. *Blood* 1997;89(6):2079–2088.
4. Silverman LR, Demakos EP, Peterson BL, et al. Randomized controlled trial of azacitidine in patients with myelodysplastic syndrome: a study of the cancer and leukemia group B. *J Clin Oncol* 2002;20(10):2429–2440.
5. Belperio PS, Rhew DC. Prevalence and outcomes of anemia in individuals with human immunodeficiency virus: a systematic review of the literature. *Am J Med* 2004;116(Suppl 7A):27S–43S.

6. Frickhoten N, Abkowitz JL, Safford M, et al. Persistent B19 parvovirus infection in patients infected with human immunodeficiency virus type 1 (HIV-1): a treatable cause of anemia in AIDS. *Ann Intern Med* 1990;113(12):926–933.

7. Rozman C, Marin P, Nomdeden B, et al. Criteria for severe aplastic anemia. *Lancet* 1987;2(8565):955–957.

8. Young NS. Acquired aplastic anemia. *Ann Intern Med* 2002;136(7):534–546.

9. Falletta JM, Woods GM, Verten JI, et al. Discontinuing penicillin prophylaxis in children with sickle cell anemia. Prophylactic Penicillin Study II. *J Pediatr* 1995;127(5):685–690.

10. Vinchinsky EP, Haberken CM, Neumayr L, et al. A comparison of conservative and aggressive transfusion regimens in the perioperative management of sickle cell disease. The Preoperative Transfusion in Sickle Cell Disease Study Group. *N Engl Med* 1995;33(4):206–213.

11. Vinchinsky EP, Neumayr LD, Earles AN, et al. Causes and outcomes of acute chest syndrome in sickle cell disease. National Acute Chest Syndrome Study Group. *N Engl J Med* 2000;342(25):1855–1865.

12. Flores G, Cunningham-Rundles C, Newland AC, et al. Efficacy of intravenous immunoglobulin in the treatment of autoimmune hemolytic anemia: results in 73 patients. *Am J Hematol* 1993;44(4):237–242.

13. Ahrens N, Kingreen D, Seltsam A, et al. Treatment of refractory autoimmune haemolytic anaemia with anti-CD20 (rituximab). *Br J Haematol* 2001;114(1): 244–245.

14. Bertentsen S, Ulvestad E, Gjertsen BT, et al. Rituximab for primary chronic cold agglutinin disease: a prospective study of 37 courses of therapy in 27 patients. *Blood* 2004;103(8):2925–2938.

15. Silliman CC, Ambruso DR, Boshkov LK. Transfusion-related acute lung injury. *Blood* 2005;105(6):2266–2273.

16. Charache S, Terrin ML, Moore RD, et al. Effect of hydroxyurea on the frequency of painful crises in sickle cell anemia. *N Engl J Med* 1995;332(20):1317–1322.

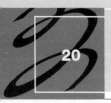

MEDICAL MANAGEMENT
OF MALIGNANT DISEASE
Mike Naughton

20

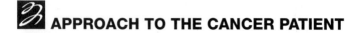

APPROACH TO THE CANCER PATIENT

GENERAL PRINCIPLES

Diagnosis

- Before treatment of a cancer patient is initiated, all patients should have a diagnosis of cancer based on tissue pathology, and, if possible, a clinical, biochemical, or radiographic marker of disease should be identified to assess the results of therapy.

Definitions

- **Stage** is a clinical or pathologic assessment of **tumor spread.** The major role of staging is to define the optimal therapy and prognosis in subsets of patients. **Treatment plans are generally determined by the stage of the tumor.** The role of local therapies, surgery, and radiation are determined by regional spread of disease. The role of systemic therapy, or chemotherapy, is also dependent on the stage of the tumor. In general, the probability of survival correlates well with tumor stage.
- The **grade** of a tumor defines its retention of characteristics compared to the cell of origin. It is designated as low, moderate, or high as the tissue loses its normal appearance. Although grade is important in determining prognosis for many tumors, it is not used as commonly as stage in defining treatment plans.
- **Performance status** is a gauge of a patient's overall functional status. Two scales are commonly used: the Karnofsky performance status scale and the Eastern Cooperative Oncology Group scale (Table 20-1). Performance status is an essential component of the evaluation of cancer patients, as it helps predict response to treatment, duration of response, and survival. For most solid tumors, patients with poor performance status are unlikely to derive significant benefit from systemic chemotherapy. However, patients with tumors that respond dramatically to chemotherapy may benefit from this treatment, even if they have poor performance status.
- Cancers are broadly characterized as "liquid" or "solid" malignancies.
  - **Leukemias and lymphomas comprise the "liquid" group.** The treatment of liquid tumors is usually chemotherapy or radiation therapy, or both.
  - The **"solid" tumors include tumors that arise from any solid organ or tissue.** Solid tumors are treated with surgery, radiation therapy, chemotherapy, or some combination of these modalities.
- **Therapy.** Cancer is in general treated with surgery, radiation, systemic chemotherapy, or a combination of these modalities.
  - **Chemotherapy** is administered in several different settings. Specific mechanisms of action and toxicities will be discussed in detail below.
    - **Induction chemotherapy** is used to achieve a complete remission.
    - **Consolidation chemotherapy** is administered to patients who initially respond to treatment.

572

| TABLE 20-1 | Performance Status |

Karnofsky performance status scale		ECOG performance status scale	
%	Definition	Grade	Definition
100	Normal; no complaints; no symptoms of disease	0	Fully active, able to carry on all predisease activity without restriction
90	Able to carry on normal activity; minor signs or symptoms of disease	1	Restricted in physically strenuous activity but ambulatory and able to carry out work of a light or sedentary nature
80	Normal activity with effort; some signs or symptoms of disease		
70	Able to care for self; unable to carry on normal activity or to do active work	2	Ambulatory and capable of all self-care but unable to carry out any work activities; up and about >50% of waking hours
60	Requires occasional care for most needs	3	Capable of only limited self-care; confined to bed or chair >50% of waking hours
50	Requires considerable assistance and frequent medical care		
40	Disabled; requires special care and assistance	4	Completely disabled; cannot carry on any self-care; totally confined to bed or chair
30	Severely disabled; hospitalization is indicated, although death is not imminent		
20	Very sick; hospitalization necessary; active supportive treatment necessary		
10	Moribund; fatal process progressing rapidly		
0	Dead		

ECOG, Eastern Cooperative Oncology Group.

- **Maintenance therapy** refers to low-dose, outpatient treatment used to prolong remissions; its use has proved effective in a few malignancies.
- **Adjuvant chemotherapy** is given after complete surgical or radiologic eradication of a primary malignancy to eliminate any unmeasurable metastatic disease.
- **Neoadjuvant chemotherapy** is given in the presence of local disease, before planned local therapy.
- **Survival data** are often reported in terms of median survival and 5-year survival, and cause confusion among patients with newly diagnosed malignancies; these data must be conveyed to the patient with caution by the treating oncologist who can help interpret these data.
  - **Median survival** equates to the period of time during which 50% of studied subjects are alive and 50% are dead.
  - **Five-year survival** means the percentage of patients studied who are alive at 5 years.

THERAPY OF SELECTED SOLID TUMORS

■ Guidelines for treatment of selected tumors are provided below.

  ▨ **Breast cancer** is the most common cause of cancer in women outside of nonmelanoma skin cancer.

  • **Approach to an undiagnosed lump in the breast.** Breast cancer develops in approximately 11% of women during their lifetime in the United States.

    ● A breast lump in a premenopausal woman is less likely to be cancerous than a breast lump in a postmenopausal woman.

    ● In a younger woman, a mass should be observed for 1 month to identify any cyclic changes that suggest benign disease.

    ● If the mass is still present, **bilateral mammography** should be performed. The accuracy of mammography to diagnose cancer in pre- and postmenopausal women is approximately 90%. **Nevertheless, a woman with a clinically suspicious lump and negative mammograms should undergo biopsy.**

  • **Surgical options.** Treatment is focused on local control and the risk of systemic spread.

    ● Local control with **tylectomy** (lumpectomy and axillary lymph node dissection) is as effective as a modified radical mastectomy. An axillary lymph node dissection should be included because it provides prognostic information and is of therapeutic value.

    ● **Sentinel lymph node mapping** and dissection allow many women to be spared full axillary dissection. In this procedure, blue dye, a radiotracer, or both are injected around the tumor bed. The lymph node(s) that pick up the dye/tracer are excised. If no cancer cells are seen in these lymph nodes, further axillary dissection can be avoided.

  • **Radiation therapy** is indicated for patients treated with tylectomy and for some individuals with axillary lymph node involvement. It can also be used for palliation of painful or obstructing metastatic lesions.

  • **Systemic therapy.** Systemic therapy is given for two reasons in the treatment of breast cancer:

    ● **Adjuvant therapy** is given to a woman who has had surgery to completely remove her tumor to reduce recurrence risk.

    ● **Palliative therapy** is given to women with metastatic breast cancer to slow the progression of their disease and to extend their lives.

    ● **Hormone therapy** is used for women with estrogen receptor (ER)– and/or progesterone receptor (PR)–positive disease.

    ● **Trastuzumab** (Herceptin) is appropriate for women with **her-2-neu–positive** breast cancer.

    ● **Anthracycline-based chemotherapy** is potentially useful in all subtypes.

  • **Adjuvant therapy.** The presence or absence of axillary lymph node metastases is the most important prognostic factor in breast cancer. All women with axillary nodal involvement should receive adjuvant therapy.

    ● Women with node-negative breast cancer should also be considered for adjuvant therapy if the tumor is >1 cm, is ER negative, or has overexpression of her-2.

    ● Chemotherapy should be considered in patients who are premenopausal, have cancers that are ER negative, or overexpress her-2.

    ● **Tamoxifen,** 20 mg PO daily for 5 years, is recommended for all ER-positive breast cancers[1] in premenopausal women.

    ● In postmenopausal women, the aromatase inhibitors **anastrozole, letrozole,** and **exemestane** have generally replaced tamoxifen for adjuvant hormone therapy.

    ● **Trastuzumab** has been found to be effective in the adjuvant treatment of women with her-2-neu–positive disease.[2]

  • **Metastatic disease.** Menopausal status, hormone receptor status, her-2-neu expression, and sites of metastatic disease dictate initial treatment.

    ● ER-negative breast cancer, lymphangitic lung disease, and liver metastasis seldom respond to hormonal manipulation and should be treated with chemotherapy.

- ER-positive disease is treated with hormonal manipulation.
  - Premenopausal women are initially treated with tamoxifen and a luteinizing hormone–releasing hormone (LHRH) agonist; postmenopausal women should receive a hormonal agent such as tamoxifen or an aromatase inhibitor. If the disease responds to hormonal therapy, subsequent disease progression may respond to other hormonal agents.
  - **Chemotherapy should be considered** if there is no response to initial hormonal therapy or if progression occurs during subsequent hormonal manipulations.
  - In her-2–overexpressing cancers, the addition of **trastuzumab** to first-line chemotherapy produced an improvement in survival compared to chemotherapy alone.[3]
  - In women with more than one osteolytic metastasis, the monthly administration of **zoledronic acid,** 4 mg IV, produces an improvement in quality of life, greater response to therapy, fewer extravertebral fractures, and possibly a prolongation in survival.[4]
- **Inflammatory and unresectable cancers.** Inflammatory breast cancer manifests as "peau d'orange" changes or erythema involving more than one-third of the chest wall. Because of the high likelihood of metastases at diagnosis, these patients and those with inoperable primary breast cancers are initially treated with chemotherapy. Subsequently, surgery and radiation therapies are used for maximal local control.

- **Lung cancer** is the most common cause of cancer death in the United States and is the most preventable given its relationship to cigarette smoking.
  - Treatment is based on the histology and stage of the disease.
  - Small-cell and non–small-cell lung cancers are treated according to whether disease is limited (confined to one hemithorax and ipsilateral regional lymph nodes) or extensive stage.
  - Whenever possible, surgical resection should be attempted for non–small-cell lung cancer because it affords the best chance of cure.
  - **Small-cell lung cancer** is often responsible for a variety of paraneoplastic syndromes in addition to local symptoms.
    - For **limited disease,** combination chemotherapy and radiation therapy result in an 85%–90% response rate, a median survival of 12–18 months, and a cure in 5%–15% of patients.
    - With **extensive disease,** the median survival is 8–9 months, and cures are rare. For patients who achieve a complete remission with chemotherapy, **prophylactic whole-brain radiation therapy** has been shown to decrease the risk of central nervous system (CNS) metastases.[5] Radiation therapy to the chest as consolidation therapy may improve survival in limited disease but is not recommended in extensive disease except for palliation of local symptoms.
  - **Non–small-cell lung cancer** (NSCLC) survival rates after resection are improved with adjuvant chemotherapy with without radiation therapy.
    - For unresectable disease confined to the lung and regional lymph nodes, radiation therapy in combination with chemotherapy is the conventional treatment.
    - In patients with metastatic disease, cisplatin-based combination chemotherapy may modestly improve survival. **Erlotinib,** a tyrosine kinase inhibitor (TKI) targeting epidermal growth factor receptor (EGFR), is approved for NSCLC.
- **Gastrointestinal (GI) malignancies** commonly present with vague symptoms and are often advanced at the time of diagnosis.
  - **Esophageal cancers** are either squamous cell (associated with cigarette smoking and alcohol use) or adenocarcinoma (arising in Barrett's esophagus).
    - **Surgical resection of the esophagus** is recommended in small primary tumors and in selected patients after chemoradiation.

- **Local control** of unresectable cancers can be achieved with combined chemotherapy and radiation therapy.[6]
- Palliation of obstructive symptoms can be accomplished by radiation therapy, dilation, prosthetic tube placement, or laser therapy.
- **Gastric cancer** is usually adenocarcinoma and can be cured with surgery in the rare patient with localized disease.
    - Adjuvant chemotherapy and concurrent radiation have been shown to improve outcomes in surgically resected gastric cancer.[7]
    - Locally advanced but unresectable cancers may benefit from concomitant chemotherapy and radiation therapy. Chemotherapy may offer palliation for metastatic disease.
- **Colon and rectal adenocarcinomas** are primarily treated by surgical resection.
    - In all patients who are undergoing surgical resection of colon or rectal cancer, a preoperative **carcinoembryonic antigen** level should be measured and followed. A persistently elevated or increasing level may indicate residual or recurrent tumor.
    - A prolonged survival in patients with colon cancer and regional lymph node involvement is seen with administration of postoperative 5-fluorouracil (FU) and levamisole for 12 months or **FU and leucovorin** (LV) for 6 months.[8]
    - The addition of oxaliplatin to the traditional FU and leucovorin improves risk reduction in stages II and III colon cancer.[9]
    - **Rectal cancer** that arises below the peritoneal reflection commonly recurs locally after surgery alone; postoperative radiation therapy and FU are recommended.
    - A number of chemotherapy agents are available for the treatment of metastatic colorectal cancer. These include FU, irinotecan, capecitabine, and oxaliplatin. In metastatic disease, the addition of irinotecan to FU/LV produces a higher likelihood of response and possible survival advantage.[10]
    - Three monoclonal antibodies have been approved for the treatment of metastatic colon cancer. Bevacizumab targets vascular endothelial growth factor (VEGF). Both cetuximab and panitumumab target EGFR.
    - Selected patients with metastases confined to the liver may be candidates for liver resection.[11]
- **Anal cancer.** Chemotherapy with concurrent radiation therapy appears to result in a higher cure rate than surgical resection and usually preserves the anal sphincter and fecal continence.[12] Surgical resection should be used only as salvage therapy.

- **Genitourinary malignancies**
    - **Bladder cancer** in the United States is usually a transitional cell carcinoma. A variety of chemical carcinogens, including those in cigarette smoke, have been implicated.
        - **Unifocal tumors confined to the mucosa should be managed with cystoscopy** and transurethral resection or fulguration, repeated at approximately 3-month intervals; multifocal mucosal disease is treated with intravesicular bacillus Calmette-Guérin, thiotepa, or mitomycin-C.
        - **Locally invasive cancers should be resected.**
        - Adjuvant chemotherapy improves survival when regional lymph node involvement is confirmed in the cystectomy specimen.
        - In metastatic or recurrent disease, the highest response rates are seen with cisplatin-containing regimens.
    - **Prostate cancer** is the most common cancer in men besides nonmelanoma skin cancer.
        - **Prostate-specific antigen** is useful as a marker for recurrence, bulk of disease, and response to therapy and may detect asymptomatic early-stage disease.
        - Local control of the primary lesion can be achieved with either prostatectomy or radiation therapy.
        - In patients with metastatic disease, bilateral orchiectomy and LHRH analogs with or without an antiandrogen produce tumor regression in approximately 85% of patients for a median of 18–24 months.

- Disease that has relapsed after hormonal therapy may respond to withdrawal of that antiandrogen.[13]
- Anthracyclines, taxanes, vinblastine, and estramustine may be of palliative value in hormone-refractory disease.
- Anemia and bone pain dominate the advanced phases of this disease and are best relieved with transfusions, growth factors, and palliative radiation therapy.
- **Renal cell cancer** is treated by surgical resection, which may be curative if disease is localized; no effective adjuvant therapy is available.
  - Chemotherapy, interferon-α, and interleukin-2 have reported response rates of 15%–30%.
  - Two new agents, **sunitinib** and **sorafanib,** have been approved for the treatment of metastatic renal cell cancer. Both agents are multitargeted TKIs. Both appear more active and better tolerated than previously available agents.
- **Testicular cancer** is considered one of the most curable malignancies and should be treated aggressively. A patient suspected of having cancer of the testis should only have tissue obtained through an inguinal orchiectomy because a transscrotal incision facilitates tumor spread to the inguinal lymph nodes.
  - The initial evaluation should include **serum α-fetoprotein and β-human chorionic gonadotropin levels** and a computed tomography (CT) scan of the abdomen and pelvis.
  - Most patients with **seminoma** should be treated with radiation therapy.
  - In **nonseminomatous germ cell cancer,** a retroperitoneal lymph node dissection should be performed for staging, except in the instance of bulky abdominal disease or pulmonary metastasis.
  - If microscopic disease is identified at surgery, two alternatives are acceptable: two cycles of postoperative chemotherapy or observation until relapse occurs followed by institution of chemotherapy.
  - With gross **metastatic disease, cisplatin-based chemotherapy** is curative for most germ cell cancers. If tumor markers normalize after chemotherapy but a radiographic mass persists, exploratory surgery should be performed. The lesion proves to be residual cancer in approximately one third of the patients. Patients with residual cancer should receive additional chemotherapy.[14]

■ Gynecologic malignancies
- **Cervical cancer.** The recognized **risk factors** are multiparity, multiple sexual partners, and infection with human papillomavirus (HPV).
  - Carcinoma in situ and superficial disease can be treated by endocervical cone biopsy.
  - Microinvasive disease is treated with an abdominal hysterectomy.
  - Advanced local disease (invasion of the cervix or local extension) is initially treated with surgery or radiation therapy, or both. The addition of chemotherapy to radiation therapy postoperatively is associated with improved survival.[15]
  - Inoperable cancer can be controlled with radiation therapy; metastatic disease is treated with cisplatin-based chemotherapy.
  - **A vaccine for HPV has recently been approved** and is being administered to young women in hopes of reducing the rates of cervical carcinoma.
- **Ovarian cancer** is primarily a disease of postmenopausal women.
  - Because symptoms are uncommon with localized disease, most patients present with advanced local disease, malignant ascites, or peritoneal metastases.
  - **Surgical staging** and treatment include an abdominal hysterectomy, bilateral oophorectomy, lymph node sampling, omentectomy, peritoneal cytology, and removal of all gross tumor. If the tumor is localized to the ovary, the surgery may be curative and further treatment is not routinely recommended. However, if microscopic foci of cancer are identified, chemotherapy is administered postoperatively.
  - The serum marker **CA-125,** although not specific, is elevated in more than 80% of women with epithelial ovarian cancer and is a sensitive indicator of response.

- After a response is achieved, a **"second-look laparotomy"** is performed to restage and remove residual tumor. Approximately one-third of the patients who are in pathologic complete remission after a second-look laparotomy are cured. Those patients who have residual cancer should receive additional chemotherapy.
- **Endometrial cancer** risks include obesity, nulliparity, polycystic ovaries, and the use of unopposed estrogens (including tamoxifen). Patients generally present with vaginal bleeding. Surgery and radiation therapy are often curative.

- **Head and neck cancer** is usually a squamous cell cancer. It may arise in a variety of sites, each of which has a different natural history.
  - Early lesions can be cured with surgery, radiation therapy, or both.
  - Despite aggressive surgical and radiation therapy, approximately 65% of patients with head and neck cancer have uncontrolled local disease.
  - The addition of chemotherapy to radiation therapy improves the survival in patients with nasopharyngeal cancers and selected patients with other primary disease sites.[16]

- **Malignant melanoma** should be considered in any changing or enlarging nevus, and suspicious lesions should be removed by **excisional biopsy.** Subsequently, a wide local excision is performed to remove possible vertical and radial spread of tumor.
  - Deeper invasion is associated with a worse prognosis.
  - **High-dose interferon** prolongs the survival of selected high-risk resected patients.[17] Systemic disease may respond to dacarbazine, interferon-α, or interleukin-2 in 10%–30% of patients.

- **Sarcomas** are tumors arising from mesenchymal tissue and occur most commonly in soft tissue or bone. Initial evaluation should include a CT scan of the chest, as hematogenous spread to the lungs is common.
  - Prognosis for **soft tissue sarcoma** is primarily determined by tumor grade and not by the cell of origin.
  - Surgical resection should be performed when feasible and may be curative.
  - In low-grade tumors, local and regional recurrence is most common, and adjuvant radiation therapy may be of benefit. High-grade tumors often recur systemically, but no advantage to the routine use of adjuvant chemotherapy has been demonstrated.
  - In metastatic disease, doxorubicin, ifosfamide, and dacarbazine produce responses in 40%–55% of patients.
  - **Osteogenic sarcomas** are treated with surgical resection followed by adjuvant chemotherapy for 1 year. Treatment of isolated pulmonary metastasis by surgical resection is associated with long-term survival.
  - **Kaposi sarcoma** in an immunocompetent patient is generally a low-grade lesion of the lower extremities that is readily treated with local radiation therapy or vinblastine. When Kaposi sarcoma complicates organ transplantation or AIDS, it is more aggressive and may arise in visceral sites. Liposomal doxorubicin alone is as effective as combination chemotherapy for palliation.[18]

- **Cancer with an unknown primary site.** Approximately 5% of cancer patients present with symptoms of metastatic disease, but no primary tumor site is identifiable on physical examination, routine laboratory studies, or chest radiography.
- The histopathologic cell type and the site of the metastasis should direct a search for the primary lesion. Immunohistochemical stains may identify specific tissue antigens that help to define the origin of the tumor and guide subsequent therapy.
  - **Cervical adenopathy** suggests cancer of the lung, breast, head and neck, or lymphoma. In this case, initial evaluation usually includes panendoscopy (nasendoscopy, laryngopharyngoscopy, bronchoscopy, and esophagoscopy) and biopsy of any suspicious lesion before excision of the lymph node. If squamous cell carcinoma is identified, the patient is presumed to have primary head and neck cancer, and radiation therapy may be curative.
  - **Midline mass in the mediastinum or retroperitoneum.** In both sexes, a midline mass in the mediastinum or retroperitoneum may be an extragonadal germ cell cancer. Elevations in α-fetoprotein or β-human chorionic gonadotropin further suggest this diagnosis. This neoplasm is potentially curable.

THERAPY OF SELECTED LYMPHOMAS/LEUKEMIAS

- **Lymphoma** is usually diagnosed by biopsy of an enlarged lymph node.
  - **Staging** of Hodgkin's disease and non-Hodgkin's lymphoma is organized into four categories.
  - **Stage I** is disease localized to a single lymph node or group.
  - **Stage II** is disease involving more than one lymph node group but confined to one side of the diaphragm.
  - **Stage III** is disease in the lymph nodes or the spleen and occurs on both sides of the diaphragm.
  - **Stage IV** is disease involving the liver, lung, skin, or bone marrow.
  - **B symptoms** include fever above $38.5°C$, night sweats that require a change in clothes, or a 10% weight loss over 6 months. These symptoms suggest bulky disease and a worse prognosis.
  - **Hodgkin's disease** usually presents with cervical adenopathy and spreads in a predictable manner along lymph node groups.
    - Treatment is based on the presenting stage of the disease; the cell type is relatively unimportant in the natural history and prognosis.
    - **Initial evaluation** includes a CT scan of the chest, abdomen, and pelvis, and bilateral bone marrow biopsies to determine the clinical stage of the disease.
    - Exploratory laparotomy with splenectomy and liver biopsy is performed only if the findings will change the disease stage and treatment.
    - **Stages I and IIA** are treated with radiation therapy or a combination of chemotherapy and radiation.
    - **Stage IIIA** disease can be treated either by radiation therapy or chemotherapy, whereas all **stage IV** patients should receive combination chemotherapy.
    - When **B symptoms** are present, chemotherapy is recommended regardless of the stage.
  - **Non-Hodgkin's lymphoma** is classified as low, intermediate, or high grade based on the histologic type. Staging evaluation is the same as for Hodgkin's disease, but non-Hodgkin's lymphoma has a less predictable pattern of spread. Advanced-stage disease (stage III or IV) is very common and can usually be diagnosed by CT scan or bone marrow biopsy; exploratory laparotomy and lymphangiography are rarely necessary.
  - **Low-grade lymphoma** often involves the bone marrow at diagnosis, but the disease has an indolent course. Because this tumor is not curable with standard chemotherapy, treatment can be delayed until the patient is symptomatic ("watch and wait").
    - Radiation therapy or an alkylating agent (e.g., cyclophosphamide) can be used to ameliorate symptoms. Radiation therapy may produce a long-term complete remission in stage I or II disease.
    - **Rituximab** produces an objective response in approximately 50% of patients with follicular lymphoma without the usual toxicities of chemotherapy.
  - **Intermediate-grade lymphoma** has a more aggressive course, usually does not involve the bone marrow at diagnosis, and can be cured with chemotherapy. Complete response rates exceed 80%.
    - Features associated with a lower likelihood of cure include an elevated lactate dehydrogenase level, stage III/IV disease, age older than 60 years, more than one extranodal site, and poor performance status.
  - **High-grade lymphoma** (Burkitt's, lymphoblastic) includes the most aggressive subtypes and has a high frequency of CNS and bone marrow involvement.
    - **Cerebrospinal fluid (CSF) cytology** should be included as part of the initial evaluation.
    - **Combination chemotherapy is the mainstay of treatment** and should include CNS prophylaxis if the CSF is cytologically free of tumor. If tumor cells are seen in the CSF, additional therapy may be indicated.
    - Prophylaxis to prevent **tumor lysis syndrome** should be initiated before induction chemotherapy.
- **Acute leukemias** may present with manifestations of cytopenias, including fatigue and dyspnea (anemia), cutaneous or mucosal hemorrhage (thrombocytopenia), and

fever/infection (neutropenia). Patients may also present with leukemic infiltration of organs, manifested as lymphadenopathy, splenomegaly (more common in acute lymphocytic leukemia), gingival hyperplasia, and skin nodules (more common in acute myeloid leukemia).

■ Leukemic blasts are usually present in the blood.

■ Bone marrow aspiration/biopsy is performed to establish the diagnosis and often shows nearly complete replacement by blasts.

■ **Flow cytometry and cytogenetics** must be performed on the bone marrow aspirate for classification and to provide prognostic information.

■ **Acute myeloid leukemia** constitutes approximately 80% of adult acute leukemia.
  - Approximately 50%–80% of patients achieve complete remission with induction chemotherapy that includes cytarabine (cytosine arabinoside [ara-C]) and daunorubicin.
  - Consolidation is given with at least one additional cycle of chemotherapy, which is typically ara-C at a dose of 10–30 times that used for induction (high-dose ara-C). High-dose ara-C consolidation results in cure in approximately 30%–40% of patients younger than 60 years.
  - Pretreatment factors associated with a low (<10%) chance for cure include preceding myelodysplastic syndrome; prior exposure to radiation, benzene, or chemotherapy; and adverse cytogenetic abnormalities.
    - For these high-risk patients, allogeneic stem cell transplant in first remission increases the likelihood of cure.

■ **Acute promyelocytic leukemia** is characterized by a chromosomal translocation (t[15;17]) that results in a hybrid protein (pml-rar).
  - Treatment with oral tretinoin (*all-trans* retinoic acid) results in complete remission in >90% of patients. After consolidation chemotherapy, approximately 75% of patients are cured.

■ **Acute lymphocytic leukemia** is predominantly a disease of childhood, with only 25% of all cases occurring in patients older than the age of 15 years.
  - For adults, induction and consolidation involve treatment with multiple chemotherapeutic agents over a period of approximately 6 months followed by at least 18 months of lower-dose maintenance chemotherapy.
  - To prevent CNS relapse, patients receive intrathecal (IT) chemotherapy and either cranial radiation or CNS penetrating chemotherapy.
  - Approximately 60%–80% of adults achieve complete remission, with about 30%–40% being cured; increasing age, higher white blood cell (WBC) count, and longer time to remission are associated with reduced survival.
  - Cytogenetics are crucial in determining prognosis, and allogeneic stem cell transplantation during the first remission should be considered in patients with a poor prognosis.

■ **Chronic lymphocytic leukemia (CLL)** usually presents with lymphocytosis, lymphadenopathy, and splenomegaly. Malignant cells resemble mature lymphocytes.
  - Treatment is similar to that for **low-grade lymphoma** except that fludarabine appears to be more active than alkylating agents.
  - Median survival is approximately 6–8 years; anemia and thrombocytopenia are associated with shortened survival. As in low-grade lymphoma, patients are treated for control of symptoms or cytopenias.
  - Because CLL is accompanied by immunodeficiency, **life-threatening infections may occur**. Therefore, febrile patients must be evaluated carefully.
  - Immune hemolytic anemia or immune thrombocytopenia may develop as complications of CLL. Treatment of these conditions is with glucocorticoids (e.g., prednisone, 1 mg/kg PO daily) or chemotherapy, or both. CLL may transform to an intermediate- or high-grade lymphoma (Richter transformation).

■ **Chronic myelogenous leukemia (CML)** presents with leukocytosis and a left shift, as well as splenomegaly. Thrombocytosis, basophilia, and eosinophilia are also common.
  - The diagnosis is confirmed by demonstration of the **Philadelphia chromosome** (t9:22), which results in production of a hybrid protein (bcr-abl).

- During the **stable phase** of the disease, leukocytosis, thrombocytosis, and splenomegaly can be controlled for several years with oral hydroxyurea, and most patients are asymptomatic.
- **Acute leukemic transformation (blast phase)** is inevitable and unpredictable, with a median time to transformation of 5–7 years. Blast phase is highly resistant to treatment and is usually fatal.
- For younger patients (40–50 years old) with HLA-identical siblings, allogeneic stem cell transplantation performed in stable phase within 1 year of diagnosis is the treatment of choice, resulting in a 50%–70% likelihood of cure.
- For older patients and for those without an HLA-identical sibling, options include unrelated donor transplant or therapy with interferon-α. The latter agent delays blast phase in some patients.
- **Imatinib** is an orally administered medication designed specifically to inhibit the bcr-abl tyrosine kinase. Because imatinib is more active and has far fewer toxicities than interferon, it is currently the first-line therapy for this disease. Even blast-phase CML or Philadelphia chromosome–positive acute leukemia may respond to imatinib. Responses in this setting are generally of relatively short duration.
- **Hairy-cell leukemia** represents 2%–3% of all adult leukemias. Clinical presentation includes splenomegaly, pancytopenia, and infection.
  - Patients are at increased risk for bacterial, viral, and fungal infections and have a unique susceptibility to atypical mycobacterial infections.
  - Bone marrow biopsy reveals infiltration by cells that have prominent cytoplasmic projections.
  - A single 7-day course of **chlorodeoxyadenosine** produces remission in more than 90% of patients. Although this drug is not curative, 5-year progression-free survival exceeds 50%.
- **Multiple myeloma** is a malignant plasma cell disorder that is usually accompanied by a serum or urine paraprotein, or both. Presenting manifestations may include hypercalcemia, anemia, lytic bone lesions with bone pain, and acute renal failure.
  - The **initial evaluation** should include a radiographic bone survey, bone marrow aspiration and biopsy, serum and urine protein electrophoresis, β_2-microglobulin, and quantitative immunoglobulins.
  - Treatment generally includes a combination of an oral alkylating agent (i.e., melphalan) and prednisone or vincristine/doxorubicin/dexamethasone.
  - Local radiation therapy can be used to relieve painful bone lesions, and **zoledronic acid**, 4 mg IV every month, decreases skeletal complications.
  - **Thalidomide**, an immunomodulatory agent, has been shown to be effective in multiple myeloma. Because thalidomide can cause severe fetal malformations, prescribing this medication requires participation in a prescriber program. Combinations of dexamethasone and thalidomide are also active in the treatment of multiple myeloma.
  - **Bortezomib** (Velcade), a proteasome inhibitor that degrades ubiquitinated proteins, has recently been approved for the treatment of multiple myeloma that has progressed despite two previous treatments. Toxicities of bortezomib are primarily thrombocytopenia and neuropathy.
  - After induction chemotherapy, consolidation with high-dose therapy and autologous stem cell transplant improves survival.

HEMATOPOIETIC STEM CELL TRANSPLANTATION

GENERAL PRINCIPLES

- Hematopoietic stem cell transplantation involves IV infusion of either hematopoietic progenitors (collected from the bone marrow by aspiration from the iliac crests) or peripheral blood stem cells (collected by apheresis after treatment of the donor with granulocyte colony-stimulating factor [G-CSF] or granulocyte-macrophage colony-stimulating factor [GM-CSF]).

Classification

- **Allogeneic** stem cells are collected from another person (the donor), whereas **autologous** stem cells are collected from the patient. For autologous transplant, peripheral blood stem cells have largely replaced bone marrow as the source of progenitors because hematologic recovery is more rapid.
- **Allogeneic stem cell transplant.** HLA-matched siblings are the most common donors, but matched unrelated donors can be identified for many patients through the National Bone Marrow Donor Registry.
  - Allogeneic transplants can be performed to restore normal hematopoiesis or immune function in patients with aplastic anemia, immunodeficiency, or hemoglobinopathies and are also used to treat resistant leukemia and lymphoma. For patients with resistant acute leukemia, allogeneic transplant is generally favored, whereas for those with resistant lymphoma, autologous transplant is usually preferred.
  - The **"preparative regimen"** is given immediately before transplant and includes chemotherapy with or without total body irradiation. For patients with nonmalignant conditions, the preparative regimen provides immunosuppression, which is needed for engraftment. For patients with resistant malignancy, the preparative regimen is designed to promote engraftment and to kill tumor cells.
  - Unlike autologous transplant, allogeneic transplants may be accompanied by a **graft versus tumor effect,** which appears to be a very important part of curing leukemia or lymphoma.
- **Autologous stem cell transplantation.** Eradication of malignancy is entirely the result of the preparative regimen, because no graft versus tumor effect can occur.
  - The major advantage of autologous transplant is that graft versus host disease (GVHD) does not occur; therefore, the risk of death from transplant-related complications is <5%.
  - Most autologous transplants are performed for relapsed lymphoma. In patients with relapsed large-cell lymphoma who achieve at least a partial response to salvage chemotherapy, cure can be achieved in 30%–50%.
  - Autologous transplant also prolongs the survival of patients with multiple myeloma and is a viable option for individuals with acute leukemia in first remission who lack a compatible sibling donor.

Complications

- **Complications of transplantation** may be the result of high-dose therapy, pancytopenia, immunodeficiency, or GVHD.
  - **Infections.** After the preparative regimen, 7–10 days of profound pancytopenia (absolute neutrophil count <100, platelets <10,000) develops in all patients. During this time nearly all patients experience fever and require empiric broad-spectrum antibiotic therapy.
    - Patients who are seropositive for herpes simplex virus should also receive acyclovir prophylaxis until neutrophil recovery.
    - **G-CSF or GM-CSF** is usually given starting on the day after transplant until neutrophil recovery.
    - Patients who have undergone autologous transplant recover immune function within 3–6 months. However, patients who undergo allogeneic transplant have profound and prolonged impairment of humoral and cell-mediated immunity that persists until GVHD resolves. Therefore, **patients who are febrile after allogeneic transplant should be cultured and immediately receive IV broad-spectrum antibiotics** even if they are not neutropenic.
    - After allogeneic transplant, patients receive long-term prophylaxis for varicella-zoster virus with acyclovir and for *Pneumocystis* with trimethoprim/sulfamethoxazole. Patients are also at risk for reactivation and systemic infection with cytomegalovirus (CMV). One strategy for preventing overt infection is to perform shell vial cultures or polymerase chain reaction assays on blood

weekly or biweekly during the period of maximal risk (1–6 months posttransplant).

- Ganciclovir or foscarnet is given if testing is positive for CMV. Patients who have undergone allogeneic transplant require reimmunization.

■ **GVHD** is an immunologic response by the donor to recipient antigens and is the major complication of allogeneic transplantation. Overall, GVHD accounts for most of the 20%–30% mortality that accompanies matched sibling transplant, with death usually resulting from infection.

- GVHD within the first 100 days of transplant (**acute GVHD**) produces a skin rash, diarrhea, and liver dysfunction. Despite prophylaxis with cyclosporine and methotrexate, significant acute GVHD occurs in 30%–50% of transplants from matched sibling donors.
- **Chronic GVHD** occurs more than 100 days after transplant and resembles an autoimmune disorder with protean manifestations, including keratoconjunctivitis sicca, lichenoid changes of the buccal mucosa, and sclerodermatous skin changes.
- After allogeneic transplant, donor T cells can mediate immunologic destruction of residual tumor cells. This "graft versus tumor effect" is unique to allogeneic transplant and plays a key role in eradicating residual malignancy.

■ **Veno-occlusive disease** (VOD) occurs in 1%–5% of patients, usually within 21 days of treatment. Risk factors include extensive prior therapy and elevated transaminase values before transplant.

- Manifestations include hyperbilirubinemia, ascites, tender hepatomegaly, and fluid retention.
- In its severe form, VOD is almost uniformly fatal. Treatment options are limited.

■ **Pulmonary complications.** CMV pneumonia usually occurs within 6 months of allogeneic transplant in patients who are seropositive or who receive transplants from seropositive donors. It is uncommon after autologous transplant. Treatment is with ganciclovir or foscarnet.

- **Interstitial pneumonitis** may complicate total body radiation or high-dose chemotherapy and is manifested by cough, dyspnea, and interstitial infiltrates that present 1–3 months after transplant. Prior chest radiotherapy is a risk factor; treatment with prednisone usually results in rapid and long-term improvement.

 COMPLICATIONS OF CANCER

■ Complications related to tumor mass

  ■ **Brain metastasis.** Patients with parenchymal brain metastasis may present with headache, mental status changes, weakness, or focal neurologic deficits. Papilledema is observed in only 25% of patients.

   - In individuals with malignancy, a CT scan of the head showing one or more round, contrast-enhancing lesions surrounded by edema is usually sufficient for the diagnosis. If cancer has not been diagnosed previously, tissue should be obtained from the brain lesion or a more accessible site before radiation therapy is initiated.
   - Therapy with **dexamethasone,** 10 mg IV or PO, should be initiated to decrease cerebral edema and should be continued at a dosage of 4–6 mg PO q6h throughout the course of radiation therapy, or longer if symptoms related to edema persist.
   - Subsequent therapy depends on the number and location of the brain lesions as well as the prognosis of the underlying cancer.
   - Patients with a chemotherapy-responsive neoplasm and a solitary accessible lesion should be considered for surgical resection. **All patients who have not received prior radiation therapy should be given whole-brain radiation therapy.**

  ■ **Meningeal carcinomatosis** should be suspected in a cancer patient with headache or cranial neuropathies. This pattern of spread is most often seen with lung or breast cancer, melanoma, or lymphoma; the diagnosis is confirmed by cytology of the CSF.

- A CT scan of the head should be performed to rule out parenchymal metastases or hydrocephalus before a lumbar puncture is performed.
- Local radiation therapy or IT chemotherapy may provide temporary relief of symptoms. Meningeal lymphoma may respond to IV ara-C.

- **Spinal cord compression** is most commonly caused by hematogenous spread of cancer to the vertebral bodies followed by expansion into the spinal canal or ischemia of the spinal cord.
  - The most common malignancies causing spinal cord compression are breast, lung, and prostate cancer, but **the diagnosis should be considered in any patient with cancer who complains of back pain.**
  - Treatment involves urgent neurosurgical and radiation oncology consultation in addition to high-dose corticosteroid therapy. **MRI** is the imaging modality of choice to assess for acute cord compression.

- **Superior vena cava obstruction** is most commonly caused by cancers that arise in or spread to the mediastinum, such as lymphoma or lung cancer. The compressed superior vena cava leads to swelling of the face or trunk, chest pain, cough, and shortness of breath. Dilated superficial veins of the chest, neck, or sublingual area suggest an engorged collateral circulation. The presence of a mass on chest radiograph or CT scan usually confirms the diagnosis.
  - **A mediastinal mass may compromise the airway.** If the histologic origin of the obstruction is unknown, tissue can be obtained for diagnosis via bronchoscopy or mediastinoscopy. Therapy is directed at the underlying disease.
  - Chemotherapy should be administered through a vein that is not obstructed by the lesion.
  - Neoplasms that are not responsive to chemotherapy are treated with radiation therapy.[19]

- **Malignant effusions**
  - **Malignant pericardial effusions** most commonly result from cancer of the breast or lung. Initial presentations range from dyspnea to acute cardiovascular collapse from cardiac tamponade requiring emergency pericardiocentesis.
    - After cardiovascular stabilization, some patients may improve with treatment if the tumor is chemotherapy sensitive.
    - When the pericardial effusion is a complication of uncontrolled disease, palliation can be achieved by pericardiocentesis with sclerosis; the effusion should be completely drained, followed by instillation of 30–60 mg bleomycin through the drainage catheter, which is subsequently clamped for 10 minutes and then withdrawn.
    - Subxiphoid pericardiotomy can be performed in patients whose effusions do not respond to other treatment.
  - **Malignant pleural effusions** develop as a result of pleural invasion by tumor or obstruction of lymphatic drainage.
    - When systemic control is impossible and reaccumulation of fluid occurs rapidly after drainage, removal of the fluid followed by instillation of a sclerosing agent into the pleural space is recommended. Resistant effusions can be controlled with pleurectomy or placement of an indwelling pleural catheter, which can drain pleural fluid as needed.
  - **Malignant ascites** is most commonly caused by peritoneal carcinomatosis and is best controlled by systemic chemotherapy. Therapeutic paracenteses can provide symptomatic relief. Intraperitoneal instillation of chemotherapy has been used but is not routinely recommended.

- **Bone metastases** may result in spontaneous fracture. Prophylactic surgical pinning and radiation therapy may be indicated. Bisphosphonates may also protect against skeletal complications from myeloma and breast cancer.[20]

- **Paraneoplastic syndromes** are complications of malignancy that are not directly caused by a tumor mass effect and are presumed to be mediated by either secreted tumor products or the development of autoantibodies. Paraneoplastic syndromes can affect virtually every organ system, and in most cases, successful treatment of the underlying malignancy eliminates these effects.

- Metabolic complications
    - **Hypercalcemia** is the most common metabolic complication in malignancy and can cause mental status changes, GI discomfort, arrhythmias, and constipation (see Chapter 3, Fluid and Electrolyte Management).
    - **Syndrome of inappropriate antidiuretic hormone (SIADH)** should be considered in a euvolemic cancer patient with unexplained hyponatremia. Although a variety of neoplasms have been described in association with SIADH, small-cell lung cancer is most often responsible. If chemotherapy is ineffective, radiation therapy may decrease the tumor mass and relieve symptoms.
    - **Cancer anorexia and cachexia** refers to the clinical syndrome of anorexia, distortion of taste perception, and loss of muscle mass. The asthenic appearance of patients is more often related to tumor type than to tumor burden. **Megestrol acetate,** 160 mg PO daily, has been used as an appetite stimulant and results in weight gain in some patients.[21] Other appetite stimulants include corticosteroids, cannabinoids, and promotility agents such as metoclopramide.
- Neuromuscular complications
    - **Polymyositis and dermatomyositis.** Dermatomyositis, more often than polymyositis, has been associated with a variety of malignancies, including non–small-cell lung cancer and colon, ovarian, and prostate cancers. In some patients, successful treatment of the underlying malignancy has resulted in resolution of the symptoms. An exhaustive search for a malignancy is not recommended because a primary malignancy is found in <20% of patients.[22]
    - **Lambert-Eaton myasthenic syndrome** is characterized by proximal muscle weakness, decreased or absent deep tendon reflexes, and autonomic dysfunction. Electromyography using high-frequency nerve stimulation may show posttetanic potentiation.
        - Small-cell lung cancer is most often associated with this syndrome, and effective chemotherapy may result in improvement. Worsening symptoms have been reported with the use of calcium channel antagonists; these agents are contraindicated in this syndrome.[23]
- **Hematologic complications.** Although cytopenias occur more often as a complication of treatment or marrow involvement with cancer, elevated counts may be explained by paraneoplastic syndromes.
    - **Erythrocytosis** is a rare complication of hepatoma, renal cell cancer, and benign tumors of the kidney, uterus, and cerebellum. Debulking the tumor with surgery or radiation therapy generally results in resolution of the erythrocytosis. Occasionally, therapeutic phlebotomy is indicated.
    - **Granulocytosis** (leukemoid reaction) in the absence of infection occurs in cancer that arises in the stomach, lung, pancreas, brain, and lymphoma. Because the neutrophils are mature and seldom exceed $100,000/mm^3$, complications are rare and intervention is generally unnecessary.
    - **Thrombocytosis** in patients with cancer may be caused by splenectomy, iron deficiency, acute hemorrhage, or inflammation; treatment is usually not necessary.
- **Thromboembolic complications.** Mucin-secreting adenocarcinomas of the GI tract and lung cancer have been associated with a "hypercoagulable state," resulting in recurrent venous and arterial thromboembolism.
    - Nonbacterial thrombotic (marantic) endocarditis, usually involving the mitral valve, may also occur.
    - Heparin anticoagulation or low molecular weight heparin should be instituted, as well as treatment of the underlying cancer. Long-term warfarin with a target international normalized ratio of 2–3 or daily low molecular weight heparin is recommended to prevent subsequent thrombi.[24]
- **Glomerular injury** resulting in renal failure has been observed as a paraneoplastic syndrome. **Minimal change disease** is often associated with lymphoma, especially Hodgkin's disease; membranous glomerulonephritis is more often seen with solid tumors. The process can be reversed with treatment of the underlying cancer.
- **Clubbing of the fingers** and **hypertrophic osteoarthropathy** (polyarthritis and periostitis of long bones) are most often observed in non–small-cell lung cancer but are also

seen with lesions that are metastatic to the mediastinum. Some improvement in the osteoarthropathy can be achieved with nonsteroidal anti-inflammatory drugs, but definitive therapy requires treatment of the underlying malignancy.

- **Fever** may accompany lymphoma, renal cell cancer, and hepatic metastasis. Once an infectious etiology for the fever has been excluded, nonsteroidal anti-inflammatory drugs (e.g., ibuprofen, 400 mg PO q6h, or indomethacin, 25–50 mg PO tid) may provide symptomatic relief.

PRINCIPLES OF CHEMOTHERAPY

- **Administration of chemotherapeutic drugs.** The advice of an oncologist and precise adherence to a treatment plan are mandatory because of the low therapeutic index of chemotherapeutic agents.
- The dosage of chemotherapy is usually based on body surface area; for some agents, dosage is determined by body weight and should be adjusted when changes in body weight occur.
- An assessment of the patient disease status, determination of side effects from the previous treatment, and a CBC should be obtained before each cycle of chemotherapy.
- Drug dosages usually must be adjusted for the following conditions: (a) neutropenia, (b) thrombocytopenia, (c) stomatitis, (d) diarrhea, or (e) limited metabolic capacity for the drug.
- **Route of administration**
  - **Oral drug administration** may be accompanied by nausea and vomiting and may require antiemetic therapy. For some agents, oral absorption is erratic and parenteral administration is preferred.
  - **IV drug administration** should be performed by experienced personnel. Care should be taken to ensure free flow of fluid to the vein, and adequate blood return should be verified before instillation of chemotherapy. Infusions should be through a large-caliber, upper extremity vein. When possible, veins of the antecubital fossa, wrist, dorsum of the hand, and arm ipsilateral to an axillary lymph node dissection should be avoided.
    - In patients with poor peripheral venous access or those who require many doses of chemotherapy, **indwelling venous catheter devices** should be considered.
  - **Intrathecal chemotherapy** is administered for the treatment of meningeal carcinomatosis or as CNS prophylaxis. Side effects include acute arachnoiditis, subacute motor dysfunction, and progressive neurologic deterioration (leukoencephalopathy). Impaired cognitive function and leukoencephalopathy occur more often when IT chemotherapy is combined with whole-brain radiation.
    - **Methotrexate,** 10–12 mg, is diluted in 5 mL preservative-free nonbacteriostatic isotonic solution. Before administration, 5–10 mL CSF should be allowed to drain; methotrexate is then injected into the spinal canal over 5–10 minutes.
    - To decrease the risk of arachnoiditis, patients should remain in a supine position for 15 minutes after the infusion is completed.
    - Slow-release cytarabine, 50 mg, or ara-C, 50–100 mg in 5–10 mL diluent, can be administered in a similar manner.[25]
  - **Intracavitary instillation** of chemotherapy may be useful in some circumstances. Thiotepa, 30–60 mg, is commonly instilled in the bladder for the treatment of bladder carcinoma. Doxorubicin and cisplatin have been given through an implanted peritoneal catheter for the treatment of peritoneal metastasis.
  - **Intra-arterial chemotherapy** is advocated as a method of achieving high drug concentrations at specific tumor sites. Although it is of theoretical advantage, there are no absolute indications for chemotherapy administered by this route.

CHEMOTHERAPEUTIC MEDICATIONS

- **Chemotherapeutic agents.** Class-specific or unique side effects are described here.
  - **Antimetabolites** exert antitumor activity by acting as pseudosubstrates for essential enzymatic reactions. Their greatest toxicity occurs in tissues that are actively replicating (e.g., GI mucosa, hematopoietic cells).
    - **Ara-C** is an analog of deoxycytidine that is most useful in hematologic neoplasms. In standard doses, myelosuppression and GI toxicity are dose limiting. In high doses, conjunctivitis is common, and prophylaxis with dexamethasone eye drops, two drops in each eye tid, should be administered. **Cerebellar ataxia, pancreatitis, and hepatitis** may also develop. If cerebellar dysfunction occurs during treatment, ara-C must be discontinued.
    - **FU** is a pyrimidine analog that is administered as an injection or as a continuous infusion.
      - When it is administered as a bolus injection, **myelosuppression is dose limiting.**
      - With infusion, stomatitis and diarrhea are dose limiting. Cerebellar ataxia has been reported with both schedules and requires discontinuation of the drug.
      - Chest pain ascribed to coronary artery vasospasm may occur with infusions and, if suspected, should be treated with a calcium channel antagonist (e.g., nifedipine) or by discontinuing the chemotherapy.[26]
      - FU can be administered over 6–8 weeks and is limited by the development of a palmar–plantar dermatologic toxicity (the **hand–foot syndrome** can be palliated with vitamin B_6, 150 mg/d). **LV** can be coadministered with FU to potentiate cytotoxicity; diarrhea is dose limiting.[27]
    - **Methotrexate** is an inhibitor of dihydrofolate reductase and has numerous toxicities. Mucositis is dose limiting.
      - **Prolonged reabsorption.** Methotrexate is polyglutamated, and these metabolites accumulate in effusions to produce substantial toxicity. Patients with effusions should either have the fluid drained before receiving methotrexate or have the dosage drastically reduced.
      - **Interstitial pneumonitis,** unrelated to cumulative dose and associated with a peripheral eosinophilia, may occur. It should be treated with glucocorticoids (e.g., prednisone, 1 mg/kg PO daily or equivalent) and precludes additional use of methotrexate.
      - **Hepatitis** may occur with long-term oral administration but may also occur after a single high dose.
      - **High-dose methotrexate** may be associated with crystalline nephropathy and renal failure. Urine alkalinization with sodium bicarbonate should be maintained to minimize this risk. **LV** is used to "rescue" normal tissue after high-dose methotrexate. The dose depends on the amount of methotrexate used, but the usual dosage is 5–25 mg IV or PO q6h for 8–12 doses, or until the serum methotrexate concentration is <50 nM.
    - **6-Mercaptopurine** is a purine analog that is partially metabolized by xanthine oxidase. To avoid increased toxicity, the dose of 6-mercaptopurine should be decreased by 75% in patients taking allopurinol. Hepatic cholestasis has also been observed.
    - **Fludarabine** is an adenosine monophosphate analog that produces myelosuppression.[28]
    - **Cladribine (2-chlorodeoxyadenosine)** is a purine substrate analog that is resistant to degradation by adenosine deaminase. Myelosuppression is predictable.[29]
    - **Gemcitabine** is a nucleoside analog that may produce fever, edema, flulike symptoms, and rash. Pneumonitis is an uncommon complication.
  - **Alkylating agents** are useful in a wide variety of malignancies. These drugs cause DNA cross linking and strand breaks. Most alkylating agents are cytotoxic to resting and dividing cells. Patients should be counseled that irreversible sterility may develop after treatment with alkylating agents. Chlorambucil, cyclophosphamide, melphalan, and mechlorethamine have been implicated in the development of acute myeloid leukemia and myelodysplasia 3–10 years after treatment.

- **Busulfan** can cause interstitial pneumonitis and gynecomastia. A reversible syndrome resembling Addison disease may develop with long-term daily oral administration.
- **Chlorambucil** is a well-tolerated orally administered drug. Myelosuppression is dose limiting and usually readily reversible.
- **Cyclophosphamide** can cause hemorrhagic cystitis; therefore, adequate hydration to maintain urine output is required during treatment. Oral cyclophosphamide should be given early in the day to ensure adequate hydration. High-dose cyclophosphamide is used as a preparative agent before stem cell transplantation; at these doses a hemorrhagic myocarditis can occur.
- **Dacarbazine** can produce a flulike syndrome consisting of fever, myalgias, facial flushing, malaise, and marked elevations of hepatic enzymes.
- **Ifosfamide** is chemically similar to cyclophosphamide, but the incidence of hemorrhagic cystitis is much higher (occurring in 20%–30% of treated patients). Administration of 2-mercaptoethanesulfonate (mesna) is recommended to lower the incidence of cystitis. Ifosfamide can also cause neurologic toxicity, including seizures.
- **Mechlorethamine (nitrogen mustard)** is a skin irritant; protective gloves and eyewear must be used during drug preparation and administration. Development of a drug rash does not prevent further use of this agent.
- **Melphalan** is available in oral and injectable forms. An idiosyncratic interstitial pneumonitis may occur, and, although usually reversible, it precludes further use of the drug.
- **Nitrosoureas (carmustine [BCNU] and lomustine [CCNU])** are lipid soluble and penetrate the blood-brain barrier. BCNU is usually administered in an ethanol solution, and toxicity from the vehicle, including giddiness, flushing, and phlebitis, may occur. Because delayed myelosuppression occurs 6–8 weeks after treatment and may be cumulative, these agents are commonly given at 8-week intervals.
- **Temozolomide** is an oral alkylating agent with activity in primary and metastatic brain tumors.
- **Thiotepa** can be administered IV with bone marrow rescue. When used intravesically, 60–90 mg is administered in 60–100 mL of water and instilled over 2 hours.

- **Antitumor antibiotics** intercalate adjacent DNA nucleotides, interrupting replication and transcription to cause strand breaks; they are cell cycle nonspecific.
- **Anthracycline antibiotics are associated with a cardiomyopathy** consisting of intractable CHF and dysrhythmias. With doxorubicin, this complication is seen in approximately 2% of patients who receive a **cumulative lifetime dose of 550 mg/m^2**. The incidence increases dramatically at higher cumulative doses. Concomitant cyclophosphamide or previous chest irradiation may potentiate this toxicity. As the cumulative dose approaches 450–550 mg/m^2, serial radionuclide ventriculography should be performed, and the anthracycline should be discontinued if LV function is compromised. Myocardial damage is related to peak serum concentrations and cumulative dosage; longer (96-hour) infusions have allowed for higher cumulative dosages.
- The cardioprotectant **dexrazoxane** has been shown to decrease the incidence and severity of the cardiomyopathy associated with doxorubicin.[30]
  - **Daunorubicin** is used in the treatment of acute leukemia. Bone marrow suppression is expected, and the dose-limiting toxicity is usually mucositis. Red urine may be caused by the drug and its metabolites.
  - **Doxorubicin** toxicity is similar to that of daunorubicin, although this drug has a broader spectrum of activity. **Liposomal doxorubicin** is indicated for Kaposi sarcoma and has similar toxicities.
  - **Mitoxantrone** is structurally similar to doxorubicin and daunorubicin but is associated with less cardiac toxicity. Mucositis and myelosuppression are dose limiting; a bluish discoloration of the urine and sclera may occur.
  - **Idarubicin** is more rapidly taken up in cells than other anthracyclines. Toxicity is similar to that of daunorubicin.

- **Bleomycin** is useful in combination chemotherapy because it is rarely myelo-suppressive. **A test dose, 1–2 mg SC, should be administered before full doses are instituted** because severe allergic reactions with hypotension may occur, especially in patients with lymphoma. **Interstitial pneumonitis,** which occasionally results in irreversible pulmonary fibrosis, is more common in patients with underlying pulmonary disease or previous lung irradiation or those who received a cumulative dose of 200 mg/m^2. Pulmonary symptoms and chest radiographs should be monitored.
- **Mitomycin-C** is associated with delayed myelosuppression that worsens with repeated use of the drug. Interstitial pneumonitis has also been observed. The **hemolytic–uremic syndrome** has been reported, is exacerbated by red blood cell (RBC) transfusions, and should be suspected in patients with sudden onset of a microangiopathic hemolytic anemia and renal failure.
- **2-Deoxycoformycin** (Pentostatin) is isolated from *Streptomyces* and acts as an inhibitor of adenosine deaminase. Myelosuppression is the chief toxicity.

- **Plant alkaloids** are naturally occurring nitrogenous bases. Most inhibit cell division through inhibition of mitotic spindle formation.
  - **Vincristine** often causes a **dose-limiting neuropathy.** Paresthesias followed by loss of deep tendon reflexes are the usual manifestations. Neuritic pain, jaw pain, diplopia, constipation, abdominal pain, and an adynamic ileus occur less often. Other adverse effects include SIADH and Raynaud phenomenon.
  - **Vinblastine** is less neurotoxic than vincristine; dosage is usually limited by myelo-suppression. At high doses, myalgias, obstipation, and transient hepatitis may occur.
  - **Etoposide (VP-16).** The major dose-limiting toxicity is myelosuppression.
  - **Teniposide (VM-26)** is a semisynthetic derivative of podophyllotoxin. Toxicities include myelosuppression, hypersensitivity reactions, alopecia, and hypotension.
  - **Paclitaxel (Taxol)** has a unique antitubulin mechanism that disrupts microtubule assembly. Because paclitaxel is dissolved in Cremophor, anaphylactoid reactions may occur and are partially related to the rate of infusion.
    - All patients should be premedicated with dexamethasone and histamine-1 (H$_1$) and H$_2$ blockers. In addition, myelosuppression, arthralgias, neuropathy, and arrhythmias may occur. An albumin-bound nanoparticle formulation of paclitaxel is now available (**Abraxane**). The albumin binding allows the drug to be delivered without the Cremophor solvent and reduces solvent-related toxicities.
  - **Docetaxel (Taxotere)** can be administered more rapidly than paclitaxel without anaphylactoid reactions. Dexamethasone, 8 mg bid for 3 days beginning the day before chemotherapy, is administered to prevent third-space fluid collections.
  - **Navelbine** may produce pain in the IV injection site.
- **Platinum-containing agents** act as intercalators, causing single- and double-strand breaks in DNA.
  - **Cisplatin** produces severe nausea and vomiting; aggressive antiemetic therapy is mandatory (see Table 20-3). The patient should be aggressively volume expanded with 1 L isotonic saline administered over 4–6 hours before and after chemotherapy to prevent renal toxicity. The dosage of cisplatin should be reduced for patients with renal insufficiency and should be withheld if the serum creatinine is >3 mg/dL.
    - Other toxicities include **hypomagnesemia and ototoxicity.**
    - Pretreatment with **amifostine** may reduce the cumulative hematologic, renal, and neurologic toxicities.[31]
  - **Carboplatin** is a cisplatin analog with less neurotoxicity, ototoxicity, and nephrotoxicity than cisplatin; myelosuppression is the dose-limiting toxicity.
  - **Oxaliplatin** is a recently approved platinum-containing agent with activity in colorectal cancer. It is associated with a sensory neuropathy.
- Other agents
  - **Hydroxyurea,** an oral agent that inhibits ribonucleotide reductase, is used in the management of the chronic phase of CML and other myeloproliferative diseases.

The dosage is adjusted according to the peripheral blood neutrophil and platelet count.

- **L-Asparaginase** hydrolyzes asparagine, depleting cells of an essential substrate in protein synthesis. Allergic or anaphylactic reactions may occur. Other toxicities include hemorrhagic pancreatitis, hepatic failure with depression of clotting factors, and encephalopathy.
- **Procarbazine** is an oral agent that inhibits DNA, RNA, and protein synthesis. It is a monoamine oxidase inhibitor, and therefore tricyclic antidepressants, sympathomimetic agents, and tyramine-containing foods should be avoided. Procarbazine has a disulfiramlike effect, and therefore ethanol should not be ingested while this medication is being administered.
- **Topotecan** is a topoisomerase I inhibitor. Myelosuppression is dose limiting.
- **Irinotecan** has a similar mechanism of action to topotecan. It can produce severe diarrhea, which can be treated with atropine and loperamide.

- **Hormonal agents** lack direct cytotoxicity. In general, they have few serious adverse effects. In disseminated disease, eventual resistance to hormonal agents should be anticipated.
  - **Tamoxifen** is a selective ER modulator. It acts as an ER antagonist in some tissues including breast and as an ER agonist on others. The usual dosage is 10 mg PO bid.
    - After 7–14 days of treatment, a **hormone flare** (increasing bone pain, erythema, and hypercalcemia) occurs in approximately 5% of women with ER-positive breast cancer and bone metastases. The symptoms abate over 7–10 days, and 75% of these patients respond to tamoxifen; therefore, palliation of pain, control of hypercalcemia, and continuation of the drug are recommended.
    - Long-term administration of tamoxifen is not associated with a systemic antiestrogen effect (vaginal atrophy, osteoporosis, or increased risk of heart disease) but is related to some estrogen effects (endometrial cancer and deep vein thrombosis).
  - **Aromatase inhibitors.** Third-generation aromatase inhibitors have become available for the treatment of postmenopausal women with hormone-responsive breast cancer. Two nonsteroidal agents, **anastrazole** (Arimidex, 1 mg/d) and **letrozole** (Femara, 2.5 mg/d), and one steroidal agent, **exemestane** (Aromasin, 25 mg/d), are available. All three agents have been found to be active in hormone-sensitive breast cancer.[32] The most common side effects of aromatase inhibitors are hot flashes and night sweats.
  - **Gonadotropin agonists.** Two LHRH agonists are used in the treatment of metastatic prostate cancer. **Leuprolide acetate** and **goserelin acetate** can be given as monthly SC depot injections, and leuprolide acetate is also available in a daily injection form. The first weeks of treatment may be associated with an initial flare in tumor symptoms, bone pain, fluid retention, hot flashes, sweats, and impotence. One should monitor for signs of neurologic dysfunction or urinary obstruction.
  - **Progestational agents. Megestrol acetate,** 40 mg PO four times daily, and **medroxyprogesterone,** 10 mg PO daily, have been used in the treatment of a variety of neoplasms. Principal toxicities include weight gain, fluid retention, hot flashes, and vaginal bleeding with discontinuation of therapy. Both agents also have been used in the treatment of cachexia associated with cancer and AIDS.
  - **Antiandrogens. Flutamide** and **bicalutamide** may produce nausea, vomiting, gynecomastia, and breast tenderness.[33] In advanced prostate cancer, withdrawal of flutamide results in tumor regression in 25% of patients.[34]

- **Targeted therapies** in the form of monoclonal antibodies and TKIs are now available.
  - **Trastuzumab** (4 mg/kg over 90 minutes week 1, then 2 mg/kg over 30 minutes weekly) should be added to the first-line chemotherapy in patients with metastatic breast cancer whose cancers overexpress her-2 as measured by gene amplification or protein expression. Its use is associated with an improved survival. As a single agent, it has modest activity and a different mechanism of action than chemotherapy.[35]

- **Rituximab,** an unconjugated antibody targeted to CD20, is administered weekly for 1 month for treatment of low-grade non-Hodgkin lymphomas that are CD20 positive. Toxicities include chills and fevers during administration and rare hypersensitivity reactions.[36]
- **Alemtuzumab** is a humanized antibody to CD52 (present on normal B and T cells) and has been used to treat CLL. Because of a high incidence of opportunistic infections from resulting immunodeficiency, prophylactic antifungals and antivirals are recommended.[37]
- **Bevacizumab** targets VEGF and is approved for the treatment of colon cancer, and has activity in breast and lung cancer. Common toxicities include hypertension and proteinuria. It has infrequently been associated with serious bleeding or clotting events and gastrointestinal perforations.
- **Cetuximab and panitumumab** target EGFR and have been approved for the treatment of colon cancer. Toxicities include infusion reactions, rash, and diarrhea.
- **Gemtuzumab** is directed against CD33 and is indicated in myeloid leukemias.
- **Ibritumomab** and **iodine 131 tositumomab** are radiolabeled antibodies indicated for the treatment of non-Hodgkin lymphoma.
- **Imatinib** is a TKI targeting the BCR-ABL fusion protein in CML, as well as c-kit in gastrointestinal stromal tumors (GISTs). It has activity in a number of less common disorders.
- **Erlotinib** is a TKI-targeting EGFR approved in NSCLC and with activity in pancreatic cancer as well. Toxicities include diarrhea and rash.
- **Sunitinib** and **sorafenib** are multitargeted TKIs approved for the treatment of renal cell carcinoma.

- **Nonspecific immunotherapy**
  - **Interferon-α** is used for hairy-cell leukemia, CML, and melanoma. Toxicity includes nausea and vomiting, flulike symptoms, and headaches. Acute toxicity may respond to acetaminophen; with continued administration these symptoms subside.
  - **Aldesleukin (interleukin-2)** can produce responses in melanoma or renal cell carcinoma; some of these remissions are durable. At high doses this agent is toxic, producing increased vascular permeability with fluid overload, hypotension, prerenal azotemia, and elevation of liver enzymes.

- **Chemopreventive agents**
  - **Retinoids** have been used as therapeutic and chemopreventive agents. Isotretinoin (13-cis-retinoic acid), 50–100 mg/m^2 PO daily for 12 months, has been shown to lower the incidence of second primary tumors in patients who were previously treated for head and neck cancer.[38] Common toxicities include dry skin, cheilitis, hyperlipidemia, and elevation of transaminases.[39]
  - **Tamoxifen,** 20 mg PO daily administered for 5 years, has been shown to decrease the incidence of breast cancer in women with a high risk of developing breast cancer.[40] **Raloxifene** has been found to have similar risk reduction benefit with a lower risk of endometrial cancer and blood clots.

COMPLICATIONS OF TREATMENT

- **Chemotherapy** often causes serious or life-threatening toxicity. The most common and predictable toxicities are to the rapidly proliferating cells of hematopoietic and mucosal tissue. Because repair of these tissues cannot be accelerated, palliation during the healing process is the primary goal.
- **Radiation therapy** toxicity is related to the location of the therapy, total dose delivered, and rates of delivery. Large-dose fractions of radiation are associated with greater toxicity to the normal tissues encompassed in the radiation field.
  - **Acute toxicity** develops within the first 3 months of therapy and is characterized by an inflammatory reaction in the tissue receiving radiation. Such toxicity may respond to anti-inflammatory agents such as glucocorticoids. Local irritations or burns in the treatment field generally resolve with time. Close observation and treatment of any

infections and palliation of symptoms such as pain, dysphagia, dysuria, or diarrhea (depending on the site of treatment) are the mainstays of supportive care until healing has occurred.
- **Subacute toxicities** between 3 and 6 months of therapy and chronic toxicity after 6 months are less amenable to therapy, as fibrosis and scarring are present. Daily **amifostine** before head and neck radiation therapy decreases the incidence of xerostomia.[41]

SPECIFIC COMPLICATIONS: TUMOR LYSIS SYNDROME

General Principles

Definition
- **Tumor lysis syndrome** occurs in patients with rapidly proliferating neoplasms that are highly sensitive to chemotherapy. Rapid tumor cell death releases intracellular contents and causes **hyperkalemia, hyperphosphatemia, and hyperuricemia.** Although reported in the treatment of a variety of malignancies, it is usually associated with **high-grade non-Hodgkin's lymphoma** and **acute leukemia.**

Diagnosis

- The diagnosis of tumor lysis syndrome is based on susceptibility, clinical suspicion, and close monitoring of laboratory data in patients at risk. Rapidly progressive hyperkalemia, hyperphosphatemia, and hyperuricemia as well as acutely worsening renal failure are the hallmarks.

Prophylaxis and Treatment

- Prophylaxis and pretreatment are paramount in preventing tumor lysis syndrome.
- During induction chemotherapy for **tumor lysis syndrome,** prophylactic measures should include **allopurinol,** 300–600 mg PO daily, and aggressive IV volume expansion (e.g., 3,000 mL/m^2/d). The addition of **sodium bicarbonate,** 50 mEq/1,000 mL IV fluid, to alkalinize the urine above a pH of 7 may prevent uric acid nephropathy and acute renal failure.
  - When hyperphosphatemia accompanies hyperuricemia, urine alkalinization should be avoided because calcium phosphate precipitation may result in renal failure.
- **Rasburicase** is a recombinant urate oxidase enzyme that catalyzes the oxidation of uric acid into allantoin, a soluble metabolite. It can be used prophylactically or in the treatment of hyperuricemia. It can be administered as a daily dose of 0.15–0.20 mg/kg/d for up to 5 days.
- Despite these preventive measures, hemodialysis may be needed for hyperkalemia, hyperphosphatemia, acute renal failure, or fluid overload.

SPECIFIC COMPLICATIONS: HEMATOLOGIC

Myelosuppression/Febrile Neutropenia

General Principles

Definition
- **The risk of infection** increases dramatically with **neutropenia** (defined as an absolute neutrophil count of **<500/mm^3**) and is directly related to the duration of the neutropenia. Fever is defined as a single core temperature reading of >38.3°C or two readings of >38.0°C spanning 1 hour. Other clinical signs of infection must be considered in this evaluation, because the inflammatory response may be muted in the absence of neutrophils. **A febrile neutropenic patient should be presumed to be infected and must be evaluated and treated promptly.**

Physical Examination

- **A complete physical examination** should be performed to locate potential sites of infection, with particular attention to indwelling catheter sites, sinuses, and the oral and perirectal areas.
  - Digital rectal examination should be avoided to prevent bacterial translocation.

Laboratory Studies

- **Cultures** of blood, urine, stool, sputum, and other foci that are susceptible to bacterial infections (e.g., fluid collections) should be collected.

Imaging

- A chest radiograph should be obtained to check for infection.

Treatment

Medications

- To guard against infection, **empiric antimicrobial treatment should be initiated immediately** after cultures are obtained. In the absence of any obvious source, the antimicrobials should provide broad coverage for Gram-negative bacilli (including *Pseudomonas aeruginosa*) and Gram-positive cocci (including α-hemolytic *Streptococcus* species). In choosing a regimen, local susceptibility patterns should also be considered. Empiric therapy may consist of an aminoglycoside and semisynthetic penicillin or a single agent such as cefepime. **Antimicrobials are continued until the neutrophil count is >500/mm³.**
  - Vancomycin should not be included in initial empiric regimens unless the patient is clinically unstable or has had a recent oxacillin-resistant *Staphylococcus aureus* infection.
  - Low-risk patients (afebrile after institution of antibiotics, negative cultures, and anticipated to recover from myelosuppression in <1 week) can be discharged on an oral broad-spectrum agent such as a fluoroquinolone or trimethoprim/sulfamethoxazole.
  - **Modification of the antimicrobial regimen** according to the culture data or clinical picture may become necessary. Additional agents to treat *Staphylococcus epidermidis*, *Clostridium difficile*, or anaerobic infections are commonly necessary based on physical examination findings and suspected foci of infection.
  - Persistent fever, in the absence of other data, usually does not warrant an empiric change in the antibacterial therapy.
  - **Empiric antifungal therapy** with amphotericin B (starting at 0.5 mg/kg and advanced to 1.0 mg/kg qd) should be added if the fever continues for longer than 72 hours.
- **Growth factors** include many cytokines that may ameliorate the myelosuppression associated with cytotoxic chemotherapy. They act on hematopoietic cells, stimulating proliferation, differentiation, commitment, and some functional activation. Because they can increase myelosuppression, they **should not be given within 24 hours of chemotherapy or radiation.**
  - **G-CSF**, given at an initial dose of 5 mcg/kg SC or IV beginning the day after the last dose of cytotoxic chemotherapy, may reduce the incidence of febrile neutropenic events. Blood counts should be monitored twice a week during therapy. Bone pain is a common toxicity that can be managed with nonnarcotic analgesics. A pegylated form of G-CSF is now available, allowing for single-dose/cycle administration at a dose of 6 mg.
  - **GM-CSF**, given subcutaneously at a dose of 250 mcg/m²/d beginning the day after the last dose of cytotoxic chemotherapy, shortens the period of neutropenia after stem cell transplant.
- Neutropenic patients should be maintained in **modified reverse isolation.** Those who enter the room should wash their hands thoroughly with antiseptic soap or an alcohol-based hand-cleaning solution. Visitors with colds should wear a mask, and those with fevers should not enter. Due to the risk of fungal infection, live plants should not be allowed in the room.

Anemia

- **Anemia** is a common side effect of multiple chemotherapeutic agents. Symptoms include fatigue, dyspnea, or lethargy. **RBC transfusions** are indicated for patients who have symptoms of anemia, active bleeding, or a hemoglobin concentration below 7–8 g/dL. Because of anecdotal reports of GVHD associated with transfusions, radiation of all blood products is generally recommended for immunosuppressed marrow transplant patients.
  - **Recombinant erythropoietin** given at a starting dose of 150 units/kg SC three times a week has been shown to improve anemia and decrease transfusion requirements in cancer patients, particularly those in whom the anemia is predominantly caused by cytotoxic chemotherapy.[42] Hematocrit should be monitored weekly during therapy, and the dosage should be adjusted accordingly.
  - **Darbepoetin alfa** is a recombinant erythropoietin with a longer half-life. It is indicated for the treatment of chemotherapy-induced anemia in patients with solid tumors and can be dosed every 2 weeks.[43]

Thrombocytopenia

- **Thrombocytopenia** is another common side effect of chemotherapeutic agents toxic to the bone marrow. Symptoms include easy bruising and bleeding, including epistaxis and gingival bleeding.
  - **Thrombocytopenia** below 10,000/mm^3 that is the result of chemotherapy should be treated with platelet transfusions to minimize the risk of spontaneous hemorrhage.
  - **Interleukin-11** was approved to reduce the duration and severity of thrombocytopenia after chemotherapy. However, limited efficacy and significant toxicity (fluid retention and atrial arrhythmias) have limited its use.
  - When prolonged thrombocytopenia is anticipated, histocompatibility testing should be performed before therapy so that HLA-matched single-donor platelets can be provided when alloimmunization makes the patient refractory to random-donor platelets.

SPECIFIC COMPLICATIONS: EXTRAVASATION

- **Extravasation** of certain chemotherapeutic agents from venous infusion sites may lead to severe local tissue injury. Offending agents are identified as **vesicants**. Initial symptoms of pain or erythema may appear within hours or may be delayed for up to 1–2 weeks. When extravasation occurs, the steps described below should be taken.
  - **Stop the chemotherapy infusion.** With the venous catheter still in place, approximately 5 mL of blood should be aspirated to remove any residual drug.

 TABLE 20-2 **Treatment of Extravasation of Selected Chemotherapeutic Agents**

Drug	Compress	Antidote
Dacarbazine	Hot	Isotonic thiosulfate IV and SC
Daunorubicin	Cold	DMSO applied topically to vein
Doxorubicin	Cold	DMSO applied topically to vein
Etoposide	Hot	Hyaluronidase (150 units/mL), 16 mL SC · 1
Mechlorethamine	—	Isotonic thiosulfate IV and SC
Mitomycin-C	—	Isotonic thiosulfate IV and SC
Vinblastine	Hot	Hyaluronidase (150 units/mL), 16 mL SC · 1
Vincristine	Hot	Hyaluronidase (150 units/mL), 16 mL SC · 1

DMSO, dimethyl sulfoxide.

■ **Certain drugs require hot or cold compresses** and may be neutralized by instillation of agents locally through the catheter and subcutaneously into the nearby tissue (Table 20-2).

■ **Observe the area closely** for signs of tissue breakdown; surgical intervention for debridement or skin grafting may be necessary. Because extravasation injuries usually result in severe pain, adequate analgesia should be supplied.[44]

SPECIFIC COMPLICATIONS: GASTROINTESTINAL

■ **Stomatitis** is an unpleasant consequence of many chemotherapeutic agents and is commonly the dose-limiting toxicity of methotrexate and FU. With simultaneous administration of radiation therapy, the toxicity is more severe. Healing generally occurs within 7–10 days of the development of symptoms. The severity of stomatitis ranges from mild (oral discomfort) to severe (ulceration, impaired oral intake, and hemorrhage).

  ▪ In mild cases of **stomatitis, oral rinses** (chlorhexidine, 15–30 mL swish and spit tid, or the combination of equal parts diphenhydramine elixir, saline, and 3% hydrogen peroxide) may provide relief. Polyvinylpyrrolidone-sodium hyaluronate gel can also be used.

  ▪ **Palifermin,** a keratinocyte growth factor analog, has been approved for use in chemotherapy-induced stomatitis.[45]

  ▪ In severe cases, IV morphine is appropriate.

  ▪ **IV fluids** should be used to supplement oral intake as needed.

  ▪ Aspiration may develop in patients with moderate or severe stomatitis; precautions should include elevation of the head of the bed and availability of a handheld suction apparatus.

  ▪ In severe or prolonged episodes, superinfection with *Candida* or herpes simplex is possible and requires appropriate diagnosis and antimicrobial intervention.

    • **Diarrhea** is the result of cytotoxicity to proliferating cells of the intestinal mucosa.

    • In some cases of **diarrhea**, IV fluids are necessary to avoid intravascular volume depletion. The use of oral opioid agents as antidiarrheals is commonly limited by abdominal cramping. Severe diarrhea associated with FU and LV has been reported to respond to octreotide, 150–500 mcg SC tid. Diarrhea secondary to irinotecan can be treated with loperamide, 4 mg PO then 2 mg q2h while awake, and 4 mg q4h during the night.

    • **Nausea and vomiting** may develop in varying degrees and frequency. Suggestions for antiemetic agent(s) are listed in Table 20-3.

SPECIFIC COMPLICATIONS: OTHER

■ **Interstitial pneumonitis** may develop as a dose-related, cumulative toxicity or as an idiosyncratic reaction. The implicated agent should be discontinued.

  ▪ With **interstitial pneumonitis**, the institution of glucocorticoids (e.g., prednisone, 1 mg/kg PO daily or equivalent) may be of some benefit. The long-term outcome, however, is unpredictable.

■ **Hemorrhagic cystitis** may develop with either cyclophosphamide or ifosfamide.

  ▪ **Hemorrhagic cystitis** is best anticipated and treated with prophylactic mesna at a dosage of at least 0.6 mg mesna to 1 mg ifosfamide. Treatment consists of continuous bladder irrigation with isotonic saline and should continue until the hematuria resolves.

 # PALLIATIVE CARE

■ **Palliative care and pain management.** Patients with cancer experience a multitude of symptoms. Studies have revealed that individuals with advanced cancer often experience

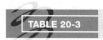

TABLE 20-3	Recommendations for Antiemetic Therapy

Phenothiazines
Prochlorperazine, 5–10 mg PO or IV q4–6h (maximum IV dose, 40 mg/d)
Prochlorperazine, 25 mg per rectum q4–6h
Chlorpromazine, 10 mg PO q4–6h
Trimethobenzamide, 100 mg PO or IM q4–6h

Serotonin receptor antagonists
Granisetron, 1 mg IV or 2 mg PO 15 min before chemotherapy
Palonsetron, 0.25 mg IV 15–30 min before chemotherapy
Ondansetron, 8–32 mg IV 15–30 min before chemotherapy or 24 mg PO or 8 mg PO tid
Dolasetron, 100 mg IV or PO 30 min before chemotherapy
Butyrophenone
Droperidol, 1–5 mg IV q4–6h
Metoclopramide, 2–3 mg/kg IV before chemotherapy and q2h for three doses

Antihistamine
Diphenhydramine, 50 mg PO or IV q4–6h

Anxiolytic
Lorazepam, 1–2 mg PO or IV tid–qid

Glucocorticoid
Dexamethasone, 10–30 mg IV before chemotherapy

NK1 Antagonist
Aprepitant 125 mg PO day 1, 80 mg PO daily days 2 and 3 (in conjunction with corticosteroids/serotonin antagonists)

ten or more symptoms, including pain, nausea, fatigue, weakness, constipation, and dyspnea. In addition to physical symptoms, patients also suffer emotionally and spiritually. Individuals with early-stage cancer experience similar symptoms, but with less frequency. The optimal management of cancer patients includes a careful assessment of symptomatology and appropriate management of these symptoms.

■ **Pain** is present at diagnosis in 5%–10% of patients with localized cancer and 60%–90% of individuals with metastases. Improved oral analgesics, use of indwelling venous access devices, development of home nursing care agencies, and public acceptance of the hospice philosophy now allow patients to receive a large portion of their palliative treatment out of the hospital. Successful treatment of the underlying disease usually provides relief of pain. Painful foci of disease that are refractory to systemic intervention can be controlled with local radiation therapy, regional nerve block, or an ablative surgical procedure. In many situations, however, analgesics are necessary (see Chapter 1, Patient Care in Internal Medicine).

■ **Mild or moderate cancer pain** may respond to nonopioid analgesics such as acetaminophen or nonsteroidal anti-inflammatory drugs. **Moderate to severe pain** almost always requires an opioid analgesic to attain significant relief. Medication administered on a prescribed schedule is more effective in maintaining analgesia than that taken intermittently once pain has developed. Several potent opioids are available in sustained-release formulations, including morphine, oxycodone hydrochloride, and fentanyl. Methadone has a long half-life and can be used as a long-lasting pain medication. Most patients with cancer pain have some combination of chronic and intermittent pain.

■ **Optimal pain management** includes a long-lasting pain medication with PRN dosing for breakthrough pain. Occasionally, infusions of morphine, 3–5 mg/hr IV, increased by 2–4 mg/hr as needed, are necessary. Under supervision, morphine drips can be used in the home setting. Morphine, as well as most other parenteral opioids, can also be administered subcutaneously. This reduces the difficulty of delivering these medications, especially in the home setting. Although tolerance and physical dependency can develop with long-term narcotic administration, **drug abuse and psychological dependency seldom occur** in the setting of chronic pain from cancer. These concerns should not compromise the patient's ability to achieve adequate analgesia.

■ **Nonopioid adjuvant pain medications.** Acetaminophen and nonsteroidal anti-inflammatory drugs may offer some relief even in the setting of severe pain, allowing a lower dose of opioid to be used. Other adjuvant pain medications include tricyclic antidepressants and antiseizure medications, which may be especially useful for neuropathic pain. The bisphosphonates may improve the treatment of bone pain.

■ **Palliative care** is defined by the World Health Organization as "the active total care of the patient whose disease is not responsive to curative intent." Palliative care focuses on the relief of symptoms and coping with the implications of advanced cancer, as most patients with advanced cancer die from their disease. Control of pain and other symptoms, as well as addressing psychological, social, and spiritual problems, is paramount (World Health Organization, Technical Report 804, 1990). A detailed overview of palliative care is beyond the scope of this chapter. The basic principles include a multidisciplinary approach to patient assessment and management. A careful and detailed assessment of symptoms, physical as well as psychological, is essential to this process, as is an assessment of the disease and patient status. This allows for realistic expectations regarding the disease process and prognosis to be determined, which in turn allows for informed decision making to formulate a plan of care.

References

1. Goldhirsch A, Glick JH, Gelber RD, et al. Meeting highlights: International Consensus Panel on the Treatment of Primary Breast Cancer. *J Natl Cancer Inst.* 1998; 90(21):1601–1608.

2. Piccart-Gebhart MJ, Procter M, Leyland-Jones B, et al. Trastuzumab after adjuvant chemotherapy in HER2-positive breast cancer. *N Engl J Med.* 2005;353(16):1659–1672.

3. Slamon DJ, Leyland-Jones B, Shak S, et al. Use of chemotherapy plus a monoclonal antibody against HER2 for metastatic breast cancer that overexpresses HER2. *N Engl J Med.* 2001;344(11):783–792.

4. Rosen LS, Gordon D, Kaminski M. Zoledronic acid versus pamidronate in the treatment of skeletal metastases in patients with breast cancer or osteolytic lesions of multiple myeloma: a phase III, double-blind, comparative trial. *Cancer J.* 2001;7(5):377–387.

5. Auperin A, Arriagada R, Pignon JP, et al. Prophylactic cranial irradiation for patients with small-cell lung cancer in complete remission. Prophylactic Cranial Irradiation Overview Collaborative Group. *N Engl J Med.* 1999;341(7):476–484.

6. Walsh TN, Noonan N, Hollywood D, et al. A comparison of multimodal therapy and surgery for esophageal adenocarcinoma. *N Engl J Med.* 1996;335(7):462–467.

7. Macdonald JS, Smalley SR, Benedetti J, et al. Chemoradiotherapy after surgery compared with surgery alone for adenocarcinoma of the stomach or gastroesophageal junction. *N Engl J Med.* 2001;345(10):725–730.

8. Moertel CG, Fleming TR, Macdonald JS, et al. Fluorouracil plus levamisole as effective adjuvant therapy after resection of stage III colon carcinoma: a final report. *Ann Intern Med.* 1995;122(5):321–326.

9. Andre T, Boni C, Mounedji-Boudiaf L, et al. Oxaliplatin, fluorouracil, and leucovorin as adjuvant treatment for colon cancer. *N Engl J Med.* 2004;350(23):2343–2351.

10. Saltz LB, Cox JV, Blanke C, et al. Irinotecan plus fluorouracil and leucovorin for metastatic colorectal cancer. Irinotecan Study Group. *N Engl J Med.* 2000;343(13):905–914.

11. Fong Y, Cohen AM, Fortner JG, et al. Liver resection for colorectal metastases. *J Clin Oncol.* 1997;15(3):938–946.

12. Martenson JA, Lipsitz SR, Lefkopoulou M, et al. Results of combined modality therapy for patients with anal cancer (E7283). An Eastern Cooperative Oncology Group study. *Cancer.* 1995;76(10):1731–1736.
13. Kelly WK, Slovin S, Scher HI. Steroid hormone withdrawal syndromes. Pathophysiology and clinical significance. *Urol Clin North Am.* 1997;24(2):421–431.
14. Einhorn LH. Treatment of testicular cancer: a new and improved model. *J Clin Oncol.* 1990;8(11):1777–1781.
15. Keys HM, Bundy BN, Stehman FB, Cisplatin, radiation, and adjuvant hysterectomy compared with radiation and adjuvant hysterectomy for bulky stage IB cervical carcinoma. *N Engl J Med.* 1999;340(15):1154–1161.
16. Calais G, Alfonsi M, Bardet E, et al. Randomized trial of radiation therapy versus concomitant chemotherapy and radiation therapy for advanced-stage oropharynx carcinoma. *J Natl Cancer Inst.* 1999;91(24):2081–2086.
17. Kirkwood JM, Strawderman MH, Ernstoff MS, et al. Interferon alfa-2b adjuvant therapy of high-risk resected cutaneous melanoma: the Eastern Cooperative Oncology Group Trial EST 1684. *J Clin Oncol.* 1996;14(1):7–17.
18. Gill PS, Wernz J, Scadden DT, et al. Randomized phase III trial of liposomal daunorubicin versus doxorubicin, bleomycin, and vincristine in AIDS-related Kaposi's sarcoma. *J Clin Oncol.* 1996;14(8):2353–2364.
19. Ahmann FR. A reassessment of the clinical implications of the superior vena caval syndrome. *J Clin Oncol.* 1984;2(8):961–969.
20. Berenson JR, Lichtenstein A, Porter L, et al. Efficacy of pamidronate in reducing skeletal events in patients with advanced multiple myeloma. Myeloma Aredia Study Group. *N Engl J Med.* 1996;334(8):488–493.
21. Tisdale MJ. Biology of cachexia. *J Natl Cancer Inst.* 1997;89(23):1763–1773.
22. Sigurgeirsson B, Lindelof B, Edhag O, et al. Risk of cancer in patients with dermatomyositis or polymyositis. A population-based study. *N Engl J Med.* 1992;326(6): 363–367.
23. McEvoy KM, Windebank AJ, Daube JR, et al. 3,4-Diaminopyridine in the treatment of Lambert-Eaton myasthenic syndrome. *N Engl J Med.* 1989;321(23):1567–1571.
24. Gould MK, Dembitzer AD, Doyle RL. Low-molecular-weight heparins compared with unfractionated heparin for treatment of acute deep venous thrombosis. A meta-analysis of randomized, controlled trials. *Ann Intern Med.* 1999;130(10):800–809.
25. Glantz MJ, LaFollette S, Jaeckle KA, et al. Randomized trial of a slow-release versus a standard formulation of cytarabine for the intrathecal treatment of lymphomatous meningitis. *J Clin Oncol.* 1999;17(10):3110–3116.
26. Freeman NJ, Costanza ME. 5-Fluorouracil-associated cardiotoxicity. *Cancer.* 1988; 61(1):36–45.
27. Petrelli N, Douglass HO Jr, Herrera L, et al. The modulation of fluorouracil with leucovorin in metastatic colorectal carcinoma: a prospective randomized phase III trial. Gastrointestinal Tumor Study Group. *J Clin Oncol.* 1989;7(10):1419–1426.
28. Chun HG, Leyland-Jones B, Cheson BD. Fludarabine phosphate: a synthetic purine antimetabolite with significant activity against lymphoid malignancies. *J Clin Oncol.* 1991;9(1):175–188.
29. Beutler E. Cladribine (2-chlorodeoxyadenosine). *Lancet* 1993;341(8836):54.
30. Shan K, Lincoff AM, Young JB. Anthracycline-induced cardiotoxicity. *Ann Intern Med.* 1996;125(1):47–58.
31. Kemp G, Rose P, Lurain J, et al. Amifostine pretreatment for protection against cyclophosphamide-induced and cisplatin-induced toxicities: results of a randomized control trial in patients with advanced ovarian cancer. *J Clin Oncol.* 1996;14(7):2101–2112.
32. Goss PE, Strasser K. Aromatase inhibitors in the treatment and prevention of breast cancer. *J Clin Oncol.* 2001;19(3):881–894.
33. Soloway MS, Matzkin H. Antiandrogenic agents as monotherapy in advanced prostatic carcinoma. *Cancer.* 1993;71(3 Suppl):1083–1088.
34. Scher HI, Kelly WK. Flutamide withdrawal syndrome: its impact on clinical trials in hormone-refractory prostate cancer. *J Clin Oncol.* 1993;11(8):1566–1572.

35. Romond EH, Perez EA, Bryant J, et al. Trastuzumab plus adjuvant chemotherapy for operable HER2-positive breast cancer. *New Engl J Med* 2005;353(16):1673–1684.

36. McLaughlin P, Grillo-Lopez AJ, Link BK, et al. Rituximab chimeric anti-CD20 monoclonal antibody therapy for relapsed indolent lymphoma: half of patients respond to a four-dose treatment program. *J Clin Oncol.* 1998;16(8):2825–2833.

37. Osterborg A, Fassas AS, Anagnostopoulos A, et al. Humanized CD52 monoclonal antibody Campath-1H as first-line treatment in chronic lymphocytic leukaemia. *Br J Haematol.* 1996;93(1):151–153.

38. Hong WK, Lippman SM, Itri LM, et al. Prevention of second primary tumors with isotretinoin in squamous-cell carcinoma of the head and neck. *N Engl J Med.* 1990; 323(12):795–801.

39. Takeshita A, Sakamaki H, Miyawaki S, et al. Significant reduction of medical costs by differentiation therapy with all-trans retinoic acid during remission induction of newly diagnosed patients with acute promyelocytic leukemia. The Japan Adult Leukemia Study Group. *Cancer.* 1995;76(4):602–608.

40. Fisher B, Costantino JP, Wickerham DL. Tamoxifen for prevention of breast cancer: report of the National Surgical Adjuvant Breast and Bowel Project P-1 Study. *J Natl Cancer Inst.* 1998;90(18):1371–1388.

41. Kemp G, Rose P, Lurain J et al. Amifostine pretreatment for protection against cyclophosphamide-induced and cisplatin-induced toxicities: results of a randomized control trial in patients with advanced ovarian cancer. *J Clin Oncol.* 1996;14(7):2101–2112.

42. Crawford J. Recombinant human erythropoietin in cancer-related anemia. Review of clinical evidence. *Oncology (Williston Park).* 2002;16(9 Suppl 10):41–53.

43. Mirtsching B, Charu V, Vadhan-Raj S, et al. Every 2 week darbepoeitin alfa is comparable to rHuEPO in treating chemotherapy induced anemia. *Oncology.* 2002;16(10 suppl 11):31–36.

44. Rudolph R, Larson DL. Etiology and treatment of chemotherapeutic agent extravasation injuries: a review. *J Clin Oncol.* 1987;5(7):1116–1126.

45. Hueber AJ, Leipe J, Roesler W. Palifermin as treatment in dose-intense conventional polychemotherapy induced mucositis. *Haematologica.* 2006;91(8 Suppl):ECR32.

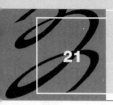

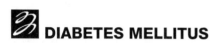 **DIABETES MELLITUS**

GENERAL PRINCIPLES

- **Diabetes mellitus (DM)** is a group of metabolic diseases characterized by hyperglycemia resulting from defects in insulin secretion, insulin action, or both.
- DM is present in 7% of the U.S. population but it is estimated that 6.2 million are undiagnosed. DM type 2 is the most common cause of death in United Sates.
- This metabolic disorder is accompanied by hypertension and hypercholesterolemia in half of the adult diabetic patients, increasing the risk for the development of diabetic-induced complications.[1]

Classification of Diabetes and Related Disorders

- DM is classified into four clinical classes[2]:
  - **Type 1 diabetes** accounts for <10% of all cases of DM and results from a cellular-mediated autoimmune destruction of the β cells of the pancreas.
    - The rate of destruction is rapid in some individuals (mainly infants and children) and slow in others (mainly adults, known as late-onset autoimmune diabetes [LADA]).
    - This form of diabetes is characterized by severe insulin deficiency. Exogenous insulin is required to control blood glucose, prevent diabetic ketoacidosis (DKA), and preserve life.
    - A transient period of insulin independence ("honeymoon phase") or reduced insulin requirement may occur early in the course of type 1 DM.
  - **Type 2 diabetes** accounts for >90% of all cases of DM. Type 2 DM is initially characterized by insulin resistance followed by failure of β cells to compensate for the increased insulin requirements.
    - It is usually a disease of adults; however, type 2 DM is being increasingly diagnosed in younger age groups.
    - Type 2 diabetes is associated with older age, obesity, family history of diabetes, history of gestational diabetes, impaired glucose metabolism, physical inactivity, and race/ethnicity. Frequency varies in different ethnic groups.
    - It is estimated that in up to 50% of affected people the disease is undiagnosed.
    - Insulin secretion is usually sufficient to prevent ketosis under basal conditions, but DKA can develop during severe stress.
  - **Other specific types of DM** include those that result from genetic defects in insulin secretion or action, exocrine pancreatic disease, pancreatectomy, endocrinopathies (e.g., Cushing syndrome, acromegaly), drugs, and other syndromes.
  - **Gestational DM** complicates approximately 4% of all pregnancies and usually resolves after delivery, although affected women remain at an increased risk for development of type 2 DM later in life.

600

- All patients with gestational diabetes should undergo a 75-g oral glucose tolerance test at 6–8 weeks postpartum to determine whether abnormal carbohydrate metabolism has persisted.
- Weight loss is encouraged to decrease the likelihood of developing diabetes mellitus after delivery.
- Patients with a history of gestational diabetes should be annually evaluated for onset of diabetes.

DIAGNOSIS

- The diagnosis of DM can be established using any of the following criteria:
  - **Plasma glucose of 126 mg/dL or greater** after an overnight fast. This should be confirmed with a repeat test.
  - **Symptoms of diabetes** and a random plasma glucose of 200 mg/dL or greater
  - **Oral glucose tolerance test** that shows a plasma glucose of 200 mg/dL or greater at 2 hours after a 75-g glucose load
- **Diagnosis of prediabetes. Impaired glucose tolerance (IGT)** and **impaired fasting glucose (IFG)** refer to intermediate states between normal glucose tolerance and DM type 2. IFG and IGT are risk factors for type 2 diabetes and micro- and macrovascular complications.
  - **IGT** is defined by a 2-hour oral glucose tolerance test plasma glucose from 140 mg/dL to 199 mg/dL.
  - **IFG** is defined by fasting plasma glucose of 100 mg/dL to 125 mg/dL.
  - Lifestyle modification is recommended for persons with IGT or IFG, but the rationale for drug therapy has not been established.

PRINCIPLES OF MANAGEMENT OF DM

- **The therapeutic goals** are alleviation of symptoms, achievement of metabolic control, and prevention of acute and long-term complications of diabetes.
  - Glycemic control is set at the same goal for type 1 and type 2 diabetes: average preprandial capillary blood glucose values of 90–130 mg/dL, postprandial capillary blood glucose values <180 mg/dL, and HbA_{1c} of <7% or as close to normal as possible while avoiding significant hypoglycemia.[2]
  - This degree of glycemic control has been associated with the lowest risk for long-term complications in patients with type 1[3] as well as type 2 DM.[4]
  - An individualized, comprehensive diabetes care plan is necessary to accomplish these goals.
- **Assessment of glycemic control consists of the following:**
  - **Self-monitoring of capillary blood glucose (SMBG)** is an important tool in preventing hypoglycemia and adjusting medications to reach glucose goals. It is recommended for all patients but especially for patients treated with insulin. SMBG should be carried out three or more times a day for patients using multiple insulin injections.
  - HbA_{1c} provides an integrated measure of blood glucose profile over the preceding 2–3 months; it should be obtained approximately every 3 months or at least twice a year in well-controlled patients. Any suspicion of a discordant HbA_{1c} level should be followed up by assessment of the self-monitoring blood glucose technique, hemoglobin level, and hemoglobin electrophoresis. Normal HbA_{1c} levels in population studies are 4%–6% using the Diabetes Control and Complications Trial (DCCT) assay.
  - **Ketonuria** grossly reflects ketonemia. All DM patients should monitor urine ketones using Ketostix or Acetest tablets during febrile illness or persistent elevated glucose (>300 mg/dL) or if signs of impending DKA (e.g., nausea, vomiting, abdominal pain) develop.
- **Patient education** is integral to successful management of diabetes. Diabetes education should be reinforced at every opportunity, particularly during hospitalization for diabetes-related complications.

- **Dietary modification.** Dietary modification provides a balanced diet to achieve adequate nutrition and maintains an ideal body weight.
  - Caloric restriction to at least 1,000–1,200 kcal/d for women and 1,200–1,600 kcal/d for men is recommended for overweight individuals.
  - Total caloric intake can be distributed as follows: 45%–65% of total caloric intake as carbohydrates, 10%–30% as protein, and <30% as total fat (<7% saturated fat) with <300 mg/d of cholesterol.
    - In patients with low-density lipoprotein (LDL) cholesterol >100 mg/dL, restrain the total fat to 25% of total calories, saturated fat to <7%, and <200 mg of cholesterol per day.
    - Patients with diabetic nephropathy are usually restricted to a protein intake of 0.8 g/kg/d. With deterioration in renal function, further restriction in protein intake (0.6 g/kg) can be considered in selected patients.
  - Monitoring the total grams of carbohydrate by using carbohydrate counting is key in the adjustment of the insulin therapy and achievement of the glycemic control. Carbohydrate allowance should be individualized based on glycemic control, plasma lipids, and weight goals.
- **Exercise** improves insulin sensitivity, reduces fasting and postprandial blood glucose, and offers numerous metabolic, cardiovascular, and psychological benefits in diabetic patients.
- **Medications** for diabetes are more effective when instituted as part of a comprehensive management approach that includes diet and exercise.

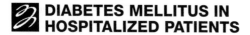 DIABETES MELLITUS IN HOSPITALIZED PATIENTS

INDICATIONS FOR HOSPITALIZATION IN DIABETIC PATIENTS

- **DKA** is characterized by a plasma glucose of >250 mg/dL in association with an arterial pH <7.30 or serum bicarbonate level of <15 mEq/L and moderate ketonuria or ketonemia.
- **Hyperosmolar nonketotic** state includes marked hyperglycemia (≥400 mg/dL) and elevated serum osmolality (>315 mOsm/kg), often accompanied by impaired mental status.
- **Hypoglycemia** is an indication if induced by a sulfonylurea drug or resulting in coma, seizures, or altered mentation.
- **Newly diagnosed type 1 DM** and newly recognized gestational DM can be an indication for hospitalization, even in the absence of ketoacidosis (see Type 1 Diabetes and Diabetic Ketoacidosis).
- **Patients with newly diagnosed type 2 DM** who meet the criteria for hospitalization often have severe hyperglycemia and may require insulin therapy for initial stabilization, even in the absence of ketoacidosis or hyperosmolar syndrome (see Type 2 Diabetes and Nonketotic Hyperosmolar Syndrome).

MANAGEMENT OF DIABETES IN HOSPITALIZED PATIENTS

- Hyperglycemia is a common finding in hospitalized patients. The prevalence of diabetes in hospitalized adults is conservatively estimated at 12%–25%. Patients presenting to hospitals may have unrecognized diabetes or hospital-related hyperglycemia.
  - HbA_{1c} can help to identify diabetes in hospitalized patients.
  - Accumulating evidence suggests that tight glycemic control improves mortality and morbidity in patients after coronary artery bypass graft (CABG), stroke, and cardiac surgery.
    - Intensive glucose control in surgical intensive care unit (ICU) patients significantly decreases in-hospital sepsis, acute renal failure requiring dialysis or hemofiltration, rate of transfusion, and polyneuropathy, and patients were less likely to require prolonged mechanical ventilation.

- However, in medical ICU patients, intensive insulin therapy significantly reduced morbidity but not the overall mortality. Mortality was only significantly decreased in medical ICU patients with intensive insulin therapy who stayed for ≥ 3 days, and hypoglycemia was identified as an independent risk factor for death in medical ICU patients.
- Therefore, caution should be applied to the widespread implementation of tight glycemic control in the ICU setting or medicine wards. Future studies are needed and the protocols should be individualized to the specific hospital environment.[5-7]

- **Glucose targets in hospitalized patients**
  - Glucose levels should be kept close to 110 mg/dL in the intensive care unit. In the noncritical care units, preprandial glucose should be kept as close to 90–130 mg/dL and maximal glucose <180 mg/dL.[8]
- **Patients hospitalized for reasons other than diabetes who are eating normally** should continue the outpatient diabetes treatment, unless specifically contraindicated.
  - The common practice of sliding scale administration of regular insulin alone, q6h, based on bedside capillary blood glucose levels, seldom gives satisfactory results; regimens that include intermediate-acting insulin along with short-acting insulin give superior glycemic control.
  - Insulin doses should be given in relation to meals and should be adjusted according to glucose levels.[9] Blood glucose should be monitored at least two to four times a day, especially in patients treated with insulin.
  - Adjustments in the next-day SC insulin dose are indicated if correction doses of insulin are frequently required. Extreme values (>300 mg/dL or <60 mg/dL) from bedside capillary blood glucose meters should be confirmed using laboratory measurements.
  - If persistent hyperglycemia is observed in febrile or sick patients, plasma ketones or urine ketone reaction by dipstick (Ketostix) or Acetest tablets should be determined and IV insulin should be considered to achieve glucose targets.
  - HbA$_{1c}$ should be measured if no recent result is available.
  - **Oral medications** for diabetes should be reviewed with regard to potential toxicities.
    - **Sulfonylureas** predispose to developing hypoglycemia in hospitalized patients not consuming their routine diet. Caution but not contraindication is recommended.
    - **Metformin** should be withheld 1 day before any diagnostic evaluation that involves the use of iodinated radiocontrast dyes. It can be restarted 48 hours after radiocontrast exposure and documentation of normal renal function. Metformin therapy should also be discontinued in the presence of sepsis, congestive heart failure (CHF), renal dysfunction, or other conditions that predispose to lactic acidosis.
    - **Thiazolidinediones** should not be administered to patients with hepatic dysfunction as indicated by elevated serum transaminases or CHF.
    - **Glucosidase inhibitors** should be continued unless the patient has gastrointestinal illness.
- **Patients hospitalized for reasons other than diabetes who are required to fast** should discontinue oral antidiabetic medications.
  - In patients requiring insulin, IV insulin infusion is recommended (see Diabetes Mellitus in Surgical Patients, Chapter 1, Patient Care in Internal Medicine). Alternative treatment for diabetics during these conditions is to administer one-half to two-thirds of the patient's long or intermediate insulin dose along with short-acting insulin by sliding scale.
  - An IV infusion of 5% dextrose in water (D5W) or dextrose in saline at 75 to 125 mL/hr should be provided to maintain plasma glucose between 90 and 180 mg/dL. Additional SC doses of short-acting insulin (1–4 units) are indicated when blood glucose levels are >200 mg/dL.
  - It is recommended that transition from insulin drip to SC insulin be done before a meal, preferably before breakfast. Insulin drip should be discontinued 30 minutes to 1 hour after patients received SC regular insulin and intermediate-acting insulin;

however, if Lispro or Aspart insulin is used, insulin drip should be discontinued after SC insulin has been administered.

■ For patients receiving glargine for basal insulin regimen, half of the basal insulin dose can be given as NPH at breakfast in addition to the usual short-acting insulin, and the total dose of glargine resumed at night.

- **Diabetic patients with emergency surgery**
  ■ Exclude DKA and neuropathy complications mimicking surgical emergencies.
  ■ Assess glycemic, acid-base, electrolyte (potassium, magnesium, and phosphate), and fluid status.
  ■ Restore circulating volume, control acidosis, and correct potassium abnormalities if surgery can be delayed.
  ■ Intravenous insulin, glucose, and potassium infusion should be administered to achieve target blood glucoses (see "Glucose targets in hospitalized patients"). Hourly glucose measurements are mandatory to adjust insulin and glucose infusions. Potassium should be monitored at least every 2 hours and replaced aggressively as required.

- **Enteral nutrition.**[10] Short-acting insulin by sliding scale should be used initially until the patient is tolerating tube feedings. When infusion rates are >30 mL/hr, start NPH or lente at half of the patient's morning preadmission dose, and then adjust the dose daily to keep glucose levels between 100 and 200 mg/dL.

- **Total parenteral nutrition (TPN).** Individuals with type II diabetes who require TPN are likely to require large amounts of insulin. See Chapter 2, Nutrition Support, for insulin management of patients on TPN.

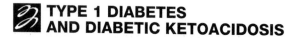

TYPE 1 DIABETES AND DIABETIC KETOACIDOSIS

GENERAL PRINICPLES

■ A comprehensive approach is necessary for successful management of type 1 DM. A team approach that includes the expertise of diabetes educators, dietitians, and other members of the diabetes care team offers the best chances of success.

TREATMENT

- **Treatment of type 1 DM** requires lifelong insulin replacement.
  ■ **Insulin preparations.** After SC injection, there is individual variability in the duration and peak activity of insulin preparations and day-to-day variability in the same subject (Table 21-1).
    • **Rapid-acting insulins** include regular insulin, lispro, insulin aspart, and glulisine. Regular insulin can be administered intravenously, intramuscularly, or subcutaneously. An IV bolus of regular insulin exerts maximum effect in 10–30 minutes and is quickly dissipated.
    • **Intermediate-acting insulins** include NPH (isophane) and lente (zinc). These insulins are released slowly from SC sites and reach peak activity after 6–12 hours, followed by gradual decline.
    • **Long-acting insulins** are absorbed more slowly than the intermediate-acting preparations. Long-acting insulins provide a steady "basal" supply of circulating insulin when administered once or twice a day. Glargine and detemir are "peakless" bioengineered human insulin analogs with an extended duration of activity. These insulins are generally administered once daily as a subcutaneous injection at bedtime, in a regimen that includes premeal regular insulin or insulin lispro. In type 1 DM patients, two injections are sometimes required for 24-hour coverage.
    • **Concentration.** Most insulins now contain 100 units/mL (U-100). A U-500 preparation is available for the rare patient with severe insulin resistance.
    • **Mixed insulin therapy.** Rapid-acting insulins (regular, lispro, and aspart) can be mixed with intermediate-acting (NPH and lente) or long-acting (ultralente)

	Approximate Kinetics of Human Insulin Preparations After Subcutaneous Injection		
TABLE 21-1			
Insulin type	**Onset of action (hr)**	**Peak effect (hr)**	**Duration of activity (hr)**
Rapid acting			
Lispro, aspart, glulisine	0.25–0.50	0.50–1.50	3–5
Regular	0.50–1.00	2–4	6–8
Intermediate acting			
NPH	1–2	6–12	18–24
Lente	1–3	6–12	18–26
Long acting			
Ultralente	4–6	10–16	24–48
Glargine	4–6	None[a]	18
Detemir	3–4		~20

[a]Insulin dosage and individual variability in absorption and clearance rates affect pharmacokinetic data. Human insulins may peak earlier and be dissipated faster than porcine or bovine insulins. Duration of insulin activity is prolonged in renal failure. After a lag time of approximately 5 hours, insulin glargine has a flat peakless effect over a 24-hour period.

insulins in the same syringe for convenience. The rapid-acting insulin should be drawn first, cross contamination should be avoided, and the mixed insulin should be injected immediately. Commercial premixed insulin preparations do not allow dose adjustment of individual components but are convenient for patients who are unable or unwilling to do the mixing themselves.

- **SC insulin delivery.** The anterior abdominal wall, thighs, buttocks, and arms are the preferred sites for SC insulin injection. Absorption is fastest from the abdomen, followed by the arm, buttocks, and thigh, probably as a result of differences in blood flow. Injection sites should be rotated within the regions rather than randomly across separate regions, to minimize erratic absorption. Exercise or massage over the injection site may accelerate insulin absorption.

- **Inhaled insulin** was recently approved. It should be administered within 10 minutes before meals. Patients have to be trained in the appropriate procedure for inhalation of insulin. The insulin is available in 1-mg and 3-mg blister packs (1 mg is equivalent to approximately 2.5–3.0 units of subcutaneously injected insulin). Typically, patients should use one or two inhalations for any given dose. Insulin has a rapid onset of action, faster than regular insulin with a duration of action between that of insulin lispro and regular insulin. Hypoglycemia, cough, and bitter taste were reported. This insulin preparation is not currently recommended in smokers or in patients with pulmonary disorders including asthma due to unclear alteration of insulin absorption.

- **Initial insulin dosage** for optimal glycemic control is approximately 0.5–1.0 units/kg/d for the average nonobese patient. A conservative total daily dose is given initially; the dose is then adjusted, using blood glucose values.
  - A regimen of **multiple daily insulin injections** is preferred to obtain optimal control.
    - This regimen provides approximately 40%–50% of the total daily dose of insulin as basal insulin supply, using one or two injections of long-acting or intermediate-acting insulin.
    - The remainder is given as three doses of rapid-acting insulin divided across the main meals, empirically or in proportion to the carbohydrate content. Typically 1 unit of insulin per 10–15 g of carbohydrate consumed is typical.
  - **The conventional insulin regimen** uses a mixture of short- and intermediate-acting insulins administered before breakfast and before the evening meal.
    - Approximately two-thirds of the total daily dose is injected in the morning and one-third in the evening.

- Approximately two-thirds of each injection comprises intermediate-acting insulin and one-third is rapid-acting insulin ("rule of thirds").
- These proportions should be modified for patients with unusual work schedules or eating patterns.
- The units of individual insulin components of each injection are then adjusted using values from preprandial and bedtime blood glucose monitoring.
- **Continuous SC insulin infusion** is a tool for intensive diabetes control in selected patients.
  - It provides 50% of total daily insulin as basal insulin and the remainder as multiple preprandial boluses of insulin, using a programmable insulin pump.
  - As with the multiple daily insulin injections regimen, the premeal insulin doses are adjusted to the carbohydrate content of each meal.
- **Sliding scale** administration of regular insulin alone to hospitalized patients, based on bedside capillary blood glucose levels, rarely achieves satisfactory glycemic control; regimens that include intermediate-acting insulin give superior results.[9]
- **Monitoring.** Blood glucose should be monitored at least four times a day (preprandially and at bedtime) in hospitalized patients with type 1 DM. The HbA_{1c} should be obtained if no recent result is available. Urine should be tested for ketones whenever hyperglycemia (>300 mg/dL) persists.

DKA

Epidemiology and Pathophysiology

- DKA, a potentially fatal complication, occurs in up to 5% of patients with type 1 DM annually; it is seen less frequently with type 2 DM. It is a manifestation of severe insulin deficiency, often in association with stress and activation of counterregulatory hormones (e.g., catecholamines, glucagon).
  - **Precipitating factors** for DKA include inadvertent or deliberate interruption of insulin therapy, sepsis, trauma, myocardial infarction, and pregnancy. DKA may be the first presentation of type 1 and, rarely, type 2 DM.

Diagnosis

- A high index of suspicion is warranted, because clinical presentation may be nonspecific.

Clinical Features

- **Clinical features** include polyuria, polydipsia, weight loss, nausea, vomiting, and vaguely localized abdominal pain.
- Tachycardia; decrease of capillary filling; rapid, deep, and labored breathing (Kussmaul respiration); and fruity breath odor are common **physical findings.**
- Prominent gastrointestinal (GI) symptoms may give rise to suspicion for intra-abdominal pathology.
- Dehydration is invariable and respiratory distress, shock, and coma can occur.

Laboratory Evaluation

- Labs will show an anion gap metabolic acidosis and positive serum ketones.
- Plasma glucose usually is elevated, but the degree of hyperglycemia may be moderate (≤300 mg/dL) in 10%–15% of patients in DKA. Pregnancy and alcohol ingestion are associated with "euglycemic DKA."
- The urine ketone reaction correlates poorly with ketonemia but is usually positive in DKA.
- Hyponatremia, hyperkalemia, azotemia, and hyperosmolality are other findings.
- Serum amylase and transaminases may be elevated.
- A focused search for a precipitating infection is always prudent.
- An electrocardiogram (ECG) should be performed to evaluate electrolyte abnormalities and for unsuspected myocardial ischemia.

Management and Treatment

■ **Management of DKA** should preferably be conducted in an ICU. **If treatment is conducted in a non-ICU setting, close monitoring by a physician is mandatory until ketoacidosis resolves and the patient's condition is stabilized.** The therapeutic priorities are fluid replacement, adequate insulin administration, and potassium repletion. Administration of bicarbonate, phosphate, magnesium, or other therapies may be advantageous in selected patients but is not a first-line consideration.

■ **IV access and supportive measures** should be instituted without delay.

■ **Fluid** deficits of several liters are common in DKA patients and can be estimated by subtracting the current weight from a recently known dry weight. The average degree of dehydration for most patients is approximately 7%–9% of body weight. Hypotension indicates a loss of >10% of body fluids.[11]

- **Initially, restoration of circulating volume** using isotonic (0.9%) saline should be accomplished. The first liter should be infused rapidly (if cardiac function is normal) and should be followed by additional fluids at a rate of 1 L/hr until the volume deficit is corrected. Hypotonic saline (0.45%) can be used in patients with severe hypernatremia (>155 mEq/L).

- The next goal is to **replenish total body water deficits**; this can be accomplished using a 0.45% saline infusion at 150–500 mL/hr if the corrected serum sodium is normal or elevated; 0.9% NaCl at a similar rate is appropriate if corrected serum sodium is low. Rate of the fluid replacement depends on the degree of dehydration and cardiac and renal status. Do not exceed a change in osmolality >3 mOsm/kg/hr. The success of the fluid replacement is judged by improvement in blood pressure, measurement of fluid balance, and clinical examination.

- **Maintenance fluid replacement** is continued until the fluid intake/output records indicate an overall positive balance similar to the estimated fluid deficit. Complete fluid replacement in a typical DKA patient may require 12–24 hours to accomplish.

■ **Insulin therapy.** Sufficient insulin must be administered to turn off ketogenesis and correct hyperglycemia.

- **An IV bolus of regular insulin,** 10–15 units (0.15 unit/kg), can be administered. This should be followed by a continuous infusion of regular insulin at an initial rate of 5–10 units/hr (or 0.1 unit/kg/hr). A solution of regular insulin, 100 units in 500 mL 0.9% saline, infused at a rate of 50 mL/hr delivers 10 units/hr of insulin.

- **A decrease in blood glucose of 50–75 mg/dL/hr** is an appropriate response; lesser decrements suggest insulin resistance, inadequate volume repletion, or a problem with insulin delivery. If insulin resistance is suspected, the hourly dose of regular insulin should be increased progressively by 50%–100% until an appropriate glycemic response is observed.

- **Excessively rapid correction of hyperglycemia** at rates >100 mg/dL/hr should be avoided to reduce the risk of osmotic encephalopathy.

- **Maintenance insulin infusion rates of 1–2 units/hr** are appropriate when serum bicarbonate rises to 15 mEq/L or higher and the anion gap has closed. Once oral intake resumes, insulin can be administered SC and the parenteral route can be discontinued. It is prudent to **give the first SC injection of insulin approximately 30 minutes before stopping the IV route.**

■ **Dextrose (5%)** in saline should be infused once plasma glucose decreases to 250 mg/dL and the insulin infusion rate should be decreased to 0.05 units/kg/hr to prevent dangerous hypoglycemia.

■ **Potassium deficit** should always be assumed or anticipated, regardless of plasma levels on admission. Insulin therapy results in a rapid shift of potassium into the intracellular compartment.

- The goal is to maintain plasma potassium in the normal range and thereby prevent the potentially fatal cardiac effects of hypokalemia. Potassium status should be documented from the outset; this includes ECG to rule out rare life-threatening hyperkalemia.

- Potassium should be added routinely to the IV fluids at a rate of 10–20 mEq/hr except in patients with hyperkalemia (>6.0 mmol/L and/or ECG evidence), renal failure, or oliguria confirmed by bladder catheterization.
- Patients who present with hypokalemia should receive higher doses of potassium, 40 mEq/hr or greater, depending on severity.
- Potassium chloride is an appropriate initial choice, but this can later be changed to potassium phosphate to reduce chloride load.

- **Monitoring of therapy**
  - Blood glucose should be monitored hourly, serum electrolytes every 1–2 hours, and arterial blood gases as often as necessary.
  - Serum sodium tends to rise as hyperglycemia is corrected; failure to observe this trend suggests that the patient is being overhydrated with free water.
  - Serial serum ketone assays are not necessary, because ketonemia lags behind clinical recovery; closure of the anion gap is a more reliable index of metabolic recovery.
  - Use of a flowchart is an efficient method of tracking clinical data (e.g., weight, fluid balance, mental status) and laboratory results during the management of DKA.
  - Continuous ECG monitoring may be required for proper management of potassium in patients with oliguria or renal failure.

- **Bicarbonate therapy** is not routinely necessary and may be deleterious in certain situations.
  - However, bicarbonate therapy may be appropriate and should be considered for DKA patients who develop (a) shock or coma, (b) severe acidosis (pH 6.9–7.1), (c) severe depletion of buffering reserve (plasma bicarbonate <5 mEq/L), (d) acidosis-induced cardiac or respiratory dysfunction, or (e) severe hyperkalemia.
  - Sodium bicarbonate, 50–100 mEq in 1 L of 0.45% saline infused over 30–60 minutes, can be given in these situations. Bicarbonate treatment should be guided by arterial pH measurement and continued until the indications are no longer present.
  - Care should be taken to avoid hypokalemia; an additional dose of potassium, 10 mEq, should be included with each infusion of bicarbonate unless hyperkalemia is present.

- **Phosphate and magnesium** stores are subnormal in DKA patients, and plasma levels (particularly phosphate) decline further during insulin therapy. The clinical significance of these changes is unclear, and routine replacement of phosphate or magnesium is not necessary.
  - In hypophosphatemic patients with compromised oral intake, the use of potassium phosphate in maintenance IV fluids can be considered (see Chapter 3, Fluid and Electrolyte Management).
  - Magnesium therapy is indicated in patients with ventricular arrhythmia and can be administered as magnesium sulfate (50%) in doses of 2.5–5.0 mL (10–20 mEq magnesium) IV.

- **IV antimicrobial therapy** should be started promptly for documented bacterial, fungal, and other treatable infections. Empiric broad-spectrum antibiotics can be started in septic patients, pending results of blood cultures (see Chapter 14, Human Immunodeficiency Virus Infection and Acquired Immunodeficiency Syndrome).

- **Complications of DKA** include life-threatening conditions that must be recognized and treated promptly.
  - **Lactic acidosis** may result from prolonged dehydration, shock, infection, and tissue hypoxia in DKA patients. Lactic acidosis should be suspected in patients with refractory metabolic acidosis and a persistent anion gap despite optimal therapy for DKA. Adequate volume replacement, control of sepsis, and judicious use of bicarbonate constitute the approach to management.
  - **Arterial thrombosis** manifesting as stroke, myocardial infarction, or an ischemic limb occurs with increased frequency in DKA. However, routine anticoagulation is not indicated except as part of the specific therapy for a thrombotic event.

- **Cerebral edema,** a dire complication of DKA, is observed more frequently in children than adults.
  - Symptoms of increased intracranial pressure (e.g., headache, altered mental status, papilledema) or a sudden deterioration in mental status after initial improvement in a patient with DKA should raise suspicion for cerebral edema.
  - Overhydration with free water and excessively rapid correction of hyperglycemia are known risk factors.
  - A fall in serum sodium or failure to rise during therapy of DKA is a clue to imminent or established overhydration with free water. Neuroimaging with a computed tomography (CT) scan can establish the diagnosis. Prompt recognition and treatment with IV mannitol is essential and may prevent neurologic sequelae in patients who survive cerebral edema.
  - **Rebound ketoacidosis** can occur due to premature cessation of insulin therapy.
- **Prevention of DKA.** Every episode of DKA suggests a breakdown in clinical communication. Diabetes education should therefore be reinforced at every opportunity, with special emphasis on (a) self-management skills during prodromal sick days; (b) the body's need for more, rather than less, insulin during such illnesses; (c) testing of urine for ketones; and (d) procedures for obtaining timely and preventive medical advice.

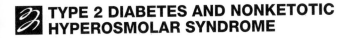

TYPE 2 DIABETES AND NONKETOTIC HYPEROSMOLAR SYNDROME

GENERAL PRINCIPLES

- Type 2 DM results from defective compensatory β-cell growth and secretory responses to insulin resistance.
- The loss of pancreatic β cells is progressive and insulin secretion is usually sufficient to prevent ketosis under basal conditions. However, type 2 DM patients can develop DKA when exposed to severe stress.
- The mechanisms underlying the β-cell loss in type 2 DM are unknown, but genetic and environmental factors are major components.

TREATMENT

- Recommended glycemic goals for patients with type 2 DM are the same as in type 1 DM.
- The achievement of these goals requires individualized therapy and a comprehensive approach that incorporates lifestyle and pharmacologic interventions. Several considerations should be taken into account before choosing oral agents (Table 21-2) in patients with type 2 DM:
  - Oral therapy should be initiated early in patients that failed glycemic control after a short-term trial of diet and exercise.
  - Monotherapy with maximum doses of insulin secretagogues, metformin, or thiazolidinediones yields comparable glucose-lowering effects.
  - The glucose-lowering effects of insulin secretagogues are observed within days, but approximately 20% of patients do not respond to these agents. In contrast, the maximum effects of metformin or thiazolidinediones may not be observed for several weeks.
  - A second or third agent including insulin should be added if no response is achieved with monotherapy.
  - Glycemic control with monotherapy is less likely to occur in patients with very high glucose readings (>240 mg/dL) at the time of diagnosis.[12] Combination therapy or insulin should be considered as first line for these patients.

| **TABLE 21-2** | | Characteristics of Oral Antidiabetic Agents | | |

Drug	Daily dosage range	Dose(s)/d	Duration of action (hr)	Main adverse effects
Insulin secretagogues sulfonylureas				
First generation				Hypoglycemia, weight gain
Tolbutamide	0.5–2.0 g	2–3	12	
Acetohexamide	0.25–1.5 g	1–2	12–24	
Tolazamide	0.1–0.5 g	1–2	12–24	
Chlorpropamide	1.25–20.0 mg	1	36–72	
Second generation				
Glyburide	5–40 mg	1–2	16–24	
Glipizide	1.8 mg	1–2	12	
Glimepiride		1	24	
Rapid acting				Hypoglycemia, weight gain
Nateglinide	60–360 mg	2–4	1–2	
Repaglinide	1–16 mg	2–4		
Biguanide				Gastrointestinal (GI) intolerance, lactic acidosis
Metformin	1.0–2.5 g	2–3	6–12	
α-Glucosidase inhibitors				GI intolerance, flatulence
Acarbose	75–300 mg	3	NA	
Miglitol	75–300 mg	3	NA	
Thiazolidinediones				Fluid retention, congestive heart failure, hepatotoxicity, weight gain
Rosiglitazone	2–8 mg	1–2	12–24	
Pioglitazone	15–45 mg	1	24	

- Because residual pancreatic β-cell function is required for the glucose-lowering effects of sulfonylureas, repaglinide, metformin, and thiazolidinediones, many patients with advanced type 2 DM do not respond satisfactorily to these agents and insulin therapy is recommended early for such patients.
- Moreover, the toxicity profile of some oral agents may preclude their use in patients with pre-existing illnesses.
- Insulin secretagogues
  - **Sulfonylureas** increase insulin secretion by binding to specific receptors in β cells. All sulfonylureas are equally effective in controlling hyperglycemia at equivalent doses.
    - These agents should be taken 30–60 minutes before food and should never be administered to fasting patients.
    - Chlorpropamide and glyburide are metabolized to an active metabolite with significant renal excretion and **should be avoided in the setting of impaired renal function and used with caution in elderly patients.**
    - Therapy should be initiated with the lowest effective dose and increased gradually over several days or weeks to the optimal dose.
    - Good responders to sulfonylurea include newly diagnosed type 2 diabetics with mild to moderate fasting hyperglycemia.
    - Hypoglycemia is more common with long-acting sulfonylureas.
    - Weight gain is also a notable adverse effect.

- **Repaglinide** is a meglitinide analog that augments food-stimulated insulin secretion with a similar glucose-lowering effect as sulfonylureas. Unlike sulfonylureas, however, the meglitinides have a very short onset of action and a short half-life.
  - Repaglinide can be used as a single agent or in combination with metformin in patients with type 2 DM.
  - The dose range is 0.5–4.0 mg PO with two to four meals daily; the drug should be taken within 30 minutes before meals and skipped if no meal is planned.
  - Adverse effects include hypoglycemia and weight gain.
- **Nateglinide**, a D-phenylalanine derivative chemically distinct from other insulin secretagogues, acts directly on the pancreatic β cells to stimulate early insulin secretion.[13]
  - It is taken 10 minutes before breakfast, lunch, and dinner and leads to significant insulin secretion within 15 minutes with a return to baseline in 3–4 hours, effectively controlling postprandial hyperglycemia. The maximum effective dosage is 120 mg.
  - There is a potential for drug interactions between nateglinide and medications affected by the cytochrome P-450 system.
  - The drug is well tolerated and the risk of hypoglycemia appears minimal.
- **Metformin**, the only biguanide in current clinical use, inhibits hepatic glucose output and stimulates glucose uptake by peripheral tissues. It is the preferred agent for patients in whom weight gain is not desirable.
  - Metformin should be taken with food and beginning with a single 500-mg or 850-mg tablet, the dose is increased slowly every 1–2 weeks until optimal glycemic effect is achieved or 2,000 mg/d is reached.
  - GI symptoms occur in 20%–30% of patients but are seldom serious and can be minimized by slow dosage titration.
  - Lactic acidosis, the most serious adverse effect, has an incidence of approximately 3 per 100,000 patient-years and a significant mortality rate. Risk factors for lactic acidosis include renal dysfunction, hypovolemia, tissue hypoxia, infection, alcoholism, and cardiopulmonary disease.
  - A serum creatinine level >1.5 mg/dL in men (>1.4 mg/dL in women) or a glomerular filtration rate of <70 mL/min are contraindications to metformin use.
  - Metformin should be discontinued at the time of the radiographic contrast procedure and not restarted for 48 hours.
  - Other situations in which metformin therapy should be avoided include cardiogenic or septic shock, congestive heart failure requiring pharmacologic therapy, severe liver disease, pulmonary insufficiency with hypoxemia, and severe tissue hypoperfusion.[14]
- **α-Glucosidase** inhibitors block polysaccharide and disaccharide breakdown and decrease postprandial hyperglycemia when administered with food. Two members of this class, acarbose and miglitol, exert maximal effects at a dosage of approximately 150 mg/d.
  - Each drug should be initiated at low doses (25 mg PO daily–tid, with food) and increased slowly in weekly steps of 25 mg to minimize GI intolerance.
  - Monotherapy with these agents seldom gives satisfactory results, but their addition to other drugs can improve glycemic control.
  - Dose-related adverse effects are diarrhea, bloating, abdominal cramping, and flatulence.
  - Acarbose has been associated with elevation in liver enzymes, and therefore periodic monitoring of transaminases is recommended.
  - Hypoglycemia in patients who are receiving regimens that include α-glucosidase inhibitors should be treated with glucose, not sucrose.
- **Thiazolidinediones** (TZDs) increase insulin sensitivity in muscle, adipose tissue, and liver. Therefore, patients with considerable endogenous insulin secretion respond better to these agents.
  - The risk of drug-induced hepatotoxicity with this class mandates close monitoring of liver function, particularly during the initial 12 months of drug exposure. Edema and cytopenia, from increased plasma volume, also occur with these agents.

- TZDs can precipitate congestive heart failure in patients who have cardiovascular disease and are in borderline compensation; therefore, therapy with these agents is not recommended in patients with significant heart disease (New York Heart Association class 3 and 4 cardiac status). Before starting TZDs, the physician should determine previous existence of cardiac disease, concomitant use of medications associated with fluid retention, edema, and shortness of breath. The risk of congestive heart failure is increased in patients with previous history of heart failure, coronary artery disease (CAD), hypertension, long-standing diabetes, left ventricular hypertrophy, pre-existing edema, edema after TZD therapy, insulin therapy, advanced age, renal failure, and aortic and mitral valve disease.[15]
- Resumption of ovulation may occur in some premenopausal women with anovulatory cycles after TZD therapy. Therefore, contraceptive practice should be reviewed to prevent unintended pregnancy. The two TZDs currently available, rosiglitazone and pioglitazone, appear to have similar efficacy on glycemia.
- **Rosiglitazone** can be used alone as an adjunct to diet and exercise or in combination with metformin or a sulfonylurea.
  - The usual starting dosage is 4 mg PO daily (or 2 mg PO bid) taken with or without food. This can be advanced to 8 mg PO daily (or 4 mg PO bid) after 12 weeks if glycemic response is inadequate.
  - Although data from clinical trials suggest a low propensity for hepatotoxicity, regular monitoring of hepatic transaminases is required in patients treated with rosiglitazone.
  - Potential drug interaction with phenobarbital, rifampin, amiodarone, and fluconazole can occur.
- **Pioglitazone** can also be used as a single agent (as an adjunct to diet and exercise) or in combination with sulfonylurea, metformin, or insulin.
  - The initial dosage is 15 mg or 30 mg PO daily, taken with or without food; this can be increased after several weeks to 45 mg PO daily for optimal effect.
  - Regular monitoring of hepatic transaminases is required during pioglitazone therapy.
  - Pioglitazone alters the levels of medications metabolized by cytochrome P-450 isoform CYP 3A4 (carbamazepine, cyclosporine, felodipine, and some oral contraceptives, among others).
- ■ **Insulin therapy** in type 2 DM is indicated in:
  - Patients in whom oral agents failed to sustain glycemic control
  - DKA
  - Nonketotic hyperosmolar crisis
  - Newly diagnosed patients with severe hyperglycemia
  - Pregnancy and other situations in which oral agents are contraindicated
- ■ **The success of insulin therapy** depends on the use of sufficient doses of insulin (0.6 to >1.0 units/kg of body weight per day) to achieve normoglycemia, rather than any specific pattern of insulin administration.
  - Once-daily injections of intermediate-acting or long-acting insulin at bedtime or before breakfast and daily or twice-daily combinations of intermediate- and short-acting insulins have all been used with good results.
  - Insulin glargine at bedtime and rapid-acting insulin at mealtimes is a good regimen to simulate physiologic insulin secretion.
  - Large doses of insulin (>100 units/d) usually are required for optimal glycemic control. Weight gain in this population can be considerable.
  - The risk of insulin-induced hypoglycemia, the most dangerous side effect, is low in this population, but its frequency increases as patients approach normal HbA_{1c} levels or when deterioration of kidney function occurs.
- ■ **Glucagonlike peptide 1 (GLP-1) agonists.** GLP-1 is an intestinal peptide that is secreted in response to food and regulates postprandial glycemia. It also protects and induces proliferation of β cells, making it an attractive alternative new therapy for diabetes.
  - Exenatide, a GLP-1 receptor agonist, has been shown to decrease postprandial hyperglycemia, reduce glucagon secretion, and induce weight loss.

- It has been approved as adjunctive therapy to sulfonylureas and/or metformin in patients who have not achieved control with these oral agents.[16,17] Data on long-term therapy with this agent are not available yet.
- Therapy should be initiated with 5 mcg twice daily and could be increased to 10 mcg after 1 month of therapy. The most common side effect is nausea.

■ **Combination therapy.** About 60% of patients on monotherapy may have worsening of metabolic control during the first 5 years of therapy, and concurrent use of two or more medications with different mechanisms of action may be necessary (United Kingdom Prospective Diabetes Study [UKPDS]).

- Dose increase and addition of agents should be performed in a short period of time until glucose control is achieved.
- Combination therapy using a secretagogue and an insulin sensitizer should be considered as first line in patients with HbA_{1c} levels ≥9. Widely used regimens include a sulfonylurea plus metformin (most common), or a TZD plus a sulfonylurea.
- Triple combination therapy has not been studied extensively and is considered somewhat controversial.
- The combination of a TZD plus insulin is less accepted because of a higher incidence of congestive heart failure exacerbations.
- Several combinations are already available (metformin-glibenclamide, rosiglitazone and metformin, and glipizide and metformin HCl).

NONKETOTIC HYPEROSMOLAR SYNDROME

General Principles

■ **Nonketotic hyperosmolar syndrome (NKHS)** is one of the most serious life-threatening complications of type 2 DM.

Epidemiology

■ Hyperosmolar hyperglycemic state occurs primarily in patients with type 2 DM, although that diagnosis may not have been known previously.
■ In 30%–40% of cases, NKHS is the initial presentation of a patient's diabetes.[18]
■ NKHS is significantly less common than DKA with an incidence of <1 case per 1,000 person-years.

Pathophysiology

■ Ketoacidosis is absent because insulin levels may effectively prevent lipolysis and subsequent ketogenesis yet are inadequate to facilitate peripheral glucose uptake and to prevent hepatic residual gluconeogenesis and glucose output.
■ Precipitating factors include stress, infection, stroke, noncompliance with medications, dietary indiscretion, and alcohol and cocaine abuse. Impaired glucose excretion is a contributory factor in patients with renal insufficiency or prerenal azotemia.

Diagnosis

Clinical Findings

■ In contrast to DKA, the onset of NKHS is usually insidious. Several days of deteriorating glycemic control are followed by increasing lethargy. Clinical evidence of severe dehydration is the rule. Some alterations in consciousness and focal neurologic deficits may be found at presentation or may develop during therapy. Therefore, repeated neurologic assessment is recommended.

Laboratory Findings

■ Clinical findings include (a) hyperglycemia, often >600 mg/dL; (b) plasma osmolality >320 mOsm/L; (c) absence of ketonemia; and (d) pH >7.3 and serum bicarbonate >20 mEq/L. Prerenal azotemia and lactic acidosis can develop. Although some patients will have detectable urine ketones, most patients do not have a metabolic acidosis. Lactic acidosis may develop from an underlying infection or other cause.

Differential Diagnosis
- The differential diagnosis of NKHS includes any cause of altered level of consciousness, including hypoglycemia, hyponatremia, severe dehydration, uremia, hyperammonemia, drug overdose, and sepsis. Seizures and acute strokelike syndromes are common presentations.

Management
- The goals of therapy are:
  - Restoration of hemodynamic stability and intravascular volume by fluid replacement
  - Correction of electrolyte abnormalities
  - Gradual correction of hyperglycemia and hyperosmolarity with fluid replacement and insulin therapy
  - Detection and treatment of underlying disease states and precipitating causes. However, such efforts should not delay fluid replacement and insulin therapy.

Treatment

- **Initial treatment** can make a difference in the frequency of complications and outcome. Therapy must be individualized based on the degree of dehydration and underlying cause (sepsis, renal and cardiac function). Rapid vein access and urinary catheterization are essential.
  - **Restoring hemodynamic stability** is the first aim. Restoration of intravascular volume should be followed by correction of total body water deficit. Compared to DKA, patients with NKHS may require as much as 10–12 L positive fluid balance over 24–36 hours to restore total deficits.
  - **Electrolyte management**
    - Although the potassium level may be initially normal or even high, all patients with NKHS are potassium depleted. Rehydration and insulin therapy usually result in hypokalemia, and this should be corrected.
    - If the initial potassium levels are low, replacement should begin immediately after urine output is ensured. Lactic acidosis requiring bicarbonate therapy may develop as a complication of NKHS or metformin therapy.
  - **Insulin therapy.** Insulin plays a secondary role in the initial management of NKHS, and fluid therapy always should precede insulin administration.
    - In patients with marked hyperglycemia (>600 mg/dL), regular insulin, 5–10 units IV, should be given immediately, followed by continuous infusion of 0.1–0.15 units/kg/hr. Lower doses of a regular insulin bolus can be used for less severe hyperglycemia.
    - Once plasma glucose decreases to 250–300 mg/dL, insulin infusion can be decreased to 1–2 units/hr and 5% dextrose should be added to the intravenous fluids. After full rehydration and clinical recovery, regular insulin can be given SC and patients can thereafter resume their usual diabetes therapy.
- **Monitoring of therapy.** Use of a flowchart is helpful for tracking clinical data and laboratory results.
  - Initially, blood glucose should be monitored every 30–60 minutes and serum electrolytes every 1–2 hours; frequency of monitoring can be decreased during recovery.
  - Neurologic status must be reassessed frequently; persistent lethargy or altered mentation indicates inadequate therapy. On the other hand, relapse after initial improvement in mental status suggests too-rapid correction of serum osmolarity.
- **Underlying illness.** Detection and treatment of any underlying predisposing illness is critical in the treatment of NKHS. Antibiotics should be administered early, after appropriate cultures, in patients in whom infection is known or suspected as a precipitant to a hyperosmolar hyperglycemic state (HHS). A high index of suspicion should be maintained for underlying pancreatitis, GI bleeding, renal failure, and thromboembolic events, especially acute myocardial infarction.

- **Complications of NKHS** include thromboembolic events (cerebral and myocardial infarction, mesenteric thrombosis, pulmonary embolism, and disseminated intravascular coagulation), cerebral edema, adult respiratory distress syndrome, and rhabdomyolysis.

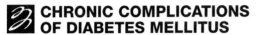 # CHRONIC COMPLICATIONS OF DIABETES MELLITUS

Prevention of long-term complications is one of the main goals of diabetes management. Appropriate treatment of established complications may delay their progression and improve quality of life.

- **Microvascular complications** include diabetic retinopathy, nephropathy, and neuropathy. These complications are directly related to hyperglycemia and can be prevented by maintaining tight glycemic control.

DIABETIC RETINOPATHY

General Principles

Epidemiology
- Diabetic retinopathy (DR) is diagnosed in 80% and 90% of type 1 diabetics after 10 and 15 years of diagnosis, respectively. DR is far less frequent in type 2 diabetics.[19]

Classification
- DR is classified in background retinopathy with or without maculopathy (microaneurysms, retinal infarcts) and proliferative retinopathy.
- **Other ocular abnormalities** associated with diabetes include cataract formation, dyskinetic pupils, glaucoma, optic neuropathy, extraocular muscle paresis, floaters, and fluctuating visual acuity. The latter is related to changes in blood glucose.
- The presence of floaters may be indicative of preretinal or vitreous hemorrhage; immediate referral for ophthalmologic evaluation is warranted.

Diagnosis

- Annual examination by an ophthalmologist is recommended at the time of diagnosis of all type 2 DM patients and at the beginning at puberty or 3–5 years after diagnosis for patients with type 1 DM. Dilated eye examination should be repeated annually by an experienced physician or ophthalmologist. Early detection is critical as therapy is more effective at these stages. In general, any diabetic with visual symptoms or abnormalities should be referred for ophthalmologic evaluation.

Treatment

- Background retinopathy usually is not associated with loss of vision. However, the development of macular edema or proliferative retinopathy (particularly new vessels near the optic disk) requires elective laser photocoagulation therapy to preserve vision. Vitrectomy is indicated for patients with vitreous hemorrhage or retinal detachment.

DIABETIC NEPHROPATHY

General Principles

Epidemiology
- Approximately 25%–45% of patients with type 1 DM develop clinically evident diabetic nephropathy during their lifetime, and this is the leading cause of end-stage renal disease (ESRD).[19] The risk of nephropathy seems to be equivalent in the two types of diabetes.[20]

Microalbuminuria

- **Microalbuminuria** precedes overt proteinuria (>300 mg albumin/d) by several years in type 1 and type 2 DM. The mean duration from diagnosis of type 1 diabetes to development of overt proteinuria is 17 years, and the time from the occurrence of proteinuria to ESRD averages 5 years. In type 2 DM, microalbuminuria can be present at the time of diagnosis.

Diagnosis

- **Screening** for microalbuminuria is mandatory because patients with nephropathy are often asymptomatic and because a number of effective intervention strategies can slow disease progression. Annual screening should be performed in type 1 patients who have had diabetes for >5 years and all type 2 diabetic patients starting at diagnosis.
- Measurement of the microalbumin-to-creatinine ratio (normal, <30 mg albumin/g creatinine) in a random urine sample is recommended for screening. At least two to three measurements within a 6-month period should be performed to establish the diagnosis.[21]

Prevention and Treatment

- **Intensive control of diabetes and hypertension** is an effective intervention for incipient or established diabetic nephropathy.
- In type 1 and type 2 patients with or without hypertension and microalbuminuria, angiotensin-converting enzyme (ACE) inhibitors delay the progression of nephropathy.
- In type 2 patients with hypertension, creatinine >1.5 mg/dL, and macroalbuminuria, angiotensin II receptor blockers (ARBs) delay progression of nephropathy.
- Nondihydropyridine calcium channel blockers, beta-blockers, or diuretics can be used in patients unable to tolerate ACE inhibitors or ARBs.[22]
- Dietary protein restriction may be beneficial in some patients.

DIABETIC NEUROPATHY

General Principles

Epidemiology

- It is the most common neuropathy in developed countries and accounts for more hospitalizations than all the other diabetic complications combined. Sensorimotor diabetic peripheral polyneuropathy is a major risk factor for foot trauma, ulceration, and Charcot arthropathy, and is responsible for 50%–75% of nontraumatic amputations.[23]

Classification

- Diabetic neuropathy can be classified in (a) subclinical neuropathy, determined by abnormalities in electrodiagnostic and quantitative sensory testing; (b) diffuse clinical neuropathy with distal symmetric sensorimotor and autonomic syndromes; and (c) focal syndromes.

Screening

- Sensation in the lower extremities should be documented at least annually, using either a light-touch monofilament or a tuning fork (frequency of 128 Hz).

Clinical Syndromes

- **Painful peripheral neuropathy** responds variably to treatment with tricyclic antidepressants (e.g., amitriptyline, 10–150 mg PO at bedtime), topical capsaicin (0.075% cream), or anticonvulsants (e.g., carbamazepine, 100–400 mg PO bid or gabapentin 1,800–3,600 mg/d). Patients should be warned about adverse effects, including sedation and anticholinergic symptoms (tricyclics), burning sensation (capsaicin), and blood dyscrasias (carbamazepine).

- **Orthostatic hypotension** is a manifestation of autonomic neuropathy, but common etiologies (e.g., dehydration, anemia, medications) should be excluded. Treatment is symptomatic: postural maneuvers, use of compressive garments (e.g., Jobst stockings), and intravascular expansion using sodium chloride, 1–4 g PO qid, and fludrocortisone, 0.1–0.3 mg PO daily. Hypokalemia, supine hypertension, and CHF are some adverse effects of fludrocortisone.
- **Intractable nausea and vomiting** in diabetes are manifestations of impaired GI motility from autonomic neuropathy. **Surveillance for DKA** is warranted in insulin-treated patients with nausea and vomiting, because interruption of insulin therapy is widespread among such patients. Other causes of nausea and vomiting should be excluded.
    - **Management of diabetic gastroenteropathy** can be challenging. Frequent, small meals (six to eight per day) of soft consistency that are low in fat and fiber provide relief for some patients. Parenteral nutrition may become necessary in some individuals. Improvement in glycemic control also is beneficial, because hyperglycemia delays gastric emptying.
    - **Pharmacologic therapy** includes the prokinetic agent metoclopramide, 10–20 mg PO (or as a suppository) before meals and at bedtime, and erythromycin, 125–500 mg PO qid. Extrapyramidal side effects (tremor and tardive dyskinesia) from the anti-dopaminergic actions of metoclopramide may limit therapy.
    - **Cyclical vomiting** that is unrelated to a GI motility disorder or other clear etiology may also occur in diabetic patients and appears to respond to amitriptyline, 25–50 mg PO at bedtime.
- **Diabetic cystopathy,** or bladder dysfunction, results from impaired autonomic control of detrusor muscle and sphincteric function. Manifestations include urgency, dribbling, incomplete emptying, overflow incontinence, and urinary retention. Recurrent urinary tract infections are common in patients with residual urine. Treatment with bethanecol, 10 mg tid, or intermittent self-catheterization may be required to relieve retention.
- **Diabetic diarrhea** should only be diagnosed after exclusion of other causes of diarrhea. The pathogenesis of diabetic diarrhea is unclear, so treatment is empiric. Repeated courses of broad-spectrum antibiotics (e.g., azithromycin, tetracycline, cephalosporins) may be beneficial; loperamide or octreotide, 50–75 mcg SC bid, can be effective in patients with intractable diarrhea.

MACROVASCULAR COMPLICATIONS OF DM

- Coronary heart disease (CHD), stroke, and peripheral vascular disease are responsible for 80% of deaths of diabetics.[24]
- Risk factors for macrovascular disease include insulin resistance, hyperglycemia, microalbuminuria, hypertension, hyperlipidemia, cigarette smoking, and obesity.
    - Aggressive risk factor reduction lowers the risk of both micro- and macrovascular complications in patients with diabetes.
        - Glycemic control should be optimized to hemoglobin A_{1c} <7 and as close to normal as possible.
        - Hypertension should be controlled to a target blood pressure of <130/80 mm Hg (or < 125/75 mm Hg in patients with proteinuria).
        - Hyperlipidemia should be treated appropriately, with a target low-density lipoprotein cholesterol level of <100 mg/dL, or < 70 mg/dL in patients with known CHD. High-density lipoprotein (HDL) cholesterol levels of >50 mg/dL, and triglyceride levels of <150 mg/dL should be achieved.
        - Cigarette smoking should be actively discouraged, and weight loss should be promoted in obese patients.
        - Aspirin, 81–325 mg/d, is of proven benefit in secondary prevention of myocardial infarction or stroke in diabetic patients.
- **Coronary artery disease**[24] occurs at a younger age and may have atypical clinical presentations in patients with diabetes.
    - Myocardial infarction carries a worse prognosis, and angioplasty gives less satisfactory results in diabetic patients.

- Cardiovascular risk factors should be assessed at least annually and treated aggressively (see Goals, above). ECG should be obtained yearly, and there should be a low threshold for ordering stress tests.
- Screening with cardiac stress test should be performed in patients with a history of peripheral or carotid occlusive disease; sedentary lifestyle; age >35 years who plans to begin a vigorous exercise program; or patients with two or more of the following CHD risk factors: dyslipidemia, hypertension, smoking, a positive family history of premature coronary disease, and the presence of micro- or macroalbuminuria.[25]
- **Management of diabetes after acute myocardial infarction**
  - Hyperglycemia (glucose >110 mg/dL), with or without a prior history of diabetes, is an independent predictor of in-hospital mortality and congestive heart failure in patients admitted for acute myocardial infarction.[26] However, the results of the studies that investigated tight glucose control with insulin in the setting of acute myocardial infarction in type 2 diabetics are inconclusive.[27–29] Nevertheless, given the consistent epidemiologic association, it is reasonable to expect that glucose-lowering effects in acute conditions could lead to clinical benefit.

Peripheral Vascular Disease

General Principles

Epidemiology

- Diabetes and smoking are the strongest risk factors for peripheral vascular disease (PVD). In diabetics, the risk of PVD is increased by age, duration of diabetes, and presence of peripheral neuropathy. PVD is a marker for systemic vascular disease involving coronary, cerebral, and renal vessels. Diabetic patients with PVD have increased risk for subsequent MI or stroke regardless of the PVD symptoms.

Clinical Presentation

- Symptoms of PVD include intermittent claudication, rest pain, tissue loss, and gangrene, but most of the patients are asymptomatic due to concomitant neuropathy.
  - Physical examination findings including diminished pulses, dependent rubor, pallor on elevation, absence of hair growth, dystrophic toenails, and cool, dry, fissured skin are signs of vascular insufficiency.

Diagnosis

- The ankle-to-brachial index (ABI) defined as the ratio of the systolic blood pressure in the ankle divided by the systolic blood pressure at the arm is the best initial diagnostic test. An ABI <0.9 by handheld 5- to 10-MHz Doppler probe has a 95% sensitivity for detecting angiogram-positive PVD.[30]
- Screening ABI should be performed in (a) diabetics older than 50 years of age, (b) diabetics younger than 50 years of age who have other PVD risk factors (e.g., smoking, hypertension, hyperlipidemia, or duration of diabetes 10 years),[31] and (c) patients with symptoms of PVD.

Treatment

- Risk factors should be controlled, with similar goals described for coronary artery disease (see Macrovascular Complications of Diabetes).
- Antiplatelets agents such as clopidogrel (75 mg/d) have additional benefits when compared to aspirin in diabetics with PVD.[31]
- Therapy for intermittent claudication could also benefit by exercise rehabilitation and cilostazol (100 mg bid). This medication is contraindicated in patients with CHF.

MISCELLANEOUS COMPLICATIONS

- **Miscellaneous complications** such as erectile dysfunction and diabetic foot ulcers have multiple etiologies.

Erectile Dysfunction

General Principles

Epidemiology
- It is estimated that 40%–60% of men with diabetes have erectile dysfunction (ED), and the prevalence varies depending on the duration of diabetes. In addition to increasing age, ED is associated with smoking, poor glycemic control, low HDL, neuropathy, and retinopathy.

Etiology
- ED in diabetics is multifactorial. It can result from nerve damage, impaired blood flow (vascular insufficiency), adverse drug effects, endocrinopathy, psychological factors, or a combination of these etiologies.

Treatment
- If endocrinologic evaluation is negative and other treatable causes have been excluded, most diabetics respond to phosphodiesterase type 5 inhibitors (sildenafil, tadalafil, vardenafil). Typical doses include sildenafil 50–100 mg or vardenafil 10 mg 1 hour prior to sexual activity, and tadalafil 10 mg/d prior to sexual activity. Glycemic control should be intensified and could be a helpful adjuvant therapy, and specialist referral should be considered if the problem persists. Cardiovascular status should be considered before starting these agents. **Sildenafil should not be used concurrently with nitrates** to prevent severe and potentially fatal hypotensive reactions.

Diabetic Foot Ulcers

General Principles

Epidemiology
- The prevalence of foot ulcers is 4%–10% and the lifetime incidence is as high as 25%.[32]

Etiology
- Causative factors include neuropathy, excessive plantar pressure, and repetitive trauma. Vascular insufficiency, poor healing, and polymicrobial infection are major contributors to ulcer formation.

Screening
- **Screening to identify patients at risk for ulcers** includes detection of loss of protective sensation by monofilament (see Peripheral Neuropathy) and peripheral vascular disease.

Treatment
- Poorly managed foot ulcers may result in limb loss from amputation. Patient education should emphasize prevention: daily foot examination, application of moisturizing lotion, use of proper footwear, and caution with self-pedicure.
- The exposed feet should be inspected and palpated at every patient encounter; significant findings, such as calluses, hammertoes or other deformities, and soft tissue lesions, should be evaluated.
- Diabetic foot infections should be treated aggressively. Proper management includes a multidisciplinary approach that includes orthopedic surgeons, specialized nursing care, and close monitoring. Revascularization should be considered as an integral part of the management of food ulcers. The presence of deep infection with abscess, cellulitis, gangrene, or osteomyelitis is an indication for hospitalization and prompt surgical drainage. Acute treatment of foot infections is dependent on severity, as outlined below.
- **Mild to moderate cellulitis.** Rest, elevation of the affected foot, and relief of pressure are essential components of treatment and should be initiated at first presentation. In localized cellulitis and new ulcers, *Staphylococcus aureus* and streptococci are the most frequent pathogens. Therapy with oral dicloxacillin, first-generation cephalosporin, amoxicillin/clavulanate, or clindamycin is recommended.

- **Moderate to severe cellulitis.** This type of involvement requires intravenous therapy and admission to the hospital. Consultation for debridement and aerobic and anaerobic cultures are necessary when necrotic tissue is present. Intravenous oxacillin/nafcillin, a first-generation IV cephalosporin, ampicillin/sulbactam, clindamycin, and vancomycin are options for therapy. Antibiotic coverage should subsequently be tailored according to the clinical response of the patient, culture results, and sensitivity testing.
- **Moderate to severe cellulitis with ischemia or significant local necrosis.** It is important to determine the presence of bone involvement and peripheral vascular disease since failure to diagnose osteomyelitis and ischemia often results in failure of wound healing.
  - Bone involvement is present if bone is seen at the base of the ulcer or is easily detected by gentle probing with a blunt sterile probe. Radiographs are not very sensitive for diagnosis and leukocyte scanning or magnetic resonance imaging offers better specificity.
  - Presence of peripheral vascular disease is suspected by absence of pedal pulses or decreased capillary filling.
  - Intravenous antibiotics, bedrest, surgical debridement, culture obtained from the base of the ulcer, and bone culture help direct antibiotic therapy.
  - Ampicillin/sulbactam and ticarcillin/clavulanate are first-line agents; piperacillin/tazobactam, clindamycin plus ciprofloxacin, ceftazidime, cefepime, cefotaxime, or ceftriaxone plus metronidazole are good alternatives for initial therapy.
  - In the presence of osteomyelitis, 20–12 weeks of intravenous antibiotic therapy is recommended. Ulcers with localized or generalized gangrene require surgical amputation.

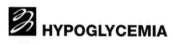 **HYPOGLYCEMIA**

DIAGNOSIS

Clinical Presentation

- Hypoglycemia is a clinical syndrome in which low serum (or plasma) glucose levels lead to symptoms of sympathoadrenal activation (sweating, anxiety, tremor, nausea, palpitations, and tachycardia) from increased secretion of counterregulatory hormones (e.g., epinephrine).
- Neuroglycopenia occurs as the glucose levels decrease further (fatigue, dizziness, headache, visual disturbances, drowsiness, difficulty speaking, inability to concentrate, abnormal behavior, confusion, and ultimately loss of consciousness or seizures).

Classification

- Hypoglycemia is uncommon in patients not treated for diabetes. Iatrogenic factors usually account for hypoglycemia in the setting of diabetes, whereas hypoglycemia in the nondiabetic population could be classified as fasting or postprandial.
  - **Iatrogenic hypoglycemia** complicates therapy with insulin or sulfonylureas and is a limiting factor to achieve glycemic control during intensive therapy in patients with DM.
    - Risk factors for iatrogenic hypoglycemia include skipped or insufficient meals, unaccustomed physical exertion, misguided therapy, alcohol ingestion, and drug overdose.
    - Recurrent episodes of hypoglycemia impair recognition of hypoglycemic symptoms, thereby increasing the risk for severe hypoglycemia (hypoglycemia unawareness).
    - Hypoglycemia unawareness results from defective glucose counterregulation with blunting of autonomic symptoms and counterregulatory hormone secretion during hypoglycemia. Seizures or coma may develop in such patients without the usual warning symptoms of hypoglycemia.

Treatment

- Isolated episodes of mild hypoglycemia may not require specific intervention. Recurrent episodes require a review of lifestyle factors; adjustments may be indicated in the content, timing, and distribution of meals, as well as medication dosage and timing. Severe hypoglycemia is an indication for supervised treatment.

  - **Readily absorbable carbohydrates** (e.g., glucose and sugar-containing beverages) can be administered orally to conscious patients for rapid effect. Alternatively, milk, candy bars, fruit, cheese, and crackers may be adequate in some patients with mild hypoglycemia. Hypoglycemia associated with acarbose or miglitol therapy should preferentially be treated with glucose. Glucose tablets and carbohydrate supplies should be readily available to patients with DM at all times.

  - **IV dextrose** is indicated for severe hypoglycemia, in patients with altered consciousness, and during restriction of oral intake. An initial bolus, 20–50 mL of 50% dextrose, should be given immediately, followed by infusion of D_5W (or $D_{10}W$) to maintain blood glucose above 100 mg/dL. Prolonged IV dextrose infusion and close observation is warranted in sulfonylurea overdose, in the elderly, and in patients with defective counterregulation.

  - **Glucagon**, 1 mg IM (or SC), is an effective initial therapy for severe hypoglycemia in patients unable to receive oral intake or in whom an IV access cannot be secured immediately. Vomiting is a frequent side effect, and therefore care should be taken to prevent the risk of aspiration. A glucagon kit should be available to patients with a history of severe hypoglycemia; family members and roommates should be instructed in its proper use.

  - **Education** regarding etiologies of hypoglycemia, preventive measures, and appropriate adjustments to medication, diet, and exercise regimens are essential tasks to be addressed during hospitalization for severe hypoglycemia.

  - **Hypoglycemia unawareness** can develop in patients who are undergoing intensive diabetes therapy. These patients should be encouraged to monitor their blood glucose frequently and take timely measures to correct low values (<60 mg/dL). In patients with very tightly controlled diabetes, slight relaxation in glycemic control and scrupulous avoidance of hypoglycemia can restore the lost warning symptoms.

- **Hypoglycemia unrelated to diabetes therapy** is an infrequent problem in general medical practice.

  - Plasma or capillary blood glucose should be obtained, whenever feasible, to confirm hypoglycemia.

  - Any patient with a serum glucose concentration <60 mg/dL should be suspected of having a hypoglycemic disorder, and further evaluation is required if the value is <50 mg/dL.

  - Absence of symptoms with these levels of glucose suggests the possibility of artifactual hypoglycemia. These levels are usually accompanied by symptoms of hypoglycemia. Detailed evaluation is usually required in a healthy-appearing patient, whereas hypoglycemia may be readily recognized as part of the underlying illness in a sick patient.[33] Major categories include fasting and postprandial hypoglycemia.

  - **Fasting hypoglycemia** can be caused by inappropriate insulin secretion (e.g., insulinoma), alcohol abuse, severe hepatic or renal insufficiency, hypopituitarism, glucocorticoid deficiency, or surreptitious injection of insulin or ingestion of a sulfonylurea.

    - These patients present with neuroglycopenic symptoms but episodic autonomic symptoms may be present. Occasionally patients with recurrent seizures, dementia, and bizarre behavior are referred for neuropsychiatric evaluation, which may delay timely diagnosis of hypoglycemia.

    - **Definitive diagnosis** of fasting hypoglycemia requires hourly blood glucose monitoring during a supervised fast lasting up to 72 hours and measurement of plasma insulin, C-peptide, and sulfonylurea metabolites if hypoglycemia (<50 mg/dL) is documented. Patients who develop hypoglycemia and have measurable plasma insulin and C-peptide levels without sulfonylurea metabolites require further evaluation for an insulinoma.

■ **Postprandial hypoglycemia** often is suspected, but seldom proven, in patients with vague symptoms that occur 1 or more hours after meals.

- **Alimentary hypoglycemia** should be considered in patients with a history of partial gastrectomy or intestinal resection in whom recurrent symptoms develop 1–2 hours after eating. The mechanism is thought to be related to too-rapid glucose absorption, resulting in a robust insulin response. These symptoms should be distinguished from dumping syndrome, which is not associated with hypoglycemia and occurs in the first hour after food intake. Thus, frequent small meals with reduced carbohydrate content may ameliorate symptoms.
- **Functional hypoglycemia.** Symptoms that are possibly suggestive of hypoglycemia, which may or may not be confirmed by plasma glucose measurement, occur in some patients who have not undergone GI surgery. This condition is referred to as "functional hypoglycemia." The symptoms tend to develop 3–5 hours after meals. Current evaluation and management of functional hypoglycemia are imprecise; some patients show evidence of IGT and may respond to dietary therapy.

References

1. Center for Disease Control and Prevention. Prevalance of diabetes. Available at: *http://www.cdc.gov/diabetes/pubs/pdf/ndfs_2005*.
2. American Diabetes Association: Standards of medical care in diabetes—2006. *Diabetes Care* 2006;29 Suppl 1:S4–42.
3. The DCCT Research Group. The effect of intensive treatment of diabetes on the development and progression of long-term complications in insulin-dependent diabetes mellitus. *N Engl J Med* 1993;329:978–986.
4. UK Prospective Diabetes Study Group. Intensive blood-glucose control with sulphonylureas or insulin compared with conventional treatment and risk of complications in patients with type 2 diabetes (UKPDS 33). *Lancet* 1998;352:837–853.
5. Moghissi ES, Hirsch IB. Hospital management of diabetes. *Endocrinol Metab Clin North Am* 2005;34:99–116.
6. Van den Berghe G, Wouters P, Weekers F, et al. Intensive insulin therapy in the critically ill patients. *N Engl J Med* 2001;345:1359–1367.
7. Van den Berghe G, Wilmer A, Hermans G, et al. Intensive Insulin Therapy in the Medical ICU. *N Engl J Med* 2006;354:449–461.
8. American College of Endocrinology Task Force on Inpatient Diabetes and Metabolic Control. Position Statement on Inpatient Diabetes and Metabolic Control. *Endocr Pract* 2004;10:77–82.
9. Queale WS, Seidler AJ, Brancati FL. Glycemic control and sliding scale insulin use in medical inpatients with diabetes mellitus. *Arch Intern Med* 1997;157:545–552.
10. McMahon MM, Rizza RA. Concise review for primary-care physicians: nutrition support in hospitalized patients with diabetes mellitus. *Mayo Clin Proc* 1996;71:587–594.
11. American Diabetes Association: Hyperglycemic crisis in diabetes (Position Statement). *Diabetes Care* 2004;27:S94–S102.
12. DeFronzo RA. Pharmacologic therapy for type 2 diabetes mellitus. *Ann Intern Med* 1999;131:281–303.
13. Hanefeld M, Dickinson S, Bouter KP, et al. Rapid and short-acting mealtime insulin secretion with nateglinide controls both prandial and mean glycemia. *Diabetes Care* 2000;23:202–207.
14. Bailey CJ, Turner RC. Metformin. *N Engl J Med* 1996;334:574–579.
15. Nesto RW, Bell D, Bonow RO, et al. Thiazolidinedione use, fluid retention, and congestive heart failure: a consensus statement from the American Heart Association and American Diabetes Association. *Diabetes Care* 2004;27:256–263.
16. Buse JB, Henry RR, Han J, et al. Effects of exenatide (exendin-4) on glycemic control over 30 weeks in sulfonylurea-treated patients with type 2 diabetes. *Diabetes Care* 2004;27:2628–2635.
17. DeFronzo RA, Ratner RE, Han J, et al. Effects of exenatide (exendin 4) on glycemic control and weight over 30 weeks in metformin treated patients with type 2 diabetes. *Diabetes Care* 2005;28:1092–1100.

18. Nugent BW. Hyperosmolar hyperglycemic state. *Emerg Med Clin North Am* 2005;23:629–648.
19. Jawa A, Kcomt J, Fonseca VA. Diabetic nephropathy and retinopathy. *Med Clin North Am* 2004;88:1001–1036.
20. Rossing P, Rossing K, Jacobsen P, et al. Unchanged incidence of diabetic nephropathy in IDDM patients. *Diabetes* 1995;44:739–743.
21. Diabetic nephropathy: American Diabetes Association. *Diabetes Care* 2003;26:S94–S98.
22. Molich ME, DeFronzo RA, Franz MJ, et al. Diabetic nephropathy. *Diabetes Care* 2004;27:S79–S83.
23. Vinik A, Mehrabyan A: Diabetic neuropathies. *Med Clin N Am* 2004;88:947–999.
24. Webster MW, Scott RS. What cardiologists need to know about diabetes. *Lancet* 1997;350 Suppl 1:SI23–SI28.
25. Weir GC, Nathan DM, Singer DE: Standards of care for diabetes (Technical Review). *Diabetes Care* 1994;17:1514–1522.
26. Capes SE, Hunt D, Malmberg K, et al. Stress hyperglycaemia and increased risk of death after myocardial infarction in patients with and without diabetes: a systematic overview. *Lancet* 2000;355:773–778.
27. Malmberg K for the DIGAMI study group. Prospective randomised study of intensive unsulin treatment on long term survival after acute myocardial infarction in patients with diabetes mellitus. *BMJ* 1997;314:1512–1515.
28. Malmberg K, Rydén L, Efendic S. Randomized trial of insulin-glucose infusion followed by subcutaneous insulin treatment in diabetic patients with acute myocardial infarction (DIGAMI study): effects on mortality at 1 year. *J Am Coll Cardiol* 1995;26:57–65.
29. Malmberg K, Ryden L, Wedel H, et al. Intense metabolic control by means of insulin in patients with diabetes mellitus and acute myocardial infarction (DIGAMI 2): effects on mortality and morbidity. *Eur Heart J* 2005;26:650–661.
30. Fowkes FGR. The measurement of atherosclerotic peripheral arterial disease in epidemiological surveys. *Int J Epidemiol* 1988;17:248–254.
31. American Diabetes Association. Peripheral arterial disease in people with diabetes. *Diabetes Care* 2003;26:3333–3341.
32. Singh N, Armstrong DG, Lipsky BA. Preventing Foot Ulcers in Patients With Diabetes. *JAMA* 2005;293:217–228.
33. Fischer KF, Lees JA, Newman JH. Hypoglycemia in hospitalized patients: causes and outcomes. *N Engl J Med.* 1986;315:1245–1250.

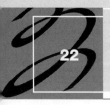

22 ENDOCRINE DISEASES
William E. Clutter

 EVALUATION OF THYROID FUNCTION

GENERAL PRINCIPLES

- The major hormone secreted by the thyroid is **thyroxine** (T_4), which is converted by deiodinases in many tissues to the more potent **triiodothyronine** (T_3). Both are bound reversibly to plasma proteins, primarily **thyroxine-binding globulin (TBG)**. Only the free (unbound) fraction enters cells and produces biological effects. T_4 secretion is stimulated by **thyroid-stimulating hormone (TSH)**. In turn, TSH secretion is inhibited by T_4, forming a negative feedback loop that keeps free T_4 levels within a narrow normal range. Diagnosis of thyroid disease is based on clinical findings, palpation of the thyroid, and measurement of plasma TSH and thyroid hormones.[1]
  - **Thyroid palpation** determines the size and consistency of the thyroid and the presence of nodules, tenderness, or a thrill.
  - **Plasma TSH is the initial test of choice in most patients with suspected thyroid disease**, except when thyroid function is not in a steady state.[2] TSH levels are elevated in very mild primary hypothyroidism and are suppressed to <0.1 microunits/mL in very mild hyperthyroidism. Thus, **a normal plasma TSH level excludes hyperthyroidism and primary hypothyroidism**. Because even slight changes in thyroid hormone levels affect TSH secretion, **abnormal TSH levels are not specific for clinically important thyroid disease.** Changes in plasma TSH lag behind changes in plasma T_4, and TSH levels may be misleading when plasma T_4 levels are changing rapidly, as during treatment of hyperthyroidism.
    - **Plasma TSH is mildly elevated** (up to 20 microunits/mL) in some euthyroid patients with **nonthyroidal illnesses** and in mild (also known as subclinical) hypothyroidism.
    - **TSH levels may be suppressed to <0.1 microunits/mL** in **severe nonthyroidal illness**, in mild (also known as subclinical) hyperthyroidism, and during treatment with dopamine or high doses of glucocorticoids. Also, TSH levels remain <0.1 microunits/mL for some time after hyperthyroidism is corrected.
    - **TSH levels are usually within the reference range in secondary hypothyroidism** and are not useful for detection of this rare form of hypothyroidism.
  - **Plasma free T_4** confirms the diagnosis and assesses the severity of hyperthyroidism when plasma TSH is <0.1 microunits/mL. It is also used to diagnose secondary hypothyroidism and adjust thyroxine therapy in patients with pituitary disease. Most laboratories measure free T_4 by analog immunoassays. Total T_4 assays are less reliable and should not be used, except when free T_4 is artifactually elevated by heparin treatment (see Table 22-1).
    - **Free T_4 measured by equilibrium dialysis** is the most reliable measure of clinical thyroid status, but results seldom are rapidly available. It is needed only in rare cases in which the diagnosis is not clear from measurement of plasma TSH and free T_4 by analog immunoassay.
  - **Effect of nonthyroidal illness on thyroid function tests.**[3] Many illnesses alter thyroid tests without causing true thyroid dysfunction (the nonthyroidal illness or euthyroid

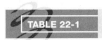

TABLE 22-1   **Effects of Drugs on Thyroid Function Tests**

Effect	Drug
Decreased free and total T$_4$	
True hypothyroidism (TSH elevated)	Iodine (amiodarone, radiographic contrast)
	Lithium
Inhibition of TSH secretion	Glucocorticoids
	Dopamine
Multiple mechanisms (TSH normal)	Phenytoin
Decreased total T$_4$ only	
Decreased TBG (TSH normal)	Androgens
Inhibition of T$_4$ binding to TBG (TSH normal)	Furosemide (high doses)
	Salicylates
Increased free and total T$_4$	
True hyperthyroidism (TSH <0.1 microunits/mL)	Iodine (amiodarone, radiographic contrast)
Inhibited T$_4$ to T$_3$ conversion (TSH normal)	Amiodarone
Increased free T$_4$ only	
Displacement of T$_4$ from TBG *in vitro* (TSH normal)	Heparin, low molecular weight heparin
Increased total T$_4$ only	
Increased TBG (TSH normal)	Estrogens, tamoxifen

T$_3$ = triiodothyronine; T$_4$ = thyroxine; TBG = thyroxine-binding globulin; TSH = thyroid-stimulating hormone.

sick syndrome). These changes must be recognized to avoid mistaken diagnosis and therapy.

- **The low T$_3$ syndrome** occurs in many illnesses, during starvation, and after trauma or surgery. Conversion of T$_4$ to T$_3$ is decreased, and plasma T$_3$ levels are low. Plasma free T$_4$ and TSH levels are normal. This may be an adaptive response to illness, and thyroid hormone therapy is not beneficial.
- **The low T$_4$ syndrome** occurs in severe illness. Plasma total T$_4$ levels fall due to decreased levels of TBG and perhaps due to inhibition of T$_4$ binding to TBG. **Plasma free T$_4$ measured by equilibrium dialysis usually remains normal.** However, when measured by commonly available analog immunoassays, free T$_4$ may be low. **TSH levels decrease early in severe illness,** sometimes to <0.1 microunits/mL. **During recovery they rise, sometimes to levels higher than the normal range** (although rarely >20 microunits/mL).
- **A number of drugs affect thyroid function tests** (Table 22-1). Iodine-containing drugs (**amiodarone** and radiographic contrast media) may cause hyperthyroidism or hypothyroidism in susceptible patients. Other drugs alter thyroid function tests, especially plasma total T$_4$, without causing true thyroid dysfunction. In general, plasma TSH levels are a reliable guide to determining whether true hyperthyroidism or hypothyroidism is present.

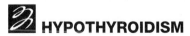

HYPOTHYROIDISM

GENERAL PRINCIPLES

Etiology

- **Primary hypothyroidism** (due to disease of the thyroid itself) accounts for >90% of cases.[4]

- Chronic lymphocytic thyroiditis (Hashimoto disease)[5] is the most common cause and may be associated with Addison disease and other endocrine deficits. Its prevalence is greater in women and increases with age.
- **Iatrogenic hypothyroidism** due to thyroidectomy or radioactive iodine (RAI, ^{131}I) therapy is also common.
- Transient hypothyroidism occurs in postpartum thyroiditis and subacute thyroiditis, usually after a period of hyperthyroidism.
- **Drugs that may cause hypothyroidism** include iodine-containing drugs, lithium, interferon-α, interleukin-2, and thalidomide.
- **Secondary hypothyroidism** due to TSH deficiency is uncommon but may occur in any disorder of the pituitary or hypothalamus. However, it rarely occurs without other evidence of pituitary disease.

Clinical Findings

- Most symptoms of hypothyroidism are nonspecific and develop gradually. They include cold intolerance, fatigue, somnolence, poor memory, constipation, menorrhagia, myalgias, and hoarseness.
- Signs include slow tendon reflex relaxation, bradycardia, facial and periorbital edema, dry skin, and nonpitting edema (myxedema). Mild weight gain may occur, but hypothyroidism does not cause marked obesity. Rare manifestations include hypoventilation, pericardial or pleural effusions, deafness, and carpal tunnel syndrome.
- Laboratory findings may include hyponatremia and elevated plasma levels of cholesterol, triglycerides, and creatine kinase. The electrocardiogram (ECG) may show low voltage and T-wave abnormalities.

DIAGNOSIS

- Hypothyroidism is readily treatable and should be suspected in any patient with compatible symptoms, especially in the presence of a diffuse goiter or a history of RAI therapy or thyroid surgery.
  - **In suspected primary hypothyroidism, plasma TSH is the best initial diagnostic test.**
    - A normal value excludes primary hypothyroidism, and a markedly elevated value (>20 microunits/mL) confirms the diagnosis.
    - Mild elevation of plasma TSH (<20 microunits/mL) may be due to nonthyroidal illness, but usually indicates **mild (or subclinical) primary hypothyroidism**, in which thyroid function is impaired but increased secretion of TSH maintains plasma free T_4 levels within the reference range. These patients may have nonspecific symptoms that are compatible with hypothyroidism and a mild increase in serum cholesterol and low-density lipoprotein cholesterol. They develop clinical hypothyroidism at a rate of 2.5% per year.
  - **If secondary hypothyroidism is suspected because of evidence of pituitary disease, plasma free T_4 should be measured.**
    - Plasma TSH levels are usually within the reference range in secondary hypothyroidism and cannot be used alone to make this diagnosis. Patients with secondary hypothyroidism should be evaluated for other pituitary hormone deficits and for a mass lesion of the pituitary or hypothalamus (see Anterior Pituitary Gland Dysfunction).
  - **In severe nonthyroidal illness,** the diagnosis of hypothyroidism may be difficult.[3] Plasma total T_4 and free T_4 measured by routine assays may be low.
    - **Plasma TSH is the best initial diagnostic test.** A normal TSH value is strong evidence that the patient is euthyroid, except when there is evidence of pituitary or hypothalamic disease or in patients treated with dopamine or high doses of glucocorticoids. Marked elevation of plasma TSH (>20 microunits/mL) establishes the diagnosis of primary hypothyroidism.
    - Moderate elevations of plasma TSH (<20 microunits/mL) may occur in euthyroid patients with nonthyroidal illness and are not specific for hypothyroidism.

Plasma free T_4 should be measured if TSH is moderately elevated, or if secondary hypothyroidism is suspected, and patients should be treated for hypothyroidism if plasma free T_4 is low. Thyroid function in these patients should be re-evaluated after recovery from illness.

THERAPY

- **Thyroxine** is the drug of choice. The average replacement dose is 1.6 mcg/kg PO daily, and most patients require doses between 75 and 150 mcg/daily. In elderly patients, the average replacement dose is somewhat lower. The need for lifelong treatment should be emphasized. Thyroxine should be taken 30 minutes before a meal, since dietary fiber interferes with its absorption, and should not be taken with medications that affect its absorption (see below).
    - **Initiation of therapy.** Young, otherwise healthy adults should be started on 100 mcg/daily. This regimen gradually corrects hypothyroidism, as several weeks are required to reach steady-state plasma levels of T_4. Symptoms begin to improve within a few weeks. In otherwise healthy elderly patients, the initial dose should be 50 mcg/daily. Patients with cardiac disease should be started on 25–50 mcg/daily and monitored carefully for exacerbation of cardiac symptoms.
    - **Dose adjustment and follow-up.**
        - **In primary hypothyroidism, the goal of therapy is to maintain plasma TSH within the normal range.** Plasma TSH should be measured 2–3 months after initiation of therapy. The dose of thyroxine then should be adjusted in 12- to 25-mcg increments at intervals of 6–8 weeks until plasma TSH is normal. Thereafter, annual TSH measurement is adequate to monitor therapy. TSH should also be measured in the first trimester of pregnancy, since the thyroxine dose requirement increases at this time. Overtreatment, indicated by a subnormal TSH, should be avoided since it increases the risk of osteoporosis and atrial fibrillation.
        - **In secondary hypothyroidism, plasma TSH cannot be used to adjust therapy.** The goal of therapy is to maintain the **plasma free T_4** near the middle of the reference range. The dose of thyroxine should be adjusted at 6- to 8-week intervals until this goal is achieved. Thereafter, annual measurement of plasma free T_4 is adequate to monitor therapy.
        - **Coronary artery disease** may be exacerbated by treatment of hypothyroidism. The dose of thyroxine should be increased slowly in patients with coronary artery disease, with careful attention to worsening angina, heart failure, or arrhythmias.
    - **Situations in which thyroxine dose requirements change.** Difficulty in controlling hypothyroidism is most often due to **poor compliance** with therapy. Observed therapy may be necessary in some cases. Other causes of increasing thyroxine requirement include:
        - **Malabsorption** due to intestinal disease or **drugs that interfere with thyroxine absorption** (e.g., **calcium carbonate, ferrous sulfate,** cholestyramine, sucralfate, aluminum hydroxide)
        - **Drug interactions that increase thyroxine clearance** (e.g., estrogen, rifampin, carbamazepine, phenytoin) or block conversion of T_4 to T_3 (**amiodarone**)
        - **Pregnancy,** in which thyroxine requirements often increase in the first trimester (see below)
        - Gradual failure of remaining endogenous thyroid function after RAI treatment of hyperthyroidism
    - **Thyroxine dose increases by an average of 50% in the first half of pregnancy.**[6] In women with primary hypothyroidism, plasma TSH should be measured as soon as pregnancy is confirmed and monthly thereafter through the second trimester. The thyroxine dose should be increased as needed to maintain plasma TSH within the normal range.
    - **Mild (or subclinical) hypothyroidism** should be treated with thyroxine if any of the following are present: (a) **symptoms compatible with hypothyroidism,** (b) a **goiter,** (c) **hypercholesterolemia** that warrants treatment, or (d) the **plasma TSH is**

>10 microunits/mL.[7] Untreated patients should be monitored annually, and thyroxine should be started if symptoms develop or serum TSH increases to >10 microunits/mL.

- **Urgent therapy** for hypothyroidism is rarely necessary. Most patients with hypothyroidism and concomitant illness can be treated in the usual manner. However, hypothyroidism may impair survival in critical illness by contributing to hypoventilation, hypotension, hypothermia, bradycardia, or hyponatremia. Little evidence supports the contention that severe hypothyroidism alone causes coma or shock; most reports of alleged "myxedema coma" predate recognition that nonthyroidal illness itself lowers thyroid hormone levels.
  - Hypoventilation and hypotension should be treated intensively, along with any concomitant diseases. Confirmatory tests (plasma TSH and free T_4) should be obtained before thyroid hormone therapy is started in a severely ill patient.
  - **Thyroxine, 50–100 mcg IV, can be given q6–8h for 24 hours,** followed by 75–100 mcg IV daily until oral intake is possible. Replacement therapy should be continued in the usual manner if the diagnosis of hypothyroidism is confirmed. No clinical trials have determined the optimum method of thyroid hormone replacement, but this method rapidly alleviates thyroxine deficiency while minimizing the risk of exacerbating underlying coronary disease or heart failure. **Such rapid correction is warranted only in extremely ill patients. Vital signs and cardiac rhythm should be monitored carefully to detect early signs of exacerbation of heart disease. Hydrocortisone, 50 mg IV q8h,** is usually recommended during rapid replacement of thyroid hormone, because such therapy may precipitate adrenal crisis in patients with adrenal failure.

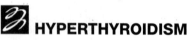

HYPERTHYROIDISM

GENERAL PRINCIPLES

Etiology

- **Graves disease**[8] causes most cases of hyperthyroidism, especially in young patients. This autoimmune disorder may also cause **proptosis** (exophthalmos) and pretibial myxedema, neither of which is found in other causes of hyperthyroidism.
- **Toxic multinodular goiter (MNG)** is a common cause of hyperthyroidism in older patients.
- Unusual causes include **iodine-induced hyperthyroidism** (usually precipitated by drugs such as **amiodarone** or radiographic contrast media), thyroid adenomas, subacute thyroiditis (painful tender goiter with transient hyperthyroidism), painless thyroiditis (nontender goiter with transient hyperthyroidism, most often seen in the postpartum period), and surreptitious ingestion of thyroid hormone. TSH-induced hyperthyroidism is extremely rare.

Clinical Findings

- Symptoms include heat intolerance, weight loss, weakness, palpitations, oligomenorrhea, and anxiety.
- Signs include brisk tendon reflexes, fine tremor, proximal weakness, stare, and eyelid lag. Cardiac abnormalities may be prominent, including sinus tachycardia, atrial fibrillation, and exacerbation of coronary artery disease or heart failure.
- **In the elderly,** hyperthyroidism may present with only atrial fibrillation, heart failure, weakness, or weight loss, and a high index of suspicion is needed to make the diagnosis.

DIAGNOSIS

- Hyperthyroidism should be suspected in any patient with compatible symptoms, as it is a readily treatable disorder that may become very debilitating.

TABLE 22-2	Differential Diagnosis of Hyperthyroidism

Type of goiter	Diagnosis
Diffuse, nontender goiter	Graves' disease or painless thyroiditis
Multiple thyroid nodules	Toxic multinodular goiter
Single thyroid nodule	Thyroid adenoma
Tender painful goiter	Subacute thyroiditis
Normal thyroid gland	Graves' disease, painless thyroiditis or factitious hyperthyroidism

- **Plasma TSH is the best initial diagnostic test,** as a TSH level >0.1 microunits/mL excludes clinical hyperthyroidism. If plasma TSH is <0.1 microunits/mL, **plasma free T_4 should be measured** to determine the severity of hyperthyroidism and as a baseline for therapy. If plasma free T_4 is elevated, the diagnosis of clinical hyperthyroidism is established.
  - **If plasma TSH is <0.1 microunits/mL but free T_4 is normal,** the patient may have clinical hyperthyroidism due to elevation of plasma T_3 alone; therefore, plasma T_3 should be measured in this case.
  - Very **mild (or subclinical) hyperthyroidism** may suppress TSH to <0.1 microunits/mL, and therefore suppression of TSH alone does not confirm that symptoms are due to hyperthyroidism.
  - TSH may also be suppressed by **severe nonthyroidal illness** (see Evaluation of Thyroid Function). A **third-generation TSH assay** with a detection limit of 0.02 microunits/mL may be helpful in patients with suppressed TSH and nonthyroidal illness. Most patients with clinical hyperthyroidism have plasma TSH levels that are <0.02 microunits/mL in such assays, whereas nonthyroidal illness rarely suppresses TSH to this degree.[2]

Differential Diagnosis

- The etiology of hyperthyroidism affects the choice of therapy. Differentiating features include (Table 22-2):
  - The presence of **proptosis** or pretibial myxedema, seen only in Graves' disease (although many patients with Graves' disease lack these signs)
  - A **diffuse nontender goiter,** consistent with Graves' disease or painless thyroiditis
  - Recent **pregnancy, neck pain, or recent iodine administration,** suggesting causes other than Graves' disease
  - In rare cases, **24-hour RAI uptake (RAIU)** is needed to distinguish Graves' disease or toxic MNG (in which RAIU is elevated) from postpartum thyroiditis, iodine-induced hyperthyroidism, or factitious hyperthyroidism (in which RAIU is very low).
  - **Thyroid imaging with ultrasound or radionuclide scan is not useful in hyperthyroidism.**

TREATMENT

Therapy[9]

- Some forms of hyperthyroidism (subacute or postpartum thyroiditis) are transient and require only **symptomatic therapy.**
  - A **β-adrenergic antagonist** (such as **atenolol** 25–100 mg daily) is used to relieve symptoms of hyperthyroidism, such as palpitations, tremor, and anxiety, until hyperthyroidism is controlled by definitive therapy, or until transient forms of hyperthyroidism subside. The dose is adjusted to alleviate symptoms and tachycardia, then reduced gradually as hyperthyroidism is controlled.

- Verapamil at an initial dose of 40–80 mg PO tid can be used to control tachycardia in patients with contraindications to β-adrenergic antagonists.
- Three methods are available for definitive therapy (none of which controls hyperthyroidism rapidly): RAI, thionamides, and subtotal thyroidectomy.
  - **During treatment, patients are followed by clinical evaluation and measurement of plasma free T_4.** Plasma TSH is useless in assessing the initial response to therapy, as it remains suppressed until after the patient becomes euthyroid.
  - Regardless of the therapy used, all patients with Graves' disease require lifelong follow-up for recurrent hyperthyroidism or development of hypothyroidism.
  - Choice of definitive therapy
    - In Graves' disease, RAI therapy is the treatment of choice for almost all patients. It is simple and highly effective, but **cannot be used in pregnancy. Propylthiouracil (PTU) should be used to treat hyperthyroidism in pregnancy.** Thionamides achieve long-term control in fewer than half of patients with Graves' disease and they carry a small risk of life-threatening side effects. Thyroidectomy should be used in patients who refuse RAI therapy and who relapse or develop side effects with thionamide therapy.
    - Other causes of hyperthyroidism. Toxic MNG and toxic adenoma should be treated with RAI (except in pregnancy). Transient forms of hyperthyroidism due to thyroiditis should be treated symptomatically with atenolol. Iodine-induced hyperthyroidism is treated with thionamides and atenolol until the patient is euthyroid. Although treatment of some patients with amiodarone-induced hyperthyroidism with glucocorticoids has been advocated, **nearly all patients with amiodarone-induced hyperthyroidism respond well to thionamide therapy.**[10]
  - RAI therapy
    - A single dose permanently controls hyperthyroidism in 90% of patients, and further doses can be given if necessary.
    - A **pregnancy test** is done immediately before therapy in potentially fertile women.
    - A 24-hour RAIU is usually measured and used to calculate the dose.
    - Thionamides interfere with RAI therapy and should be stopped at least 3 days before treatment. If iodine treatment has been given, it should be stopped at least 2 weeks before RAI therapy.
    - Most patients with Graves' disease are treated with 8–10 mCi, although treatment of toxic MNG requires higher doses.
    - **Follow-up.** Usually, several months are needed to restore euthyroidism. Patients are evaluated at 4- to 6-week intervals, with assessment of clinical findings and plasma free T_4.
      - **If thyroid function stabilizes within the normal range,** the interval between follow-up visits is gradually increased to annual intervals.
      - **If symptomatic hypothyroidism develops,** thyroxine therapy is started (see Hypothyroidism).
      - **If symptomatic hyperthyroidism persists after 6 months, RAI treatment is repeated.**
    - Side effects
      - **Hypothyroidism** occurs in most patients within the first year and continues to develop at a rate of approximately 3% per year thereafter.
      - Because of the release of stored hormone, a slight rise in plasma T_4 may occur in the first 2 weeks after therapy. This development is important only in **patients with severe cardiac disease,** which may worsen as a result. Such patients should be treated with thionamides to restore euthyroidism and to deplete stored hormone before treatment with RAI.
      - No convincing evidence has been found that RAI has a clinically important effect on the course of Graves' eye disease.
      - It does not increase the risk of malignancy. No increase in congenital abnormalities has been found in the offspring of women who conceive after RAI therapy, and the radiation exposure to the ovaries is low, comparable to that from common diagnostic radiographs.

- **Thionamides.**[11] Methimazole and PTU inhibit thyroid hormone synthesis. PTU also inhibits extrathyroidal deiodination of T_4 to T_3. Once thyroid hormone stores are depleted (after several weeks to months), T_4 levels decrease. These drugs have no permanent effect on thyroid function. **In the majority of patients with Graves' disease, hyperthyroidism recurs within 6 months after therapy is stopped.** Spontaneous remission of Graves' disease occurs in approximately one-third of patients during thionamide therapy and, in this minority, no other treatment may be needed. Remission is more likely in mild, recent-onset hyperthyroidism and if the goiter is small.
  - **Initiation of therapy.** Before starting therapy, patients must be warned of side effects and precautions. Usual starting doses are PTU, 100–200 mg PO tid, or methimazole, 10–40 mg PO daily; higher initial doses can be used in severe hyperthyroidism.
  - **Follow-up.** Restoration of euthyroidism takes up to several months.
    - Patients are evaluated at 4-week intervals with assessment of clinical findings and plasma free T_4. If plasma free T_4 levels do not fall after 4–8 weeks, the dose should be increased. Doses as high as PTU, 300 mg PO qid, or methimazole, 60 mg PO daily, may be required.
    - Once the plasma free T_4 level falls to normal, the dose is adjusted to maintain plasma free T_4 within the normal range.
    - No consensus exists on the optimal duration of therapy, but periods of 6 months to 2 years are used most commonly. Patients must be monitored carefully for recurrence of hyperthyroidism after the drug is stopped.
  - **Side effects** are most likely to occur within the first few months of therapy.
    - Minor side effects include rash, urticaria, fever, arthralgias, and transient leukopenia.
    - **Agranulocytosis** occurs in 0.3% of patients treated with thionamides. Other life-threatening side effects include **hepatitis**, vasculitis, and drug-induced lupus erythematosus. These complications usually resolve if the drug is stopped promptly.
    - **Patients must be warned to stop the drug immediately if jaundice or symptoms suggestive of agranulocytosis develop (e.g., fever, chills, sore throat)** and to contact their physician promptly for evaluation. Routine monitoring of the white blood cell (WBC) is not useful for detecting agranulocytosis, which develops suddenly.
- **Subtotal thyroidectomy.** This procedure provides long-term control of hyperthyroidism in most patients.
  - Surgery may trigger a perioperative exacerbation of hyperthyroidism, and patients should be prepared for surgery by one of two methods.
    - **A thionamide** is given until the patient is nearly euthyroid (see section. IV.D). **Supersaturated potassium iodide (SSKI),** 40–80 mg (one to two drops) PO bid, is then added 1–2 weeks before surgery. Both drugs are stopped postoperatively.
    - **Atenolol** (50–100 mg daily) is started 1–2 weeks before surgery. The dose of atenolol is increased, if necessary, to reduce the resting heart rate below 90 beats/min and is continued for 5–7 days postoperatively. SSKI is dosed as above.
  - **Follow-up.** Clinical findings and plasma free T_4 and TSH should be assessed 4–6 weeks after surgery.
    - If thyroid function is normal, the patient is seen at 3 and 6 months, then annually.
    - If symptomatic hypothyroidism develops, thyroxine therapy is started (see Hypothyroidism).
    - Mild hypothyroidism after subtotal thyroidectomy may be transient, and asymptomatic patients can be observed for a further 4–6 weeks to determine whether hypothyroidism will resolve spontaneously.
    - Hyperthyroidism persists or recurs in 3%–7% of patients.
  - **Complications** of thyroidectomy include **hypothyroidism** in 30%–50% of patients and **hypoparathyroidism** in 3%. Rare complications include permanent vocal cord

paralysis, due to recurrent laryngeal nerve injury, and perioperative death. The complication rate appears to depend on the experience of the surgeon.

- **Mild (or subclinical) hyperthyroidism** is present when the plasma TSH is suppressed to <0.1 microunits/mL but the patient has no symptoms that are definitely caused by hyperthyroidism, and plasma levels of free T_4 and T_3 are normal.[7]
    - Subclinical hyperthyroidism increases the risk of **atrial fibrillation** in patients older than 60 years and those with heart disease, and predisposes to **osteoporosis** in postmenopausal women; it should be treated in these groups of patients.
    - Asymptomatic young patients with mild Graves' disease can be observed for spontaneous resolution of hyperthyroidism, or the development of symptoms or increasing free T_4 levels that warrant treatment.
- **Urgent therapy** is warranted when hyperthyroidism exacerbates heart failure or acute coronary syndromes, and in rare patients with severe hyperthyroidism complicated by fever and delirium. Concomitant diseases should be treated intensively, and confirmatory tests (serum TSH and free T_4) should be obtained before therapy is started.
    - **PTU, 300 mg PO q6h**, should be started immediately.
    - **Iodide (SSKI, one to two drops PO q12h)** should be started 1 hour after the first dose of PTU, to inhibit thyroid hormone secretion rapidly.
    - **Propranolol**, 40 mg PO q6h (or an equivalent dose IV), should be given to patients with angina or myocardial infarction, and the dose should be adjusted to prevent tachycardia. Propranolol may benefit some patients with heart failure and marked tachycardia but can further impair left ventricular systolic function. In patients with clinical heart failure, it should be given only with careful monitoring of left ventricular function.
    - Plasma free T_4 is measured every 4–6 days. When free T_4 approaches the normal range, the doses of PTU and iodine are gradually decreased. RAI therapy should be scheduled 2 weeks after iodine is stopped.
- **Hyperthyroidism in pregnancy.**[12] If hyperthyroidism is suspected, plasma TSH should be measured. Plasma TSH declines in early pregnancy, but rarely to <0.1 microunits/mL.
    - If TSH is <0.1 microunits/mL, the diagnosis should be confirmed by measurement of plasma free T_4.
    - RAI is contraindicated in pregnancy, and therefore patients should be treated with PTU. The dose should be adjusted at 4-week intervals to maintain the plasma free T_4 near the upper limit of the normal range. The dose required often decreases in the later stages of pregnancy.
    - Atenolol, 25–50 mg PO daily, can be used to relieve symptoms while awaiting the effects of PTU.
    - The fetus and neonate should be monitored carefully for hyperthyroidism.

EUTHYROID GOITER

GENERAL PRINCIPLES

- The diagnosis of euthyroid goiter is based on palpation of the thyroid and evaluation of thyroid function. If the thyroid is enlarged, the examiner should determine whether the enlargement is **diffuse or multinodular, or whether a single palpable nodule is present.** All three forms of euthyroid goiter are common, especially in women.
- Thyroid scans or ultrasonography provide no useful additional information about goiters that are diffuse or multinodular by palpation and should not be performed in these patients.
- Furthermore, 30%–50% of people have nonpalpable thyroid nodules that are detectable by ultrasound. These nodules rarely have any clinical importance, but their incidental discovery may lead to unnecessary diagnostic testing and treatment.[13]

DIFFUSE GOITER

- Almost all euthyroid diffuse goiters in the United States are due to **chronic lympho-cytic thyroiditis (Hashimoto's thyroiditis).**[5] Since Hashimoto thyroiditis may also cause hypothyroidism, plasma TSH should be measured even in patients who are clinically euthyroid.
- Small diffuse goiters usually are asymptomatic, and therapy is seldom required.
- Symptomatic diffuse goiters may shrink with suppression of plasma TSH to the lower part of the normal range by thyroxine therapy. If thyroxine is not given, the patient should be monitored regularly for the development of hypothyroidism.

MULTINODULAR GOITER

- Multinodular goiter (MNG) is common in older patients, especially women. Most patients are asymptomatic and require no treatment.
- In a few patients, **hyperthyroidism** (toxic MNG) develops (see Hyperthyroidism).
- In rare patients, the gland compresses the trachea or esophagus, causing dyspnea or dysphagia, and treatment is required. Thyroxine treatment has little if any effect on the size of MNGs. RAI therapy reduces gland size and relieves symptoms in most patients. Subtotal thyroidectomy can also be used to relieve compressive symptoms.
- Evaluation for thyroid carcinoma with needle biopsy is warranted if one nodule is disproportionately enlarged.

SINGLE THYROID NODULES

- **Single palpable thyroid nodules** are usually benign, but about 5% are thyroid carcinomas.[14]
- Clinical findings that increase the likelihood of carcinoma include the presence of cervical lymphadenopathy, a history of radiation to the head or neck in childhood, and a family history of medullary thyroid carcinoma or multiple endocrine neoplasia syndromes type 2A or 2B. A hard fixed nodule, recent nodule growth, or hoarseness due to vocal cord paralysis also suggests malignancy.
- However, most patients with thyroid carcinomas have none of these risk factors, and all **palpable single thyroid nodules should be evaluated with needle aspiration biopsy.**[15] Patients with thyroid carcinoma should be managed in consultation with an endocrinologist.
- Nodules with benign cytology should be re-evaluated periodically by palpation. Thyroxine therapy has little or no effect on the size of single thyroid nodules and is not indicated.[16]
- Radionuclide thyroid scans cannot distinguish benign from malignant nodules and should not be performed. The management of nonpalpable thyroid nodules discovered incidentally by ultrasound is controversial.[17]

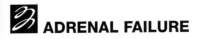 ADRENAL FAILURE

GENERAL PRINCIPLES

Etiology

- Adrenal failure may be due to disease of the adrenal glands (**primary adrenal failure, Addison's disease**), with deficiency of both cortisol and aldosterone and elevated plasma adrenocorticotropic hormone (ACTH), or to ACTH deficiency caused by disorders of the pituitary or hypothalamus (**secondary adrenal failure**), with deficiency of cortisol alone.
  - Primary adrenal failure[18] is most often due to **autoimmune adrenalitis,** which may be associated with other endocrine deficits (e.g., hypothyroidism).

- Infections of the adrenal gland such as **tuberculosis** and **histoplasmosis** also may cause adrenal failure.
- **Hemorrhagic adrenal infarction** may occur in the postoperative period, in coagulation disorders and hypercoagulable states, and in sepsis. Adrenal hemorrhage often causes abdominal or flank pain and fever; computed tomography (CT) scan of the abdomen reveals high-density bilateral adrenal masses.
- Adrenal failure may develop in patients with AIDS, caused by disseminated cytomegalovirus, mycobacterial or fungal infection, and adrenal lymphoma.
- Less common etiologies include adrenoleukodystrophy that causes adrenal failure in young males, and drugs such as ketoconazole and etomidate that inhibit steroid hormone synthesis and can cause adrenal failure.

■ **Secondary adrenal failure** is due most often to **glucocorticoid therapy**; ACTH suppression may persist for a year after therapy is stopped. Any disorder of the pituitary or hypothalamus can cause ACTH deficiency, but other evidence of these disorders is usually obvious.

CLINICAL FINDINGS

■ Clinical findings in adrenal failure are nonspecific, and without a high index of suspicion, the diagnosis of this potentially lethal but readily treatable disease is easily missed.

   ■ Symptoms include **anorexia, nausea, vomiting, weight loss, weakness, and fatigue.** **Orthostatic hypotension** and **hyponatremia** are common.

   ■ Usually, symptoms are chronic, but **shock** may develop suddenly, and is fatal unless promptly treated. Often, this adrenal crisis is triggered by illness, injury, or surgery. All these symptoms are due to cortisol deficiency and occur in both primary and secondary adrenal failure.

   ■ **Hyperpigmentation** (due to marked ACTH excess) and **hyperkalemia** and **volume depletion** (due to aldosterone deficiency) occur only in primary adrenal failure.

DIAGNOSIS[19]

■ Adrenal failure should be suspected in patients with hypotension, weight loss, persistent nausea, hyponatremia, or hyperkalemia.

   ■ **The cosyntropin (Cortrosyn) stimulation test** is used for diagnosis. Cosyntropin, 250 mcg, is given IV or IM, and **plasma cortisol is measured 30 minutes later.** The normal response is a stimulated plasma cortisol >20 mcg/dL. This test detects primary and secondary adrenal failure, except within a few weeks of onset of pituitary dysfunction (e.g., shortly after pituitary surgery; see Anterior Pituitary Gland Dysfunction).

   ■ **The distinction between primary and secondary adrenal failure** is usually clear.

   - Hyperkalemia, hyperpigmentation, or other autoimmune endocrine deficits indicate primary adrenal failure, whereas deficits of other pituitary hormones, symptoms of a pituitary mass (e.g., headache, visual field loss), or known pituitary or hypothalamic disease indicate secondary adrenal failure.
   - If the cause is unclear, the **plasma ACTH** level distinguishes primary adrenal failure (in which it is markedly elevated) from secondary adrenal failure.
   - Most cases of primary adrenal failure are due to autoimmune adrenalitis, but other causes should be considered. Radiographic evidence of adrenal enlargement or calcification indicates that the cause is infection or hemorrhage.
   - Patients with secondary adrenal failure should be tested for other pituitary hormone deficiencies and should be evaluated for a pituitary or hypothalamic tumor (see Anterior Pituitary Gland Dysfunction).

THERAPY[20]

■ **Adrenal crisis** with hypotension must be treated immediately. Patients should be evaluated for an underlying illness that precipitated the crisis.

- If the diagnosis of adrenal failure is known, hydrocortisone, 100 mg IV q8h, should be given, and **0.9% saline with 5% dextrose** should be infused rapidly until hypotension is corrected. The dose of hydrocortisone is decreased gradually over several days as symptoms and any precipitating illness resolve, then changed to oral maintenance therapy. Mineralocorticoid replacement is not needed until the dose of hydrocortisone is <100 mg/d.

- If the diagnosis of adrenal failure has not been established, a single dose of dexamethasone, 10 mg IV, should be given, and a rapid infusion of 0.9% saline with 5% dextrose should be started. A **Cortrosyn stimulation test** should be performed. Dexamethasone is used because it does not interfere with measurement of plasma cortisol. After the 30-minute plasma cortisol measurement, hydrocortisone, 100 mg IV q8h, should be given until the test result is known.

- **Maintenance therapy** in all patients with adrenal failure requires cortisol replacement with prednisone; most patients with primary adrenal failure also require replacement of aldosterone with fludrocortisone.

  - **Prednisone, 5 mg PO every morning,** should be started. The dose is then adjusted with the goal being the lowest dose that relieves the patient's symptoms, to prevent osteoporosis and other signs of Cushing syndrome. Most patients require doses between 4 mg PO every morning and 5 mg PO every morning and 2.5 mg every evening. Concomitant therapy with rifampin, phenytoin, or phenobarbital accelerates glucocorticoid metabolism and increases the dose requirement.

  - **During illness, injury, or the perioperative period, the dose of prednisone must be increased.**
    - For minor illnesses, the patient should double the dose for 3 days. If the illness resolves, the maintenance dose is resumed.
    - **Vomiting requires immediate medical attention,** with IV glucocorticoid therapy and IV fluid. Patients can be given a 4-mg vial of dexamethasone to be self-administered IM for vomiting or severe illness if medical care is not immediately available.
    - **For severe illness or injury,** hydrocortisone, 50 mg IV q8h, should be given, with the dose tapered as severity of illness wanes. The same regimen is used in **patients undergoing surgery,** with the first dose of hydrocortisone given preoperatively. The dose can be tapered to maintenance therapy by 2–3 days after uncomplicated surgery.

  - **In primary adrenal failure, fludrocortisone, 0.1 mg PO daily,** should be given, along with liberal salt intake. The dose is adjusted to maintain blood pressure (BP; supine and standing) and serum potassium within the normal range; the usual dosage is 0.05–0.2 mg PO daily.

  - **Patients should be educated in management of their disease,** including adjustment of prednisone dose during illness. They should wear a medical identification tag or bracelet.

CUSHING'S SYNDROME

GENERAL PRINCIPLES

- Cushing's syndrome[21] is most often **iatrogenic,** due to therapy with glucocorticoid drugs.
- **ACTH-secreting pituitary microadenomas (Cushing's disease)** account for 80% of cases of endogenous Cushing's syndrome.
- **Adrenal tumors and ectopic ACTH secretion** account for the remainder.

CLINICAL FINDINGS

- Findings include truncal obesity, rounded face, fat deposits in the supraclavicular fossae and over the posterior neck, hypertension, hirsutism, amenorrhea, and depression.

More specific findings include thin skin, easy bruising, reddish striae, proximal muscle weakness, and osteoporosis.
- Diabetes mellitus develops in some patients.
- Hyperpigmentation or hypokalemic alkalosis suggests Cushing's syndrome due to ectopic ACTH secretion.

DIAGNOSIS

- **Diagnosis** is based on increased cortisol excretion and lack of normal feedback inhibition of ACTH and cortisol secretion.[22]
    - The best initial test is the **24-hour urine cortisol** measurement test. Alternatively, an **overnight dexamethasone suppression test** (1 mg dexamethasone given PO at 11:00 p.m.; plasma cortisol measured at 8:00 a.m. the next day; normal range: plasma cortisol <2 mcg/dL) may be performed. Both tests are very sensitive, and a normal value virtually excludes the diagnosis. If the overnight dexamethasone suppression test is abnormal, 24-hour urine cortisol should be measured.
    - If the 24-hour urine cortisol excretion is more than four times the upper limit of the reference range in a patient with compatible clinical findings, the diagnosis of Cushing's syndrome is established.
    - In patients with milder elevations of urine cortisol, a **low-dose dexamethasone suppression test** should be performed. Dexamethasone, 0.5 mg PO q6h, is given for 48 hours, starting at 8:00 a.m.. Urine cortisol is measured during the last 24 hours, and plasma cortisol is measured 6 hours after the last dose of dexamethasone. Failure to suppress plasma cortisol to <2 mcg/dL and urine cortisol to less than the normal reference range is diagnostic of Cushing's syndrome.
    - Testing should not be done during severe illness or depression, which may cause false-positive results. Phenytoin therapy also causes a false-positive test by accelerating metabolism of dexamethasone.
    - Random plasma cortisol levels are not useful for diagnosis, because the wide range of normal values overlaps those of Cushing's syndrome. After the diagnosis of Cushing's syndrome is made, tests to determine the cause are best done in consultation with an endocrinologist.

 INCIDENTAL ADRENAL NODULES

GENERAL PRINCIPLES

- Adrenal nodules are a common incidental finding on abdominal imaging studies.
- Most incidentally discovered nodules are benign adrenocortical tumors that do not secrete excess hormone, but the differential diagnosis includes adrenal adenomas causing Cushing's syndrome or primary hyperaldosteronism, pheochromocytoma, adrenocortical carcinoma, and metastatic cancer.[23]

EVALUATION

- The imaging characteristics of the nodule may suggest a diagnosis but are not specific enough to obviate further evaluation.[24]
    - **In patients without a known malignancy elsewhere,** the diagnostic issues are whether a **syndrome of hormone excess** or an **adrenocortical carcinoma** is present. Patients should be evaluated for hypertension, symptoms suggestive of pheochromocytoma (episodic headache, palpitations, and sweating) and signs of Cushing's syndrome (see Cushing's Syndrome).
        - **Plasma potassium and dehydroepiandrosterone sulfate** should be measured, and an **overnight dexamethasone suppression test** should be performed.

- Pheochromocytoma should be tested for by either **plasma fractionated metanephrines** or **24-hour urine catecholamines and metanephrines.**[25]
- Patients who have **potentially resectable cancer elsewhere** and in whom an adrenal metastasis must be excluded may require needle biopsy of the nodule.
  - **Pheochromocytoma should be excluded before biopsy.**

MANAGEMENT[26]

- Patients with hypertension and hypokalemia should be evaluated for primary hyperaldosteronism in consultation with an endocrinologist.
- An abnormal overnight dexamethasone suppression test should be evaluated further (see Cushing's Syndrome).
- If clinical or biochemical evidence of a pheochromocytoma is found, the nodule should be resected after appropriate α-adrenergic blockade with phenoxybenzamine.
- Elevation of plasma dehydroepiandrosterone sulfate or a large nodule suggests adrenocortical carcinoma. A policy of resecting all nodules >4 cm in diameter appropriately treats the great majority of adrenal carcinomas while minimizing the number of benign nodules that are removed unnecessarily.[27]
- Most incidental nodules are <4 cm in diameter, do not produce excess hormone, and do not require therapy. At least one **repeat imaging procedure** 3–6 months later is recommended to ensure that the nodule is not enlarging rapidly (which would suggest an adrenal carcinoma).

 # ANTERIOR PITUITARY GLAND DYSFUNCTION

GENERAL PRINCIPLES

- The anterior pituitary gland secretes **prolactin, growth hormone,** and four **trophic hormones:** corticotropin (ACTH), thyrotropin (TSH), and the gonadotropins, luteinizing hormone and follicle-stimulating hormone. Each trophic hormone stimulates a specific target gland.
- Anterior pituitary function is regulated by hypothalamic hormones that reach the pituitary via portal veins in the pituitary stalk. **The predominant effect of hypothalamic regulation is to stimulate secretion of pituitary hormones, except for prolactin,** which is inhibited by hypothalamic dopamine production.
- **Secretion of trophic hormones is also regulated by negative feedback** by their target gland hormone, and the normal pituitary response to target hormone deficiency is increased secretion of the appropriate trophic hormone.
- **Anterior pituitary dysfunction** can be caused by disorders of either the pituitary or hypothalamus.
  - **Pituitary adenomas** are the most common pituitary disorder. They are classified by size and function.
    - **Microadenomas** are <10 mm in diameter and cause clinical manifestations only if they produce excess hormone. They are too small to produce hypopituitarism or mass effects.
    - **Macroadenomas** are >10 mm in diameter and may produce any combination of pituitary hormone excess, hypopituitarism, and mass effects (headache, visual field loss).
    - **Secretory adenomas** produce prolactin, growth hormone, or ACTH.
    - **Nonsecretory macroadenomas** may cause hypopituitarism or mass effects.
    - **Nonsecretory microadenomas** are common incidental radiographic findings, seen in approximately 10% of the normal population, and do not require therapy.[28]
  - **Other pituitary or hypothalamic disorders,** such as head trauma, pituitary surgery or radiation, and postpartum pituitary infarction (Sheehan's syndrome) may cause hypopituitarism. Other tumors of the pituitary or hypothalamus (e.g., craniopharyngioma,

metastases), inflammatory disorders (e.g., sarcoidosis, histiocytosis X), and infections (e.g., tuberculosis) may cause hypopituitarism or mass effects.

CLINICAL FINDINGS

- Pituitary and hypothalamic disorders may present in several ways.
  - In **hypopituitarism** (deficiency of one or more pituitary hormones), gonadotropin deficiency is most common, causing amenorrhea in women and androgen deficiency in men. Secondary hypothyroidism or adrenal failure rarely occurs alone. Secondary adrenal failure causes deficiency of cortisol but not of aldosterone; hyperkalemia and hyperpigmentation do not occur, although life-threatening adrenal crisis may develop.
  - **Hormone excess** most commonly results in **hyperprolactinemia,** which can be due to a secretory adenoma or to nonsecretory lesions that damage the hypothalamus or pituitary stalk. Growth hormone excess (**acromegaly**) and ACTH and cortisol excess (**Cushing's disease**) are caused by secretory adenomas.
  - **Mass effects** due to pressure on adjacent structures, such as the optic chiasm, include **headaches** and **loss of visual fields or acuity.** Hyperprolactinemia also may be due to mass effect. **Pituitary apoplexy** is sudden enlargement of a pituitary tumor due to hemorrhagic necrosis.
  - Asymptomatic pituitary adenomas
    - If a microadenoma is found on imaging done for another purpose, the patient should be evaluated for clinical evidence of hyperprolactinemia, Cushing's disease, or acromegaly.
      - Plasma prolactin should be measured, and tests for acromegaly and Cushing's syndrome should be performed if symptoms or signs of these disorders are evident.
      - If no pituitary hormone excess exists, therapy is not required. Whether such patients need repeat imaging is not established, but the risk of enlargement is clearly small.[28]
    - Incidental discovery of a macroadenoma is unusual. Patients should be evaluated for hormone excess and hypopituitarism. Most macroadenomas should be treated since they are likely to grow further.

DIAGNOSIS OF HYPOPITUITARISM

- Hypopituitarism may be suspected in the presence of clinical signs of target hormone deficiency (e.g., hypothyroidism) or pituitary mass effects.
  - **Laboratory evaluation** for hypopituitarism begins with evaluation of **target hormone function,** including **plasma free T_4** and a **Cortrosyn stimulation test** (see Adrenal Failure).
    - If recent onset of secondary adrenal failure is suspected (within a few weeks of evaluation), the patient should be treated empirically with glucocorticoids and should be tested later, since the Cortrosyn stimulation test cannot detect secondary adrenal failure of recent onset.
    - In men, **plasma testosterone** should be measured. The best evaluation of gonadal function in women is the **menstrual history**.
  - If a target hormone is deficient, its trophic hormone is measured to determine whether target gland dysfunction is secondary to hypopituitarism. An elevated trophic hormone level indicates primary target gland dysfunction. In hypopituitarism, trophic hormone levels are not elevated and are usually within (not below) the reference range. Thus, **pituitary trophic hormone levels can be interpreted only with knowledge of target hormone levels,** and **measurement of trophic hormone levels alone is useless in the diagnosis of hypopituitarism.** If pituitary disease is obvious, target hormone deficiencies may be assumed to be secondary, and trophic hormones need not be measured.

■ Anatomic evaluation of the pituitary gland and hypothalamus is done best by magnetic resonance imaging (**MRI**). However, hyperprolactinemia and Cushing's disease may be caused by microadenomas too small to be seen with current techniques. The prevalence of incidental microadenomas should be kept in mind when interpreting MRIs. Visual acuity and **visual fields** should be tested when imaging suggests compression of the optic chiasm.

TREATMENT OF HYPOPITUITARISM

■ Deficient target hormones should be replaced.
  ■ Secondary adrenal failure should be treated immediately, especially if patients are to undergo surgery (see Adrenal Failure).
  ■ Treatment of secondary hypothyroidism should be monitored by measurement of **plasma free T$_4$** (see Hypothyroidism).
  ■ Infertility due to gonadotropin deficiency may be correctable, and patients who wish to conceive should be referred to an endocrinologist.
  ■ Treatment of growth hormone deficiency in adults has been advocated by some, but the benefits, risks and cost effectiveness of this therapy are not established.[29]
  ■ Treatment of pituitary macroadenomas generally requires transsphenoidal surgical resection, except for prolactin-secreting tumors.

HYPERPROLACTINEMIA[30]

General Principles

■ In women, the most common causes of pathologic hyperprolactinemia are prolactin-secreting pituitary **microadenomas** and **idiopathic hyperprolactinemia** (Table 22-3).
■ In men, the most common cause is a prolactin-secreting **macroadenoma.**
■ Hypothalamic or pituitary lesions that cause deficiency of other pituitary hormones often cause hyperprolactinemia.
■ **Medications** are an important cause in both men and women.[31]

Clinical Findings

■ In women, hyperprolactinemia causes **amenorrhea** or irregular menses and **infertility.** Only approximately half of these women have **galactorrhea.** Prolonged estrogen deficiency increases the risk of **osteoporosis.**
■ In men, hyperprolactinemia causes **androgen deficiency** and **infertility** but not gynecomastia; **mass effects and hypopituitarism** are common.

 TABLE 22-3   **Major Causes of Hyperprolactinemia**

Pregnancy and lactation
Prolactin-secreting pituitary adenoma (prolactinoma)
Idiopathic hyperprolactinemia
Drugs (e.g., phenothiazines, metoclopramide, risperidone, verapamil)
Interference with synthesis or transport of hypothalamic dopamine
    Hypothalamic lesions
    Nonsecretory pituitary macroadenomas
Primary hypothyroidism
Chronic renal failure

Diagnosis

- **Hyperprolactinemia is common in young women,** and plasma **prolactin should be measured in women with amenorrhea,** whether or not galactorrhea is present. Mild elevations should be confirmed by repeat measurements.
- The history should include medications and symptoms of pituitary mass effects or hypothyroidism.
- Laboratory evaluation should also include **plasma TSH** and a **pregnancy test** in women.
- Prolactin levels of >200 ng/mL occur only in prolactinomas, and levels between 100 and 200 ng/mL strongly suggest this diagnosis. Levels <100 ng/mL may be due to any cause except prolactin-secreting macroadenoma, and such levels in a patient with a large pituitary mass indicate that it is a nonfunctioning tumor rather than a prolactinoma.
- Testing for hypopituitarism is needed only in patients with a macroadenoma or hypothalamic lesion. **Pituitary imaging** should be performed in most cases, as large nonfunctional pituitary or hypothalamic tumors may present with hyperprolactinemia.

Therapy

- **Microadenomas and idiopathic hyperprolactinemia.**
  - Most patients are treated because of **infertility** or to prevent **estrogen deficiency and osteoporosis.**
  - Some women may be observed without therapy by periodic follow-up of prolactin levels and symptoms. In most patients, hyperprolactinemia does not worsen, and prolactin levels sometimes return to normal. Enlargement of microadenomas is rare.
  - The **dopamine agonists bromocriptine** and **cabergoline** suppress plasma prolactin and restore normal menses and fertility in most women.
    - Initial dosages are bromocriptine, 1.25–2.5 mg PO at bedtime with a snack, or cabergoline, 0.25 mg twice a week.
    - Plasma prolactin levels are initially obtained at 2- to 4-week intervals, and doses are adjusted until the lowest dose required to maintain prolactin in the normal range is reached. In general, the maximally effective doses are bromocriptine 2.5 mg tid and cabergoline 1.5 mg twice a week.
    - **Side effects** include **nausea** and **orthostatic hypotension,** which can be minimized by increasing the dose gradually, and usually resolve with continued therapy. Side effects are less severe with cabergoline.
    - Initially, patients should use barrier contraception, as fertility may be restored quickly.
      - **Women who want to become pregnant** should be managed in consultation with an endocrinologist.
      - **Women who do not want to become pregnant** should be followed with clinical evaluation and plasma prolactin levels every 6–12 months. Every 2 years, plasma prolactin should be measured after bromocriptine has been withdrawn for several weeks, to determine whether the drug is still needed. Follow-up imaging studies are not warranted unless prolactin levels increase substantially.
    - Transsphenoidal resection of prolactin-secreting microadenomas is used only in the rare patient who does not respond to or cannot tolerate dopamine agonists. Prolactin levels usually return to normal, but up to one-half of patients experience relapse.
- **Prolactin-secreting macroadenomas** should be treated with a dopamine agonist, which usually suppresses prolactin levels to normal, reduces tumor size, and improves or corrects abnormal visual fields in 90% of cases.
  - If mass effects are present, the dose should be increased to maximally effective levels over a period of several weeks. Visual field tests, if initially abnormal, should be repeated 4–6 weeks after therapy is started.
  - Pituitary imaging should be repeated 3–6 months after initiation of therapy. If tumor shrinkage and correction of visual abnormalities are satisfactory, therapy can be continued indefinitely, with periodic monitoring of plasma prolactin levels.

■ The full effect on tumor size may take more than 6 months. Further pituitary imaging is probably not warranted unless prolactin levels rise despite therapy.

■ **Transsphenoidal surgery** is indicated to relieve mass effects and to prevent further tumor growth if the tumor does not shrink or if visual field abnormalities persist during dopamine agonist therapy. However, the likelihood of surgical cure of hyperprolactinemia due to a macroadenoma is low, and most patients require further therapy with a dopamine agonist.

■ **Women with prolactin-secreting macroadenomas should not become pregnant** unless the tumor has been resected surgically, as the risk of symptomatic enlargement during pregnancy is 15%–35%. Barrier contraception is essential during dopamine agonist treatment.

ACROMEGALY[32]

General Principles

■ Acromegaly is the syndrome caused by growth hormone excess in adults and is due to a growth hormone–secreting pituitary adenoma in the vast majority of cases.

■ Clinical findings include thickened skin and enlargement of hands, feet, jaw, and forehead. Arthritis or carpal tunnel syndrome may develop, and the pituitary adenoma may cause headaches and vision loss. Mortality from cardiovascular disease is increased.

Diagnosis

■ **Plasma insulinlike growth factor I (IGF-1)**, which mediates most effects of growth hormone, is the best diagnostic test. Marked elevations establish the diagnosis.
  ■ If IGF-1 levels are only moderately elevated, the diagnosis can be confirmed by giving 75 mg glucose orally and measuring serum growth hormone q30min for 2 hours. Failure to suppress growth hormone to <1 ng/mL confirms the diagnosis of acromegaly. Once the diagnosis is made, the pituitary should be imaged.

Therapy

■ The treatment of choice is transsphenoidal resection of the pituitary adenoma. Most patients have macroadenomas, and complete tumor resection with cure of acromegaly often is impossible. If IGF-1 levels remain elevated after surgery, radiotherapy is used to prevent regrowth of the tumor and to control acromegaly.
  ■ The somatostatin analog **octreotide** in depot form can be used to suppress growth hormone secretion while awaiting the effect of radiation. A dose of 10–30 mg IM monthly suppresses IGF-1 to normal in most patients.[33] Side effects include cholelithiasis, diarrhea, and mild abdominal discomfort.
  ■ **Pegvisomant** is a new growth hormone antagonist that lowers IGF-1 to normal in almost all patients.[34] The dose is 10–30 mg SC daily. Few side effects have been reported, but patients should be monitored for pituitary adenoma enlargement and transaminase elevation.

METABOLIC BONE DISEASE

OSTEOMALACIA

■ Osteomalacia is characterized by defective mineralization of osteoid. Bone biopsy reveals increased thickness of osteoid seams and decreased mineralization rate, assessed by tetracycline labeling.

General Principles

Etiologies

- Dietary vitamin D deficiency
- **Malabsorption** of vitamin D and calcium due to intestinal, hepatic, or biliary disease.
- Disorders of vitamin D metabolism (e.g., renal disease, vitamin D–dependent rickets)
- Vitamin D resistance
- Chronic hypophosphatemia
- Renal tubular acidosis
- Hypophosphatasia
- Therapy with anticonvulsants, fluoride, etidronate, or aluminum compounds.

Clinical Findings

- Clinical findings include diffuse skeletal pain, proximal muscle weakness, waddling gait, and propensity to fractures.
- Radiographic findings include osteopenia and radiolucent bands perpendicular to bone surfaces (pseudofractures or Looser zones).
- Serum alkaline phosphatase is elevated. Serum phosphorus, calcium, or both may be decreased.

Diagnosis

- Osteomalacia should be suspected in a patient with osteopenia, elevated serum alkaline phosphatase, and either hypophosphatemia or hypocalcemia.
- **Serum 25-hydroxyvitamin D** (25[OH]D) levels may be low, establishing the diagnosis of vitamin D deficiency or malabsorption.
- Radiography of the chest, pelvis, and hips may reveal characteristic pseudofractures.

Treatment

- **Dietary vitamin D deficiency** can initially be treated with vitamin D, 50,000 IU PO weekly for several weeks, to replete body stores, followed by long-term therapy with 400–1,000 International Units/d. Preparations include calcium supplements that contain vitamin D (Os-Cal + D, 125 International Units/250- or 500-mg tablet), many multivitamins (400 International Units/tablet), and vitamin D drops (200 International Units/drop or 8,000 International Units/mL).
- **Malabsorption of vitamin D** may require therapy with high doses, ranging from 50,000 International Units PO per week to 50,000 International Units PO daily. The dose should be adjusted to maintain serum 25(OH)D levels within the normal range. Calcitriol 0.5–2.0 mcg PO daily can also be used. Calcium supplements, 1 g PO daily–tid, may also be required. Serum 25(OH)D, serum calcium, and 24-hour urine calcium should be monitored every 3–6 months to avoid hypercalcemia or hypercalciuria. If the underlying disease responds to therapy, the dose of vitamin D must be reduced accordingly.

PAGET'S DISEASE[35]

General Principles

- Paget's disease of bone is a focal skeletal disorder characterized by rapid, disorganized bone remodeling. It usually occurs after age 40 and most often affects the pelvis, femur, spine, and skull.
- Clinical manifestations include bone pain and deformity, degenerative arthritis, pathologic fractures, neurologic deficits due to nerve root or cranial nerve compression (including deafness), and, rarely, high-output heart failure and osteogenic sarcoma.
- Most patients are asymptomatic, with disease discovered incidentally because of elevated serum alkaline phosphatase or a radiograph taken for other reasons.

Diagnosis

■ The radiographic appearance is usually diagnostic. A bone scan will reveal areas of skeletal involvement which can be confirmed by radiography. Serum alkaline phosphatase is elevated, reflecting the activity and extent of disease. Serum and urine calcium are usually normal but may increase with immobilization, as after a fracture.

MANAGEMENT

■ **Indications for therapy** include (a) bone pain due to Paget's disease, (b) nerve compression syndromes, (c) pathologic fracture, (d) elective skeletal surgery, (e) progressive skeletal deformity, (f) immobilization hypercalcemia, and (g) asymptomatic involvement of weight-bearing bones or the skull.
■ **Bisphosphonates** inhibit excessive bone resorption, relieve symptoms, and restore serum alkaline phosphatase to normal in most patients. The effectiveness of therapy is monitored by measuring serum alkaline phosphatase. Patients are treated with a course of therapy with **alendronate**, 40 mg/d for 6 months, or **risedronate**, 30 mg/d for 2 months. Serum alkaline phosphatase is monitored every 3 months. Therapy can be repeated when serum alkaline phosphatase rises above normal. Bisphosphonates may cause esophagitis, and are not recommended in patients with renal insufficiency.

References

1. Ladenson PW, Singer PA, Ain KB, et al. American Thyroid Association guidelines for detection of thyroid dysfunction [erratum in *Arch Intern Med.* 2001;161:284]. *Arch Intern Med.* 2000;160:1573–1575.
2. Ross DS. Serum thyroid-stimulating hormone measurement for assessment of thyroid function and disease. *Endocrinol Metab Clin North Am.* 2001;30:245–264.
3. Langton JE. Brent GA. Nonthyroidal illness syndrome : evaluation of thyroid function in sick patients. *Endocrinol Metab Clin North Am.* 2002;31:159–172.
4. Roberts CG, Ladenson PW: Hypothyroidism. *Lancet* 2004;363:793–803.
5. Pearce EN, Farwell AP, Braverman LE. Thyroiditis. *N Engl J Med.* 2003;348:2646–2655.
6. Alexander EK, et al. Timing and magnitude of increases in levothyroxine requirements during pregnancy in women with hypothyroidism. *N Engl J Med* 2004;351:241–249.
7. Surks MI, Ortiz E, Daniels GH, et al. Subclinical Thyroid Disease: Scientific Review and Guidelines for Diagnosis and Management. *JAMA* 2004;291:228–238.
8. Weetman AP. Graves' disease. *N Engl J Med.* 2000;343:1236–1248.
9. Cooper DS. Hyperthyroidism. *Lancet* 2003;362:459–468.
10. Osman F, Franklyn JA, Sheppard MC, et al. Successful treatment of amiodarone-induced thyrotoxicosis. *Circulation* 2002;105:1275–1277.
11. Cooper DS. Antithyroid drugs. *N Engl J Med* 2005;352:905–917.
12. Him Beau SH, Mandel SJ. Thyroid Disorders During Pregnancy. *Endocrinol Metab Clin N Am* 2006;35:117–136.
13. Burguera B, Gharib H. Thyroid incidentalomas. Prevalence, diagnosis, significance, and management. *Endocrinol Metab Clin North Am* 2000;29:187–203.
14. Sherman SI. Thyroid carcinoma. *Lancet.* 2003;361:501–511.
15. Hegedüs L. The thyroid nodule. *N Engl J Med.* 2004;351:1764–1771.
16. Richter B, Neises G, Clar C. Pharmacotherapy for thyroid nodules. A systematic review and meta-analysis. *Endocrinol Metab Clin North Am* 2002;31:699–722.
17. Topliss D. Thyroid incidentaloma: the ignorant in pursuit of the impalpable. *Clin Endocrinol* 2004;60:18–20.
18. Arlt W, Allolio B. Adrenal Insufficiency. *Lancet* 2003;361:1881–1893.
19. Dorin RI, Qualls CR, Crapo LM. Diagnosis of adrenal insufficiency. *Ann Intern Med* 2003;139:194–204.
20. Coursin DB and Wood KE. Corticosteroid Supplementation for Adrenal Insufficiency. *JAMA* 2002;287:236–240.
21. Newell-Price J et al. Cushing's syndrome. *Lancet* 2006;367:1605–1617.

22. Raff H, Findling JW. A physiologic approach to diagnosis of the Cushing syndrome. *Ann Intern Med* 2003;138:980–991.

23. Mansmann G, Lau J, Balk E., et al. The Clinically Inapparent Adrenal Mass: Update in Diagnosis and Management. *Endocr Rev* 2004;25:309–340.

24. Udelsman R, Fishman EK. Radiology of the adrenal. *Endocrinol Metab Clin North Am* 2000;29:27–42.

25. Sawka AM, Jaeschke R, Singh JR, et al. A comparison of biochemical tests for pheochromocytoma: measurement of unfractionated plasma metanephrines compared with the combination of 24-hour urinary metanephrines and catecholamines. *J Clin Endocrinol Metab* 2003;88:553–558.

26. Grumbach MM, Biller BM, Braunstein GD, et al. Management of the clinically inapparent adrenal mass ("incidentaloma"). *Ann Intern Med* 2003;138:424–429.

27. Management approaches to adrenal incidentalomas: a view from Rochester, Minnesota. *Endocrinol Metab Clin North Am* 2000;29:159–185.

28. Aron DC, Howlett TA. Pituitary incidentalomas. *Endocrinol Metab Clin North Am* 2000;29:205–221.

29. Isley, WL. Growth Hormone Therapy for Adults: Not Ready for Prime Time?. *Ann Intern Med* 2002;137:190–196.

30. d Gillam MP, Molitch ME, Lombardi GC. Advances in the Treatment of Prolactinomas. *Endocr Rev* 2006;27:485–534.

31. Molitch ME. Medication-induced hyperprolactinemia. *Mayo Clin Proc* 2005;80:1050–1057.

32. Stockigt JR. Free thyroid hormone measurement. A critical appraisal. *Endocrinol Metab Clin North Am* 2001;30:265–289.

33. Freda PU. Somatostatin Analogs in Acromegaly. *J Clin Endocrinol Metab* 2002;87:3013–3018.

34. Clemmons DR, Chihara K, Freda PU, et al. Optimizing control of acromegaly: integrating a growth hormone receptor antagonist into the treatment algorithm. *J Clin Endocrinol Metab* 2003;88:4759–4767.

35. Whyte MP. Paget's Disease of Bone. *N Engl J Med* 2006 Aug 10;355:593–600.

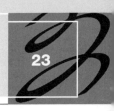

THERAPEUTIC APPROACHES TO RHEUMATIC DISEASE

- The etiology of most rheumatologic disorders is unknown. Therapeutic approaches in rheumatology are largely palliative. Such approaches involve either local or systemic administration of analgesic, anti-inflammatory, immunomodulatory, or immunosuppressive drugs. Because the same procedures and medications are used for most of the rheumatologic disorders, they are discussed as a group rather than separately under each disorder.

JOINT ASPIRATION AND INJECTION

- **Indications.** Joint aspiration should be performed (a) when an effusion is present in a single joint and its etiology is unclear, (b) for symptomatic relief in a patient with a known arthritis diagnosis, and (c) to monitor the response to therapy in patients with infectious arthritis. Analysis of synovial fluid should include a cell count, microscopic examination for crystals, Gram stain, and culture. Intra-articular glucocorticoid therapy can be used to suppress inflammation when only one or a few peripheral joints are inflamed and infection has been excluded. The joint should be aspirated to remove as much fluid as possible before glucocorticoid injection. Glucocorticoid preparations include methylprednisolone acetate, triamcinolone acetonide, and triamcinolone hexacetonide. The dose used is arbitrary, but the following guidelines based on volume are useful: large joints (knee, ankle, shoulder), 1–2 mL; medium joints (wrists, elbows), 0.5–1.0 mL; and small joints of the hands and feet, 0.25–0.5 mL. Lidocaine (or its equivalent), up to 1 mL of a 1% solution, can be mixed in a single syringe with the glucocorticoid to promote immediate relief but is not generally used in the digits.
- **Technique.** The site of aspiration should be cleansed with povidone-iodine solution. Topical ethylchloride spray can be used as a local anesthetic. The site can also be infiltrated with local anesthetic in preparation for the procedure, particularly if there is little or no joint effusion or if there is notable joint space narrowing.
    - **Knee.** (See Fig. 23.1) The leg should be positioned by gently flexing the knee 10–15 degrees. A rolled towel can be placed in the popliteal fossa to support the knee and allow the quadriceps to relax. The joint is then entered either medially or laterally, immediately beneath the undersurface of the patella.
    - **Ankle.** (See Fig. 23.2) Aspiration should be performed with the patient supine and the foot perpendicular to the leg. Medial aspiration is performed immediately medial to the extensor hallucis longus tendon, which can be identified by alternately flexing and extending the great toe. A lateral approach can also be used by introducing the needle just distal to the fibula.
    - **Wrist.** (See Fig. 23.3) Aspiration is performed on the dorsum of the wrist between the distal radius and carpus with the wrist joint flexed slightly. The point of entry for lateral aspiration is just distal to the end of the radius, between the extensor tendons of the thumb. Medial aspiration can also be performed between the distal ulna and the carpus.

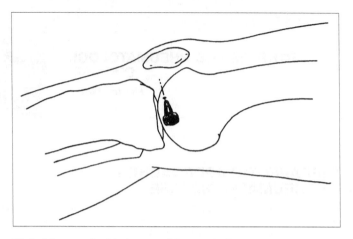

Figure 23-1. Arthrocentesis of the knee: medial approach. [Reproduced with permission from JR Beary III, CL Christian, NA Johanson (eds). *Manual of Rheumatology and Outpatient Orthopedic Disorders* (2nd ed). Boston: Little, Brown, 1987.]

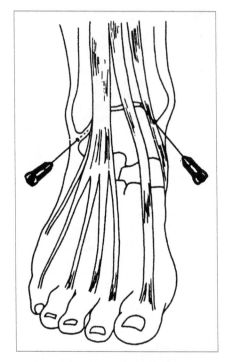

Figure 23-2. Arthrocentesis of the ankle: medial and lateral approaches. [Reproduced with permission from JR Beary III, CL Christian, NA Johanson (eds). *Manual of Rheumatology and Outpatient Orthopedic Disorders* (2nd ed). Boston: Little, Brown, 1987.]

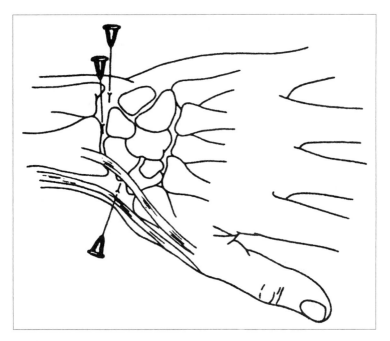

Figure 23-3. Arthrocentesis of the wrist: medial, dorsal, and lateral approaches. [Reproduced with permission from JR Beary III, CL Christian, NA Johanson (eds). *Manual of Rheumatology and Outpatient Orthopedic Disorders* (2nd ed). Boston: Little, Brown, 1987.]

- **Joints of the hands and feet.** Small joints of the hands and feet are entered similarly by introducing the needle from the dorsal surface immediately beneath the extensor tendon from either the medial or the lateral side. Because these joints yield only very small amounts of fluid, flushing aspirate from the syringe with saline may increase the yield when analysis for crystals is attempted.
- Contraindications
  - **Infection overlying the site to be injected is an absolute contraindication.**
    - Significant hemostatic defects and bacteremia are relative contraindications to joint aspiration and injection.
- Complications
  - Postinjection synovitis may develop rarely as a result of phagocytosis of glucocorticoid ester crystals. Such reactions usually resolve within 48–72 hours. More persistent symptoms suggest the possibility of iatrogenic infection, which occurs very rarely (in <0.1% of patients).
  - **Localized skin depigmentation and atrophy** may result after glucocorticoid injection. Accelerated deterioration of bone and cartilage also may occur when frequent injections are administered over an extended period. Therefore, any single joint should be injected no more frequently than every 3–6 months.

NONSTEROIDAL ANTI-INFLAMMATORY DRUGS

- **Therapeutic effects.** These drugs exert their effects by inhibiting the constitutive (COX-1) and inducible (COX-2) isoforms of cyclooxygenase, producing a mild to moderate anti-inflammatory and analgesic effect. Individual responses to these agents are variable: If one drug is not effective during a 2- to 3-week trial, another should be tried.

- Side effects
    - **Gastrointestinal (GI) toxicity** manifests clinically as dyspepsia, nausea, vomiting, or GI bleeding. Nausea and dyspepsia often respond to the addition of a histamine-2 (H_2)-blocking agent or proton pump inhibitor or to a change in nonsteroidal anti-inflammatory drugs (NSAIDs). Direct GI irritation can be minimized by administration after food, by the use of enteric-coated preparations, and by use of the lowest effective dose. However, all NSAIDs have a systemic effect on the GI mucosa, resulting in increased permeability to gastric acid. Most serious GI bleeds during NSAID use occur without prior GI symptoms. **Risk factors for GI bleed** include a history of duodenal-gastric ulceration, age, smoking, ethanol use, and concomitant use of corticosteroids. **Misoprostol,** a synthetic prostaglandin E analog, decreases the risk of NSAID-induced gastric or duodenal ulceration but may cause diarrhea and is an abortifacient. An alternative is high-dose **famotidine,** 40 mg PO bid, or **omeprazole,** 20 mg daily. Diarrhea due to NSAIDs is rare except for the fenamates (e.g., meclofenamic acid, mefenamic acid).
    - **Acute renal failure** is the most common form of renal toxicity, and nephrotic syndrome and acute interstitial nephritis may also occur. **Risk factors** for acute renal failure include pre-existing renal dysfunction, congestive heart failure (CHF), cirrhosis with ascites, **and concomitant angiotensin-converting enzyme (ACE) inhibitor or angiotensin-receptor blockers.** Periodic monitoring of renal function is recommended, particularly in elderly patients.
    - **Platelet dysfunction** can be caused by all NSAIDs, and particularly aspirin, which is a covalent inhibitor of cyclooxygenase. NSAIDs should be used cautiously or avoided in patients with a bleeding diathesis or those who are taking warfarin, and should be discontinued 5–7 days before surgical procedures.
    - **Hypersensitivity reactions** are often seen in patients with a history of asthma, nasal polyps, or atopy. NSAIDs may cause a variety of type I hypersensitivity-like reactions, including urticaria, asthma, and anaphylactoid shock, presumably by increasing leukotriene synthesis. Patients with a hypersensitivity reaction to one NSAID should avoid all NSAIDs and selective COX-2 inhibitors.
    - **Other side effects. Central nervous system** (CNS) toxicity (headaches, dizziness, dysphoria, confusion, aseptic meningitis) is uncommon. Tinnitus and deafness can complicate NSAID use, particularly with high-dose salicylates. **Blood dyscrasias** including aplastic anemia have been observed as isolated case reports with ibuprofen, piroxicam, indomethacin, and phenylbutazone. **Dermatologic reactions** and **elevations in transaminases** have also been described. **Acid-base imbalance** is seen with high doses of salicylates. Nonacetylated salicylates have been reported to have less toxicity but also may be less effective. The use of NSAIDs, in general, may be associated with an increased risk for **cardiovascular thrombotic events.**

SELECTIVE COX-2 INHIBITORS

- **Therapeutic effects.** These agents exhibit selective inhibition of COX-2, thereby inhibiting inflammation while preserving the homeostatic functions of constitutive COX-1–derived prostaglandins. Their anti-inflammatory and analgesic efficacy are similar to that of traditional NSAIDs.
- Side effects
    - **GI symptoms** and **GI ulcerations** are reduced with these agents in comparison to NSAIDs.
    - **Platelet function** is not impaired, making selective COX-2 inhibitors a good anti-inflammatory option for patients with thrombocytopenia, hemostatic defects, or chronic anticoagulation. In patients who are taking warfarin, however, the international normalized ratio (INR) should be monitored after the addition of a COX-2 inhibitor, as with any medication change. In addition, there has been controversy as to whether the inhibition of prostacyclin but not thromboxane by these agents may promote clotting slightly.
    - **Fluid retention** has been noted with high-dose rofecoxib therapy, and renal function should be monitored in patients at risk of NSAID-induced acute renal failure.

- Patients with hypersensitivity reactions to NSAIDs should not use a COX-2 inhibitor, and individuals with a sulfonamide allergy should not use celecoxib.
- **An increased risk for myocardial infarction** has been associated with the use of COX-2 inhibitors. The association is strongest for rofecoxib.

GLUCOCORTICOIDS (TABLE 23-1)

- **Therapeutic effects.** Glucocorticoids exert a pluripotent anti-inflammatory effect via the inhibition of inflammatory mediator gene transcription.
- **Preparations, dosages, and routes of administration.** The goal of glucocorticoid therapy is to suppress disease activity with the minimum effective dosage. Prednisone (PO) and methylprednisolone (IV) are generally the preferred drugs because of cost and half-life considerations. IM absorption is variable and therefore is not advised. The dose, route, and frequency of administration are determined by the type of disease and the severity of the disease manifestations. The following are **relative anti-inflammatory potencies** of common glucocorticoid preparations: cortisone, 0.8; hydrocortisone, 1; prednisone, 4; methylprednisolone, 5; dexamethasone, 25.
- **Side effects.** Adverse effects are related to dosage and duration of administration and, except for cataracts and osteopenia, can be minimized by alternate-day administration once the disease is controlled (twice the daily dose given every other day).
  - **Adrenal suppression.** Glucocorticoids suppress the hypothalamic-pituitary-adrenal axis. Patients who have received more than 10 mg prednisone (or the equivalent) daily for several weeks may have some degree of axis suppression for up to 1 year after cessation of therapy. Adrenal suppression is minimized by dosing in the morning and using a single daily low dose of a short-acting preparation, such as prednisone, for a short period. In patients who are receiving chronic glucocorticoid therapy, hypoadrenalism (anorexia, weight loss, lethargy, fever, and postural hypotension) may occur at times of severe stress (e.g., infection, major surgery) and should be treated with stress doses of glucocorticoids. Mineralocorticoid activity, however, is preserved. These patients should wear a medical-alert bracelet or carry identification.

| **TABLE 23-1** | **Corticosteroids and Immunomodulatory and Immunosuppressive Drugs** |

Generic name	Tablet size (mg)	Starting dose (mg)	Dose interval	Maximum daily or interval dose (mg)
Prednisone	1, 2.5, 5, 10, 20, 50	5–20 (low), 1–2 mg/kg (high)	Daily	—
Methylprednisolone (IV)	—	500	bid for 3–5 d	—
Methotrexate	2.5	7.5	Weekly	25
Sulfasalazine	500	500	bid	3,000
Hydroxychloroquine	200	200	bid	400
Leflunomide	10, 20	20	Daily	20[a]
Azathioprine	50 (scored)	1.5 mg/kg	Daily	2.5–3.0 mg/kg[b]
Cyclophosphamide	25, 50	1.0–1.5 mg/kg	Daily	2.5–3.0 mg/kg[b]
Cyclophosphamide (IV)	—	0.5–1.0 g/m²	Monthly	—[b,c]
Cyclosporine	25, 50, 100	2–3 mg/kg	Daily	5 mg/kg

[a]Treatment can be begun with a loading dose of 100 mg/d for 3 days.
[b]Titrate peripheral white blood cell count to 3,500–4,500 cells/mcL (with neutrophils >1,000).
[c]The addition of 2-mercaptoethanesulfonate (mesna) is recommended.

- **Immunosuppression.** Glucocorticoid therapy reduces resistance to infections. **Bacterial infections** in particular are related to the dosage of glucocorticoids and are a major cause of morbidity and mortality. Thus, minor infections may become systemic, quiescent infections may be activated, and organisms that usually are nonpathogenic may cause disease. Local and systemic signs of infection may be partially masked, although fever associated with infection generally is not suppressed completely by glucocorticoids. When possible, a skin test for tuberculosis should be placed before glucocorticoid therapy is instituted, and, if it is positive, appropriate prophylaxis is indicated (see Chapter 13, Treatment of Infectious Diseases).
- **Endocrine abnormalities.** Possible endocrine abnormalities include a cushingoid habitus and hirsutism. Hyperglycemia may be induced or aggravated by glucocorticoids but usually is not a contraindication to therapy. Insulin therapy may be required, although ketoacidosis is rare. Fluid and electrolyte abnormalities include hypokalemia and sodium retention, which may induce or aggravate hypertension.
- **Musculoskeletal problems**
  - **Osteopenia** with vertebral compression fractures is common among patients who are receiving long-term glucocorticoid therapy. Supplemental calcium, 1.0–1.5 g/d PO, should be given along with vitamin D, **400–800 units daily PO**, as soon as steroid therapy is begun. A bisphosphonate may be indicated in postmenopausal women or in men or premenopausal women who are at high risk for osteopenia, and calcitonin can be considered for those who cannot tolerate a bisphosphonate. Determination of baseline bone density is appropriate in these patients. A judicious exercise program may be beneficial in stimulating bone formation.
  - **Steroid myopathy** generally involves the hip and shoulder girdle musculature. Muscles are weak but not tender and, in contrast to inflammatory myositis, serum creatine kinase, aldolase, and electromyography are normal. The myopathy usually resolves slowly with a reduction in glucocorticoid dosage and an aggressive exercise program.
  - **Ischemic bone necrosis** (aseptic necrosis, avascular necrosis) caused by glucocorticoid use often is multifocal, most commonly affecting the femoral head, humeral head, and tibial plateau. Early changes can be demonstrated by bone scan or magnetic resonance imaging (MRI). Early surgical intervention with core decompression remains controversial.
- **Other adverse effects.** Changes in **mental status** ranging from mild nervousness, euphoria, and insomnia to severe depression or psychosis may occur. **Ocular effects** include increased intraocular pressure (sometimes precipitating glaucoma) and the formation of posterior subcapsular cataracts. **Hyperlipidemia, menstrual irregularities,** increased perspiration with **night sweats,** and **pseudotumor cerebri** also may occur.

IMMUNOMODULATORY AND IMMUNOSUPPRESSIVE DRUGS

- These agents can be used to treat rheumatologic disorders (Table 23-1). This group of drugs includes a number of pharmacologically diverse agents that exert anti-inflammatory or immunosuppressive effects. Often, such agents are referred to as *disease-modifying antirheumatic drugs.* They are characterized by a delayed onset of action and the potential for serious toxicity. Consequently, they should be prescribed with the guidance of a rheumatologist or other physician who is experienced in their use and given only to well-informed, cooperative patients who are willing to comply with meticulous follow-up.
- **Methotrexate,** a purine inhibitor and folic acid antagonist, is used to treat synovitis and myositis and may improve the leukopenia of Felty syndrome.
  - **Dosage and administration.** Typically, methotrexate is administered as a single PO dose once a week starting with 7.5 mg. Clinical response is usually noted in 4–8 weeks. If no response is attained after 6–8 weeks of therapy, the dosage can be increased by 2.5- to 5.0-mg increments every 2–4 weeks to a maximum of 25 mg/wk or until improvement is observed. Dosages above 20 mg/wk are generally given by SC injection to promote absorption. Methotrexate in a dosage of 7.5–17.5 mg/wk is

also used in a treatment regimen for rheumatoid arthritis (RA) in combination with sulfasalazine, 500 mg bid, and hydroxychloroquine, 200 mg bid.

- **Contraindications and side effects.** Methotrexate is **teratogenic** and should not be used during pregnancy. It should also be avoided in patients with significant hepatic or renal impairment. **Folic acid supplementation** at a dosage of 1–2 mg daily may reduce methotrexate toxicity without impeding its efficacy. Concomitant use of trimethoprim/sulfamethoxazole should be avoided.
  - **Minor side effects** include GI intolerance, stomatitis, rash, headache, and alopecia.
  - **Bone marrow suppression** may occur, particularly at higher doses. Blood and platelet counts should be obtained before initiation, monthly during the first 3–4 months, and every 6–8 weeks thereafter. Macrocytosis may herald serious hematologic toxicity and is an indication for folate supplementation, dose reduction, or both.
  - **Cirrhosis** may occur rarely with long-term use. Aspartate transaminase (AST), alanine transaminase (ALT), and serum albumin should be measured every 4–8 weeks. Liver biopsy should be performed if the AST is elevated in five of nine determinations or if the serum albumin level falls below the normal range. Alcohol consumption increases the risk of methotrexate hepatotoxicity.
  - **Hypersensitivity pneumonitis** may occur but usually is reversible. Patients with pre-existing pulmonary parenchymal disease may be at increased risk.
  - **Rheumatoid nodules** may develop or worsen, paradoxically, in some patients on methotrexate.
- **Sulfasalazine** is useful for treating synovitis in the setting of RA and the seronegative spondyloarthropathies.
  - **Dosage.** The initial dosage is 500 mg PO daily, with increases in 500-mg increments weekly until a total daily dose of 2,000–3,000 mg (given in evenly divided doses) is reached. Clinical response usually occurs in 6–10 weeks.
  - **Contraindications and side effects. Sulfasalazine should not be used in patients with glucose-6-phosphate dehydrogenase deficiency or sulfa allergy.** Nausea is the principal adverse effect and can be minimized by the use of the enteric-coated preparation of the drug. Hematologic toxicity including a reduction in any cell line and aplastic anemia rarely occurs. However, periodic monitoring of blood and platelet counts is warranted.
- **Hydroxychloroquine** is an antimalarial agent that is used to treat dermatitis, alopecia, and synovitis in systemic lupus erythematosus (SLE) and mild synovitis in RA.
  - **Dosage.** Hydroxychloroquine typically is given at a dosage of 4–6 mg/kg PO daily (200–400 mg) after meals to minimize dyspepsia and nausea.
  - **Contraindications and side effects. Hydroxychloroquine should not be used in patients with porphyria, glucose-6-phosphate dehydrogenase deficiency, or significant hepatic or renal impairment.** It is probably safe during pregnancy. The most common side effects are allergic skin eruptions and nausea. Serious ocular toxicity occurs but is rare with currently recommended dosages. Ophthalmologic evaluation should be performed every 12–18 months.
- **Leflunomide** is a pyrimidine inhibitor that has been approved for the treatment of RA.
  - **Dosage and administration.** Treatment is begun with 10 or 20 mg PO daily. A loading dose of 100 mg for 3 days can be used. Clinical response is generally seen within 4–8 weeks.
  - **Contraindications and side effects.** Leflunomide is **teratogenic** and has a very long half-life. Women who plan to become pregnant must discontinue the drug and complete a course of elimination therapy with cholestyramine, 8 g PO tid for 11 days. Plasma levels should then be verified to be <0.02 mg/L on two separate tests at least 14 days apart before pregnancy is considered. Leflunomide is **contraindicated** in patients with significant hepatic dysfunction or in those who are receiving rifampin. **GI side effects** are the most common. **Diarrhea** occurs in up to 20% of patients and may require discontinuation of the drug. Dosage reduction to 10 mg/d may provide relief while maintaining efficacy, and loperamide can be used for symptomatic relief. **Elevations in serum transaminase levels** may occur, and transaminase levels

should be measured at baseline and then monitored monthly. The dosage should be reduced for confirmed twofold elevations, and greater elevations should be treated with cholestyramine and discontinuation of leflunomide. **Rash** and **alopecia** may occur during therapy

- **Azathioprine** is an antimetabolite that is used to treat refractory synovitis or myositis. It can also be used as a steroid-sparing agent.
  - **Dosage.** Therapy is initiated at 1.5 mg/kg/d PO, given as a single dose or in two divided doses. The dosage can be increased at 8- to 12-week intervals to a maximum of 2.5–3.0 mg/kg/d as long as the white blood cell (WBC) count remains at or above 3,500–4,500 cells/microliters with more than 1,000 neutrophils. The dosage of azathioprine should be reduced by 60%–75% if it is given concomitantly with allopurinol, which blocks its metabolic degradation.
  - **Side effects.** Adverse effects of azathioprine include an increased incidence of infection, nausea, rare hepatotoxicity, and potential long-term oncogenicity.
- **Mycophenolate mofetil** is an inhibitor of inosine monophosphate dehydrogenase used to treat lupus nephritis and, occasionally, as a steroid-sparing agent.
  - **Dosage.** Treatment is initiated at 1 g PO daily and can be increased to 2 g/d if the WBC remains at or above 3,500–4,500 cells/microliters.
  - **Side effects.** The most common adverse effects with mycophenolate mofetil are nausea, diarrhea, and vomiting. Leukopenia and an increased frequency of opportunistic infections have also been reported.
- **Cyclophosphamide,** an alkylating agent, is used to treat life-threatening manifestations of SLE and vasculitis.
  - **Dosage and administration.** Cyclophosphamide can be administered either daily (low-dose PO therapy) or intermittently (high-dose IV bolus therapy). The latter route is probably less toxic but also less immunosuppressive. Oral therapy is initiated at a daily morning dose of 1.0–1.5 mg/kg and can be increased to a maximum of 2.5–3.0 mg/kg/d to obtain a WBC count of 3,500–4,500 cells/microliters, with more than 1,000 neutrophils. Peripheral WBC counts should be checked 10–14 days after each dosage change and monthly when on a stable dose. IV therapy is initiated at a dosage of 0.5–1.0 g/m^2 every 1–3 months. The goal of therapy is to achieve a nadir WBC count of 3,500–4,500 cells/microliters, with more than 1,000 neutrophils, 10–14 days after infusion.
  - **Side effects.** Adverse effects include an increased incidence of infection, hemorrhagic cystitis, GI toxicity (nausea, vomiting), gonadal suppression and sterility, alopecia, pulmonary interstitial fibrosis, and oncogenicity (particularly bladder carcinoma). Patients should be encouraged to take the medication in the morning with a lot of fluid, to void frequently, and to void before going to bed to minimize the risk of hemorrhagic cystitis. With IV therapy, sodium 2-mercaptoethanesulfonate (**mesna**) and large volumes of fluid can be given concomitantly to minimize the risk of hemorrhagic cystitis. Mesna can be administered concomitantly with the cyclophosphamide infusion and repeated 3 and 6 hours later. Each mesna dose should be 20% of the total cyclophosphamide dose. **Antiemetics** may be necessary with high-dose IV therapy. The use of trimethoprim/sulfamethoxazole three times a week for *Pneumocystis carinii* prophylaxis should be considered
- **Cyclosporine** is occasionally used to treat refractory synovitis. Therapy is initiated at a dose of 2–3 mg/kg/d PO. The dose can be increased to as high as 5 mg/kg/d, but **renal toxicity** is the usual limiting factor. The dosage should be reduced if the serum creatinine level increases more than 30% or if hypertension develops. Other toxicities include hirsutism, anemia, liver dysfunction, and oncogenicity.

ANTICYTOKINE THERAPIES

New treatments directed at specific cytokines have been developed.

- **Tumor necrosis factor (TNF) inhibitors** have been approved for treatment of RA and seronegative spondyloarthropathies, and have also been useful in some forms of vasculitis. In general, these agents are used in patients with moderate to severe RA who have failed a trial of one or more disease-modifying antirheumatic drugs as listed above. Three preparations are currently available, with similar efficacy and toxicity profiles.

■ **Etanercept** is a fusion protein that consists of the ligand-binding portion of the human TNF receptor linked to the Fc portion of human immunoglobulin (Ig) G. It binds to TNF, blocking its interaction with cell surface receptors, thus inhibiting the inflammatory and immunoregulatory properties of TNF. This preparation is given in a dosage of 25 mg SC twice a week or 50 mg SC weekly.

■ **Infliximab** is a chimeric monoclonal antibody that binds specifically to human TNF-α, blocking its proinflammatory and immunomodulatory effects. It is given by IV infusion in conjunction with methotrexate to reduce production of neutralizing antibodies against infliximab. The recommended treatment regimen includes infliximab infusions of 3 mg/kg at initiation, at 2 and 6 weeks, and every 8 weeks thereafter, along with methotrexate at a dose of at least 7.5 mg/wk.

■ **Adalimumab** is a recombinant human IgG-1 monoclonal antibody that is specific to human TNF-α. It can be given in a dosage of 40 mg SC every other week. Some patients form antiadalimumab antibodies, and their regimen may include weekly injections of adalimumab or the addition of low-dose methotrexate. The effect of these agents on RA synovitis can be dramatic, with responsive patients reporting the onset of symptomatic benefits within 1–2 weeks. In addition to their symptomatic benefits, these agents appear to retard joint damage significantly.

■ **Contraindications and side effects**

  • **Serious infections and sepsis,** including fatalities, have been reported during the use of TNF-blocking agents. These drugs are contraindicated in patients with acute or chronic infections, and if serious infection or sepsis occurs, the drug should be stopped. Those with a history of recurrent infections and those with underlying conditions that may predispose to infection should be treated with caution and counseled to be vigilant for signs and symptoms of infection. Upper respiratory and sinus infections are most common. Tuberculosis has also been noted, and a tuberculin skin test and chest radiograph should be obtained before beginning therapy. Patients who are undergoing elective surgical procedures can omit the last dose of the drug that is scheduled to be given before surgery, as well as the next dose scheduled to follow the surgery. These agents are also contraindicated in patients with congestive heart failure.

  • **Local injection site reactions** are common with etanercept and adalimumab, particularly during the first month of therapy. These reactions are generally self-limited and do not require discontinuation of therapy. Serious systemic allergic reactions are rare but may occur with infliximab infusions.

  • **Other adverse effects** may include induction of antinuclear antibodies and, rarely, a lupuslike illness. A demyelinating disorder has been described, as well as exacerbations of pre-existing multiple sclerosis. It is unclear whether the frequency of occurrence of lymphoma may be increased in patients who receive these agents.

■ **Inhibitors of interleukin-1α (IL-1).** Currently, only one inhibitor of interleukin is available for patients with rheumatic diseases, but several more are in development.

  ■ **Anakinra** is a recombinant form of the naturally occurring IL-1– receptor antagonist that is approved for use in RA. It blocks binding of IL-1 to its receptor, thus inhibiting the proinflammatory and immunomodulatory actions of IL-1.

  • This agent is given in a **dosage** of 100 mg SC daily. Like the TNF blockers, it should not be prescribed to patients with ongoing or recurrent infections.

  • **Adverse effects** include an increased frequency of bacterial infections and injection site reactions.

  • **Anakinra should not be used in conjunction with a TNF blocker because of enhanced risk of serious infection and neutropenia.**

PLASMAPHERESIS

■ Until concomitant therapy with glucocorticoids or immunosuppressives has taken effect, plasmapheresis has been used on an investigational basis in life-threatening situations to control various rheumatic diseases. It is an impractical long-term therapy, and its short-term use remains controversial. A new approach, pheresis across a column bound with staphylococcal protein A, the **Prosorba** column, has been approved for treatment of RA.

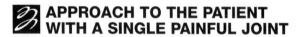

APPROACH TO THE PATIENT WITH A SINGLE PAINFUL JOINT

DIAGNOSIS

Physical Examination

- The first step for diagnosis for a patient with a single painful joint is to **identify the structure involved.** Pain that arises from periarticular (e.g., tendon, bursa), muscular, and neurologic structures may be perceived as joint pain.

Differential Diagnosis

- If the pain arises in the joint itself and a single joint is involved, the major disorders in the differential diagnosis are **trauma, infection,** and **crystalline arthritis.**

Imaging

- **Radiographs** of the joint may be useful in documenting trauma or pre-existing joint disease. The presence of chondrocalcinosis on the radiograph suggests pseudogout but is not diagnostic (see Crystal-Induced Synovitis). Radiographs are usually normal in acute infectious or crystalline arthritis.

Diagnostic Procedures

- **Synovial fluid** should be aspirated in all patients with a monarticular arthritis who do not have a pre-existing diagnosis that is consistent with the clinical picture. Polyarticular disorders such as RA or lupus (SLE) occasionally present initially as monarthritis, but when a single joint is inflamed out of proportion to other joints in what is typically a polyarticular disorder, infection must be excluded. Synovial fluid cell counts above 5,000 nucleated cells/microliters suggest an inflammatory etiology. Counts above 50,000 cells/microliters may indicate infection, particularly if 75% or more of the cells are polymorphonuclear.

TREATMENT

- Management is based on the results of radiographs and synovial fluid analysis. Trauma or internal derangement of the joint can be managed by immobilization of the joint and consultation with an orthopedic surgeon.

INFECTIOUS ARTHRITIS AND BURSITIS

GENERAL PRINCIPLES

Classification

- **Infectious arthritis** is generally categorized into gonococcal and nongonococcal disease.

Etiology

■ **Nongonococcal infectious arthritis** in adults tends to occur in patients with previous joint damage or compromised host defenses. In contrast, **gonococcal arthritis** causes one-half of all septic arthritis in otherwise healthy, sexually active young adults.

DIAGNOSIS

Clinical Presentation

■ The usual presentation is with fever and an acute monarticular arthritis, although multiple joints may be affected by hematogenous spread of pathogens.

Laboratory Studies

■ A joint fluid leukocyte count is useful diagnostically and as a baseline for serial studies to evaluate response to treatment. Cultures of blood and other possible extra-articular sites of infection also should be obtained.

Diagnostic Procedures

■ **Joint fluid examination,** including Gram stain of a centrifuged pellet, a joint fluid leukocyte count, and cultures are mandatory to make a diagnosis and to guide management.

TREATMENT

■ **IV antimicrobials** provide good serum and synovial fluid drug concentrations.
  ▪ Oral or intra-articular antimicrobials are not appropriate as initial therapy.
■ **An NSAID or a selective COX-2 inhibitor** (see Therapeutic Approaches to Rheumatic Disease) is often useful to reduce pain and increase joint mobility but should not be used until response to antimicrobial therapy has been demonstrated by symptomatic and laboratory improvement.
■ **Surgical drainage** or arthroscopic lavage and drainage are indicated for (a) a septic hip; (b) joints in which either the anatomy, large amounts of tissue debris, or loculation of pus prevent adequate needle drainage (most commonly the shoulder); (c) septic arthritis with coexistent osteomyelitis; (d) joints that do not respond in 3–5 days to appropriate therapy and repeated arthrocenteses; and (e) prosthetic joint infection.
■ **General supportive** measures include splinting of the joint, which may help to relieve pain. However, prolonged immobilization can result in joint stiffness.
■ **Hospitalization** is indicated to ensure drug compliance and careful monitoring of the clinical response.
■ **Repeated arthrocenteses** should be performed daily or as often as necessary to prevent reaccumulation of fluid. Arthrocentesis is indicated to (a) remove destructive inflammatory mediators, (b) reduce intra-articular pressure and promote antimicrobial penetration into the joint, and (c) monitor response to therapy by documenting sterility of synovial fluid cultures and steadily decreasing leukocyte counts.

NONGONOCOCCAL SEPTIC ARTHRITIS

General Considerations

Etiology

■ Nongonococcal septic arthritis is caused most often by *Staphylococcus aureus* (60%) and *Streptococcus* species. Gram-negative organisms are less common except with IV drug abuse, neutropenia, concomitant urinary tract infection, and postoperative patients.

Diagnosis

■ Diagnosis is made with a carefully performed Gram stain, which reveals the organism in approximately 50% of patients.

Treatment

■ **Initial therapy** is based on the clinical situation.
  ▪ With a positive Gram stain, antibiotic coverage can be focused accordingly.
  ▪ With a nondiagnostic Gram stain, antibiotics should be chosen to cover *S. aureus*, *Streptococcus* species, and *Neisseria gonorrhoeae* in otherwise healthy patients, whereas broad-spectrum antibiotics are appropriate in immunosuppressed patients.
  ▪ IV antimicrobials usually are given for at least 2 weeks, followed by 1–2 weeks of oral antimicrobials, with the course of therapy tailored to the patient's response.

GONOCOCCAL ARTHRITIS

General Principles

Epidemiology
■ Gonococcal arthritis is more common than nongonococcal septic arthritis.

Diagnosis

Clinical Presentation
■ The clinical spectrum of disease often includes migratory or additive polyarthralgias, followed by tenosynovitis or arthritis of the wrist, ankle, or knee and asymptomatic dermatitis on the extremities or trunk.

Laboratory Studies
■ In contrast to nongonococcal septic arthritis, Gram staining of synovial fluid and cultures of blood or synovial fluid often are negative.
  ▪ Bacteriologic assessment of the throat, cervix, urethra, and rectum may aid in establishing the diagnosis.

Treatment

■ **Initial treatment is with an IV antibiotic** for the first 1–3 days, generally ceftriaxone, 1 g IV daily, or ceftizoxime, 1 g IV q8h. Response to IV antibiotics is usually noted within the first 24–36 hours of treatment. After clinical improvement is noted, therapy is continued with an oral antibiotic to complete 7–10 days of treatment. Ciprofloxacin, 500 mg PO bid, or amoxicillin/clavulanate, 500–850 mg PO bid, can be used. Treatment of coexisting *Chlamydia* infection should also be considered.

NONBACTERIAL INFECTIOUS ARTHRITIS

■ **Nonbacterial infectious arthritis** is common with many viral infections, especially hepatitis B, rubella, mumps, infectious mononucleosis, parvovirus, enterovirus, and adenovirus.
■ It is generally self-limiting, lasting for <6 weeks, and responds well to a conservative regimen of rest and NSAIDs.
■ Arthralgias (often severe) or a reactive arthritis can also be a manifestation of HIV infection.
■ A variety of fungi and mycobacteria can cause septic arthritis and should be considered in patients with chronic monoarticular arthritis.

SEPTIC BURSITIS

Diagnosis

- Usually involving the olecranon or prepatellar bursa, it can be differentiated from septic arthritis by localized, fluctuant superficial swelling and by relatively painless joint motion (particularly extension).
- Most patients have a history of previous trauma to the area or an occupational predisposition (e.g., "housemaid's knee," "writer's elbow").
- *S. aureus* is the most common pathogen of septic bursitis.

Treatment

- Septic bursitis should be treated with aspiration, which can be repeated if fluid reaccumulates. Oral antibiotics and outpatient management are usually appropriate, and surgical drainage is rarely indicated.
- Preventive measures (e.g., knee pads) should be used in patients with occupational predispositions to septic bursitis.

LYME DISEASE

General Principles

Etiology
- Lyme disease is caused by the tick-borne spirochete *Borrelia burgdorferi.*

Diagnosis

- Typical manifestations begin with an erythematous annular rash (erythema migrans) and flulike symptoms.
- Arthralgias, myalgias, meningitis, neuropathy, and cardiac conduction defects may follow in weeks to a few months. Months later, an intermittent or chronic arthritis in one or a few joints, characteristically including the knee, may develop in untreated patients.
- The diagnosis is based mainly on the clinical picture and exposure in an endemic area.

Laboratory Studies
- Unfortunately, serologic studies often give false-negative or false-positive results, and patients may remain seropositive for years following treatment.

Treatment

- Antibiotic therapy is required.
- NSAIDs are a useful adjunct for arthritis.

Risk Management
- A vaccine against Lyme disease is safe and effective but was withdrawn from the market by the manufacturer due to limited demand.

CRYSTAL-INDUCED SYNOVITIS

GENERAL PRINCIPLES

Definition

- Deposition of microcrystals in joints and periarticular tissues results in **gout, pseudogout,** and **apatite disease.**

Epidemiology

■ **Primary gouty arthritis.** Men are much more commonly affected than women; most premenopausal women with gout have a family history of the disease.

Classification

■ The clinical phases of gout can be divided into (a) asymptomatic hyperuricemia, (b) acute gouty arthritis, and (c) chronic arthritis.
■ **Asymptomatic hyperuricemia** (uric acid levels >8 mg/dL in men and >7 mg/dL in women)

Etiology

■ **Primary gouty arthritis** is characterized by hyperuricemia that is usually due to under-excretion of uric acid (90% of cases) rather than to overproduction. Urate crystals may be deposited in the joints, SC tissues (tophi), and kidneys.
■ **Secondary gout,** like primary gout, can be caused by either defective renal excretion or overproduction of uric acid. Intrinsic renal disease, diuretic therapy, low-dose aspirin, nicotinic acid, cyclosporine, and ethanol all interfere with renal excretion of uric acid. Starvation, lactic acidosis, dehydration, pre-eclampsia, and diabetic ketoacidosis also can induce hyperuricemia.
■ **Pseudogout** results when calcium pyrophosphate dihydrate crystals deposited in bone and cartilage are released into synovial fluid and induce acute inflammation. **Risk factors** include older age, advanced osteoarthritis (OA), neuropathic joint, gout, hyperparathyroidism, hemochromatosis, diabetes mellitus, hypothyroidism, and hypomagnesemia.

DIAGNOSIS

Clinical Presentation

■ **Acute gouty arthritis** presents as an excruciating attack of pain, usually in a single joint of the foot or ankle. Occasionally, a polyarticular onset can mimic RA.
■ **Chronic gouty arthritis.** With time, acute gouty attacks occur more frequently, asymptomatic periods are shorter, and chronic joint deformity may appear. Overproduction of uric acid occurs in myeloproliferative and lymphoproliferative disorders, hemolytic anemia, polycythemia, and cyanotic congenital heart disease.
■ **Pseudogout** may present as an **acute monarthritis or oligoarthritis** mimicking gout or as a **chronic polyarthritis** resembling RA or OA. Usually the knee or wrist is affected, although any synovial joint can be involved.
■ **Apatite disease** may present with periarthritis or tendonitis, particularly in patients with chronic renal failure. An episodic oligoarthritis also may occur.

History

■ Acute gouty arthritis attacks can be precipitated by surgery, dehydration, fasting, binge eating, or heavy ingestion of alcohol. Although the acute gouty attack will subside spontaneously over several days, prompt treatment can abort the attack within hours.

Laboratory Studies

■ A definitive diagnosis of gout or pseudogout is made by finding intracellular crystals in joint fluid examined with a compensated polarized light microscope. Urate crystals, which are diagnostic of gout, are needle shaped and strongly negatively birefringent. The calcium pyrophosphate dihydrate crystals seen in pseudogout are pleomorphic and weakly positively birefringent. Hydroxyapatite complexes, diagnostic of apatite disease, and basic calcium phosphate complexes can be identified only by electron microscopy and mass spectroscopy. In most cases, the arthritides associated with these compounds are suspected clinically but never confirmed.

■ **Acute gouty arthritis.** The serum uric acid level is normal in 30% of patients with acute gout and, if elevated, should not be manipulated until an attack has resolved.

■ Apatite disease should be suspected when no crystals are present in the synovial fluid.

Imaging

■ Erosive arthritis may be seen.

TREATMENT

■ **Asymptomatic hyperuricemia** is not routinely treated because of expense, potential drug toxicity, and the low risk for adverse outcome from the hyperuricemia itself.

■ **Management of secondary gout** includes treatment of the underlying disorder and allopurinol therapy.

■ The treatment of **apatite disease** is similar to that for pseudogout.

Medications

■ Acute gout
  ■ NSAIDs are the treatment of choice due to ease of administration and low toxicity. Clinical response may require 12–24 hours, and initial doses should be high, followed by rapid tapering over 2–8 days (see Therapeutic Approaches to Rheumatic Disease). One approach is to use indomethacin, 50 mg PO q6h for 2 days, followed by 50 mg PO q8h for 3 days and then 25 mg PO q8h for 2–3 days. The long-acting NSAIDs generally are not recommended for acute gout. Selective COX-2 inhibitors appear to have similar efficacy.
  ■ Glucocorticoids are useful when NSAIDs are contraindicated. An intra-articular injection of glucocorticoids produces rapid dramatic relief. Alternatively, prednisone, 40–60 mg PO daily, can be given until a response is obtained and then should be tapered rapidly.
  ■ Colchicine is most effective if given in the first 12–24 hours of an acute attack and usually brings relief in 6–12 hours. In view of the efficacy and tolerability of a short course of NSAIDs, colchicine is not commonly used to treat gout but is useful when NSAIDs or glucocorticoids are contraindicated or not tolerated.
    • **Oral administration** is often associated with severe GI toxicity. The dosage during an acute attack is 0.5–0.6 mg (one tablet) q1–2h for three dosages started at the first sign of the attack. Alternatively, colchicine 0.6 mg bid in addition to an NSAID can be used. The previous dosage regimen of 0.5–0.6 mg (one tablet) q1–2h or 1.0–1.2 mg q2h until symptoms abate, GI toxicity develops, or the maximum dose of 6 mg in a 24-hour period is reached is not recommended as primary treatment for most cases due to toxicity.
    • **IV colchicine** is not recommended for general use and its administration in almost all circumstances is questionable.
■ Chronic gouty arthritis
  ■ Colchicine (0.5–0.6 mg PO daily or bid) can be used prophylactically for acute attacks. The dosage needs to be adjusted in patients with renal insufficiency. Colchicine 0.6 mg every other day or every 3 days should be considered in patients with a creatinine clearance between 10 and 34 mL/min. Aspirin (uricoretentive), diuretics, large alcohol intake, and foods high in purines (sweetbreads, anchovies, sardines, liver, and kidney) should be avoided. The serum uric acid level should be lowered if arthritic attacks are frequent, renal damage is present, or serum or urine uric acid levels are elevated consistently. **Maintenance colchicine, 0.5–0.6 mg PO bid, should be given a few days before manipulation of the uric acid level to prevent precipitation of an acute attack.** If no attacks occur after the uric acid has been maintained in the normal range for 6–8 weeks, colchicine can be discontinued.

- **Allopurinol,** a xanthine oxidase inhibitor, is effective therapy for hyperuricemia in most patients.
  - **Dosage and administration.** The initial dosage is usually 300 mg PO daily. Daily doses can be increased by 100 mg every 2–4 weeks to achieve the minimum maintenance dosage that will keep the uric acid level within the normal range. In patients with impaired renal function, the daily dose should be reduced by 50 mg for each 20-mL/min decrease in the creatinine clearance. For patients with a creatinine clearance below 20 mL/min, the starting dosage is 100 mg every other or every third day. The daily dose should be decreased also in patients with hepatic impairment. The concomitant use of a uricosuric agent may hasten the mobilization of tophi. If an acute attack occurs during treatment with allopurinol, it should be continued at the same dosage while other agents are used to treat the attack.
  - **Side effects. Hypersensitivity reactions** from a minor skin rash to a diffuse exfoliative dermatitis associated with fever, eosinophilia, and a combination of renal and hepatic injury occur in up to 5% of patients. Patients who have mild renal insufficiency and are receiving diuretics are at greatest risk. **Severe cases are potentially fatal** and usually require glucocorticoid therapy. Allopurinol may potentiate the effect of oral anticoagulants and blocks metabolism of azathioprine and 6-mercaptopurine, necessitating a 60%–75% reduction in dosage of these cytotoxic drugs.
- **Febuxostat,** a new class of uric acid–lowering drug, is a nonpurine selective inhibitor of the xanthine oxidase that is expected to be available soon in the United States.
- **Uricase** catabolizes uric acid to the more soluble compound, allantoin. It is available in the United States for the treatment of tumor lysis syndrome.
- **Uricosuric drugs** lower serum uric acid levels by blocking renal tubular reabsorption of uric acid. A 24-hour measurement of creatinine clearance and urine uric acid should be obtained before therapy is started, as these drugs are **ineffective with glomerular filtration rates of** <50 mL/min. They are also not recommended for patients who already have high levels of urine uric acid (800 mg/24 hours) because of the risk of urate stone formation. This risk can be minimized by maintaining a high fluid intake and by alkalinizing the urine. If these drugs are being used when an acute gouty attack begins, they should be continued while other drugs are used to treat the acute attack.
  - **Probenecid**
    - Initial dosage is 500 mg PO daily, which can be raised in 500-mg increments every week until serum uric acid levels normalize or urine uric acid levels exceed 800 mg/24 hours. The maximum dose is 3,000 mg/d. Most patients require a total of 1.0–1.5 g/d in two to three divided doses.
    - Salicylates and probenecid are antagonistic and should not be used together.
    - Probenecid decreases renal excretion of penicillin, indomethacin, and sulfonylureas.
    - Side effects are minimal.
  - **Sulfinpyrazone** has uricosuric efficacy similar to that of probenecid; however, it also inhibits platelet function. The initial dosage of 50 mg PO bid can be increased in 100-mg increments weekly until serum uric acid levels normalize, to a maximum dose of 800 mg/d. Most patients require 300–400 mg/d in three to four divided doses.
- **Pseudogout**
  - As in gout, the therapy of choice for most patients is a brief high-dose course of an **NSAID** (see Therapeutic Approaches to Rheumatic Disease).
  - **Oral corticosteroids** can be used and **colchicine** also may relieve symptoms promptly, but toxicity limits its use. Dosage and administration are similar to the ones used in the treatment of gout.
  - Maintenance daily PO colchicine may diminish the number of recurrent attacks. Allopurinol or uricosuric agents have no role in treating pseudogout.
  - Aspiration of the inflammatory joint fluid often results in prompt improvement and intra-articular injection of glucocorticoids may hasten the response.

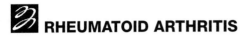 **RHEUMATOID ARTHRITIS**

GENERAL PRINCIPLES

Definition

- RA is a systemic disease of unknown etiology that is characterized by symmetric inflammatory polyarthritis, extra-articular manifestations (rheumatoid nodules, pulmonary fibrosis, serositis, vasculitis), and serum rheumatoid factor in up to 80% of patients.

DIAGNOSIS

Clinical Presentation

- The course of RA is variable but tends to be chronic and progressive.
- **Sjogren's syndrome,** characterized by failure of exocrine glands, occurs in a subset of patients with RA, producing sicca symptoms (dry eyes and mouth), parotid gland enlargement, dental caries, and recurrent tracheobronchitis.
- **Felty's syndrome,** the triad of RA, splenomegaly, and granulocytopenia, also occurs in a small subset of patients, and these patients are at risk for recurrent bacterial infections and nonhealing leg ulcers.
- Approximately 70% of patients show irreversible joint damage on radiography within the first 3 years of disease. Work disability is common, and life span is shortened by between 3 and 12 years.
- **Reactive depression and sleep disorders** are often encountered in patients with rheumatic diseases.

TREATMENT

- Most patients can benefit from an early aggressive treatment program that combines medical, rehabilitative, and surgical services designed with three distinct goals: (a) early suppression of inflammation in the joints and other tissues, (b) maintenance of joint and muscle function and prevention of deformities, and (c) repair of joint damage to relieve pain or improve function.

Behavioral

- **Acute care** of inflammatory arthritides involves joint protection and pain relief. Proper joint positioning and splints are important elements in joint protection. Heat is a useful analgesic.
- **Subacute disease** therapy should include a gradual increase in passive and active joint movement.
- **Chronic care** encompasses instruction in joint protection, work simplification, and performance of activities of daily living. Adaptive equipment, splints, orthotics, and mobility aids may be useful. Specific exercises designed to promote normal joint mechanics and to strengthen affected muscle groups are useful. Overall cardiac conditioning also improves functional status.
- **Sicca symptoms** (dry eyes and mouth) can be treated symptomatically with artificial tears and saliva. Assiduous dental and ophthalmologic care is recommended, and drugs that suppress lacrimal–salivary secretion further should be avoided.

Medications

- **NSAIDs or selective COX-2 inhibitors** (see Therapeutic Approaches to Rheumatic Disease) are used as the initial therapy for RA and as an adjunct to immunomodulatory–immunosuppressive therapy. A longer-acting NSAID may facilitate patient compliance.

- **Glucocorticoids** are not curative and probably do not alter the natural history of RA; however, they are among the most potent anti-inflammatory drugs available (see Therapeutic Approaches to Rheumatic Disease). Unfortunately, once systemic glucocorticoid therapy has been initiated, few RA patients are able to discontinue it completely.
  - **Indications** for glucocorticoids include (a) symptomatic relief while waiting for a response to a slow-acting immunosuppressive or immunomodulatory agent, (b) persistent synovitis despite adequate trials of NSAIDs and immunosuppressive or immunomodulatory agents, and (c) severe constitutional symptoms (e.g., fever and weight loss) or extra-articular disease (vasculitis, episcleritis, or pleurisy).
  - **Oral administration** of prednisone 5–20 mg daily usually is sufficient for the treatment of synovitis, whereas severe constitutional symptoms or extra-articular disease may require up to 1 mg/kg PO daily. Although alternate-day glucocorticoid therapy reduces the incidence of undesirable side effects, some patients do not tolerate the increase in symptoms that may occur on the off day.
  - **Intra-articular administration** may provide temporary symptomatic relief when only a few joints are inflamed (see Therapeutic Approaches to Rheumatic Disease). The beneficial effects of intra-articular steroids may persist for days to months and may delay or negate the need for systemic glucocorticoid therapy.
- **Immunomodulatory and immunosuppressive agents** appear to alter the natural history of RA by retarding the progression of bony erosions and cartilage loss. Because RA may lead to substantial long-term disability (and is associated with increased mortality), the current trend is to initiate therapy with such agents early in the course of RA (see Therapeutic Approaches to Rheumatic Disease). Once a clinical response has been achieved, the chosen drug usually is continued indefinitely at the lowest effective dosage to prevent relapse.
  - **Indications** for the use of immunomodulatory or immunosuppressive agents include (a) active synovitis that does not respond to conservative management (e.g., NSAIDs); (b) rapidly progressive, erosive arthritis; and (c) dependence on steroids to control synovitis.
  - **Selection** of an immunomodulatory or immunosuppressive agent is tailored to the character of the patient's disease, taking into account the potential toxicity of these agents (see Therapeutic Approaches to Rheumatic Disease) (Table 23-1). **Methotrexate** typically is the initial choice for moderate to severe RA. **Hydroxychloroquine or sulfasalazine** can be used as the initial choice in very mild RA. If response to the initial agent is unsatisfactory after an adequate trial (or if limiting toxicity supervenes), an alternate agent, such as **leflunomide, a TNF or IL-1 blocker, or azathioprine**, can be used. **Rituximab,** a monoclonal antibody directed against the B-cell surface molecule CD20, causes depletion of B cells and has been shown to be effective in cases of severe rheumatoid arthritis not responding to conventional treatment. It is U.S. Food and Drug Administration (FDA) approved to be used routinely for RA. **Abatacept** is a fusion protein comprising the CTLA4 molecule and the Fc portion of IgG1. It blocks selective costimulation of T cells.
- **Combinations of immunomodulatory–immunosuppressive agents** can be used if the patient has a partial response to the initial agent.
  - Common combination therapies include methotrexate with either hydroxychloroquine, sulfasalazine, or both (see Therapeutic Approaches to Rheumatic Disease). For severe RA, methotrexate has been combined with leflunomide, azathioprine, or cyclosporin A. Such combinations may lead to synergistic or unexpected toxicities and should be used with appropriate caution.
- **Reactive depression and sleep disorders** are often encountered in patients with rheumatic diseases. Judicious use of antidepressants and sedatives may improve the functional status of selected patients.
- Sicca symptoms
  - **Pilocarpine** in a dosage of up to 5 mg PO qid may provide symptomatic relief.

Surgery

- **Corrective surgical procedures,** including synovectomy, total joint replacement, and joint fusion, may be indicated in patients with RA to reduce pain and to improve function.

- Carpal tunnel syndrome is common, and surgical repair may be curative if local injection therapy is unsuccessful.
- **Synovectomy** may be helpful if major involvement is limited to one or two joints and if a 6-month trial of medical therapy has failed, but usually it is only of temporary benefit.
- Prophylactic synovectomy and débridement of the ulnar styloid should be considered for patients with severe wrist disease to prevent rupture of the extensor tendons.
- Other procedures that may be beneficial include **total joint replacement** of the hip and knee joints, resection of metatarsal heads in patients with bunion deformities, and subluxation of the toes. Reconstructive hand surgery may be useful in carefully selected patients.
- **Surgical fusion of joints** usually results in freedom from pain but also in total loss of motion; this is tolerated well in the wrist and thumb.
- Cervical spine fusion of C1 and C2 is indicated for significant cervical subluxation (>5 mm) with associated neurologic deficits.
  - Patients with RA undergoing elective surgical procedures should have a lateral cervical spine radiograph in flexion and extensions performed to screen for this subluxation.

Referrals

- Rehabilitative therapy should be managed by a team of physicians, physical and occupational therapists, nurses, social workers, and psychologists. This approach may benefit patients with any form of arthritis.

Patient Education

- **Patient education,** including pamphlets and support groups, is available in many communities through local chapters of the Arthritis Foundation.

Complications

- Patients with RA and a single joint inflamed out of proportion to the rest of the joints must be evaluated for coexistent septic arthritis. This complication occurs with increased frequency in RA and carries a 20%–30% mortality.

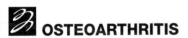 **OSTEOARTHRITIS**

GENERAL PRINCIPLES

Definition

- **OA, or degenerative joint disease,** is characterized by deterioration of articular cartilage, with subsequent formation of reactive new bone at the articular surface. The joints affected most commonly are the distal and proximal interphalangeal joints of the hands, hips, knees, and cervical and lumbar spine.

Epidemiology

- The disease is more common in the elderly but may occur at any age, especially as a sequel to joint trauma, chronic inflammatory arthritis, or congenital malformation. OA of the spine may lead to spinal stenosis (neurogenic claudication), with aching or pain in the legs or buttocks on standing or walking.

TREATMENT

Medications

- **Acetaminophen** in a dosage of up to 1,000 mg up to qid is the initial pharmacologic treatment.
- **Low-dose NSAIDs or selective COX-2 inhibitors** are the next step, followed by full-dose treatment (see Therapeutic Approaches to Rheumatic Disease). However, because this patient population is often elderly and may have concomitant renal or cardiopulmonary disease, NSAIDs should be used with caution. NSAID-induced GI bleeding also is increased in the elderly population.
- **Glucosamine sulfate,** 1,500 mg PO daily, may reduce symptoms as well as the rate of cartilage deterioration. **Intra-articular glucocorticoid injections** often are beneficial but probably should not be given more than every 3–6 months (see Therapeutic Approaches to Rheumatic Disease).
- Systemic steroids and narcotic analgesics should be avoided, although the μ-opioid agonist **tramadol** may be useful as an alternative analgesic agent.
- **Topical capsaicin** may provide symptomatic relief with minimal toxicity.
- Synthetic and naturally occurring hyaluronic acid derivatives (**Hyalgan, Synvisc**) can be administered intra-articularly. They reduce pain and improve mobility.

Surgery

- When serious disability results from severe pain or deformity, **surgery** can be considered. Total hip or knee replacement usually relieves pain and increases function in selected patients.
- **Laminectomy and spinal fusion** should be reserved for patients who have severe disease with intractable pain or neurologic complications. Lumbar spinal stenosis may require extensive decompressive laminectomy for relief of symptoms.

Nonoperative

- **Nonpharmacologic approaches** may complement drug treatment of arthritis. Activities that involve excessive use of the joint should be identified and avoided. Brief periods of rest for the involved joint can relieve pain. Poor body mechanics should be corrected and malalignments such as pronated feet may be aided by orthotics. An exercise program to prevent or correct muscle atrophy can also provide pain relief. When weight-bearing joints are affected, support in the form of a cane, crutches, or a walker can be helpful, as well as weight reduction and wearing soft-soled shoes. Consultation with occupational and physical therapists may be helpful.
- **OA of the spine** may cause radicular symptoms from pressure on nerve roots and often produces pain and spasm in the paraspinal soft tissues.
  - Physical supports (cervical collar, lumbar corset), local heat, and exercises to strengthen cervical, paravertebral, and abdominal muscles may provide relief in some patients.
- **Epidural steroid injections** may reduce radicular symptoms.

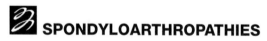 **SPONDYLOARTHROPATHIES**

GENERAL PRINCIPLES

Definition

- The **spondyloarthropathies** are an interrelated group of disorders characterized by one or more of the following features: (a) spondylitis, (b) sacroiliitis, (c) enthesopathy (inflammation at sites of tendon insertion), and (d) asymmetric oligoarthritis. Extra-articular features of this group of disorders may include inflammatory eye disease, urethritis, and mucocutaneous lesions. The spondyloarthropathies aggregate in families, where they are associated with HLA-B27.

ANKYLOSING SPONDYLITIS

Diagnosis

Clinical Presentation

- **Ankylosing spondylitis (AS)** clinically presents as inflammation and ossification of the joints and ligaments of the spine and of the sacroiliac joints.
    - Hips and shoulders are the peripheral joints that are most commonly involved. Progressive fusion of the apophyseal joints of the spine occurs in many patients and cannot be predicted or prevented.

Treatment

Behavioral

- Physical therapy emphasizing extension exercises and posture is recommended to minimize possible late postural defects and respiratory compromise.
- Patients should be instructed to sleep supine on a firm bed without a pillow and to practice postural and deep-breathing exercises regularly.
- Cigarette smoking should be discouraged strongly.

Medications

- **Nonsalicylate NSAIDs,** such as indomethacin, are used to provide symptomatic relief, and **selective COX-2 inhibitors** are also effective (see Therapeutic Approaches to Rheumatic Disease).
- **Methotrexate and sulfasalazine** provide benefit in some patients (see Therapeutic Approaches to Rheumatic Disease) (Table 23-1).
- **TNF blockade** has been shown to be of benefit even in some patients with apparent fixed deformities.
- Glucocorticoids and immunosuppressive therapy have been used occasionally in patients who do not respond to other agents.

Surgery

- Many patients develop osteoporosis in the fused spondylitic spine and are at risk of spinal fracture. Surgical procedures to correct some spine and hip deformities may result in significant rehabilitation in carefully selected patients.

Referrals

- **Acute anterior uveitis** occurs in up to 25% of patients with AS and should be managed by an ophthalmologist. Generally, this problem is self-limited, although glaucoma and blindness are unusual secondary complications.

ARTHRITIS OF INFLAMMATORY BOWEL DISEASE

General Principles

- **Arthritis of inflammatory bowel disease** occurs in 10%–20% of patients with Crohn's disease or ulcerative colitis and is similar to that of AS. It may also occur in some patients with intestinal bypass and diverticular disease.

Diagnosis

Clinical Presentation

- Clinical features include **spondylitis, sacroiliitis,** and **peripheral arthritis,** particularly in the knee and ankle. Although peripheral joint disease may correlate with the activity of the colitis, spinal disease does not.

Diagnostic Procedures

■ Joint aspiration may be useful to exclude an associated septic arthritis, but antimicrobials are not effective in the management of sterile synovitis associated with colitis.

Treatment

Medications

■ As in AS, **NSAIDs** (other than salicylates) are the treatment of choice, and **selective COX-2 inhibitors** are also effective. However, GI intolerance of NSAIDs may be increased among this group of patients, and misoprostol may cause unacceptable diarrhea (see Therapeutic Approaches to Rheumatic Disease).

■ **Sulfasalazine** also may be beneficial for this form of arthritis (see Therapeutic Approaches to Rheumatic Disease) (Table 23-1).

■ Local **injection of glucocorticoids** and **physical therapy** are useful adjunctive measures.

REITER SYNDROME AND REACTIVE ARTHRITIS

General Principles

Epidemiology

■ Reiter syndrome is seen predominantly in young men and may occur with increased frequency in patients infected with HIV. *Chlamydia* infection has been implicated in some patients.

Etiology

■ A reactive arthritis may follow dysentery caused by *Shigella flexneri*, *Salmonella* species, *Yersinia enterocolitica*, or *Clostridium difficile* infections.

Diagnosis

Clinical Presentation

■ The clinical syndrome consists of **asymmetric oligoarthritis, urethritis, conjunctivitis,** and characteristic **skin and mucous membrane lesions.** The syndrome is usually transient, lasting from 1 to several months, but recurrences associated with varying degrees of disability are common.

■ Articular manifestations are identical to those of Reiter syndrome; extra-articular manifestations may occur but tend to be mild.

Treatment

Medications

■ Conservative therapy is indicated for control of pain and inflammation in these diseases.

■ Spontaneous remissions are common, making evaluation of therapy difficult.

■ **NSAIDs** (especially indomethacin) are often useful, and **selective COX-2 inhibitors** also provide relief (see Therapeutic Approaches to Rheumatic Disease).

■ **Sulfasalazine** or **methotrexate** may be of benefit in some patients (see Therapeutic Approaches to Rheumatic Disease) (Table 23-1).

■ In unusually severe cases, **glucocorticoid therapy** may be required to prevent rapid joint destruction (see Therapeutic Approaches to Rheumatic Disease) (Table 23-1).

■ Prolonged antibiotic therapy (such as doxycycline, 100 mg PO bid) may be beneficial in Reiter syndrome that is related to *Chlamydia*.

Referrals

■ **Conjunctivitis** usually is transient and benign, but ophthalmologic referral and treatment with topical or systemic glucocorticoids are indicated for **iritis.**

PSORIATIC ARTHRITIS

General Principles

Epidemiology
■ Seven percent of patients with psoriasis have some form of inflammatory arthritis.

Classification
■ Five major patterns of joint disease occur: (a) asymmetric oligoarticular arthritis, (b) distal interphalangeal joint involvement in association with nail disease, (c) symmetric rheumatoidlike polyarthritis, (d) spondylitis and sacroiliitis, and (e) arthritis mutilans.

Treatment

Medications
■ **NSAIDs,** particularly indomethacin, are used to treat the arthritic manifestations of psoriasis, in conjunction with appropriate measures for the skin disease.
■ **Selective COX-2 inhibitors** are also effective (see Therapeutic Approaches to Rheumatic Disease).
■ **Intra-articular glucocorticoids** may be useful in the oligoarticular form of the disease, but injection through a psoriatic plaque should be avoided. Severe skin and joint diseases generally respond well to **methotrexate** (see Therapeutic Approaches to Rheumatic Disease) (Table 23-1).
■ **Sulfasalazine, leflunomide, TNF-α blockers,** and **hydroxychloroquine** (see Therapeutic Approaches to Rheumatic Disease) (Table 23-1) may also have disease-modifying effects in polyarthritis.

Complications
■ When reconstructive joint surgery is performed, colonization of psoriatic skin with *S. aureus* increases the risk of wound infection.

SYSTEMIC LUPUS ERYTHEMATOSUS

GENERAL PRINCIPLES

Definition
■ SLE is a multisystem disease of unknown etiology that primarily affects women of child-bearing age.

Pathophysiology
■ Autoantibodies to nuclear and other autoantigens are the hallmark of disease.

DIAGNOSIS

Clinical Presentation
■ The course of this disease is highly variable and unpredictable.
■ Disease manifestations are protean, ranging in severity from fatigue, malaise, weight loss, arthritis or arthralgias, fever, photosensitivity, rashes, and serositis to potentially life-threatening thrombocytopenia, hemolytic anemia, nephritis, cerebritis, vasculitis, pneumonitis, myositis, and myocarditis.
■ Patients with lupus have accelerated coronary and peripheral vascular disease, which should be managed aggressively.

TREATMENT

Medications

- **NSAIDs** usually control SLE-associated arthritis, arthralgias, fever, and serositis but not fatigue, malaise, or major organ system involvement. The response to **selective COX-2 inhibitors** is similar (see Therapeutic Approaches to Rheumatic Disease). Hepatic and renal toxicities of the NSAIDs appear to be increased in SLE. NSAIDs should be avoided in patients with active nephritis.

- **Hydroxychloroquine** (see Therapeutic Approaches to Rheumatic Disease) (Table 23-1) may be effective in the treatment of rash, photosensitivity, arthralgias, arthritis, alopecia, and malaise associated with SLE and in the treatment of **discoid and subacute cutaneous lupus erythematosus.** Skin lesions may begin to improve within a few days, but joint symptoms may require 6–10 weeks to subside. The drug is not effective for treating fever or renal, CNS, and hematologic problems.

- **Glucocorticoid therapy** (see Therapeutic Approaches to Rheumatic Disease) (Table 23-1)
  - **Indications** for systemic glucocorticoids include (a) life-threatening manifestations of SLE, such as glomerulonephritis, CNS involvement, thrombocytopenia, and hemolytic anemia; and (b) debilitating manifestations of SLE (fatigue, rash) that are unresponsive to conservative therapy.
  - **Dosage.** Patients with severe or potentially life-threatening complications of SLE should be treated with prednisone, 1–2 mg/kg PO daily, which can be given in divided doses. After disease is controlled, prednisone should be tapered slowly, the dosage being reduced by no more than 10% every 7–10 days. More rapid reduction may result in relapse. Alternate-day therapy may reduce many of the adverse effects of long-term glucocorticoid therapy. **IV pulse therapy** in the form of methylprednisolone, 500 mg IV q12h for 3–5 days, has been used in SLE in such life-threatening situations as rapidly progressive renal failure, active CNS disease, and severe thrombocytopenia. Patients who do not show improvement with this regimen probably are unresponsive to steroids, and other therapeutic alternatives must be considered. A course of oral prednisone should follow completion of pulse therapy. Electrolytes should be monitored in patients who receive high-dose steroids.

- **Immunosuppressive therapy** (see Therapeutic Approaches to Rheumatic Disease) (Table 23-1)
  - **Indications** for immunosuppressive therapy in SLE include (a) such life-threatening manifestations of SLE as glomerulonephritis, CNS involvement, thrombocytopenia, and hemolytic anemia; and (b) the inability to reduce corticosteroid dosage or severe corticosteroid side effects.
  - **Choice of an immunosuppressive** is individualized to the clinical situation. Often, **cyclophosphamide** is used for life-threatening manifestations of SLE. High-dose IV pulse cyclophosphamide may be less toxic but also less immunosuppressive than is low-dose daily PO cyclophosphamide. **Azathioprine** and **mycophenolate mofetil** are used more often as steroid-sparing agents but may not be as effective as cyclophosphamide in treating nephritis. **Rituximab**, a monoclonal antibody directed against the B-cell surface molecule CD20, causes depletion of B cells and has been shown to be effective in cases of severe SLE not responding to conventional treatment.

Nonoperative

- **Conservative therapy** is warranted if the patient's manifestations are mild.
- **General supportive measures** include adequate sleep and avoidance of fatigue, as mild disease exacerbations may subside after a few days of bed rest.
- For patients with photosensitive rashes, sunscreens with a sun protection factor of 30 or greater; protective clothing, such as a hat and long sleeves; and avoidance of sun exposure are recommended. Isolated skin lesions may respond to topical glucocorticoids.

Special Therapy

- **Transplantation and chronic hemodialysis** have been used successfully in SLE patients with renal failure. Clinical and serologic evidence of disease activity often disappears when renal failure ensues. The survival rate in these patients is equivalent to that of patients with other forms of chronic renal disease. Recurrence of nephritis in the allograft rarely occurs.

SPECIAL CONSIDERATIONS

- **Pregnancy in SLE.** An increased incidence of second-trimester spontaneous abortion and stillbirth has been reported in some women with antibodies to cardiolipin or the lupus anticoagulant. Neonatal lupus may occur in offspring of anti-Ro/SSA positive mothers. SLE patients may experience an exacerbation in the activity of their disease in the third trimester or peripartum period. Differentiation between active SLE and pre-eclampsia often is difficult. Women whose SLE is in good control when they become pregnant are less likely to have a flare of disease during pregnancy.

 # SYSTEMIC SCLEROSIS

GENERAL PRINCIPLES

Definition

- **Systemic sclerosis (scleroderma)** is a systemic illness of unknown etiology characterized by thickening and hardening of the skin and visceral organs. Most of the manifestations of scleroderma have a vascular basis (Raynaud's phenomenon, telangiectasias, nailfold capillary changes, early edematous skin changes, nephrosclerosis), but frank vasculitis rarely is seen.

Classification

- The label *scleroderma* includes diffuse scleroderma and limited scleroderma (formerly known as the **CREST syndrome:** calcinosis, Raynaud's phenomenon, esophageal dysmotility, sclerodactyly, telangiectasias).

DIAGNOSIS

Clinical Presentation

- **Diffuse scleroderma** is characterized by extensive skin disease, the potential for hypertensive "renal crisis," and shortened survival. Internal organs are affected.
    - **GI involvement.** Decreased motility of bowel segments can occur, leading to bacterial overgrowth, malabsorption, diarrhea, and weight loss.
    - **Renal involvement.** The appearance of hypertension and renal insufficiency, often associated with a microangiopathic hemolytic anemia, signals a poor prognosis.
    - **Cardiopulmonary involvement.** Patchy myocardial fibrosis can result in CHF or arrhythmias. Pulmonary involvement includes pleurisy with effusion, interstitial fibrosis, pulmonary hypertension, and cor pulmonale.
- **Limited scleroderma,** in contrast, may be associated with primary pulmonary hypertension or biliary cirrhosis and has skin thickening that is limited to the face and the distal forearms and hands. GI involvement is seen.

Laboratory Studies

- Up to 70% of patients with limited scleroderma have anticentromere antibody, which is not seen in individuals with diffuse scleroderma.

TREATMENT

Nonoperative

- No curative therapy for scleroderma exists; instead, treatment focuses on particular organ involvement in a problem-oriented manner.
  - **Skin and periarticular changes.** No therapeutic agent is clearly effective for these cutaneous manifestations, although penicillamine or methotrexate is sometimes used. **Physical therapy** is important to retard and reduce joint contractures.
  - **GI involvement**
    - Reflux esophagitis generally responds to standard therapy (e.g., H_2-receptor antagonists, proton pump inhibitors, and promotility agents.)
    - Treatment with broad-spectrum antimicrobials in a rotating sequence including **metronidazole** often improves the malabsorption. Metoclopramide may reduce bloating and distention.
    - Occasionally, esophageal strictures require mechanical esophageal dilation.
    - Rarely, severe constipation or intestinal pseudo-obstruction may occur.
  - **Renal involvement.** Aggressive blood pressure control with **ACE inhibitors** may delay or prevent the onset of uremia, particularly in patients with a serum creatinine of <3 mg/dL. Angiotensin-receptor blockade does not appear to be as effective.
  - **Cardiopulmonary involvement.** Coronary artery vasospasm can cause angina pectoris and may respond to calcium channel antagonists. Pulmonary involvement includes pleurisy with effusion, interstitial fibrosis, pulmonary hypertension, and cor pulmonale. Standard therapies for these conditions are used. Patients with rapidly progressive pulmonary parenchymal disease may benefit from a course of cyclophosphamide.

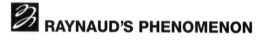 **RAYNAUD'S PHENOMENON**

GENERAL PRINCIPLES

Definition

- **Raynaud's phenomenon** is a reversible vasospasm of the digital arteries that can result in ischemia of the digits.

TREATMENT

Medications

- Most pharmacologic approaches have had limited success.
  - **Calcium channel antagonists** (e.g., nifedipine) are the preferred initial agents, although they may exacerbate gastroesophageal reflux and constipation in these patients.
  - Alternative vasodilators, such as prazosin, occasionally are helpful, but significant side effects, especially orthostatic hypotension, may preclude their use.
  - Daily low-dose aspirin therapy is often prescribed for its antiplatelet effects.
  - **Sympathetic ganglion blockade** with a long-acting anesthetic agent may be useful when a patient has progressive digital ulceration that fails to improve with conservative therapy.

Surgery

- Surgical digital sympathectomy may be beneficial.

Patient Education

- Patients must be instructed to avoid exposure of the entire body to cold, protect the hands and feet from cold and trauma, and discontinue cigarette smoking.

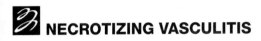

NECROTIZING VASCULITIS

GENERAL PRINCIPLES

Definition

- Necrotizing vasculitis is characterized by inflammation and necrosis of blood vessels leading to tissue damage. This diagnosis includes a broad spectrum of disorders that have various causes and involve vessels of different types, sizes, and locations.

Pathophysiology

- The immunopathogenic process often involves immune complexes.

Etiology

- Although in most cases the inciting antigen has not been identified, vasculitic syndromes have been associated with chronic hepatitis B and C.

DIAGNOSIS

Clinical Presentation

- Table 23-2 summarizes clinical features and diagnostic and treatment approaches to the most common forms of vasculitis. **Clinical features** are diverse and depend in part on the size of the vessel involved. Systemic manifestations including fever and weight loss are also common. The response to therapy and the long-term prognosis of these disorders are highly variable.

Differential Diagnosis

- Vasculitis "mimics" should be considered, including bacterial endocarditis, HIV, atrial myxoma, paraneoplastic syndromes, cholesterol emboli, and cocaine and amphetamine use.

TREATMENT

Medications

- **Glucocorticoids** are the usual initial therapy and are beneficial in most vasculitides (see Therapeutic Approaches to Rheumatic Disease) (Table 23-1). Although vasculitis that is limited to the skin may respond to lower doses of corticosteroids, the initial dosage for visceral involvement should be high (prednisone, 1–2 mg/kg/d). **If life-threatening manifestations are present,** a brief course of high-dose pulse therapy with methylprednisolone, 500 mg IV q12h for 3–5 days, should be considered.
- **Immunosuppressives,** in particular oral cyclophosphamide, often are used in the initial management of necrotizing vasculitis, especially when major organ system involvement (e.g., lung, kidney, or nerve) is present (see Therapeutic Approaches to Rheumatic Disease) (Table 23-1).

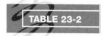

TABLE 23-2	Clinical Features and Diagnostic and Treatment Approaches to Vasculitis		
Vasculitic syndrome	**Clinical features**	**Diagnostic approach**	**Treatment**
Large-vessel involvement			
Giant-cell arteritis	Headache	Temporal artery biopsy	Prednisone, 60–80 mg/d
	Jaw claudication		
Takayasu arteritis	Finger ischemia	Aortic arch arteriogram	Prednisone, 60–80 mg/d
	Arm claudication		
Medium-vessel involvement			
Polyarteritis nodosa	Skin ulcers	Skin biopsy	Prednisone, 60–100 mg/d
			Cyclophosphamide, 1–2 mg/kg/d, can be added
	Nephritis	Renal biopsy	
	Mononeuritis multiplex	Sural nerve biopsy	
	Mesenteric ischemia	Mesenteric angiogram	
		Hepatitis B, C testing	
Wegener's granulomatosis	Sinusitis	c-ANCA	Prednisone, 60–100 mg/d *and* cyclophosphamide, 1–2 mg/kg/d
	Pulmonary infiltrates	Lung biopsy	
	Nephritis		
Microscopic polyangiitis	Pulmonary infiltrates	p-ANCA	Prednisone, 60–100 mg/d
	Nephritis	Renal biopsy	Cyclophosphamide, 1–2 mg/kg/d, can be added
Vasculitis in SLE or RA	Skin ulcers	Skin or sural nerve biopsy	Prednisone, 60–80 mg/d
	Polyneuropathy		
			Cyclophosphamide, 1–2 mg/kg/d, can be added
Small-vessel involvement			
Hypersensitivity vasculitis	Palpable purpura	Skin biopsy	Prednisone, 20–60 mg/d
			Discontinue inciting drug
Henoch-Schönlein purpura	Palpable purpura	Skin biopsy	Supportive treatment
	Nephritis	Renal biopsy	Prednisone, 20–60 mg/d, may be needed
	Mesenteric ischemia		

c-ANCA, cytoplasmic antineutrophil cytoplasmic antibodies; p-ANCA, perinuclear antineutrophil cytoplasmic antibodies; RA, rheumatoid arthritis; SLE, systemic lupus erythematosus.

- **Trimethoprim/sulfamethoxazole** can be used in variants of Wegener's granulomatosis limited to the upper airway and may also be useful in preventing relapse, but is not sufficient treatment for systemic disease. This drug is also used for *P. carinii* prophylaxis in patients who are receiving cyclophosphamide.
- The use of **biologic agents** is under study and may provide further therapeutic options in the near future.

Referrals

- **Management** should include consultation with a physician experienced in the treatment of these disorders. Treatment should be tailored to the severity of organ system involvement.

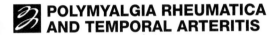 # POLYMYALGIA RHEUMATICA AND TEMPORAL ARTERITIS

DIAGNOSIS

Clinical Presentation

- **Polymyalgia rheumatica (PMR)** presents in elderly patients as proximal limb girdle pain, morning stiffness, and constitutional symptoms.
- **Temporal arteritis (TA)** is a form of vasculitis that presents with headache, scalp tenderness, jaw or tongue claudication, vision disturbances (including blindness), stroke, and, in up to 40% of patients, symptoms of PMR.

Laboratory Studies

- PMR: elevated erythrocyte sedimentation rate (ESR)
- TA: elevated ESR (often >100)

Surgical Diagnostic Procedures

- The diagnosis of TA should be confirmed by **temporal artery biopsy,** which is not altered by 3–5 days of prednisone therapy.

TREATMENT

Medications

- PMR
  - If PMR is present without evidence of TA, **prednisone,** 10–15 mg PO daily, usually produces dramatic clinical improvement within a few days.
  - The ESR should return to normal during initial treatment, but subsequent therapeutic decisions should be based on ESR and clinical status.
  - Glucocorticoid therapy can be tapered gradually to a maintenance dosage of 5–10 mg PO daily but should be continued for at least 1 year to minimize the risk of relapse.
  - NSAIDs may facilitate reduction in prednisone dosage.
- TA
  - Patients who are suspected of having TA should be treated promptly with **prednisone,** 1–2 mg/kg/d PO daily, to prevent irreversible blindness.
  - High-dose steroid therapy should be continued until symptoms have abated and the ESR has returned to normal. The dosage then should be tapered gradually to 10–20 mg, with close monitoring of the ESR and clinical status, and should be maintained for 1–2 years.

CRYOGLOBULIN SYNDROMES

GENERAL PRINCIPLES

Definition

- Cryoglobulins are serum proteins that reversibly precipitate in the cold.

Classification

- Cryoglobulinemia is traditionally categorized as monoclonal (formerly type 1) or poly-clonal (mixed; formerly types 2 and 3).

Etiology

- Patients with **monoclonal cryoglobulinemia** usually have an underlying lymphoprolifer-ative disorder such as myeloma or lymphoma.
- The majority of patients with **mixed cryoglobulinemia** have hepatitis C; the remainder of cases are found in association with autoimmune disorders such as SLE or RA, or are idiopathic.

DIAGNOSIS

Clinical Presentation

- Symptoms are related to hyperviscosity (blurring of vision, digital ischemia, headache, lethargy) and respond to treatment of the underlying disorder, although plasmapheresis can be used in the acute setting.
- Clinical manifestations of mixed cryoglobulinemia are mediated by immune complex deposition (arthralgias, purpura, glomerulonephritis, and neuropathy).

TREATMENT

- **Therapy** for secondary cryoglobulinemic states is directed at the underlying disease.

Medication

- Treatment of hepatitis C with interferon-α and ribavirin effectively reduces cryoglobu-lins, although they may recur when treatment is stopped.
- Prednisone or immunosuppressive agents can be used to treat cryoglobulinemia due to SLE or RA but may exacerbate hepatitis C.

 POLYMYOSITIS AND DERMATOMYOSITIS

GENERAL PRINCIPLES

Definition

- Polymyositis (PM) is an inflammatory myopathy that presents as weakness and occa-sionally tenderness of the proximal musculature.
- Dermatomyositis (DM) is PM with a concomitant rash.

Classification

- PM–DM can occur in three forms: (a) alone, (b) in association with any of the other autoimmune diseases, or (c) with a variety of neoplasms.

DIAGNOSIS

Laboratory Studies

- PM: elevated muscle enzyme levels (creatine kinase, aldolase, AST)
- Certain subsets of disease are associated with myositis-specific antibodies such as Jo-1 and signal recognition particle. These antibodies have therapeutic and prognostic implications, and therefore levels should be measured in all patients.

Imaging

- PM: abnormal electromyogram

Surgical Diagnostic Procedure

- PM: muscle biopsy

TREATMENT

Medications

- Prednisone
  - When PM–DM occurs without associated disease, it usually responds well to **prednisone**, 1–2 mg/kg PO daily (see Therapeutic Approaches to Rheumatic Disease) (Table 23-1).
  - Systemic complaints, such as fever and malaise, respond to therapy first, followed by muscle enzymes and, finally, muscle strength.
  - Once serum enzyme levels normalize, the prednisone dosage should be reduced slowly to maintenance levels of 10–20 mg PO daily or 20–40 mg PO every other day.
  - The appearance of steroid-induced myopathy and hypokalemia may complicate therapeutic assessment.
- IV infusion of **immunoglobulin** may hasten improvement of severe dysphagia.
- PM–DM associated with neoplasia tends to be less responsive to glucocorticoid therapy but may improve after removal of an associated malignant tumor.
- Patients who do not respond or cannot tolerate the side effects of glucocorticoids may respond to methotrexate or azathioprine (see Therapeutic Approaches to Rheumatic Disease) (Table 23-1).
- The use of **biologic agents** is under study and may provide further therapeutic options in the near future.

Special Therapy

- **Physical therapy** is essential in the management of myositis. Bed rest with active assisted range of motion is appropriate during very active disease, with more active exercise prescribed to improve strength once inflammation has been controlled.

Risk Management

- Risk factors for malignancy in the setting of myositis include the presence of DM, cutaneous vasculitis, male sex, and advanced age.
- Screening for common neoplasms, such as colon, lung, breast, and prostate cancer, should be considered in these patients.

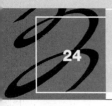

NEUROLOGIC DISORDERS
Kelvin A. Yamada and Sylvia Awadalla

ALTERATIONS IN CONSCIOUSNESS

GENERAL PRINCIPLES

Definition

- **Coma** is a state of complete behavioral unresponsiveness to external stimulation in which the patient lies with the eyes closed. Because some causes of coma may lead to irreversible brain damage, expeditious evaluation and treatment must proceed concurrently. The need for neurosurgical intervention must be determined promptly.
- Acute confusional states (**delirium**) result from diffuse or multifocal cerebral dysfunction and are characterized by impaired attention, concentration, and memory; fluctuations of consciousness; disorientation and hallucinations; incoherent speech; and agitation.

Anatomy and Pathophysiology

- Coma results from diffuse or multifocal dysfunction of both cerebral hemispheres or of the reticular activating system in the brainstem. Unilateral cerebral lesions (e.g., stroke or tumor) rarely impair consciousness unless they produce sufficient mass effect to compress the opposite hemisphere (midline shift or subfalcine herniation) or the brainstem (transtentorial herniation). Mass lesions in the posterior fossa cause coma by compressing the brainstem. Metabolic disorders impair consciousness by diffuse effects on both cerebral hemispheres.

Etiology and Differential Diagnosis

- Etiologies for delirium include those listed in Table 24-1 and also medication effect or withdrawal (also consider serotonin syndrome and neuroleptic malignant syndrome), drug intoxication or withdrawal (see Alcohol Withdrawal, and Chapter 1, Patient Care in Internal Medicine), endocrine disease (i.e., thyroid disorders, diabetes, Cushing's disease), acute intermittent porphyria, confusional migraine, and complex partial seizures. Mild systemic illness commonly produces delirium in an elderly or demented patient, especially in combination with new medications, fever, or sleep deprivation. Structural lesions such as in Table 24-1 can cause acute confusion but must be distinguished from aphasia (secondary to transient ischemic attack [TIA], stroke, trauma, seizure, abscess, etc.) and transient global amnesia. Acute psychosis can mimic acute delirium, but confusion and depressed consciousness are usually less prominent.

676

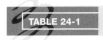

TABLE 24-1	Causes of Stupor and Coma

Diffuse or metabolic
Central nervous system infection/inflammation (vasculitis)
Diabetic ketoacidosis
Drugs and toxins
Global cerebral ischemia
Head trauma
Hypercalcemia
Hypernatremia
Hypertensive encephalopathy
Hypoglycemia
Hyponatremia
Hypoxemia or hypercapnia
Liver failure
Renal failure
Sepsis
Subclinical seizures/postictal state
Thiamine deficiency

Structural lesions, supra- or infratentorial
Abscess
Epidural/subdural hematoma
Hemorrhage/aneurysm
Hydrocephalus
Stroke
Tumor
Venous occlusion

DIAGNOSIS

Clinical Presentation and History

- Initial assessment should focus on development and progression of altered consciousness, history of trauma, seizures, medications, alcohol or drug use, and existing medical conditions.
- If trauma has or may have occurred, **immobilize the spine immediately** while arranging radiographs to identify or exclude fracture or instability.

Physical Examination

- Search for signs of systemic illness associated with coma (e.g., cirrhosis, hemodialysis shunt, rash of meningococcemia) or signs of head trauma (e.g., lacerations, periorbital or mastoid ecchymosis, hemotympanum).
- The physical and neurologic examination may reveal systemic illness (e.g., pneumonia) or neurologic signs (meningismus or paralysis) to narrow the differential diagnosis.
- The neurologic examination (see Neurologic Examination of Patients with Alteration in Consciousness) should localize structural lesions and diagnose brain herniation, **which must be recognized and treated immediately** (serial examinations should be performed to detect and intervene if clinical deterioration occurs).

Neurologic Examination of Patients with Alteration in Consciousness

- **Level of consciousness** can be assessed semiquantitatively and followed by all levels of caregivers with the Glasgow Coma Scale (Table 24-2). Scores range from 3 (unresponsive) to 15 (normal).

TABLE 24-2	Glasgow Coma Scale

Eye opening	
Spontaneous	4
To voice	3
To painful stimulation	2
None	1
Best verbal response	
Oriented	5
Confused	4
Inappropriate words	3
Unintelligible sounds	2
None	1
Best motor response	
Follows commands	6
Localizes pain	5
Withdraws from pain	4
Flexor response	3
Extensor response	2
None	1

- Respiratory rate and pattern:
  - Cheyne-Stokes respirations (rhythmic crescendo–decrescendo hyperpnea alternating with periods of apnea) occur in metabolic coma and supratentorial lesions, as well as in chronic pulmonary disease and congestive heart failure (CHF).
  - Hyperventilation is usually a sign of metabolic acidosis, hypoxemia, pneumonia, or other pulmonary disease but may be caused by upper brainstem injury.
  - Apneustic breathing (long pauses after inspiration), cluster breathing (breathing in short bursts), and ataxic breathing (irregular breaths without pattern) are signs of brainstem injury and warn of impending respiratory arrest.
- Pupil size and light reactivity
  - Anisocoria (asymmetric pupils) in a patient with altered mental status requires diagnosis and treatment, or exclusion, of uncal herniation. Anisocoria may be physiologic or produced by mydriatics (e.g., scopolamine, atropine).
  - Small but reactive pupils are seen in narcotic overdose, metabolic encephalopathy, and thalamic or pontine lesions.
  - Midposition fixed pupils imply midbrain lesions and occur in transtentorial herniation.
  - Bilaterally fixed and dilated pupils are seen with severe anoxic encephalopathy or intoxication with drugs such as scopolamine, atropine, glutethimide, or methyl alcohol.
- Eye movements
  - The oculocephalic (doll's eyes) test is performed (if no cervical injury is present) by quickly turning the head laterally or vertically. In coma with intact brainstem oculomotor function, eyes move conjugately opposite the direction of head movement.
  - The oculovestibular (cold caloric) test is used if cervical trauma is suspected or if eye movements are absent with the oculocephalic test. Verify intact tympanic membrane and patent auditory canal. Elevate the head 30 degrees above horizontal, patient supine. Lavage external auditory canal with 10–50 mL ice water. In coma with intact brainstem oculomotor function, eyes move conjugately toward the lavaged ear. Vertical gaze can be assessed with simultaneous lavage of both ears (cold water, eyes depress, warm eyes elevate).
    - Absence of all eye movements indicates a bilateral pontine lesion or drug-induced ophthalmoplegia (e.g., barbiturates, phenytoin, paralytics).

- Disconjugate gaze suggests a brainstem lesion.
- A gaze preference conjugately to one side suggests a unilateral pontine or frontal lobe lesion. An associated hemiparesis and oculocephalic and oculovestibular tests help localize the lesion. In pontine lesions gaze preference is toward the paretic side, and eyes may move toward but do not cross midline. In frontal lobe lesions gaze preference is away from the paresis, and eyes move conjugately across midline to both sides.
- Impaired vertical eye movement occurs in midbrain lesions, central herniation. Conjugate depression and impaired elevation suggest a tectal lesion (pinealoma) or hydrocephalus.

■ **Motor responses** help to assess the level of impaired consciousness (see also Table 24-2). Asymmetric motor responses (spontaneous or stimulus induced) have localizing value.

■ **Herniation** occurs when mass lesions or edema cause shifts in brain tissue. Prompt diagnosis and treatment are necessary to prevent irreversible brain damage and death.

   ■ **Nonspecific signs and symptoms of increased intracranial pressure** include headache, nausea, vomiting, hypertension, bradycardia, papilledema, sixth nerve palsy, transient visual obscurations, and alterations in consciousness.

   ■ **Uncal herniation** is caused by unilateral supratentorial lesions and may progress rapidly. The earliest sign is a dilated pupil ipsilateral to the mass, diminished consciousness, and hemiparesis, first contralateral to the mass and later ipsilateral to the mass (Kernohan notch syndrome).

   ■ **Central herniation** is caused by medial or bilateral supratentorial lesions. Signs include progressive alteration of consciousness, Cheyne-Stokes or normal respirations followed later by central hyperventilation, midposition and unreactive pupils, loss of upward gaze, and posturing of the extremities.

   ■ **Tonsillar herniation** occurs when pressure in the posterior fossa forces the cerebellar tonsils through the foramen magnum, compressing the medulla. Signs include altered level of consciousness and respiratory irregularity or apnea.

Laboratory Studies

■ Check glucose, electrolytes, blood urea nitrogen (BUN), complete blood count (CBC), calcium, magnesium, thyroid function tests, arterial blood gases (ABGs), bacterial cultures, liver enzymes, ammonia, prothrombin time (PT), activated partial thromboplastin time (PTT), and blood type and screen. Blood and urine should be sent for toxicologic/drug analysis. A urinalysis should be performed. Urine porphobilinogens to screen for porphyria can be obtained in selected cases.

■ **Lumbar puncture** is indicated whenever central nervous system (CNS) infection is considered and when subarachnoid hemorrhage (SAH) is clinically suspected but not confirmed by neuroimaging. **One should not perform lumbar puncture if a mass lesion or midline shift is present on computed tomography (CT) scan.** In such cases, if CNS infection is suspected, appropriate broad-spectrum antibiotics and acyclovir should be administered without lumbar puncture.

■ **Cerebrospinal fluid (CSF) studies** include cell count, protein, glucose, Gram stain, bacterial cultures, and polymerase chain reaction for pathogens (particularly herpes simplex). Rapid detection of bacterial antigens (particularly if antibiotics have been given), acid-fast stain, India ink stain, cryptococcal antigen, and fungal and viral cultures are often indicated.

Imaging

■ **If trauma has or may have occurred, immobilize the spine** immediately while arranging radiographs to identify or exclude fracture or instability.

■ After the patient is stabilized, **a head CT scan** should be obtained to distinguish operable lesions (e.g., cerebellar hematoma) from inoperable lesions (e.g., pontine hemorrhage).

Monitoring

- Vital signs, electrocardiogram (ECG), and oximetry should be continuously monitored. Airway and mental status (e.g., Glasgow Coma Scale) should be frequently assessed.
- Electroencephalogram (EEG) is necessary for diagnosis of subclinical seizures (nonconvulsive status epilepticus).
- Some EEG features are characteristic (though not necessarily diagnostic) of certain conditions:
  - Generalized periodic complexes in postanoxic encephalopathy (also keep in mind prion disease), periodic lateralized epileptiform discharges (PLEDs) in encephalitis [e.g., herpes simplex virus (HSV)], triphasic waves in hepatic or uremic encephalopathy, and β activity or voltage suppression in barbiturate or other sedative intoxications.

Differential Diagnosis

See Etiologies.

TREATMENT

- Ensure adequate airway and ventilation, administer oxygen as needed, and maintain normal body temperature.
- Establish secure IV and adequate circulation.
- Arterial, central venous, and intracranial pressure may need to be monitored and treated depending on clinical circumstances.

Medications

- IV thiamine (100 mg), followed by dextrose (50 mL 50% dextrose in water = 25 g dextrose), should be administered. Thiamine is administered first because dextrose administration in thiamine-deficient patients may precipitate Wernicke encephalopathy.
- IV naloxone (opiate antagonist), 0.01 mg/kg, should be administered if opiate intoxication is suspected (coma, respiratory depression, small reactive pupils). Naloxone may provoke opiate withdrawal syndrome in addicted patients.
- Flumazenil (benzodiazepine antagonist), 0.2 mg IV, may reverse benzodiazepine intoxication, but its duration of action is short, and additional doses may be needed. Flumazenil can cause seizures.
- In delirious patients, sedatives should be avoided if possible, but if necessary low doses of lorazepam (1 mg) or chlordiazepoxide (25 mg) can be used. A quiet, well-lit room with close observation is necessary. Restraints are sometimes needed for patient safety and should be carefully adjusted and checked periodically to prevent excessive constriction.

Nonoperative Management

- **If herniation is identified,** treatment consists of measures to lower intracranial pressure while surgically treatable etiologies are identified or excluded.
  - Endotracheal intubation is usually performed to enable hyperventilation to a PCO_2 of 25–30 mm Hg, which reduces intracranial pressure within minutes by cerebral vasoconstriction. Bag-mask ventilation can be performed if manipulation of the neck is precluded by possible or established spinal instability. Reduction of PCO_2 below 25 mm Hg is not recommended because it may reduce cerebral blood flow excessively.
  - Administration of mannitol IV, 1–2 g/kg over 10–20 minutes, osmotically reduces brain free water via elimination by the kidneys. The effect peaks at 90 minutes.
  - Dexamethasone, 10 mg IV, followed by 4 mg IV q6h, reduces the edema surrounding a tumor or abscess.
- Coagulopathy (see Chapter 19, Anemia and Transfusion Therapy) should be corrected if intracranial hemorrhage is diagnosed and before surgical treatment or invasive

procedures (e.g., lumbar puncture) are performed. Each patient's circumstances should be carefully assessed before therapeutic anticoagulation is reversed.

Operative Management

- Surgical evacuation of epidural, subdural, or intraparenchymal (e.g., cerebellar) hemorrhage, shunting for acute hydrocephalus, may be life saving, but clinical circumstances dictate the need for, and urgency of, intervention. Some structural lesions are not amenable to surgical treatment.

Referrals

- Neurologic and neurosurgical consultations are frequently indicated.

Results

- If the initial evaluation yields no diagnosis, a metabolic or toxic etiology is most likely.
- In general, admit patient to an intensive care unit (ICU) with continued supportive care while pursuing additional diagnostic studies.

SPECIAL CONSIDERATIONS

Brain Death

- Brain death occurs from irreversible brain injury sufficient to permanently eliminate all cortical and brainstem function. Because the vital centers in the brainstem sustain cardiovascular and respiratory functions, brain death is incompatible with survival despite mechanical ventilation and cardiovascular and nutritional supportive measures. Brain death is distinguished from persistent vegetative state, in which the absence of higher cortical function is accompanied by intact brainstem function. Patients in a persistent vegetative state are unable to think, speak, understand, or meaningfully respond to visual, verbal, or auditory stimuli, yet with nutritional and supportive care their cardiovascular and respiratory functions can sustain viability for many years.
- The first step in establishing the diagnosis of brain death is to establish an irreversible and untreatable etiology for the brain injury. Examples include global ischemia (cardiac arrest), asphyxia (near-drowning), intracranial hemorrhage with uncal or central herniation, and severe head trauma with diffuse cerebral edema. Contributing factors that may be reversible, such as hypoxia, hypotension, and hypothermia, and medications that depress consciousness (e.g., barbiturates, benzodiazepines, opiates) must be corrected.
- The neurologic examination is the critical element of the diagnosis.
  - The patient is comatose.
  - There is no response to visual, auditory, or painful stimulation.
  - There is no respiratory effort; the patient requires mechanical ventilation.
    - The oxygen apnea test is used to confirm apnea without mechanical ventilation. After increasing the FIO_2 to increase PO_2, the patient is removed from the ventilator and observed for respiratory effort. If there is no respiratory effort when the PCO_2 rises above 50 mm Hg, apnea is established.
    - Arterial or venous blood gas is conveniently obtained if arterial or central IV catheters are in place.
    - This part of the exam is usually reserved for last because patients are often unstable and the apnea test may produce cardiopulmonary arrest. The possibility that cardiopulmonary arrest may occur must be carefully considered.
  - The pupils are not reactive.
  - There are no eye movements by oculocephalic maneuver or by caloric stimulation.
  - Corneal and gag reflexes are absent.
  - There is no spontaneous movement and there is no motor response to noxious external stimulation.

- Ancillary diagnostic studies are useful, but not required in most cases. Some hospitals adopt brain death criteria requiring certain supportive diagnostic studies, which reduce the time interval between confirmatory evaluations.
  - If an EEG is used it should be performed using guidelines established by the American Board of Clinical Neurophysiology for performing EEG to establish electrocerebrosilence (ECS), which is the absence of brain-derived electrical activity.
  - Radionuclide brain scan demonstrates absence of cerebral blood flow.
  - Somatosensory-evoked potentials demonstrate absence of subcortical and cortical responses with intact peripheral nerve responses.
  - Conventional angiography shows absent cerebral blood flow.
- If brain death is established by the initial evaluation, a repeat evaluation is performed 6–24 hours after the initial exam to confirm the persistent absence of brainstem function. If the second exam confirms brain death, the attending physician has sufficient evidence to pronounce the patient brain dead. Life support measures may be continued by discretion of the attending physician to allow informing the family and exploring the patient's advanced directives such as organ transplantation.

Alcohol Withdrawal

- **Alcohol withdrawal** typically occurs when illness or hospitalization interrupts alcohol intake and deserves emphasis because severe forms carry significant mortality.
- Tremulousness, irritability, anorexia, and nausea characterize minor alcohol withdrawal. Symptoms usually appear within a few hours after reduction or cessation of alcohol consumption and resolve within 48 hours. Treatment includes a well-lit room, reassurance, and the presence of family or friends. Thiamine, 100 mg IM, followed by 100 mg PO daily; multivitamins containing folic acid; and a balanced diet as tolerated should be administered. Chlordiazepoxide (25–100 mg PO q6h) with dosage adjusted until the patient is calm may reduce the incidence of seizures and delirium tremens.[1] Serial evaluation for signs of major alcohol withdrawal is essential; social circumstances dictate whether this should be done at home or in the hospital.
- Alcohol withdrawal seizures, typically one or a few brief generalized convulsions, occur 12–48 hours after cessation of ethanol intake. Antiepileptic drugs are not indicated for typical alcohol withdrawal seizures. Other causes for seizures (see Seizures) must be excluded. If hypoglycemia is present, thiamine should be administered before glucose.
- Severe withdrawal or delirium tremens consists of tremulousness, hallucinations, agitation, confusion, disorientation, and autonomic hyperactivity (fever, tachycardia, diaphoresis), typically occurring 72–96 hours after cessation of drinking. Symptoms generally resolve within 3–5 days. Delirium tremens complicates 5%–10% of cases of alcohol withdrawal, with mortality up to 15%. Other causes of delirium must be considered in the differential diagnosis (see Table 24.1). One should administer supportive management as follows:
  - Chlordiazepoxide is an effective sedative for delirium tremens, 100 mg IV or PO q2–6h as needed (maximum dose, 500 mg in the first 24 hours). One-half the initial 24-hour dose can be administered over the next 24 hours; the dosage can be reduced by 25–50 mg/d each day thereafter. Longer-lasting benzodiazepines facilitate smoother tapering, but shorter-acting agents (i.e., lorazepam, 1–2 mg PO or IV q6–8h as needed) may be desirable in older patients and those with reduced drug clearance. In patients with severe hepatic failure, oxazepam (15–30 mg PO, q6–8h as needed), which is excreted by the kidney, can be used instead of chlordiazepoxide.
  - Maintenance of fluid and electrolyte balance is important. Alcoholic patients are susceptible to hypomagnesemia, hypokalemia, hypoglycemia, and fluid losses, which may be considerable due to fever, diaphoresis, and vomiting.
  - Other drugs have been used to treat alcohol withdrawal, including clonidine, atenolol, haloperidol, carbamazepine, clomethiazole, and others. Controlled studies and careful evaluation of the indications for the individual patient must dictate their use for alcohol withdrawal.

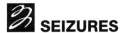
SEIZURES

GENERAL PRINCIPLES

Definition

- Generalized convulsive status epilepticus consists of sustained unconsciousness and continuous or intermittent generalized convulsive seizure activity. Convulsive seizure activity lasting 10 minutes continuously, or intermittently without recovery of consciousness, warrants IV anticonvulsant therapy.

Anatomy and Pathophysiology

- Generalized convulsions indicate that seizure activity involves thalamocortical connections and both cerebral hemispheres. Insufficient oxygenation, ventilation, and perfusion in conjunction with increased metabolic demand result in organ injury and further metabolic derangements. Stopping seizures enables restoring vital functions with appropriate supportive measures. Focal seizures arise from a localized brain region, and may or may not affect consciousness.

Classification

- Generalized convulsive status epilepticus may begin with focal or generalized seizures. Refractory status epilepticus refers to ongoing seizures despite adequate treatment with a benzodiazepine, fosphenytoin, and/or barbiturate. **Focal motor seizures or nonconvulsive status epilepticus at onset may herald refractory status epilepticus.**[2] Nonconvulsive status epilepticus includes complex partial status epilepticus, in which there is alteration of consciousness and automatisms, and absence status epilepticus, in which there is loss of consciousness without generalized convulsive activity.

Mechanisms of Injury

- Persistent seizures produce brain injury, cardiovascular and respiratory insufficiency, and other life-threatening complications.

DIAGNOSIS

Clinical Presentation and History

- Query for history of epilepsy, trauma, medical historical information including preexisting medical conditions, current medications, drug allergies, and possible precipitating events.

Physical Examination

- Convulsive seizures are usually easily identified. Rigors, extrapyramidal movement disorders, or pseudoseizures may mimic seizures.

Laboratory Studies

- Laboratory analysis should include glucose, electrolytes, calcium, magnesium, ABG, CBC, BUN, creatinine, alanine transaminase (ALT), antiepileptic drug levels if indicated, urinalysis, and urine drug screen toxicology.
- CSF analysis is often indicated to diagnose infectious etiologies [Gram stain, cultures, HSV or other polymerase chain reaction (PCR), latex agglutination].

Imaging

- Neuroimaging is usually indicated to identify structural etiologies.

Monitoring

- EEG is not required for initial diagnosis and management of generalized convulsive status epilepticus, but is essential after seizures stop to exclude conversion to nonconvulsive status epilepticus. EEG is needed for managing refractory status epilepticus.

Differential Diagnosis

- A specific etiology is often associated with status epilepticus, and its treatment may influence successful management of seizures. Acute structural causes include CNS infections (e.g., bacterial meningitis, herpes encephalitis), trauma, stroke (usually embolic), tumor, inflammatory processes (e.g., CNS, lupus). Nonstructural precipitants include hypoglycemia, electrolyte abnormalities (e.g., hyponatremia, hypocalcemia), uremia, anoxia, sepsis, drug toxicity or withdrawal (particularly acute withdrawal of benzodiazepines, barbiturates, and antiepileptic drugs), and drug intoxication (e.g., cocaine, methamphetamine). In epileptic patients an acute febrile illness or subtherapeutic antiepileptic drug levels (noncompliance, drug interaction, etc.) may initiate status epilepticus.

TREATMENT

- Ongoing and repetitive generalized convulsive seizure activity warrants aggressive anticonvulsant therapy and supportive care. Evaluation and treatment must proceed concurrently.
- Initial management includes placement of an oral or nasopharyngeal airway and administration of supplemental oxygen. Bag-mask ventilation and seizure cessation by anticonvulsants may enable airway establishment, but airway compromise in a convulsing patient typically necessitates neuromuscular blockade to establish an airway by endotracheal intubation. Vital signs, oximetry, and continuous ECG should be monitored. Two large-bore IV lines (one dextrose free) should be placed and rapid blood glucose checked. Thiamine (100 mg) should be given intravenously followed by 50 mL of 50% dextrose. Bed padding reduces traumatic injury.

MEDICATIONS

- Parenteral anticonvulsants should be promptly and systematically administered to patients with persistent generalized convulsive seizures.[3] If a patient stops convulsing and recovers consciousness, it is safer to administer loading doses of anticonvulsants orally. Failure to stop seizures after two anticonvulsants constitutes refractory status epilepticus, which has higher mortality and requires intubation, critical care support, ICU and EEG monitoring, and often general anesthetics.
- **Lorazepam** (0.1 mg/kg at 2 mg/min up to 8 mg) is the preferred initial treatment; diazepam (0.2 mg/kg at 5 mg/min up to 20 mg) is an alternative. Short duration of action requires concomitant administration of maintenance anticonvulsants. Respiratory depression may require intubation and assisted ventilation.
  - **Phenytoin** is the preferred maintenance anticonvulsant after benzodiazepine administration for convulsive status epilepticus. The preferred parenteral formulation is fosphenytoin, a phosphate ester prodrug of phenytoin. Fosphenytoin is converted in vivo in equimolar concentrations to phenytoin. The loading dose for phenytoin in status epilepticus is 20 mg/kg. Fosphenytoin should be ordered in long-hand expressed as phenytoin equivalents (PEs), the dose being 20 mg PE/kg. Fosphenytoin produces less venous irritation and sclerosis than phenytoin. The maximum infusion rate for fosphenytoin is 150 mg PE/min, for phenytoin 50 mg/min in saline (no dextrose, phenytoin precipitates in dextrose solutions). Peak phenytoin levels are comparable and occur after similar durations with either formulation, but shorter

infusion time for fosphenytoin (about 10 minutes for a 75-kg patient) allows preparation of the next anticonvulsant infusion if seizure activity continues (~15 mg/kg IV phenytoin produced a postinfusion serum level of approximately 30 mcg/mL[4]). Phenytoin sodium should be administered through an easily flushing large-bore IV with dextrose-free saline. Although fosphenytoin can be administered IM, this route is undesirable in an emergent situation. Blood pressure (BP) and cardiac rhythm should be monitored continuously for hypotension and heart block, which often resolve when the administration rate is reduced. Phenytoin is contraindicated in heart block.

- **Phenobarbital** (20 mg/kg loading dose at 50 mg/min) should be given if seizures continue after phenytoin loading. Respiratory depression caused by benzodiazepines combined with phenobarbital usually necessitates intubation and mechanical ventilation. There is no strict dose when phenobarbital is used to stop recalcitrant seizures; 5 mg/kg doses can be repeated until seizures stop. Within 1 hour of administration, 15 mg/kg IV phenobarbital produced a postinfusion serum level of approximately 30 mcg/mL.[4] As with phenytoin, arrhythmias and hypotension may occur during administration, requiring continuous ECG and BP monitoring. Parenteral valproic acid is an alternative, loading dose 30 mg/kg.

- **Continuous anticonvulsant infusion** for refractory status epilepticus requires intensive care and EEG monitoring, and may be a preferable option over phenytoin and barbiturates in some patients (e.g., cardiac failure/arrhythmia). Options include **midazolam** (0.2 mg/kg load followed by 0.75–10 mcg/kg/min infusion) or **propofol** (2 mg/kg load followed by 30–250 mcg/kg/min infusion). Barbiturate coma or general anesthesia with neuromuscular blockade may be required.

Referrals

- Neurologic consultation may be helpful for managing status epilepticus, and for evaluation and management of new-onset seizures. The diagnostic approach to a patient with spontaneously terminating seizures with recovery of consciousness is similar to that for status epilepticus, except that depending on the circumstances outpatient evaluation may be appropriate.

Counseling and Patient Education

- Patients with epilepsy should not drive, swim unsupervised, bathe in a bathtub of standing water, use motorized tools, or be in position to fall from heights during a seizure. Other restrictions may require consideration.

Follow-Up

- After seizures stop, anticonvulsant drugs are usually continued during diagnostic evaluation, except for benzodiazepines (maintenance phenytoin, 4–7 mg/kg/d; phenobarbital, 1–5 mg/kg/d, IV or PO bid).
- The need for long-term anticonvulsant therapy and conversion to an oral regimen (ideally monotherapy) must be individually determined.
- Correctable causes for seizures (e.g., hyponatremia, drug toxicity) do not require long-term anticonvulsant therapy.

 # CEREBROVASCULAR DISEASE

GENERAL PRINCIPLES

Definition

- Stroke is a medical emergency that requires rapid diagnosis and treatment.
- The hallmark of **stroke** is the abrupt onset of neurologic deficits that correspond to interruption of vascular supply to a specific brain region. A stroke may be **ischemic,**

resulting from the occlusion of an artery within the brain, or **hemorrhagic**, resulting from the rupture of an artery in the brain. Fluctuation of functional deficits after stroke onset, reversible deficits known as **TIAs** (deficits resolve within 24 hours), and reversible ischemic neurologic deficits (deficits resolve within a week) suggest that tissue at risk for infarction may be rescued by re-establishing perfusion.

Etiology

- Atherosclerotic cerebrovascular disease usually affects large arteries.
- Cardiogenic embolism accounts for about 20% of strokes.
- The location of intracerebral hemorrhage may suggest **etiology.**
  - The most common **etiology of SAH** is a ruptured saccular or "berry" aneurysm, which results from defects in the arterial media and internal elastic lamina of large arteries. Other types of aneurysms include fusiform aneurysms (probably secondary to atherosclerosis) and mycotic aneurysms (from septic embolism).
  - Putaminal/thalamic hemorrhage is usually due to chronic systemic hypertension.
  - Amyloid angiopathy typically causes lobar hemorrhages and is a common etiology in the elderly.
- Head trauma, anticoagulants or other drugs (including L-asparaginase, cocaine, or amphetamines), aneurysm, arteriovenous malformation, tumor, blood dyscrasia, hemoglobinopathy, angiopathy, or vasculitis are other etiologies for hemorrhagic stroke.

DIAGNOSIS

Clinical Presentation and History

- The onset and progression of symptoms and contributory events (e.g., head trauma or seizure) assist diagnosis.
  - Prior TIA symptoms (e.g., transient monocular loss of vision, aphasia, dysarthria, paresis, or sensory disturbance) suggest atherosclerotic vascular disease, the most common cause for stroke.
  - A history of neck trauma warrants evaluation for extracerebral arterial dissection.
  - Cardiac arrhythmia or valvular disease, connective tissue disease, and sickle cell anemia are medical conditions associated with stroke.
  - Migraine with aura can mimic stroke and is a risk factor for stroke.
  - In epileptic patients, ictal paralysis is rare, but postictal paralysis (Todd's paralysis) is common after a focal seizure.
  - Stroke risk factors such as hypertension, diabetes, smoking, postpartum state, illicit IV drug use, and medications such as oral contraceptives may suggest the diagnosis and influence management.
- **SAH** may present with only **sudden onset of severe headache**. Lethargy or coma, fever, vomiting, seizures, and low back pain may also be present.

Physical Examination

- A careful **neurologic examination** reliably establishes the anatomic location of a stroke.
- In general, **carotid artery** distribution strokes (anterior circulation) produce combinations of functional deficits (hemiparesis, hemianopsia, cortical sensory loss, often with aphasias or agnosias) contralateral to the affected hemisphere
- **Vertebral-basilar** strokes (posterior circulation) produce unilateral or bilateral motor/sensory deficits, usually accompanied by cranial nerve and brainstem signs.
- **Horner's syndrome** (ptosis, miosis, anhidrosis) contralateral to an acute hemiparesis suggests carotid dissection.
- Nuchal rigidity and retinal hemorrhages (subhyaloid) suggest SAH.
- **General physical examination** may provide clues that indicate specific diagnostic tests and therapy.
  - **With embolic stroke** search for murmur of mitral or aortic stenosis, and evidence of systemic emboli in the fundi, conjunctivae, nail beds, fingers, and palms.

■ Fever raises concern for infectious etiologies. Meningismus, seizures, or altered mental status suggests meningitis or encephalitis. Septic emboli from bacterial endocarditis can cause meningitis or cerebral or parameningeal abscess.

■ The patient should be examined for evidence of neurocutaneous disease (neurofibromatosis and tuberous sclerosis) and vasculitis (e.g., systemic lupus erythematosus).

Monitoring

■ Vital signs, including oximetry and continuous ECG, should be monitored.

Laboratory Studies

■ Laboratory studies include CBC with differential and platelet count, PT/international normalized ratio (INR), activated PTT, electrolyte panel, blood glucose, and ABGs (if indicated). Urinalysis should be performed to evaluate for hematuria. Erythrocyte sedimentation rate, antinuclear antibody, anticardiolipin antibody, hemoglobin electrophoresis, lipid profile, or other specific tests may be required as indicated to establish a specific diagnosis.

■ ECG (for atrial fibrillation) and a chest radiograph should be obtained.

■ Diagnostic lumbar puncture is indicated if meningitis/encephalitis is suspected. Lumbar puncture must not be performed if there is risk for precipitating brain herniation. Imaging should be performed prior to lumbar puncture to exclude a mass lesion that could predispose to brain herniation (see Alterations in Consciousness).

■ In some patients, **lumbar puncture** is necessary to confirm the diagnosis of SAH. Bloody CSF should be centrifuged immediately and examined for **xanthochromia** (yellow color). Xanthochromia results from red blood cell (RBC) lysis and takes several hours to develop, indicating SAH rather than traumatic lumbar puncture.

■ CSF analysis for malignant cells, special cultures, preps (e.g., acid-fast bacilli stain, India ink preparation), or antibody titers (e.g., VDRL) is helpful in the identification of carcinomatous or less common infectious etiologies.

Imaging

■ Head **CT scan** most rapidly differentiates intracerebral hemorrhage from ischemic stroke.

■ Magnetic resonance imaging (MRI) scan is the most sensitive imaging study for stroke diagnosis. Diffusion weighted sequences detect stroke earliest.

■ **Head CT scan is diagnostic** of subarachnoid hemorrhage, demonstrating blood in the sulci and cisternae in 90% of SAH patients in the first 24 hours.

■ MR angiography is a useful noninvasive test to evaluate large arteries and veins.

■ Carotid Doppler studies enable noninvasive estimation of carotid stenosis.

■ Cerebral angiography
  ▦ Definitive study for vascular malformation
  ▦ Often necessary prior to endarterectomy
  ▦ Necessary for presurgical evaluation of saccular aneurysms

■ Transthoracic two-dimensional echocardiography is helpful to demonstrate intracardiac thrombi, valve vegetations, valvular stenosis or insufficiency, and right-to-left shunting (contrast echocardiogram). In some patients, transesophageal echocardiography is necessary to evaluate the left atrium for thrombi.

TREATMENT

■ **The most important aspect of stroke management is rapid diagnosis.**

Medications

■ Recombinant tissue plasminogen activator (**rt-PA**) is the only proven therapy for acute ischemic stroke, but patients must be selected carefully, and administration of rt-PA must commence within 3 hours of stroke onset. Other treatments, including intra-arterial thrombolysis, are available at some centers under research protocols.

- **rt-PA** therapy should be considered when a nonhemorrhagic ischemic infarct has been demonstrated and infectious etiologies are excluded while one continues to pursue a specific diagnosis. rt-PA treatment increases risk for symptomatic brain hemorrhage, but with comparable 3- and 12-month mortality versus placebo. **Strict adherence to the Stroke Council of the American Stroke Association/American Heart Association guidelines is recommended.**[5,6] Exclusion criteria include stroke onset longer than 3 hours; recent surgery, head trauma, or gastrointestinal (GI) or urinary hemorrhage; seizure at stroke onset; bleeding disorder or anticoagulation with prolonged PT/PTT (patients on anticoagulants with INR ≤ 1.7 can be treated with rtPA); and severe uncontrolled hypertension (systolic >185, diastolic >110 mm Hg). The rt-PA dose is 0.9 mg/kg up to a maximum of 90 mg, with the first 10% (maximum, 9 mg) given IV over 1 minute, then the remaining 90% (maximum, 81 mg) given by infusion pump over 1 hour. Aspirin, heparin, and warfarin are not given during the first 24 hours. Systolic BP should be maintained at <185 and diastolic BP at <110 mm Hg to reduce the patient's risk for hemorrhagic transformation.
- **Aspirin** reduces **atherosclerotic stroke** morbidity and mortality, and is recommended for acute and long-term treatment at doses 50–325 mg/d.[7,8] Other antiplatelet aggregating drugs are available or are under study, and may be alternatives for certain patients.
- **Heparin**, low molecular weight heparin, and warfarin anticoagulant treatment is controversial, and is not generally recommended for ischemic stroke.[5]
- Treatment of **intracranial hemorrhage** consists of supportive care and gradual reduction in BP. Vascular autoregulation is unpredictably impaired in patients with chronic hypertension and intracerebral hemorrhage. **Higher than normal systemic BP may be required to maintain cerebral perfusion.** Therefore, BP is gradually reduced over days, with careful observation for worsening neurologic deficits, which may reflect cerebral ischemia.
- **Treatment** of SAH depends on etiology. Saccular aneurysms are usually treated surgically. Supportive measures include bed rest, sedation, analgesia, and laxatives to prevent sudden increases in intracranial pressure or BP. **Avoid hypotension**, as it may worsen ischemic deficits. Only extreme elevations in BP (diastolic >130 mm Hg) should be treated, and reduction of BP should be gradual, with careful monitoring of BP and the neurologic examination. Nimodipine, a calcium channel blocker, improves outcome in SAH patients and may reduce the incidence of associated cerebral infarction with few side effects. Recommended dosage is 60 mg PO q4h, for 21 days, initiated within 4 days of presentation. Volume expansion, induced hypertension, and balloon dilation can occasionally be used to reverse neurologic deterioration due to vasospasm.
- Appropriate antimicrobial and antiviral drugs should be administered for presumed CNS infection, including situations when lumbar puncture is not performed.

Surgery

- **Carotid endarterectomy** decreases the risk of stroke and death in patients with recent TIAs or nondisabling strokes and ipsilateral high-grade (70%–99%) carotid stenosis.[9] Carotid endarterectomy for asymptomatic high-grade carotid stenosis ($\geq 60\%$) reduces the relative risk of stroke provided that the surgical/angiography complication rate is $<3\%$.[10] Stroke risk factor reduction and antiplatelet therapy are important components of postoperative management.[11]
- **Surgical consultation is indicated for cerebellar hematomas**, because brainstem compression or obstructive hydrocephalus may develop, and immediate hematoma evacuation or ventricular shunting may be life saving. Evacuation of deep cerebral hematomas is rarely beneficial.
- Saccular aneurysms causing SAH are usually treated surgically.

Special Therapy

- Treatment of **cardiogenic embolus**. Anticoagulation with warfarin is indicated to prevent recurrent embolic strokes due to atrial fibrillation, target INR 2–3 (see Chapter

18, Disorders of Hemostasis). The target INR is 2.5–3.5 for anticoagulation for mechanical heart valves. Systemic hypertension is a relative contraindication to long-term anticoagulation because of increased risk for intracranial hemorrhage.

- **Modification of risk factors,** including systemic hypertension, diabetes, smoking, and elevated lipids reduce risk for stroke. Blood pressure reduction even in normotensive stroke patients is beneficial.[12] Oral contraceptives may need to be discontinued in women with stroke.

Complications

- **Complications** of SAH include rebleeding (20% at 2 weeks), vasospasm with ischemic deficits (days 4–14), hydrocephalus, seizures, and hyponatremia.

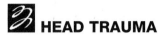 # HEAD TRAUMA

GENERAL PRINCIPLES

Mechanisms of Injury

- Closed head injuries are most common. Impact may produce axonal injury (when impact is orthogonal to axon tracts or with rotational injuries).
- Impact of the brain on the skull may produce contusion or hemorrhage (in the direction of initial impact, "coup injury;" when the brain surface impacts the skull opposite the site of impact, "contrecoup injury").
- Penetrating injuries (including depressed skull fracture) or foreign objects cause brain injury directly.
- Secondary ischemia, cytotoxic edema, excitotoxicity, and inflammatory responses may contribute to ongoing brain injury.
- Development of increased intracranial pressure may compromise cerebral perfusion.

DIAGNOSIS

Clinical Presentation and History

- **History** should include the temporal course of all symptoms, particularly loss of consciousness, occurrence of a lucid interval (which suggests expanding hematoma), and amnesia (which is related to the severity of the blow).
- Concussion is defined as a closed head injury with posttraumatic confusion, amnesia, and normal neurologic exam and radiographic studies.
- Intracerebral hematomas may be present initially or develop within a contusion.
- Epidural hematoma is usually associated with skull fractures across a meningeal artery and may cause precipitous deterioration after a lucid interval. Deterioration often follows the classic uncal herniation syndrome (see Alterations in Consciousness).
- Chronic subdural hematoma is most common in aged, debilitated, and alcoholic individuals and in anticoagulated patients. Antecedent trauma is often minimal. Symptoms tend to be nonspecific (e.g., headache, confusion, lethargy) and can fluctuate.
- Skull fractures increase the risk of epidural hemorrhage and meningitis. Basilar skull fracture is often a clinical diagnosis (see below).

Physical Examination

- Carefully search for penetrating wounds and other injuries, particularly of the neck.
- Hemotympanum, postauricular hematoma (Battle's sign), periorbital hematoma ("raccoon eyes"), and CSF otorrhea/rhinorrhea are indicative of **basilar skull fracture.**

- Neurologic examination should focus on the level of consciousness (see Alterations in Consciousness and Table 24-2), focal deficits, and signs of herniation. **Serial examinations must be performed and documented to identify neurologic deterioration.**

Imaging

- **Noncontrast head CT scan** best identifies intracranial hemorrhage and contusion.
  - A lenticular-shaped extra-axial hematoma is characteristic of epidural hematoma.
  - Bone window views may locate fractures.
- Skull and facial radiographs may be necessary to demonstrate some fractures.
- **Cervical radiographs must be performed to exclude fracture or dislocation.**

Monitoring

- Awake, alert patients with concussion are observed in the hospital for 24 hours with hourly neurologic assessment to detect delayed deterioration. Some patients are observed at home by a reliable adult with instructions for frequent checks and criteria for return.
- Continuously monitor vital signs, oximetry, and ECG. Arterial pressure monitoring in conjunction with intracranial monitoring may be needed to optimize cerebral perfusion.

Surgical Diagnostic Procedures

- In some cases of closed head injury complicated by increased intracranial pressure, intracranial pressure monitoring assists medical management.

TREATMENT

- **Ensure adequate airway, oxygenation, ventilation, and circulation.**
- **Immobilize the neck** in a hard cervical collar to avoid spinal cord injury from manipulating an unstable or fractured cervical spine.
- Avoid nasal intubation in patients with facial fractures; emergency tracheotomy may be necessary.
- Avoid hypoventilation and systemic hypotension, which may reduce cerebral perfusion.
- Secure IV access and continuously monitor vital signs, oximetry, and ECG.
  - Avoid hypotonic fluids.
  - Institute modest fluid restriction, maintaining perfusion and urine output.
- Anticipate and conservatively treat increased intracranial pressure:
  - Head midline and elevated 30 degrees. Steroids are not indicated for head injury.
  - In the mechanically ventilated patient, modest hyperventilation (PCO_2 ~35 mm Hg) reduces intracranial pressure by cerebral vasoconstriction; excessive hyperventilation may reduce cerebral perfusion.
- **Brain herniation requires immediate countermeasures** (see Alterations in Consciousness).

Surgery

- **Neurosurgical consultation** is indicated for patients with contusion, intracranial hematoma, cervical fracture, skull fractures, penetrating injuries, or focal neurologic deficits.
  - **Emergency evacuation** of acute epidural and subdural hematomas may be life saving.
  - **Do not move foreign objects** in penetrating head injuries.
  - Surgical stabilization of spinal injuries may be indicated.
  - Evacuation of chronic subdural hematoma is determined by the symptoms and degree of mass effect.
- **If surgery appears imminent** (severe or multiple injuries, intracranial hematoma), restrict oral intake (NPO) and perform preoperative laboratory analysis.

Complications

- **Neurologic deterioration** after head injury of any severity requires an immediate repeat head CT scan to differentiate between an expanding hematoma that necessitates surgery from diffuse cerebral edema that requires monitoring and reduction of intracranial pressure.

 # ACUTE SPINAL CORD DYSFUNCTION

GENERAL PRINCIPLES

Definition

- The hallmark of spinal cord dysfunction is demonstration of a level below which motor, sensory, and autonomic function is interrupted, due to the spinal cord's segmental functional organization. Rapid diagnosis and treatment may reverse or prevent progression of functional deficits.
- **Traumatic spinal cord injury** may be obvious from the history or initial examination but must also be excluded in patients who are unconscious, confused, or inebriated when the history regarding trauma is unknown.
- **Spinal cord concussion** refers to posttraumatic spinal cord symptoms and signs that resolve rapidly (hours to days).

Anatomy and Pathophysiology

- **Spinal cord compression** typically presents with back pain at the level of compression (some lesions are painless), progressive difficulty in walking, sensory impairment, and urinary retention with overflow incontinence. Rapid deterioration may occur.
- **Transverse myelitis or myelopathy** present with symptoms and signs similar to cord compression.

Etiology

- Etiologies of spinal cord compression include tumor (primary or metastatic), herniated disk, epidural abscess, hematoma, and vascular malformation.
- Transverse myelitis occurs with enteroviruses, herpes zoster, tuberculosis or other granulomatous disease, syphilis, and systemic lupus erythematosus.
- Transverse myelopathy is caused by infarction (cardiogenic, fibrocartilaginous, or gaseous embolus; hypotension; aortic dissection or surgery) and multiple sclerosis.

Mechanisms of Injury

- Spinal cord syndromes occur most commonly after spinal trauma, in which direct or indirect impact and vascular and inflammatory alterations contribute to the neurologic dysfunction.
- Vascular insults during circulatory insufficiency or from thromboembolism may also cause spinal cord syndromes.

DIAGNOSIS

Clinical Presentation, History, and Neurologic Examination

- Acute presentations suggest traumatic or vascular insults, while a subacute course suggests an enlarging mass lesion or infectious process.
- **Examination** helps localize the level of dysfunction (remember that there might be multiple lesions).

- **Radicular signs** (lancinating pain, paresthesias, and numbness in the dermatomal distribution of a nerve root, with weakness and decreased tone and reflexes in muscles supplied by the root) imply inflammation or compression of the nerve root. Tenderness to spinal percussion over the lesion may be present.
- **Myelopathic** signs are the hallmark of spinal cord syndromes.
  - Complete bilateral flaccid paralysis (quadriplegia or paraplegia) and loss of all sensation (anesthesia) below a dermatomal level with areflexia and sphincter dysfunction (urinary retention loss of rectal tone) constitute a complete spinal cord syndrome.
  - Hypotonia and areflexia are typically diminished below acute lesions (spinal shock).
  - Bilateral weakness (quadriparesis or paraparesis) and a level of sensory loss, a horizontal band of dysesthesia at the lesion level, hypertonia and hyperreflexia below the lesion, and extensor plantar responses (Babinski signs) constitute an incomplete spinal cord syndrome. These findings are typical of subacute progressive lesions (spinal stenosis, tumor, abscess, etc.).
  - Urinary retention commonly accompanies spinal cord compression.
- Unilateral cord lesions may result in contralateral pain and temperature loss, with ipsilateral weakness and proprioceptive loss (**Brown-Séquard's syndrome**).
- Anterior spinal artery ischemia produces bilateral symptoms and signs, sparing dorsal column function (proprioception and vibratory sensation).
- **Cauda equina syndrome** from compression of the lower lumbar and sacral roots produces sensory loss in a saddle distribution, flaccid leg weakness, decreased reflexes, and urinary/bowel incontinence.
- After traumatic spinal cord injury, search for injury to other systems.
- Serial exams are important in partial spinal cord syndromes to detect acute deterioration.

Laboratory Studies

- Inflammatory and infectious etiologies often require CSF analysis for pleocytosis, malignant cells, and abnormal protein/glucose, and tests for specific pathogens. Generally imaging should be performed first. Lumbar puncture should be performed with caution (see Neurosurgical Consultation under Imaging, below).
- Serum studies may help establish some etiologies.

Imaging

- The presence and extent of spinal cord injuries should be confirmed with neuroimaging. Plain radiographs of the spine may reveal metastatic disease, osteomyelitis, discitis, fractures, or dislocation.
- Emergent MRI scan or myelography with CT scan helps confirm the exact level and extent of the lesion(s). Imaging should include the entire spine.
- **Neurosurgical consultation should be obtained before myelography,** because occasionally acute postmyelography decompensation occurs with compressive lesions, requiring emergent decompressive laminectomy. For the same reason, lumbar puncture for diagnosis of infection, inflammation, or carcinomatous meningitis should follow exclusion of a compressive lesion.

Monitoring

- Vital signs should be continuously monitored, and adequate oxygenation and perfusion ensured.

TREATMENT

- Support vital functions. **Respiratory insufficiency** from cervical cord injuries requires immediate airway control and ventilatory assistance, without manipulation of the neck. Bag-mask ventilation, blind nasal intubation, or tracheostomy may be required.

- Immobilization, especially of the neck, is essential to prevent further injury while the patient's condition is stabilized and radiographic and neurosurgical assessment of the injuries is performed.
- Perform preoperative evaluation.
- Anticipate autonomic dysfunction.
  - **Autonomic instability** may lead to fluctuating vital signs and BP. Hypotension may require vasopressors (dopamine or dobutamine). α-Adrenergic agonists increase BP but reduce cardiac output and impair spinal cord perfusion. Fluid resuscitation alone usually results in pulmonary edema.

Medications

- Treatable infections require appropriate antibiotics. Herpes zoster (suggested by a vesicular rash) should be treated with acyclovir.
- **Dexamethasone**, 10 mg IV followed by 4 mg IV q6h, is given for compressive lesions, and sometimes for transverse myelitis or spinal cord infarction, although benefit has not been proved for all etiologies.
- For traumatic spinal cord injury **methylprednisolone**, 30 mg/kg IV bolus, followed by an infusion of 5.4 mg/kg/hr for 24 hours when initiated within 3 hours of injury, and infusion for 48 hours when initiated within 3–8 hours of injury, may improve neurologic recovery.[13]

Surgery

- **Neurosurgical consultation should be obtained** because many causes for spinal cord compression are surgically treatable. Penetrating injury, foreign bodies, comminuted fractures, misalignment, and hematoma usually require surgical treatment.

Special Therapy

- **Emergent radiation therapy** combined with high-dose steroids is usually indicated for cord compression due to malignancy and generally requires a histologic diagnosis.
- **Anticipatory acute and long-term supportive care** is important for patients with spinal cord dysfunction. Airway security should be confirmed frequently. Pulmonary and urinary infections, skin breakdown at pressure points, joint contractures, and irregular bowel and bladder elimination are common problems. Bladder distention can cause sympathetic overactivity (headache, tachycardia, diaphoresis, hypertension) as a result of autonomic dysreflexia.

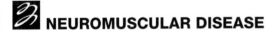

NEUROMUSCULAR DISEASE

GUILLAIN-BARRÉ'S SYNDROME

General Principles

Definitions
- **Guillain-Barré's syndrome (GBS)** is an acute inflammatory polyneuropathy typically following (few days to few weeks) viral infection, vaccination (e.g., influenza), and surgery.

Classification
- The demyelinating type is most common.
- Axonal type
  - Certain axolemma antibodies may differentiate axonal subtypes affecting motor fibers (acute motor axonal neuropathy) from those affecting motor and sensory fibers (acute motor-sensory axonal neuropathy).[14]
- Miller-Fischer variant consists of ophthalmoparesis, ataxia, and areflexia.

Etiology

- GBS is probably immune mediated, via antibodies to peripheral myelin or axonal antigens.

Diagnosis

Clinical Presentation and History

- Presentation of GBS is typically a rapidly progressive, symmetric ascending paralysis, often following a viral illness (Epstein-Barr virus, cytomegalovirus), gastroenteritis (especially *Campylobacter jejuni*, often axonal), surgical procedure, or immunization (influenza).

Physical Examination

- GBS typically presents with progressive, symmetric ascending paralysis. Fever and asymmetric weakness are useful findings that suggest alternative diagnoses.
- Cranial nerves, especially the facial nerves, may be involved.
- Proximal weakness may be pronounced.
- Sensory symptoms are often present, but objective sensory loss is uncommon.
- Reflexes are hypoactive or absent, and loss of reflexes on serial exams is a useful diagnostic feature.

Laboratory Studies

- CSF protein is usually elevated, without pleocytosis (occasionally increased lymphocytes present, but usually <20 cells/microliter).
- Nerve conduction test demonstrating absent H reflexes, prolonged F-wave latencies, slowed conduction velocities, and conduction block support the diagnosis of GBS. These may be normal early in the course.
- Creatine kinase may be elevated.

Imaging

- Imaging is not usually indicated.

Monitoring

- Frequently monitor vital signs, especially ventilation (negative inspiratory pressure) and blood pressure.

Differential Diagnosis

- Differential diagnosis includes postdiphtheritic paralysis, tick paralysis, botulism, arsenic neuropathy, and acute intermittent porphyria.
- Acute paralysis from poliovirus, HIV, West Nile virus, and polio-type illness from enteroviruses usually have fever and CSF pleocytosis. Paralysis is often asymmetric.

Treatment

Medications

- Plasmapheresis and IV immunoglobulin are comparably effective in improving outcome and shortening duration when administered early to patients who cannot walk or have respiratory failure.[15,16]
- Fewer complications may occur with IV immunoglobulins (IGs).
- Indications for treatment in mild forms of stable and improving GBS are less clear.

Special Therapy

- Treatment is supportive.
- Follow **respiratory function closely**, including oximetry, vital capacity (VC), and inspiratory force (IF). Hypoxemia, acidosis, and declining VC (<10–15 mL/kg) and IF (<25 cm H_2O) are indications for ventilatory assistance (see Chapter 9, Pulmonary Disease).
- Paroxysmal hypertension should not usually be treated with antihypertensive medications, but if indicated titratable short-acting agents are preferred (see Chapter 4, Hypertension).

- Hypotension is usually caused by decreased venous return and peripheral vasodilation. Mechanically ventilated patients are particularly prone to hypotension. Treatment consists of intravascular volume expansion; occasionally vasopressors may be required (see Chapter 8, Critical Care).
- **Cardiac arrhythmias** (bradyarrhythmias, including sinus arrest, complete heart block, or tachyarrhythmias) may be a serious complication in GBS; therefore, continuous ECG monitoring is necessary. Hypoxia and electrolyte abnormalities should be excluded as causes of cardiac arrhythmias.
- Corticosteroids and immunosuppressive drugs are not recommended.
- Prevention of exposure keratitis, venous thrombosis, and vigilance for hyponatremia (including syndrome of inappropriate diuretic hormone [SIADH]) should be priorities. Consider deep venous thrombosis prophylaxis.

Referrals
- Rehabilitation may be required during recovery.

MYASTHENIA GRAVIS

General Principles

Definitions
- **Myasthenia gravis (MG)** is an autoimmune disorder that involves antibody-mediated disruption of postsynaptic nicotinic acetylcholine receptors at the neuromuscular junction of skeletal muscle.

Classification
- MG usually involves skeletal muscle diffusely.
- Ocular MG is confined to eyelid and oculomotor function.

Diagnosis

Clinical Presentation and History
- MG is more common in women (typically third decade) than men (typically fifth to sixth decade).
- Clinical course is variable; spontaneous remissions and exacerbations may occur. Progressive deterioration is more likely to occur in the first 3 years.
- Typical symptoms are fatigable weakness (especially worse after exercise and better after rest), but chronic, fixed weakness may occur.
- **Myasthenic crisis** consists of respiratory failure or the need for airway protection, and occurs in approximately 10% of MG patients. Patients with bulbar and respiratory muscle weakness are particularly prone to respiratory failure, which may develop rapidly and unexpectedly.
- Respiratory infection, surgery (e.g., thymectomy), medications (e.g., aminoglycosides, quinine, beta blockers, lithium), pregnancy, and thyroid dysfunction can precipitate crisis or exacerbate symptoms.
- MG is often associated with thymus hyperplasia; 10% may have malignant thymoma.

Physical Examination
- **Presenting signs** include ptosis, diplopia, dysarthria, hypophonia, dysphagia, extremity weakness, and respiratory difficulty. Fatigability on examination is a useful diagnostic feature.
- Carefully evaluate the airway, handling of secretions, ventilation, and the work of breathing; negative inspiratory flow (NIF) is useful at the bedside to assess ventilatory status.
- Autonomic instability may produce blood pressure lability.

Laboratory and Diagnostic Studies

- ABGs, thyroid function tests, CBC, electrolytes, and calcium are helpful in the acutely ill MG patient.
- Blood **acetylcholine receptor antibody** level remains a highly sensitive and very specific assay and is the diagnostic test of choice. Antimuscle specific kinase (MuSK) antibody is detected in a small proportion of patients.
- **Repetitive nerve stimulation** (2–5 Hz) typically shows >10% decrement in the amplitude of the compound muscle action potential (CMAP) in MG. In botulism and the Eaton-Lambert's syndrome, the response is incremental with fast repetitive nerve stimulation (20–50 Hz).
- **Edrophonium (Tensilon test)** often produces a marked temporary improvement of strength in myasthenic patients. However, its utility as a diagnostic tool in MG is limited by a high incidence of false positives.
- Autoimmune thyroiditis is associated with MG; thyroid function tests should be performed.

Imaging

- **Chest CT** is indicated to identify thymoma.
- Chest radiograph

Monitoring

- Vital signs, ECG, oximetry, and negative inspiratory flow should be monitored in the acutely ill MG patient.

Differential Diagnosis

- Differential diagnosis includes presynaptic neuromuscular junction dysfunction in botulism, caused by the toxin produced by *Clostridium botulinum,* and the Eaton-Lambert syndrome, a paraneoplastic syndrome associated with carcinoma.

Treatment

- Treatment of MG follows no specific protocol; management depends upon symptoms, lifestyle, and response to treatment.
- **Myasthenic crisis** requires prompt recognition and aggressive support.
  - Monitor pulmonary function closely. Respiratory support follows the guidelines given in Chapter 8, Critical Care.
  - Eliminate precipitating medications; treat infections and metabolic derangements.
  - Anticholinesterases should be temporarily withdrawn from patients who are receiving ventilation support; this avoids uncertainties about overdosage ("cholinergic crisis") and avoids cholinergic stimulation of pulmonary secretions.
  - Steroids, IVIG, or plasmapheresis may be helpful.
  - Thymectomy is not part of the emergency treatment of MG.

Medications

- **Anticholinesterase** drugs can produce symptomatic improvement in all forms of MG.
- **Pyridostigmine** should be started at 30–60 mg PO tid–qid and subsequently titrated to the minimum required for symptom relief. Dose frequency is individually determined by response and side effects; some patients require dosing every 2–3 hours. Extended-release formulation is useful for the evening dose to reduce morning weakness.
- **Neostigmine** methylsulfate as a continuous IV infusion at one–forty-fifth the total daily dose of pyridostigmine over 24 hours can be substituted for patients who are not able to take medications orally.
- **Immunosuppressive** drugs are typically used when additional benefit is needed after cholinesterase inhibitors.
  - High-dose **prednisone** (50 mg daily) is frequently used to achieve rapid improvement, but **hospitalization is advised because initial exacerbation of weakness often occurs.** Initiating therapy at a lower dose (20 mg daily) followed by dose titration may avoid worsening symptoms. The goal is to identify an effective daily dose, maintain stable improvement, and then taper to an alternate-day regimen. Additional dose reductions

can be made gradually. Potential risks of steroid treatment need to be weighed against observed clinical benefit on an individual basis.

- **Azathioprine,** 1–2 mg/kg PO daily, is an alternative drug for patients who do not respond to steroids or cannot take them. Onset of benefit may require months of treatment. **Side effects** include leukopenia, pancytopenia, infection, GI irritation, and abnormal liver function tests.
- **Cyclosporine A** has been shown to be effective in MG in a double-blind, placebo-controlled clinical trial.[17]
- **Cyclophosphamide** and IV **human immunoglobulin** may be beneficial in selected refractory patients.
- Curariform medications are absolutely contraindicated in MG.

Surgery
- Thymoma is an absolute indication for thymectomy.
- **Thymectomy** may induce remission or reduce medication dependence. Generally thymectomy is considered for moderate to severe generalized MG, early in the course of the disease, and if medical treatment is unsatisfactory.
- Thymectomy is typically performed electively when the patient is stable and MG is under optimal medical treatment.
- In children, adults older than 60 years, and isolated ocular MG, thymectomy is controversial.

Special Therapy
- **Plasmapheresis** is used to treat acute exacerbations, impending crisis, and disabling myasthenia refractory to other therapies. Plasmapheresis is used before surgery when postoperative deterioration is possible (e.g., before thymectomy). Benefits are temporary, and no consensus has been reached about exact indications and protocol. Hypotension and thromboembolism are potential complications.

Patient Education
- Avoid triggering medications.
- Be aware of triggering illnesses.

Complications
- Cholinergic crisis
- Autonomic dysfunction

OTHER NEUROMUSCULAR DISORDERS

General Principles

Etiologies of Muscular Weakness
- **Myopathies** (ethanol, steroids, cholesterol-lowering drugs, hypothyroidism) may present with rapidly progressive proximal muscle weakness. **Critical illness myopathy,** increasingly recognized in patients with critical illness, is commonly associated with use of steroids and neuromuscular blocking agents. Polymyositis and dermatomyositis should also be considered, particularly if muscle pain is prominent (see Chapter 23, Arthritis and Rheumatologic Diseases).
- **Rhabdomyolysis** may produce rapid muscle weakness, and has multiple etiologies including various medications or toxic effects [e.g., antipsychotics, cholesterol-lowering drugs ("**statins**"), selective serotonin uptake inhibitors (**SSRIs**), alcohol, etc.] or less commonly secondary to strenuous exercise or metabolic myopathy. Complications include hyperkalemia, myoglobinuria, elevated creatine kinase, and renal failure (see Chapter 11, Renal Disease, for management).
- **Botulism** is a disorder of the neuromuscular junction caused by ingestion of an exotoxin produced by *Clostridium botulinum*. The exotoxin interferes with release of acetylcholine from presynaptic terminals at the neuromuscular junction. **Symptoms** begin within 12–36 hours of ingestion and include autonomic dysfunction (xerostomia,

blurred vision, bowel and bladder dysfunction) followed by cranial nerve palsies and weakness. Management includes removing nonabsorbed toxin with cathartics; neutralizing absorbed toxin with equine trivalent antitoxin, one vial IV and one vial IM (after normal intradermal horse serum sensitivity test); and supportive care.

NEUROMUSCULAR DISORDERS WITH RIGIDITY

- **Neuroleptic malignant syndrome** is associated with drugs such as haloperidol, phenothiazines, lithium, and reserpine. **Typical features** include fever, obtundation, and muscular rigidity, with elevated creatine kinase and myoglobinuria. **Treatment** includes discontinuing precipitating drug(s), cooling, monitoring and supporting vital functions (arrhythmias, shock, hyperkalemia, acidosis, renal failure), and administering dantrolene (2 mg/kg IV; additional doses q5min up to 10 mg/kg total can be given). Oral bromocriptine can be used in mild cases.
- **Serotonin syndrome** (triad of mental status change, autonomic over activity, and muscular rigidity) results from excessive serotonergic activity, especially following recent dosage changes of SSRIs, monoamine oxidase inhibitors (MAOIs), and tricyclic antidepressants (TCAs). Fever, tremor, and clonus are common signs. Treatment includes aggressive supportive care as above, cyproheptadine, and benzodiazepines.
- Acute development of high fever, obtundation, and muscular rigidity following triggering factors (e.g., halothane anesthesia) characterize **malignant hyperthermia syndrome.** Ryanodine receptor mutations that predispose to abnormal elevation in intracellular calcium triggered by certain anesthetics are the genetic basis for some cases of malignant hyperthermia syndrome. Certain muscle disorders (central core disease, Duchenne's muscular dystrophy) are also at risk. Serum creatine kinase is markedly elevated. Renal's failure from myoglobinuria and cardiac arrhythmias from electrolyte imbalance can be life threatening. Successful **management** requires prompt recognition of the syndrome, discontinuation of the offending anesthetic agent, aggressive supportive care that focuses on oxygenation/ventilation, circulation, correction of acid-base and electrolyte derangements, and dantrolene sodium, 1–10 mg/kg/d, to reduce muscular rigidity.
- **Tetanus** typically presents with generalized muscle spasm (especially trismus) caused by the exotoxin (tetanospasmin) from *Clostridium tetani.* The organism usually enters the body through wounds; onset typically occurs within 14 days of an injury (range, 2–54 days). Mortality may be as high as 50%–60%. **Patients who are unvaccinated or have reduced immunity are at risk, underscoring the importance of prevention by tetanus toxoid boosters following wounds.** Tetanus may occur in drug abusers who inject subcutaneously. **Management** consists of supportive care, particularly airway control (laryngospasm) and treatment of muscle spasms (benzodiazepines, barbiturates, analgesics, and sometimes neuromuscular blockade). Cardiac arrhythmias and fluctuations in BP can occur. The patient should be kept in quiet isolation, sedated but arousable. **Specific measures** include wound debridement; **penicillin G**, 2 million units IV q6h for 10 days (tetracycline, 2 g/d, or erythromycin, 2 g/d, is an alternative in penicillin-allergic patients); and human **tetanus immunoglobulin** (3,000–10,000 units) distributed intramuscularly among several sites proximal to the suspected source of exotoxin. **Active immunization is needed after recovery** (see Appendix D, Immunizations and Post-Exposure Therapies).

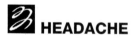 **HEADACHE**

GENERAL PRINCIPLES

Definitions

- Headache is a common symptom in hospitalized patients, and frequently a presenting symptom in emergency departments. The objective in these settings is to distinguish primary headache syndromes (most commonly migraine), which is treated symptomatically, from secondary headache, which warrants establishment of a specific etiology and treatment. The evaluation and management of primary headache syndromes are typically performed in the outpatient setting; the focus here will be on emergent aspects of diagnosis and treatment.

Classification

- **Primary headache syndromes** include **migraines** with (classical) or without (common) aura, **tension** headaches, and **cluster** headaches. Posttraumatic, exertional, cough- and cold-induced, and fleeting ice pick (stabbing) headaches are also considered within the same category after underlying structural lesions have been excluded. The mechanisms of primary headache syndromes are poorly understood but probably include release of calcitonin gene–related peptide and a disturbance in serotonergic neurotransmission. Examination should reveal normal findings during asymptomatic intervals in patients with primary headache syndromes, although transient (usually evolving over several minutes and any one symptom should not last continuously >60 minutes) neurologic deficits including visual field defects, aphasia, and hemiparesis may complicate migraine with aura. The evolution and slower development of neurologic deficits distinguish migraine from the typically abrupt onset of deficits with stroke or TIA.
- **Secondary headaches** have specific etiologies, and symptomatic features vary depending on the underlying pathology. For example, **SAH** causes abrupt onset of severe pain with neck stiffness. Frontal lobe **tumors** may be asymptomatic until very large, producing headache by compression or traction of pain-sensitive structures such as blood vessels or meninges. In contrast, small tectal tumors cause headache from obstructive hydrocephalus and intracranial hypertension. Headaches from intracranial hypertension may wake the patient from sleep and are worse with postural changes and in the morning upon arising from sleep.
- **Temporal arteritis** typically begins after 50 years of age, which is uncommon for the onset of migraines. Focal neurologic signs suggest an underlying structural lesion, but as mentioned above, transient focal neurologic deficits can occur in migraine. Diplopia from sixth nerve palsy in intracranial hypertension from any cause is considered a false localizing sign (i.e., not necessarily indicating a focal structural lesion).

Etiology and Differential Diagnosis

- Primary headaches are diagnosed by clinical features and exclusion of secondary etiologies.
- Intracranial etiologies of secondary headache include subdural hematoma, intracerebral hematoma, SAH, arteriovenous malformation, brain abscess, meningitis, encephalitis, vasculitis, obstructive hydrocephalus, and cerebral ischemia or infarction. Benign intracranial hypertension (pseudotumor cerebri) presents with headache, papilledema, diplopia, and elevated CSF pressure (>20 cm H_2O, relaxed lateral decubitus position). Extracranial causes include giant-cell arteritis, sinusitis, glaucoma, optic neuritis, dental disease (including temporomandibular joint syndrome), and disorders of the cervical spine. Systemic causes include fever, viremia, hypoxia (including CO poisoning, measure carboxyhemoglobin), hypercapnia, systemic hypertension, allergy, anemia, caffeine withdrawal, and vasoactive or toxic chemicals (nitrites). Depression is a common cause of long-standing, treatment-resistant headaches. Specific inquiry about vegetative signs of depression and exclusion of other causes help to support this diagnosis.

DIAGNOSIS

Clinical Presentation and History

- Physical examination and laboratory studies are important in diagnosis of secondary headache etiologies.

■ Neuroimaging is generally not indicated for primary headache syndromes, but may be required to exclude secondary etiologies in cases that have not been previously diagnosed, or that present atypical features. Remember that secondary etiologies for headache may occur in patients with established primary headaches, and may be difficult to distinguish in an acute setting.

TREATMENT

Medications

■ **Acute treatment of migraine,** the most common primary headache syndrome, is directed at aborting the headache. This is easier at onset and often very difficult when the attack is well established. Patients have often used nonprescription analgesics (acetylsalicylic acid [ASA], acetaminophen, NSAIDs) and oral prescription medications (isometheptene, butalbital with aspirin or acetaminophen), which are first-line treatments most effective early in the course of an attack. Emergent treatments include serotonin agonists and other parenteral medications. Long-term treatment additionally involves prophylactic medications. It is important to review a patient's use of all medications as they may influence acute management.

■ **Triptans** (serotonin receptor $5HT_{1B}$ and $5HT_{1D}$ agonists) are effective abortive medications available in multiple formulations and may be effective even in a protracted attack. Triptans should not be used in patients with coronary artery disease, cerebrovascular disease, uncontrolled hypertension, hemiplegic migraine, or vertebrobasilar migraine.

   ■ **Sumatriptan,** 6 mg SC, can be repeated in 1 hour (maximum, two shots per 24 hours), 5 or 20 mg nasal (maximum daily dose, two sprays, with minimum interval between doses of 2 hours), or 25–100 mg PO can be repeated in 2 hours (maximum daily dose, 200 mg).

   ■ **Zolmitriptan,** 2.5–5.0 mg PO or 5.0 mg nasal can be repeated in 2 hours (maximum dose, 10 mg/24 hours).

   ■ **Rizatriptan,** 5–10 mg, can be repeated every 2 hours as needed (maximum dose, 30 mg/24 hours). If on propranolol, rizatriptan dose is reduced to 5 mg PO and can be repeated every 2 hours (maximum of 15 mg/24 hours).

   ■ **Almotriptan,** 6.25–12.5 mg PO, can be repeated in 2 hours (maximum of 25 mg/24 hours).

   ■ **Eletriptan,** 40 mg PO, can be repeated in 2 hours (maximum of 80 mg/24 hours).

   ■ **Naratriptan,** 1.0–2.5 mg PO, can be repeated in 4 hours (maximum dose, 5 mg/24 hours).

   ■ **Frovatriptan,** 2.5 mg, can be repeated in 2 hours (maximum of 7.5 mg/24 hours).

   ■ Sometimes headache recurs within 24 hours after complete resolution. *Triptans should not be taken within 24 hours of other triptans, isometheptene, or ergot derivatives.*

■ **Dihydroergotamine** (DHE) is a potent venoconstrictor with minimal peripheral arterial constriction. Cardiac precautions are indicated in those with a history of angina, peripheral vascular disease, or elderly patients. A dose of 1–2 mg IM or SC can abort a migraine headache before it reaches peak intensity. If an attack has climaxed, 5–10 mg prochlorperazine can be given IV, followed immediately by 0.2 mg DHE IV given over 3 minutes. If tolerated, another 0.8 mg DHE IV is given. This relieves the primary headache in the majority of cases. For intractable migraines (status migrainosus), DHE can be given q8h with IV metoclopramide.[18] DHE 45 NS is administered intranasally, one spray in each nostril. It can be repeated in 15 minutes. The maximum recommended dose is four sprays per day.

■ **Ergotamine** is a vasoconstrictive agent effective for aborting migraine headaches, particularly if administered during the prodromal phase. Ergotamine should be taken at symptom onset in the maximum dose tolerated by the patient; nausea often limits the dose. Rectal preparations are better absorbed than oral agents. The initial oral dose is 2–3 mg PO. Additional doses of 1–2 mg can be taken every 30 minutes, up to a total dose of 8–10 mg, but these rarely succeed when an initial dose has failed. Rectal (2 mg) administration should be tried in patients who are unresponsive to oral delivery or when emesis prevents oral administration. Dosages that exceed 16 mg/wk should be used cautiously to avoid toxicity, which includes angina pectoris, limb claudication, and ergotamine headache and dependency.

- **Other agents** may be used in the acute treatment of recalcitrant headaches:
  - **Ketorolac tromethamine**, 30–60 mg IM or IV
  - **Prochlorperazine**, 5–10 mg IV, may terminate migraine and helps alleviate nausea. Acute dystonic reactions and hypotension are potential side effects.
  - **Opiate analgesics** (see Chapter 1, Patient Care in Internal Medicine), usually meperidine 50 mg IM or IV. Chronic daily headaches should not be treated with narcotic analgesics to prevent addiction and tachyphylaxis.
- **Treatment of secondary headaches** is directed at the primary etiology, such as surgical treatment of cerebral aneurysm causing SAH, evacuation of subdural hematoma, or shunting obstructive hydrocephalus. Diagnostic lumbar puncture for benign intracranial hypertension and meningitis (especially aseptic) often relieves the headache and CSF pressure measurement helps guide CSF removal until it is within a normal range (e.g., 10 cm H_2O). Alternatively, postural headache after lumbar puncture (**"post lumbar puncture headache"**) may occur.

Surgery

- Surgery is indicated to treat certain secondary etiologies, including cerebral aneurysm causing SAH, evacuation of subdural hematoma, or shunting obstructive hydrocephalus. Neurosurgical consultation is indicated as there are multiple factors that determine the necessity, timing, and type of surgery that should be performed.

References

1. Mayo-Smith MF. Pharmacological management of alcohol withdrawal. A meta-analysis and evidence-based practice guideline. American Society of Addiction Medicine Working Group on Pharmacological Management of Alcohol Withdrawal. *JAMA* 1997;278:144–151.
2. Mayer SA, Claassen J, Lokin J, et al. Refractory status epilepticus: frequency, risk factors, and impact on outcome. *Arch Neurol* 2002;59:205–210.
3. Lowenstein DH. Treatment options for status epilepticus. *Curr Opin Pharmacol* 2005; 5:334–339.
4. Treiman DM, Meyers PD, Walton NY, et al. A comparison of four treatments for generalized convulsive status epilepticus. Veterans Affairs Status Epilepticus Cooperative Study Group. *N Engl J Med* 1998;339:792–798.
5. Adams H, Adams R, Del Zoppo G, et al. Guidelines for the early management of patients with ischemic stroke: 2005 guidelines update a scientific statement from the Stroke Council of the American Heart Association/American Stroke Association. *Stroke* 2005;36:916–923.
6. Adams HP Jr, Adams RJ, Brott T, et al. Guidelines for the early management of patients with ischemic stroke: a scientific statement from the Stroke Council of the American Stroke Association. *Stroke* 2003;34:1056–1083.
7. Collaborative meta-analysis of randomised trials of antiplatelet therapy for prevention of death, myocardial infarction, and stroke in high risk patients. *BMJ* 2002;324: 71–86.
8. The International Stroke Trial (IST): a randomised trial of aspirin, subcutaneous heparin, both, or neither among 19435 patients with acute ischaemic stroke. International Stroke Trial Collaborative Group. *Lancet* 1997;349:1569–1581.
9. Beneficial effect of carotid endarterectomy in symptomatic patients with high-grade carotid stenosis. North American Symptomatic Carotid Endarterectomy Trial Collaborators. *N Engl J Med* 1991;325:445–453.
10. Endarterectomy for asymptomatic carotid artery stenosis. Executive Committee for the Asymptomatic Carotid Atherosclerosis Study. *JAMA* 1995;273:1421–1428.

11. Biller J, Feinberg WM, Castaldo JE, et al. Guidelines for carotid endarterectomy: a statement for healthcare professionals from a special writing group of the Stroke Council, American Heart Association. *Stroke* 1998;29:554–562.

12. Randomised trial of a perindopril-based blood-pressure-lowering regimen among 6,105 individuals with previous stroke or transient ischaemic attack. *Lancet* 2001;358:1033–1041.

13. Bracken MB, Shepard MJ, Collins WF, et al. A randomized, controlled trial of methylprednisolone or naloxone in the treatment of acute spinal-cord injury. Results of the Second National Acute Spinal Cord Injury Study. *N Engl J Med* 1990;322: 1405–1411.

14. Hughes RA, Cornblath DR. Guillain-Barré syndrome. *Lancet* 2005;366:1653–1666.

15. Ropper AH, Kehne SM. Guillain-Barré syndrome: management of respiratory failure. *Neurology* 1985;35:1662–1665.

16. Bril V, Ilse WK, Pearce R, et al. Pilot trial of immunoglobulin versus plasma exchange in patients with Guillain-Barré syndrome. *Neurology* 1996;46:100–103.

17. Tindall RS, Phillips JT, Rollins JA, et al. A clinical therapeutic trial of cyclosporine in myasthenia gravis. *Ann NY Acad Sci* 1993;681:539–551.

18. Raskin NH. Repetitive intravenous dihydroergotamine as therapy for intractable migraine. *Neurology* 1986;36:995–997.

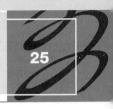

MEDICAL EMERGENCIES
Daniel Goodenberger

GENERAL PRINCIPLES

- Medical emergencies may not allow time for orderly information gathering and formulation of a narrow differential diagnosis before the initiation of therapy.
- **The first responsibility** is to provide basic life support (i.e., maintenance of an intact airway, adequate ventilation, and circulation; see Chapter 8, Critical Care).

 ACUTE UPPER AIRWAY OBSTRUCTION

GENERAL PRINCIPLES

- Airway obstruction in the awake patient without ventilation:
    - The most likely causes are a foreign body (usually food) and angioedema.
    - Other causes include infection or posttraumatic hematoma.
    - History is often unavailable.
- Airway obstruction in an unconscious patient without intact ventilation:
    - Such a situation may be due to obstruction by the tongue, or it may be caused by a foreign body, trauma, infection, or angioedema.
    - A history usually is unavailable except from paramedics or relatives.

DIAGNOSIS

Clinical Presentation

- In the **conscious patient:**
    - Manifestations may include stridor, impaired or absent phonation, sternal or suprasternal retractions, display of the universal choking sign, and respiratory distress.
    - Look for urticaria, angioedema, fever, or evidence of trauma.
- The **unconscious patient:**
    - The patient may have labored breathing or apnea.
    - Suspect airway obstruction in a nonbreathing patient who is difficult to ventilate.

Physical Examination

- Partial obstruction in the awake patient with adequate ventilation:
    - Rapidly take a history, focusing on the causes just listed.
    - Perform a directed physical examination, looking for airway swelling, trismus, pharyngeal obstruction, respiratory retractions, angioedema, stridor, wheezing, and grossly swollen lymph nodes and masses in the neck.
    - Treatment is aimed at the underlying disease process; observe the patient carefully and be prepared to intervene to maintain an airway.

- Airway obstruction in an unconscious patient without intact ventilation:
  - Examination reveals an unresponsive patient with no air movement or paradoxical respiratory efforts.
  - Examine the upper airway visually for evidence of obstruction as part of the resuscitative effort.

Imaging

- Partial obstruction in the awake patient with adequate ventilation:
  - **Soft tissue radiography** of the neck (posteroanterior and lateral views) is less sensitive and specific than is direct examination but may be a valuable adjunct. Such radiography should be performed in the emergency department as a portable study, as the patient should not be left unattended.
  - **Rapid computed tomography (CT)** of the airway with constant attendance is an alternative approach where available.

Other Diagnostic Procedures

- Partial obstruction in the awake patient with adequate ventilation:
  - If the patient's condition is stable, perform indirect **laryngoscopy** or **fiberoptic nasopharyngolaryngoscopy**. A careful examination is unlikely to cause acute airway obstruction in an adult.

Differential Diagnosis

- Trauma to the face and neck, foreign body, infection (croup, epiglottitis, Ludwig angina, retropharyngeal abscess, and diphtheria), tumor, angioedema, laryngospasm, anaphylaxis, retained secretions, or blockage of the upper airway by the tongue (in the unconscious patient)

TREATMENT

Nonoperative

- Therapy is directed at **rapid relief of obstruction** to prevent cardiopulmonary arrest and anoxic brain damage.
  - **Airway obstruction in the awake patient without ventilation:**
    - Perform the **Heimlich maneuver** (subdiaphragmatic abdominal thrust) repeatedly until the object is expelled from the airway or patient becomes unconscious (see Chapter 8, Critical Care). Up to half of patients may require a second technique (i.e., back slaps, chest thrusts) for success.[1]
  - **Airway obstruction in an unconscious patient without intact ventilation:**
    - Perform the head tilt–chin lift maneuver if cervical spine trauma is not suspected. Perform a jaw thrust if cervical spine trauma is suspected.
    - If these maneuvers are effective, place an oral or nasal airway. If they are ineffective, attempt to ventilate the patient with a bag-valve-mask apparatus. If these attempts are also unsuccessful, rapidly examine the oropharynx and hypopharynx. Avoid a blind finger sweep if it is possible to examine the airway directly using a laryngoscope and McGill forceps (if necessary) to remove a foreign body.
    - If laryngoscopy cannot be performed immediately and a foreign body is suspected, perform **the supine Heimlich maneuver** (straddling the supine patient and applying repeated subdiaphragmatic thrusts). Chest thrusts may generate higher airway pressures and be successful when abdominal thrusts have failed.
    - Substitute chest thrusts if the patient is very obese or is in late pregnancy.

Operative

- **Airway obstruction in an unconscious patient without intact ventilation:**
  - Failure of the supine Heimlich maneuver should prompt an attempt at direct laryngoscopy and endotracheal intubation.
  - Establish a surgical airway if the patient cannot be intubated.
  - If a surgeon is not immediately available, perform needle cricothyrotomy using a 12- to 14-gauge over-the-needle catheter with high-flow oxygen (15 L/min from a 50-psi wall source).
  - **Cricothyrotomy** (see Chapter 8, Critical Care) is a preferred alternative.

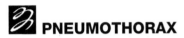 **PNEUMOTHORAX**

GENERAL PRINCIPLES

- Pneumothorax may occur spontaneously or as a result of trauma.
- **Primary spontaneous pneumothorax** occurs without obvious underlying lung disease.
- **Secondary spontaneous pneumothorax** results from underlying parenchymal lung disease, including chronic obstructive pulmonary disease, interstitial lung disease, necrotizing lung infections, *Pneumocystis jiroveci* pneumonia, and cystic fibrosis.
- **Traumatic pneumothoraces** may occur as a result of penetrating or blunt chest wounds.
- **Iatrogenic pneumothorax** occurs after thoracentesis, central line placement, transbronchial biopsy, transthoracic needle biopsy, and barotrauma from mechanical ventilation and resuscitation.

DIAGNOSIS

History

- The patient typically complains of ipsilateral chest or shoulder pain, usually of abrupt onset. An occasional patient may experience dyspnea alone. Recent chest trauma or a medical procedure may suggest the diagnosis.

Clinical Presentation

- Dyspnea is usually present, and the patient sometimes has a cough.
- Symptoms related to an underlying pulmonary disease process may be seen or a history of recent trauma obtained.

Physical Examination

- Examination of the patient with a small pneumothorax may be normal.
- There may be decreased breath sounds, decreased vocal fremitus, and a more resonant percussion note.
- With a larger pneumothorax or with underlying lung disease, there may be tachypnea and respiratory distress. The affected hemithorax may be noticeably larger (due to decreased elastic recoil of the collapsed lung) and relatively immobile during respiration.
- If the pneumothorax is very large, and particularly if it is under tension, the patient may exhibit severe distress, diaphoresis, cyanosis, and hypotension. The patient may have signs of recent procedures or trauma.
- In addition, there may be indications of underlying lung disease such as clubbing or fever.
- If the pneumothorax is the result of penetrating trauma or pneumomediastinum, subcutaneous emphysema may be felt.

Imaging

- A chest **radiograph** will reveal a separation of the pleural shadow from the chest wall. A small pneumothorax is more easily seen on a film taken during expiration. Air travels to the highest point in a body cavity; thus, a pneumothorax in a supine patient may be detected as an unusually deep costophrenic sulcus and excessive lucency over the upper abdomen caused by the anterior thoracic air. This is particularly important in the critical care unit, where radiographs of the mechanically ventilated patient are often obtained with the patient supine.
- Although tension pneumothorax is a clinical diagnosis, radiographic correlates include mediastinal and tracheal shift away from the pneumothorax and depression of the ipsilateral diaphragm.

Other Tests

- An **electrocardiogram** (ECG) may reveal diminished anterior QRS amplitude and an anterior axis shift. In extreme cases, tension pneumothorax may cause electromechanical dissociation.

TREATMENT

- Treatment depends on cause, size, and degree of physiologic derangement. **A small, primary, spontaneous pneumothorax** without a continued pleural air leak may resolve spontaneously. Air is resorbed from the pleural space at roughly 1.5% daily, and therefore a small (~15%) pneumothorax is expected to resolve without intervention in approximately 10 days.
  - Confirm that the pneumothorax is **not increasing in size** (repeat the chest radiograph in 6 hours if there is no change in symptoms) and send the patient home if he or she is asymptomatic (apart from mild pleurisy). Obtain follow-up radiographs to confirm resolution of the pneumothorax in 7–10 days. Air travel is proscribed during the follow-up period, as a decrease in ambient barometric pressure results in a larger pneumothorax.
  - If the pneumothorax is **small but the patient is mildly symptomatic,** far from home, or unlikely to cooperate with follow-up, admit the patient and administer high-flow oxygen; the resulting nitrogen gradient will speed resorption.
  - If the pneumothorax is **larger than 15%–20% or is more than mildly symptomatic,** insert a small thoracostomy tube [No. 8 French (Fr.) over a needle] in the second interspace in the midclavicular line; the air can be manually aspirated with a stopcock attached to a one-way (Heimlich) valve, or, if necessary, connected to suction.[2] If the bronchopleural fistula has sealed, cough or Valsalva results in re-expansion with the one-way valve. Most such patients should be hospitalized. If the pneumothorax fails to expand or if there is a continuous large air leak, arrange for insertion of a larger tube with suction.
  - **Pleural sclerosis** to prevent recurrence is recommended by some experts but in most cases is not used after a first episode unless a persistent air leak is present.
  - **Doxycycline** or a **talc slurry** can be used via chest tube for patients who wish to avoid surgery or who are at high surgical risk (see Pleural Effusion, in Chapter 9, Pulmonary Disease). Apical bullectomy via thoracoscopy accompanied by pleural sclerosis has a higher success rate (78%–91% vs. 95%–100%).[2]
- **Individuals with a secondary spontaneous pneumothorax** usually are symptomatic and require lung re-expansion.
  - Often a bronchopleural fistula persists, and a larger thoracostomy tube and suction are required.
  - If no associated effusion is present, a No. 24–28 Fr. tube is recommended; if fluid is present, choose a larger tube (No. 34–36 Fr.). Attach the thoracostomy tube to a three-bottle suction system or the commercial equivalent (Pleur-evac, Genzyme

Biosurgery, Cambridge, MA) and apply 20 cm H_2O suction. Large air leaks may require greater suction.
- ▦ **Consult a pulmonologist** about pleural sclerosis for persistent air leak and to prevent recurrence.
- ▦ **Surgery** may be required for persistent air leak and should be considered for high-risk patients for prevention of recurrence.
- ■ **Iatrogenic pneumothorax**
  - ▦ Iatrogenic pneumothorax generally is caused either by introducing air into the pleural space through the parietal pleura (e.g., thoracentesis, central line placement) or by allowing intrapulmonary air to escape through breach of the visceral pleura (e.g., transbronchial biopsy). Often no further air leak occurs after the initial event.
  - ▦ If the pneumothorax is small and the patient is minimally symptomatic, it can be managed conservatively. If the procedure that caused the pneumothorax required sedation, admit the patient, administer oxygen, and repeat the chest radiograph in 6 hours to ensure the patient's stability. If the patient is completely alert and the chest radiograph shows no change, the patient can be discharged.
  - ▦ If the patient is symptomatic or if the pneumothorax is too large for expectant care, a pneumothorax catheter with aspiration or a one-way valve usually is adequate and can often be removed the following day.
  - ▦ Iatrogenic pneumothorax due to barotrauma from mechanical ventilation almost always has a persistent air leak and should be managed with a chest tube and suction.
- ■ **Tension pneumothorax**
  - ▦ Tension pneumothorax results from continued accumulation of air in the chest that is sufficient to shift mediastinal structures and impede venous return to the heart, resulting in hypotension, abnormal gas exchange, and, ultimately, cardiovascular collapse.
  - ▦ It can occur as a result of barotrauma due to mechanical ventilation, a chest wound that allows ingress but not egress of air, or a rent in the visceral pleura that behaves in the same way ("ball-valve" effect).
  - ▦ Suspect tension pneumothorax when a patient experiences hypotension and respiratory distress on mechanical ventilation or after any procedure in which the thorax is pierced by a needle. When the clinical situation and physical examination strongly suggest this diagnosis, decompress the affected hemithorax immediately with a 14-gauge needle attached to a fluid-filled syringe. Release of air with clinical improvement confirms the diagnosis. Seal any chest wound with an occlusive dressing and arrange for placement of a thoracostomy tube.

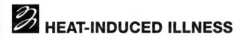

HEAT-INDUCED ILLNESS

HEAT CRAMPS

- ■ Heat cramps occur in unacclimatized individuals who engage in vigorous exercise in a hot environment; no published evidence has shown unequivocally that they are a result of salt depletion and hypotonic fluid replacement.[3]
- ■ Cramps typically occur in large muscle groups, most often in the legs.
- ■ **Diagnosis** is made on examination. The patient has moist cool skin, a normal body temperature, and minimal distress.
- ■ **Treatment** consists of resting the patient in a cool environment and giving salt replacement.
  - ▦ Administer 1/2–1 tsp salt or a 650-mg sodium chloride tablet in 500 mL water PO or use a commercially available, oral, balanced electrolyte replacement solution.
  - ▦ IV therapy rarely is required, but 2 L normal saline administered over several hours resolves symptoms.

HEAT EXHAUSTION

- Heat exhaustion occurs in unacclimatized individuals who exercise in the heat and is partly a result of loss of salt and water.
- The patient notes headache, nausea, vomiting, dizziness, weakness, irritability, and cramps. The patient is diaphoretic, demonstrates piloerection, has postural hypotension, and has normal or minimally increased core temperature.
- **Treatment** consists of resting the patient in a cool environment, accelerating heat loss by fan evaporation, and repleting fluids with salt-containing solutions.
  - If the patient is not vomiting and has stable blood pressure (BP), an oral, commercial, balanced salt solution is adequate.
  - If the patient is vomiting or hemodynamically unstable, check electrolytes and give 1–2 L 0.9% saline IV.
  - The patient should avoid exercise in a hot environment for 2–3 additional days.

HEAT SYNCOPE

- Heat syncope affects unacclimatized individuals.
- Exercise in a hot environment results in peripheral vasodilation and pooling of blood, with subsequent loss of consciousness. The affected individual regains consciousness promptly when supine, and the body temperature is normal. These factors separate this syndrome from heat stroke.
- **Treatment** consists of rest in a cool environment, fluid repletion, and a more gradual approach to building exercise endurance.

HEAT STROKE

General Principles

- Heat stroke occurs in two varieties, each with high core temperature, which causes direct thermal tissue injury. Secondary effects include acute renal failure from rhabdomyolysis. Even with rapid therapy, mortality may reach 76% for body temperatures of $41.1°C$ ($106°F$) or higher.
- **Classic heat stroke**
  - Classic heat stroke occurs after several days of heat exposure.
  - **Individuals at risk** include those who are chronically ill, dehydrated, elderly, or obese; those who have chronic cardiovascular disease; those who abuse alcohol; and those who use sedatives, hypnotics, α-adrenergic antagonists, diuretics, anticholinergics, or antipsychotics.
  - Abuse of phencyclidine, cocaine, and amphetamines also may contribute.
  - **Risk factors** include high humidity and lack of air-conditioning.
  - More than 50% may have infection at presentation.[4]
  - Typically, these patients have **core temperatures higher than $40.5°C$ ($105°F$) and are comatose and anhidrotic.**
- **Exertional heat stroke**
  - Exertional heat stroke occurs rapidly in unacclimatized and unfit individuals who exercise in conditions of high ambient temperature and humidity.
  - Those **at risk** include athletes, soldiers, and laborers, particularly if they lack access to water. Some of the risks associated with classic heat stroke may also be present, and certain congenital diseases that impair sweating may contribute. The core temperature may be lower than $40.5°C$; 50% of patients are still sweating at presentation.
  - Individuals with exertional heat stroke are more likely than are those with classic heat stroke to have **disseminated intravascular coagulation (DIC), lactic acidosis, and rhabdomyolysis.**

Diagnosis

- Diagnosis is based on the history of exposure or exercise, a core temperature usually of 40.6°C (105°F) or higher, and changes in mental status ranging from confusion to delirium and coma.

Differential Diagnosis
- Malignant hyperthermia after exposure to anesthetic agents
- Neuroleptic malignant syndrome associated with antipsychotic drugs
  - It is worth noting that neuroleptic malignant syndrome and malignant hyperthermia are both accompanied by severe muscle rigidity.
- Anticholinergic poisoning
- Sympathomimetic toxicity (including cocaine)
- Severe hyperthyroidism
- Sepsis
- Meningitis
- Cerebral malaria
- Encephalitis
- Hypothalamic dysfunction due to stroke or hemorrhage
- Brain abscess

Treatment

- **Immediate cooling** is necessary.
  - The best method of cooling is controversial. No study has directly compared ice water application with tepid spray. However, ice water lowers body temperature twice as quickly and is the procedure chosen when exertional heat stroke is anticipated (long-distance races, military training).[5,6]
  - Wrap the patient in sheets that are continuously wetted with ice water.
  - If response is insufficiently rapid, submerge the patient in ice water, recognizing that this may interfere with resuscitative efforts.[7]
  - Most emergency facilities that do not care for large numbers of heat illness cases are not equipped for this treatment. In that case, mist the patient continuously with tepid water (20°–25°C). Cool the patient with a large electric fan with maximum body surface exposure.
  - Ice packs at points of major heat transfer, such as the groin, axillae, and chest, may further speed cooling.
  - If severely elevated core temperature does not respond to these maneuvers, **gastric lavage with ice water** may be helpful, although this treatment is controversial.[8]
  - Cold peritoneal lavage is not more effective than evaporative cooling.
- **Dantrolene sodium** does not appear to be effective for the treatment of heat stroke.[9] However, if malignant hyperthermia due to anesthetic agent is diagnosed, give dantrolene, 2 mg/kg IV repeated q5 min as necessary for symptom relief to a total of 10 mg/kg, followed by 1–2 mg/kg qid for 3–4 days. Treat **neuroleptic malignant syndrome** with dantrolene in the same way, but add bromocriptine, 2.5–5.0 mg PO or per gastrostomy tube q8h.
- If it is necessary to treat **severe hypertension**, nitroprusside may be preferable, as it promotes more rapid heat loss via peripheral vasodilation.
- Shivering and vasoconstriction impair cooling and should be prevented by administration of **chlorpromazine**, 10–25 mg IM, or **diazepam**, 5–10 mg IV.
- Monitor core temperatures continuously by rectal probe. Tympanic membrane temperature measurement does not correlate well with rectal temperature and may be affected by environmental conditions.[10,11] Oral temperatures are unreliable and are frequently incorrectly low.
- Discontinue cooling measures when the core temperature reaches 39°C (102.2°F), which should ideally be achieved within 30 minutes. A temperature rebound may occur in 3–6 hours and should be retreated.

- For **hypotension, administer crystalloids;** if refractory, treat with vasopressors and monitor hemodynamics. Avoid pure α-adrenergic agents, as they cause vasoconstriction and impair cooling. Administer crystalloids cautiously to normotensive patients.

Patient Monitoring
- Laboratory studies should include complete blood count (CBC); partial thromboplastin time; prothrombin time; fibrin degradation products; electrolytes; blood urea nitrogen (BUN); creatinine, glucose, calcium, and creatine kinase levels; liver function tests; arterial blood gases (ABGs); urinalysis; and ECG.
- Monitor the cardiac rhythm continuously. If an infectious etiology is suspected, obtain appropriate cultures. If a central nervous system (CNS) etiology is considered likely, CT imaging followed by spinal fluid examination is appropriate.

Complications
- Treat **rhabdomyolysis** or urine output of <30 mL/hr with adequate volume replacement, mannitol (12.5–25 g IV), and bicarbonate (44–100 mEq/L in 0.45% normal saline) to promote osmotic diuresis and urine alkalinization. Despite these measures, **renal failure** may still complicate 5% of cases of classic heat stroke and 25% of cases of exertional heat stroke.
- **Hypoxemia and acute respiratory distress syndrome (ARDS)** may occur. Treat as described in Chapter 8, Critical Care.
- Treat seizures with diazepam and phenytoin.
- Provide supportive care for hepatic injury, congestive heart failure (CHF), and coagulopathy.

COLD-INDUCED ILLNESS

GENERAL PRINCIPLES
- Exposure to the cold may result in several different forms of injury.
- Risk factors are accelerated heat loss, which is promoted by exposure to high wind or by immersion.
- Extended cold exposure may result from alcohol or drug abuse, injury or immobilization, and mental impairment.

CHILBLAINS
- Chilblains are among the mildest form of cold injury and result from exposure of bare skin to a cold, windy environment (33°–60°F).
- The ears, fingers, and tip of the nose typically are injured, with itchy, painful erythema on rewarming.
- **Treatment** involves rapid rewarming (see Frostnip), moisturizing lotions, and analgesics and instruct the patient to avoid re-exposure.

IMMERSION INJURY (TRENCH FOOT)
- Immersion injury is caused by prolonged immersion (longer than 10–12 hours) at a temperature <50°F.
- Treat by rewarming followed by dry dressings. Treat secondary infections with antibiotics.

FROSTNIP

- Frostnip is the mildest form of frostbite.
- It occurs most frequently on the distal extremities, the nose, or the ear.
- It is marked by tissue blanching and decreased sensitivity.
- **Rapid rewarming,** in a water bath at 104°–108°F (40°–42°C), is the treatment of choice for all forms of frostbite. The water temperature should never be hotter than 112°F.

SUPERFICIAL FROSTBITE

- Superficial frostbite involves the skin and subcutaneous tissues.
- Areas with first-degree involvement are white, waxy, and anesthetic; have poor capillary refill; and are painful on thawing. Second-degree involvement is manifested by clear or milky bullae.
- The **treatment of choice** is rapid rewarming. Immerse the affected body part for 15–30 minutes; hexachlorophene or povidone-iodine can be added to the water bath. Narcotic analgesics may be necessary for rewarming pain. No deep injury ensues, and healing occurs in 3–4 weeks.

DEEP FROSTBITE

General Principles

- Deep frostbite involves death of skin, subcutaneous tissue, and muscle (third degree) or deep tendons and bones (fourth degree).

Diagnosis

- The tissue appears frozen and hard.
- On rewarming, there is no capillary filling.
- Hemorrhagic blisters form, followed by eschars. Healing is very slow, and demarcation of tissue with autoamputation may occur.
- Diabetes mellitus, peripheral vascular disease, an outdoor lifestyle, and high altitude are additional **risk factors.** More than 90% of deep frostbite occurs at temperatures <6.7°C (44°F) with exposures longer than 7–10 hours.

Treatment

- The treatment is rapid rewarming as described above. **Rewarming should not be started until there is no chance of refreezing.**
- Administer analgesics (IV opioids) as needed.
- Admit the patient to a surgical service.
- **Elevate** the affected extremity, prevent weight bearing, separate the affected digits with cotton wool, prevent tissue maceration by using a blanket cradle, and prohibit smoking.
- Update tetanus immunization.
- Intra-arterial vasodilators, heparin, dextran, prostaglandin inhibitors, thrombolytics, and sympathectomy are not routinely justified.
- Use antibiotics only for documented infection.
- Amputation is undertaken only after full demarcation has occurred.

HYPOTHERMIA

General Principles

Definition

- Hypothermia is defined as a core temperature of <35°C (95°F).
- Classification of severity by temperature is not universal. One scheme defines hypothermia as mild at 34°–35°C, moderate at 30°–34°C, and severe at <30°C.

Etiology
- The most common cause of hypothermia in the United States is cold exposure due to alcohol intoxication.
- Another common cause is cold water immersion.

Diagnosis

Differential Diagnosis
- Cerebrovascular accident
- Drug overdose
- Diabetic ketoacidosis
- Hypoglycemia
- Uremia
- Adrenal insufficiency
- Myxedema

Monitoring
- Monitor core temperature.
- A standard oral thermometer registers only to a lower limit of $35°C$. Monitor the patient continuously with a rectal probe with a full range of $20°–40°C$.
- Equal efficacy of ear thermistor monitoring has **not** been demonstrated.

Clinical Presentation
- Presentation varies with the temperature of the patient at presentation. All organ systems can be involved.
- CNS effects
    - At temperatures **below 32°C**, mental processes are slowed and the affect is flattened.
    - At $<32.2°C$ ($90°F$), the ability to shiver is lost, and deep tendon reflexes are diminished.
    - At **28°C**, coma often supervenes.
    - **Below 18°C**, the electroencephalogram (EEG) is flat. On rewarming from severe hypothermia, central pontine myelinolysis may develop.
- Cardiovascular effects
    - After an initial increased release of catecholamines, there is a decrease in cardiac output and heart rate with relatively preserved mean arterial pressure. ECG changes, manifest initially as sinus bradycardia with T-wave inversion and QT-interval prolongation, may progress to atrial fibrillation at temperatures of $<32°C$.
    - Osborne waves (J-point elevation) may be visible, particularly in leads II and V_6.
    - An increased susceptibility to ventricular arrhythmias occurs at temperatures **below 32°C**.
    - At temperatures of $<30°C$, the susceptibility to ventricular fibrillation is increased significantly, and unnecessary manipulation or jostling of the patient should be avoided.
    - A decrease in mean arterial pressure may also occur, and, at temperatures of $<28°C$, progressive bradycardia supervenes.
- Respiratory effects
    - After an initial increase in minute ventilation, respiratory rate and tidal volume decrease progressively with decreasing temperature.
    - ABGs measured with the machine set at $37°C$ should serve as the basis for therapy without correction of pH and carbon dioxide tension (PCO_2).[12,13]
- Renal manifestations
    - Cold-induced diuresis and tubular concentrating defects may be seen.

Laboratory Studies
- Basic laboratory studies should include CBC; coagulation studies; liver function tests; BUN; electrolytes; creatinine, glucose, creatine kinase, calcium, magnesium, and amylase levels; urinalysis; ABGs; and ECG.

- Obtain toxicology screen if mental status alteration is more profound than expected for temperature decrease.
- Serum potassium often is increased.
- Elevated serum amylase may reflect underlying pancreatitis.
- Hyperglycemia may be noted but should not be treated, as rebound hypoglycemia may occur with rewarming.
- DIC may also occur.

Imaging
- Obtain chest, abdominal, and cervical spine radiographs to evaluate all patients with a history of trauma or immersion injury.

Treatment

Medications
- Administer supplemental oxygen.
- Give **thiamine** to most patients with cold exposure, as exposure due to alcohol intoxication is common.
- Administration of **antibiotics** is a controversial issue; many authorities recommend antibiotic administration for 72 hours, pending cultures. In general, those patients with hypothermia due to exposure and alcohol intoxication are less likely to have a serious underlying infection than are those who are elderly or who have an underlying medical illness.

Special Therapy
- **Rewarming.** The patient should be rewarmed with the goal of increasing the temperature by 0.5°–2.0°C/hr, although the rate of rewarming has not been shown to be related to outcome.
- **Passive external rewarming**
    - This method depends on the patient's ability to shiver.
    - It is effective only at core temperatures of **32°C or higher.**
    - Remove wet clothing, cover patient with blankets in a warm environment, and monitor.
- **Active external rewarming**
    - Application of heating blankets (40°–45°C) or warm bath immersion. This type of therapy has been feared to cause paradoxical core acidosis, hyperkalemia, and decreased core temperature, as cold stagnant blood returns to the central vasculature,[14] although Danish naval research supports arm and leg rewarming as effective and safe.[15]
    - Pending further investigation, active rewarming is best reserved for young, previously healthy patients with acute hypothermia and minimal pathophysiologic derangement.
- **Active core rewarming is preferred for treatment of severe hypothermia,** although few data are available on outcomes.[16]
    - **Heated oxygen** is the initial therapy of choice for the patient whose cardiovascular status is stable. This therapeutic maneuver can be expected to raise core temperatures by 0.5°–1.2°C/hr.[17] Administration through an endotracheal tube results in more rapid rewarming than delivery via face mask. Administer heated oxygen through a cascade humidifier at a temperature of 45°C or lower.
    - **IV fluids** can be heated in a microwave oven or delivered through a blood warmer; give fluids only through peripheral IV lines.
    - **Heated nasogastric or bladder lavage** is of limited efficacy because of low exposed surface area and is reserved for the patient with cardiovascular instability.
    - **Heated peritoneal lavage** with fluid warmed to 40°–45°C is more effective than is heated aerosol inhalation, but it should be reserved for patients with cardiovascular

instability. Only those who are experienced in its use should perform heated peritoneal lavage, in combination with other modes of rewarming.

- Closed thoracic lavage with heated fluid by thoracostomy tube has been recommended but is unproved.[18]
- **Hemodialysis** can be used for the severely hypothermic, particularly when due to an overdose that is amenable to treatment in this way.
- **Extracorporeal circulation** (cardiac bypass) is used only in hypothermic individuals who are in cardiac arrest; in these cases, it may be dramatically effective.[19] Extracorporeal circulation may raise the temperature as rapidly as 10°–12°C/hr but must be performed in an intensive care unit (ICU) or operating room.

Resuscitation
- Maintain airway and administer oxygen.
- If intubation is required, the most experienced operator should perform it (see Airway Management and Tracheal Intubation in Chapter 8, Critical Care).
- Conduct **cardiopulmonary resuscitation (CPR)** in standard fashion. Perform simultaneous vigorous core rewarming; as long as the core temperature is severely decreased, it should not be assumed that the patient cannot be resuscitated. Reliable defibrillation requires a core temperature of 32°C or higher; prolonged efforts (to a core temperature of 35°C) may be justified because of the neuroprotective effects of hypothermia. **Do not begin CPR if an organized ECG rhythm is present,** as inability to detect peripheral pulses may be due to vasoconstriction, and CPR may precipitate ventricular fibrillation.
- Do not perform Swan-Ganz catheterization, as it may precipitate ventricular fibrillation.
- If ventricular fibrillation occurs, begin CPR as per the advanced cardiac life support (ACLS) protocol. Amiodarone may be administered as per the protocol, although there is no evidence to support its use or guide dosage; some experts suggest reducing the maximum cumulative dose by half. Avoid procainamide because it may precipitate ventricular fibrillation and increase the temperature that is necessary to defibrillate the patient. Rewarming is key.
- Monitor ECG rhythm, urine output, and, possibly, central venous pressure in all patients with an intact circulation.

Disposition
- Admit patients with an underlying disease, physiologic derangement, or core temperature <32°C, preferably to an ICU.
- Discharge individuals with mild hypothermia (32°–35°C) and no predisposing medical conditions or complications when they are normothermic and an adequate home environment can be ensured.

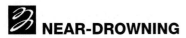

NEAR-DROWNING

GENERAL PRINCIPLES

Definition
- Near-drowning is defined as survival for at least 24 hours after submersion in a liquid medium.

Etiology
- Risk factors include youth, inability to swim, alcohol and drug use, barotrauma (in scuba diving), head and neck trauma, and loss of consciousness associated with epilepsy, diabetes, syncope, or dysrhythmias.

Pathophysiology

- Much has been made of the differences in pathophysiology between fresh- and salt-water drownings. However, the **major insults** [i.e., hypoxemia and tissue hypoxia related to ventilation-perfusion (V/Q) mismatch, acidosis, and hypoxic brain injury with cerebral edema] are common to both.
- Hypothermia, pneumonia, and, rarely, DIC, acute renal failure, and hemolysis also may occur.

DIAGNOSIS

Laboratory Studies

- Obtain serum electrolytes, CBC, and ABGs. Monitor the cardiac rhythm continuously. Obtain blood alcohol level and drug screen if the mental status is not normal.

Imaging

- Obtain chest radiograph.

Other

- Obtain ECG.

TREATMENT

Resuscitation

- Begin with resuscitation, focusing on airway management and ventilation with 100% oxygen.
- Establish an IV line with 0.9% saline or lactated Ringer solution.
- The Heimlich maneuver is not indicated unless upper airway obstruction is present.[21]
- **Immobilize the cervical spine,** as trauma may be present.
- **Treat hypothermia** vigorously (see Cold-Induced Illness).

Medications

- **Reserve antibiotics for documented infection.** Pneumonia may be due to water-borne organisms such as *Pseudomonas*, *Aeromonas*, and *Proteus*.
- **Prophylactic glucocorticoids** have no role.[21]

Complications

- Cerebral edema
  - Cerebral edema may occur suddenly within the first 24 hours and is a major cause of death. Treatment of cerebral edema does not appear to increase survival,[22] and intracranial pressure monitoring does not appear to be effective. Nevertheless, if cerebral edema occurs, hyperventilate the patient to a PCO_2 not lower than 25 mm Hg (to avoid excessive vasoconstriction), and administer mannitol (1–2 g/kg q3–4h) or furosemide (1 mg/kg IV q4–6h).
  - Treat seizures aggressively with **phenytoin.**
  - The routine administration of glucocorticoids is not recommended.
  - Hypothermia or barbiturate "coma" is not indicated.[23]
  - It may be necessary to sedate and paralyze the patient to reduce oxygen consumption and facilitate intracranial pressure management.

- Pulmonary complications
  - Administer 100% oxygen initially, titrating thereafter by ABGs.
  - Intubate the patient endotracheally and begin mechanical ventilation with positive end-expiratory pressure (PEEP) if the patient is apneic, is in severe respiratory distress, or has oxygen-resistant hypoxemia.
  - Administer bronchodilators if bronchospasm is present.
  - Artificial surfactant has not been shown to be useful.[24,25]
- Metabolic complications
  - **Manage metabolic acidosis** with mechanical ventilation, sodium bicarbonate (if the pH is persistently <7.2), and BP support.

Disposition

- Admit patients who have survived severe episodes of near-drowning to an ICU. Non-cardiogenic pulmonary edema may still develop in those individuals with less severe immersions.
- Admit any patient with pulmonary signs or symptoms, including cough, bronchospasm, abnormal ABGs or oxygen saturation as measured by pulse oximetry (SpO_2), or abnormal chest radiograph.
- Observe the asymptomatic patient with a questionable or brief water immersion for 4–6 hours and discharge the patient if the chest radiograph and ABGs are normal.[26] However, if a documented long submersion, unconsciousness, initial cyanosis or apnea, or even a brief requirement for resuscitation has occurred, the patient must be admitted for at least 24 hours.

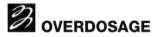 # OVERDOSAGE

GENERAL PRINCIPLES

- **Recognition of poisoning and medication overdose** requires a high index of suspicion and careful clinical evaluation. In the most recent year for which information is available, more than 2.4 million toxic exposures occurred in the United States, resulting in 1,183 deaths.[27] Of these exposures, nearly 200,000 were suicidal (accounting for over half the deaths), about 46,000 due to drug abuse, and over 9,000 malicious (e.g., date-rape drugs).

DIAGNOSIS

History

- Up to 50% of all initial poisoning histories may be incorrect. The ingestion of multiple drugs is common.
- Seek identification of the drug or drugs ingested and their dosages from the patient's family or friends, private physician, pharmacist, and paramedical personnel. Obtain supporting materials (e.g., pill bottles) and clues regarding the timing of ingestion.
- Recognition of specific toxic syndromes is often helpful in directing initial management (Table 25-1).

Clinical Presentation

- Pay particular attention to vital signs, neurologic status, pupillary reactions, cardiovascular response, abdominal findings, and unusual odors and excreta.

Laboratory Studies

- ABGs, serum electrolytes, and acid-base abnormalities may suggest a particular toxin.
- Order baseline screening of liver and kidney function.
- Screening of blood, urine, and gastric aspirate for specific toxic agents is important, but, in most cases, therapy must proceed before such results are available.
- Perform a pregnancy test in women of child-bearing years

Imaging

- **Abdominal radiography** may be useful in detecting retained pills (such as iron).

Other

- Obtain an **ECG** and monitor the cardiac rhythm continuously until the ingested agent is identified and thereafter as appropriate.

Resources

- Although the computerized Poisindex (2006; Micromedex, Greenwood Village, CO) system is helpful, seek additional specific advice from the regional poison control center.

TREATMENT

- **Supportive care** is crucial. **Maintain a patent airway** and adequate ventilation. Intubate the trachea if airway protection is required.
- **Hypotension** usually responds to IV fluids, although vasopressors may be required in refractory cases or in the presence of pulmonary edema. Use dopamine in most situations; choose norepinephrine for overdoses with α antagonists (phenothiazines) and tricyclic antidepressants (due to the proarrhythmic effect of dopamine).
- **Arrhythmias** may be related to cardiac or autonomic effects; treatment depends on the toxin.
- **CNS depression** or coma occurs frequently.
    - When present, administer **naloxone** (2 mg IV) for possible narcotic overdose, give 50% dextrose in water (50 mL IV) or determine finger-stick glucose immediately, administer **thiamine** (100 mg IV push) for possible Wernicke-Korsakoff's syndrome, and give **oxygen** for possible carbon monoxide intoxication.
    - Give **flumazenil** for known or suspected benzodiazepine overdose. However, do not give it for unknown overdoses, as this agent may precipitate seizures in cyclic antidepressant overdose. Also, avoid flumazenil administration in patients who have ingested drugs that are known to cause seizures (cocaine, lithium, theophylline, isoniazid, cyclosporine) or who are known to have a pre-existing seizure disorder.[28]

Prevention of Further Drug Absorption

- Principles
    - Prevention of further drug absorption has traditionally been thought to be facilitated by gastric emptying (gastric lavage, induced emesis), followed by administration of activated charcoal.
        - Gastric emptying procedures, if used, should be initiated within 1 hour of the ingestion.
        - Because most adult overdose patients present several hours after toxic ingestion and because the use of syrup of ipecac may delay subsequent therapy, administration of activated charcoal alone is recommended as the primary gastrointestinal (GI) decontamination procedure for most patients.[29]
    - No difference in outcome appears to occur whether gastric emptying plus charcoal or charcoal administration alone is used.[30,31] Theoretic exceptions may include phenothiazine overdose (delayed gastric emptying) and drugs that form gastric concretions.

TABLE 25-1 Toxic Syndromes and Possible Causes

Syndrome	Manifestations	Possible causes
Acquired hemoglobinopathies	Dyspnea, cyanosis, confusion or lethargy, headache	Carbon monoxide Methemoglobinemia (nitrites, phenazopyridine) Sulfhemoglobinemia
Anion-gap metabolic acidosis	Variable	Methanol Ethanol Ethylene glycol Paraldehyde Iron Isoniazid Salicylate Vacor Cyanide
Anticholinergic	Dry mouth and skin, blurred vision, mydriasis, tachycardia, generalized sunburnlike rash or flushing of skin, hyperthermia, abdominal distention, urinary urgency or retention, confusion, hallucinations, delusions, excitation, or coma	Atropine and other belladonna alkaloids Antihistamines Tricyclics Phenothiazines Jimson seeds
Cholinergic	Hypersalivation, bronchorrhea, bronchospasm, urination or defecation, neuromuscular failure, lacrimation	Acetylcholine Organophosphate insecticides Bethanechol Methacholine Wild mushrooms

Syndrome	Clinical features	Agents
Cyanide	Nausea, vomiting, collapse, coma, bradycardia, no cyanosis, decreased arteriovenous O_2 difference with severe metabolic acidosis	Cyanide Amygdalin
Extrapyramidal	Dysphoria and dysphagia, trismus, oculogyric crisis, rigidity, torticollis, laryngospasm	Prochlorperazine Haloperidol Chlorpromazine and other antipsychotics Other phenothiazines
Narcotic	Central nervous system depression, respiratory depression, miosis, hypotension	Morphine and heroin Codeine Propoxyphene Other synthetic and semisynthetic opiates
Salicylism	Fever, hyperpnea, respiratory alkalosis or mixed acid-base disturbance, hypokalemia, tinnitus	Aspirin Other salicylate products
Sympathomimetic	Excitation, hypertension, cardiac arrhythmias, seizures	Amphetamines Cocaine Caffeine Aminophylline β Agonists, inhaled or injected

Source: Modified from Quick G, Crocker PJ. Toxic emergency: agent unknown. *Emerg Decisions* 1986;7:44. Reprinted with permission from Physicians World/Thomson Healthcare, Secaucus, NJ.

- **Activated charcoal**
  - Treatment adsorbs most drugs, preventing further absorption from the GI tract. Exceptions include alkalis, arsenic and other heavy metals, hydrocarbons, cyanide, ethanol (EtOH) and other alcohols, lithium, ferrous sulfate, carbamate, and mineral acids. It is not indicated for these ingestions.
    - Activated charcoal also promotes efflux of selected drugs (theophylline, phenobarbital, and carbamazepine) from the blood into the bowel lumen.
  - Do not use activated charcoal when bowel obstruction or perforation is present or when endoscopy is contemplated.
  - When repeated dosing is used, no more than a single dose of sorbitol or other cathartic should be given. Although **multidose charcoal** has been shown to increase selected drug elimination significantly, it has not yet been demonstrated in a controlled study to reduce mortality in poisoned patients.
  - It is indicated in ingestions of life-threatening amounts of carbamazepine, phenobarbital, theophylline, quinine, dapsone, paraquat, and Amanita phalloides.[33,34] It may be of use in overdoses of amitriptyline, cyclosporine, dextropropoxyphene, diazepam, digitoxin, digoxin, disopyramide, methotrexate, nadolol, phencyclidine, phenylbutazone, phenytoin, piroxicam, sotalol, and valproate. Its use in salicylate overdose is controversial.
  - Give an initial dose of 50–100 g and repeat that dose every 4 hours until the patient's condition and laboratory parameters improve. Prehospital administration further enhances recovery. Evidence to support its use more than 1 hour after toxic ingestion is unavailable, and many experts do not recommend its administration after that interval.[32] If the patient is obtunded or has an absent gag reflex, the **airway must be protected;** endotracheal intubation may be necessary.
- **Ipecac**
  - Because there is no evidence to show that administration of **ipecac** improves outcome and there is some evidence to suggest an increase in complications,[35] and because of its many contraindications, routine use in the emergency center has largely been abandoned.[36]
  - **Contraindications** to ipecac use include decreased level of consciousness, absent gag reflex, caustic ingestion, convulsions or exposure to a substance that is likely to cause convulsions, and medical conditions that make emesis unsafe. Do not give ipecac for ingestion of unknown toxins, as aspiration may occur if coma or seizures develop.
- **Gastric lavage**
  - Gastric lavage should not be used routinely in the management of the poisoned patient. Exceptions include ingestions of a life-threatening amount of toxin when the patient presents within 60 minutes[37] or when concretions are believed to be present. Use a large orogastric tube (No. 28–36 Fr.) for these patients.
  - **Contraindications** include corrosive ingestion. Lavage should not be performed with an unprotected airway if the patient has lost airway protective reflexes or has ingested hydrocarbons with a high aspiration potential. In these cases, lavage should be performed only **after endotracheal intubation.** Lavage with 200-mL boluses of warm saline, repeated until the effluent is clear, and follow this by instillation of activated charcoal.
- The use of a **cathartic** is not supported by clinical evidence and is therefore not routinely recommended.[38] If used, give no more than a single dose.
  - Acceptable forms:
    - Magnesium citrate, 4 mL/kg (300 mL maximum)
    - Sorbitol, 1–2 g/kg (150 g maximum)
    - Magnesium or sodium sulfate, 25–30 g
    - Do not give magnesium salts to patients with renal failure.
- **Whole-bowel irrigation**
  - Commercially available polyethylene glycol bowel preparation solution should not be used routinely in the management of the poisoned patient,[39] as there is no conclusive evidence that it improves outcomes.
  - **Exceptions** can be considered for toxic ingestions of sustained-release drugs such as β-adrenergic antagonists, calcium channel antagonists, lithium, and theophylline.

Evidence is insufficient either to support or exclude its use for iron ingestion with radiographically persistent tablets in the GI tract or body packing with heroin or cocaine.
- It is contraindicated in the presence of bowel obstruction, ileus, intestinal perforation, and hemodynamic instability and should not be administered to a patient with a compromised unprotected airway.
- Administer 1–2 L/hr to a total of 10 L; it can be discontinued earlier if the rectal effluent is clear. Obtain an abdominal radiograph to document clearance of iron or drug-containing packets.
- **Endoscopic or surgical removal, or both**
  - These should be considered only for ingestion of life-threatening agents that have not been or cannot be effectively removed by the above measures, such as button batteries lodged in the esophagus and pharmacobezoars of highly toxic materials and for cocaine body packers with severe toxicity due to rupture of a packet.
  - Endoscopy should not be performed to remove unruptured drug packets, as this intervention may result in rupture and greater toxicity.

Removal of Absorbed Drugs

- Removal can be achieved by enhancement of renal excretion and extracorporeal methods.
  - **Use forced diuresis only when specifically indicated** because of the risk of causing acid-base disturbances, electrolyte abnormalities, and cerebral or pulmonary edema. Do not attempt forced diuresis in patients with renal insufficiency, cardiac disease, or existing electrolyte abnormalities. Few data support the efficacy of this procedure in improving survival.
  - **Forced alkaline diuresis,** achieving a urinary pH of 7.5–9.0, promotes excretion of drugs that are weak acids, such as salicylates, barbital, and phenobarbital. Administer a solution of sodium bicarbonate, 44–100 mEq, added to 1 L 0.45% saline, at 250–500 mL/hr for the first 1–2 hours. Concomitant administration of potassium chloride may be necessary to treat diuresis-induced hypokalemia and to achieve urinary alkalinization. Exercise great care to avoid excessive volume expansion, especially in the elderly. Administer maintenance alkaline solution and diuretics to maintain a urinary output of 2–3 mL/kg/hr.
  - **Forced acid diuresis** is not recommended for any agent.

Extracorporeal Removal of Specific Toxins by Hemodialysis or Hemoperfusion

- Hemodialysis or hemoperfusion may be used when:
  - Clinical deterioration persists despite intensive supportive therapy
  - Blood levels reach potentially lethal concentrations
  - A risk of lethal delayed effects exists
  - Renal or hepatic failure impairs clearance of toxin. Common toxins that can be removed by hemodialysis include toxic alcohols, salicylates, theophylline, and lithium. Generally, compounds with low molecular weight, small volume of distribution, and low degree of protein binding of drug are amenable to removal by hemodialysis.

Antidotes

- **Specific antidotes** are available that neutralize or prevent the toxic effect of certain drugs (Table 25-2). For information on the pharmacokinetics of the offending agent and specific treatment guidelines, contact the regional poison control center immediately if the drug that was ingested is known.

Disposition

- Observe even those patients with apparently trivial overdoses of potentially toxic agents for at least **4 hours** before contemplating their discharge. Do not discharge any patient

TABLE 25-2 Antidotes

Poison or toxic sign	Antidote	Adult dosage
Acetaminophen	N-Acetylcysteine	140 mg/kg PO, followed by 70 mg/kg q4h for 17 doses
Anticholinesterases	Atropine sulfate	15 mg IV (IM, SC) q15min PRN to drying of secretions
	Pralidoxime (2-PAM) chloride[a]	1 g IV (PO) over 15–30 min q8–12h three doses PRN
Benzodiazepines	Flumazenil	0.2 mg (2 mL) IV over 30 sec, followed by 0.3 mg at 1-min intervals to a total dose of 3 mg
Carbon monoxide	Oxygen	100%, hyperbaric
Cyanide	Amyl nitrite[b] followed by	Inhalation pearls for 15–30 sec every min
	Sodium nitrite[b] followed by	300 mg (10 mL 3% solution) IV over 3 min, repeated in half dosage in 2 hr if persistent or recurrent signs of toxicity
	Sodium thiosulfate	12.5 g (50 mL 25% solution) IV over 10 min, repeated in half dosage in 2 hr if persistent or recurrent signs of toxicity
Digoxin	Antidigoxin Fab' fragments	Acute ingestion: Dose (vials) = [ingested digoxin (mg)] × 0.8]/0.5
		Chronic ingestion: Dose (vials) = [serum level (ng/mL) × weight (kg)]/100, infused in 0.9% saline over 15–30 min; repeat if toxicity persists
Ethylene glycol (EG)	Fomepizole	15 mg/kg IV, followed by 10 mg/kg IV q12h for four doses, followed by 15 mg/kg IV q12h until the EG level <20 mg/dL
	Ethanol[c]	0.6 g/kg in D5W IV (PO) over 30–45 min, followed initially by 110 mg/kg/hr to maintain a blood level of 100–150 mg/dL
Extrapyramidal signs	Diphenhydramine hydrochloride	25–50 mg IV (IM, PO) PRN
	Benztropine mesylate	1–2 mg IV (IM, PO) PRN
Heavy metals (e.g., arsenic, copper, gold, lead, mercury)	Chelators[d]	
	Calcium disodium edetate (EDTA)	1 g IV (IM) over 1 hr q12h
	Dimercaprol (BAL)	2.5–5.0 mg/kg IM q46h
	Penicillamine	250–500 mg PO q6h
	2,3-Dimercaptosuccinic acid (DMSA, Succimer)	10 mg/kg PO tid × 5 d, then bid × 14 d

	Deferoxamine mesylate	1 g IM (IV at a rate 15 mg/kg/hr if hypotension) q8h PRN
Iron		
Isoniazid (INH)	Pyridoxine	Amount equal to estimated INH ingestion up to 5 g over 30–60 min; any remainder by IV drip over 12 hr
Methanol	Ethanol[c]	See Ethylene glycol
Methemoglobinemia	Methylene blue	1–2 mg/kg (0.1–0.2 mL/kg 1% solution) IV over 5 min, repeated in 1 hr PRN
Opioids	Naloxone hydrochloride	0.4–2.0 mg IV (IM, SC, endotracheally) PRN
Warfarin and related drugs	Vitamin K1 (phytonadione)	10 mg IM, SC, or IV[e]
	Fresh frozen plasma	Variable

D$_5$W, 5% dextrose in water.
Note: This table is only a guide. Antidote usage and dosage depend on the specific clinical situation. The regional poison control center should be contacted for specific therapeutic recommendations.

[a]Pralidoxime is indicated in severe organophosphate poisoning with muscle weakness or fasciculations or respiratory depression.
[b]Nitrites may have an antidotal effect in hydrogen sulfide poisoning.
[c]The requisite ethanol dose depends on prior alcohol use, liver function, and dialysis. Consult the regional poison control center for assistance.
[d]The use of a specific chelating agent or combination of agents depends on the heavy metal involved and on the clinical situation.
[e]Caution should be used when giving vitamin K1 IV. It should be given over 20 minutes.

who has taken an intentional overdose without formal psychiatric consultation and assessment of disposition.

- Refer individuals who experience inadvertent recreational drug overdose for counseling and, possibly, detoxification.
- Patients who are considered potentially suicidal require constant one-on-one supervision while on the medical service.

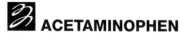 **ACETAMINOPHEN**

GENERAL PRINCIPLES

- Acetaminophen is a common ingredient in many analgesic and antipyretic preparations. Because of this, ingredients of over-the-counter medications taken in overdose should be examined carefully.
- Hepatic toxicity is due to depletion of hepatic **glutathione** and subsequent accumulation of a toxic intermediate metabolite, N-acetyl-p-benzoquinoneimine. Toxicity usually occurs after acute ingestion of more than 140 mg/kg, or at least 7.5 g. Precise determination of probable toxicity can be obtained by plotting a plasma acetaminophen level (drawn at least 4 hours after ingestion) on a nomogram in relation to the time since ingestion (Fig. 25-1). However, nearly half of hospitalizations for acetaminophen toxicity are due to toxicity from chronic ingestion, which is increased in those with excess alcohol intake.[40]
- The nomogram does not provide useful information regarding toxicity of chronic ingestion, however. In this instance, treatment is recommended if there is evidence of liver toxicity and the acetaminophen level is >10 mcg/mL. If in doubt, consult with an expert in clinical toxicology or hepatology, or both.
- The nomogram is also of uncertain usefulness in acute overdose of sustained-release products. In this latter situation, the Rocky Mountain Poison Center recommends that a second drug level be obtained 4–6 hours after the first; if either level falls in the possibly toxic range, antidotal therapy is advised.[41]

DIAGNOSIS

- **Symptoms** during the first 24 hours include anorexia, vomiting, and diaphoresis.
- Hepatic enzymes begin to rise 24–36 hours after ingestion and peak (aspartate aminotransferase earliest) 72–96 hours after ingestion. Recovery starts after approximately 4 days unless hepatic failure develops.

TREATMENT

- **Treatment** includes supportive measures and GI decontamination.
- Gastric lavage is not indicated.
- Do not administer ipecac, as its use delays administration of the specific antidote.
- Administer activated charcoal as soon as possible after the ingestion. Charcoal appears to provide an additional hepatoprotective effect.[42]
- When the history suggests that a toxic dose has been ingested, do not wait for return of the blood acetaminophen level to administer the first dose of **acetylcysteine (Mucomyst)**, a specific antidote that acts as a glutathione substrate. This antidote is most effective in preventing hepatotoxicity if given within 8 hours of ingestion and is recommended up to 24 hours; it may be helpful when administered up to 36 hours after the event if hepatotoxicity is evident.[43]
    - The initial dose is 140 mg/kg diluted to a 5% solution in a soft drink, juice, or water, given PO or by gastric tube; **it can be given simultaneously with charcoal** without impairment of its efficacy.
    - Subsequent administration (70 mg/kg q4h for a total of 17 doses) is directed by the initial plasma acetaminophen level. **If a toxic level is detected, give the full 17 doses;** if

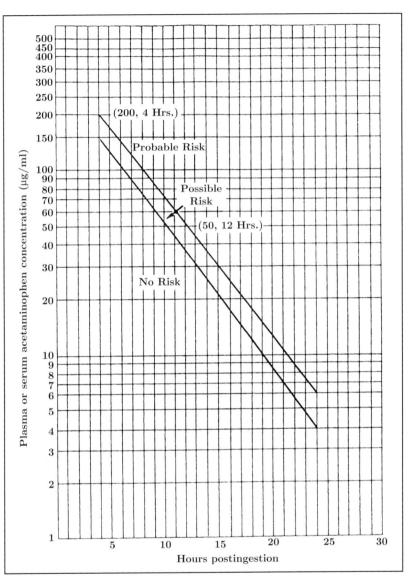

Figure 25-1. Nomogram for acetaminophen hepatotoxicity. (Adapted from Rumack BH, Peterson RC, Koch GG, et al. Acetaminophen overdose: 662 cases with evaluation of oral acetylcysteine treatment. *Arch Intern Med* 1981;141:380.)

not, no further antidote is indicated. If vomiting occurs <1 hour after administration of the antidote, repeat the dose.

- If vomiting is repetitive and interferes with acetylcysteine administration, use metoclopramide or droperidol, or administer acetylcysteine via a fluoroscopically placed nasoduodenal tube over a period of 30–60 minutes.

- IV acetylcysteine is now U.S. Food and Drug Administration (FDA) approved and available commercially as **Acetadote®**. It should be considered for those who cannot or will not take oral acetylcysteine or who have bowel obstruction, GI bleeding, or fulminant hepatic failure.
  - It should be considered for use in the pregnant patient. The initial dosage is 150 mg/kg IV over 1 hour in 200 mL 5% dextrose in water (D_5W), followed by 50 mg/kg in 500 mL over 4 hours, followed by 100 mg/kg in 500 mL over 16 hours.
  - Side effects include bronchospasm, rash, flushing, and anaphylactoid reaction and are generally dose related. Flushing requires no treatment; treat urticaria with diphenhydramine. Give albuterol and corticosteroids for bronchospasm. Treat angioedema with diphenhydramine, epinephrine, and corticosteroids. Consider administration of IV cimetidine. Administration of acetylcysteine can be safely resumed 1 hour after successful treatment.[44]
- Obtain baseline aspartate transaminase (AST), alanine transaminase (ALT), bilirubin level, BUN, and prothrombin time or international normalized ratio (INR) and repeat these readings at least daily for 3 days. Obtain hepatology consultation for consideration of orthotopic liver transplantation if there is biochemical evidence of hepatic failure. Transplantation is considered if the pH is <7.3 after 24 hours or the prothrombin time is >100 seconds (international normalized ratio >6.5) and grade 3–4 coma is present and the creatinine is >3.4 mg/dL.

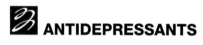

ANTIDEPRESSANTS

CYCLIC ANTIDEPRESSANTS

General Principles

- Traditional tricyclic antidepressants include amitriptyline, imipramine, desipramine, nortriptyline, doxepin, and protriptyline.
- Pharmacologic actions include central and peripheral anticholinergic activity, depression of myocardial contractility, slowing of intraventricular and atrioventricular conduction, and CNS effects that are similar to those of phenothiazines. Despite the widespread use of the much safer selective serotonin reuptake inhibitor antidepressants, overdose with cyclic antidepressants is still the third-leading cause of drug overdose–related death in the United States.[27]
- Overdoses of <20 mg/kg cause few fatalities; 35 mg/kg is the approximate median lethal dose, and overdoses in excess of 50 mg/kg are likely to result in death.
- Next-generation cyclic antidepressants include amoxapine and loxapine (tricyclics with diminished cardiovascular toxicity but increased propensity to severe seizures), maprotiline (a tetracyclic with greater seizure proclivity and cardiovascular toxicity similar to that of older tricyclics), mianserin (a tetracyclic with low propensity for cardiovascular or neurologic toxicity), and trazodone (a noncyclic with minimal cardiovascular and CNS toxicity).
- Still newer antidepressants include mirtazapine, venlafaxine, bupropion, and nefazodone. Limited data suggest that mirtazapine is relatively nontoxic in overdose.[45] Venlafaxine is also relatively nontoxic in overdose.

Diagnosis

Clinical Presentation

- **Clinical manifestations** include evidence of cholinergic blockade (mydriasis, ileus, urinary retention, and hyperpyrexia).
  - **Cardiovascular toxicity** occurs as a result of anticholinergic, catecholamine-related, quinidinelike, and α-antagonist effects; these effects result in supraventricular and ventricular arrhythmias, including torsades de pointes, conduction blocks, hypotension, hypoperfusion, and pulmonary edema.

■ **CNS manifestations** range from initial agitation to confusion, stupor, and coma. Seizures may occur, and the resultant metabolic acidosis may worsen cardiac toxicity.

■ Symptoms of bupropion overdose include labored breathing, salivation, arched back, ataxia, and convulsions. Symptoms of nefazadone overdose include drowsiness, vomiting, hypotension, tachycardia, incontinence, and coma.

Laboratory Studies

■ Laboratory studies aid in assessing the severity of the condition and in monitoring progress. Plasma levels correlate poorly with severity of symptoms, although blood levels >1,000 ng/mL have a higher risk of cardiac toxicity. ABGs are useful for ensuring adequate gas exchange and for monitoring alkalinization. ECGs showing limb-lead QRS duration of >100 ms are predictive of seizures; duration >160 ms predicts ventricular dysrhythmias; a terminal 40-ms QRS axis that is more rightward than 120 degrees is even more sensitive.[46,47]

Treatment

■ The course of therapy includes supportive measures and GI decontamination.

■ Do not administer ipecac syrup, as obtundation may occur rapidly and promote aspiration.

■ Gastric lavage theoretically may be performed regardless of the time of presentation, as cyclic antidepressants delay gastric emptying; however, clinical studies do not show a difference in patients treated in this way versus those given activated charcoal only.[48]

■ Repetitive administration of activated charcoal, 50 g PO or per tube q2–4h, is not routinely recommended.

■ Forced diuresis and hemodialysis are not indicated. Resin or charcoal hemoperfusion removes <1%–3% of body burden, but this reduction may be associated with improvement of life-threatening cardiac or CNS complications.

■ **Continuous cardiac monitoring is mandatory.** Cyclic antidepressants are protein bound in an alkaline environment and are toxic in an acid environment. Cardiac (and CNS) toxicity therefore is enhanced by metabolic or respiratory acidosis. Initiate treatment prophylactically, as toxic complications often are refractory to therapy once they have developed.

■ Induce **alkalinization** with IV sodium bicarbonate, 1–2 mEq/kg, to maintain an arterial pH of 7.45–7.55. Such an alkaline pH is effective in preventing and treating hypotension, arrhythmias (ventricular and supraventricular), and conduction disturbances. If the patient is intubated, hyperventilate to a PCO_2 of no lower than 25 mm Hg and an arterial pH of 7.45–7.55, as this is an effective means of alkalinization and avoids the administration of large amounts of sodium.

■ Manage ventricular arrhythmias refractory to alkalinization with lidocaine or phenytoin (see Chapter 7, Cardiac Arrhythmias). **Type Ia antiarrhythmics** (procainamide, quinidine, or disopyramide) **are contraindicated** because of additive toxicity. Treat torsades de pointes with magnesium, isoproterenol, and atrial overdrive pacing (see Chapter 7, Cardiac Arrhythmias). Do not use physostigmine unless all other measures for life-threatening arrhythmias have failed. Use temporary ventricular pacing for complete heart block. Treat hypotension that is unresponsive to alkalinization with norepinephrine and fluid administration.

■ **CNS complications.** Alkalinization does not reverse CNS complications. Physostigmine (2 mg IV over 1 minute) reverses CNS depression rapidly in patients with pure cyclic antidepressant overdose. However, because repeated doses are necessary and physostigmine may cause dysrhythmias and seizures, its use is not recommended for coma. Supportive care of coma usually is adequate. Treat seizures with diazepam and phenytoin (see Chapter 24, Neurologic Disorders). Barbiturates are preferred over phenytoin for drug-induced seizures by some but not all authorities. Status epilepticus should be treated aggressively, including the use of high-dose barbiturates, paralysis, and general anesthesia, to prevent permanent neurologic damage. Treat hyperthermia by cooling.

- **Respiratory depression.** Treat this commonly occurring complication with endotracheal intubation and mechanical ventilation. Pulmonary edema and aspiration also are common.
- **Disposition.** Patients should be admitted to an ICU if they have a depressed level of consciousness, respiratory depression, hypotension, arrhythmia, conduction blocks (including QRS >100 ms), or seizures. Observe any asymptomatic individual with a normal ECG in the emergency department and perform cardiac monitoring of such a patient for 6 hours. If the patient remains asymptomatic, the ECG remains normal, and bowel sounds are normal, the patient may safely undergo assessment for psychiatric disposition. If any signs or symptoms are present, the patient must be admitted. **Caution is imperative:** 25% of fatalities occur in patients who are awake and alert at the time of presentation, and three-fourths of these patients are in normal sinus rhythm. After a patient's admission, criteria for discharge from an ICU include normal mental status, absence of all cyclic antidepressant symptoms, and no ECG abnormalities (including sinus tachycardia) for 24 hours. Significant arrhythmias rarely develop in a patient who meets all these criteria.

SELECTIVE SEROTONIN REUPTAKE INHIBITORS

- Commonly available selective serotonin reuptake inhibitors (SSRIs) include fluoxetine, sertraline, paroxetine, fluvoxamine, and citalopram.

Diagnosis

- **Symptoms** are usually minimal.
  - Patients may become agitated or drowsy or, occasionally, confused.
  - Ataxia, vertigo, tremor, delusions, or hallucinations may occur, as may nausea and emesis.
  - Seizures are rare, occurring most often after fluoxetine or citalopram overdose.[49,50]
  - Tachycardia is noted frequently; however, ECG changes and significant cardiovascular toxicity are uncommon, although severe citalopram overdose may have QT prolongation. Fatalities are rare.[51]
  - Simultaneous ingestion of these drugs with tricyclic antidepressants may raise plasma levels of the tricyclic. If they are ingested with other drugs that cause serotonin release, such as clomipramine, monoamine oxidase inhibitors, and l-tryptophan, the serotonin syndrome may result.

Treatment

- **Avoid emesis.** GI lavage may be considered if the patient presents <1 hour after ingestion. Administer activated charcoal. Although cardiovascular and CNS toxicity rarely occur, obtain an ECG as a baseline.
- Admit patients who have taken large overdoses to a medical floor, particularly if they are symptomatic or if there is coingestion. Treat seizures with diazepam and phenytoin.
- If the patient is asymptomatic and medically stable after 6 hours of observation, psychiatric evaluation and disposition assessment can be made safely.

SEROTONIN SYNDROME

- Serotonin syndrome occurs most frequently after ingestion of two or more drugs that increase serotonin levels by different mechanisms.
- Examples include monoamine oxidase inhibitors, l-tryptophan, amphetamines, cocaine, 3,4-methylenedioxymethamphetamine (MDMA), fenfluramine, serotonin reuptake inhibitors, tricyclic antidepressants, sumatriptan, amantadine, levodopa, and bromocriptine.

Symptoms

- Symptoms include agitation, confusion, hallucinations, myoclonus, diaphoresis, tremor, shivering, nystagmus, diarrhea, and fever. Drowsiness may progress to coma. Seizures may occur.
- Autonomic effects include tachycardia, hypertension, tachypnea, mydriasis, flushing, salivation, abdominal pain, hyperreflexia, and diarrhea.
- **Hyperthermia** is characteristic. Rigidity, trismus, and opisthotonus may be present.
- Severe complications include DIC, rhabdomyolysis and renal failure, respiratory failure, and ARDS.

Treatment

- Treatment is supportive with the administration of activated charcoal.
- Emesis should not be induced.
- Consider benzodiazepines for agitation.
- Treat hyperthermia with cooling.
- Diazepam and phenytoin can be given for seizures.
- Hypertension can be treated with sedation and, if necessary, nitroprusside. If IV saline is unsuccessful for hypotension, administer norepinephrine.
- Protect the airway and provide ventilatory support for respiratory failure.
- Consider the administration of cyproheptadine, 4–8 mg q1–4h, until improvement occurs or a total of 32 mg is given.

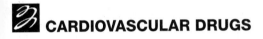

CARDIOVASCULAR DRUGS

β-ADRENERGIC ANTAGONISTS

General Principles

- **Symptoms** usually occur within 2 hours of ingestion.
- Cardiovascular manifestations include bradycardia, atrioventricular block, hypotension, and depression of cardiac function, which results in CHF. Sotalol may cause QT prolongation and torsades de pointes. Bradycardia occurs early but does not predict more serious cardiac disturbances.
- Although some β_1-specific agents may have little respiratory effect at the standard dosage in patients with asthma or chronic obstructive pulmonary disease, severe bronchospasm may result from ingestion of any β-adrenergic antagonist, because β_1 selectivity is lost at high doses.
- CNS manifestations include drowsiness, coma, hypoventilation, and seizures (caused most frequently by propranolol).
- Nausea and vomiting may occur, and mesenteric ischemia may be severe, particularly with propranolol ingestion, as a result of decreased cardiac output and unopposed α-agonist activity.
- β-Adrenergic antagonist overdose may cause hypoglycemia by blockade of counterregulatory mechanisms and may also make the appreciation of hypoglycemic symptoms more difficult.
- Renal failure may occur as a result of hypotension.

Diagnosis

Laboratory Studies

- Measurement of serum drug levels is not useful. Obtain serum glucose and electrolyte levels. Record a baseline ECG and monitor cardiac activity continuously.

Treatment

- Establish an IV line before any other therapy is undertaken.
- Consider gastric lavage if the patient is seen within 1 hour of ingestion of a potentially life-threatening amount, and administer activated charcoal. A second dose of activated charcoal for sustained-release preparation overdose has been recommended by some because of the theoretical potential for drug desorption, but there is no clinical evidence to support this.
- **Do not give syrup of ipecac** because of the rapidity with which cardiac compromise may occur. Moreover, the increase in vagal tone associated with emesis may promote cardiovascular collapse.
- If the patient becomes bradycardic or has other manifestations of a vagal reaction, administer up to 2 mg atropine IV.
- Consider multidose charcoal for sotalol ingestion.
- Treat hypotension with IV saline; hemodynamic monitoring may be necessary to gauge optimal fluid resuscitation.
  - **Glucagon** (50–150 mcg/kg IV over 1 minute, followed by 1–5 mg/hr in 5% dextrose) increases cardiac contractility and heart rate and is the drug of first choice for β-adrenergic antagonist overdose.
  - Isoproterenol (2–20 mcg/min) may be useful, but high doses (200 mcg/min) may be necessary.
  - If the BP does not improve or falls, add norepinephrine.
  - Use epinephrine with caution, particularly with propranolol overdoses, because of the propensity for hypertension and reflex bradycardia.
  - Calcium chloride 10%, 10 mL IV, may also be useful for refractory propranolol overdose.
  - Consider intra-aortic balloon pump for refractory hypotension.
- For torsades de pointes associated with sotalol overdose, isoproterenol, magnesium, and overdrive pacing may be useful (see Chapter 7, Cardiac Arrhythmias). A pacemaker may be necessary for severe bradycardia or heart block that is unresponsive to medications.
- Use β-adrenergic agonists and theophylline for bronchospasm.
- Treat seizures with IV benzodiazepine followed by IV phenytoin.
- Treat hypoglycemia with IV glucose and, if resistant, IV glucagon.
- Severe respiratory depression may require mechanical ventilation.
- Dialysis may be useful in removal of nadolol, sotalol, atenolol, and acebutolol but is ineffective for propranolol, metoprolol, and timolol.
- **Disposition.** Obtain a baseline ECG and monitor the patient's rhythm for at least 6 hours, even in the absence of symptoms. If any cardiovascular, respiratory, or neurologic symptoms are present, admit the patient to an ICU for therapy and continuous monitoring. If, however, no toxic symptoms have occurred 6 hours after ingestion, disposition guided by psychiatric consultation can be made safely.

CALCIUM CHANNEL ANTAGONISTS

General Principles

- Manifestations of calcium channel antagonist overdose depend on the drug ingested. Hypotension is common, as are nausea and vomiting.
- Severe bradycardia, atrioventricular block, and asystole are most common after verapamil and diltiazem overdose and less common with the dihydropyridines (e.g., nifedipine, nicardipine, amlodipine), which are more likely to cause reflex tachycardia.
- Pulmonary edema is most likely to occur after verapamil overdose, as is hypocalcemia. Lethargy, confusion, and coma are common. Seizures are most often due to verapamil, less common with diltiazem, and rare with nifedipine. Hyperglycemia occurs frequently.
- Cardiovascular manifestations usually are apparent within 1–5 hours after ingestion and may persist for more than 24 hours.

- Sustained-release preparations, particularly verapamil, may cause rhythm disturbances up to 7 days after ingestion.

Diagnosis

Laboratory Studies
- Obtain serum calcium, magnesium, electrolyte, and glucose levels.
- Blood levels of the drugs are not generally available or useful.

Other
- Obtain an ECG and monitor the cardiac rhythm. Monitor oxygenation by pulse oximetry, and obtain a chest radiograph.

Treatment

- Gastric decontamination
  - **Avoid inducing emesis** because of the potential for rapid cardiovascular collapse and aspiration.
  - If the patient presents soon after ingestion, consider gastric lavage followed by administration of charcoal.
  - Consider gastroscopy or whole-bowel irrigation with polyethylene glycol solution for removal of retained sustained-release tablets.
  - A second dose of activated charcoal for sustained-release preparation overdose has been recommended by some because of the theoretical potential for drug desorption, but there is no clinical evidence to support this.
- Medications
  - **Treat hypotension** with IV 0.9% saline; if resistant, give IV dopamine.
  - Administer 10% **calcium chloride** (10–20 mL IV) for hypotension, bradycardia, or heart block. Repeat at 10-minute intervals three to four times as necessary.
  - Calcium gluconate (3 g) is preferred when the patient is severely acidotic. A calcium gluconate drip at up to 2 g/hr can be titrated to BP, with monitoring of ECG and serum calcium.
  - **Glucagon** (50–150 mcg/kg IV over 1 minute followed by 1–5 mg/hr) may also be useful for heart block and hypotension.
  - Insulin infusion, 0.1–1.0 unit/kg/hr with sufficient dextrose to maintain a normal blood glucose, has also been reported to be successful.
  - If hypotension is resistant to the preceding measures, arrange for placement of an intra-aortic balloon pump.
  - Atropine (up to 2 mg IV) can also be given for **bradycardia or atrioventricular block,** although it rarely is successful.
  - Isoproterenol is a less desirable alternative.
  - Place a transvenous pacemaker for medication-resistant heart block.
- Treat seizures with an IV benzodiazepine (diazepam or lorazepam; see Chapter 24, Neurologic Disorders) and phenytoin.
- Hemodialysis and hemoperfusion are not useful to accelerate drug removal.
- **Disposition.** Admit all patients who have cardiovascular symptoms or seizures or who have ingested a sustained-release preparation to an ICU for continuous cardiovascular monitoring. If the patient has taken a non–sustained-release preparation and is asymptomatic, obtain a baseline ECG and monitor ECG rhythm for at least 8 hours. If, at that point, the patient is completely asymptomatic and has a normal ECG, consider discharge after psychiatric consultation.

DIGOXIN

See Chapter 7, Cardiac Arrhythmias, for details; for doses of Fab' fragments, see Table 25-2.

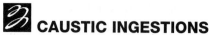 CAUSTIC INGESTIONS

ALKALINE INGESTIONS

- Substances include liquid and crystalline lye, automatic dishwasher detergents, oven cleaners, hair relaxers, and some toilet bowl cleaners.
- Strong alkali solutions, such as liquid drain cleaner, are the agents most commonly associated with injury.

Diagnosis

Symptoms and Signs

- Deep tissue injury in the aerodigestive tract is common. Oral burns are common and may cause drooling. A lack of oral burns does not exclude esophageal injury. The overall rate of esophageal injury for alkali ingestions is 30%–40%; such injury is suggested by vomiting, drooling, or stridor.
- Esophageal perforation may occur and result in mediastinitis. Esophageal stricture may develop as a late complication.
- Gastric injury and perforation also may occur and are much more likely with liquid lye ingestions, as the lye passes rapidly into the stomach.
- Crystalline lye ingestion may lead to severe upper airway injury with stridor and airway obstruction that necessitate rapid intervention.
- Other symptoms of alkaline ingestion include oral pain, odynophagia, chest pain, abdominal pain, nausea, and vomiting.

Imaging

- Obtain chest and abdominal radiographs for evidence of perforation (pneumomediastinum, pleural effusion, and pneumoperitoneum).

Laboratory Studies

- Obtain CBC, electrolytes, BUN, creatinine, and coagulation parameters.
- If there are signs suggesting severe burns or perforation, type and cross-match blood.

Treatment

- Immediately rinse the oral cavity copiously with cold water.
- Do not induce emesis because it may increase injury.
- Charcoal administration, cathartic administration, and gastric lavage are **not** indicated. Administration of charcoal obscures anatomic detail for subsequent endoscopy.
- Diluents are controversial and may induce emesis. Poisindex[52] currently recommends administration of diluents (no more than 8 oz milk or water), although other experts strongly disagree, and an update on the Poisindex consensus has not been reported since 1988.
- Do not attempt to neutralize the alkaline agent with a weak acid, as this results in an exothermic reaction and increases tissue damage.
- Protect the airway and administer oxygen. Endotracheal intubation or early tracheostomy may be required.
- Avoid use of a nasogastric tube.
- Establish an IV line and give fluids guided by vital signs.
- Monitor the cardiac rhythm and oximetry.
- Glucocorticoid treatment of esophageal burns in an attempt to prevent stricture is controversial and generally not recommended.
- Prophylactic antibiotics are not appropriate.

Referrals

- If the patient exhibits drooling, stridor, or odynophagia, consult a gastroenterologist to arrange for immediate endoscopy; otherwise, it can be deferred 12–24 hours.
- Obtain surgical consultation.
- **Disposition** will depend on the results of the evaluation above.

Follow-Up

- Obtain a barium swallow after 2–4 weeks to assess for esophageal stricture.

ACIDS

General Principles

- Common household acids include most toilet bowl cleaners, drain cleaners, metal cleaners, battery acid, and swimming pool cleaners.
- Tissue injury is generally less deep than that produced by alkaline agents.
- Gastric and esophageal injuries including perforation are common. Pyloric stricture may result.

Diagnosis

- **Symptoms** include oral pain, drooling, odynophagia, and abdominal pain.
- Severe cases may have respiratory distress, DIC, hemolysis, and systemic acidosis.

Imaging
- Obtain an upright chest radiograph to detect perforation.

Laboratory Studies
- Obtain CBC, prothrombin time, partial thromboplastin time, platelet count, electrolytes, BUN, and creatinine.
- In severe burns, type and cross-match.

Treatment

- Wash mouth out copiously with cold water.
- Diluent administration often is recommended (with the same caveats as noted above for alkaline ingestions) but has no demonstrated clinical efficacy.
- Neutralization with a weak base is contraindicated.
- **Induction of emesis, gastric lavage, and charcoal administration are all contraindicated, and a nasogastric tube should be avoided.**
- Establish IV access and administer fluids guided by vital signs.
- Sucralfate (1 g q6h) may decrease symptoms but does not appear to decrease complications or perforation.
- The administration of glucocorticoids is controversial, but their use probably is of no added benefit. Prophylactic antibiotics are not recommended.

Referrals

- Unsuspected esophageal and gastric burns and duodenal injury are commonly seen with endoscopy, which should be performed by a GI consultant within 24 hours. The likelihood of stricture formation (pyloric or esophageal) and perforation depends on the severity of ingestion.
- Obtain surgical consultation.

Follow-Up

- Obtain upper GI radiograph after 2–4 weeks.

ETHANOL AND OTHER ALCOHOLS

ETHANOL (EtOH)

General Principles

- The toxicity of ethanol (EtOH) is dose related, but tolerance varies widely.
- Blood levels >100 mg/dL are associated with ataxia.
- At 200 mg/dL, patients are drowsy and confused.
- At levels >400 mg/dL, respiratory depression is common and death is possible.

Diagnosis

Laboratory Studies

- Obtain electrolytes, glucose level, serum osmolality, and blood EtOH level.
- The blood EtOH level can be rapidly estimated by calculating the osmolal gap (measured osmolality minus calculated osmolality, or measured osmolality minus [2 Na (mEq/L) + (urea [mg/dL])/2.8 + (glucose [mg/dL])/18]). **The standard formula for blood EtOH level in mg/dL equals 4.6 times the osmolal gap,**[53] in the absence of other low molecular weight toxins. However, multipliers ranging from 2.7[54] to 3.7[55] have been reported using linear regression from actual in vivo measurements in humans; thus, if the standard multiplier is used, the patient may appear to have a residual osmolal gap, implying the presence of another toxin such as methanol (MeOH) or ethylene glycol (EG) when there is none.

Treatment

- If the patient's mental status is severely depressed, insert an endotracheal tube before performing gastric lavage if the patient presents <1 hour after ingestion.
- Charcoal is not helpful due to the rapid absorption of EtOH from the stomach.
- Hemodialysis may be useful for life-threatening overdoses.
- Administer 100 mg **thiamine IV** followed by 50 mL 50% dextrose in water IV to any **comatose alcoholic patient.**
- Admit patients with alcohol intoxication if they have severe underlying illness or significant alcoholic ketoacidosis or if ventilatory support is required.
- Observe other patients until they are sober (blood alcohol level <100 mg/dL) or can be discharged to the care of a responsible sober adult.
- If the patient's mental status is more abnormal than would be expected for the blood alcohol level, consider additional toxicology testing and head CT.

ISOPROPYL ALCOHOL

General Principles

- Most rubbing alcohol is 70% isopropyl alcohol (IPA). IPA is more toxic than EtOH at any blood level (50 mg/dL = intoxication, 100–200 mg/dL = stupor and coma). Respiratory depression and hypotension occur at high blood levels.
- Other symptoms include nausea, vomiting, and abdominal pain.

Diagnosis

- Workup commonly reveals ketosis without acidosis (IPA is metabolized to acetone).
- Metabolic acidosis, if present, is usually related to associated hypotension.
- IPA concentration in the blood can be measured directly or can be estimated in the same fashion as for EtOH, substituting a multiplier of 6.0 for 4.6. Absence of an osmolal gap

does not exclude IPA ingestion. Measure plasma glucose, as hypoglycemia may occur, particularly in children.
- If diagnosis is in doubt, obtain blood levels of other toxic alcohols and determine acid-base status with ABGs.

Treatment

- Do not induce emesis, as mental status may decline rapidly, with subsequent aspiration.
- Gastric lavage followed by charcoal administration may be useful if performed within 60 minutes of ingestion. Protect the airway.
- For cutaneous exposures, wash the skin and remove contaminated clothes. Maintain an adequate airway and support BP.
- Hemodialysis is reserved for patients with persistent hypotension despite supportive therapy.

METHANOL

General Principles

- Methanol (MeOH) is in gas-line antifreeze, carburetor fluid, duplicator fluid, and wind-shield washer fluid.
- Sterno Canned Heat fuel contains EtOH and MeOH, and the EtOH that is present may delay manifestations of MeOH toxicity.
- The toxicity of MeOH is due to its conversion by alcohol dehydrogenase to formaldehyde and then by acetaldehyde dehydrogenase to formic acid. Initial symptoms may include lethargy and confusion, followed by an apparent hangover.

Diagnosis

Clinical Presentation

- MeOH toxicity presents with headache, visual symptoms (blurring, diminished acuity, and whiteness in the visual field), nausea, vomiting, abdominal pain, tachypnea, and respiratory failure.
- Coma and convulsions may occur in severe MeOH intoxication. The range of toxic ingestion is 15–400 mL
- Symptoms may be delayed 18–24 hours.

Physical Examination

- Typically, examination reveals an uncomfortable patient who may be remarkably tachypneic with decreased visual acuity; optic disk hyperemia may be hard to appreciate.

Laboratory Studies

- Obtain CBC, electrolytes, BUN, creatinine, amylase, urinalysis, EtOH, and MeOH levels, as well as ABGs, which reveal a severe anion-gap metabolic acidosis. Development of the acidosis may be delayed 18 hours or more, until the accumulation of toxic metabolites; coingestion of alcohol may prolong this phase for many hours.
- In general, pH and acid-base status are better predictors of toxicity than is the absolute MeOH level.
- The MeOH level (in mg/dL) can be estimated in the same way as for EtOH, substituting a multiplier of 3.2 for 4.6. However, the absence of an osmolal gap does not rule out MeOH intoxication, and for the reasons noted above, EtOH intoxication may result in an apparent osmolal gap that is greater than anticipated, leading to temporary misdiagnosis of intoxication with MeOH or another osmotically active toxin.

Treatment

- Do not induce emesis.
- Consider gastric lavage if the patient is seen <1 hour after ingestion. Charcoal does not absorb significant amounts of MeOH.
- Give **folinic acid** (leucovorin), 1 mg/kg (maximum, 50 mg) IV, followed by folic acid, 1 mg/kg IV q4h for six doses, to increase the metabolism of formate.
- Administering IV **NaHCO$_3$** for severe acidosis may reduce permanent vision damage.
- **4-Methylpyrazole** (**fomepizole;** an alcohol dehydrogenase antagonist)[56] is FDA approved for the treatment of MeOH toxicity, although no direct comparison with EtOH has been made. Nevertheless, it is more easily administered than EtOH and does not cause depression of mental status or hypoglycemia. Although much more expensive, it is now the antidote of choice.
  - In the United States, emergency orders may be placed with Jazz Pharmaceuticals, (800) 359–4304.
  - Administer fomepizole for the following indications: peak MeOH level >20 mg/dL, while awaiting levels for an ingestion suspected of being MeOH, or an anion-gap metabolic acidosis after suspicious ingestion.
  - The dosage is 15 mg/kg IV followed by 10 mg/kg IV q12h for four doses. This should be followed by 15 mg/kg IV q12h until the MeOH level is <20 mg/dL. During hemodialysis, the dosing interval should be changed to q4h (Table 25-3).
- **EtOH delays metabolism of MeOH to its toxic metabolites** by competing for alcohol dehydrogenase and can be used in situations in which fomepizole is unavailable or contraindicated.
  - Administer EtOH for the following indications: peak MeOH level >20 mg/dL, while awaiting levels for an ingestion suspected of being MeOH, or an anion-gap metabolic acidosis after suspicious ingestion.
  - The **loading dose of EtOH** is 7.6–10 mL/kg of a 10% solution, given IV, or 0.8–1 mL/kg of 95% alcohol, administered PO in orange juice. EtOH for infusion is available as stock 5% or 10% solutions in D$_5$W; the latter is preferred. EtOH (10%) for IV infusion can also be prepared by removing 100 mL D$_5$W from a 1-L bag and replacing it with 100 mL absolute alcohol. Maintenance dosage varies depending on previous alcohol exposure (Table 25-4).
  - The goal is achievement of a blood alcohol level of 100–130 mg/dL to saturate the available alcohol dehydrogenase and prevent formation of MeOH's toxic metabolites. Check EtOH levels 1 hour after the loading dose and at least two to three times a day during maintenance infusion (some authorities recommend hourly levels). It is ultimately less hazardous to the patient to have blood alcohol levels that are too high than too low. Monitor blood glucose levels, as hypoglycemia may occur. Administer EtOH continuously until the MeOH level is <10 mg/dL, the formate level is

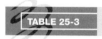

TABLE 25-3 **Fomepizole Administration During Dialysis**

Time from last dose	Dose
Beginning of dialysis	
<6 hr	None
>6 hr	Give next scheduled dose
During dialysis	Maintenance dose q4h
At conclusion of dialysis	
<1 hr	None
1–3 hr	One-half of next scheduled dose
>3 hr	Give next scheduled dose

| **TABLE 25-4** | Maintenance Ethanol Dosage Regimens for Ethylene Glycol and Methanol Intoxication | | | |

	10% ethanol IV (mL/kg/hr)	40% ethanol PO (mL/kg/hr)	95% ethanol PO (mL/kg/hr)	Hemodialysis with 10% ethanol IV[a] (mL/kg/hr)
Moderate drinker	1.4	0.3	0.15	3.3
Chronic drinker	2.0	0.4	0.2	3.9
Nondrinker	0.8	0.2	0.1	2.7

[a]Dialysate bath concentration of 100 mg/dL preferable.
Source: Modified with permission from Kuffner E, Hurlbut KM. Methanol (management/treatment protocol). In: Rumack BH, Spoerke DG, eds. Poisindex Information System. Denver: Micromedex, 2003.

<1.2 mg/dL, there is resolution of acidosis, CNS symptoms abate, and a normal anion gap is restored.

■ This implies regular monitoring of electrolytes, BUN, creatinine, and ABGs. If MeOH levels cannot be readily measured, administer EtOH for at least 9 days without dialysis (or 1 day with dialysis) and until clinical findings resolve.[57] Every effort should be made to move the patient to a center where levels and dialysis are available.

Special Therapy

■ **Hemodialysis** generally is indicated for an MeOH level that exceeds 50 mg/dL, severe and resistant acidosis, renal failure, or visual symptoms. Adjust fomepizole and ethanol doses as shown in Tables 25-3 and 25-4.

ETHYLENE GLYCOL AND DIETHYLENE GLYCOL

General Principles

■ Ethylene glycol is used commonly in antifreeze and windshield deicer. Various metabolites are responsible for toxicity.

Diagnosis

Clinical Presentation
■ The initial syndrome resembles alcohol intoxication.
■ Vomiting is common.
■ CNS depression, seizures, or coma may occur.
■ CHF and pulmonary edema may occur 12–36 hours after ingestion. Death is most likely in this stage.
■ Oliguric renal failure (from oxalate crystal deposition) may occur 24–72 hours after ingestion. Associated flank pain may be prominent.

Laboratory Studies
■ Obtain electrolyte, BUN, and creatinine levels; serum osmolality; ABGs; urinalysis; and EtOH and EG levels.
■ Findings include a severe metabolic acidosis with an anion gap (which may be delayed for hours until accumulation of toxic metabolites occurs), an osmolal gap, and oxalate and hippurate crystalluria in addition to hematuria and proteinuria.
■ Serum level can be calculated from the osmolal gap as for EtOH, using a multiplier of 6.2.

- Fluorescein often is added to antifreeze, and urine fluorescence detected with a Wood lamp up to 6 hours after ingestion is diagnostic,[58] although the accuracy of this has been disputed.[59]

Treatment

- Do not induce emesis.
- Neither gastric lavage nor charcoal administration is likely to be effective but can be considered if the patient presents within 1 hour of ingestion, particularly if the ingestion is mixed with other toxins that are amenable to gastric decontamination.
- Avoid magnesium salt cathartics because of the likelihood of renal failure.
- **Correct life-threatening acidosis** with IV sodium bicarbonate pending dialysis; administration for lesser severity is not justified. Administer 1–3 mEq/kg IV and titrate to achieve a normal pH. Monitor the calcium level, as hypocalcemia may result.
- **4-Methylpyrazole (fomepizole)**[60,61] is FDA approved for use in EG poisoning. Indications include an EG level >20 mg/dL, a suspected EG ingestion (while levels are being awaited), or an anion-gap metabolic acidosis with a history of EG ingestion, regardless of level. The dosing is similar to the treatment of MeOH poisoning. Treatment with 4-methylpyrazole should continue until the EG level is <20 mg/dL.[62]
- **IV EtOH** (although not FDA approved and never studied prospectively; Table 25-4) can be used as an alternative when fomepizole is unavailable or contraindicated (hypersensitivity). It is dosed in the same manner as for MeOH intoxication. It should be continued until the EG level is <10 mg/dL, with no symptoms and a normal pH. An EtOH level of at least 100 mg/dL should be maintained. If levels are unavailable, infusion should be continued for at least 3 days, or 1 day with dialysis. Every effort should be made to transfer the patient safely to a facility with the capacity to measure EG levels and perform dialysis.
- **Administer pyridoxine** (100 mg IV daily) to promote the conversion of glyoxylate to glycine and **thiamine** (100 mg IV daily) to promote the formation of nontoxic α-hydroxy-beta-ketoadipic acid.

Special Therapy

- **Dialysis** is highly effective in severe cases. Fomepizole dosage is adjusted as in Table 25-3. EtOH infusion should be continued at higher doses (Table 25-4) during dialysis.
  - Indications are glycol level >50 mg/dL (unless the patient is being given 4-methylpyrazole and the patient is asymptomatic with a normal pH), electrolyte abnormalities that are unresponsive to standard therapy, deteriorating vital signs despite supportive therapy, renal failure, or a pH of <7.25–7.30 that is unresponsive to therapy.[62]
  - Discontinue when the glycol level is <10 mg/dL, the glycolic acid level is undetectable, and the acidosis, clinical status, and anion gap have returned to normal.
  - When levels cannot be measured easily, continue EtOH administration for at least 3 days without hemodialysis (or for 1 day with hemodialysis) and until clinical findings resolve, whichever is longer.[63] Measure EtOH levels after the loading dose and two to three times a day during maintenance therapy.

HYDROCARBONS

GENERAL PRINCIPLES

- Morbidity and mortality usually are attributed to **pulmonary aspiration.** Low viscosity (e.g., kerosene, gasoline, and liquid furniture polish) is associated with greater aspiration potential. Motor oil, transmission oil, mineral oil, baby oil, and suntan oil usually are nontoxic.

DIAGNOSIS

Clinical Presentation

- Hydrocarbon ingestions are characterized by GI upset, pulmonary aspiration, and CNS alterations.
- Clinical manifestations usually are apparent within the first 6 hours and include vomiting, chest or abdominal pain, cough, dyspnea, low-grade fever, arrhythmias, an altered sensorium, seizures, and radiographic evidence of aspiration pneumonitis or pulmonary edema.

Imaging

- Obtain a chest radiograph.

TREATMENT

- **Treatment of nontoxic hydrocarbon ingestion** is not required in the absence of symptoms. These agents have high aspiration potential but are associated with little or no GI absorption. Gastric emptying is never necessary.
- **Treatment of toxic hydrocarbon ingestion** is begun by **removing contaminated clothing** and **washing the affected skin** to prevent dermatitis and percutaneous absorption.
- Provide **supplemental oxygen** to patients with significant aspiration injuries.
- **Gastric emptying,** although controversial, is recommended for ingestion of toxic hydrocarbons, particularly halogenated hydrocarbons (trichloroethylene, carbon tetrachloride, methylene chloride) or those that contain toxic additives (e.g., heavy metals, insecticides, nitrobenzene, aniline, or camphor), although some authorities recommend only administration of activated charcoal. Other potentially toxic hydrocarbons (gasoline, benzene, kerosene, lighter fluid, paint thinner, and toluene), except for large suicidal ingestions, do not require gastric emptying.
- If **gastric emptying** is performed, this is one of the few potential indications for ipecac, as aspiration appears to be less frequent with the use of ipecac than after gastric lavage. Therefore, in alert patients with a very strong indication, consider inducing emesis with ipecac, 30 mL PO. Perform **gastric lavage** after intubation with a cuffed endotracheal tube in any patient with CNS depression, a depressed gag reflex, or seizures.
- Prophylactic antibiotics or glucocorticoids are not indicated.

Monitoring

- Observe the patient for at least 6 hours after gastric decontamination.
- Hospitalize patients who are lethargic or have pulmonary symptoms or an abnormal pulmonary examination, ABGs, or chest radiograph.
- Patients who remain asymptomatic with a normal chest radiograph after 6 hours may be discharged.

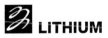 **LITHIUM**

GENERAL PRINCIPLES

- **Lithium** is administered as a carbonate or citrate salt for the treatment of psychiatric disease, principally bipolar disorder. Overdose often is suicidal.
- Excretion is renal. States of dehydration and sodium uptake promote lithium retention and toxicity, as does thiazide diuretic use.

Classification

- Symptoms are loosely related to blood level in acute overdose. Therapeutic blood levels range between 0.6 and 1.2 mEq/L.
- At <2.5 mEq/L, symptoms are mild and consist of tremor, ataxia, nystagmus, and lethargy.
- Between 2.5 and 3.5 mEq/L, the patient may be agitated and confused and have fasciculations, nausea, vomiting, and diarrhea.
- Levels >3.5 mEq/L are associated with seizures, coma, cardiac arrhythmias, hypotension, noncardiogenic pulmonary edema, nephrogenic diabetes insipidus, and death. Levels associated with severe symptoms may be lower in those with chronic ingestion.

DIAGNOSIS

Laboratory Studies

- Obtain electrolytes, creatinine, and lithium level.
  - Electrolytes may reveal a low anion gap with elevated bicarbonate, and there may be evidence of diabetes insipidus.
  - Lithium levels should be measured repetitively until at least two sequential levels show continued decline.

Monitoring

- Obtain an ECG and monitor the patient continuously while he or she is being evaluated and treated.

TREATMENT

- Consider gastric lavage if the patient presents within 1 hour of ingestion.
- Charcoal does not bind lithium; **sodium polystyrene sulfonate** (15 g PO qid or 30–50 g per rectum) can decrease absorption.[64]
- Sustained-release preparations may form concretions. If levels continue to rise despite treatment, perform whole-bowel irrigation with commercial polyethylene glycol solution, 2 L/hr for 5 hours.
- Establish IV access and hydrate with 0.9% saline to achieve euvolemia. Avoid dehydration, as this promotes renal lithium reabsorption.
- Treat arrhythmias in standard fashion (see Chapter 7, Cardiac Arrhythmias).
- Criteria for **dialysis** are inexact. **Consult a nephrologist** for consideration of hemodialysis (preferably with a bicarbonate rather than acetate bath) for the following indications: blood level >3.5–4.0 mEq/L after an acute ingestion, chronic toxicity with a blood level >2.5 mEq/L, worsening mental status, seizures, dysrhythmias, pulmonary edema, and renal failure.
  - The goal is achievement of a sustained level of 1 mEq/L 8 hours after dialysis, which may necessitate prolonged or repeated dialysis.

METHEMOGLOBINEMIA (ACQUIRED)

GENERAL PRINCIPLES

- Methemoglobinemia can be caused by nitrites, nitroprusside, nitroglycerin, chlorates, sulfonamides, aniline dyes, nitrobenzene, antimalarials, and phenazopyridine.
- Methemoglobinemia has also been reported after benzocaine topical anesthesia for endoscopy as well as other topical anesthetics[65] and after dapsone therapy.[66]

DIAGNOSIS

Symptoms

- Symptoms include headache, fatigue, lethargy, dyspnea, tachycardia, and dizziness. The patient may be hypotensive due to the vasodilating properties of nitrates as well as tissue hypoxia. Seizures may occur.
- Severity correlates with methemoglobin level. Blood levels exceeding 50% indicate severe toxicity, often associated with CNS depression, seizures, coma, and arrhythmias; levels higher than 70% are often fatal.

Laboratory

- Obtain CBC, electrolytes, ABGs, and methemoglobin level.
- The diagnosis is suggested in patients with a normal oxygen tension (as measured by ABGs) and generalized cyanosis (corresponding to a methemoglobin level of 15% or more) that does not respond to oxygen.
- Blood with that level of methemoglobin placed on white filter paper appears chocolate colored when exposed to room air as compared to blood from a normal control.
- Measured arterial oxygen saturation that is much lower than that calculated for the alveolar oxygen tension also is suspicious for methemoglobinemia.
- Obtain an ECG and monitor the cardiac rhythm continuously.

TREATMENT

- Give 100% oxygen.
- Do not give ipecac because seizures may occur and promote aspiration.
- Consider gastric lavage (with airway protection) if the patient presents within 1 hour of ingestion or has coma or seizures.
- Administer activated charcoal.
- If signs of hypoxia are present or if the methemoglobin level exceeds 30%, administer methylene blue, 1–2 mg/kg in a 1% solution IV over 5 minutes.
  - The dose can be repeated in 1 hour if signs of hypoxia persist and q4h thereafter to a maximum dose of 7 mg/kg.
- Treat seizures with a benzodiazepine and phenytoin in addition to methylene blue.
- Treat hypotension with IV fluids and, if resistant, with dopamine.
- Hyperbaric oxygen and exchange transfusion are extreme measures for severely symptomatic patients.

Disposition

- Hospitalize the patient in an ICU if he or she is symptomatic or if the methemoglobin level is >20%.

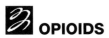 **OPIOIDS**

DIAGNOSIS

Symptoms

- Symptoms of opioid overdose are respiratory depression, a depressed level of consciousness, and miosis. However, the pupils may be dilated with acidosis or hypoxia or after overdoses with meperidine or diphenoxylate plus atropine. Overdose with α-methylfentanyl ("China white") may result in negative toxicology screens.

Special Considerations

■ Heroin may be adulterated with scopolamine, cocaine, or caffeine, complicating the clinical picture. Less common complications include hypotension, bradycardia, and pulmonary edema.

■ Be aware of body packers, who smuggle heroin in their intestinal tracts. Deterioration of latex or plastic containers may result in drug release and death.[70]

Laboratory Studies

■ Drug levels and other standard laboratory tests are of little use. **Pulse oximetry** and **ABGs** are useful for monitoring respiratory status.

Radiology

■ Chest radiograph should be obtained if pulmonary symptoms are present.

TREATMENT

■ Treatment includes airway maintenance, ventilatory and circulatory support, and prevention of further drug absorption.

■ **Emesis is contraindicated.**

■ **Gastric lavage** can be considered for oral ingestions that present within 1 hour; administer activated charcoal.

■ **Whole-bowel irrigation** may be safe and effective for body packers; surgery is not indicated except for obstruction. Endoscopic removal should not be attempted due to the danger of rupture.

■ **Naloxone hydrochloride** specifically reverses opioid-induced respiratory and CNS depression and hypotension. The initial dose is 2 mg IV; large doses may be required to reverse the effects of propoxyphene, diphenoxylate, buprenorphine, or pentazocine.

■ In the absence of an IV line, naloxone can be administered sublingually,[67] via endotracheal tube, or intranasally.[68] Isolated opioid overdose is unlikely if there is no response to a total of 10 mg naloxone. Repetitive doses may be required (duration of action is 45 minutes), and this should prompt hospitalization despite the patient's return to an alert status.

■ **Methadone overdose** may require therapy for 24–48 hours, whereas levo-α-acetylmethadol may require therapy for 72 hours. A continuous IV drip that provides two-thirds of the initial dose of naloxone hourly, diluted in D_5W, may be necessary to maintain an alert state.[69]

■ Ventilatory support should be provided for the patient who is unresponsive to naloxone and for pulmonary edema.

Disposition

■ If the patient is alert and asymptomatic for 6 hours after an oral ingestion and a single dose of naloxone, or for 4 hours after a single treatment for an IV overdose, he or she can be discharged safely.

■ Body packers should be admitted to an ICU for close monitoring of the respiratory rate and level of consciousness and remain so until all packets have passed, as documented by CT.

ORGANOPHOSPHATES

GENERAL PRINCIPLES

- Organophosphates are responsible for a number of human poisonings, particularly in developing countries. **Parathion** and **malathion** are the most common insecticides involved; they often are contained in hydrocarbon solvent.
- Suicidal ingestion and agricultural exposure, including dermal absorption, occur. "**Nerve gases**" used in terrorist biowarfare are anticholinesterases, such as sarin.

DIAGNOSIS

Symptoms

- **Toxic manifestations** are due to inhibition of acetylcholinesterase in the nervous system.
- **Muscarinic manifestations** include miosis, increased lacrimation, blurred vision, bronchospasm, bronchorrhea, diaphoresis, salivation, bradycardia, urinary incontinence, and increased GI motility, manifested by cramps, nausea, vomiting, and diarrhea.
- Among the **nicotinic manifestations** are muscle weakness and cramps, muscle fasciculations, hypotension, and respiratory paralysis.
- **CNS toxicity** is characterized by anxiety, slurred speech, mental status changes (e.g., delirium, coma, and seizures), and respiratory depression.

Complications

- Complications of ingestion include pulmonary edema, aspiration pneumonia, chemical pneumonitis, delayed polyneuropathy, and ARDS.
- Nonketotic hyperglycemia and glucosuria are common.
- Hyperamylasemia may reflect pancreatitis.
- Red cell cholinesterase and plasma pseudocholinesterase levels are decreased; activities of <50% of baseline are associated with poor outcome.

Laboratory Studies

- Obtain CBC, electrolytes, ABGs, and plasma and red cell cholinesterase levels.

Other

- Obtain chest radiograph and ECG.

Monitoring

- Monitor ABGs and ECG; QTc prolongation is associated with a worse prognosis.

TREATMENT

- Apply measures to support ventilation and circulation, decontaminate the skin (the medical team should wear rubber gloves, aprons, and shoe covers if there is major skin contamination), and consider gastric lavage for oral poisonings if presentation is within 1 hour of ingestion; **induction of emesis is contraindicated.**
- Administer **activated charcoal.**
- **Atropine** (preservative free, to avoid benzyl alcohol toxicity with large doses) is the drug of choice for organophosphate toxicity.

- Give an initial dose of 1 mg IV; if the patient experiences no adverse effects, repeat a dose of 2 mg q15min until atropinization (as manifested by drying of secretions, tachycardia, flushing, dry mouth, and dilated pupils) occurs.
- The average patient requires approximately 40 mg/d, but larger doses (500–1,500 mg/d) may be necessary. Intermittent administration may have to be continued for at least 24 hours until the organophosphate is metabolized.
- Severe cases may require several days or more of therapy, because of slow regeneration of acetylcholinesterase activity. Atropine does not reverse the muscle weakness.

- Give **pralidoxime,** 1–2 g IV in 100 mL normal saline over 30 minutes, which reactivates the cholinesterase and counteracts weakness, muscle fasciculations, and respiratory depression. Repeat administration q6–12h to a maximum of 12 g in 24 hours. An alternative is continuous infusion at 500 mg/hr as needed for several days. Unlike organophosphates, carbamate intoxications do not irreversibly inhibit cholinesterase, and thus pralidoxime is not usually required and may worsen symptoms.
- Treat **seizures** with a **benzodiazepine** and **phenytoin;** if severe seizures require muscle relaxants, **do not use succinylcholine,** which may result in prolonged paralysis.
- **Hemoperfusion** should be considered for severe parathion overdoses, although there is little objective evidence to support its use.
- Support respiratory failure with **mechanical ventilation.**

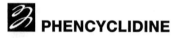 **PHENCYCLIDINE**

GENERAL PRINCIPLES

Definition

- **Phencyclidine** is a dissociative anesthetic and is available illicitly, mislabeled as LSD, mescaline, psilocybin, and tetrahydrocannabinol. Frequency of use varies widely by geographic region and is frequent in some urban areas but uncommon in many other parts of the United States.

DIAGNOSIS

Symptoms

- Symptoms that occur even with small ingestions include agitation, hallucinations, bizarre or violent behavior, hypertension, tachycardia, and horizontal or vertical nystagmus.
- Patients are relatively impervious to pain and may be catatonic or self-destructive and difficult to subdue.
- Stupor progressing to coma, hypertension, hyperpyrexia, hypertonicity, and bronchospasm characterizes moderate ingestions.
- Massive ingestions may lead to hypotension, respiratory failure, rhabdomyolysis, and acute tubular necrosis. Hypoglycemia is common, and death may occur.

Laboratory Studies

- Monitor electrolytes, creatinine, and creatine phosphokinase (CPK). Drug levels are not useful.

TREATMENT

- Treatment is primarily supportive.
- Minimize sensory input and remove potentially injurious objects from the area.
- **Ipecac is contraindicated.**

- Gastric lavage may provoke violent behavior and is recommended only in severe poisonings and only after the airway has been protected.
- **Repeated charcoal administration** also may interrupt enterogastric and enterohepatic circulations but has not been demonstrated to have an effect on outcome.
- Use **diazepam** to control agitation; give haloperidol if the agitation is severe.
- Treat dystonic reactions with **diphenhydramine.**
- Control adrenergic manifestations (e.g., hypertension) with β-adrenergic blockade if bronchospasm is not present; sodium nitroprusside may be required in severe cases.
- Seizures are uncommon in adults; treat with **benzodiazepines** and **phenytoin.** Consider discharging any patient with low-dose intoxication from the emergency department after his or her symptoms resolve and psychiatric consultation has been obtained. Hospitalize patients with more severe intoxication.
- **Acid diuresis is no longer recommended.**
- **Avoid restraints,** as they may increase rhabdomyolysis.
- Treat hyperthermia with cooling and hydration.

Disposition

- Consider discharge after low-dose ingestion after symptoms resolve and psychiatric consultation has been obtained.
- Hospitalize those with more severe overdose.

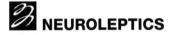

NEUROLEPTICS

GENERAL PRINCIPLES

- Neuroleptics are antipsychotics.

PHENOTHIAZINES

- Phenothiazines that are used commonly include chlorpromazine, thioridazine, prochlorperazine, perphenazine, trifluoperazine, fluphenazine, mesoridazine, haloperidol (a butyrophenone), and thiothixene.

Diagnosis

Clinical Presentation

- Overdoses are characterized by agitation or delirium, which may progress rapidly to coma. Pupils may be mydriatic and deep tendon reflexes are depressed. Seizures and disorders of thermoregulation, particularly hyperthermia, may occur.
- Hypotension (due to strong α-adrenergic antagonism), tachycardia, arrhythmias (including torsades de pointes), and depressed cardiac conduction occur.

Laboratory Studies

- Measuring blood levels is not helpful.
- Radiographs may reveal pill concretions that are present in the stomach despite apparently effective gastric emptying.

Monitoring

- Monitor the cardiac rhythm continuously.

Treatment

- Treatment includes airway protection, respiratory and hemodynamic support, and administration of activated charcoal.

- Emesis is contraindicated.
- Consider gastric lavage, which may be effective hours later due to delayed gastric emptying caused by the phenothiazines.
- Consider whole-bowel irrigation for ingestion of sustained-release formulations.
- Monitor the cardiac rhythm.
- Treat ventricular arrhythmias with lidocaine and phenytoin; class Ia agents (e.g., procainamide, quinidine, disopyramide) are contraindicated; avoid sotalol.
- Treat hypotension with IV fluid administration and α-adrenergic vasopressors (norepinephrine). Dopamine is an acceptable alternative. Paradoxic vasodilation may occur in response to epinephrine administration because of unopposed β-adrenergic response in the setting of strong α-adrenergic antagonism.
- Recurrent torsades de pointes may require magnesium, isoproterenol, or overdrive pacing (see Chapter 7, Cardiac Arrhythmias).
- Treat seizures with diazepam and phenytoin.
- Treat dystonic reactions with benztropine, 1–4 mg, or diphenhydramine, 25–50 mg, IM or IV.
- Treat hyperthermia with cooling. Forced diuresis, hemodialysis, and hemoperfusion are not useful.
- Frank neuroleptic malignant syndrome may complicate use of these agents, and should be treated as described above.
- Admit those patients who have ingested a significant overdose for cardiac monitoring for at least 48 hours.

ATYPICAL NEUROLEPTICS

CLOZAPINE

Diagnosis

Clinical Presentation

- Overdose is characterized by altered mental status, ranging from somnolence to coma. Anticholinergic effects occur, including blurred vision, dry mouth (although hypersalivation may occur in overdose), lethargy, delirium, and constipation. Seizures occur in a minority of overdoses. Coma may occur.
- Physical manifestations include hypotension, tachycardia, fasciculations, tremor, and myoclonus. Agranulocytosis may result. ECG abnormalities are unusual, but atrioventricular block may occur. Serious dysrhythmias rarely occur.

Laboratory Studies

- Obtain WBC and liver function tests; follow the WBC weekly for 4 weeks. Clozapine levels are not useful.

Treatment

- Induction of emesis is contraindicated.
- Perform gastric lavage if the patient presents within 1 hour of ingestion.
- Give activated charcoal.
- Treat hypotension with crystalloids; if resistant, treat with norepinephrine or dopamine.
- Treat seizures with benzodiazepines and phenytoin.
- Provide ventilatory support for respiratory failure.
- No evidence has been shown that forced diuresis, hemodialysis, or hemoperfusion is beneficial
- Filgrastim can be given for agranulocytosis.
- Admit and monitor patients with severely symptomatic overdoses for 24 hours or more.

OLANZAPINE

Diagnosis

Clinical Presentation

- Overdose is characterized by somnolence, slurred speech, ataxia, vertigo, nausea, and vomiting.[71]
- Anticholinergic effects occur, including blurred vision, dry mouth, and tachycardia.
- Seizures are uncommon. Coma may occur.
- Physical manifestations include hypotension, tachycardia, and pinpoint pupils that are unresponsive to naloxone. Serious dysrhythmias rarely occur.

Treatment

- Induction of emesis is contraindicated.
- Consider gastric lavage if presentation is within 1 hour of ingestion.
- Give activated charcoal.
- Treat hypotension with fluids and, if ineffective, norepinephrine or dopamine.
- Give benzodiazepines and phenytoin for seizures.
- Provide ventilatory support for respiratory failure, which occurs uncommonly.

RISPERIDONE, ZIPRASIDONE, AND QUETIAPINE

- These agents are newer atypical antipsychotics with limited information about overdose.

Diagnosis

Clinical Effects

- These include CNS depression, tachycardia, hypotension, and electrolyte abnormalities. QRS and QTc prolongation have occurred with each, but clinically significant ventricular dysrhythmias are uncommon.

Laboratory Studies

- Monitor electrolytes, liver function, and ECG with continuous telemetry.

Treatment

- Do not induce emesis.
- Consider gastric lavage if presentation is within 1 hour of ingestion.
- Administer activated charcoal.
- Monitor and provide support for respiratory depression.
- Treat hypotension with fluids, and if severe and persistent, **norepinephrine** in preference to dopamine.
- Treat ventricular dysrhythmias with **sodium bicarbonate** to maintain a pH of 7.45–7.55, and avoid Ia antiarrhythmics (procainamide, quinidine, and disopyramide).
- Diuresis, hemodialysis, and hemoperfusion do not appear to be useful.

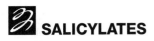 **SALICYLATES**

GENERAL PRINCIPLES

- **Salicylate** toxicity may result from acute ingestion or chronic intoxication. Toxicity is usually mild after acute ingestions of <150 mg/kg, moderate after ingestions of 150–300 mg/kg, and generally severe with overdoses of 300–500 mg/kg.
- Toxicity from chronic ingestion typically is due to intake of >100 mg/kg/d over a period of several days and usually occurs in elderly patients with chronic underlying illness. Diagnosis often is delayed in this group of patients, and mortality is approximately

25%. Significant toxicity due to chronic ingestion may occur with blood levels lower than those associated with acute ingestions.

DIAGNOSIS

Symptoms

- Nausea, vomiting, tinnitus (implying levels >30 mg/dL), hyperpnea, and malaise can occur. Fever suggests a poor prognosis in adults.
- Severe intoxications are associated with lethargy, convulsions, and coma, which may result from cerebral edema.
- Noncardiogenic pulmonary edema occurs in up to 30% of adults and is more common with chronic ingestion, cigarette smoking, neurologic symptoms, and older age.
- Severe overdoses are manifested by tachypnea, dehydration, pulmonary edema, altered mental status, seizures, coma, or a total dose >300 mg/kg.

Laboratory Studies

- Obtain CBC, electrolytes, BUN, creatinine blood glucose levels, and prothrombin and partial thromboplastin times. Prothrombin time prolongation is common.
- **Hypoglycemia,** common in children, is rare in adults.
- **ABGs** may reveal an early respiratory alkalosis, followed by metabolic acidosis. Approximately 20% of patients exhibit either respiratory alkalosis or metabolic acidosis alone.[72] Most adults with pure salicylate overdose have a primary metabolic acidosis and a primary respiratory alkalosis. After mixed overdoses, respiratory acidosis may become prominent.[73]
- **Blood levels** must be drawn 6 hours or more after acute ingestion of salicylates to allow prediction of severity of intoxication and patient disposition (Fig. 25-2). Obtaining earlier levels is appropriate in severely intoxicated patients, to guide intervention. Levels >70 mg/dL at any time represent moderate to severe intoxication; levels >100 mg/dL are very serious and often fatal. This information is useful only for acute overdoses; estimation of severity is invalidated by the use of enteric-coated aspirin or chronic ingestion. Bicarbonate levels and pH are more useful than salicylate levels as prognostic indicators in chronic intoxication.

TREATMENT

- Consider **gastric lavage** if presentation is within 1 hour of ingestion.
- Administer **activated charcoal.**
  - **Multidose charcoal** may be useful in severe overdose[74] but is not routinely recommended.
- **Alkaline diuresis** is indicated for salicylate blood levels that are >40 mg/dL.
  - Administer 88 or 100 mEq (two ampules) sodium bicarbonate in 1,000 mL D_5W at a rate of 10–15 mL/kg/hr if the patient is clinically volume depleted until urine flow is achieved.
  - Maintain alkalinization using the same solution at 2–3 mL/kg/hr, and monitor urine output, urine pH (target pH, 7–8), and serum potassium. Achievement of **alkaline diuresis** often requires the simultaneous administration of at least 20 mEq/L **potassium chloride.**
  - Because there is little evidence of improved outcome with alkaline diuresis, and because older patients may have cardiac, renal, and pulmonary comorbidity, **avoid vigorous fluid therapy in the elderly,** as pulmonary edema is more likely to occur in this population.
- Although acetazolamide causes urine alkalinization, the associated acidemia increases salicylate toxicity, and therefore it must not be used.
- Treat **cerebral edema** with hyperventilation and osmotic diuresis.

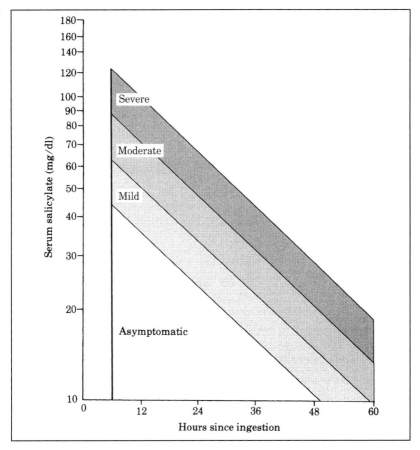

Figure 25-2. Severity of salicylate intoxication. (Adapted from Done AK. Salicylate intoxication. *Pediatrics* 1960;26:800.)

- Treat seizures with a **benzodiazepine** (diazepam, 5–10 mg IV q15min up to 50 mg) followed by **phenobarbital,** 15 mg/kg IV.
- **Hemodialysis** is indicated for blood levels >100–130 mg/dL after acute intoxication but may be useful with chronic toxicity when levels are as low as 40 mg/dL if other indications for dialysis exist. Among these are refractory acidosis, severe CNS symptoms, progressive clinical deterioration, pulmonary edema, and renal failure.
- **Treatment of pulmonary edema** may also require mechanical ventilation with a high fraction of inspired oxygen concentration and PEEP.
- **The elderly are at high risk.** Repeated blood levels that fail to decline should prompt contrast radiography of the stomach; concretions should be subjected to bicarbonate lavage and multidose charcoal, and whole-bowel irrigation should be considered.

Monitoring

- **Patients with minor symptoms** (nausea, vomiting, tinnitus), an acute ingestion of <150 mg/kg, and a first blood level of <65 mg/dL can be treated in the emergency department. Blood levels should be repeated q2h until they show a decline. These patients often are medically stable for discharge, and their disposition can be determined based on psychiatric evaluation.

■ Admit moderately symptomatic patients for at least 24 hours.
■ Admit patients with severe overdoses to an ICU.

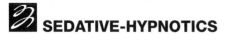

SEDATIVE-HYPNOTICS

BARBITURATES

General Principles

■ Toxic manifestations of barbiturates vary with the amount of ingestion, type of drug, and length of time since ingestion.
■ Toxicity can occur with lower doses of the short-acting barbiturates (e.g., butabarbital, hexobarbital, secobarbital, and pentobarbital) than of the long-acting barbiturates (e.g., phenobarbital, barbital, mephobarbital, and primidone), but fatalities are more common with the latter.

Diagnosis

Clinical Presentation

■ Mild intoxication resembles alcohol intoxication. Moderate intoxication is characterized by greater depression of mental status, response only to painful stimuli, decreased deep tendon reflexes, and slow respirations. Severe intoxication causes coma and a loss of all reflexes (except the pupillary light reflex).
■ Plantar reflexes are extensor. Characteristic bullae ("barb burns") may be seen over pressure points and on the dorsum of the fingers.[75] Hypothermia and hypotension may occur. In severe cases, no electrical activity is seen on an EEG.

Treatment

■ Maintain a patent airway and adequate ventilation.
■ Do not induce emesis.
■ Perform **gastric lavage** if presentation occurs within 1 hour of ingestion.
■ **Administer multidose activated charcoal.** Multidose activated charcoal markedly decreases the half-life of phenobarbital.
■ **Forced alkaline diuresis,** similar to that used for salicylate intoxication, is effective in enhancing phenobarbital excretion, but not that of short-acting barbiturates. Its use should be reserved for severe, life-threatening intoxication.
■ **Hemoperfusion** may be effective for excretion of phenobarbital and short-acting barbiturates. Hemoperfusion is used rather than hemodialysis because of better drug removal but is reserved for patients with stage IV coma with increased blood levels and refractory hemodynamic compromise.
■ Treat hypotension with crystalloid administration. If this fails, administer norepinephrine or dopamine.

BENZODIAZEPINES

General Principles

■ Most overdoses are the result of attempts at self-harm. Fatalities are rare; mixed overdoses are common.
■ An exception is **flunitrazepam** (Rohypnol, "roofies"), which is ten times as potent as diazepam. It is mixed with low-quality heroin and used to soften the effects of cocaine. It is also mixed with alcohol as a "date rape" drug. Effects are similar to those of

other benzodiazepines. It may cause hallucinations, and mixing with alcohol increases respiratory depression. It often is not detected on standard toxicology screens.

Diagnosis

- Symptoms include drowsiness, dysarthria, ataxia, slurred speech, and confusion. Severe overdoses may result in coma and respiratory depression.

Treatment

- Do not induce emesis.
- Consider gastric lavage if presentation is within 1 hour of ingestion.
- Administer activated charcoal.
- Provide general supportive measures for hypotension and bradycardia.
- Rarely, respiratory depression may require intubation.
- **Flumazenil**, a benzodiazepine antagonist, reverses toxicity without causing respiratory depression.
  - Administer 0.2 mg (2 mL) IV over 30 seconds, followed by 0.3 mg at 1-minute intervals to a total dose of 3 mg.
  - If no response is observed after such treatment, benzodiazepines are unlikely to be the cause of the patient's sedation.
  - If a partial response has occurred, give additional 0.5-mg increments to a total of 5 mg. Rarely, as much as a 10-mg total dose may be necessary for full reversal. If no IV access is available, the drug can be administered by endotracheal tube.
  - Treat recurrence of sedation or respiratory depression by repeating the preceding regimen or by continuous infusion of 0.1–0.5 mg/hr.
  - **If mixed overdose with cyclic antidepressants is suspected or the patient has a known history of seizure disorder, flumazenil should not be used.**
  - Forced diuresis and hemodialysis are ineffective.

γ-HYDROXYBUTYRATE

General Principles

- γ-Hydroxybutyrate (GHB) is an endogenous short-chain fatty acid that occurs naturally in the body; this until recently illegal substance is not detected by standard toxicology screens. It has emerged as an important intoxicant.
- It is now available legitimately, under severely controlled circumstances, for the treatment of narcolepsy as **Xyrem.**®
- It is often sold to participants at large dance parties ("raves") and has been responsible for mass intoxications,[76] though use may be decreasing.[77] It has also been used as a "date rape" drug. Synonyms include, but are not limited to, "liquid Ecstasy," "liquid E," "grievous bodily harm," "Georgia home boy," "soap," "salty water," and "organic Quaaludes."

Diagnosis

- Symptoms include ataxia, nystagmus, somnolence progressing to coma, vomiting, and random clonic movements of the face and extremities.
  - EEG recording supports the belief that these represent myoclonus and not true seizures. Respiratory depression may progress to apnea.

Treatment

- Absorption is very rapid, and lavage and activated charcoal administration are of little use.
- Do not induce emesis.
- The drug is not antagonized by naloxone or flumazenil.
- Experimental but no clinical evidence has been found to support the administration of physostigmine, and its use is not recommended.

- Administer oxygen and protect the airway; monitor oxygenation.
- Drug levels are not usually available, and the drug is not detected on routine toxicology screens.
- Obtain electrolytes and glucose and establish an IV line.
- Stimulation, including endotracheal intubation, may stimulate violently aggressive behavior.
- Give atropine for persistent symptomatic bradycardia.
- Treat hypotension with IV fluids; pressors are rarely necessary.
- Obtain an ECG and monitor the cardiac rhythm continuously.
- Intoxication is usually short lived; coma typically lasts for 1–2 hours, and full recovery often occurs within 8 hours. Stable asymptomatic patients can be discharged after 6 hours of observation. Admit any patient who is still clinically intoxicated after 6 hours.[78]

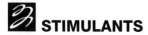 **STIMULANTS**

AMPHETAMINES

Diagnosis

Clinical Presentation
- Symptoms include hyperactivity, irritability, delirium, hallucinations, psychosis, mydriasis, hyperpyrexia, flushing, diaphoresis, hypertension, arrhythmias, vomiting, and diarrhea.
- Less common manifestations include acute renal failure secondary to rhabdomyolysis, seizures, CNS hemorrhage, coma, myocardial infarction, aortic dissection, and circulatory collapse.

Treatment

- Administer activated charcoal.
- **Induction of emesis is contraindicated,** as it may induce seizures.
- Perform gastric lavage only for recent large ingestions.
- Establish an IV line.
- Monitor electrolytes, renal function, and CPK.
- Obtain an ECG and monitor the cardiac rhythm.
- Treat agitation with **diazepam;** physical restraints may increase the occurrence of rhabdomyolysis.
- Treat hallucinations and psychosis with **haloperidol. Droperidol,** 2.5–5.0 mg IV, may be superior to benzodiazepines for sedation.[79] However, it may cause QT prolongation and torsades de pointes; therefore, its use should be reserved for severe agitation that is resistant to benzodiazepines, and continuous cardiac monitoring should be used.
- Treat severe hypertension with nitroprusside or a β-adrenergic antagonist; phentolamine can also be considered (see Chapter 4, Hypertension).
- Diazepam is the initial drug of choice for seizures, followed by phenytoin or phenobarbital.
- Arrhythmias usually respond to propranolol or lidocaine.
- Monitor core temperature. Hyperthermia may require cooling blankets, evaporative cooling, or paralysis; if unsuccessful, dantrolene or bromocriptine may be useful. Hemodialysis is not clearly effective.
- Treat rhabdomyolysis as outlined in Chapter 11, Renal Diseases.
- Admit patients with moderate to severe symptoms or with abnormal vital signs.

3-4 METHYLENEDIOXYMETHAMPHETAMINE (MDMA, "ECSTASY")

- MDMA has been a popular drug of abuse associated with "rave" culture. Surveys have shown that nearly 40% of college students have used it at least once.
- It is often used in association with prolonged vigorous dancing, causing dehydration and contributing to hyperthermia.

Diagnosis

Clinical Presentation
- Symptoms include hypertension, tachycardia, dilated pupils, diaphoresis, and trismus.
- Severe intoxications may result in hyperthermia, DIC, muscle rigidity, myoclonus, rhabdomyolysis, acute renal failure, and occasionally the syndrome of inappropriate antidiuretic hormone secretion. Supraventricular and ventricular arrhythmias may occur. Initial confusion and agitation may progress to coma and seizures.

Laboratory Studies
- Toxicology screens are unreliable. Initiation of therapy is based on presumptive diagnosis according to history and presentation. Monitor electrolytes, BUN, creatinine, liver function tests, CBC, coagulation studies, and CPK.

Treatment

- Therapy at present is based on case reports and reviews.[80]
- Do not induce emesis, as coma and seizures may occur abruptly.
- Gastric lavage is useful only if initiated within 1 hour of ingestion.
- Administer activated charcoal.
- Establish an IV line and maintain hydration.
- Treat agitation with benzodiazepines, with preparation to protect the airway and support ventilation.
- β-Adrenergic antagonists may be useful in treatment of tachycardia and hypertension. Severe hypertension may require nitroprusside.
- Treat seizures with benzodiazepines followed by phenytoin or phenobarbital.
- Treat ventricular arrhythmias with lidocaine, phenytoin, or esmolol.
- Cool the hyperthermic patient with evaporative cooling; consider dantrolene administration.
- Treat rhabdomyolysis supportively (see Chapter 11, Renal Diseases).

COCAINE

Diagnosis

Clinical Presentation
- Symptoms include short-lived CNS and sympathetic stimulation, hypertension, tachypnea, tachycardia, and mydriasis. Depression of the higher nervous centers ensues rapidly and may result in death.
- **Mortality** may also result from drug-induced seizures, subarachnoid hemorrhage, stroke, or direct cardiac effects (e.g., coronary artery spasm, myocardial injury, and precipitation of lethal arrhythmias).[81]
- **Myocardial infarction** may be precipitated in individuals without underlying heart disease. Rhabdomyolysis may occur, precipitating renal failure.
- **Pulmonary edema** may develop abruptly after an individual smokes the free alkaloid form of cocaine ("free base") or its heated bicarbonate precipitant ("crack"). Pneumomediastinum may occur after smoking crack and may progress to pneumothorax. Other pulmonary complications include alveolar hemorrhage, obliterative bronchiolitis, hypersensitivity pneumonitis, and asthma.[82] Bowel ischemia and necrosis may occur.

- Special situations include **body packing,** in which "mules" swallow multiple cocaine-containing packets, often latex condoms. Rupture of one or more may result in severe symptoms or death. **Body stuffers** may ingest crack cocaine that is unwrapped or wrapped only in a layer of cellophane, to avoid arrest. Their course is generally benign, presumably due to poor absorption.

Laboratory

- Obtain CBC, electrolytes, urinalysis, and CPK.
- Urine screen may be useful to confirm the diagnosis; drug levels are not useful.
- Obtain an ECG and monitor the cardiac rhythm continuously.
- Obtain abdominal radiographs to detect cocaine-containing packets in the intestinal tract of suspected body packers; Gastrografin®-enhanced CT may be more sensitive.

Treatment

- Maintain a patent airway and support respiration and circulation.
- Avoid β-adrenergic antagonists in patients with myocardial ischemia or infarction, as they allow unopposed α-adrenergic vasospasm.[83]
  - **Labetalol** may be preferable, and **phentolamine** may be useful in selected cases.
- Myocardial ischemia and infarction should be managed as outlined in Chapter 5, Ischemic Heart Disease.
- **Nitroglycerin** can be used for ischemic pain.
- Treat ventricular arrhythmias with **lidocaine;** β-adrenergic antagonists may be useful in those without myocardial ischemia.
- Use **benzodiazepines** to decrease the stimulatory effect of cocaine and to treat seizures initially. Follow with phenytoin or phenobarbital for longer-term seizure control.
- Treat noncoronary manifestations of adrenergic stimulation with **labetalol;** severe or sustained hypertension may require treatment with **nitroprusside.**
- Treat rhabdomyolysis and hypotension supportively.
- Hyperthermia may require a cooling blanket, evaporative cooling, sedation, or paralysis.
- Diuresis and dialysis are not useful.
- For body packers with retained packets, perform gentle catharsis with charcoal and psyllium; mineral oil may dissolve latex packets and precipitate toxicity.
  - Admit such patients to an ICU for monitoring, as rupture may be rapidly fatal.
  - Whole-bowel irrigation and surgery probably are rarely necessary, although they have been recommended; surgery is clearly indicated only for bowel obstruction.
  - Attempts at endoscopy are contraindicated, as rupture may result.
  - Obtain repeated radiographs until the packets are no longer visible. With appropriate care, mortality is <1%.
- Body stuffers have a generally benign course. Abdominal radiography is almost invariably negative. Nearly three-fourths of patients remain asymptomatic, and most of the rest have only mild to moderate symptoms. Only 4% have severe toxicity, including seizures, dysrhythmias, and death.[84,85] Close observation is nevertheless warranted.

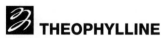 **THEOPHYLLINE**

GENERAL PRINCIPLES

Classification

- Nausea and vomiting are the most common symptoms of theophylline toxicity and are associated with serum levels >20 mg/mL.
- **Moderate toxicity** is largely due to relative epinephrine excess and includes tachycardia, arrhythmias, tremors, and agitation.
- **Severe toxicity** is most common at serum levels >90 mg/mL in the acutely intoxicated, usually younger individual.

- **Severe toxicity** results in hallucinations, seizures (which may be refractory to standard therapy), dysrhythmias (including sinus tachycardia, atrial fibrillation, supraventricular tachycardia, and ventricular tachycardia and fibrillation), and hypotension.
- **Seizures** and **cardiac toxicity** are likely at serum levels >60 mg/mL in the chronically intoxicated and might occur at even lower levels.
- **Rhabdomyolysis** occurs occasionally.[86] The severity of intoxication is modified by chronicity, age of the patient, and the presence of comorbid diseases.

DIAGNOSIS

Laboratory Studies

- Obtain theophylline levels q2h until a plateau is reached. The peak level may be delayed significantly after the ingestion of sustained-release theophylline preparations, with toxic levels persisting 50–60 hours after ingestion.
- Check potassium, electrolyte, glucose, CPK, calcium, and magnesium levels; BUN; and ABGs.
- Obtain a baseline ECG and maintain continuous cardiac monitoring.
- Acid-base abnormalities include respiratory alkalosis and metabolic acidosis. Hypokalemia, hyperglycemia, hypercalcemia, and hypophosphatemia may be present.

TREATMENT

- Establish an IV line and perform gastric lavage if the patient has taken a potentially life-threatening acute ingestion. Consider lavage also after a large ingestion of a sustained-release preparation, as a bezoar may form.
- Avoid the use of ipecac because of the potential for seizures and aspiration.
- Administer activated charcoal. Multidose charcoal decreases the half-life of theophylline by 50%, although it has not been clearly shown to improve outcome.
- Consider whole-bowel irrigation with polyethylene glycol solution for overdoses with sustained-release preparations and blood levels that continue to rise despite therapy.
- Treat severe nausea with **metoclopramide,** 10–60 mg IV, or **ondansetron,** 0.15 mg/kg IV (8–10 mg in the average individual). **Do not use phenothiazines** because of their propensity to lower the seizure threshold.
- Treat hypotension with **IV crystalloids** and, if resistant, with **dopamine.**
- **Phenobarbital** is preferred to phenytoin for seizure prophylaxis in the severely poisoned patient. The treatment of choice for seizures is a benzodiazepine followed by phenobarbital (10 mg/kg loading dose at 50 mg/min, followed by up to a total of 30 mg/kg at a rate of 50 mg/min, followed by 1–5 mg/kg/d to maintain therapeutic plasma levels). Because of the cardiovascular and respiratory depressant activities of barbiturates, careful management of the airway and cardiovascular status are mandatory. For those patients who are refractory to phenobarbital therapy, obtain anesthesiology consultation for administration of pentobarbital; muscle paralysis and general anesthesia can be considered.
- Arrhythmias should be treated as they would be in nonintoxicated patients. β-adrenergic antagonists may be particularly useful but may precipitate bronchospasm in asthmatics. Because of its short half-life, IV esmolol usually is safer.
- **Hemoperfusion** (charcoal or resin) is preferable to hemodialysis because of faster drug removal and is indicated for:
  - Intractable seizures or life-threatening cardiovascular complications, regardless of drug level.
  - A theophylline level that approaches or exceeds 100 mg/mL after an acute overdose.
  - A theophylline level >60 mg/mL in acute intoxication, with increasing symptoms, and a patient who is intolerant of oral charcoal administration.
  - A theophylline level >60 mg/mL in chronic intoxication without life-threatening symptoms.
  - A theophylline level >40 mg/mL in a patient with chronic intoxication and CHF, respiratory insufficiency, hepatic failure,[87] or age older than 60 years.

Disposition

- Admit patients who have chronic intoxication, acute ingestion of sustained-release formulations, acute ingestions with levels that fail to fall or are rising despite therapy, or worsening symptoms.
- Those with levels that are falling to <20 mg/mL and whose symptoms are resolving can be discharged.

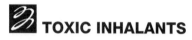 **TOXIC INHALANTS**

GENERAL PRINCIPLES

- Toxic inhalants comprise a variety of noxious gases and particulate matter that are capable of producing local irritation, asphyxiation, and systemic toxicity.
- In the management of exposure victims, identification of the offending agent is critical, and the regional poison control center must be contacted for specific therapeutic guidelines.

IRRITANT GASES

- Irritant gases produce cutaneous burns, mucosal irritation, laryngotracheitis, bronchitis, pneumonitis, bronchospasm, and pulmonary edema (which may be delayed up to 24 hours after exposure).
- The more water-soluble gases (e.g., chlorine, ammonia, formaldehyde, sulfur dioxide, ozone) primarily produce inflammation of the eyes, throat, and upper respiratory tract, whereas the less soluble gases (e.g., phosgene, nitrogen dioxide) tend to cause more damage to the terminal airways and alveoli. Household exposure may result from inadvertent mixture of bleach (sodium hypochlorite) with toilet bowl cleaner (sulfuric acid), which produces chlorine gas, or of bleach with ammonia, which produces chloramine gas.

Treatment

- Maintain a patent airway and adequate oxygenation.
- Treat bronchospasm with bronchodilators. Severe cough may require narcotic antitussives. Treat noncardiogenic pulmonary edema with oxygen, mechanical ventilation, and PEEP as needed (see Chapter 8, Critical Care).
- Treat skin burns by copious irrigation, removal of contaminated clothing, and tetanus prophylaxis (see Appendix F, Immunizations and Postexposure Therapies), if needed. Irrigate the eyes immediately and copiously with water or saline if the patient has had chemical contact.
- Obtain ophthalmologic consultation for caustic eye burns.

Risk Management

- Because the development of pulmonary edema may be delayed, observe asymptomatic patients with normal ABGs and chest radiographs for at least 6 hours.
- Hospitalize patients with symptoms or signs of upper airway edema or pulmonary involvement.

SIMPLE ASPHYXIANTS

- These include acetylene, argon, ethane, helium, hydrogen, nitrogen, methane, butane, neon, carbon dioxide, natural gas, and propane, all of which cause hypoxia by displacing oxygen from the inspired air.
- Morbidity and mortality are related to the extent and duration of the hypoxia.

Treatment

- Supplemental oxygen
- Supportive care for symptomatic patients

SYSTEMIC TOXIC INHALANTS

- These are gases that are capable of producing prominent systemic toxicity; they include hydrogen sulfide, methyl bromide, organophosphates, carbon monoxide, and hydrogen cyanide.
- Treatment consists of supportive care and specific therapy directed toward the offending agent.

Carbon Monoxide

- Poisoning usually occurs in poorly ventilated areas in which carbon monoxide (CO) is released by fires, combustion engines, or faulty stoves or heating systems. Intoxication is seasonal, with more cases occurring in winter.
- CO displaces oxygen from hemoglobin, shifts the oxyhemoglobin dissociation curve to the left, and depresses cellular respiration by inhibiting the cytochrome oxidase system.
- Direct binding to cardiac myoglobin depresses cardiac function. Toxic manifestations are a consequence of tissue hypoxia.

Diagnosis

- Symptoms correlate imperfectly with the carboxyhemoglobin level.
    - Carboxyhemoglobin levels of 20%–40% are associated with dizziness, headache, weakness, disturbed judgment, nausea and vomiting, and diminished visual acuity. These symptoms and seasonality frequently lead to a misdiagnosis of influenza. Examination may reveal retinal hemorrhages.
    - Levels of 40%–60% are associated with tachypnea, tachycardia, ataxia, syncope, and seizures. The ECG may reveal ST-segment changes, conduction blocks, and atrial or ventricular arrhythmias.
    - Levels >60% are associated with coma and death. Cherry-red coloration of the lips or skin is a relatively rare, late manifestation. Late complications include basal ganglia infarction and parkinsonism. Less severe, delayed neuropsychiatric symptoms also may occur.

Laboratory Studies

- Obtain electrolytes, CPK, ABGs, and an ECG, and monitor the cardiac rhythm continuously.
- Arterial oxygen tension usually is normal; thus, the diagnosis of carbon monoxide poisoning requires a high level of suspicion and direct measurement of arterial oxygen saturation or carbon monoxide (carboxyhemoglobin) levels. Standard pulse oximetry is not reliable.

Treatment

- Administer **100% oxygen** by tight-fitting mask or endotracheal tube. The latter ensures tissue oxygen delivery and decreases the half-life of carboxyhemoglobin from 4–5 hours to 90 minutes. Measure carboxyhemoglobin levels q2–4h, and continue oxygen administration until blood levels are <10%.
- **Hyperbaric oxygen** (3 atm) has been strongly recommended for patients who have been unconscious at any time and present with neurologic signs or symptoms, ECG changes consistent with ischemia, severe metabolic acidosis, rhabdomyolysis, pulmonary edema, or shock. Hyperbaric treatment of patients who have minor or no symptoms but who have carboxyhemoglobin levels of >25%–30% is controversial, as is treatment in pregnancy.
- Hyperbaric oxygen appears to improve long-term neurologic outcome.[88] Consult with an expert in the field when indications are unclear. In no case should patients be transferred to a hyperbaric oxygen facility until their condition is stabilized. Treat seizures

with diazepam and phenytoin (see Chapter 24, Neurologic Disorders). Arrhythmias and rhabdomyolysis are treated as described elsewhere.

Hydrogen Cyanide

- Hydrogen cyanide may be present in industrial fumigants, insecticides, and products of combustion of synthetics and plastics. It may be generated as a byproduct of phencyclidine manufacture.
- It has a characteristic bitter almond odor. Toxic amounts are absorbed rapidly through the bronchial mucosa and alveoli, and symptoms usually appear seconds after inhalation. Concentrations of 0.2–0.3 mg/L air are almost immediately fatal.
- Oral exposures to **potassium cyanide** may be due to rodenticides, insecticides, silver polish, artificial fingernail remover (acetonitrile), film developer, laboratory reagents, and amygdalin.

Diagnosis

- Symptoms include headache, palpitations, dyspnea, and mental status depression, which may progress quickly to coma, seizures, and death. ECG changes include atrial fibrillation, ventricular ectopy, and abnormal ventricular repolarization.
- Severe lactic acidosis is present, and venous oxygen content is higher than normal and may approach arterial oxygen content. Do not delay initiation of therapy for measurement of whole-blood cyanide levels.

Treatment

- Treatment focuses on conversion of hemoglobin to methemoglobin, which binds to the cyanide ion, sparing vital oxidative enzymes.
  - **Amyl nitrite** (one broken pearl held under the nostril for 15–30 sec/min, repeated every minute, with a new pearl q3min) produces a methemoglobin level of approximately 5%. This should be followed as rapidly as possible with 10 mL 3% **sodium nitrite** IV (0.3 g over 3–5 minutes). If the response is inadequate, one-half of the dose of sodium nitrite should be repeated in 30 minutes. The goal is a measured methemoglobin level of 30%.
  - Give **sodium thiosulfate** (50 mL of a 25% solution IV) immediately after the sodium nitrite, as it converts the cyanide into thiocyanate, which is excreted in the urine. Repeat one-half the dose in 30 minutes if the response is inadequate.
  - **Administer 100% oxygen** at all times during treatment to ensure adequate tissue oxygen delivery despite methemoglobinemia.
  - Do not give methylene blue for methemoglobin levels <70%, as cyanide may be released.
  - In the event of life-threatening methemoglobinemia, consider exchange transfusion.
  - Monitor the cardiac rhythm continuously.
  - For severe persistent acidosis (pH <7.2), **administer sodium bicarbonate,** 1 mEq/kg, after the preceding measures have been undertaken.
  - In the event of oral ingestion, empty the stomach by gastric lavage after the preceding measures have been undertaken. Do not induce emesis. Rapid absorption makes administration of activated charcoal of dubious utility.
  - The efficacy of hyperbaric oxygen is controversial but can be considered for those who respond poorly to conventional therapy.
  - The FDA recently approved hydroxycobalamin for the treatment of cyanide poisoning (Cyanokit®). Experience in Europe for more than ten years shows that this is a safe and effective alternative to the above regimen. The dose is 5 grams (two vials) in 100 mL normal saline IV over 15 minutes; if the response is inadequate, a second dose of 5 grams may be administered over 15 minutes (for a patient in extremis) to 2 hours (for the less severely affected). Dicobalt ethylenediaminetetra-acetic acid (dicobalt EDTA) and dimethylaminophenol are antidotes that are not available in the United States. If dicobalt EDTA is available, the dose is 300–600 mg (20–40 mL) IV over 1–5 minutes, followed by a 50-mL flush with D_5W. An additional 300 mg can be given in 5 minutes if the clinical response is inadequate.

Hydrogen Sulfide

- Hydrogen sulfide is a colorless gas with a characteristic rotten-egg odor. It is found in mines and sewers as well as petrochemical, agricultural (liquid manure processing), and tanning industries.

Diagnosis

- Exposure to low concentrations of hydrogen sulfide causes mucous membrane and eye irritation and vision changes.
- Higher concentrations cause cyanosis, confusion, pulmonary edema, coma, and convulsions. Rapid death occurs in approximately 6% of cases.

Treatment

- Therapy is similar to that used for hydrogen cyanide. Oxygen therapy at 100% and nitrites are used, but thiosulfate is not. The efficacy of nitrites is controversial.[89]
- Flush the mucous membranes with saline or water. Consider hyperbaric oxygenation for severe intoxication.

Smoke Inhalation

- This is the cause of death in more than 50% of fire-related fatalities. Thermal injury usually is confined to the upper airway because of the rapid cooling of inhaled gases that occurs proximal to the larynx.
- Toxic gases released by fire include carbon dioxide, carbon monoxide, hydrogen chloride, phosgene, chlorine, benzene, isocyanate, hydrogen cyanide, aldehydes, oxides of sulfur and nitrogen, ammonia, and numerous organic acids.
- Carbon monoxide accounts for 80% of mortality in the first 12 hours. The other toxins produce epithelial injury that results in airway edema, increased capillary permeability, and mechanical obstruction from desquamated tissue and secretions.
- Patients who have lost consciousness, have been exposed to a large quantity of smoke in a closed space, have suffered prolonged inhalation or steam exposure, were involved in an explosion, were with other persons who died or were severely injured, or have sustained facial burns or singed nasal vibrissae are at risk for development of respiratory complications, which may be delayed in onset for up to 3 days.

Diagnosis

Clinical Presentation

- Asphyxiation, expectoration of carbonaceous sputum, hoarseness, dyspnea from upper airway edema, stridor, bronchospasm, and noncardiogenic pulmonary edema are characteristic features of smoke inhalation.
- Upper airway burns may also be noted.
- Neurologic manifestations include stupor and coma.
- Late complications include bacterial pneumonia and pulmonary embolism.

Evaluation

- Obtain CBC, electrolytes, ABGs, chest radiograph, ECG, and carboxyhemoglobin level.
- High-risk patients should undergo upper airway endoscopy to rule out any life-threatening airway injury immediately; bronchoscopy rarely provides additional therapeutically useful information.
- A positive xenon scan predicts increased mortality but is rarely justified.
- Carboxyhemoglobin levels that exceed 15% are indicative of severe exposure.

Treatment

- **Scrupulous airway care is essential,** with frequent suctioning as needed.
- Endotracheal intubation is required in patients who display evidence of significant upper airway edema or respiratory insufficiency.
- Bronchoscopy may be necessary to remove endotracheal debris. Administer **humidified oxygen** to all patients.
- Give bronchodilators for bronchospasm.

- Treat ARDS with mechanical ventilation and PEEP. High-frequency flow interruption ventilation has been reported to be effective[90] but is not widely available and requires additional confirmation.
- Prophylactic antibiotics and glucocorticoids are not indicated.
- Treat specific intoxications (e.g., cyanide and carbon monoxide poisoning) appropriately. Suspect cyanide intoxication if coma and significant lactic acidosis are present.

Disposition

- Patients who have experienced minor smoke inhalation, who are asymptomatic at 4–6 hours, and who exhibit none of the risk factors just listed can be safely discharged home.
- Admit asymptomatic patients who have any risk factors for potential respiratory complications for a minimum of 24 hours.
- Admit patients who have symptoms, significant laboratory abnormalities, or an abnormal alveolar-arterial oxygen gradient to an ICU.

References

1. 2005 American Heart Association Guidelines for Cardiopulmonary Resuscitation and Emergency Cardiovascular Care. *Circulation* 2005;112(Supp 24):IV19–IV34.
2. Baumann MH, Strange C, Heffner JE, et al. Management of spontaneous pneumothorax: an American College of Chest Physicians Delphi consensus statement. *Chest* 2001;119:590.
3. Noakes TD. Fluid and electrolyte disturbances in heat illness. *Int J Sports Med* 1998;19:S146.
4. Dematte JE, O'Mara K, Buescher J, et al. Near-fatal heat stroke during the 1995 heat wave in Chicago. *Ann Intern Med* 1998;129:173.
5. Eichner ER. Treatment of suspected heat illness. *Int J Sports Med* 1998;19(Supp 2): S150.
6. Gaffin SL, Gardner JW, Flinn SD. Cooling methods for heatstroke victims. *Ann Intern Med* 2000;132:678.
7. Armstrong LE, Crago AE, Adams R, et al. Whole-body cooling of hyperthermic runners: comparison of two field therapies. *Am J Emerg Med* 1996;14:355.
8. White JD, Riccobene E, Nucci R, et al. Evaporation versus iced gastric lavage treatment of heatstroke: comparative efficacy in a canine model. *Crit Care Med* 1987;15:748.
9. Bouchama A, Cafege A, Deval EB, et al. Ineffectiveness of dantrolene sodium in the treatment of heatstroke. *Crit Care Med* 1991;19:176.
10. Briner WW. Tympanic membrane vs. rectal temperature measurement in marathon runners. *JAMA* 1996;276:194.
11. Hansen RD, Amos D, Leake B. Infrared tympanic temperature as a predictor of rectal temperature in warm and hot conditions. *Aviat Space Environ Med* 1996;67:1048.
12. Swain JA. Hypothermia and blood pH. A review. *Arch Intern Med* 1998;148:1643.
13. Delaney KA, Howland MA, Vassalo S, et al. Assessment of acid-base disturbances in hypothermia and their physiologic consequences. *Ann Emerg Med* 1989;18:72.
14. Golden FS, Hervey GR, Tipton MJ. Circum-rescue collapse: collapse, sometimes fatal, associated with rescue of immersion victims. *J Royal Naval Med Serv* 1991;77:139.
15. Vanggaard L, Eyolfson D, Xu X, et al. Immersion of distal arms and legs in warm water (AVA rewarming) effectively rewarms mildly hypothermic humans. *Aviat Space Environ Med* 1999;70:1081.
16. Weinberg AD. The role of inhalation re-warming in the early management of hypothermia. *Resuscitation* 1998;36:101.
17. Miller JW, Danzl DF, Thomas DM. Urban accidental hypothermia: 135 cases. *Ann Emerg Med* 1980;9:456.
18. Hall KN, Syverud SN. Closed thoracic cavity lavage in the treatment of severe hypothermia in human beings. *Ann Emerg Med* 1990;19:204.
19. Walpoth BH, Walpoth-Aslan BN, Mattle HP, et al. Outcome of survivors of accidental deep hypothermia and circulatory arrest treated with extracorporeal blood warming. *N Engl J Med* 1997;337:1500.

20. Rosen P, Stoto M, Harley I. The use of the Heimlich maneuver in near-drowning: Institute of Medicine report. *J Emerg Med* 1995;13:397.

21. Gonzales-Rothi R. Near-drowning: consensus and controversies in pulmonary and cerebral resuscitation. *Heart Lung* 1987;16:474.

22. Bohn DJ, Biggar WD, Smith CR, et al. Influence of hypothermia, barbiturate therapy, and intracranial pressure monitoring on morbidity and mortality after near-drowning. *Crit Care Med* 1986;14:529.

23. Nussbaum E, Maggi JC. Pentobarbital therapy does not improve neurologic outcome in nearly drowned, flaccid-comatose children. *Pediatrics* 1988;81:630.

24. Anker AL, Santora T, Spivey W. Artificial surfactant administration in an animal model of near-drowning. *Acad Emerg Med* 1995;2:204.

25. Perez-Benavides F, Riff E, Franks C. Adult respiratory distress syndrome and artificial surfactant replacement in the pediatric patient. *Pediatr Emerg Care* 1995;11:153.

26. Pratt FD, Haynes BE. Incidence of "secondary drowning" after saltwater submersion. *Ann Emerg Med* 1986;15:1048.

27. Watson WA, Litovitz TL, Rodgers GC, et al. 2004 Annual Report of the American Association of Poison Control Centers toxic exposure surveillance system. *Am J Emerg Med* 2005;23:589.

28. Spivey WH. Flumazenil and seizures: analysis of 43 cases. *Clin Ther* 1992;14:292.

29. Tenenbein M, Cohen S, Sitar DS. Efficacy of ipecac-induced emesis, orogastric lavage, and activated charcoal for acute drug overdose. *Clin Ther* 1992;14:292.

30. Kulig K, Bar-Or D, Cantrill SV, et al. Management of acutely poisoned patients without gastric emptying. *Ann Emerg Med* 1985;14:562.

31. Pond SM, Lewis-Driver DJ, Williams GM, et al. Gastric emptying in acute overdose: a prospective randomized controlled trial. *Med J Aust* 1995;163:345.

32. Chyka M, Seger D. Position statement: single-dose activated charcoal. *J Toxicol Clin Toxicol* 1997;35:721.

33. Anonymous. Position statement and practice guidelines on the use of multi-dose activated charcoal in the management of acute poisoning. *J Toxicol Clin Toxicol* 1999;37:731.

34. Jones AL, Volans G. Management of self-poisoning. *BMJ* 1999;319:1414.

35. Albertson TE, Derlet RW, Foulke GE, et al. Superiority of activated charcoal alone compared with ipecac and activated charcoal in the treatment of acute toxic ingestions. *Ann Emerg Med* 1989;18:56.

36. Anonymous. Position paper: ipecac syrup. *J Toxicol Clin Toxicol* 2004;42:133.

37. Vale JA, Kulig K. Position paper: gastric lavage. *J Toxicol Clin Toxicol* 2004;42:933.

38. Anonymous. Position paper: cathartics. *J Toxicol Clin Toxicol* 2004;42:243.

39. Anonymous. Position paper: whole bowel irrigation. *J Toxicol Clin Toxicol* 2004;42:843.

40. Bond GR, Hite LK. Population-based incidence and outcome of acetaminophen poisoning by type of ingestion. *Acad Emerg Med* 1999;6:1115–1120.

41. Acetaminophen. In: Poisindex® System [Internet database]. Greenwood Village, CO: Thomson Micromedex. Updated periodically.

42. Buckley NA, Whyte IM, O'Connell DL, et al. Activated charcoal reduces the need for N-acetylcysteine treatment after acetaminophen (paracetamol) overdose. *J Toxicol Clin Toxicol* 1999;37:753.

43. Harrison PM, Keays R, Bray GP, et al. Improved outcome of paracetamol-induced fulminant hepatic failure by late administration of acetylcysteine. *Lancet* 1990;335:1572.

44. Bailey B, McGuigan MA. Management of anaphylactoid reactions to intravenous N-acetylcysteine. *Ann Emerg Med* 1998;31:710.

45. Bremner JD, Wingard P, Walshe TA. Safety of mirtazapine in overdose. *J Clin Psychiat* 1998;59:233.

46. Boehnert MT, Lovejoy FH Jr. Value of the QRS duration versus the serum drug level in predicting seizures and ventricular arrhythmias after an acute overdose of tricyclic antidepressants. *N Engl J Med* 1985;313:474.

47. Wolfe TR, Caravati EM, Rollins DE. Terminal 40-ms frontal plane QRS axis as a marker for tricyclic antidepressant overdose. *Ann Emerg Med* 1989;18:348.

48. Bosse GM, Barefoot JA, Pfeifer MP, et al. Comparison of three methods of gut decontamination in tricyclic antidepressant overdose. *J Emerg Med* 1995;13:203.
49. Borys DJ, Setzer SC, Ling LJ, et al. Acute fluoxetine overdose: a report of 234 cases. *Am J Emerg Med* 1992;10(2):115–120.
50. Grundemar L, Wohlfart B, Lagerstedt C, et al. Symptoms and signs of severe citalopram overdose. *Lancet* 1997;349:1602.
51. Barbey JT, Roose SP. SSRI safety in overdose. *J Clin Psychiat* 1998;59(Suppl 15):42.
52. Alkalis. In: Poisindex® System [Internet database]. Greenwood Village, CO: Thomson Micromedex. Updated periodically.
53. Ethanol. In: Poisindex® System [Internet database]. Greenwood Village, CO: Thomson Micromedex. Updated periodically.
54. Weiss M, Thurnheer U. The osmotic gap in the diagnosis of alcoholic intoxication. *Schweiz Medizin Woch J Suisse Med* 1988;118:845.
55. Purssell RA, Pudek M, Brubacher J, et al. Derivation and validation of a formula to calculate the contribution of ethanol to the osmolal gap. *Ann Emerg Med* 2001;38:653.
56. Brent J, McMartin K, Phillips S, et al. Methylpyrazole for Toxic Alcohols Study Group. Fomepizole for the treatment of methanol poisoning. *N Engl J Med* 2001;344(6):424–429.
57. Methanol. In: Poisindex® System [Internet database]. Greenwood Village, CO: Thomson Micromedex. Updated periodically.
58. Winter ML, Ellis MD, Snodgrass WR. Urine fluorescence using a Wood's lamp to detect the antifreeze additive sodium fluorescein: a qualitative adjunctive test in suspected ethylene glycol ingestions. *Ann Emerg Med* 1990;19:633.
59. Wallace KL, Suchard JR, Curry SC, et al. Diagnostic use of physicians' detection of urine fluorescence in a simulated ingestion of sodium fluorescein-containing antifreeze. *Ann Emerg Med* 2001;38:49.
60. Jacobsen D. New treatment for ethylene glycol poisoning. *N Engl J Med* 1999;340:879.
61. Brent J, McMartin K, Phillips S, et al. Fomepizole for the treatment of ethylene glycol poisoning. Methylpyrazole for Toxic Alcohols Study Group. *N Engl J Med* 1999;340:832.
62. Barceloux DG, Krenzelok EP, Olson K, et al. American Academy of Clinical Toxicology Practice Guidelines on the Treatment of Ethylene Glycol Poisoning. Ad Hoc Committee. *J Toxicol Clin Toxicol* 1999;37:537–560.
63. Ethylene glycol. In: Poisindex® System [Internet database]. Greenwood Village, CO: Thomson Micromedex. Updated periodically.
64. Tomaszewski C, Musso C, Pearson JR, et al. Lithium absorption prevented by sodium polystyrenesulfonate in volunteers. *Ann Emerg Med* 1992;21:1308.
65. Khan NA, Kruse JA. Methemoglobinemia induced by topical anesthesia: a case report and review. *Am J Med Sci* 1999;318:415.
66. Ward KE, McCarthy MW. Dapsone-induced methemoglobinemia. *Ann Pharmacother* 1998;32:549.
67. Maio RF, Gaukel B, Freeman B. Intralingual naloxone injection for narcotic-induced respiratory depression. *Ann Emerg Med* 1987;16:572.
68. Ashton H, Hassan Z. Best evidence topic report. Intranasal naloxone in suspected opioid overdose. *Emerg Med J* 2006;23:221.
69. Goldfrank L, Weisman RS, Errick JK, et al. A dosing nomogram for continuous infusion intravenous naloxone. *Ann Emerg Med* 1986;15:566.
70. Wetli CV, Rao A, Rao VJ. Fatal heroin bodypacking. *Am J Forensic Med Pathol* 1997;18:312.
71. O'Malley GF, Seifert S, Heard K, et al. Olanzapine overdose mimicking opioid intoxication. *Ann Emerg Med* 1999;34:279.
72. Gabow PA. How to avoid overlooking salicylate intoxication. *J Crit Illness* 1986;1:77.
73. Gabow PA, Anderson RJ, Potts DE, et al. Acid-base disturbances in the salicylate-intoxicated adult. *Arch Intern Med* 1978;138:1481.
74. Vertrees JE, McWilliams BC, Kelly HW. Repeated oral administration of activated charcoal for treating aspirin overdose in young children. *Pediatrics* 1990;85:594.
75. Dunn C, Held JL, Spitz J, et al. Coma blisters: report and review. *Cutis* 1990;45:423.

76. Eckstein M, Henderson SO, DelaCruz P, et al. Gammahydroxybutyrate (GHB): report of a mass intoxication and review of the literature. *Prehosp Emerg Care* 1999;3:357.

77. Anderson IB, Kim SY, Dyer JE, et al. Trends in gamma-hydroxybutyrate (GHB) and related drug intoxication: 1999 to 2003. *Ann Emerg Med* 2006;47:177.

78. Li J, Stokes SA, Woeckener A. A tale of novel intoxication: a review of the effects of gamma-hydroxybutyric acid with recommendations for management. *Ann Emerg Med* 1998;31:729.

79. Richards JR, Derlet RW, Duncan DR. Methamphetamine toxicity: treatment with a benzodiazepine versus a butyrophenone. *Eur J Emerg Med* 1997;4:130.

80. Schwartz RH, Miller NS. MDMA (ecstasy) and the rave: a review. *Pediatrics* 1997;100:705.

81. Isner JM, Estes NA, Thompson PD, et al. Acute cardiac events temporally related to cocaine abuse. *N Engl J Med* 1986;315:1438.

82. Ettinger NA, Albin RJ. A review of the respiratory effects of smoking cocaine. *Am J Med* 1989;87:664.

83. Lange RA, Cigarroa RG, Flores ED, et al. Potentiation of cocaine-induced coronary vasoconstriction by beta-adrenergic blockade. *Ann Intern Med* 1990;112:897.

84. Sporer KA, Firestone J. Clinical course of crack cocaine body stuffers. *Ann Emerg Med* 1997;29:596.

85. June R, Aks SE, Keys N, et al. Medical outcome of cocaine bodystuffers. *J Emerg Med* 2000;18:221.

86. Titley OG, Williams N. Theophylline toxicity causing rhabdomyolysis and acute compartment syndrome. *Intens Care Med* 1992;18:129.

87. Cooling DS. Theophylline toxicity. *J Emerg Med* 1993;11:415.

88. Weaver LK, Hopkins RO, Chan KJ, et al. Hyperbaric oxygen for acute carbon monoxide poisoning. *N Engl J Med* 2002;347:1057.

89. Hall AH, Rumack BH. Hydrogensulfide poisoning: an antidotal role for sodium nitrite? *Veterin Hum Toxicol* 1997;39:152.

90. Lentz CW, Peterson HD. Smoke inhalation is a multilevel insult to the pulmonary system. *Curr Opin Pulm Med* 1997;3:321.

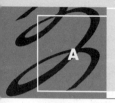

BARNES-JEWISH HOSPITAL LABORATORY REFERENCE VALUES

$\mathcal{R}$eference values for the more commonly used laboratory tests are listed in the following table. These values are given in the units currently used at Barnes-Jewish Hospital and in Système International (SI) units, which are used in many areas of the world. Individual reference values can be population and method dependent.

TABLE A-1 Lab Reference Values

Test	Current units	Factor[a]	SI units
Common serum chemistries			
Albumin	3.6–5.0 g/dL	10	36–50 g/L
Ammonia (plasma)	9–33 mcmol/L	1	9–33 mcmol/L
Bilirubin			
Total[b]	0.3–1.1 mg/dL	17.1	5.13–18.80 mcmol/L
Direct	0–0.3 mg/dL	17.1	0–5.1 mcmol/L
Blood gases (arterial)			
pH	7.35–7.45	1	7.35–7.45
PO_2	80–105 mm Hg	0.133	10.6–14.0 kPa
PCO_2	35–45 mm Hg	0.133	4.7–6.0 kPa
Calcium			
Total	8.6–10.3 mg/dL	0.25	2.15–2.58 mmol/L
Ionized	4.5–5.1 mg/dL	0.25	1.13–1.28 mmol/L
CO_2 content (plasma)	22–32 mmol/L	1	22–32 mmol/L
Ceruloplasmin	18–46 mg/dL	0.063	1.5–2.9 mcmol/L
Chloride	97–110 mmol/L	1	97–110 mmol/L
Cholesterol[c]			
Desirable	<200 mg/dL	0.0259	<5.18 mmol/L
Borderline high	200–239 mg/dL	0.0259	5.18–6.19 mmol/L
High	≥240 mg/dL	0.0259	6.22 mmol/L
HDL cholesterol[c]	>35 mg/dL	0.0259	>0.91 mmol/L
Copper (total)	75–145 mg/dL	0.157	11.8–22.8 mmol/L
Creatinine[b]			
Male, age 4–20 yr	0.2–1.2 mg/dL	88.4	18–106 mcmol/L
Female, age 4–20 yr	0.2–1.2 mg/dL	88.4	18–106 mcmol/L
Male, age 20–69 yr	0.7–1.5 mg/dL	88.4	62–133 mcmol/L
Female, age 20–69 yr	0.6–1.4 mg/dL	88.4	53–124 mcmol/L
Male, age ≥70 yr	0.7–1.7 mg/dL	88.4	62–150 mcmol/L
Female, age ≥70 yr	0.6–1.5 mg/dL	88.4	53–133 mcmol/L
Ferritin			
Male adult	20–323 ng/mL	2.25	45–727 pmol/L
Female adult	10–291 ng/mL	2.25	23–655 pmol/L

(continued)

TABLE A-1 Lab Reference Values (*continued*)

Test	Current units	Factor[a]	SI units
Folate			
Plasma	3.1–12.4 ng/mL	2.27	7.0–28.1 nmol/L
Red cell	186–645 ng/mL	2.27	422–1,464 nmol/L
Glucose, fasting (plasma)	65–109 mg/dL	0.055	3.58–6.00 mmol/L
Haptoglobin	30–220 mg/dL	0.01	0.3–2.2 g/L
Hemoglobin A1c (estimated)	4.0%–6.0%	0.01	0.04–0.06
Iron (total) (age >13 yr)			
Male	45–160 mcg/dL	0.179	8.1–31.3 mcmol/L
Female	30–160 mcg/dL	0.179	5.4–31.3 mcmol/L
Iron-binding capacity	220–420 mcg/dL	0.179	39.4–75.2 mcmol/L
Transferrin saturation	20%–50%	0.01	0.2–0.5
Lactate (plasma)	0.7–2.1 mmol/L	1	0.7–2.1 mmol/L
Magnesium	1.3–2.2 mEq/L	0.5	0.65–1.10 mmol/L
Osmolality	275–300 mOsm/kg	1	275–300 mmol/kg
Phosphate	2.5–4.5 mg/dL	0.323	0.8–11.45 mmol/L
Potassium (plasma)	3.3–4.9 mmol/L	1	3.3–4.9 mmol/L
Protein, total (plasma)	6.5–8.5 g/dL	10	65–85 g/L
Sodium	135–145 mmol/L	1	135–145 mmol/L
Triglycerides, fasting[c]	<250 mg/dL	0.0113	<2.8 mmol/L
Troponin I			
Normal	0.1 ng/mL	100	60 ng/L
Indeterminant	0.1–1.4 ng/mL	100	70–140 ng/L
Abnormal	≥1.5 ng/mL	100	≥150 ng/L
Urea nitrogen	8–25 mg/dL	0.357	2.9–8.9 mmol/L
Uric acid[b]	3–8 mg/dL	59.5	179–476 mcmol/L
Vitamin B12	180–1,000 pg/mL	0.738	133–738 pmol/L
Common serum enzymatic activities			
Aminotransferases			
Alanine (ALT, SGPT)	7–53 International Units/L	0.01667	0.12–0.88 mckat/L
Aspartate (AST, SGOT)	11–47 International Units/L	0.01667	0.18–0.78 mckat/L
Amylase	25–115 International Units/L	0.01667	0.42–1.92 mckat/L
Creatine kinase			
Male	30–200 International Units/L	0.01667	0.50–3.33 mc/kat/L
Female	20–170 International Units/L	0.01667	0.33–2.83 mc/kat/L
MB fraction	0–7 International Units/L	0.01667	0–0.12 mc/kat/L
Gamma-glutamyl transpeptidase (GGT)			
Male	11–50 International Units/L	0.01667	0.18–0.83 mckat/L
Female	7–32 International Units/L	0.01667	0.12–0.53 mckat/L
Lactate dehydrogenase[b]	100–250 International Units/L	0.01667	1.67–4.17 mckat/L
Lipase	<100 International Units/L	0.01667	<1.67 mckat/L
5′-Nucleotidase	2–16 International Units/L	0.01667	0.0–30.27 mckat/L
Phosphatase, acid	0–0.7 International Units/L	16.67	0–11.6 nkat/L
Phosphatase, alkaline[d]			
Age 10–15 yr	130–550 International Units/L	0.01667	2.17–9.17 mc/kat/L
Age 16–20 yr	70–260 International Units/L	0.01667	1.17–4.33 mc/kat/L
Age >20 yr	38–126 International Units/L	0.01667	0.13–2.10 mc/kat/L
Common serum hormone values[e]			
ACTH, fasting (8 am, supine)	<60 pg/mL	0.22	<13.2 pmol/L
Aldosterone[f]	10–160 ng/L	2.77	28–443 mmol/L
Cortisol (plasma, morning)	6–30 mg/dL	0.027	0.16–0.81 mcmol/L

(*continued*)

TABLE A-1 Lab Reference Values (*continued*)

Test	Current units	Factor[a]	SI units
FSH			
Male	1–8 International Units/L	1	1–8 International Units/L
Female			
Follicular	4–13 International Units/L	1	4–13 International Units/L
Luteal	2–13 International Units/L	1	2–13 International Units/L
Midcycle	5–22 International Units/L	1	5–22 International Units/L
Postmenopausal	20–138 International Units/L	1	20–138 International Units/L
Gastrin, fasting	0–130 pg/mL	1	0–130 ng/L
Growth hormone, fasting			
Male	<5 ng/mL	1	<5 mcg/L
Female	<10 ng/mL	1	<10 mcg/L
17-Hydroxyprogesterone			
Male adult	<200 ng/dL	0.03	<6.6 nmol/L
Female			
Follicular	<80 ng/dL	0.03	<2.4 nmol/L
Luteal	<235 ng/dL	0.03	<8.6 nmol/L
Postmenopausal	<51 ng/dL	0.03	<1.5 nmol/L
Insulin, fasting	315 microunits/L	7.18	144 pmol/L
LH			
Male	2–12 International Units/L	1	2–12 International Units/L
Female			
Follicular	1–18 International Units/L	1	1–18 International Units/L
Luteal	20 International Units/L	1	20 International Units/L
Midcycle	24–105 International Units/L	1	24–105 International Units/L
Postmenopausal	15–62 International Units/L	1	15–62 International Units/L
Parathyroid hormone	12–72 pg/mL	—	—
Progesterone			
Male	<0.5 ng/mL	3.18	<1.6 nmol/L
Female			
Follicular	0.1–1.5 ng/mL	3.18	0.32–4.80 nmol/L
Luteal	2.5–28.0 ng/mL	3.18	8–89 nmol/L
First trimester	9–47 ng/mL	3.18	29–149 nmol/L
Third trimester	55–255 ng/mL	3.18	175–811 nmol/L
Postmenopausal	<0.5 ng/mL	3.18	<1.6 nmol/L
Prolactin			
Male	1.6–18.8 ng/mL	1	1.6–18.8 mcg/L
Female	1.4–24.2 ng/mL	1	1.4–24.2 mcg/L
Renin activity (plasma)[g]	0.9–3.3 ng/mL/hr	0.278	0.25–0.91 ng/(L sec)
Testosterone, total			
Male	270–1,070 ng/dL	0.0346	9.3–37.0 nmol/L
Female	6–86 ng/dL	0.0346	0.2–13.0 nmol/L
Testosterone, free			
Male	9–30 ng/dL	0.0346	0.3–11.0 pmol/L
Female	0.3–1.9 ng/dL	0.0346	0.001–30.26 pmol/L
Thyroxine, total (T4)	4.5–12.0 mcg/dL	12.9	58–155 nmol/L
Thyroxine, free	0.7–1.8 ng/dL	12.9	10.3–34.8 pmol/L
uptake[h]	30%–46%	0.01	0.3–0.46
Triiodothyronine (T3)	45–132 ng/dL	0.0154	0.91–2.70 nmol/L
T4 index[i]	1.5–4.5	1	1.5–4.5
TSH	0.35–6.20 microunits/mL	1	0.35–6.20 microunits/L

(*continued*)

TABLE A-1 Lab Reference Values (*continued*)

Test	Current units	Factor[a]	SI units
Vitamin D, 1,25-dihydroxy	15–60 pg/mL	2.4	36–144 pmol/L
Vitamin D, 25-hydroxy	10–55 ng/mL	2.49	25–137 nmol/L
Common urinary chemistries			
Delta-aminolevulinic acid	1.5–7.5 mg/d	7.6	11.4–53.2 mcmol/d
Amylase	0.04–0.30 International Units/min	16.67	0.6–75.00 nkat/min
	60–450 Units/24 hr		
Calcium	50–250 mg/d	0.250	1.25–6.25 mmol/d
Catecholamines	<540 mcg/d	—	—
Dopamine	65–400 mcg/d	—	—
Epinephrine	<20 mcg/d	5.5	<110 nmol/d
Norepinephrine	15–80 mcg/d	5.9	88.5–472.0 nmol/d
Copper	15–60 mcg/d	0.0157	0.24–0.95 mcmol/d
Cortisol, free	9–53 mcg/d	2.76	25–146 nmol/d
Creatinine			
Male	0.8–1.8 g/d	8.84	7.1–15.9 mmol/d
Female	0.6–1.5 g/d	8.84	5.3–13.3 mmol/d
5-Hydroxyindoleacetic acid	<6 mg/d	5.23	<47 mcmol/d
Metanephrine	<1.3 mg/d	5.46	<7.1 mcmol/d
Oxalate			
Male	7–44 mg/d	11.4	80–502 mcmol/d
Female	4–31 mg/d	11.4	46–353 mcmol/d
Porphyrins			
Coproporphyrin			
Male	0–96 mcg/d	1.53	0–110 nmol/d
Female	0–60 mcg/d	1.54	0–92 nmol/d
Uroporphyrin			
Male	0–46 mcg/d	1.2	0–32 nmol/d
Female	0–22 mcg/d	1.2	0–26 nmol/d
Protein	0–150 mg/d	0.001	0–0.150 g/d
Vanillylmandelic acid (VMA)	<8 mg/d	5.05	<40 mcmol/d
Common hematologic values			
Coagulation			
Bleeding time[j]	2.5–9.5 min	60	150–570 sec
Fibrin degradation products	<8 mcg/mL	—	—
Fibrinogen[k]	150–400 mg/dL	0.01	1.5–4.0 g/L
Partial thromboplastin time (activated)	24–34 sec	1	24–34 sec
Prothrombin time[l]	10.5–14.5 sec	1	10.5–14.5 sec
INR	0.78–1.22	—	—
Thrombin time	11.3–18.5 sec	1	11.3–18.5 sec
CBC			
Hematocrit			
Male	40.7%–50.3%	0.01	0.407–0.503
Female	36.1%–44.3%	0.01	0.361–0.443
Hemoglobin			
Male	13.8–17.2 g/dL	0.620[m]	8.56–10.70 mmol/L
Female	12.1–15.1 g/dL	0.620	7.50–9.36 mmol/L
Erythrocyte count			
Male	$4.5–5.7 \times 10^6$/microliters	1	$4.55.7 \times 10^{12}$/L
Female	$3.9–5.0 \times 10^6$/microliters	1	$3.9–5.0 \times 10^{12}$/L

(*continued*)

TABLE A-1 Lab Reference Values (*continued*)

Test	Current units	Factor[a] SI units	
Mean corpuscular hemoglobin	26.7–33.7 pg/cell	0.062	1.66–2.09 fmol/cell
Mean corpuscular hemoglobin concentration	32.7–35.5 g/dL	0.620	20.3–22.0 mmol/L
Mean corpuscular volume	80.0–97.6 mcm^3	1	80.0–97.6 fL
Red cell distribution width	11.8%–14.6%	0.01	0.118–0.146
Leukocyte profile			
Total	$3.8–9.8 \times 10^3$/microliters	1	$3.8–9.8 \times 10^9$/L
Lymphocytes	$1.2–3.3 \times 10^3$/microliters	1	$1.2–3.3 \times 10^9$/L
Mononuclear cells	$0.2–0.7 \times 10^3$/microliters	1	$0.2–0.7 \times 10^9$/L
Granulocytes	$1.8–6.6 \times 10^3$/microliters	1	$1.8–6.6 \times 10^9$/L
Platelet count	$140–440 \times 10^3$/microliters	1	$140–440 \times 10^9$/L
Erythrocyte sedimentation rate			
Male, <50 yr	0–15 sec		
Male, >50 yr	0–20 sec		
Female, <50 yr	0–20 sec		
Female, >50 yr	0–30 sec		
Reticulocyte count			
Adults	0.5%–1.5%	0.01	0.005–0.015
Children	2.5%–6.5%	0.01	0.025–0.065
Immunology testing			
Complement (total hemolytic)[n]	118–226 units/mL		
C3	75–165 mg/dL	0.01	0.85–1.85 g/L
C4	12–42 mg/dL	0.01	0.12–0.54 g/L
Immunoglobulin			
IgA	70–370 mg/dL	0.01	0.70–3.70 g/L
IgM	30–210 mg/dL	0.01	0.30–2.10 g/L
IgG	700–1450 mg/dL	0.01	7.00–14.50 g/L
Therapeutic agents			
Amitriptyline (+ nortriptyline)	150–250 mcg/L		
Carbamazepine	4–12 mg/L	4.23	17–51 mcmol/L
Clonazepam	10–50 mcg/mL	3.17	32–159 nmol/L
Cyclosporine (whole blood)	183–335 ng/mL		Exact range depends on the type of transplant
Digoxin	0.8–2.0 mcg/L	1.28	1.0–2.6 nmol/L
Disopyramide	2–5 mg/L	2.95	6–15 mcmol/L
Ethosuximide	40–75 mg/L	7.08	283–531 mcmol/L
Imipramine	150–300 mcg/L	3.57	536–1071 nmol/L
Desipramine	100–300 mcg/L	3.75	375–1,125 nmol/L
Lithium	0.6–1.3 mmol/L	1	0.6–1.3 mmol/L
Nortriptyline	50–150 mcg/L	3.8	190–665 nmol/L
Phenobarbital	10–40 mg/L	4.3	43–172 mcmol/L
Phenytoin (diphenylhydantoin)	10–20 mg/L	3.96	40–79 mcmol/L
Primidone			
Primidone	5–15 mg/L	4.58	23–69 mcmol/L
Phenobarbital	1–5 mcg/L	4.3	6–9 mcmol/L
Procainamide	4–10 mg/L	4.23	17–42 mcmol/L
Procainamide + N-acetylprocainamide	6–20 mg/L		
Quinidine	2–5 mg/L	3.08	6.2–15.4 mcmol/L
Salicylate[o]	20–290 mg/L	0.0072	0.14–2.10 mmol/L

(*continued*)

TABLE A-1	Lab Reference Values (*continued*)

Test	Current units	Factor[a]	SI units
Theophylline	10–20 mg/L	5.5	55–110 mcmol/L
Valproic acid	50–100 mg/L	6.93	346–693 mcmol/L
Antimicrobials			
Amikacin			
Trough	1–8 mg/L	1.71	1.7–13.7 mcmol/L
Peak	20–30 mg/L	1.71	34–51 mcmol/L
5-Fluorocytosine			
Trough	20–60 mg/L		
Peak	50–100 mg/L		
Gentamicin			
Trough	0.5–2.0 mg/L	2.09	1.0–4.2 mcmol/L
Peak	6–10 mg/L	2.09	12.5–20.9 mcmol/L
Ketoconazole			
Trough	1 mg/L	—	—
Peak	1–4 mg/L	—	—
Sulfamethoxazole			
Trough	75–120 mg/L	—	—
Peak	100–150 mg/L	—	—
Tobramycin			
Trough	0.5–2.0 mg/L	2.14	1.1–4.3 mcmol/L
Peak	6–10 mg/L	2.14	12.8–21.4 mcmol/L
Trimethoprim			
Trough	2–8 mg/L	—	—
Peak	5–15 mg/L	—	—
Vancomycin			
Trough	5–15 mg/L	0.69	3.5–10.4 mcmol/L
Peak	20–40 mg/L		13.8–27.0 mcmol/L

ACTH, adrenocorticotropic hormone; fL, femtoliter; fmol, femtomole; FSH, follicle-stimulating hormone; HDL, high-density lipoprotein; INR, international normalized ratio; katal, mole/sec; kPa, kilopascal; LH, luteinizing hormone; μkat, microkatal; nkat, nanokatal; pmol, picomole; TSH, thyroid-stimulating hormone.

[a]A more complete list of multiplication factors for converting conventional units to SI units can be found in *Ann Intern Med* 1967;106:114, and in *The SI for the Health Professions.* Geneva: World Health Organization, 1977.

[b]Variation occurs with age and gender. This range includes both genders and persons older than 5 yr.

[c]National Institutes of Health Congress Development Panel on Triglycerides, HDL, and Coronary Artery Diseases, *JAMA* 1993;269:505.

[d]Higher values (up to 350 μU/mL) can be normal in persons younger than 20 yr.

[e]Because most hormones are measured by immunologic techniques and because hormones may vary in molecular weight (e.g., gastrin), most are expressed as mass/L. The reference ranges are method dependent.

[f]Supine, normal unit diet; in the upright position, the reference range is 40–310 ng/L.

[g]High-sodium diet, supplemented with sodium, 3 g/d.

[h]Replaces T_3 resin uptake.

[i]$T_4 \cdot$ (T uptake).

[j]Template modified after Ivy.

[k]Determined by the Clauss method.

[l]Normal ranges for prothrombin times vary according to the reagent used. Therefore, we report an INR with all prothrombin times ordered.

[m]This factor assumes a unit molecular weight of 16,000; assuming a unit molecular weight of 64,500, we have a multiplication factor of 0.156.

[n]CH_{50} is the reciprocal of dilution of sera required to lyse 50% of sheep erythrocytes.

[o]Therapeutic range for treatment of rheumatoid arthritis (see Chapter 23, Arthritis and Rheumatologic Diseases).

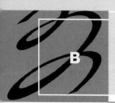

PREGNANCY AND MEDICAL THERAPEUTICS
Amber R. Cooper and Gilad A. Gross

$\mathcal{U}$sing medications during pregnancy or lactation always creates discussion between the patient and the physician. There is a continuous balance among treating a maternal condition for the safety of the mother, treating a maternal condition for the safety of the fetus, and potential drug toxicity to the fetus.

- It is important to remember that the risk to the embryo or fetus changes throughout gestation, such that many of the more teratogenic medications can be relatively safe during certain parts of the pregnancy or during lactation.
- Many factors play a role in the possible teratogenic nature of a medication, such as the genetic susceptibility of the fetus, maternal ability to absorb and metabolize medications, other environmental factors, the developmental stage of the embryo or fetus, dose and duration of exposure, activity of metabolites, and drug–drug interactions.
- Placental transport is very important and occurs more readily with medications that are of low molecular weight, lipid soluble, nonpolar, and nonprotein bound.

Gestational timing of medications is very important.

- There is thought to be an "all-or-none" phenomenon for an embryo during the first 2 weeks after conception. It is during this time that exposure to a teratogen is believed to either cause enough damage to the embryo that death or a spontaneous miscarriage occurs, or no damage or sufficient repair occurs such that there are no lasting effects. This is a common period of fetal exposure, given that many women may not yet know they are pregnant.
- The first trimester is the very important time of organogenesis, during which both adequate control of maternal disease states (e.g., diabetes), and limiting exposure to teratogens (e.g., radiation exposure and many medications) are equally important and may require consultation with an obstetrician or maternal fetal medicine specialist.
- The remainder of pregnancy is a period of cell growth and differentiation that can be inhibited by certain medications in varying doses and duration of exposure.
- Finally, lactation represents a time during which certain medications may be transported to the fetus through breast milk. The cellular mechanisms through which this occurs are different than during placental transport, and certain medications (e.g., warfarin) that can be teratogenic or cause disastrous complications when passage occurs in utero can be very safe during lactation, given transportation in only an inactive form.

One final consideration when reviewing drugs in pregnancy and lactation is the confounding factors that are involved in the epidemiologic data reporting and the extrapolation of risk from animal studies. There are many resources for healthcare professionals on teratogens in pregnancy (see later discussion). Yet, much of our human teratogenic database comes from observational/epidemiologic studies, case reports, retrospective case-control studies or registries. There are some data derived from prospective cohort studies or registries. Although the teratogenic potential of a medication is crucial to its risk/benefit profile, pregnant or nursing women are rarely, if ever, included in clinical trials for this information to be obtained at the time of distribution. We rely heavily on postmarketing surveillance of medications because, inevitably, pregnant women will be exposed to various medications. On the other hand, we must carefully analyze much of this retrospective reporting. As expected, there can be a significant amount of recall bias from parents who deliver a child with an unfortunate outcome or anomaly. Biologic plausibility is not always known even though a possible association between a medication and a teratogenic effect is reported. In addition, much of our toxicity data are extrapolated from animal data. Some consider a drug to pose a low risk to humans if the toxic dose in animals is >10 times the dose in humans (Scialli et al. 2004). Yet, even though some drugs are teratogenic in animals, they may be safe in humans and vice versa. Of the countless medications marketed to patients, there are only approximately 20 drugs, especially anticonvulsants, antineoplastic medications, and retinoids, that have been shown to have significantly increased teratogenic risk at clinically relevant human doses (Schardein 2000). Finally, long-term effects of medications on a fetus in utero or a neonate through breast milk are often unknown, or there has not yet been a sufficient length of follow-up. Many of the associations between a particular medication and an adverse fetal or neonatal risk are not uncovered until decades later, after thousands of children are affected, as with diethylstilbestrol (DES), warfarin, angiotensin-converting-enzyme (ACE) inhibitors, or thalidomide.

Table B-1 lists commonly used medications and their risk in pregnancy. By no means is this table all-inclusive. Its purpose is to be a ready reference for practitioners of various specialties when prescribing drug therapy to pregnant women or women of reproductive age, in which case an unknown or unplanned pregnancy should always be considered. The drugs are classified according to their risk factor category (A, B, C, D, or X; as described in detail later). Although the definitions for each category are used by the Food and Drug Administration (FDA), most of the medications listed are assigned to a category by their manufacturer. Although most category assignments are in agreement with the literature and prescribing physicians, there are some differing opinions. One should consider each medication with respect to the specific nature of the condition requiring treatment and have a low threshold to consult the literature or a specialist should any questions arise. For women with significant medical conditions or complicated medication profiles, consultation with an obstetrician or maternal fetal medicine specialist should always be considered.

Teratogen Database Resources:

- **National Library of Medicine:**
  www.nlm.nih.gov
- **Reproductive Toxicology Center**
  REPROTOX® is available to residents in training without charge:
  www.reprotox.org
- **Shepard's Catalog of Teratogenic Agents**
  FDA Reviewer Guidance: Evaluating the Risks of Drug Exposure in Human Pregnancies:
  www.fda.gov/cber/gdlns/rvrpreg.htm
- **A list of pregnancy exposure registries:**
  http://www.fda.gov/womens/registries/default.htm

Risk Factor Categories:

- **Category A:** Controlled studies in women fail to demonstrate a risk to the fetus in the first trimester, there is no evidence of a risk in later trimesters, and the possibility of fetal harm appears remote. Very few drugs have sufficient safety profiles, and therefore the table excludes this category. The only medications classified as category A are each of the vitamins when used in Recommended Dietary Allowance (RDA)-recommended doses, levothyroxine, the antiemetic doxylamine, and the electrolytes potassium citrate, potassium chloride, and potassium gluconate.
- **Category B:** Either animal studies have not demonstrated a fetal risk but there are no controlled studies in pregnant women, or animal studies have shown an adverse effect that was not confirmed in controlled studies in women in the first trimester, and there is not evidence of a risk in the later trimesters.
- **Category C:** Either studies in animals have revealed adverse effects on the fetus (teratogenic or embryocidal or other) and there are no controlled studies in women, or studies in women and animals are not available. These drugs should only be given if the potential benefit justifies the potential risk to the fetus.
- **Category D:** There is positive evidence of human fetal risk, but the benefits from use in pregnant women may be acceptable despite the risk, as if the drug is needed in a

TABLE B-1 Pregnancy and Medical Therapeutics

Class of medication	Category B	Category C	Category D	Category X
Analgesics	Acetaminophen Diclofenac* Hydromorphone* Ibuprofen* Indomethacin* Meperidine* Methadone* Naproxen* Oxycodone* Oxymorphone*	Triptans (antimigraine) Aspirin* Butalbital Butorphanol* Celecoxib* Codeine* Fentanyl* Hydrocodone* Ketorolac* Morphine* Propoxyphene* Sufentanil* Tramadol	*	Dihydroergotamine Ergotamine
Anesthetics	Halothane Isoflurane Ketamine Lidocaine (local) Propofol Ropivacaine (local)	Nitrous oxide Sevoflurane		
Antibiotics	Azithromycin Aztreonam Cephalosporins Clavulanate Clindamycin Ethambutol Meropenem Metronidazole Penicillins Polymyxin B Sulbactam Tazobactam Vancomycin	Gentamycin Bacitracin Chloramphenicol Chloroquine Clarithromycin Dapsone Imipenem-cilastatin Isoniazid Linezolid Pyrazinamide Quinolones** Rifampin Spectinomycin Sulfonamides Trimethoprim	Quinine Streptomycin Tetracyclines	
Anticonvulsants	Magnesium sulfate	Ethosuximide Gabapentin Lamotrigine Levetiracetam Oxcarbazepine Topiramate Zonisamide	Carbamazepine Clonazepam Diazepam Phenobarbital Phenytoin Primidone Valproic acid	
Antidepressants/ antipsychotics/ anxiolytics	Buproprion Buspirone Zolpidem	Aripiprazole Chlorpromazine Clozapine Haloperidol Olanzapine Quetiapine Risperidone SSRIs[a] TCAs Thioridazine Ziprasidone	Alprazolam Chlordiazepoxide Clonazepam Diazepam Lithium Lorazepam Midazolam Oxazepam	Other benzodiazepines

(*continued*)

TABLE B-1 Pregnancy and Medical Therapeutics (*continued*)

Class of medication	Category B	Category C	Category D	Category X
Antifungals	Amphotericin B Clotrimazole	Caspofungin Fluconazole Griseofulvin Ketoconazole Miconazole Nystatin Terconazole		
Antihistamines	Cetirizine Chlorpheniramine Diphenhydramine Loratadine Meclizine	Fexofenadine Hydroxyzine Promethazine		
Antilipemics	Cholestyramine Colestipol Niacin[b]	Clofibrate Gemfibrozil		Statins
Antiretrovirals[c]	Atazanavir Didanosine Emtricitabine Ritonavir Saquinavir Tenofovir	Efavirenz Indinavir Lamivudine Lopinavir Nevirapine Zidovudine		
Antivirals	Acyclovir Famciclovir Valacyclovir	Amantadine Foscarnet Ganciclovir Oseltamivir Rimantadine		
Bisphosphonates		Alendronate Ibandronate Risedronate	Pamidronate	
Cardiovascular drugs	Methyldopa Hydrochlorothiazide[d]	Acetazolamide Adenosine Calcium-channel blockers Clonidine Digoxin Esmolol Flecainide Hydralazine Isosorbides Labetalol[d] Metoprolol[d] Minoxidil Nitroglycerin (B/C) Nitroprusside Prazosin Propranolol[d] Terazosin	ACE Inhibitors Amiodarone ARBs Atenolol	
Dermatology	Azelaic acid Clindamycin Erythromycin	Benzoyl peroxide Tretinoin (topical)	Doxycycline	Isotretinoin

(*continued*)

TABLE B-1   Pregnancy and Medical Therapeutics (*continued*)

Class of medication	Category B	Category C	Category D	Category X
Gastrointestinal	Cimetidine Famotidine Lactulose Lansoprazole Loperamide Meclizine Mesalamine Metoclopramide Ondansetron Opium tincture Orlistat Pantoprazole Ranitidine Sucralfate Ursodiol	Docusate Droperidol Kaolin Mineral oil Omeprazole Prochlorperazine Promethazine Senna Simethicone		Misoprostol
Hematologic	Argatroban Clopidogrel Dalteparin Dypyridamole Enoxaparin Lepirudin	Alteplase Epoetin alfa Filgrastim Heparin Pentoxifylline Streptokinase	Aminocaproic acid	Warfarin
Hormones	Acarbose Desmopressin Insulin Metformin Somatostatin Troglitazone Vasopressin Micronized progesterone	Adrenal hormones[e] Calcitonin Glipizide Glyburide Melatonin Repaglinide Rosiglitazone Tolbutamide	Methimazole Propylthiouracil Tamoxifen Hydroxyprogesterone[f]	Danazol Estrogens Iodide[131] Leuprolide Mifepristone Testosterone
Respiratory	Acetylcysteine Budesonide Cromolyn sodium Ipratropium Montelukast Zafirlukast	Albuterol Corticosteroids (inhaled) Dextromethorphan Guaifenesin Salmeterol Theophylline		
Urologic	Oxybutynin Phenazopyridine	Tolterodine Trospium		

ACE, angiotensin-converting enzyme; ARB, angiotensin-receptor blockers; SSRI, selective serotonin reuptake inhibitor; TCA, tricyclic antidepressant.

*All of these can be considered category D if used in large doses or for prolonged duration.

**Although classified as category C by the manufacturer, use with caution, given concern for floroquinolone-induced fetal cartilage damage. This is somewhat controversial, but most obstetricians avoid their use in pregnancy.

[a]Recent data suggest that there may be concern for increased risk of persistent pulmonary hypertension with exposure in the latter half of pregnancy or neonatal withdrawl syndrome—although usually self-limited—with exposure in the third trimester. Fluoxitine is the most studied and has been followed the longest, and setraline still has a good safety profile. Much of this is still hotly debated in the literature.

[b]Considered category C if used in doses for lipid treatment or above RDA doses.

[c]Efavirenz is generally not recommended in the first trimester. Consider consultation with a specialist who has experience in HIV and pregnancy because there are specific recommendations for treating HIV in pregnancy that differ from nonpregnant treatment regimens.

[d]There is concern for use of beta-blockers in the second and third trimesters given reports of intrauterine growth restriction and reduced placental weights, although labetalol has the most safety data of the class. Diuretics should not be used to treat gestational hypertension.

[e]Adrenal hormones (e.g., cortisol, dexamethasone, hydrocortisone, and prednisone) are generally regarded as category C, although some argue that one should try to avoid use during the first trimester, given some concern for teratogenic data in animals and human epidemiologic studies.

[f]Avoid in the 1st trimester. The American college of Obstetrics & Gynecology (ACOG) supports its use in pregnancy if history of spontaneous preterm delivery.

life-threatening situation or for serious diseases for which safer drugs are ineffective or cannot be used.

■ **Category X:** Studies in animals or humans have demonstrated fetal abnormalities or there is evidence of fetal risk based on human experience, and the risk of the use of the drug in pregnant women clearly outweighs any possible benefit. These drugs are contraindicated in women who are or may become pregnant.

Suggested Readings

Brent RL. The complexities of solving the problem of human malformations. *Clin Perinatol* 1986;13:491.

Briggs GG, Freeman RK, Yaffe SJ. *Drugs in Pregnancy and Lactation*, 7th ed. Philadelphia: Lippincott, Williams & Wilkins, 2005.

Forfar JO, Nelson MM. Epidemiology of drugs taken by pregnant women: drugs that may affect the fetus adversely. *Clin Pharmacol Ther* 1973;14:632.

Hogge W, Prosen T. Principles of teratology, UpToDate, March 15, 2006. Schardein JL. *Chemically Induced Birth Defects*, 3rd ed. New York: Marcel Dekker, 2000.

Scialli A, et al. *Birth Defects Res* [Part A] 2004;70:7.

Simpson JL, Golbus MS. Principles of Teratology. In: *Genetics in Obstetrics and Gynecology*, Simpson JL, Golbus MS (eds). Philadelphia: W.B. Saunders, 1992.

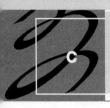

C IMMUNIZATIONS AND POSTEXPOSURE THERAPIES

Alexis M. Elward and Victoria J. Fraser

TABLE C-1   Routine Adult Immunizations

Vaccine	Persons for whom indicated	Dose	Contraindications
Hepatitis A	Travelers to endemic areas, homosexual men, military personnel, illicit drug users, patients with clotting factor disorders, chronic liver disease, occupational risk for infection (i.e., researchers)	1.0 mL IM (repeated in 6–18 mo for extended immunity) Age ≥18 yr HAVRIX: 1440 ELU/dose VAQTA: 50 U/dose	Severe allergic reaction to vaccine or to vaccine component
Hepatitis B	Everyone	1 mL IM (in the deltoid) at 0, 1, and 6 mo (higher dose for immunocompromised and dialysis patients)	Severe allergic reaction to vaccine or to vaccine component
Influenza	Everyone ≥50 yr, high-risk patients,[a] women who will be in second or third trimester of pregnancy during influenza season, health care workers (consider offering to everyone)	0.5 mL IM every fall	Severe allergic reaction to vaccine or to vaccine component, including egg protein
Pneumococcus	Everyone ≥65 yr, high-risk patients[a] ≥2 yr old, anatomic or functional asplenia, CSF leak	0.5 mL IM once (repeated after ≥5 yr for highest-risk patients)	Severe allergic reaction to vaccine or to vaccine component
Tetanus/diphtheria booster (adult Td)	Everyone	0.5 mL q10 yr (or a single booster at age 50)	Severe allergic reaction to vaccine or to vaccine component
Varicella	All susceptible persons, especially (1) health care workers, (2) persons who live/work in environments where VZV transmission is likely,[b] (3) adolescents and adults living with children, (4) nonpregnant women of childbearing age, (5) international travelers	0.5 mL SC	Severe allergic reaction to vaccine or to vaccine component Pregnancy, HIV infected other than CDC class N1 deficiency or A1, primary immunodeficiency, neoplasms affecting bone marrow or lymphatic system[c]

(continued)

TABLE C-1	Routine Adult Immunizations (continued)		

Vaccine	Persons for whom indicated	Dose	Contraindications
Measles	Persons entering college, U.S. travelers to foreign countries, health care workers	0.5 mL SC	Pregnancy, history of sensitivity to eggs or neomycin; severe immunosuppression
Meningococcus	During outbreaks of serogroup C,[d] consider for college freshmen living in dormitories; indicated for patients with terminal complement component deficiencies, functional or anatomic asplenia, travelers to countries where *Neisseria meningitidis* is hyperendemic (i.e., sub-Saharan Africa)	0.5 mL SC	Severe allergic reaction to vaccine or to vaccine component
Haemophilus influenzae type b (Hib)	All children <5 yr, persons with functional or anatomic asplenia, sickle cell anemia,[e] HIV, Hodgkin's lymphoma[f]	Schedule depends on age; see *MMWR Morb Mortal Wkly Rep* 40(RR-07), 1991	Severe allergic reaction to vaccine or vaccine component

CDC, Centers for Disease Control and Prevention; CSF, cerebrospinal fluid; ELU, ELISA units; HAVRIX, hepatitis A vaccine, inactivated; Td, adult tetanus-diphtheria booster; VAQTA, hepatitis A vaccine, inactivated; VZV, varicella-zoster virus.

[a]High-risk patients are those with chronic pulmonary, cardiovascular, metabolic, or renal diseases or hemoglobinopathies, or immunosuppressed or institutionalized persons.

[b]Teachers of young children, day care employees, residents/staff in institutional settings, college students, correctional institution inmates/staff members, military personnel.

[c]Research protocol available through vaccine manufacturer for use in patients with acute lymphocytic leukemia who meet eligibility criteria.

[d]Outbreak is defined as ≥3 probable or confirmed cases within ≤3 months for a primary attack rate of ≥10 cases/100,000 population.

[e]Limited data on antibody response; consider giving >1 dose.

[f]Give dose ≥2 weeks before chemotherapy or ≥3 months after the end of chemotherapy [*MMWR Morb Mortal Wkly Rep* 42(RR-04), 1993].

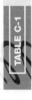

TABLE C-2 **Passive Immunization**

Disease	Indications and dosage
Diphtheria	Suspected respiratory tract diphtheria: diphtheria antitoxin (DAT—equine source), 20,000–120,000 Units IM (IV for serious illness) after cultures taken (given in addition to antibiotics). Not routinely recommended for household contacts given significant risk of anaphylaxis (7%) and serum sickness (5%) and equivalent efficacy of antimicrobial prophylaxis (benzathine penicillin, 1.2 million units IM ×1, or erythromycin, 1 g/daily in divided doses ×7–10 days).
Hepatitis A	**Postexposure:** within 14 daily of known exposure of high-risk persons [unvaccinated household and sexual contacts of infected individual; coworkers of infected food handlers; all staff and children at day care centers where ≥1 case has occurred or when cases occur in ≥2 households of center attendees; consider for family members of diapered children who attend such a day care center during outbreaks (cases in ≥3 families)]: IG, 0.02 mL/kg IM.[a] IG not indicated for casual contacts (e.g., office coworkers).
Hepatitis B	**Preexposure:** Vaccine prophylaxis preferred (Table C-1). **Postexposure:** see Table C-5.
Measles	For nonimmune contacts within 6 days of exposure: IG, 0.25 mL/kg (maximum 15 mL) for normal host; 0.5 mL/kg (maximum 15 mL) for immuno-
Measles	compromised patients. MMR vaccine may provide some protection if given within 72 hr of initial exposure.
Rabies	See Table C-4.
Tetanus	See Table C-3.
Varicella	Vaccine, 0.5 mL SC within 3 days of exposure (possibly effective up to 5 days postexposure) or varicella-zoster IG, 1 vial (125 units) IM for each 10 kg body weight (minimum, 125 Units; maximum, 625 units) within 96 hr of exposure (optimal if given within 48 hr) [*MMWR Morb Mortal Wkly Rep* 45 (RR-11):1–25, 1996].

DAT, direct antiglobulin test; MMR, measles, mumps, rubella.
[a]Anaphylaxis has been reported after injection of IG in IgA-deficient persons. Live attenuated vaccines [MMR, varicella-zoster virus (VZV)] should be delayed after administration of IG (3 mo for MMR, 5 mo for VZV). Patients who received MMR within 2 wk before IG or VZV within 3 wk before IG should be revaccinated.

 TABLE C-3 **Tetanus Prophylaxis**

History of tetanus immunization (doses)	Clean, minor wounds		Other wounds	
	Give Td	**Give TIG**	**Give Td**	**Give TIG**
Unknown or <3 doses	Yes	No	Yes	Yes
≥3 doses	No if dose within 10 yr; otherwise yes	No	Yes unless last dose within 5 yr	No

Td, adult tetanus-diphtheria booster; TIG, tetanus immune globulin, 250 units IM, given concurrently with Td at a separate site.

MANAGEMENT OF RABIES

- **Preexposure vaccination** is indicated for persons in high-risk groups, including laboratory workers, veterinarians, animal handlers, and international travelers.[a]
  - The **dose** is three 1.0-mL injections of human diploid cell vaccine (HDCV),[b] rabies vaccine adsorbed, or purified chick embryo cell vaccine IM (deltoid) on days 0, 7, and 21 or 28.
  - **Contraindications.** Intradermal HDCV should not be given to travelers taking antimalarial prophylaxis (IM should be used instead).
  - **Research laboratory and vaccine production workers** should have serum rabies antibody testing every 6 months; spelunkers, veterinarians and staff, animal control and wildlife officers in areas where rabies is enzootic, and laboratory workers who perform rabies diagnostic testing should have serum rabies antibody testing every 2 years.
  - **Preexposure booster vaccination** should be given to people in the above groups to maintain serum titer corresponding to complete neutralization at a 1:5 serum dilution by the rapid fluorescent focus inhibition test.
- **Postexposure rabies therapy.** See Table C-4.
  - For **bats and wild animals**, capturing and sacrificing the animal and performing immunofluorescence on brain tissue provide definitive determination of the animal's rabies status. Except in cases of bites or scratches on the head or neck or bat exposure, it is reasonable to wait for diagnostic testing on the animal before instituting postexposure therapy. If diagnostic testing on animal brain tissue is negative, no postexposure therapy is necessary.
  - For **bites or scratches on the head or neck**, postexposure therapy should be instituted immediately because of proximity to the central nervous system and potentially shorter incubation period.
  - **Any bat exposure warrants therapy.** Potential bat exposures also warrant therapy if there is any possibility of an unobserved bite or scratch (i.e., person sleeping in a room, unattended child, demented or obtunded adult).

---

[a] If contact with potentially rabid animals and limited access to medical care are likely.
[b] HDCV can also be given intradermally; the intradermal dose is 0.1 mL on days 0, 7, and 21 or 28.

TABLE C-4 **Postexposure Rabies Therapy**

Species	Condition of animal at time of attack	Treatment of exposed[a] persons
Domestic cat, dog, ferret	Healthy and available for 10 days of observation	None unless animal develops rabies
	Rabid or suspected rabid	RIG and vaccine[b]
	Unknown	Contact public health department
Bat[a]	Any	RIG and vaccine[b]
Wild skunk, fox, coyote, raccoon, or other carnivore	Unknown; to be regarded as rabid unless proven negative by laboratory testing	RIG and vaccine[b]
Wild or domestic rodents (squirrels, rats, mice) and lagomorphs (rabbits, hares)	Unknown: rarely infected with rabies	Contact local health department

RIG, rabies immunoglobulin.

[a]Exposure: bites or scratches, or animal saliva contaminating abrasions, open wounds, or mucous membranes *except for bats.* **Any bat exposure or potential bat exposures warrants therapy.**

[b]RIG: Administer once to previously unvaccinated persons, 20 International Units/kg; best if done immediately (can be given through seventh day after first dose of vaccine administered). Full dose should be infiltrated around wound(s); inject remaining RIG IM at site distant from vaccine administration. **Do not** administer RIG in same syringe or at same anatomic site as vaccine. Previously vaccinated persons (those who received one of the recommended regimens of human diploid cell vaccine, rabies vaccine adsorbed, or purified chick embryo cell vaccine and had a documented rabies antibody titer): two IM 1.0-mL doses of vaccine, days 0 (immediately) and 3.

Vaccine: Five 1-mL doses on days 0, 3, 7, 14, and 28 IM in deltoid (anterolateral aspect of thigh acceptable for children). Gluteal area should not be used, as this results in lower neutralizing antibody titers.

| TABLE C-5 | Blood-Borne Pathogen Postexposure Guidelines[a] |

Pathogen	Treatment
HIV[b]	For percutaneous injury (e.g., bloody needle-stick) or prolonged, excessive exposure of mucous membrane or nonintact skin to blood, blood-contaminated fluids, or potentially infectious material (e.g., cerebrospinal fluid, amniotic fluid), one of the following drug regimens for 4 wk (determine based on resistance in source patient and geographic area): (1) zidovudine, 200 mg PO tid (or 300 mg PO bid), plus lamivudine (3TC), 150 mg PO bid, or (2) 3TC, 150 mg PO bid, plus stavudine (d4T), 40 mg PO bid, or (3) didanosine, 400 mg PO daily, plus d4T, 40 mg PO bid. For highest-risk exposure (e.g., large blood volumes, high HIV viral load, hollow-bore needle), indinavir, 800 mg PO tid, or nelfinavir, 750 mg PO tid, or abacavir; 300 mg PO bid, or efavirenz, 600 mg PO at bed time, can be added; consult with experts in occupational health or infectious diseases[c]; occupational health follow-up essential [*MMWR Morb Mortal Wkly Rep* 50(RR-11);1–42, 2001]. For exposures to other material (e.g., urine), therapy is not recommended.
Hepatitis B	For percutaneous injury with blood or blood-contaminated fluids: Unvaccinated health care worker: Administer hepatitis B immunoglobulin (HBIG), 0.06 mL/kg IM, within 96 hr of exposure; start hepatitis B vaccine series. Vaccinated health care worker: Check anti-HBs titer. If ≥10 International Units/mL, no therapy. If <10 International Units/mL, give HBIG, 0.06 mL/kg, and booster dose of vaccine or 2 doses of HBIG 1 mo apart (this preferred for health care workers known not to have responded to second vaccine series).
Hepatitis C	Immunoglobulin not effective. Ensure occupational health follow-up for baseline and subsequent follow-up testing.

[a]All blood and body fluid exposures should be reported to the occupational health department. Source patients should be tested for HIV (with consent), hepatitis B surface antigen (HbsAg), and hepatitis C antibody (anti-HCV).
[b]For exposure to patients with known HIV or at high risk for HIV, post-exposure prophylaxis should be started as soon as possible (preferably within 1–2 hr, because there is less evidence for efficacy in preventing transmission after 24–36 hr).
[c]Other antiretrovirals may be indicated if there is a high likelihood that the source patient has drug resistance to components of the standard regimen. If therapy is started for a patient with suspected HIV, it can be stopped if the patient's HIV antibody test is negative, unless there is a high suspicion of acute HIV illness.

POSTEXPOSURE PROPHYLAXIS RESOURCES

- National Clinicians Postexposure Hotline — Telephone: 1-888-448-4911
  http://www.ucsf.edu/hivcntr

- CDC (for reporting HIV sero-conversions in health care workers with and without postexposure prophylaxis) — Telephone: 1-800-893-0485

- Antiretroviral Pregnancy Registry — Telephone: 1-800-258-4263
  http://www.apregistry.com

- US FDA (for reporting unusual or severe toxicity to antiretroviral agents) — Telephone: 1-800-322-1088
  http://www.fda.gov/medwatch
- Hepatitis Hotline — Telephone: 1-888-443-7232
  http://www.cdc.gov/hepatitis

TABLE C-6 **Postexposure Prophylaxis for Centers for Disease Control and Prevention (CDC) Class A Bioterrorism Agents**[a]

Pathogen	Treatment
Anthrax	For inhalational exposure, the ACIP recommends that the CDC make vaccination with three doses of AVA available under an investigational drug protocol, to be given 0.5 mL SC at 0, 2, and 4 wk[b]; anthrax vaccine is not currently licensed for use in postexposure prophylaxis. If vaccine is given, one of the following antibiotic regimens is recommended ×7–14 days after the third dose of vaccine. If antibiotics alone are used, they should be continued for 60 days [*MMWR Morb Mortal Wkly Rep* 51(45):1024–1026, 2002]. After exposure to cutaneous or GI anthrax, consider using one of the following antibiotic regimens for 7–14 daily: Adults: Ciprofloxacin, 500 mg PO q12h *or* doxycycline, 100 mg PO q12h Children: Ciprofloxacin, 10–15 mg/kg PO q12h or Doxycycline: >8 yr and >45 kg: 100 mg PO q12h >8 yr and ≤45 kg: 2.2 mg/kg/dose PO q12h ≤8 yr 2.2 mg/kg/dose PO q12h
Botulinum toxin	Close observation of exposed person, treat with equine antitoxin at first sign of illness
Pneumonic plague	For close contacts (<2 m), doxycycline, 100 mg PO q12h, or ciprofloxacin, 500 mg PO q12h for 7 days is preferred (see above for pediatric dosing); chloramphenicol, 25 mg/kg/dose q6h is alternative (not used in children <2 yr old); watch closely for fever or cough, promptly initiate parenteral therapy with streptomycin, 1 g IM q12h, or gentamicin in symptomatic patients
Tularemia	If attacks identified during early incubation period: ciprofloxacin or doxycycline, PO ×14 days (see above for dosing); if attack unrecognized until multiple people ill, observe exposed closely, initiate parenteral therapy at first sign of illness
Smallpox	Vaccinate[c] ideally within 3 days of exposure; vaccination 4–7 days after exposure may offer some protection

ACIP, Advisory Committee on Immunization Practices; AVA, anthrax vaccine adsorbed.
[a]In the event of a bioterrorism attack, the latest recommendations can be accessed via the US Centers for Disease Control and Prevention internet site: http://www.bt.cdc.gov.
[b]The efficacy of alternative dosing schedules is currently under investigation. Contraindications to vaccination are a previous history of anthrax infection or a history of anaphylaxis after AVA or any vaccine components.
[c]An individualized assessment of risks and benefits of vaccination must be made. In general, vaccination for contacts of smallpox cases is recommended even in the presence of usual contraindications (history of or presence of eczema; atopic dermatits; other acute, chronic, or exfoliative skin conditions; immunosuppression; pregnancy or intent to become pregnant within 4 wk; breast-feeding; age <1 yr). If an exposed person declines vaccination, the alternative strategy is isolation for 19 d.

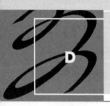

INFECTION CONTROL AND ISOLATION RECOMMENDATIONS

Victoria J. Fraser and Alexis M. Elward

■ **Standard precautions** should be practiced on **all patients at all times** to minimize the risk of nosocomial infection (previously called *body substance isolation* or *universal precautions*).

■ **Perform hand hygiene,** preferably with an alcohol-based rub or foam, before and after direct patient contact, after contact with the environment, between caring for different patients, and after removing gloves. Soap and water should be used for visibly contaminated hands.

■ **Wear gloves** when direct contact with moist body substances (e.g., blood, sputum, urine, pus, stool) is anticipated.

■ **Wear a gown** when clothing is likely to be soiled by a body fluid.

■ **Wear a mask and goggles or glasses** when splashes of a body fluid are anticipated (e.g., during most invasive procedures).

■ **Specific isolation categories.** In addition to precautions that should be followed for all patients, certain diseases, depending on their mode of spread, **require additional isolation precautions.** Categories and indications for their use may vary slightly among different hospitals. Contact an infection control specialist if there is any uncertainty about what type of isolation a patient might need. The following categories are those suggested by the Centers for Disease Control and Prevention.

■ **Airborne precautions**
  • Use a negative-pressure room.
  • Keep doors closed.
  • Wear a **respirator, grade N95 or better,** certified by the National Institute for Occupational Safety and Health (**not a surgical mask**) if entering the room of a patient who is suspected of having tuberculosis.
  • For patients with measles or varicella (e.g., chickenpox) infections, immune persons may enter the room without a mask. Nonimmune persons ideally should not enter the room of such patients, but, if it is absolutely necessary that they enter, they should wear a mask.
  • If patient transport is absolutely necessary, the patient should wear a **surgical** mask.
  • Instruct the patient to cover his or her mouth when coughing or sneezing, even if alone.

■ **Droplet precautions**
  • Keep doors closed.
  • Wear a surgical mask if entering the room.
  • Discard mask **after** leaving the room.
  • If patient transport is absolutely necessary, the patient should wear a **surgical** mask.

■ **Contact precautions**
  • Wear a gown and gloves to enter the room.
  • Use a dedicated stethoscope and thermometer.
  • Remove gown and gloves before leaving the room.

■ Perform hand hygiene with an alcohol-based rub or foam or antimicrobial soap before leaving the room.

■ **Isolation for specific infections and duration of isolation.** See Tables D-1 and D-2.

| TABLE D-1 | Isolation for Specific Infections and Duration of Isolation |

Isolation type and diseases	Duration of isolation
Airborne	
Tuberculosis (TB)	Until TB is ruled out with three negative acid-fast bacilli smears on consecutive days. (If patient has documented or strongly suspected TB, isolation for hospitalized patients should continue for at least 2 wk of therapy with a good clinical response; however, patients can be discharged during this time if proper follow-up has been arranged with the local health department.)
Measles	4 days after start of rash or for duration of illness if patient is immunocompromised
Chickenpox[a]/disseminated zoster[a]	Until all lesions are crusted. (Note: Nonimmune persons are potentially contagious days 8–21 after exposure to varicella-zoster virus.)
Severe acute respiratory syndrome (strict isolation: airborne, contact, and eye/nose protection)	Duration of illness
Avian influenza	Duration of illness
Droplet	
Adenovirus (pneumonia)	Duration of illness
Diphtheria (pharyngeal)	Until cultures are negative (at least 24 hr after stopping antibiotics)
Influenza	Duration of illness
Meningitis	24 hr after start of therapy for known or suspected *Neisseria meningitidis* or *Haemophilus influenzae*; this is prudent for all meningitis initially
Mumps[a]	9 days after onset of swelling
Mycoplasma	Duration of illness
Parvovirus B19[b]	7 days for aplastic crisis or for duration of illness if patient is immunosuppressed
Pertussis	5 days after start of therapy
Plague (pneumonic)	72 hr after start of therapy
Rubella[b]	7 days after onset of rash; for congenital rubella place infant on contact precautions during any admission until 1 yr of age unless nasopharyngeal and urine cultures are negative after age 3 mo
Streptococcal pharyngitis, pneumonia, or scarlet fever in infants and young children	24 hr after start of therapy
Contact	
Acute infectious diarrhea	Duration of illness
Abscess/draining wound	Duration of illness
Clostridium difficile	Until diarrhea resolves or treatment is completed
Enterovirus	Duration of illness
Herpes simplex (neonatal, primary or disseminated mucocutaneous, severe)	Duration of illness
Hepatitis A	Until 1 wk after onset of symptoms

(continued)

TABLE D-1 Isolation for Specific Infections and Duration of Isolation (*continued*)

Isolation type and diseases	Duration of isolation
Parainfluenza	Duration of illness
Respiratory syncytial virus (infants, young children, and immunocompromised adults)	Duration of illness
Scabies	24 hr after start of therapy
Viral conjunctivitis ("pink eye")	Duration of illness
Oxacillin-resistant *Staphylococcus aureus*	Duration of hospitalization and future hospitalizations[c]
Vancomycin-resistant or intermediate-sensitive *S. aureus*	Duration of hospitalization and future hospitalizations[c]
Vancomycin-resistant enterococci	Duration of hospitalization and future hospitalizations[c]
Multidrug-resistant gram-negative bacteria	Duration of hospitalization and future hospitalizations[c]

[a]Nonimmune persons should stay out of room if possible.
[b]Nonimmune pregnant women should stay out of room (Barnes-Jewish Hospital policy, not an official Centers for Disease Control and Prevention recommendation).
[c]Unless criteria for discontinuing isolation have been met; consult hospital infection control specialists for specific criteria.

TABLE D-2 Isolation for Centers for Disease Control and Prevention Class A[a] Agents of Bioterrorism

Isolation type and agent	Duration of isolation
Airborne	
Smallpox[b]	Duration of hospitalization or until scabs fall off
Viral hemorrhagic fevers[c]	Duration of hospitalization
Droplet	
Pneumonic plague (*Yersinia pestis*)	Until 72 hr after start of antimicrobial therapy
Contact	
Cutaneous anthrax	Until lesions resolve
Standard precautions	
Inhalational anthrax	Duration of hospitalization
Botulism	Duration of hospitalization
Tularemia	Duration of hospitalization

[a]Six class A agents have been identified by the Centers for Disease Control and Prevention. Criteria for inclusion in class A are easily disseminated or transmitted person to person, high mortality, potential for major public health impact, potential for public panic and social disruption, and requirement for special action for public health preparedness.
[b]Contact precautions should be used in handling items potentially contaminated by infectious lesions.
[c]Lassa, Marburg, Ebola, Congo-Crimean. Droplet isolation can be used if the patient does not have prominent coughing, vomiting, diarrhea, or hemorrhaging. Private rooms with potential for conversion of air flow to negative pressure are recommended at admission to avoid later patient transport to negative-pressure isolation.

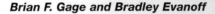
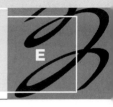

CLINICAL EPIDEMIOLOGY
Brian F. Gage and Bradley Evanoff

E

TREATMENT

Clinical Trials

- A **double-blind, randomized controlled trial** is the **gold standard** to evaluate a new treatment. After enrolling consenting patients, such trials typically assign one-half of the participants to receive the experimental therapy and one-half to receive the standard of care (often with a placebo). Participants are then followed prospectively until they experience the end point of interest or until trial termination. **End points** can be a clinical outcome (e.g., an adverse event); a surrogate outcome, such as a significant change in a laboratory value (e.g., cholesterol); or a clinical measurement (e.g., BP).
- When interpreting the results of clinical trials, **clinicians should evaluate validity** by asking the following key questions:
  - Was the assignment of patients to treatments randomized?
  - Were all patients who entered the trial properly accounted for and attributed at its conclusion?
  - Was follow-up complete?
  - Were patients analyzed in the groups to which they were randomized?
  - Were patients, health workers, and study personnel blind to treatment?
  - Were the groups similar at the start of the trial?
  - Aside from the experimental intervention, were the groups treated equally?
- To quantify the risks and benefits of a therapy, clinicians use standard epidemiologic concepts.
  - **Patient-years** is the product of the number of patients multiplied by their length of observation in years.
  - **Incidence rate** can be calculated by dividing the number of adverse events by the number of patient-years.
  - **Absolute risk reduction (ARR)** is the difference between two incidence rates: $\text{Rate}_{\text{thearpy}} - \text{Rate}_{\text{control}}$.
  - **Number needed to treat (NNT)** is the number of patients that have to receive the therapy to prevent one adverse event. NNT can be calculated by taking the reciprocal of ARR (1/ARR).
  - **Relative risk (RR)** is the ratio of the rate in the experimental group divided by the rate in the control group: $\text{Rate}_{\text{therapy}}/\text{Rate}_{\text{control}}$. Studies that compare rates using time-to-event analyses (e.g., Cox proportional hazard regression) often report the **hazard rate**, which is similar to the RR.
  - **Relative risk reduction (RRR)** is 1 – RR.

Observational Studies

- Most medical treatments have not been evaluated by double-blinded, randomized, controlled trials. For ethical or logistical reasons, observational studies provide the best currently available data for many important questions. Common observational study designs include cohort and case-control studies.
- With few exceptions (e.g., nested case-control studies), incidence rates are not available from case-control studies. Thus, the RR and related terms cannot be calculated directly from such trials. However, a similar measure, **the odds ratio (OR)**, can be calculated

787

TABLE E-1	2 × 2 Table for an Observational Study	
	Disease status	
Exposure	**Present**	**Absent**
Exposed	a	b
Not exposed	c	d

from a case-control study. The OR is calculated from a standard 2 × 2 table (Table E-1) as ad/bc. The results of logistic regression analyses, commonly presented in the medical literature, are also expressed as ORs. For rare events, the OR accurately estimates the RR.

DIAGNOSTIC TESTS

- Clinicians can use clinical epidemiology to help interpret the results of a physical examination finding or diagnostic test. These tests are described in terms of sensitivity and specificity (Table E-2).
- In most cases, clinicians can obtain the sensitivity and specificity from the text of a journal article; however, these values can easily be calculated from raw data using a 2 × 2 table (Table E-3) and the following definitions:
  - **Sensitivity** is the proportion of diseased persons who have a positive test. Sensitivity is also called the **true positive rate** and can be calculated from a/(a + c).
  - **Specificity** is the proportion of nondiseased persons who have a negative test. Specificity is also called the **true negative rate** and can be calculated from d/(b + d).
  - **Positive predicitive value** is the proportion of people with a positive test who have the disease, as calculated by a/(a + b).
  - **Negative predictive value** is the proportion of people with a negative test who are free of disease, as calculated by d/(c + d).
- Before applying these results to patient care, clinicians should critically evaluate the studies about the diagnostic test by asking the following key questions (*JAMA* 271:389, 1994):
  - Was there an independent, blind comparison with a reference standard?
  - Did the study include an appropriate spectrum of patients to whom the diagnostic test will be applied?
  - Did the results of the test being evaluated influence the decision to perform the reference standard?
  - Were the methods for performing the test described in sufficient detail to permit replication?
  - Will the reproducibility of the test results and its interpretation be satisfactory in my setting?
  - Will the results change my management?
  - Will patients be better off as a result of the test?
    Clinician can calculate the posttest probability of a disease based on the pretest probability, the results of the test, and sensitivity and spcificity of the test.

Likelihood Ratios

- The **likelihood ratio** (LR) is the likelihood that a given test result would be expected in a patient with the target disorder compared to the likelihood that a given test result would be expected in a patient without this disorder. The LR can be used to assess the value of a diagnostic test, sign, or symptom. The LR of a positive test (LR+) can be calculated as sensitivity/(1 − specificity). High LRs (>5) make the target disorder substantially more likely in people exhibiting a given result, whereas low LRs (<0.2)

TABLE E-2 Common Diagnostic Tests at Barnes-Jewish Hospital

Test	Disease	Threshold	Sensitivity (%)	Specificity (%)
B-Natriuretic peptide[a]	Heart failure	>100 pg/mL	90	76
		>150 pg/mL	85	83
Serial troponin I[b]	Myocardial infarction	>1.0 ng/mL	90–100	83–96
Ferritin[c]	Iron-deficiency anemia	≤18 ng/mL	55	99
		≤45 ng/mL	82	90
D-Dimer, microlatex agglutination assay[d]	DVT or PE	>500 ng/mL	96	39
Helical CT (spiral CT)[e]	PE	2 mm cuts on CT scan	70–80	91
Prostate-specific antigen	Prostate cancer	≥4 ng/mL	18–46	91–98
Ventilation-perfusion scan[g]	PE	High probability	41	97
		High or intermediate probability	82	52
		Any abnormal result (high, intermediate, or low probability)	98	10

DVT, deep venous thrombosis; PE, pulmonary embolism.
[a] *N Engl J Med* 347:161, 2002.
[b] *Ann Emerg Med* 37:478, 2001.
[c] *Am J Med* 88:205, 1990.
[d] *Thromb Haemost* 84:770, 2000.
[e] *Ann Intern Med* 135:88, 2001.
[f] *N Engl J Med* 349:335, 2003.
[g] *JAMA* 263:2753, 1990.

make the disease substantially less likely. Likelihood ratios of approximately 1 add no useful clinical information.
- The LR is also useful because it allows direct calculation of the posttest odds of disease (posttest odds = pretest odds × LR). In this way, it gives information analogous to the positive or negative predictive values discussed above.

TABLE E-3 2 × 2 Table for a Diagnostic Test

	Disease status	
Test status	**Present**	**Absent**
Test +	a	b
Test −	c	d

- Use of the LR requires the use of **odds of disease** rather than the more familiar probability of disease. Prior probability of disease can be easily converted to pretest odds [pretest odds = prior probability/(1 − prior probability)] and posttest odds can be easily converted to posterior probability [posterior probability = posttest odds/(1 + posttest odds)]. Lists of likelihood ratios for various clinical tests and signs, as well as nomograms and calculators to simplify the use of LR, can be found at www.cebm.utoronto.ca/glossary/lrs.htm.

Receiver Operator Characteristic (ROC) Curve

- The **ROC curve** is a method to plot the discriminatory power of a test using sensitivity and specificity data. The curve plots the sensitivity and specificity of a given test at differing cut points for defining an abnormal test result. The curve thus allows direct visualization of the trade-off between sensitivity and specificity. The upper left-hand corner of the curve represents perfect sensitivity and specificity; the cut points that most closely approach this corner have the greatest discriminant ability. The upper right-hand corner maximizes sensitivity at the expense of poor specificity, whereas the lower left-hand corner maximizes specificity at the expense of sensitivity. Calculation of the area under the ROC curve also allows comparison between two different tests to see which has the greater ability to discriminate between patients with and without a disorder (Fig. E-1).

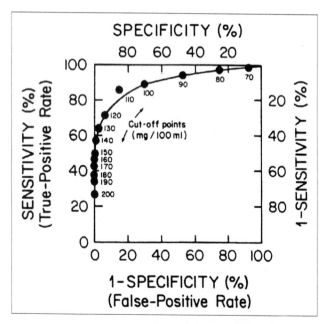

Figure E-1. A receiver operator characteristic curve. The accuracy of 2-hour postprandial blood sugar as a diagnostic test for diabetes mellitus. (Data from *Diabetes Program Guide,* Public Health Service Publication No. 506, 1960.)

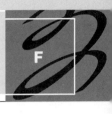

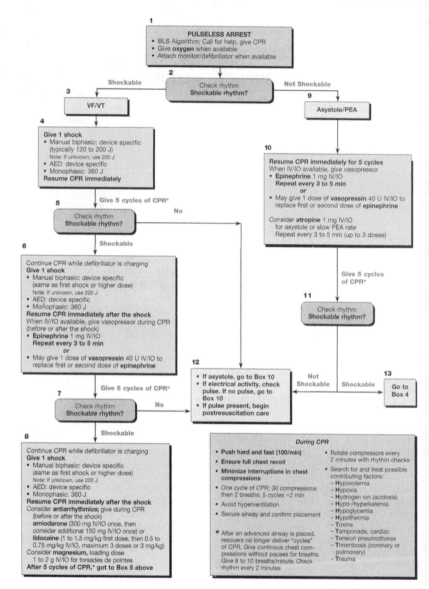

Figure F-1. Advanced Caridac Life Support Pulseless Arrest algorithm. From American Heart Association in collaboration with the International Liaison Committee on Resuscitation. Guidelines 2005 for cardiopulmonary resuscitation and emergency cardiovascular care. Part 7.2: Management of cardiac arrest. *Circulation* 2005;112(24 Suppl):IV58–IV66.

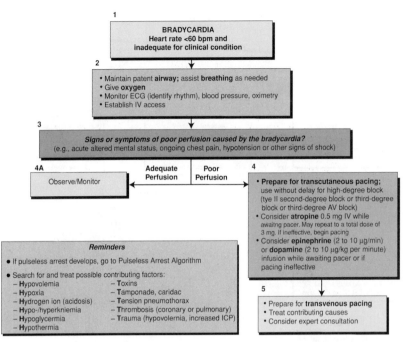

Figure F-2. Bradycardia algorithm. AV, atrioventricular; bpm, beats per minute; ECG, electrocardiogram; IV, intravenous. From American Heart Association in collaboration with the International Liaison Committee on Resuscitation. Guidelines 2005 for cardiopulmonary resuscitation and emergency cardiovascular care. Part 7.2: Management of symptomatic bradycardia and tachycardia. *Circulation* 2005;112(24 Suppl):IV67–IV87.

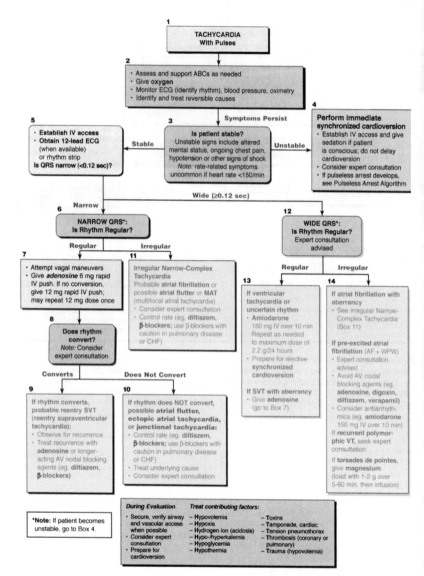

Figure F-3. Advanced Caridac Life Support Tachycardia algorithm. From American Heart Association in collaboration with the International Liaison Committee on Resuscitation. Guidelines 2005 for cardiopulmonary resuscitation and emergency cardiovascular care. Part 7.2: Management of symptomatic bradycardia and tachycardia. *Circulation* 2005;112(24 Suppl):IV67–IV87.]

NOTE: Italic *f* indicates an illustration; *t* indicates a table.

A

Abacavir (ABC), 412t
Abatacept, for rheumatoid arthritis, 662
Abciximab
  for platelet disorders, 524
  for unstable angina/non–ST-segment
    elevation MI, 135, 136t
Abdominal compartment syndrome, acute
    renal failure from, 321
Abdominal infections, 384–385
Abscess, hepatic, 498–499
Absolute risk reduction (ARR), 787
Accelerated idioventricular rhythm, after
    MI, 150
Accelerated junctional rhythm, after MI,
    150
Acebutolol, for syncope, 222
Acetaminophen
  for osteoarthritis, 664
  overdose of, 722t, 724–726, 725f
  for pain, 7
Acetazolamide
  for hyperphosphatemia from renal
    insufficiency, 86
  for metabolic acidosis, 99
Acetylcysteine, for acetaminophen
    overdose, 724–726
Acetylene, 756–757
Achalasia, 447
Acid-base abnormalities. *See also specific
    disorders*
  from mechanical ventilation, 234
Acid-base homeostasis, 91
Acidemia, 91
Acid ingestions, 733
Acidosis, metabolic, 91, 93t, 94t, 95–98
  anion-gap, from overdose, 718t
  compensatory responses to, expected, 94t
  diagnosis of, 96
  etiology of, 93t, 95–96
  from mechanical ventilation, 234
  treatment of, 96–98, 332
Acidosis, respiratory, 91, 93t, 99–100
Acid suppression, for peptic ulcer disease,
    450

Acquired immunodeficiency syndrome
    (AIDS), 408–428. *See also* Human
    immunodeficiency virus (HIV)
  characteristics of, 408
  diagnosis of, 408–409
  diarrhea with, 466
  opportunistic infections in, 417–428
    bacterial, 420–421
    definition of, 417
    fungal, 423–425
    monitoring of, 417
    mycobacterial, 421–423
    neoplasms, 427–428
    protocols for medications for,
      417–418
    protozoal, 426–427
    viral, 418–420
  treatment of, 409–417
    antiretroviral drugs in, 411–413,
      412t–413t (*See also specific drugs*)
    antiretroviral drug interactions
      with, 411, 413, 415t
    other drug interactions with, 416t
    antiretroviral therapy in, 410–411,
      410t
    complications of, 413, 415, 417
    general principles of, 410t
    immunizations in, 409–410
    non-nucleoside analog reverse
      transcriptase inhibitors in, 411,
      413t
    nucleoside analog reverse transcriptase
      inhibitors in, 411, 412t
    patient education in, 413
    protease inhibitors in, 411, 414t
    protocol in, 413
Acquired inhibitors of coagulation factors,
    528
Acromegaly, 641
Activated charcoal. *See* Charcoal, activated
Activated partial thromboplastin (aPTT),
    512
Acute chest syndrome, in sickle cell disease,
    564
Acute colonic pseudo-obstruction, 456–457